NKCA	natural killer cell activity
NMJ	neuromuscular junction
NMS	neuromuscular spindle
NT	neurotransmitter
OBLA	onset of blood lactate accumulation
OP	oxidative phosphorylation
OTS	overtraining syndrome
P_A	pressure in the alveoli
P_ACO_2	partial pressure of carbon dioxide in the alveoli
P_AO_2	partial pressure of oxygen in the alveoli
P_B	barometric pressure
P_G	partial pressure of a gas
P_i	inorganic phosphate
P	pressure
$PaCO_2$	partial pressure of carbon dioxide in arterial blood
PaO_2	partial pressure of oxygen in arterial blood
PC	phosphocreatine
PCO_2	partial pressure of carbon dioxide
PFK	phosphofructokinase
pH	hydrogen ion concentration
PN_2	partial pressure of nitrogen
PNF	proprioceptive neuromuscular facilitation
PNS	peripheral nervous system
PO_2	partial pressure of oxygen
PP	peak power
PRO	protein
PvO_2	partial pressure of oxygen in venous blood
$PvCO_2$	partial pressure of carbon dioxide in venous blood
$\dot{Q}$	cardiac output
R_a	rate of appearance
R_d	rate of disappearance
R	resistance
RBC	red blood cells
RDA	recommended daily allowance
RER	respiratory exchange ratio
RH	relative humidity
RHR	resting heart rate
RM	repetition maximum
RMR	resting metabolic rate
ROM	range of motion
RPE	rating of perceived exertion
RPP	rate pressure product
RQ	respiratory quotient
RV	residual volume
$SaO_2\%$	percent saturation of arterial blood with oxygen
$SbO_2\%$	percent saturation of blood with oxygen
$SvO_2\%$	percent saturation of venous blood with oxygen
SBP	systolic blood pressure
SO	slow, oxidative muscle fibers
SR	sarcoplasmic reticulum
SSC	stretch shortening cycle

ST	slow-twitch muscle fibers
STPD	standard temperature and pressure, dry air
SV	stroke volume
T	temperature
Tamb	ambient temperature
TC	total cholesterol
Tco	core temperature
TEF	thermic effect of feeding
TEM	thermic effect of a meal
TExHR	target exercise heart rate
$TEx\dot{V}O_2$	target exercise oxygen consumption
TG	triglycerides
TLC	total lung capacity
TPR	total peripheral resistance
Tre	rectal temperature
Tsk	skin temperature
Ttym	tympanic temperature
URTI	upper respiratory tract infection
$\dot{V}_A$	alveolar ventilation
V_D	volume of dead space
$\dot{V}_E$	volume of expired air
V_G	volume of a gas
$\dot{V}_I$	volume of inspired air
V_T	tidal volume
$\dot{V}$	volume per unit of time
V	volume
VAT	visceral abdominal tissue
VC	vital capacity
$\dot{V}CO_2$	volume of carbon dioxide produced
VEP	ventricular ejection period
VFP	ventricular filling period
VLDL	very low density lipoprotein
$\dot{V}O_2$	volume of oxygen consumed
$\dot{V}O_2max$	maximal volume of oxygen consumed
$\dot{V}O_2peak$	peak volume of oxygen consumed
$\dot{V}O_2R$	oxygen consumption reserve
VT	ventilatory threshold
$v\dot{V}O_2max$	velocity at maximal oxygen consumption
W/H	waist to hip ratio
WBC	white blood cells
WT	weight

Icon Identification Guide

Short-term, light to moderate submaximal aerobic

Long-term, moderate to heavy submaximal aerobic

Incremental aerobic to maximum

Static

Dynamic resistance

Free Student Aid.

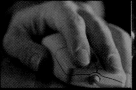

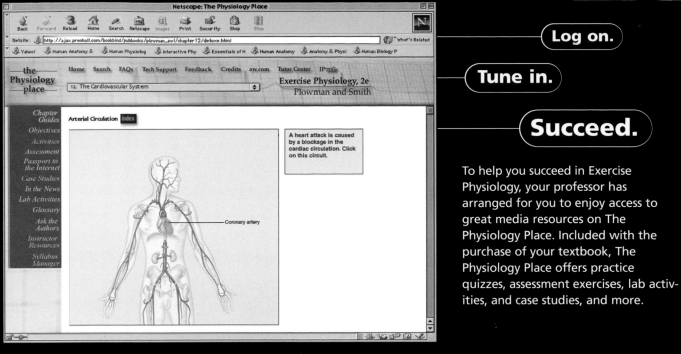

To help you succeed in Exercise Physiology, your professor has arranged for you to enjoy access to great media resources on The Physiology Place. Included with the purchase of your textbook, The Physiology Place offers practice quizzes, assessment exercises, lab activities, and case studies, and more.

Here's your personal ticket to success:

How to log on to The Physiology Place

1. Go to www.physiologyplace.com.
2. Click *Exercise Physiology for Health, Fitness, and Performance, Second Edition.*
3. Click "Register Here."
4. Scratch off the silver foil coating below to reveal your pre-assigned access code.
5. Enter your pre-assigned access code exactly as it appears below.
6. Complete the online registration form to create your own personal Login Name and Password.
7. Once your personal Login Name and Password are confirmed by email, go back to www.physiologyplace.com, type in your new Login Name and Password, and click "Enter."

Your Access Code is:

Got technical questions?

For technical support, please visit www.aw.com/techsupport and complete the appropriate online form. Technical support is available Monday-Friday, 9 a.m. to 6 p.m. Eastern Time (US and Canada).

What your system needs to use these media resources:

WINDOWS™
- 250 MHz
- Windows-98/NT/2000/XP
- 32 MB RAM installed, 64 preferred
- 800x600 screen resolution
- Thousands of colors
- Browsers: Internet Explorer 5.0 and higher; Netscape 4.7, 7.0
- Plug-ins: Flash player, QuickTime

NOTE: Use of Netscape 6.0 and 6.1 are not recommended due to a known compatibility issue between Netscape 6.0 and 6.1 and the Flash and Shockwave plug-ins.

MACINTOSH™
- 233 MHz PowerPC
- OS 9.2 or higher
- 32 MB RAM minimum
- 800x600 screen resolution
- Thousands of colors.
- Browsers: Internet Explorer 5.0; Netscape 4.7
- Plug-ins: Flash player, QuickTime

NOTE: Use of Netscape 6.0 and 6.1 are not recommended due to a known compatibility issue between Netscape 6.0 and 6.1 and the Flash and Shockwave plug-ins.

Important: Please read the License Agreement, located on the launch screen before using **The Physiology Place**. By using the web site, you indicate that you have read, understood, and accepted the terms of this agreement.

Exercise Physiology
for Health, Fitness, and Performance

Related Benjamin Cummings Kinesiology Titles

Bishop, *Fitness through Aerobics,* Fifth Edition (2002)

Bishop/Aldana, *Step Up to Wellness: A Stage-Based Approach* (1999)

Carr/Metzler, *Soccer: Mastering the Basics with the Personalized Sports Instruction System (A Workbook Approach)* (2001)

Darst/Pangrazi, *Dynamic Physical Education for Secondary School Students,* Fourth Edition (2002)

Darst/Pangrazi, *Lesson Plans for Dynamic Physical Education for Secondary School Students,* Fourth Edition (2002)

Freeman, *Physical Education and Sport in a Changing Society,* Sixth Edition (2001)

Fronske, *Teaching Cues for Sport Skills,* Second Edition (2001)

Fronske/Wilson, *Teaching Cues for Basic Sports Skills for Elementary and Middle School Children* (2002)

McGown/Fronske/Moser, *Coaching Volleyball: Building a Winning Team* (2001)

Metzler, *Badminton: Mastering the Basics with the Personalized Sports Instruction System (A Workbook Approach)* (2001)

Metzler, *Golf: Mastering the Basics with the Personalized Sports Instruction System (A Workbook Approach)* (2001)

Metzler, *Racquetball: Mastering the Basics with the Personalized Sports Instruction System (A Workbook Approach)* (2001)

Metzler, *Tennis: Mastering the Basics with the Personalized Sports Instruction System (A Workbook Approach)* (2001)

Mosston/Ashworth, *Teaching Physical Education,* Fifth Edition (2002)

Pangrazi, *Dynamic Physical Education for Elementary School Children,* Thirteenth Edition (2001)

Pangrazi, *Lesson Plans for Dynamic Physical Education for Elementary School Children,* Thirteenth Edition (2001)

Poole/Metzler, *Volleyball: Mastering the Basics with the Personalized Sports Instruction System (A Workbook Approach)* (2001)

Powers/Dodd, *Total Fitness: Exercise, Nutrition, and Wellness,* Second Edition (1999)

Schmottlach/McManama, *Physical Education Activity Handbook,* Tenth Edition (2002)

Silva/Stevens, *Psychological Foundations of Sport* (2002)

Check out these and other Benjamin Cummings kinesiology titles at: www.aw.com/bc.

Exercise Physiology

for Health, Fitness, and Performance

Second Edition

Sharon A. Plowman
Northern Illinois University

Denise L. Smith
Skidmore College

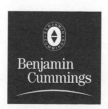

Benjamin
Cummings

San Francisco Boston New York
Cape Town Hong Kong London Madrid Mexico City
Montreal Munich Paris Singapore Sydney Tokyo Toronto

Publisher: Daryl Fox
Acquisitions Editor: Deirdre McGill
Project Editor: Susan Teahan
Publishing Assistant: Michelle Cadden
Managing Editor: Wendy Earl
Production Editor: Leslie Austin
Cover and Text Design: Kathleen Cunningham
Copy Editor: Sally Peyrefitte
Proofreader: Martha Ghent
Compositor: The Left Coast Group
Photo Researcher: Diane Austin
Manufacturing Buyer: Stacey Weinberger
Marketing Manager: Sandra Lindelof

Cover Photographs: © Don Mason/CORBIS (rock climber) and © 1998–2001 EyeWire, Inc. (EKG background)

Library of Congress Cataloging-in-Publication Data
Plowman Sharon A.
    Exercise physiology for health, fitness, and performance / Sharon A. Plowman, Denise
L. Smith.—2nd ed.
        p. cm.
    Includes bibliographical references and index.
    ISBN 0-8053-5349-6
     1. Exercise—Physiological aspects. I. Smith, Denise L. II. Title.

QP301 .P585 2002
612´.044—dc21

2001059861

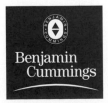

ISBN 0-8053-5349-6

3 4 5 6 7 8 9 10–QWV–06 05 04

www.aw.com/bc

To our teachers and students,
past, present, and future:
sometimes one and the same.

Brief Contents

Metabolic System

Neuromuscular–Skeletal System

Cardiovascular–Respiratory System

Contents

Preface

The second edition of *Exercise Physiology for Health, Fitness, and Performance* builds upon and expands the strengths of the first edition. The purpose for the second edition, however, remains unchanged from that of the first edition. That is, the goal is to present concepts in a clear and comprehensive way that will allow students to apply the principles of exercise physiology in the widest variety of possible work situations. The primary audience is kinesiology and physical education majors and minors, including students in traditional teaching preparation programs (with or without a coaching emphasis) and students in exercise and sport science tracts where the goal is to prepare for careers in fitness, rehabilitation, athletic training, or physical therapy.

As with other textbooks in the field, a great deal of information is presented. Most of the information has been summarized and conceptualized based on research. However, we have occasionally included specific research studies to illustrate certain points, believing that students need to develop an appreciation for research and the constancy of change that research precipitates. **Focus on Research** boxes have been added to this second edition to highlight important new basic and applied studies in exercise physiology as well as relevant experimental design considerations. The chapters are thoroughly referenced and a complete list of references, in scientific format, is provided at the end of each chapter. These references should prove to be a useful resource for students to explore topics in more detail for laboratory reports or term projects.

The body of knowledge in exercise physiology is extensive and growing every day. Each individual faculty member must determine what is essential for his or her students. To this end, we have tried to allow for choice and flexibility, particularly in the organization and content of the book.

A Unique Integrative Approach

The intent of this textbook is to present the body of knowledge based on the traditions of exercise physiology but in a way that is not bound by those traditions. Instead of proceeding from a unit of basic science, through one or more units of applied science, to a final unit of special populations or situations (which can lead to the false sense that scientific theories and applications can and should be separated), we have chosen a completely integrative approach to make the link between basic theories and applied concepts both strong and logical.

Flexible Organization

Two chapters are included in the introductory unit of the second edition. The first explains the text organization, provides an overview of exercise physiology, and establishes the basic concepts that will be covered in each unit. The new second chapter describes the neuroendocrine control of exercise and links these systems to the stress response and the problem of overtraining. Three major units follow the introductory: metabolic system, cardiovascular–respiratory system, and neuromuscular–skeletal system. Although the units are presented in this order, each unit is intended to stand alone and has been written in such a way that it may be taught before or after each of the other two. Figure 1.1 depicts the circular integration of the units. Unit openers and graphics throughout the text reinforce this concept.

Consistent Sequence of Presentation

To lay a solid pedagogical foundation, the chapters in each unit follow a consistent sequence of presentation: basic anatomy and physiology, the measurement and meaning of variables important to understanding exercise physiology, exercise responses, training principles and adaptations, and special applications, problems, and considerations.

Basic Sciences It is assumed that the students using this text will have had a basic course in anatomy, physiology, chemistry, and math. However, it is also acknowledged that reviewing specific aspects of these courses is essential for many students. Some students do not need this review and for them the basic chapters can be de-emphasized.

Measurement Inclusion of the measurement sections serves two purposes—to identify how the variables most frequently used in exercise physiology are obtained and to contrast criterion or laboratory test results with field test results. Criterion or laboratory test results are essential for accurate determination and understanding of the exercise responses and training adaptations, but field test results are often the only items available to the professional in school or health club settings.

Exercise Responses and Training Adaptations   The chapters or sections on exercise responses and training adaptations present the definitive and core information for exercise physiology. Exercise response chapters are organized by exercise modality and intensity. Specifically, physiological responses to the following five categories of exercise (based on the duration, intensity, and type of muscle contraction) are presented: (1) short-term, light to moderate submaximal aerobic exercise; (2) long-term, moderate to heavy submaximal aerobic exercise; (3) incremental aerobic exercise to maximum; (4) static exercise; and (5) dynamic resistance exercise. Training principles for the prescription of exercise are presented for each physical fitness component: aerobic and anaerobic metabolism, body composition, cardiovascular and muscular strength, endurance, and flexibility. These principles are followed by the training adaptations that will result from a well prescribed training program.

Special Applications   The special applications chapters always relate the unit topic to health-related fitness and then deal with such diverse topics as altitude, thermoregulation, and immunology (Cardiovascular–Respiratory Unit); making weight and eating disorders (Metabolic Unit); and anabolic steroids (Neuromuscular–Skeletal Unit). **Focus on Application** boxes emphasize how research and underlying exercise physiology principles are relevant to the world of the practitioner.

Complete Integration of Age Groups and Sexes

A major departure from tradition in the organization of this text is the complete integration of information relevant to all age groups and both sexes. In the past, there was good reason to describe evidence and derive concepts based on information from male college students and elite male athletes. These were the populations most involved in physical activity and sport, and they were the groups most frequently studied. As more women, children, and elderly began participating in sport and fitness programs, information became available on these groups. Chapters on females, children, and the elderly were added to the back of exercise physiology texts as supplemental material. However, most physical education and exercise professionals will be dealing with both males and females, children and adolescents in school settings, average middle-aged adults in health clubs or fitness centers, and the elderly in special programs. Very few will be dealing strictly with college-age students, and

fewer still will work with elite athletes. This does not mean that information based on the young adult male populations has been excluded or even de-emphasized. However, it does mean that it is time to move coverage of the groups who make up most of the population from the back of the book and integrate information about males and females at various ages throughout the text.

Pedagogical Considerations

Most of the pedagogical techniques used in this textbook are straightforward. These techniques include a list of learning objectives at the beginning of each chapter as well as a chapter summary, review questions, and references at the end of each chapter. Another pedagogical aid is the use of a running glossary. Terms are boldfaced and defined in the text where they first appear as well as highlighted in definition boxes to emphasize the context in which the terms are used. A glossary is also included in the back matter of the book. Embedded within the chapter summaries are references to related *Interactive Physiology*® animated tutorials that review a particular topic. The *Interactive Physiology*® sampler CD is provided with the purchase of this text, and the full *Interactive Physiology*® *7-System Suite* tutorial is available with a discount when bundled with the text.

To aid the student, a complete list of commonly used symbols and abbreviations with their meanings is printed on the front endpapers of the text. Each chapter contains a multitude of tables, graphs, charts, diagrams, and photographs to underscore the pedagogy and enhance the visual appeal of the text.

Unique Color-Coding

A unique aspect of the graphs is color-coding, which allows for quick recognition of the condition represented. For exercise response patterns, each exercise type has its own shaded background color and a representative icon. A key to color-coding and icons are fully presented to the reader in Chapter 1. Similarly, training adaptations are presented on a specific tinted background. Finally, the most frequent comparisons (training status, sex, and age) have consistent line or bar profile colors, providing visual guides that allow for tracking of specific groups throughout the text.

Active Learning

Throughout the text, **A Question of Understanding** boxes engage the student in active learning beyond just reading. In some instances, the boxes require students to work through problems that address their understanding of the material. In other instances, students are asked to interpret a set of circumstances or deduce an answer based on previously presented information. Where appropriate, equations are highlighted and examples worked out in the text. Each chapter ends with a set of essay review questions.

Appendices

Appendix A provides information on the metric system, units, symbols, and conversions both within and between the metric and English systems. Appendix B offers supplementary material, consisting of three parts that deal with aspects of oxygen consumption calculation. Appendix C contains an executive summary of *Physical Activity and Health: A Report of the Surgeon General*. Answers to **A Question of Understanding** boxes are presented in Appendix D.

New to the Second Edition

For the second edition, two new chapters have been added to *Exercise Physiology for Health, Fitness, and Performance. Chapter 2: Neuroendocrine Control of Exercise* offers basic anatomy and physiology of the neural and hormonal systems as well as comprehensive coverage of the effects of exercise and training on the nervous and hormonal systems. Immunology has been expanded to chapter length; *Chapter 17: The Immune System in Health and Disease* emphasizes interaction between the immune system, acute exercise responses, training adaptations, maladaptations, and disease.

Several new pedagogical features are offered in the new edition. **Focus on Research** boxes in every chapter explore new findings in the field. **Focus on Application** boxes throughout the text relate basic concepts, principles, or specific research findings to situations, concerns, or recommendtions relevant to using the information that is presented. The new section, **Passport to the Internet,** references web sites related to specific topics covered in each chapter. References to *Interactive Physiology® CD-ROM*, a richly detailed graphic and animated tutorial program, are offered in chapter summaries and are indicated by the icon **IP** . An *Interactive Physiology®* sampler CD is included with each copy of the text as well.

Supplements

A comprehensive set of ancillary materials designed to facilitate classroom preparation and ease the transition into a new text is available to adopters of *Exercise Physiology for Health, Fitness, and Performance.*

- The *Instructor's Guide and Test Bank*, prepared by Sharon A. Plowman, Denise L. Smith, and their colleague Patricia Fehling, is a comprehensive teaching tool that provides chapter-by-chapter outlines, suggested laboratory activities, review questions, and a test bank with multiple choice and fill-in-the-blank questions. For the second edition, the *Instructor's Guide and Test Bank* offers a synopsis of each chapter, cross references to the *Laboratory Manual*, and media references for the *Interactive Physiology® CD-ROM* and *The Physiology Place* companion web site. ISBN: **0-8053-5343-7**

- The *Computerized Test Bank* is a cross-platform CD-ROM in Tamarack TestGen-EQ 3.0 and contains all of the questions found in the printed test bank. Tests can be generated with a user-friendly interface that allows for easy viewing, editing, sorting, and adding of questions. To help navigation through the program, the *Computerized Test Bank* is packaged with a *User's Manual*. ISBN: **0-8053-5344-5**

- The *Transparencies (acetates)* are expanded for the second edition to 280 sheets. Included are graphs, charts, schematic figures, and anatomical art from the text. ISBN: **0-8053-5345-3**

- The **PowerPoint®** **presentation slides** correspond to the organization of content in the textbook. Created for each chapter of the text is a lecture slide show that highlights key concepts and incorporates graphs, charts, figures, exercise modality icons, and the color-coding system. ISBN: **0-321-10662-8**

- *The Physiology Place* **web site,** which is located at www.physiologyplace.com, offers book-specific chapter quizzes, interactive learning activities, case studies, lab activities, web links, and more. In addition to student resources, *The Physiology Place* includes a password-protected instructor's resource section with figures and tables from the book, and an electronic version of the *Instructor's Guide*. A 12-month subscription to *The Physiology Place* is included with every new copy of the text.

- **Laboratory Manual.** The *Laboratory Manual,* which includes 21 separate labs, is designed specifically to accompany this text. It provides experiments to showcase the physiological responses to the five categories of exercise, compares and contrasts criterion tests with field tests, and emphasizes practical applications such as the caloric cost of activities and muscle soreness. New test items (such as the Field Anaerobic Shuttle Test) have been included in the second edition. Student activities guide the analysis and interpretation of the obtained data. Each lab presents the instructor a number of choices to meet the specific needs of a particular class, available equipment, and/or meeting time. ISBN: **0-321-10658-X**

- **Student Study Guide.** New with the second edition of the text is the *Student Study Guide for Exercise Physiology for Health, Fitness, and Performance.* The study guide is intended to assist the student in identifying key concepts in exercise physiology and in the organization of material. It may also be used for self-testing. Each chapter begins with a learning task for definitions and includes true-false and multiple choice questions. As the material allows, diagrams, tables, and matching items are also included. ISBN: **0-321-10660-1**

Acknowledgments

The completion of this textbook required the help of many people. A complete list of individuals is impossible, but four groups to whom we are indebted must be recognized for their meritorious assistance. The first group is our families and friends who saw less of us than either we or they desired due to the constant time demands. Their support, patience, and understanding were much appreciated. The second group contains our many professional colleagues, known and unknown, who critically reviewed the manuscript at several stages and provided valuable suggestions for revisions along with a steady supply of encouragement. This kept us going. The third group is our students, who provided much of the initial motivation for undertaking the task. Some went far beyond that and provided meaningful feedback by using the text in manuscript form. The final group is the editors and staff at Benjamin Cummings, particularly our Project Editor, Susan Teahan, and our Production Editor, Leslie Austin, whose faith in the project and commitment to excellence in its production are responsible for the finished product you now see. We thank you all.

The following reviewers provided excellent feedback and criticism throughout the development of the text. To the following we offer grateful acknowledgment of expertise and thorough review:

Rosemary Lindle
University of Maryland
Ed Heath
Utah State University
Michael Rogers
Wichita State University
Karen Gallagher
Brown Medical School
Patricia Eisenman
University of Utah
Joan Finn
Southern Connecticut State University
Don Tarara
High Point University
John Daniel
Texas Tech University
Michelle Fisher
Montclair State University
R.O. Ruhling
George Mason University
David Hill
University of North Texas
Janice Herring
California State University–Stanislaus
Cheryl Cohen
Western Illinois University

Sharon A. Plowman
Denise L. Smith

About the Authors

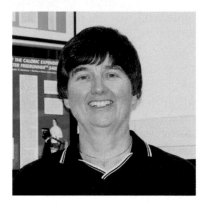

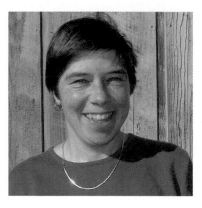

SHARON A. PLOWMAN earned her Ph.D. at the University of Illinois at Urbana–Champaign under the tutelage of Dr. T. K. Cureton Jr. She is a professor in the Department of Kinesiology and Physical Education and Director of the Exercise Physiology Laboratory at Northern Illinois University. Dr. Plowman has taught for 34 years including classes in exercise physiology, stress testing, and exercise bioenergetics. She has published over sixty-five scientific and research articles in the field as well as numerous applied articles on physical fitness with emphasis on females and children in such journals as *ACSM's Health & Fitness Journal; Annals of Nutrition and Metabolism; Human Biology; Medicine and Science in Sports & Exercise; Pediatric Exercise Science;* and *Research Quarterly for Exercise and Sport.* She is a co-author with M. H. Anshel (ed.) et al. of the *Dictionary of the Sport and Exercise Sciences* (1991).

Dr. Plowman is a Fellow in the American College of Sports Medicine, and served on the Board of Trustees of that organization from 1980–1983. In 1992 she was elected an Active Fellow by the American Academy of Kinesiology and Physical Education. She serves on the Advisory Council for FITNESS-GRAM®. The American Alliance for Health, Physical Education, Recreation and Dance (AAHPERD) recognized her with the Mable Lee Award in 1976 and the Physical Fitness Council Award in 1994. Dr. Plowman received the Excellence in Teaching Award (at Northern Illinois University at the department level in 1974 and 1975 and at the university level in 1975) and the Distinguished Alumni Award from the Department of Kinesiology at the University of Illinois at Urbana-Champaign in 1996.

DENISE L. SMITH is an Associate Professor in the Department of Exercise Science, Dance and Athletics and Director of the Human Performance Laboratory at Skidmore College. With a Ph.D. in kinesiology and specialization in exercise physiology from the University of Illinois at Urbana–Champaign, Dr. Smith has taught for over 11 years, including classes in anatomy and physiology, cardiorespiratory aspects of human performance, neuromuscular aspects of human performance, and research design. Much of her research is focused on the physiological effects of firefighting, particularly the cardiovascular strain associated with firefighting. She has published in such journals as *Aviation, Space and Environmental Medicine; Ergonomics; European Journal of Applied Physiology; Journal of Applied Physiology; Journal of Cardiopulmonary Rehabilitation;* and *Medicine and Science in Sports & Exercise.*

Dr. Smith is a Fellow in the American College of Sports Medicine and has served as secretary for the Occupational Physiology Interest Group and as a member of the National Strategic Health Initiative Committee. She has also served on the executive board and as an officer for the MidAtlantic Regional Chapter of ACSM. Since 1994 she has been a visiting professor at the University of Illinois Fire Service Institute at Urbana–Champaign.

Introductory

Unit

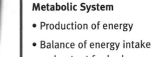

Cardiovascular–Respiratory System

Circulation:

- Transportation of oxygen and energy substrates to muscle tissue
- Transportation of waste products

Respiration:

- Intake of air into body
- Diffusion of oxygen and carbon dioxide at lungs and muscle tissue
- Removal of carbon dioxide from body

Metabolic System

- Production of energy
- Balance of energy intake and output for body composition and weight control

Neuromuscular–Skeletal System

- Locomotion (exercise)
- Movement brought about by muscular contraction (under neural stimulation acting on bony levers of skeletal system)

This text is organized into units according to the basic physiological systems that support human movement: metabolic, cardiovascular–respiratory, and neuromuscular–skeletal. Within each unit, a pattern of presentation is established. Chapter 1 introduces the pattern and emphasizes common terminology, graphic depictions, and interpretive considerations that are used to describe the body's acute response to exercise and chronic adaptation to exercise training. Chapter 1 also introduces the training principles that must be properly applied in order to achieve training adaptations. Although a systems approach is taken in this book, the exercise responses and training adaptations are obviously not isolated in the human body. Control and coordination occur by the nervous and hormonal systems. The basic functioning of these two systems is presented in Chapter 2, as well as their possible role in maladaptation if the training principles are ignored or improperly applied. Mastery of the Introductory Unit content will facilitate learning of the material in subsequent units.

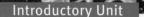

Chapter 1

The Warm-Up

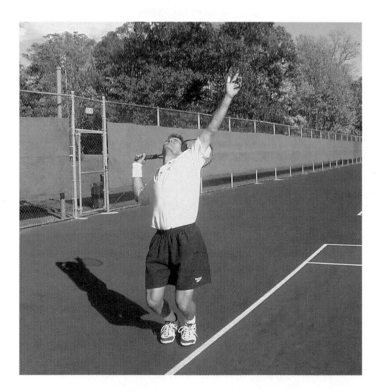

After studying the chapter, you should be able to

- Describe what exercise physiology is and discuss why you need to study it.
- Identify the organizational structure of this text.
- Differentiate between exercise responses and training adaptations.
- List and explain the five categories of exercise whose responses are documented throughout this book.
- List and explain the factors that must be considered in interpreting the exercise response.
- Describe the graphic patterns that physiological variables may exhibit in response to different categories of exercise and as a result of adaptation to training.
- List and explain the training principles.
- Describe the differences and similarities between health-related and sport-specific physical fitness.
- Define and explain periodization.

What Is Exercise Physiology and Why Study It?

In a 1966 science fiction movie called *Fantastic Voyage* (CBS/Fox), a military medical team is miniaturized in a nuclear-powered submarine and injected through a hypodermic needle into the carotid artery. Anticipating an easy float into the brain, where they plan to remove a blood clot by laser beam, they are both awed and imperiled by what they see and what befalls them. They see erythrocytes turning from an iridescent blue to vivid red as oxygen bubbles replace carbon dioxide; nerve impulses appear as bright flashes of light; and when air pressure is lost, all they need to do is tap into an alveolus. Not all of their encounters are so benign, however: They are sucked into a whirlpool caused by an abnormal fistula between the carotid artery and jugular vein. They have to get the outside team to stop the heart so that they will not be crushed by its contraction. They are jostled about by the conduction of sound waves in the inner ear. They are attacked by antibodies. And finally, their submarine is destroyed by a white blood cell—they are, after all, foreign bodies to the natural defense system. Of course, in the end, the "good guys" on the team escape through a tear duct, and all is well.

Although the journey you are about to take through the human body will not be quite so literal, nor anywhere near as dangerous, it should be just as incredible and probably more fascinating, for it goes beyond the basics of anatomy and physiology into the realm of the moving human. The body is capable of great feats, whose limits and full benefits in terms of exercise and sport are still unknown.

Consider these events and changes, all of which have probably taken place within the life span of your parents.

- President Dwight D. Eisenhower suffered a heart attack on September 23, 1955 (Raab, 1966). At that time 6 weeks of bed rest and a lifetime of curtailed activity was normal medical treatment and advice (Hellerstein, 1979). Eisenhower's rehabilitation, including a return to golf, was, if not revolutionary, certainly progressive. Today, cardiac patients are mobilized within days and frequently train for and safely run marathons.

- The 4-min mile was considered an unbreakable limit until May 6, 1954, when Roger Bannister ran the mile in 3:59.4. Hundreds of runners (including some high school boys) have since accomplished that feat. The men's world record for the mile, which was set in 1999, is 3:43.13. The women's mile record, of 4:12.56 set in 1996, is approaching the old 4-min "barrier."

- The 800-m run was banned from the Olympics from 1928 to 1964 for women because females were "too weak and delicate" to run such a "long" distance. In the 1950s when the 800-m run was reintroduced for women in Europe, ambulances were stationed at the finish line, motors running, to carry off the casualties (Ullyot, 1976). In 1963 the women's world marathon record (then not an Olympic sport for women) was 3:37.07, a time now commonly achieved by females not considered to be elite athletes. The women's world record (set in 2001) was 2:18.47, an improvement of 1:18:20 (36.3%).

- In 1954 Kraus and Hirschland published a report indicating that American children were less fit than European children (Kraus and Hirschland, 1954). At that time being *fit* was defined as being able to pass the Kraus-Weber test of minimal muscular fitness, which consisted of one each of the following: bent-leg sit-up; straight-leg sit-up; standing toe touch; double-leg lift, prone; double-leg lift, supine; and trunk extension, prone. Today, physical fitness is more broadly defined in terms of both physiology and age span and is even more sought after.

These changes and a multitude of others that we readily accept as a normal part of our daily lives have come about as a combined result of formal medical and scientific research and informal experimentation by individuals with the curiosity and courage to try new things.

These events and changes also typify the concerns with which the broad area of exercise physiology deals—that is, athletic performance, physical fitness, and rehabilitation. **Exercise physiology** can be defined as both a basic and an applied science that describes, explains, and uses the body's response to exercise and adaptation to exercise training to maximize human physical potential.

Any single course or textbook cannot, of course, provide all the information a prospective professional will need. However, a knowledge of exercise physiology and an appreciation for basing practice on research findings goes a long way in setting professionals in the field apart from mere practitioners. It is one thing to be able to lead step aerobic routines. It is

---

Exercise Physiology A basic and an applied science that describes, explains, and uses the body's response to exercise and adaptation to exercise training to maximize human physical potential.

another to be able to design routines based on predictable short- and long-term responses of given class members, to be able to evaluate those responses, and then to be able to modify the sessions as needed. Thus, it is important for students of exercise science and physical education who are intent on becoming respected professionals in any of the related fields to learn exercise physiology in order to:

1. Understand how the basic physiological functioning of the human body is modified by short- and long-term exercise and the mechanisms that bring about these changes. Unless one knows what responses are normal, it is not possible to recognize an abnormal response or adjust to it.

2. Provide quality physical education programs in the schools that stimulate children and adolescents both physically and intellectually. Students need to understand how physical activity can benefit them, why they take physical fitness tests, and what to do with fitness test results in order to become lifelong exercisers.

3. Be able to apply the results of scientific research to maximize health, rehabilitation, and/or athletic performance in a variety of subpopulations.

4. Be able to respond accurately to questions and advertising claims, as well as recognize and react to myths and misconceptions that appear in relation to exercise. Good advice should be based on scientifically determined evidence.

Overview of the Text

So that students can accomplish the goals just outlined, this textbook has been divided into three units: metabolic system, cardiovascular-respiratory system, and neuromuscular-skeletal system. Within each unit the following format is followed.

1. basic information
    a. anatomical structures
    b. physiological function, including regulatory mechanisms
    c. laboratory techniques and variables typically measured
2. exercise responses
3. training
    a. application of the training principles
    b. adaptations to training
4. special applications, problems, and considerations

The first part of each unit deals with the basic anatomical and physiological structures and functions necessary to understand the material that follows. The next part of each unit deals with the acute responses to exercise. This is followed by a specific application of the training principles and the adaptations that typically occur if the training principles are applied correctly. Finally, each unit ends with one or more special application topics, such as thermal concerns, weight control/body composition, and osteoporosis.

This integrated approach is intended to provide fairly immediate relevance in applying the basic information. More information continues to be available on college-age males or elite male athletes than on any other portion of the population. Wherever possible, though, we have attempted to expand beyond this base and to compare both sexes, not only as young or middle-aged adults but also as children and adolescents at one end of the age spectrum and as the elderly at the other.

Each unit is intended to be independent of the other two, although the body obviously functions as a whole. The separation is designed to provide each individual faculty member flexibility in determining the sequence of his or her course. It is possible to start with any unit and proceed in any order through the other two. This concept is represented by the circle in Figure 1.1.

Figure 1.1 also illustrates two other important points: (1) all of the systems respond to exercise in an integrated fashion, and (2) the responses of the systems are interdependent. The metabolic system is responsible for producing cellular energy, in the form of adenosine triphosphate (ATP). ATP is then used for muscular contraction. In order for the cells (including muscle cells) to produce ATP, they must be supplied with oxygen and fuel (foodstuffs). The respiratory system is responsible for bringing oxygen into the body via the lungs, and the cardiovascular system is responsible for distributing that oxygen and fuel to the cells of the body via the blood pumped by the heart through the blood vessels. During exercise, all of these functions must be increased.

Each unit is divided into chapters as the length and depth of the material dictates. Each chapter begins with a list of learning objectives. The objectives will help you get an overall picture of what is to be presented and to understand what you should be learning in the chapter. Definitions are highlighted in boxes as they are introduced. Each chapter ends with a summary and review questions. Scattered throughout the text are Research and Application focus boxes as well as Question of Understanding boxes. The latter are problems for you to complete; answers to these are presented in Appendix D by page number. When appropriate, worked-out calculations

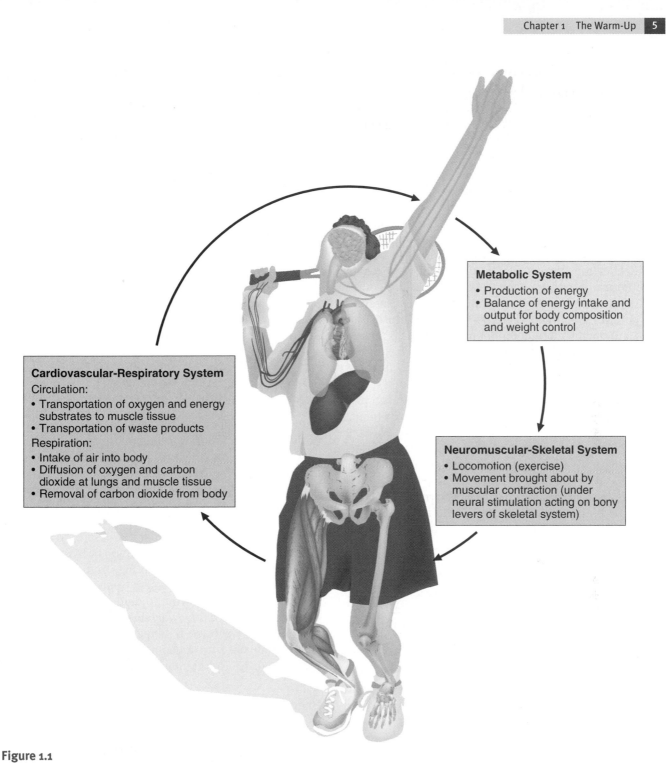

Metabolic System
• Production of energy
• Balance of energy intake and output for body composition and weight control

Cardiovascular-Respiratory System
Circulation:
• Transportation of oxygen and energy substrates to muscle tissue
• Transportation of waste products
Respiration:
• Intake of air into body
• Diffusion of oxygen and carbon dioxide at lungs and muscle tissue
• Removal of carbon dioxide from body

Neuromuscular-Skeletal System
• Locomotion (exercise)
• Movement brought about by muscular contraction (under neural stimulation acting on bony levers of skeletal system)

Figure 1.1
Schematic Representation of Text Organization

are presented in examples. The appendices and end-papers provide supplemental information. For example, Appendix A contains a listing of the basic physical quantities, units of measurement, and conversions within the Système International d'Unités (SI or metric system of measurement commonly used in scientific work) and between the metric and English measurement systems. In the front of the book, you will find a list of the symbols and abbreviations used throughout the book, along with their definitions. You may need to refer to these appendices frequently if these symbols and measurement units are new to you.

The field of exercise physiology is a dynamic area of study with many practical implications. At the very least, over the next few months you should gain an appreciation for the tremendous range over which the human body can function. At the very best, you will become better prepared as a professional for the safe and effective execution of the responsibilities of your chosen field. Somewhere along the way, you will probably also learn something about yourself. Enjoy the voyage.

The Exercise Response

Let's begin with some definitions and concepts that are basic to all of the units and thus need to be established right away. **Exercise** is a single acute bout of bodily exertion or muscular activity that requires an expenditure of energy above resting level and generally results in voluntary movement. Exercise sessions are generally planned and structured to improve or maintain one or more components of physical fitness. The term *physical activity* generally connotes movement in which the goal (often to sustain daily living or recreation) is different from physical fitness, but which also requires the expenditure of energy and often provides health-related benefits. For example, walking to school or work is physical activity; walking around a track at a predetermined heart rate is exercise. However, from a physiological standpoint both bring about changes (both acute and chronic). Therefore, the terms *exercise* and *physical activity* are used interchangeably in this textbook. Where the amount of exercise can actually be measured, the terms *workload* or *work rate* may be used as well.

Exercise disrupts the homeostatic state or dynamic equilibrium of the body. These homeostatic disruptions or changes represent the body's response to exercise. An **exercise response** is the pattern of change that physiological variables exhibit during a single acute bout of physical exertion. A *physiological variable* is any measure of bodily function that changes or varies under different circumstances. Heart rate is a variable with which you are undoubtedly already familiar. You probably also know that heart rate increases during exercise. However, to state simply that heart rate increases during exercise does not describe the full pattern of the response. For example, the heart rate response to a 400-m sprint is different from the heart rate response to a 50-mi bike ride. To fully describe the response of heart rate or any other variable, we must first have more information about the exercise itself. Three factors need to be considered to determine or describe the acute response to exercise:

1. the exercise modality,
2. the exercise intensity, and
3. the exercise duration.

Exercise Modality

Exercise modality (or **mode**) means the type of activity or the particular sport. For example, rowing has a very different effect on the cardiovascular-respiratory system than does football. Modalities are often classified by the type of energy demand (aerobic or anaerobic), the major muscle action (continuous and rhythmical, dynamic resistance, or static), or a combination of energy system and muscle action. Walking, cycling, and swimming are examples of continuous, rhythmical aerobic activities; jumping, sprinting, and weight lifting are anaerobic and/or dynamic resistance activities. Thus, when you are trying to determine the effects of exercise on a particular variable, you must first know what type of exercise is being performed. The basic terminology used throughout the text will be primarily *aerobic, static,* and *dynamic resistance* exercise.

Exercise Intensity

Exercise intensity is most easily described as maximal or submaximal. Of these, **maximal (max) exercise** is the most straightforward; it simply refers to the highest intensity, greatest load, or longest duration an individual is capable of doing. Motivation plays a large part in the achievement of maximal levels of exercise. Most maximal values are reached at the endpoint of an *incremental exercise test to maximum;* that is, the exercise task begins at a level the individual is comfortable with and gradually increases until he or she can do no more. The values for the physiological variables measured at this time are labeled as max; for example, maximum heart rate is symbolized as HRmax.

Exercise A single acute bout of bodily exertion or muscular activity that requires an expenditure of energy above resting level and that in most, but not all, cases results in voluntary movement.

Exercise Response The pattern of homeostatic disruption or change that physiological variables exhibit during a single acute bout of physical exertion.

Exercise Modality or Mode The type of activity or sport; usually classified by energy demand or type of muscle action.

Maximal (max) Exercise The highest intensity, greatest load, or longest duration exercise of which an individual is capable.

Focus on Research

Cardiovascular Responses to Exercise

Ogawa, T., et al.: Effects of aging, sex, and physical training on cardiovascular responses to exercise. *Circulation.* 86:494–503 (1992).

Exercise professionals, and indeed many exercise participants, have long been interested in how characteristics of the participants influence the body's response to exercise. In this study, the authors investigated the effects of age, sex, and physical training on cardiovascular responses to exercise. To accomplish this objective, the authors separated 110 healthy subjects into eight groups based on three variables: age (young [mid 20s] or old [mid 60s]), gender (male or female), and physical training (trained or untrained). The table below identifies the eight groups based on these three subject characteristics.

	Men	*Women*
Young	Trained (TR)	Trained (TR)
	Untrained (UT)	Untrained (UT)
Old	Trained (TR)	Trained (TR)
	Untrained (UT)	Untrained (UT)

Results of this study are shown in the figure at the right, which depicts for each group the systolic blood pressure responses to incremental treadmill tests to maximum. Examining these data reveals the following information:

1. Systolic blood pressure response to incremental exercise to maximum was significantly greater in older persons than in younger persons. This is true for men and women, regardless of training status.
2. Maximal systolic blood pressure was significantly lower in trained women than in untrained women.

Although the authors investigated many variables, we discuss only systolic blood pressure, because our purpose is not to examine the cardiovascular results so much as to demonstrate how exerciser characteristics affect exercise response. Throughout this book, exercise response is discussed in terms of age, sex, and physical training. This study provides an excellent example of how researchers investigate the impact of exerciser characteristics (including age, sex, and training status) on the exercise response of a given variable. It is important for exercise professionals to appreciate this relationship so that they can recognize normal and abnormal responses to exercise and respond accordingly.

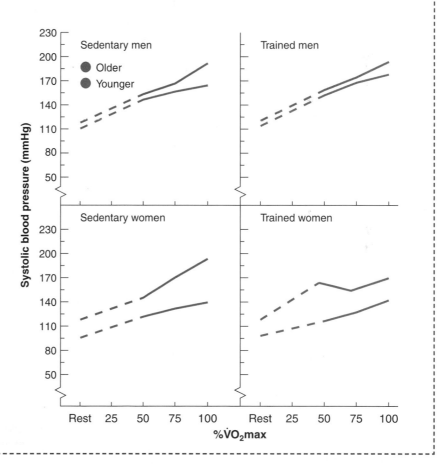

Submaximal exercise may be described in one of two ways. The first involves a *set load,* which is a load that is known or is assumed to be below an individual's maximum. This load may be established by some physiological variable, such as working at a specific heart rate (perhaps 150 b·min^{-1}); at a specific work rate (for example, 600 kgm·min^{-1} on a cycle ergometer), or for a given distance (perhaps a 1-mi run). Such a load is called an **absolute workload.** If an

> **Absolute Submaximal Workload** A set exercise load performed at any intensity from just above resting to just below maximum.

Table 1.1
Absolute and Relative Submaximal Workloads

| | Absolute Workload | | Relative Workload | |
	Maximal Lift	# of Times 80 lb Can Be Lifted	75% of Maximal Lift	# of Times 75% Can Be Lifted
Gerry	160	12	120	10
Pat	100	6	75	10
Terry	80	1	60	10

absolute workload is used, and the individuals being tested vary in their fitness level, then some individuals will be challenged more than others. Generally, those who are more fit in terms of the component being tested will be less challenged and so will score better than those who are less fit and more challenged. For example, suppose the exercise task is to lift 80 lb in a bench press as many times as possible. As illustrated in Table 1.1, if the individuals tested were able to lift a maximum of 160, 100, and 80 lb once, respectively, it would be anticipated that the first individual could do more repetitions than anyone else. Similarly, it would be expected that the second individual could do more repetitions than the third and that the third individual could do only one repetition. The assumption that the load was submaximal for all individuals would not be upheld, because Terry could only lift the weight one time (making it a maximal lift for Terry). However, the use of an absolute load does allow for a ranking among individuals in a single exercise bout and is most often the type of task used in physical fitness screenings or tests.

The second way to describe submaximal exercise is as a percentage of the maximum. Thus, a load may be set at a percentage of maximal heart rate, a percentage of the maximal ability to use oxygen, or a percentage of a maximal workload. This value is called a **relative workload** because it is prorated or relative to each individual. It is both the intent and expectation that all individuals will then be equally challenged by the task and that the same amount of time or number of repetitions can be completed by most, if not all, individuals. For example, for the individuals described in the previous paragraph, suppose that the

----

Relative Submaximal Workload A workload above resting but below maximum that is prorated to each individual; typically set as some percentage of maximum.

----

task now is to lift 75% of the maximal load as many times as possible. Now the individuals will be lifting 120, 75, and 60 lb, respectively. If each person is equally motivated, there should be no meaningful difference in the total number of repetitions each can perform. Relative workloads are occasionally used in physical fitness testing. They are more frequently used to describe exercises that are light, moderate, or heavy in intensity or to give guidelines for exercise prescription.

Unfortunately, there is no universal agreement as to what constitutes light, moderate, or heavy intensity, but in general this book uses the following classification descriptors:

Low or light	≤ 54% of maximum
Moderate	55–69% of maximum
Hard or heavy	70–89% of maximum
Very hard or very heavy	90–99% of maximum
Maximal	100% of maximum
Supramaximal	> 100% of maximum

Maximum is defined variously in terms of workload, heart rate, oxygen consumption, weight lifted a specific number of repetitions, or force exerted in a voluntary contraction. Where results are reported from specific studies, these percentages and definitions of maximum may vary slightly.

Exercise Duration

Exercise duration is simply a description of the length of time the muscular action continues. Duration may vary from as short a time as 1–3 seconds for an explosive action, such as a jump, to as long as 12 hours for a full triathlon (3.2-km [2-mi] swim, 160-km [100-mi] bicycle ride, and 42.2-km [26.2-mi] run). In general, the shorter the duration, the higher the intensity, and vice versa. Thus, the amount of homeostatic disruption is a function of both the duration and intensity of the exercise.

Exercise Categories

In this textbook we have combined the descriptors of exercise modality, intensity, and duration into five primary categories of exercise for which the exercise response patterns are described and discussed:

1. *Short-term, light to moderate submaximal aerobic exercise.* Exercises of this type are rhythmical and continuous in nature, utilize aerobic energy, and are performed at a constant workload for 10–15 minutes at approximately 30–69% of maximal work capacity.

2. *Long-term, moderate to heavy submaximal aerobic exercise.* Exercises in this category also

Table 1.2
Color and Icon Interpretation

Component	Color		Component	Color	Icon
Sex			**Exercise Response Pattern**		
Male	▭		Basic or generic	▭	
Female	▭		Short-term, light to moderate submaximal aerobic	▭	🚶
Age Group			Long-term, moderate to heavy submaximal aerobic	▭	🎿
Young (< 20 years)	▭		Incremental aerobic to maximum	▭	🚣
Adult (20–50 years)	▭				
Elderly (50+ years)	▭		Static	▭	🏋
Status					
Untrained	▭		Dynamic resistance	▭	🏋
Trained	▭		Training adaptations		

utilize rhythmical and continuous muscle action. Although predominantly aerobic, anaerobic energy utilization may be involved. The duration is generally between 30 minutes and 4 hours at constant workload intensities ranging from 55–89% of maximum.

3. *Incremental aerobic exercise to maximum.*   Incremental exercises start at light loads and proceed by a predetermined sequence of progressively increasing workloads to an intensity that the exerciser cannot sustain or increase further. This point becomes the maximum (100%). The early stages are generally light and aerobic, but as the exercise bout continues, anaerobic energy involvement becomes significant. Each workload is called a stage, and each stage may last from 1 to 10 minutes, although 3 minutes is most common. Incremental exercise bouts typically last between 5 and 30 minutes for total duration.

4. *Static exercise.*   Static exercises involve muscle contractions that produce an increase in muscle tension and energy expenditure but do not result in meaningful movement. Static contractions are measured as some percentage of the muscle's **maximal voluntary contraction (MVC),** the maximal force that the muscle can exert. The intent is for the workload to remain constant, but fatigue sometimes makes that impossible. The duration is inversely related to the percentage of maximal voluntary contraction (% MVC) that is being held, but generally ranges from 2 to 10 minutes.

5. *Dynamic resistance exercise.*   Exercises of this type utilize muscle contractions that exert sufficient force to overcome the resistance presented to the muscle, so that movement occurs, as in weight lifting. Energy is supplied by both aerobic and anaerobic processes, but anaerobic is the more dominant source. The workload is constant and can be based on some percentage of the maximal weight the individual can lift **(1-RM)** or a resistance that can be lifted for a specified number of times. The number of repetitions, not time, is the measure of duration.

Occasionally, a sixth type of exercise will be described: exercise of very short duration (30 seconds to 3 minutes) and high intensity. Activities of this type are anaerobic and very often supramaximal.

Exercise Response Patterns

Throughout the textbook, the exercise response patterns for the five categories of exercise just described are depicted both graphically and verbally. For ease of recognition, background colors and icons have been selected to represent each category of exercise. In addition, line or bar colors have been selected for each population to differentiate age, sex, or training status on graphs. The various colors and icons are depicted in Table 1.2. Figure 1.2 presents six of the most

> **Maximal Voluntary Contraction (MVC)** The maximal force that the muscle can exert.
>
> **1-RM** The maximal weight that an individual can lift once during a dynamic resistance exercise.

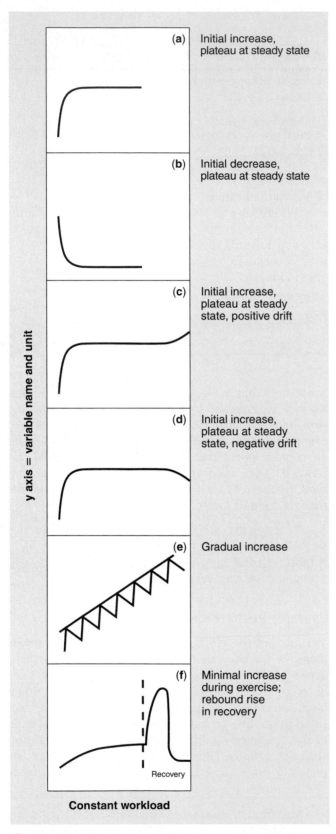

(a) Initial increase, plateau at steady state

(b) Initial decrease, plateau at steady state

(c) Initial increase, plateau at steady state, positive drift

(d) Initial increase, plateau at steady state, negative drift

(e) Gradual increase

(f) Minimal increase during exercise; rebound rise in recovery

Recovery

y axis = variable name and unit

Constant workload

Figure 1.2
Graphic Patterns and Verbal Descriptors for Constant Workload/Work Rate Exercise Responses

frequent graphic patterns resulting from a constant workload, that is, all of the exercise categories except incremental exercise to maximum. Frequent incremental exercise patterns are depicted in Figure 1.3. The verbal descriptors used throughout the book are included on the graphs in both figures and in the following paragraphs. Note that each time an exercise response is described, the baseline, or starting point against which the changes are compared, is the resting value for the variable.

The patterns showing an initial increase or decrease with a plateau at steady state (Figure 1.2a and 1.2b) are the most common responses to *short-term, light to moderate submaximal aerobic exercise.* Patterns that include a drift (Figure 1.2c and 1.2d) typically occur as a result of *long-term, moderate to heavy submaximal aerobic exercise.* The gradual increase, despite no change in the external workload pattern (Figure 1.2e), is frequently seen during dynamic resistance exercise as the sawtooth pattern, which results from the sequential lifting and lowering of the weight. Other categories of exercise may result in the more simple, smooth gradual increase exemplified by the straight slanted line. Minimal change during exercise with a rebound rise in recovery is almost exclusively a static exercise response (Figure 1.2f).

As the title of the graph states, all of the patterns of response presented in Figure 1.3 routinely result from incremental exercise to maximum. Panel f shows two versions of the U-shaped pattern. You may see either a complete or truncated (shortened) U, either upright or inverted.

Exercise Response Interpretation

To interpret the response of selected variables to any of the exercise categories, keep in mind the following:

1. characteristics of the exerciser,
2. appropriateness of the selected exercise,
3. accuracy of the selected exercise, and
4. environmental and experimental conditions.

Characteristics of the Exerciser

Certain characteristics of the exerciser can make a difference in the magnitude of the exercise response. The basic pattern of the response will be similar, but the magnitude of the response can vary with the sex, age (child/adolescent, adult, elderly), and/or physiological status, such as health and training level of the individual. Where possible, these differences in response will be pointed out.

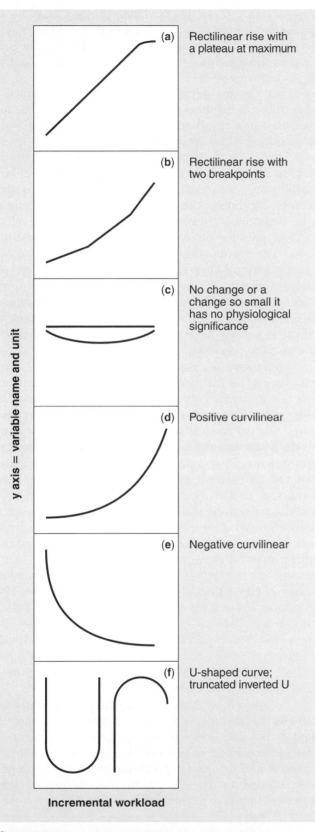

Figure 1.3
Graphic Patterns and Verbal Descriptors for Incremental Workload/Work Rate Exercise Responses

Appropriateness of the Selected Exercise

The exercise test used should match the physiological system or physical fitness component you are most interested in evaluating. For example, you cannot determine cardiovascular endurance utilizing dynamic resistance exercise. However, if your goal is to determine how selected cardiovascular variables respond to dynamic resistance exercise, then, obviously, that is the type of exercise that must be used.

The modality used within each exercise category should also match the intended outcome. For example, if the goal is to demonstrate changes in cardiovascular-respiratory fitness for individuals training on a stationary cycle, then an incremental dynamic exercise to maximum test should be conducted on a cycle ergometer, not a treadmill or other piece of equipment.

Accuracy of the Selected Exercise

The most accurate tests are called **criterion tests;** they represent a standard against which other tests are evaluated. Most criterion tests are **laboratory tests**—precise, direct measurements of physiological function that usually involve monitoring, collection, and analysis of expired air, blood, or electrical signals—and require expensive equipment and trained technicians. Not all laboratory tests, however, are criterion tests.

Field tests are tests that can be conducted almost anywhere, such as school gymnasia, playing fields, or health clubs. Field tests are often performance-based and estimate the values measured by the criterion test. The mile run is a field test used to assess cardiovascular-respiratory fitness, which is more directly and accurately measured by maximal oxygen consumption ($\dot{V}O_2$max). Both laboratory and field tests will be discussed in this text.

> **Criterion Test** The standard against which other tests are judged.
>
> **Laboratory Test** Precise, direct measurement of physiological functions for the assessment of exercise responses or training adaptations; usually involves monitoring, collection, and analysis of expired air, blood, or electrical signals.
>
> **Field Test** A test that can be conducted anywhere; is performance-based and estimates the values measured by the criterion test.

Environmental and Experimental Conditions

Many physiological variables are sensitive to environmental conditions, most notably temperature, relative humidity (RH), and barometric pressure. Normal responses typically occur at neutral conditions (approximately 20–29°C [68–84°F]; < 50%; and 630–760 mmHg, respectively). Likewise, when a response to exercise is described, the assumption is that the exerciser had adequate sleep, was not ill, had not recently eaten or exercised, and was not taking any prescription or nonprescription drugs or supplements. If any of these assumed conditions is not met, the expected exercise response might not occur.

Training

Health-Related versus Sport-Specific Physical Fitness

Training is a consistent or chronic progression of exercise sessions designed to improve physiological function for better health or sport performance. There are two main goals for exercise training: (1) health-related physical fitness and (2) sport-specific physical fitness, sometimes called athletic fitness.

In this textbook the concept of **health-related physical fitness** means that portion of physical fitness which is directed toward the prevention of or rehabilitation from disease as well as the development of a high level of functional capacity for the necessary and

---

Training A consistent or chronic progression of exercise sessions designed to improve physiological function for better health or sport performance.

Health-Related Physical Fitness That portion of physical fitness directed toward the prevention of or rehabilitation from disease as well as the development of a high level of functional capacity for the necessary and discretionary tasks of life.

Hypokinetic Diseases Diseases caused by and/or associated with lack of physical activity.

Sport-Specific Physical Fitness That portion of physical fitness which is directed toward optimizing athletic performance.

Physical Fitness A physiological state of well-being that provides the foundation for the tasks of daily living, a degree of protection against hypokinetic disease, and a basis for participation in sport.

---

discretionary tasks of life. Thus, the goal may be to participate minimally in an activity to achieve some health benefit before a disease state occurs. The goal may be to participate in a substantial amount of activity to improve or maintain a high level of physical fitness. Or the goal may be to participate in an activity that allows a disabled individual to recover and/or attain the maximal function possible. All goals should be attained while avoiding injury.

Three components of health-related physical fitness are generally recognized: cardiovascular-respiratory endurance, body composition, muscular fitness (strength, muscular endurance, and flexibility). Figure 1.4 shows that the components of health-related physical fitness form the core of physical fitness. The relationship between each of these fitness components and hypokinetic disease will be described in the appropriate units of the text. For now it is sufficient to know that **hypokinetic diseases** are diseases which are caused by and/or associated with a lack of physical activity. Health-related physical fitness is important for everyone.

Sport-specific physical fitness has a more narrow focus; it is that portion of physical fitness directed toward optimizing athletic performance. To develop this type of fitness program, you must first analyze the physiological demands of the sport. Second, you must evaluate where the athlete is in terms of these requirements. Once you know both of these elements, you can develop a specifically designed individualized program. This program should work the specific musculature involved while achieving a proper balance between agonistic and antagonistic muscle groups; use the muscles in the biomechanical patterns of the sport; match the metabolic requirements; and incorporate any motor fitness attributes that are needed at a starting level that is appropriate for the athlete. The demands of the sport will not change to accommodate the athlete. The athlete must be the one to meet the demands of the sport if reasonable success is desired. Figure 1.4 shows that sport-specific athletic fitness builds on the core of health-related physical fitness and expands from there.

Putting all of these elements together, **physical fitness** may be defined as a physiological state of well-being that provides the foundation for the tasks of daily living, a degree of protection against hypokinetic disease, and a basis for participation in sport (American Alliance for Health, 1988). The key to achieving physical fitness is physical activity.

Training Principles

Although there is much we do not know about training, and new techniques of training are always

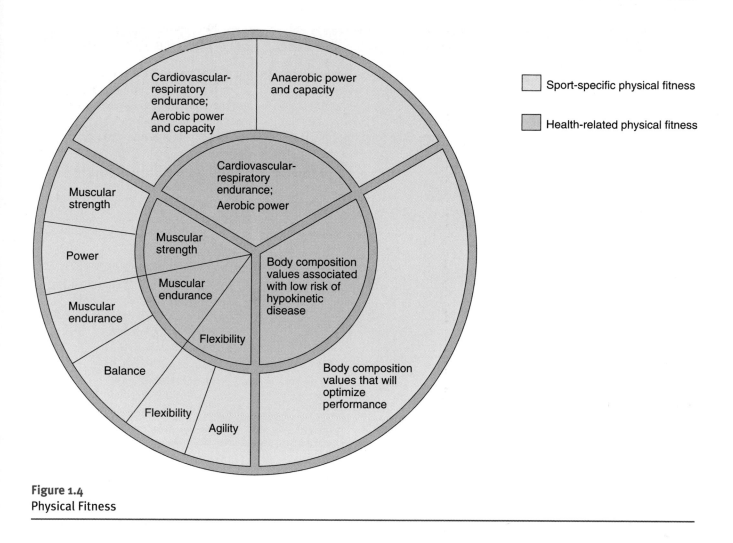

Figure 1.4
Physical Fitness

appearing, there are eight well-established fundamental guidelines that should form the basis for the development of any training program. These **training principles** are defined and briefly discussed here. The specific details for applying each principle, as well as the anticipated results or adaptations, will be discussed in connection with each physiological system in the units that follow.

1. *Specificity.* This principle is sometimes called the SAID principle, which stands for "specific adaptations to imposed demands"; that is, what you do is what you get.

Thus, when you develop a training program, you must first determine the goal. Fitness programs for children and adolescents will differ from those for the elderly. Physical fitness programs for nonathletes

will vary from fitness programs for athletes. Athletic training programs will vary by sport, by event, or even by position within the same sport.

Second, you must be able to analyze the goal in terms of its physiological requirements. What system is being stressed: the cardiovascular-respiratory, the metabolic, or the neuromuscular-skeletal? What is the major energy system involved? What motor fitness attributes (agility, balance, flexibility, strength, power, muscular endurance) need to be developed? The closer the training program matches the answers to these questions, the greater the chance for success.

2. *Overload.* To overload is to place a demand on the body greater than that to which it is accustomed. To determine what an overload might be, you must first evaluate each individual on the critical physiological variables discussed under specificity. Then, three factors must be considered: frequency—the number of training sessions on a daily or weekly basis; intensity—the level of work, energy expenditure, or physiological response in relation to the maximum; and duration—the amount of time spent

---

Training Principles Fundamental guidelines that form the basis for the development of an exercise training program.

Focus on Application

✳ The Surgeon General's Report on Physical Activity and Health

The role of the Office of the Surgeon General is to focus the country's attention on important public health issues. In 1996 the U.S. Department of Health and Human Services released a publication titled *Physical Activity and Health: A Report of the Surgeon General*. This landmark report both acknowledged the major role that physical activity plays in relation to health and called attention to the growing epidemic of inactivity in the U.S. population. A summary of the Surgeon General's report is included in Appendix C. Much of this report is based on the body of knowledge of exercise physiology that you will be studying in this text.

The overwhelming message of the Surgeon General's report is that Americans can make meaningful improvements in their health and quality of life by including moderate but regular physical activity into their normal living routines. Statistics compiled by the Centers for Disease Control and Prevention (CDC) in the year 2000 (on data collected in 1998) from answers to the question "During the past month, did you participate in any physical activity? Yes or No?" The "No" responses are presented in the figure below. These results clearly show that far too many Americans remain inactive. Despite the compelling scientific, medical, and public health data and both educational and media promotions, the current generation of exercise scientists, physical educators, and related health workers has much to do. ✳

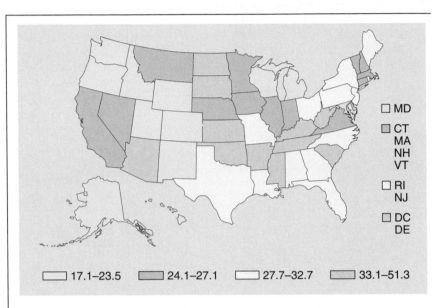

Legend: □ 17.1–23.5   ▨ 24.1–27.1   □ 27.7–32.7   ▨ 33.1–51.3

Boxes labeled: MD; CT MA NH VT; RI NJ; DC DE

Percentage of Adults Who Reported No Leisure-Time Physical Activity

Despite the proven benefits of being physically active, more than 60% of American adults do not engage in levels of physical activity necessary to provide health benefits. More than one-fourth are not active at all in their leisure time. Activity decreases with age and is less common among women than men and among those with lower income and less education.

Insufficient physical activity is not limited to adults. Information gathered through CDC's Youth Risk Behavior Surveillance System indicates that more than a third of young people aged 12–21 years do not regularly engage in vigorous physical activity. Daily participation in high school physical education classes dropped from 42% in 1991 to 27% in 1997.

Source: CDC, Behavioral Risk Factor Surveillance System, 1998.

---

training per session or per day. **Training volume** indicates the *quantity* or amount of overload (frequency times duration), whereas *training intensity* represents the *quality* of overload.

3. *Rest/Recovery/Adaptation.* Adaptation is the change in physiological function that occurs in response to training. Adaptation occurs during periods of rest, when the body recovers from the acute

> **Training Volume** The quantity of training overload calculated as frequency times duration.

homeostatic disruptions and/or residual fatigue and, as a result, compensates to above-baseline levels of physiological functioning. This is sometimes called *supercompensation* (Bompa, 1999; Freeman, 1996). Thus, it is vitally important that exercisers receive sufficient rest between individual exercise training sessions, after periods of increased training overload, and both before and after competition. Adaptation allows the individual to either do more work or do the same work with a smaller disruption of baseline values. Keeping records and retesting individuals are generally necessary to determine the degree of adaptation.

4. *Progression.* Progression is the change in overload in response to adaptation. Progression implies that the increments in training load are small, controlled, and flexible. Progression should not be thought of as a continuous unbroken increase in training overload. The best progression occurs in a series of steps (which is called steploading), in which every third or fourth change is actually a slight decrease in training load (Bompa, 1999; Freeman, 1996). This stepdown allows recovery, which leads to adaptation. Complete the Question of Understanding box below. Check your answer in Appendix D.

A Question of Understanding

Below are three patterns that represent overload and progression for a general conditioning phase for an athlete. Select the one that is best, and justify your response.

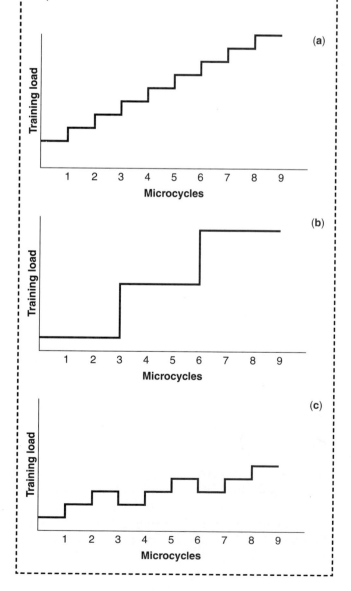

5. *Retrogression/Plateau/Reversibility.* Progress is rarely linear, predictable, or consistent. When an individual's adaptation or performance levels off or gets worse, a plateau has been reached or retrogression has occurred, respectively. Plateaus must be interpreted relative to the training regimen. Too much time spent doing the same type of workout using the same equipment in the same environment can lead to a plateau. Either too little or too much competition can lead to a plateau. Plateaus are a normal consequence of a maintenance overload and may also occur normally, even during a well-designed and well-implemented steploading progression. Variety and rest may help a person move beyond these plateaus. However, if a plateau continues for some time or if other signs and symptoms appear, then the plateau may be an early warning signal of overtraining. Retrogression may signal overtraining. Reversibility is the reversal of achieved physiological adaptations that occurs when training stops (detraining).

6. *Maintenance.* Maintenance refers to sustaining the achieved adaptation with the most efficient use of time and effort. At this point the individuals have reached an acceptable level of physical fitness or training. The amount of time and effort required to maintain the individuals' adaptation depends on the systems involved; it is higher, for example, in the cardiovascular system than in the neuromuscular system. In general, intensity is the key to maintenance; that is, as long as exercise intensity is maintained, frequency and duration of exercise may be decreased without losing positive adaptations.

7. *Individualization.* Individuals both require personalized exercise prescriptions based on their fitness levels and goals and adapt differently to the same training program. The same training overload may improve physiological performance in one individual, maintain physiological and performance levels in a second individual, and result in maladaptation and decrease in performance in a third. A major reason for these differences is lifestyle, particularly nutritional and sleep habits, stress levels, and substance use (such as tobacco or alcohol). Finally age, sex, genetics, and disease conditions all affect individual exercise prescriptions and adaptations.

8. *Warm-Up/Cool-Down.* A warm-up prepares the body for activity by elevating the body temperature. Conversely, a cool-down allows for a gradual return to normal body temperature. The best type of warm-up is specific to the activity that will follow and individualized so as not to produce fatigue.

A nonphysiological consideration is needed at this point. Except at a military boot camp, it is very difficult to force anyone to train. Therefore, some motivation is needed. Thus, it is important that there be an element of fun in any training program. Intersperse games, variations, and special events, and make normal training sessions as enjoyable as possible.

Periodization

Once a training program is designed, it should be applied in a pattern that will be most beneficial. Such a pattern is called the *training cycle* or *periodization*. **Periodization** is a plan for training based on a manipulation of the fitness components and training principles; the objective is to peak the athlete's performance for the competitive season or some part of it. An individual training for any level of health-related physical fitness should also utilize periodization to build in cycles of harder or easier training and/or emphasize one component or another to prevent boredom.

Figure 1.5 is an example of how periodization might be arranged for an athlete, in this case a basketball player whose season lasts approximately 4.5 months. This is intended as an example only, because periodization depends on individual situations and abilities. In Figure 1.5, the time frame of 1 year—presented as 52 weeks (outer circle)—has been divided into four phases or cycles: the general preparatory phase (sometimes labeled *off-season*), the specific preparatory phase (also known as *preseason*); the competitive (or *in-season*) phase; and the transition (*active rest*) phase (Bompa, 1999; Freeman, 1996; Kearney, 1996). Each phase is typically divided into macrocycles that may vary in length from 2–6 weeks. A macrocycle is further divided into microcycles lasting 1 week (Fry, et al., 1992; Kibler and Chandler, 1994). Each type of cycle aims for an optimal mixture of work and rest. Macrocycles and microcycles have five basic goals or patterns: developmental; shock; competitive, or maintenance; tapering, or unloading; and transition, or regeneration (Bompa, 1999).

In Figure 1.5, the first macrocycle (Figure 1.5a) represents a developmental cycle, which is specific to the preparatory stages and is designed to improve either general or specific fitness attributes, such as strength, progressively. Overloading is achieved by a stepwise progression from low to medium to high by gradually increasing the load for three cycles,

---

> **Periodization** Plan for training based on a manipulation of the fitness components with the intent of peaking the athlete for the competitive season or varying health-related fitness training in cycles of harder or easier training.

---

followed by a regeneration cycle back to the level of the second load. This second load level then becomes the base for the next loading cycle. This is what is meant by *steploading*.

Shock cycles, illustrated in Figure 1.5b, are used primarily during the preparatory phases and are designed to increase training demands suddenly. They should always be followed by a regeneration cycle which consists of a drastically reduced training load.

Competitive cycles (Figure 1.5c) are based on maintaining physiological fitness while optimizing performance on game days. Obviously, competitive macrocycles and microcycles occur during the competitive phase.

Tapering or unloading regeneration cycles (Figure 1.5d) involve systematic decreases in overload to facilitate a physiological fitness peak (Bompa, 1999). As noted, regeneration cycles are used both as breaks between other cycles and to form the basis of the active transition phase (Figure 1.5e) (Bompa, 1999; Freeman, 1996; Kibler and Chandler, 1994). They are intended to remove fatigue, emphasize relaxation, and prevent overtraining. Transition phases are just as valuable for the fitness participant as the athlete. Microcycles are further subdivided into daily workouts or lesson plans. Depending on the maturity and experience of the athlete and the level of competition, a training day may entail one, two, or three work-outs (Bompa, 1999).

The general preparatory, or off-season, phase should be preceded by a sport-specific fitness evaluation to guide both the general and specific preparatory training programs. Another evaluation might be conducted prior to the season if desired, or evaluations might be conducted systematically throughout the year to determine how the individual is responding to training and to make any necessary adjustments. All evaluation testing should be done at the end of a regeneration cycle so that fatigue is not a confounding factor. The off-season is a time of general preparation when the health-related physical fitness components are emphasized to develop cardiovascular-respiratory endurance (an aerobic base), flexibility, and muscular strength and endurance. Any needed changes in body composition should be addressed during this phase (Kibler and Chandler, 1994). An aerobic base is important for all athletes, even those whose event is primarily anaerobic. A high aerobic capacity allows the individual to work at a higher intensity before accumulating large quantities of lactic acid and becoming fatigued. A high aerobic capacity also allows the individual to recover faster, which is important both in and of itself and for allowing for a potentially greater total volume of work during interval sessions (Bompa, 1999).

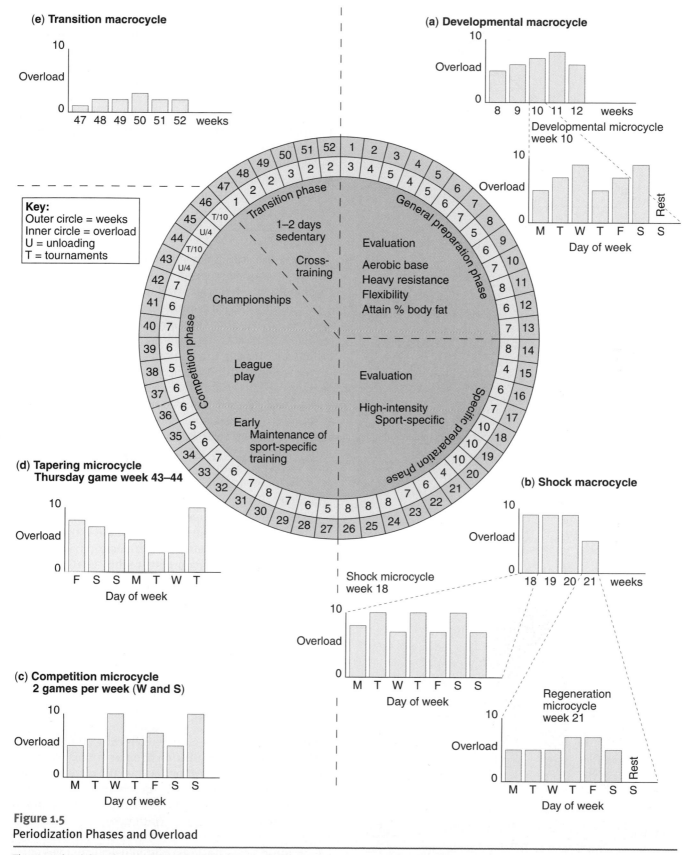

Figure 1.5
Periodization Phases and Overload

The annual training plan consists of four phases: the general preparatory phase; the specific preparatory phase; the competitive phase; and the transition phase. Overload is rated on a scale of 0 (complete rest) to 10 (maximal) on the inner circle.

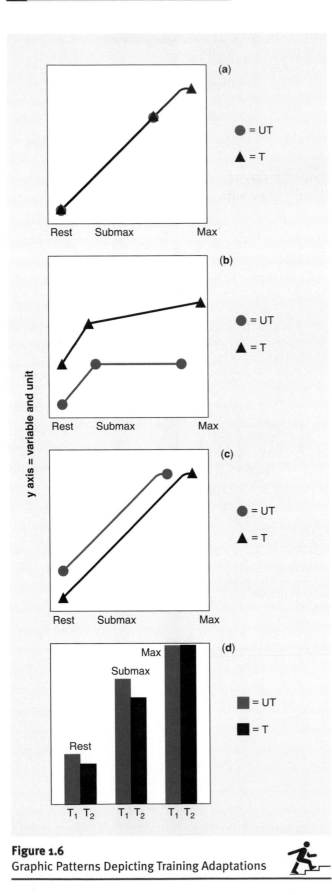

Figure 1.6
Graphic Patterns Depicting Training Adaptations

General preparation may occupy most of the year for a fitness participant. During this general preparatory phase, overload progresses by steps in both intensity and volume (frequency times duration), with volume typically being relatively more important than intensity (Bompa, 1999). During the preseason phase, the athlete shifts to specific preparation for the fitness and physiological components needed to succeed in the intended sport. The training program at this time is very heavy and generally occupies the 6–8 weeks prior to the first competition. About midway through the specific preparatory phase, intensity may surpass volume in importance. This will vary with the physiological demands of particular sports (Kibler and Chandler, 1994).

Once the athlete begins the competition phase, the early emphasis shifts to maintaining the sport-specific fitness that was developed during the preseason. Although both volume and intensity may be maintained, any heavy work that is done should immediately follow a competition instead of directly preceding one. During the late season, when the most important competitions are usually held (such as conference championships or bowl games), the athlete should do only a minimum of training or taper gradually by decreasing training volume but maintaining intensity so that he or she is rested without being detrained. For particularly important contests, both training volume and intensity might be decreased to peak for a maximal effort (Kibler and Chandler, 1994).

The transition phase begins immediately after the last competition of the year. The athlete should take a couple days of complete rest and then participate in active rest using noncompetitive physical activities that are not his or her primary sport. This type of activity is often called *cross-training*. In this transition phase, neither training volume nor intensity should exceed low levels (Kibler and Chandler, 1994).

Where possible throughout this text, periodization will be considered in the application of the training principles.

Training Adaptations

Training brings about changes typically labeled *adaptations*. **Training adaptations** represent adjustments that promote optimal functioning. Whereas exercise responses use resting values as the baseline, training adaptations are evaluated against the same condition

> **Training Adaptations** Physiological changes or adjustments resulting from an exercise training program that promote optimal functioning.

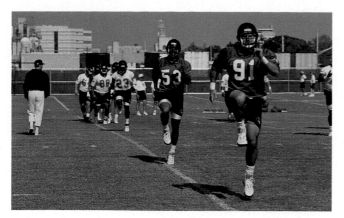

Figure 1.7
Training to Improve Physiological Function and Skill for Improved Performance

as opposed to training. Training adaptations may be presented as exercise response patterns using a line graph, as in Figure 1.6a to 1.6c, or simply as specific values using a bar graph, as in Figure 1.6d. The background graph color for training adaptations is included in Table 1.2 on page 9.

Training results in adaptations that are either an increase, a decrease, or unchanged in relation to the untrained state. For example, in Figure 1.6a, there is no difference between the trained and untrained conditions either at rest or during submaximal exercise. However, the trained group increased at maximum over the untrained. In Figure 1.6b, training resulted in an increase at rest, during submaximal exercise, and at maximum. Figures 1.6c and 1.6d describe the same adaptations using both a line and bar graph to show how each might look. On the bar graph, T_1 indicates evaluation results before the training, and T_2 represents evaluation results after training. Both types of graphs indicate that training resulted in a decrease at rest and submaximal work, but no change at maximum.

Training adaptations at rest show more variation than either submaximal or maximal changes; increases, decreases, and no change are all common. In general, if the exercise test is an absolute submaximal test, the physiological responses will probably be decreased after training. If the exercise test is a relative submaximal test, the physiological responses will probably show no change after training. And if the comparison is made at maximal effort, most physiological responses will be increased. These results do not hold for all variables that are measured but are general patterns.

The predominant way of looking at training adaptations is that not only do they result from the chronic application of exercise but also that they themselves represent *chronic changes.* Such adaptations become greater with harder training, are thought to exist as long as the training continues, and gradually return to baseline values when training stops (detraining). In point of fact, not all training adaptations follow this standard pattern. Some benefits occur only immediately after the exercise session. These effects are called *last-bout effects* and should not be confused with the exercise response. For example, a last-bout effect occurs with blood pressure levels. The acute response of blood pressure to continuous aerobic endurance exercise is an increase in systolic blood pressure but no change in diastolic blood pressure. The last-bout effect in individuals with high blood pressure is a decrease below their resting level for up to 3 hours after exercise. After 3 hours, the high resting values return. In some cases the last-bout effect can be augmented. That is, for a period of one to several weeks the positive change occurring after the exercise bout can be increased. In the example just referred to, the decrease in systolic blood pressure after several weeks would be more than the initial decrease. However, the adjustments that can occur are finite. Once the level of the *augmented last-bout effect* is reached, no further increase in training will bring about additional benefit (Haskell, 1994). This may be the reason why reductions in high blood pressure that occur with training rarely result in normal resting values.

Thus, the adaptations that result from training can occur on three levels: (1) a chronic change, (2) a last-bout effect, and (3) an augmented last-bout effect. The majority of the training adaptations will be dealt with in this book as if they are chronic changes.

Summary

1. The purpose of this chapter has been both to acquaint you with the general organization of the text and to provide background information that will help you interpret and understand the information that will subsequently be presented.

2. The response to exercise, which is always a disruption in homeostasis, depends upon the exercise modality, the exercise intensity, and the exercise duration. Interpretation of exercise responses must consider characteristics of the exerciser (age, sex, training status), appropriateness of the exercise test used (match between the intended physiological system and outcome), accuracy of the selected exercise (criterion or field test), and environmental and experimental conditions (temperature, relative humidity, barometric pressure, and subject preparation).

3. The baselines against which the exercise-caused disruptions of homeostasis are compared are normal resting values of the measured variables.
   a. Constant workloads/work rates that are aerobic most frequently result in a small initial increase in the measured variable with a plateau at steady state if intensity is light to moderate and duration is short; if the intensity is moderate to heavy and the duration is long, aerobic workloads/work rates result in a large increase with a plateau at steady state that evolves into a positive or negative drift. Constant dynamic resistance exercise exhibits a seesaw pattern of gradual increase. Sustained static contraction often results in no change or a change so small that it has no physiological significance during the exercise but a rebound rise in recovery.
   b. Incremental exercise to maximum most frequently results in either a rectilinear rise (with or without breakpoints) or a curvilinear rise (positive, negative, or U-shaped).

4. Health-related physical fitness is composed of components representing cardiovascular-respiratory endurance, metabolism, and muscular fitness (strength, muscular endurance, and flexibility).

5. Sport-specific physical fitness should build on health-related physical fitness, adding motor fitness attributes (such as agility, balance, and power) and anaerobic power and capacity, as needed.

6. Eight general training principles provide guidance for establishing and applying training programs: specificity, overload, rest/recovery/adaptation, progression, retrogression/plateau/reversibility, maintenance, individualization, and warm-up/cool-down.

7. Periodization provides a timeline for the planning of training programs that cycles through four phases or cycles: the general preparatory phase (off-season), the specific preparatory phase (pre-season), the competitive phase (in-season), and the transition phase (active rest).

8. To prescribe a training program:
   a. analyze the physiological demands of the physical fitness program, rehabilitation, or sport goal;
   b. evaluate the individual relative to the established physiological demands; and
   c. apply the training principles relative to the established physiological demands in periodization cycles that allow for a steploading pattern of varying levels of exercise and rest or recovery.

9. Exercise training brings about adaptations in physiological function. The baselines against which training adaptations are compared are the corresponding pretraining conditions.

10. Training adaptations may occur on at least three levels: a last-bout effect, an augmented last-bout effect, or a chronic change.

Review Questions

1. Define *exercise physiology, exercise,* and *exercise training.*

2. Graph the most frequent responses a physiological variable might exhibit in response to a constant workload/work rate. Verbally describe these responses.

3. Graph the most frequent responses a physiological variable might exhibit in response to an incremental exercise to maximum. Verbally describe these responses.

4. Differentiate between an absolute and relative submaximal workload/work rate, and give an example other than weight lifting.

5. Fully describe an exercise situation, including all elements that are needed to accurately evaluate the exercise response.

6. Compare the components of health-related physical fitness with those of sport-specific physical fitness.

7. List and explain the training principles.

8. Diagram and give an example of periodization for a sport of your choice.

9. Differentiate between the three levels of training adaptation, and state which level of adaptation is most common.

For further review and additional study tools, go to The Physiology Place (www.physiologyplace.com) and the Student Study Guide for Exercise Physiology for Health, Fitness, and Performance *by Sharon A. Plowman and Denise L. Smith.*

Passport to the Internet

Visit the following Internet sites to explore further topics and issues related to general exercise physiology. To visit an organization's web site, go to www.physiologyplace.com and click on "Passport to the Internet."

American College of Sports Medicine Home page of the professional organization for individuals interested in sports medicine and exercise science. Spend some time exploring this site and discovering the multitude of resources available.

National Library of Medicine Visit the world's largest biomedical library for resources on everything from medical history to biotechnology. This site also provides connections to major medical links, such as Medline.

World Health Organization Explore health topics as they affect people throughout the world, and investigate various information sources and reports as they relate to issues in exercise science.

Centers for Disease Control and Prevention: Surgeon General's Report on Physical Activity and Health Access the complete contents of *Physical Activity and Health: A Report of the Surgeon General.* You can download the full report or portions of it, as well as connect to related government sites dedicated to addressing the concerns raised in the Surgeon General's report.

References

American Alliance for Health, Physical Education, Recreation and Dance: *Physical Best: A Physical Fitness Education and Assessment Program.* Reston, VA: Author (1988).

Bompa, T. O.: *Periodization: Theory and Methodology of Training.* Champaign, IL: Human Kinetics (1999).

Centers for Disease Control and Prevention: *Physical Activity and Good Nutrition: Essentials for Good Health: At a Glance 2000.* http://www.cdc.gov/needphp/dnpa/dnpaaag.htm (2000).

Freeman, W. H.: *Peak When It Counts: Periodization for American Track & Field* (3rd ed.). Mountain View, CA: Tafnews Press (1996).

Fry, R. W., A. R. Morton, & D. Keast: Overtraining in athletes: An Update. *SportsMedicine.* 12(1):32–65 (1991).

Fry, R. W., A. R. Morton, & D. Keast: Periodisation and the prevention of overtraining. *Canadian Journal of Sports Science.* 17(3):241–248 (1992).

Haskell, W. L.: Health consequences of physical activity: Understanding and challenges regarding dose response. *Medicine and Science in Sports and Exercise.* 26(6):649–660 (1994).

Hellerstein, H. K.: Cardiac rehabilitation: A retrospective view. In M. L. Pollock & D. H. Schmidt (eds.), *Heart Disease and Rehabilitation.* Boston: Houghton Mifflin, 511–514 (1979).

Kearney, J. T.: Training the Olympic athlete. *Scientific American.* 274(6):52–63 (1996).

Kibler, W. B., & T. J. Chandler: Sport-specific conditioning. *American Journal of Sports Medicine.* 22(3):424–432 (1994).

Kraus, H., & R. Hirschland: Minimum muscular fitness tests in school. *Research Quarterly.* 25:178–188 (1954).

Ogawa, T., R. J. Spina, W. H. Martin, W. M. Kohrt, K. B. Schectman, & J. O. Holloszy: Effects of aging, sex, and physical training on cardiovascular responses to exercise. *Circulation.* 86:494–503 (1992).

Raab, W.: Heart attack—Number one killer of Americans. In *The Healthy Life: How Diet and Exercise Affect Your Heart and Vigor.* New York: Time Incorporated (1966).

Ullyot, J.: *Women's Running.* Mountain View, CA: World Publications (1976).

U.S. Department of Health and Human Services: *Physical Activity and Health: A Report of the Surgeon General.* Atlanta, GA: U.S. Department of Health and Human Services, Centers for Disease Control and Prevention, National Center for Chronic Disease Prevention and Health Promotion (1996).

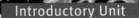

Chapter 2

Neuroendocrine
Control of Exercise

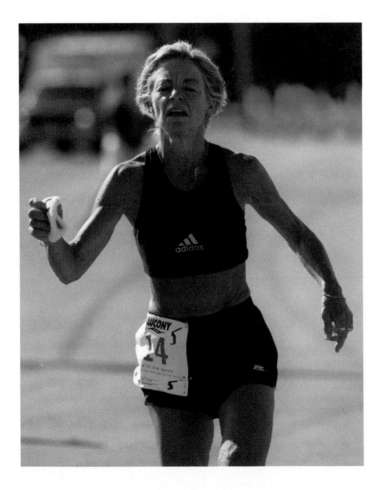

After studying the chapter, you should be able to

- Identify and briefly describe the role of the two systems involved in maintaining homeostasis.
- Identify changes that may occur in a target cell as a result of the binding of a neurotransmitter or hormone to a cell receptor (receptor activation).
- Describe the structure of the nervous system.
- Identify the regions of a neuron and discuss the importance of each region.
- Describe the roles of the somatic and autonomic nervous systems as they relate to movement and regulating the exercise response.
- Identify the primary hormones involved in regulating the exercise response and describe the exercise response of these hormones.
- Identify the adaptations that occur in the hormonal system as a result of exercise training.
- Describe Selye's theory of stress and its applications to exercise and training.
- Differentiate between overreaching and overtraining.
- Identify the causes of the overtraining syndrome (OTS) and indicate how to prevent and treat it.

Introduction

You know from your own experience that when you exercise certain changes take place in your body. The most obvious change—contraction of the muscles—you initiate consciously by activating the nervous system, which in turn signals the muscles to contract. You may also be aware of other changes, such as an increased breathing rate, increased heart rate, and increased sweating; these responses you do not consciously initiate. Still other changes—fuel mobilization, enzyme actions, and energy utilization—occur during exercise without conscious initiation, or even awareness of their occurrence. These changes are all part of an ongoing internal effort to maintain balance. *Homeostasis,* the dynamic state of equilibrium of the internal functioning of the body at rest, is controlled and coordinated by the nervous and endocrine systems of the body. Furthermore, these two complementary and often overlapping systems regulate the body's response to a disruption in homeostasis, such as the disruption created by exercise. The nervous

system is the fast-acting regulator of the body, whereas the endocrine system is the slow-acting regulator. The two systems interact and overlap in multiple ways to support exercise. Because these two systems function so closely together, they are often referred to as the *neuroendocrine* (or *neurohormonal*) system. This chapter examines the role of the nervous system in initiating exercise and the role of the neuroendocrine system in regulating the body's responses to exercise. Because the neuroendocrine system controls each of the systems in the body, including those presented in this book (cardiorespiratory, metabolic, and neuromusculoskeletal), the basic principles of neuroendocrine control become critical in understanding exercise response, training adaptations, and the integrated nature of all the systems included in the study of exercise physiology.

Both the nervous system and the endocrine system rely on chemical messengers to communicate with target cells. Figure 2.1 depicts the cells of the

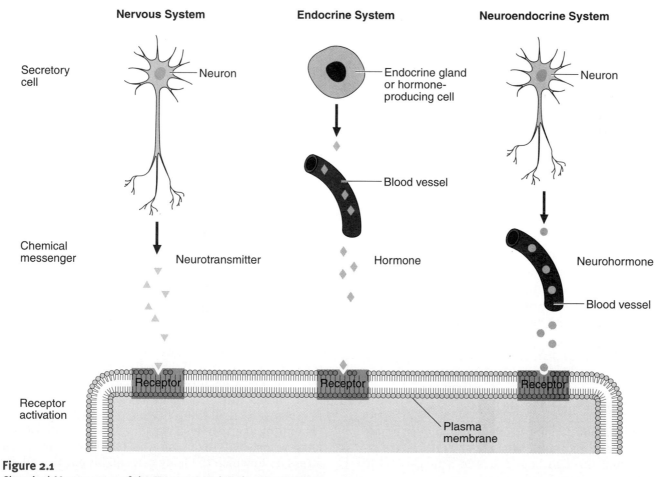

Figure 2.1
Chemical Messengers of the Nervous and Endocrine Systems

Table 2.1
Outline of Nervous and Endocrine Systems

	Nervous System	Endocrine System
Basic Structure	Central and peripheral nervous system composed of neurons	Endocrine gland/tissue, which releases hormones
Chemical Messenger	Neurotransmitter (NT)	Hormones
Mechanism of Chemical Release	Action potential in axon causes release of NT	Endocrine gland/tissue secretes hormone into blood/body fluid
Chemical/Receptor Binding	NT binds to receptor on target cell because of complementary shape and affinity	Hormone binds to receptor on target cell because of complementary shape and affinity
Mechanism of Action	Change in membrane permeability Second messenger system Direct gene activation	Second messenger system Direct gene activation

Role in Exercise	1. Contraction of skeletal muscle
	2. Regulation of cardiovascular-respiratory systems
	3. Coordination with endocrine system to
	  • Mobilize fuel for energy production
	  • Transport fuel, oxygen, and waste
	  • Maintain fluid and electrolyte balance
	  • Maintain thermal balance
		1. Regulate metabolic system
		  • Mobilize fuel for energy production
		  • Increase rate at which fuel is broken down to produce ATP
		  • Maintain blood glucose levels
		2. Regulate cardiovascular system
		  • Transport fuel, oxygen, and waste
		  • Maintain fluid and electrolyte balance
		  • Maintain thermal balance

nervous and endocrine system and the chemical messengers they use. Neurons are the secretory cells that release **neurotransmitters** at the site of the target cell. Endocrine glands, or hormone-producing tissues, release **hormones** into the bloodstream (or body fluid), which transports the hormone to the target cell. If a neuron releases a chemical substance into the bloodstream, this substance is called a *neurohormone.*

The effect of the chemical messengers (neurotransmitters, hormones, and neurohormones) on a target cell is mediated by the substance's binding to a receptor on (or in) the target cell. The chemical messenger binds to the receptor because of the comple-

mentary shape of the messenger and the receptor. Thus, chemical messengers bind only to very specific receptors. The messenger-receptor binding is known as *receptor activation,* and results in one or more changes within the target cell:

1. change in permeability, electrical state or transport properties of the cell;

2. change in enzyme activity of the cell (altering metabolism);

3. change in secretory activity of the cell;

4. muscle contraction; and

5. protein synthesis.

The first two sections of this chapter describe the nervous system and the endocrine system, respectively, and how each responds to exercise and adapts to training. Table 2.1 provides an overview of the nervous and endocrine systems and a framework for comparing the two systems. The third section of the chapter presents exercise and exercise training as stressors to which the body can exhibit positive adaptation or negative maladaptation.

> **Neurotransmitters** Chemical messengers that allow neurons to communicate with target cells of either other neurons or effector organs.
>
> **Hormones** Chemical substances that originate in glandular tissue (or cells) and are transported through body fluids to a target cell to influence physiological activity.

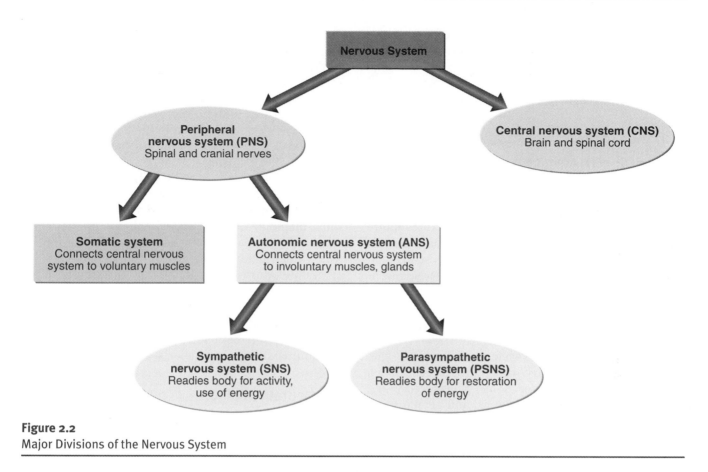

Figure 2.2
Major Divisions of the Nervous System

The Nervous System

The nervous system is a fast-acting control system that regulates a virtually endless list of bodily functions. In general, the nervous system has three primary functions:

1. monitoring the internal and external environment through sensory receptors,

2. integrating the information it has received, and

3. initiating and coordinating a response by activating muscles (skeletal, smooth, and cardiac) and glands (including endocrine glands).

These functions are accomplished by the cells of the nervous system (neurons) that communicate with each other and with effector organs (muscle and glands). Communication *within* a neuron occurs by electrical signals (action potentials). Communication *between* neurons or between neurons and an *effector organ* (e.g., skeletal muscle) occurs by *chemical signals (neurotransmitters).*

The Basic Structure of the Nervous System

As shown in Figure 2.2, the nervous system can be structurally divided into the *central nervous system* (CNS), which consists of the brain and spinal cord, and the *peripheral nervous system* (PNS), which consists of everything outside the CNS. The PNS contains afferent and efferent neurons. *Afferent* neurons relay information about the internal and external environment (from sensory receptors in the periphery) to the CNS. The CNS integrates information it receives from afferent neurons and initiates a response by activating the efferent division. *Efferent* neurons relay signals from the CNS to *effector* organs in the periphery.

The efferent division is further subdivided into the somatic and autonomic nervous systems. The *somatic (or motor) system* sends signals from the CNS to skeletal muscle to initiate muscle contraction and thus movement. Although we may not always achieve the desired result from such movement (think about your last golf outing), the somatic system is under voluntary control. The autonomic nervous system (ANS) is involuntary, meaning we do not consciously control its activity. The *autonomic nervous system* carries information from the CNS to cardiac muscle, smooth muscle, and endocrine glands, thereby providing subconscious neural regulation of the internal environment of the body. The ANS has two branches, which work in opposition to each other by dual innervation. The *sympathetic nervous system* (SNS) supports activities associated with the "fight or flight" response and is vital in controlling the body's response to exercise. The *parasympathetic nervous system* (PSNS) supports activities associated with "rest and digest" and is vital in the process of recovering from exercise.

Activation of the Nervous System

The somatic nervous system may be activated by conscious thought or by afferent input from the periphery. Afferent signals that are involved in regulating nervous control of muscle contraction rely on different types of sensory receptors: mechanoreceptors (pressure, stretch, or contraction) and proprioceptors (spatial orientation), located primarily in skeletal muscle, tendons, and joints. Activation of these receptors often results in a reflex movement. A *reflex* is a rapid, involuntary movement in response to a stimulus. (Details of reflex action and voluntary movement are provided in Chapter 22.)

The autonomic nervous system is activated by specialized external sensory receptors (touch, taste, sound, sight, smell, and/or pain), thermoreceptors, proprioceptors, mechanoreceptors, and chemoreceptors (which monitor blood levels of specific chemicals).

The Nerve Cell

The neuron, or nerve cell, is the functional unit of the nervous system. In addition to the afferent and efferent neurons described above, there are also connection or *association* neurons within the central nervous system. Neurons vary considerably in size and shape, depending on their function and location in the body. However, the neurons described in this text generally contain three distinct regions. The *dendrites* are highly branched extensions of the neuron that represent the receptor sites that receive information and convey it to the cell body. The *cell body* is the control center. It integrates the information that it receives from the dendrites and, if the signal is strong enough (at or above threshold level), passes it along to the axon. A cluster of cell bodies in the CNS is called a *nucleus;* a cluster of cell bodies in the PNS is called a *ganglion.*

The *axon* of a motor neuron is a single extension of the neuron. The axon has two important functions: conducting the action potential and secreting the neurotransmitter. An action potential causes the axon to release a *neurotransmitter* (a chemical signal) from its axon terminal. It is through the release of neurotransmitters that neurons communicate with one another. The length of axons vary according to the part of the body that is being innervated, but they may be very long. The axons that extend from the spinal cord

to the feet may be over a meter in length. A long axon is called a nerve fiber, and a bundle of axons is called a *nerve.* The axon may be myelinated (wrapped with Schwann cells) or unmyelinated.

Nerve cells have the functional characteristic of *irritability* (the ability to respond to a stimulus), and that characteristic is evident in the dendrites and cell body. Nerve cells also have the characteristic of *conductivity* (the transmission of an electrical impulse from one location to another). It is the axon that conducts an electrical impulse. In general, large-diameter nerves conduct an impulse faster than small-diameter nerves. A myelin sheath protects and electrically insulates axons and speeds up the rate at which electrical impulses can be conducted (Kapit, et al., 2000; Marieb, 2001; Van de Graaff and Fox, 1989). For example, the nerve conduction velocity in an unmyelinated neuron is in the range of 13.5–22.5 miles per hour; in a myelinated skeletal muscle neuron of the same diameter, the speed is 135–225 miles per hour (Robergs and Roberts, 1997)!

The Neural Impulse

An **impulse** is a charge transmitted through certain tissue that results in the stimulation or inhibition of physiological activity. The impulse carried by a neuron is an electrical impulse, called the *action potential.* Neurons, and all cells, possess an electrical resting membrane potential. The resting membrane potential is measured by comparing the electrical charge on the inside of the cell to the charge on the outside of the cell (Figure 2.3). This resting potential is the result of the unequal distribution of positively and negatively charged particles called *ions.* Negatively charged ions (anions [An^-]) predominate along the inside of the cell membrane and attract positively charged ions (cations) along the outside of the cell membrane. In a typical neuron at rest, sodium (Na^+) and chloride (Cl^-) ions predominate extracellularly. Potassium ions (K^+) and negatively charged protein anions predominate intracellularly.

The cell membrane itself is composed of proteins floating in a fluid bilayer of lipids. The membrane is permeable, or capable of allowing ions to pass through it, some by diffusion and some through specific protein channels. Channels may be passive (always open so that they allow a leakage) or active (requiring a chemical or electrical change to open their gates).

> **Impulse** An electrical charge transmitted through certain tissue that results in the stimulation or inhibition of physiological activity.

At rest, potassium (K^+) "leaks" out through passive channels, and a sodium-potassium pump, which actively transports sodium out across the membrane and potassium back into the cell, removes three sodium ions from the cell for each two potassium ions it brings into the cell. Thus, at rest there is a net loss of positive ions from the interior of the cell, making the interior negatively charged (-65 to -85 microvolts) with respect to the exterior (Figure 2.3a). Thus, the resting neuron is said to be *polarized*.

When a sufficient stimulus (usually a chemical stimulus from other neurons) is applied to the cell, sodium (Na^+) channels open, and positive ions flow into the neuron. Polarity is reversed; that is, the cell is *depolarized*, meaning that the inside of the cell is now positive relative to the outside (Figure 2.3b). This process takes about 1 millisecond, at which time the sodium gates close and potassium gates open. Potassium exits the cell, bringing about *repolarization*, or a return to a net negative charge inside. Sodium is returned to the outside of the cell and potassium to the inside by the sodium-potassium pump, which restores the ionic balance and resting membrane potential. This sequence of events is repeated down the length of the axon. The reversal of polarity or change in electrical potential across a nerve membrane that generates an electrical current is an **action potential.** The propagation of an action potential along the axon of a neuron is the mechanism by which electrical signals are sent within a neuron (Kapit, et al., 2000; Marieb, 2001; Van de Graaff and Fox, 1989).

Nerve Communication and Responses

Once generated in the axon, the action potential moves along the entire length of the axon, causing a neurotransmitter to be released from the terminal end of the axon. The terminal end of the axon communicates with other neurons, muscle cells, or glands across junctions known as **synapses.** If the synapse is between a neuron and a muscle cell, it is known as a *neuromuscular junction.*

The dominant form of synapse is a chemical synapse, which involves the release of a neurotransmitter from the neuron. (The sequence of events involved in the release of a neurotransmitter at the

---

Action Potential The reversal of polarity or change in electrical potential across a nerve membrane that generates an electrical current.

Synapses The gap, or junction, between terminal ends of the axon and other neurons, muscle cells, or glands.

(a) Resting (Polarized) State

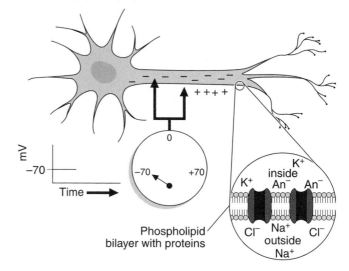

(b) Action Potential

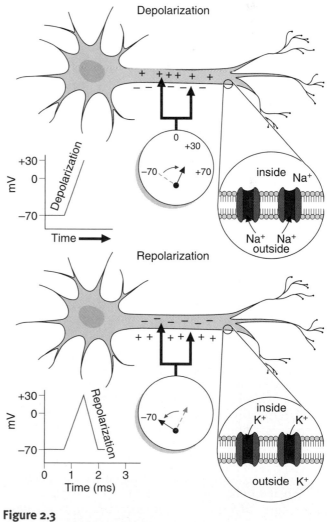

Figure 2.3
Generation of Action Potential

(a) Resting (polarized) state. (b) Action potential.

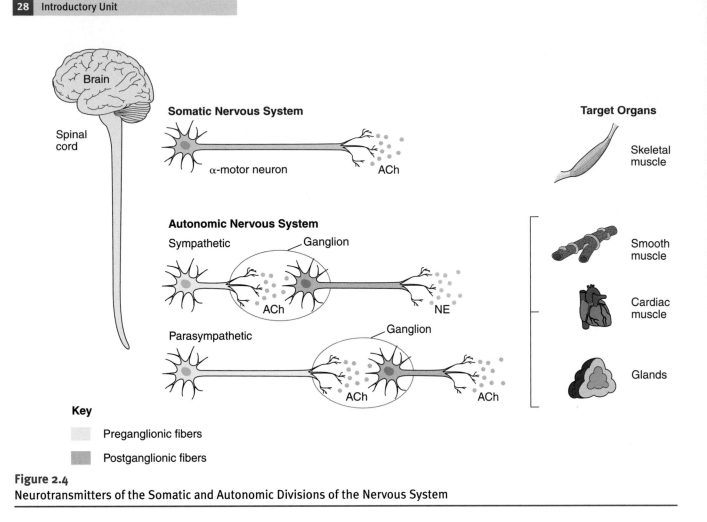

Figure 2.4
Neurotransmitters of the Somatic and Autonomic Divisions of the Nervous System

neuromuscular junction is discussed more fully in Chapter 22.) Acetylcholine (ACh) is the neurotransmitter released from somatic motor neurons, parasympathetic and sympathetic preganglionic fibers, and parasympathetic postganglionic fibers (Figure 2.4). Acetylcholine is always excitatory to skeletal muscle, but may be inhibitory or excitatory to target cells of the autonomic nervous system (smooth muscle, cardiac muscle, glands), depending on the receptors on the target cell to which it binds. Norepinephrine (NE) is the neurotransmitter released by sympathetic postganglionic neurons. NE is also inhibitory or excitatory depending on the receptors to which it binds. Neurons that release ACh are called *cholinergic* fibers; neurons that release NE are called *adrenergic* fibers (Kapit, et al., 2000; Marieb, 2001; Van de Graaff and Fox, 1989).

The response of the target organ depends not only on the neurotransmitter, but also on the receptor with which it binds. There are two types of cholinergic receptors (*nicotinic* and *muscarinic*) and two types of adrenergic receptors (alpha [α] and beta [β]), which are further subdivided into α_1, α_2, β_1, and β_2.

Although target organs tend to have either nicotinic or muscarinic receptors, they may have both types of adrenergic receptors. For example, the heart has β_1 adrenergic receptors and muscarinic cholinergic receptors. Binding of NE to the β_1 receptors results in an increased rate and force of contraction in the heart. Binding of ACh to the muscarinic receptors results in precisely the opposite response: a decreased rate and force of contraction. Smooth muscle surrounding blood vessels in skeletal muscle have α, β, and nicotinic receptors (Guyton, 1996; Kapit, et al., 2000; Marieb, 2001; Van de Graaff and Fox, 1989).

Role of the Nervous System in Exercise

Both the somatic nervous system and the autonomic nervous system play important roles in controlling and/or regulating the body's response to exercise.

Role of the Somatic Nervous System

The role of the somatic nervous system in exercise is straightforward. Skeletal muscle will not contract unless it receives a signal from a motor neuron. The action potential in the neuron causes the neuron to release its neurotransmitter that acts as the signal to initiate contraction. Hence, the somatic nervous system directly regulates exercise. (A detailed explanation of the events involved in muscle contraction is given in Chapter 19.)

Role of the Autonomic Nervous System

The role of the autonomic nervous system in regulating the exercise response is very diverse. As previously stated, the exercise response is mediated primarily through the sympathetic branch of the nervous system. As summarized in Figure 2.5, the primary functions of the sympathetic branch of the ANS during exercise are to

1. enhance cardiorespiratory function,
2. regulate blood flow and maintain blood pressure,
3. maintain thermal balance, and
4. increase fuel mobilization for the production of energy.

Autonomic nerve fibers innervate the respiratory system and the heart. Stimulation of the SNS causes a decrease in airway resistance facilitating movement of air into and out of the lungs. Stimulation of the SNS also increases heart rate and force of contraction, causing an increase in the amount of blood ejected from the heart and an increase in blood pressure. The increase in cardiac pumping is important for transporting fuel and oxygen necessary to support muscular contraction and for transporting waste products that build up as a result of contraction and must be eliminated from the body.

The ANS is important in redirecting blood flow during exercise and in maintaining blood pressure. These functions are achieved by controlling the diameter of blood vessels. Sympathetic nerve stimulation causes blood vessels in nonworking muscles to vasoconstrict (decrease in diameter). This makes more blood available to support contracting muscles.

The ANS helps maintain thermal balance by controlling blood flow to the skin (where heat can be more easily dissipated from the surface of the body) and by regulating sweat glands. The evaporation of sweat is the primary mechanism for heat loss during most exercise.

Sympathetic nerve stimulation causes the adrenal medulla to release epinephrine (E) and norepinephrine (NE). These hormones reinforce the effect of NE from the sympathetic nervous system on the systems described above and stimulate adipose cells to release fatty acids and the liver to release glucose.

Cardiorespiratory Function
Bronchial Dilation
- ↓ resistance to airflow
- ↑ airflow
Increased heart rate
Increased force of contraction
- ↑ cardiac output
- ↑ blood pressure

Blood Flow/Blood Pressure
Vasoconstriction in nonworking muscle
- allows blood flow to be directed to working muscle
- helps maintain blood pressure

Thermoregulation
Increased sweating
Vasodilation—increased blood flow to the skin

Fuel Mobilization
Adipose cells release fatty acids
Liver cells release glucose

Figure 2.5
Primary Results of Sympathetic Nerve Stimulation during Exercise

The increased free fatty acids and glucose are used as fuel to produce energy to support muscle contraction. Further details about the role of the autonomic nervous system in regulating the exercise response are provided in the relevant chapters throughout the text.

In addition to the activation of the sympathetic nervous system described above, the parasympathetic nervous system is simultaneously inhibited during exercise. The inhibition of the parasympathetic nervous system is often referred to as parasympathetic withdrawal.

Neural Exercise Responses

Neural responses are not typically measured in exercise situations. It is usually the *result* of neural activation (i.e., muscle contraction, increased heart rate, and so forth) that matters, not the activation itself. There is a measure, however, that attempts to quantify the activation of the sympathetic nervous system during exercise. Mean sympathetic nerve activity (MSNA) measures electrical activity in the peroneal nerve and serves as an index of sympathetic excitation (Vallbo, 1979).

Electrical activity in the muscle (EMG) is sometimes used as an index of somatic nervous system activation because the muscle will not contract unless it is stimulated by a somatic motor neuron. Thus, an increase in muscle electrical activity indirectly reflects an increase in somatic nerve activity.

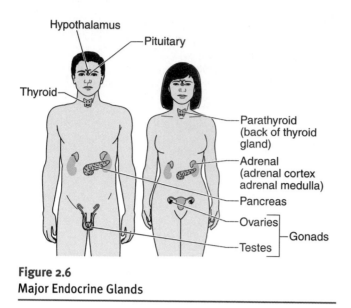

Figure 2.6
Major Endocrine Glands

Training Adaptations in the Nervous System

Exercise training results in consistent and readily recognized changes in the muscular system. Endurance training results in muscle fibers that are more resistant to fatigue, and resistance training results in muscle fibers that are stronger. Although many of these changes are due to alterations within the muscle cell (including metabolic changes and changes in the size of the muscle cell), adaptations also occur in the motor neurons supplying the muscle fibers (McComas, 1996). The adaptations that occur in the nervous system help to optimize the control of the muscles involved in exercise (Sale, 1992). For example, endurance training may lead to changes in the structure and function of the neuromuscular junction (Deschenes, et al., 1994). Resistance training increases the number of motor units recruited and the frequency of the nerve stimulation. As a result, agonist muscles (those principally responsible for the movement) are more fully activated, and synergistic muscles (muscles that support the agonists) and antagonist muscles (muscles opposing the movement) are more appropriately activated (Sale, 1992) or relaxed.

The Endocrine System

The endocrine system, along with the nervous system, regulates the body's response to exercise. Although many hormones display a change in blood concentrations during exercise, this book concentrates only on those hormones that play a primary role in regulating the exercise response or training adaptations. The primary role of the hormonal system during exercise is to help regulate the metabolic and cardiovascular systems (Bunt, 1986).

The Basic Structure of the Endocrine System

The endocrine system is composed of a series of ductless glands, other tissues, and the *hormones* they secrete. Hormones are chemical substances that originate in glandular tissue (or cells) and that are transported through body fluids to a target cell to influence physiological activity (Guyton, 1996; Kapit, et al., 2000; Marieb, 2001; Van de Graaff and Fox, 1989). The major endocrine glands involved in exercise or training (Figure 2.6) include the hypothalamus, pituitary, thyroid, parathyroid, adrenal, pancreas, and gonads (ovaries and testes.) Other tissues that secrete hormones include the heart, kidneys, liver, and gastrointestinal tract, as well as endothelial, immunological, and adipose cells. Hormones released from ductless glands are released directly into the bloodstream and travel throughout the body. Hormones released from tissue cells are excreted into the surrounding extracellular fluid, from which they may diffuse into nearby cells. Although a complete inventory and description of all hormones is beyond the scope of this book, Table 2.2 lists those hormones directly involved in regulating exercise responses, training adaptations, or other topics covered in this text.

Activation of the Endocrine System

Secretion of Hormones Endocrine glands and tissues can be activated to secrete hormones in three ways: neural, hormonal, or humoral (Marieb, 2001). Regardless of the type, the activation of an endocrine gland always depends on a chemical signal. Furthermore, the synthesis and release of most hormones are regulated by *negative feedback* mechanisms; that is, the output (in this case the hormone, or a variable controlled by the hormone) shuts off the original stimulus or reduces its intensity. Negative feedback mechanisms cause the variable to change in a direction that is opposite to the original change, returning the variable to its "set point" and thus helping to maintain homeostasis (Marieb, 2001).

Neural activation occurs directly when a neuron releases a neurotransmitter that signals the endocrine tissue to release a hormone. For example, sympathetic neurons release the neurotransmitter norepinephrine (NE), which stimulates the adrenal medulla to release the hormones epinephrine (E) and NE.

Hormonal activation literally means that one hormone (sometimes called hormone-releasing factor) stimulates another gland to release a hormone in a *feed forward control system*. Hormones that stimulate the release of another hormone are called *trophic* hormones. The hypothalamus secretes numerous

Table 2.2
Hormones Involved in Regulating Exercise

Site Produced (Endocrine Gland/Tissue)	Hormone(s)	Selected Functions Relative to Exercise Physiology
Adipose tissue	Leptin	Food intake, metabolic rate
Adrenal gland		
• Adrenal cortex	Cortisol	Metabolism; stress response; immune function; anti-inflammatory; catabolic to muscle tissue
	Aldosterone	Na^+, K^+, and acid secretion by kidneys; fluid balance
• Adrenal medulla	Epinephrine, norepinephrine	Metabolism; cardiovascular function; stress response
Gonads		
• Ovaries (female)	Estrogen	Fat deposition; bone remodeling
	Progesterone	Catabolic to muscular tissue; bone remodeling
• Testes (male)	Testosterone	Bone and muscle growth and development
Hypothalamus	Hypophysiotrophic hormones (general)	Controls secretions of hormones of anterior pituitary (in general): see anterior pituitary
	• Corticotrophin-releasing hormone (CRH)	Stimulates anterior pituitary (APIT) to secrete adrenocorticotrophic hormone (ACTH)
	• Thyrotrophin-releasing hormone (TRH)	Stimulates APIT to secrete thyroid-stimulating hormone (TSH)
	• Growth hormone-releasing hormone (GHRH)	Stimulates APIT to secrete growth hormone (GH)
	• Growth hormone-inhibiting hormone (GHIH)	Inhibits secretion of GH
	• Gonadotrophin-releasing hormone (GnRH)	Stimulates APIT to secrete luteinizing hormone (LH) and follicle-stimulating hormone (FSH)
	Production of antidiuretic hormone (ADH), which is released by posterior pituitary gland	Water retention; fluid balance
Kidneys	Erythropoietin	Erythrocyte (RBC) production
Leukocytes (WBC) and endothelial cells	Cytokines	Immune function
Liver	Somatomedins (insulin-like growth factors [IGF])	Anabolic to muscle tissue
Pancreas	Insulin, glucagon	Metabolism; regulates blood glucose levels
Parathyroid	Parathyroid hormone (PTH)	Plasma Ca^{2+}, PO_4^- levels
Pituitary		
• Anterior	Growth hormone (GH)	Bone and muscle growth; metabolism; stimulates IGF release
	Thyroid-stimulating hormone (TSH)	Secretion of hormones from thyroid gland
	Adrenocorticotrophic hormone (ACTH)	Secretion of hormones from adrenal cortex
• Posterior	Follicle-stimulating hormone (FSH) and luteinizing hormone (LH)	Sex hormone secretion
	Antidiuretic hormone (ADH, also called vasopressin)	Water excretion by kidney; fluid balance; cardiovascular function
Thyroid	Thyroxine (T_4) triiodothyronine (T_3)	Metabolic rate
	Calcitonin	Plasma Ca^{2+} levels

trophic hormones, including corticotrophin-releasing hormone (CRH). CRH in turn stimulates the anterior pituitary to release adrenocorticotrophic hormone (ACTH). ACTH then stimulates the adrenal cortex to release cortisol (the long-term stress hormone). When hormones from one gland cause the target gland to secrete a hormone, which affects yet another gland, it is called an *axis*. The example given above describes the hypothalamus-pituitary-adrenal axis (Marieb, 2001).

Humoral refers to blood or other body fluids. Hence, *humoral activation* refers to stimulation of an endocrine gland by blood levels of nutrients, electrolytes, water, ions, or other factors. For example, the pancreas responds to blood levels of glucose (a nutrient) by releasing the hormone insulin. Likewise, the thyroid gland and parathyroid glands are stimulated to release calcitonin and parathyroid hormone, respectively, in response to blood levels of calcium (an electrolyte).

Blood Hormone Levels The plasma concentration of a hormone depends on several factors, including

1. the rate at which the hormone is secreted;

2. the rate at which it is broken down and removed from the blood; and

3. for some hormones, the effective, or biologically active, amount, that is, how much of the hormone is bound to a protein versus how much is circulating in the free or unbound state.

Hormones can be secreted in pulsatile (or rhythmic), circadian (day/night or 24-hr periodization), entropic (random moment-to-moment variation), or cyclical (often monthly) patterns as well as on demand. Some hormones act instantaneously; others require minutes to hours to days before their impact is manifested. Hormones can be broken down and cleared from the body by the kidney, liver, or target cells. In addition, many hormones (primarily the steroids) circulate in blood bound to protein. However, in order to interact with a receptor, the hormone must be unbound, or "free." In these cases, it is the amount of free hormone, not the total amount circulating, that determines the biological effectiveness of the hormone.

In addition to the factors listed above, hormonal blood levels are affected by disease, temperature, altitude, nutritional status, age, sex, exercise, hydration level, and training status.

Extent of Cellular Response As stated earlier, hormones affect a target cell by binding to a receptor on, or in, the target cell. This binding requires comple-

mentary shapes between the hormone and the receptor. The hormone-receptor binding is known as *receptor activation*. The extent of cellular response to receptor activation depends on three factors (Marieb, 2001; Vander, et al., 2001):

1. the blood levels of the hormone,

2. the relative number of receptors, and

3. the strength (affinity) of the bond between the hormone and receptor.

Factors influencing the blood level of the hormone are described in the preceding section. The number of receptors on a cell for any given hormone can vary over time. Hormone-receptor binding often destroys the receptor; as a result, replacement receptors are needed. High-affinity receptors produce a more pronounced hormonal effect than low-affinity receptors. High blood levels of a hormone may cause either an increase in the number of receptors (*up regulation*) or a decrease in the number of receptors (*down regulation*). Up regulation increases the cell's ability to bring about the hormone-specific cellular response; down regulation prevents the target cells from overreacting to persistently high hormonal levels. Low blood levels of a hormone may also result in up regulation. The more receptors, the lower the hormone concentration required to obtain any given physiological response.

Mechanism of Action

Most hormones are divided into two major classifications based on their chemical structure: *amino acid–based hormones* and *steroid-based hormones*. Amino acid–based hormones range in size from very small amino acid derivatives (including the *amines*—epinephrine and norepinephrine—and thyroxine), to short chains of amino acids (the *peptides*) to long chains of amino acids (*proteins*). Steroid-based hormones are derived from cholesterol and include only those hormones secreted from the adrenal cortex (aldosterone and cortisol) and gonads (estrogen and testosterone) (Marieb, 2001; Vander, et al., 2001).

Once a hormone binds to a receptor on a target cell, a response is initiated. The sequence of steps that occurs from receptor activation to cellular response is complex and is known as the *signal transduction pathway* or *mechanism of action*. There are two pathways or mechanisms of hormonal action (Figure 2.7) (Guyton, 1996; Kapit, et al., 2000; Marieb, 2001; Van de Graaff and Fox, 1989; Vander, et al., 2001):

1. second messenger system and

2. direct gene activation.

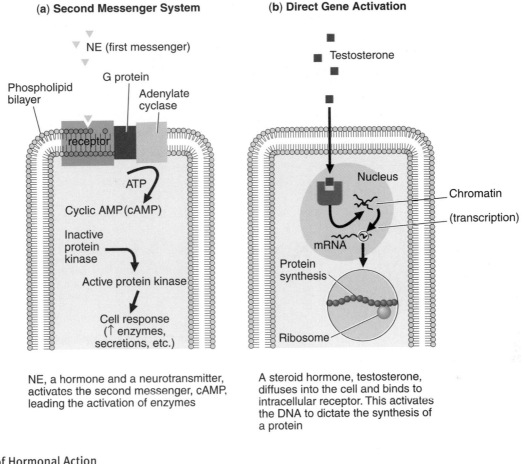

(a) Second Messenger System

NE (first messenger)

Phospholipid bilayer

G protein

Adenylate cyclase

receptor

ATP

Cyclic AMP (cAMP)

Inactive protein kinase

Active protein kinase

Cell response
(↑ enzymes, secretions, etc.)

NE, a hormone and a neurotransmitter, activates the second messenger, cAMP, leading the activation of enzymes

(b) Direct Gene Activation

Testosterone

Nucleus

Chromatin

(transcription)

mRNA

Protein synthesis

Ribosome

A steroid hormone, testosterone, diffuses into the cell and binds to intracellular receptor. This activates the DNA to dictate the synthesis of a protein

Figure 2.7
Mechanisms of Hormonal Action

Second Messenger System   Because they are lipid insoluble and cannot diffuse into a cell, amino acid–based hormones exert their influence primarily through a *second messenger system*. The second messenger mechanism begins when the amino acid–based hormone, known as the *first messenger* because it is delivering a chemical message from another tissue, binds to its specific receptor on the cell membrane (Figure 2.7a). The binding of the first messenger to the receptor activates another membrane protein (G protein), which in turn activates an enzyme called adenyl cyclase. Adenyl cyclase catalyzes the breakdown of adenosine triphosphate (ATP) to cyclic adenosine monophosphate (cAMP). Cyclic AMP is the second messenger and initiates a *cascade* of chemical reactions. It changes a protein kinase enzyme in the cell from an inactive to an active form. The activated protein kinase continues the process by acting on other enzymes that are in the cell. The result is either a stimulation or activation of the activity of those enzymes. The specific effects depend on the cell and the particular enzyme activated (Marieb, 2001; Van de Graaff and Fox, 1989; Vander, et al., 2001).

Although cAMP is the most important second messenger or mechanism, it is not the only one. The calcium-calmodulin system is another. In this case, when the first messenger binds to the membrane receptor, the G protein activates a Ca^{2+} ion channel. When the calcium concentration intracellularly reaches a sufficient level, it activates another cellular protein called calmodulin. The calmodulin, as the second messenger, now proceeds precisely as cAMP did and initiates the cascade of chemical reactions, starting with the activation of protein kinase, which in turn modifies the actions of other enzymes in the cell.

Direct Gene Activation   Steroid hormones, and a few protein hormones, are lipid soluble and diffuse easily into target cells. Once inside the cell, they operate by *direct gene activation*. Lipid-soluble hormones enter the cell and bind to receptors either in the nucleus or in the cell cytoplasm (forming a complex that must then migrate into the nucleus) (Figure 2.7b). The activated hormone-receptor complex signals the chromatin portion of the DNA, a gene, to be transcribed to messenger RNA (mRNA). The mRNA carries the code

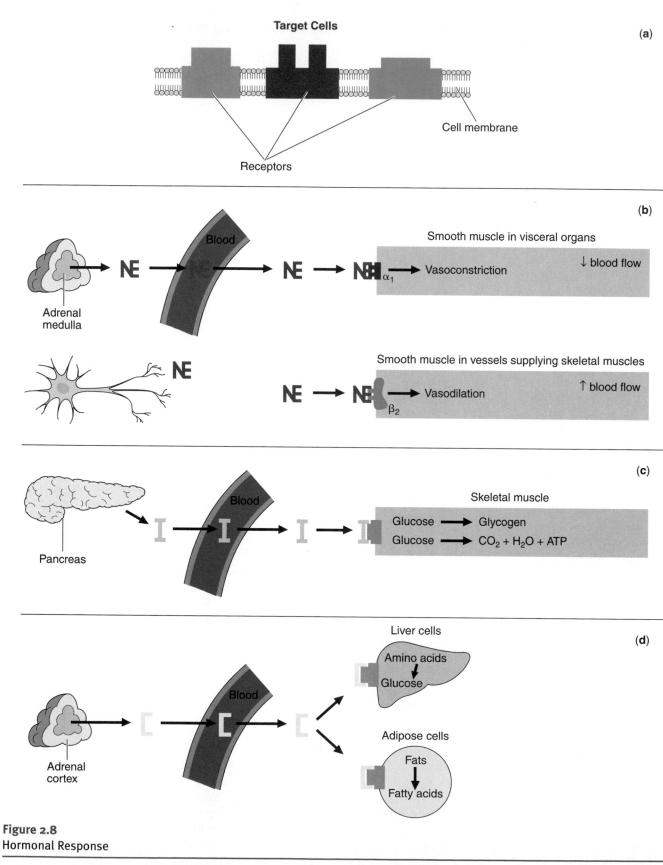

Figure 2.8
Hormonal Response

from the nucleus to the cytoplasm where a specific protein is synthesized. The protein produced may be a muscle filament or an enzyme that regulates cell metabolism (Marieb, 2001; Van de Graaff and Fox, 1989; Vander, et al., 2001).

Hormonal Communication and Responses

Figure 2.8 summarizes several basic principles essential to understanding how hormone-receptor binding functions within the human organism:

- *A target cell may (and usually does) have many different receptor types.* It is helpful to remember that a cell is a complicated structure and that a cell membrane will have many different types of receptors expressed on its surface (Figure 2.8a). Furthermore, as noted earlier, the number of any given receptor may change over time based on cell needs.

- *A hormone may have different functions in different target cells, depending on the specific receptor to which it binds* (Figure 2.8b). For example, when norepinephrine (NE) binds to α_1 receptors on smooth muscle, it causes vasoconstriction (a decrease in vessel diameter), whereas when norepinephrine binds to β_2 receptors on smooth muscle it causes vasodilation (an increase in vessel diameter). Figure 2.8b reinforces the point that NE is both a neurotransmitter (released from sympathetic neurons) and a hormone (released from the adrenal medulla).

- *A hormone may have several different functions within a cell* (Figure 2.8c). For example, when insulin binds to receptors on skeletal muscle cells, it may cause several things to happen, depending on the metabolic conditions within the cell. These include an increase in the uptake of glucose into the cell, the formation of glycogen from glucose (by a process known as *glycogenesis*), or an increase in the rate at which glucose is broken down to produce ATP within the cell (glycolysis) (Marieb, 2001).

- *A hormone may affect multiple target cells* (Figure 2.8d). For example, when cortisol binds to receptors on the membrane of liver cells, it causes glycogen to be broken down into glucose (by the process known as *glycogenolysis*). Thus, glucose levels in the blood increase, and glucose can be used as a fuel for active muscle cells and nervous tissue. However, when cortisol binds to receptors on adipose cells, it stimulates the breakdown of fats into free fatty acids and glycerol (by the process known as *lipolysis*). Thus, free fatty acid levels in the blood increase and can be used as a fuel for active muscle cells.

Interaction of Hormones

Many cellular responses require the joint action of many hormones. In a *synergistic response,* the combined effect of the hormones may be greater than the sum of the individual effects. In a *complementary response,* both or all hormones are needed to accomplish the task. *Permissive* hormones facilitate or potentiate the actions of another hormone, making the response more effective. In some situations, the actions of one hormone oppose another. These hormones are said to be *antagonistic.*

Role of the Endocrine System in Exercise

The role of the endocrine system during an acute bout of exercise is predominantly to regulate the metabolic and cardiovascular systems (Bunt, 1986). The following sections provide an overview of how the endocrine system helps regulate the metabolic and cardiovascular systems. The role of the individual hormones will be covered in greater detail as they relate to the systems of the body (metabolic, cardiorespiratory, neuromuscular). For now, it is important to understand the general functions of hormones in regulating the body's response to exercise.

Hormonal Regulation of Metabolism

The goals of the endocrine system relative to the metabolic system are to

1. mobilize fuel for the production of ATP energy needed to support muscle contraction, and

2. maintain blood glucose levels (because neural tissue can use only glucose to produce energy).

Glucagon, epinephrine, norepinephrine, growth hormone, and cortisol operate together under the permissive influence of triiodothyronine (T_3) to accomplish the first goal. Glucagon and insulin act antagonistically; glucagon levels increase and insulin levels are simultaneously suppressed during exercise. As shown in Figure 2.9, glucagon, NE, E, growth hormone (GH), and cortisol affect three primary target cells: adipose, liver, and skeletal muscle cells. When these hormones bind to receptors on adipose cells, fat storage is inhibited and fat mobilization and uptake enhanced. When these hormones bind to receptors on the liver, glycogen (chains of glucose molecules chemically linked together) is broken down to glucose, and additional glucose is synthesized from other sources, such as alanine (an amino acid), glycerol, or lactate. When these hormones bind to receptors on skeletal

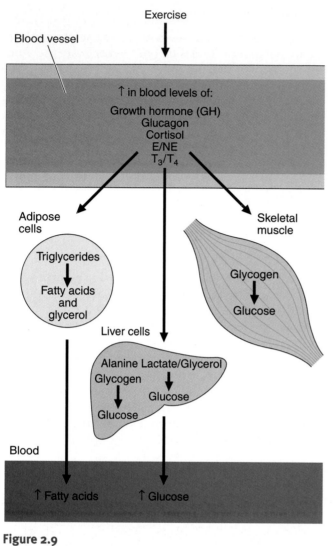

Figure 2.9
Effect of Metabolic Hormones

muscle, stored glycogen is broken down to glucose. These hormones also cause skeletal muscles to increase their uptake and utilization of fatty acids.

Hormonal Regulation of Cardiovascular Function

The goals of the hormonal system relative to cardiac function are to

1. enhance cardiac function,
2. distribute blood to active tissues, and
3. maintain blood pressure by stabilizing fluid and electrolyte balance.

Enhanced cardiac function and distribution of blood to the working musculature are primarily accomplished by E and NE, reinforcing the actions of NE as a neurotransmitter. Two hormones predomi-

nate in the stabilization or maintenance of fluid and electrolyte balance: antidiuretic hormone (ADH, sometimes called vasopressin), and aldosterone. These hormones act on the kidneys to increase water resorption and retain or excrete specific electrolytes (Bunt, 1986). By maintaining fluid and electrolyte balance, these hormones positively affect blood volume and blood pressure as well.

Hormonal Responses to Exercise

It should be fairly obvious that the action of most of the aforementioned hormones increases during exercise (with insulin being the exception). Without an increase in hormonal secretion, the enhanced functions just described would not occur. What is not so obvious is the pattern of response seen in blood concentrations of each of these hormones to exercises of different intensities, durations, and metabolic demands. The following section presents what is known about hormonal response patterns in relation to the five categories of exercise introduced in Chapter 1:

1. short-term light to moderate submaximal aerobic exercise,
2. long-term moderate to heavy submaximal aerobic exercise,
3. incremental aerobic exercise to maximum,
4. static exercise, and
5. dynamic resistance exercise.

In many instances, the hormonal responses for all five categories of exercise have not been identified. In general, much more is known about long-term moderate to heavy aerobic exercise and incremental exercise to maximum than other categories of exercise. As you read this section, keep in mind that changes in blood concentration of hormones may not simply indicate an increase in secretion, because hormonal levels are affected by changes in clearance rates, blood volume, receptor-binding turnover, and other factors (Bunt, 1986; Kraemer, 1992a).

Although it might seem overwhelming to consider *how* different hormones respond to various categories of exercise, it is important to appreciate *that* there are differences in the hormonal response based on the type of exercise performed. Indeed, many of the metabolic and cardiorespiratory variables discussed in subsequent chapters will be determined, in large part, by the endocrine responses described here. The graphs in Figure 2.10–2.13 may well be an important reference as you proceed through the textbook. In fact, we have included this information early in the textbook precisely because it helps explain how the other systems respond to exercise.

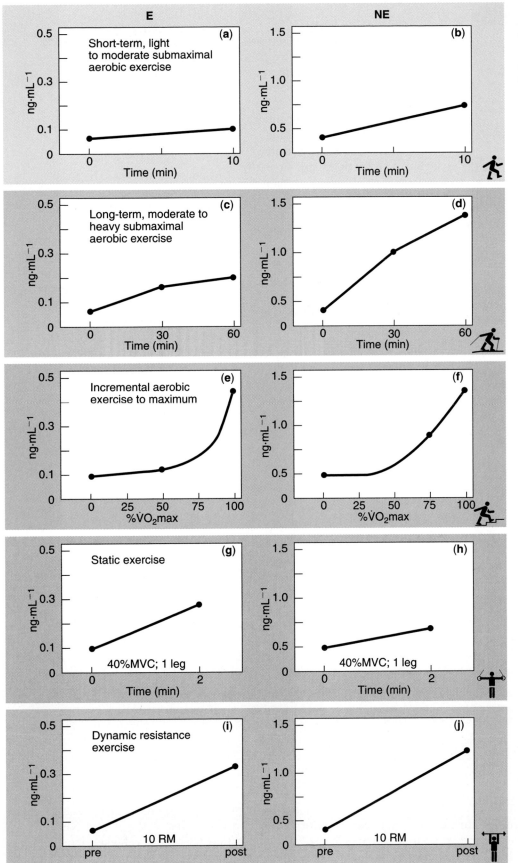

Figure 2.10
E and NE Responses to Various Categories of Exercise

Sources: Galbo, 1983; Kraemer, 1988.

Focus on Research

Hormonal Response to Resistance Exercise

Bush, J. A., et al. Exercise and recovery responses of adrenal medullary neurohormones to heavy resistance exercise. *Medicine and Science in Sports and Exercise.* 31(4):554–559 (1999).

The response of the adrenal medullary hormones, epinephrine (E) and norepinephrine (NE), have been relatively well studied. However, little has been known about the response of these hormones to the stress of heavy resistance exercise. Therefore, Bush and colleagues designed a study to examine the effect of dynamic resistance exercise on the response of the adrenal medullary hormones immediately after different protocols of resistance exercise and during recovery. Each participant was involved in 2 days of testing: on one day, participants performed a high-force protocol (using a 10-repetition maximum [RM]), and on the other day, participants performed a high-power protocol (using 15 repetitions). The total work performed on the 2 days was equal. Blood was drawn at four different times: prior to each resistance training session, immediately postexercise (0-min recovery), after 15 minutes of recovery, and after 4 hours of recovery. The concentration of norepinephrine and epinephrine in the plasma at each time period with the two protocols is shown in the figures below.

Statistical analysis revealed the following:

1. Norepinephrine was significantly higher postexercise for both protocols.
2. Epinephrine increased significantly following the exercise for both protocols and returned to near baseline levels by 15 minutes of recovery.

Results from this study indicate that heavy resistance exercise activates the adrenal medulla. Because the activation of the sympathetic nervous system, the "fight or flight" response, is thought to be an important mediator of acute stress, the elevation of norepinephrine and epinephrine after a bout of heavy resistance exercise suggests that the neuroendocrine system helps regulate the body's response to the stress of resistance exercise. Furthermore, the similar response of NE and E in the two protocols suggests that, as long as the total work is equated, subtle differences in mean force and mean power characteristics of a workout do not affect this hormonal response one way or the other.

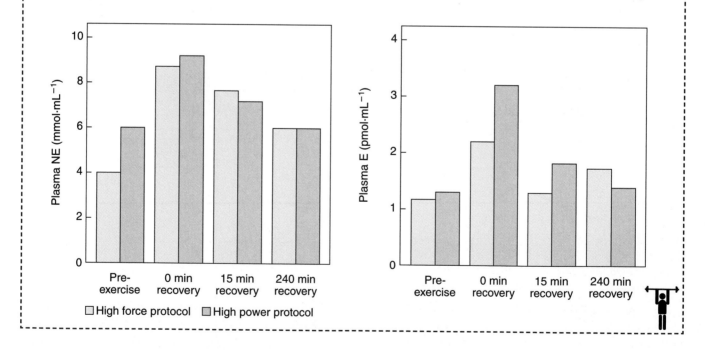

Epinephrine and Norepinephrine (Catecholamines)

Epinephrine (E) and norepinephrine (NE) are released when the sympathetic nervous system is activated. These hormones have widespread actions throughout the body and affect both the metabolic and cardiorespiratory responses to exercise. When interpreting the responses of the E and NE to exercise, remember that NE is also released from sympathetic nerve endings. Because neural stimulation occurs more quickly than endocrine response, the initial increase in NE is from the sympathetic nervous system. Both E and NE are later released from the adrenal medulla. In this light, it should not be surprising that NE shows an elevation at lower workloads than E and that blood levels are generally higher for NE than E (Galbo, 1983). Minimal increases in both E and NE are seen during short-term light to moderate submaximal aerobic exercise (Figures 2.10a and 2.10b). During long-term moderate to heavy submaximal aerobic exercise, the increase is time dependent and gradual if energy is supplied aerobically up to the point of fatigue (Figures 2.10c and 2.10d). Incremental aerobic exercise to maximum elicits positive exponential increases in both E and NE (Figures 2.10e and 2.10f), clearly indicating that a lower limit of submaximal intensity must be exceeded before a response is achieved and that above that point the increase in hormonal level is intensity dependent. The E and NE response to static exercise (Figures 2.10g and 2.10h) is larger than during dynamic resistance exercise of equal heart rate or aerobic energy demand (oxygen consumption), and the rise in plasma E seems to be larger relative to NE than during aerobic exercise (Galbo, 1983). The response of E and NE to dynamic resistance exercise appears to be related to the force of muscle contraction, the amount of muscle tissue stimulated, and the amount of rest between repetitions. Rapid, large increases occur similar to heavy anaerobic sprint responses (Figures 2.10i and 2.10j) (Kraemer, 1988).

Metabolic Hormones

The exercise responses of the metabolic hormones have been studied most extensively during long-term moderate to heavy submaximal aerobic exercise and incremental aerobic exercise to maximum. Therefore, what is known about the exercise response of these hormones applies primarily to these categories of exercise. Although plasma levels are presented for each hormone, keep in mind that changes in levels may not reflect changes in secretion, but rather changes in clearance rates. The responses might also reflect autonomic nervous system changes.

Insulin and Glucagon Insulin operates to store fuel, whereas glucagon's role is to mobilize fuel. Therefore, in general, the responses of these two hormones are close to mirror images of each other. However, it is the ratio of glucagon to insulin that primarily controls fuel mobilization. During short-term light to moderate submaximal aerobic exercise, insulin exhibits a small initial decline before leveling off, and glucagon a small initial rise before leveling off (Galbo, 1983).

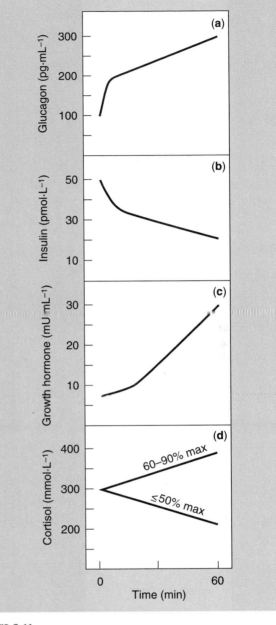

Figure 2.11

Hormonal Responses to Long-Term Moderate to Heavy Submaximal Aerobic Exercise

Sources: Galbo, 1983; Sutton, et al., 1990.

Long-term moderate to heavy submaximal aerobic exercise elicits an increase in glucagon, followed by a gradual increase (Figure 2.11a) and a complementary initial drop in insulin followed by gradual decline (Figure 2.11b) (Galbo, 1983). During incremental exercise to maximum, glucagon increases in a positively exponential manner. The increase in glucagon is proportionally greater as exercise intensity increases than is the decline in insulin

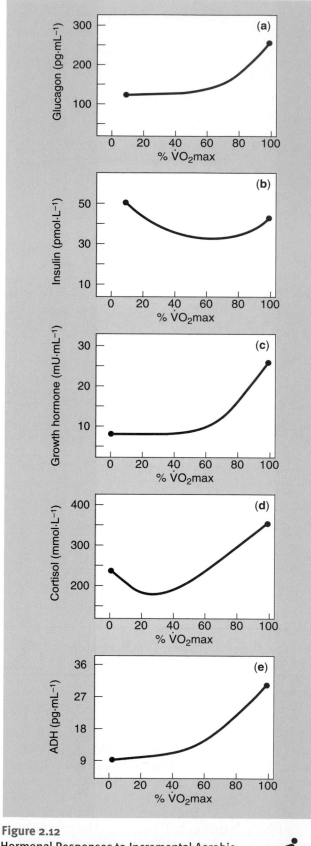

Figure 2.12
Hormonal Responses to Incremental Aerobic Exercise to Maximum

Sources: Galbo, 1983; Sutton, et al., 1990; Wade, 2000.

(Figures 2.12a and 2.12b). Indeed, at high workloads (>60 $\dot{V}O_2$max) plasma insulin levels begin to rise again, resulting overall in a truncated U-shaped curve that remains below resting levels. Neither static activity nor short-term high-intensity exercise (such as sprinting or dynamic resistance exercise) appears to elicit changes in either insulin or glucagon, because fuel demands for these activities do not require extensive mobilization.

Growth Hormone   As a protein hormone, growth hormone (GH) has a slow rate of response, secretion, and clearance (Galbo, 1983). This means that there is a delay between the onset of exercise and changes in blood hormonal levels. The greater the intensity of the exercise, the shorter the delay period. Short-term light to moderate submaximal aerobic exercise and static exercise are too brief for any changes to become apparent. A short but high-intensity exercise will show a peak value, but its manifestation can be anywhere from 15 to 30 minutes into recovery.

Long-term moderate to heavy submaximal aerobic exercise shows a gradual increase in GH over a period of 30 to 60 min (Figure 2.11c) (Galbo, 1983). However, if the activity is continued for much longer durations, as in a marathon, GH concentrations will return to near baseline levels. The GH response to incremental aerobic exercise to maximum (Figure 2.12c) indicates that GH concentration increases with increasing workloads in a positive exponential fashion after allowing for the initial delay.

GH release is increased during and following resistance exercise. High total work and short rest periods are associated with a much larger increase in GH than low total work volume and long rest periods (Kraemer, 1992a).

Cortisol   Like growth hormone, the steroid-based cortisol is a slow-acting hormone. It is difficult to generalize a pattern of exercise response because there is an initial delay in exercise-enhanced concentrations and because in short duration and/or low to moderate intensity activity, clearance of the hormone exceeds secretion. This means that although secretion may have increased, blood concentrations actually decrease (Sutton, et al., 1990). This outcome can be seen in Figure 2.11d, which depicts cortisol response to long-term moderate to heavy exercise. Work intensity less than or equal to 50% of $\dot{V}O_2$max results in a steady decrease in blood cortisol level, whereas intensity loads from approximately ~60–90% of $\dot{V}O_2$max elicit a gradual rise in blood cortisol level as time continues, despite a constant workload. The truncated U pattern for incremental exercise to maximum seen in

Figure 2.12d reinforces the importance of intensity to the cortisol response. Indeed, the exercise increase in cortisol may not occur until anaerobic metabolism makes a significant contribution to the total energy supply. Anaerobic exercise elicits greater increases in cortisol than aerobic exercise, even at the same total work output, probably owing to the greater intensity (Kraemer, 1992a; Kraemer, 1988). Dynamic resistance exercise has been shown to cause large increases both during and after high-intensity sessions, probably owing to its large anaerobic component. Cortisol levels in the blood remain elevated for up to several hours after exercise.

Thyroid and Parathyroid Hormone   It is not possible to describe the pattern of thyroid and parathyroid hormonal responses to the different categories of exercise (Galbo, 1983). Numerous studies have reported no change in blood concentrations of triiodothyronine (T_3) or thyroxine (T_4). However, it is possible that free T_3 and free T_4 change without resulting in changes in the total concentration of thyroid hormone; the lack of change in concentration does not mean a lack of change in turnover (Berent and Wartofsky, 2000). Little more can be concluded than that with long-term heavy aerobic exercise, free T_4 increases slightly, while free T_3 declines gradually with time. There are not enough data to draw any conclusions regarding calcitonin or parathyroid hormone responses to exercise.

Fluid Balance Hormones

Changes in renin, antidiuretic hormone and aldosterone—known as *fluid balance hormones*—occur parallel to each other. They highly correlate with changes in NE and have similar time courses. Figure 2.12e depicts the positive exponential response of incremental exercise to maximum of ADH (Wade, 2000).

Hormonal Adaptations to Training

Training programs are not consciously designed to bring about adaptations in the hormonal system. There are no research-based training principles to follow and few systematic attempts to vary intensity, duration, frequency, length of training period, and modality in large numbers of subjects. Some of the available information has been derived from cross-sectional studies where untrained (or sedentary) individuals have been compared to trained (or fit) individuals. Some information has also been derived from testing individuals before and after a training period. The greatest amount of information and agreement relates to hormonal responses to an absolute submax-

imal aerobic exercise training program that is long term and moderate to heavy in intensity. This section describes those changes and, where information is available, indicates training adaptations that result from resistance training programs. It is important to understand that adaptations in one hormone may impact plasma levels of another, or changes in receptor sensitivity may not be reflected in circulating hormone levels. Furthermore, adaptations in sympathetic nervous system responses may be the cause of changes in hormonal levels. As with hormonal responses to exercise, training adaptations in the metabolic, cardiorespiratory, and neuromuscular systems are often the result of adaptations in the endocrine system.

Adaptations Related to Metabolic Function

Most of what is known regarding hormonal training adaptations is based on evidence from studies that compare the response of individuals to a prolonged bout of exercise before and after exercise training (Figure 2.13). The major hormones involved in fuel mobilization (glucagon, insulin, NE, E, cortisol) all show a dampening effect as a result of exercise training; that is, the change from resting levels that occurs during exercise represents a smaller disruption of homeostasis than in the untrained state (Bunt, 1986). Given that endurance training decreases the sympathetic nervous system response to an absolute workload, it is to be expected that epinephrine and norepinephrine show muted responses (Figure 2.13a). The decline in insulin is less in the trained than in the untrained state (Figure 2.13b). The rise in glucagon is also less: so much less that 60 min of submaximal exercise may not be long enough or intense enough to require a glucagon response in a trained individual (Figure 2.13c) (Coggan and Williams, 1995; Sutton, et al., 1990). An increase in insulin sensitivity compensates for these changes. Growth hormone and cortisol exhibit the same dampening effect, although, interestingly, both of these appear to have higher resting levels in the aerobically trained than untrained individuals (Figure 2.13d and 2.13e). Resistance-trained individuals appear to have unchanged resting GH concentrations (Kraemer, 1992a).

Adaptations Related to Cardiovascular Function

Neither of the hormones primarily responsible for fluid and electrolyte balance (ADH and aldosterone) show any clear training adaptation. The thyroid hormones adapt with an enhanced turnover rate, but too little is known about parathyroid hormone to draw any conclusion.

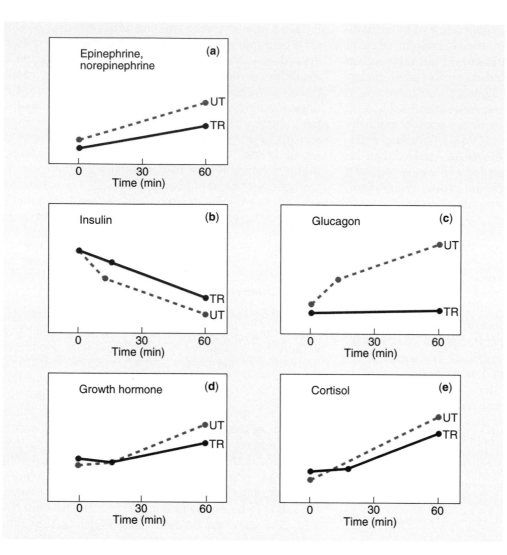

Figure 2.13
Training Adaptations Exhibited during Long-Term Submaximal Aerobic Exercise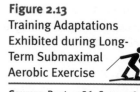

Sources: Bunt, 1986; Coggan & Williams, 1995; Kjaer & Lange, 2000; Sutton, et al., 1990.

Maximal values obtained at the end of incremental exercise have revealed increased levels of E, NE, and cortisol. Higher values reflect the trained individual's ability to do more high-intensity work (Bunt, 1986; Kjaer and Lange, 2000; Sutton, et al., 1990).

Hormones Related to Muscle, Bone, and Adipose Tissue

Hormones involved in the structure and function of muscle, bone, and adipose cells are beyond the immediate goals of supporting acute exercise; however, they may be important during recovery and thus facilitate overall training adaptations (Bunt, 1986; Kraemer, 1992b). Tissue repair mechanisms are activated during recovery after all exercise sessions. Hormones that impact muscle, bone, and adipose tissue include growth hormone, somatomedins or insulin-like growth factors (IGF), testosterone, estrogen, progesterone, calcitonin, parathyroid hormone, and leptin.

Muscle The impact of GH on protein synthesis is mediated through IGF. Growth hormone stimulates the release of IGF from the liver, and both muscle and connective tissue produce IGF. Specific effects of IGF include amino acid uptake, muscle synthesis, connective tissue (collagen) synthesis, bone and cartilage growth, and maintenance of fat-free muscle mass. There is no clear pattern of response of IGF to acute exercise, although there is some indication of an early (at about 10 min of exercise) increase in IGF that is unrelated to intensity and declines with increasing duration of exercise. It has been hypothesized that IGF initially decreases as a result of training but that after an unknown length of time (probably longer than 5 weeks), resting levels of both GH and IGF increase, indicating an anabolic (tissue growth) internal environment (Eliakim, et al., 2000).

Testosterone is responsible for the high ratio of muscle mass to fat mass that occurs in the male at adolescence. Testosterone stimulates the release of

GH and influences neural factors contributing to anabolic processes. During and following high-intensity dynamic aerobic and resistance exercise, testosterone levels are elevated and remain so for a couple of hours during recovery. Prolonged exercise results in an initial increase, followed by a return to baseline or below as the duration extends into recovery (Cumming, 2000). The impact of chronic training on testosterone is controversial, possibly reflecting the level of training. Moderate training results in an increase, and extreme training a decrease (Urhausen and Kindermann, 2000). Together, a training increase in testosterone and growth hormone could contribute to increases in muscle mass (Kraemer, 1992b).

Bone Estrogen, progesterone, testosterone, GH, IGF, calcitonin, and parathyroid hormone (PTH) are important for bone formation, resorption, and turnover. Acute dynamic aerobic and resistance exercise results in elevated blood levels of estrogen and progesterone. Moderate exercise training appears to result in elevated resting levels of estrogen and progesterone, whereas severe training results in decreased resting levels. Male and female athletes have been reported to have lower PTH levels and higher bone mineral density than nonathletes (Chilibeck, 2000). The role of PTH, calcitonin, and estrogen in bone health is detailed in this text in Chapter 18.

Adipose Tissue Estrogen, testosterone, and leptin are important in determining body fat content. Estrogen and progesterone stimulate female fat deposition. Obese individuals have elevated leptin levels, a plasma protein associated with the obese gene. Testosterone may suppress leptin in an acute bout of exercise. Training has been shown to suppress leptin levels (Gleim and Glace, 2000).

Exercise and Training as Stressors

Individuals in the professional fields that depend on exercise and training typically think of exercise and training as universally positive factors. However, both acute exercise and chronic training are stressors.

Selye's Theory of Stress

A *stressor* is any activity, event, or impingement that causes stress. **Stress** is defined most simply as a disruption in body homeostasis and all attempts by the body to regain homeostasis. Selye, however, defines stress more completely as "the state manifested by a specific syndrome that consists of all the nonspecifically induced changes within a biological system." The biological system here is the human body. The specific syndrome is the *General Adaptation Syndrome* (GAS), a step-by-step description of the bodily reactions to a stressor. It consists of three major stages (Selye, 1956):

1. the Alarm-Reaction: Shock and Countershock;
2. the Stage of Resistance; and
3. the Stage of Exhaustion.

In the Alarm-Reaction stage, the body responds to a stressor with a disruption of homeostasis (shock). It immediately attempts to regain homeostasis (countershock). If the body is able to adjust, the response is mild and advantageous to the organism; the stage of resistance or adaptation ensues. If the stress becomes chronic or the acquired adaptation is lost, the body enters the stage of exhaustion. At this point the nonspecifically induced changes, which are apparent during the Alarm-Reaction but disappear during the Stage of Resistance, become paramount. These changes are labeled the *triad of symptoms* and include enlargement of the adrenal glands, shrinkage of thymus and lymphatic tissue, and bleeding ulcers of the digestive tract. Specifically induced changes directly related to the stressor may also occur; for example, if the stressor is cold, the body may shiver. Ultimate exhaustion is death (Selye, 1956).

Both the neural and the hormonal regulatory systems are involved in the stress response system, as shown in the schematic outline in Figure 2.14. The primarily neural component is called the *brain stem (locus ceruleus)–sympathetic nervous system* pathway, shown on the left. The primarily hormonal component is called the *hypothalamus-pituitary-adrenal axis* and is the pathway on the right.

When the individual is presented with a stressor, the hypothalamus coordinates the response. The hypothalamus is both a neural structure and an endocrine gland. Thus, it can orchestrate the body's response by stimulating both the sympathetic nervous system and the endocrine glands.

The sympathetic nerve fibers originate in the brain stem and travel throughout the body to a variety of target sites. The sympathetic nerve fibers also go to

---

Stress The state manifested by the specific syndrome that consists of all the nonspecifically induced changes within a biological system; a disruption in body homeostasis and all attempts by the body to regain homeostasis.

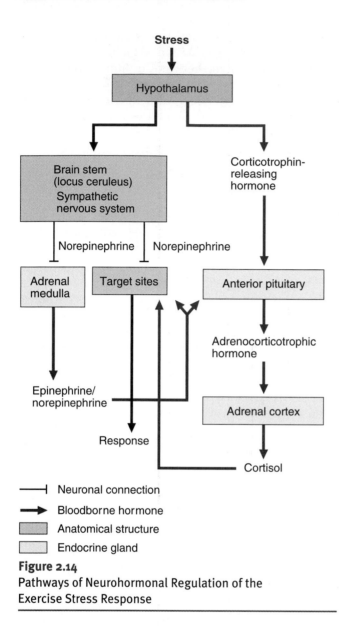

Figure 2.14
Pathways of Neurohormonal Regulation of the Exercise Stress Response

and control the adrenal medulla. Norepinephrine (NE) is released by sympathetic nerve fibers, and both norepinephrine and epinephrine (E) are secreted by the adrenal medulla. The NE released from the sympathetic nerve endings and from the adrenal medulla is the same chemical. However, when NE is released by the nerves, it is considered to be a neurotransmitter; when it is released by the adrenal medulla, it is considered to be a hormone. The NE and E secreted by the adrenal medulla circulate in the bloodstream to the target sites, where they mimic and reinforce the actions of the sympathetic nerve fibers that innervate these same target sites, for example, in elevating the heart rate. This response pattern is often referred to as *sympathoadrenal activation*. Both NE and E may also influence other endocrine glands, as indicated by

the connecting line to the anterior pituitary gland in Figure 2.14 (Chrousos and Gold, 1992).

The hypothalamus directly regulates endocrine glands both neurally and hormonally through a series of releasing factors, sometimes called *releasing hormones*. In the generic stress response, corticotrophin-releasing hormone (CRH) is released by the hypothalamus and stimulates the anterior pituitary to secrete adrenocorticotrophic hormone (ACTH). ACTH in turn stimulates the adrenal cortex to release cortisol, which acts on specific target sites.

Selye's Theory of Stress Applied to Exercise and Training

In the context of Selye's theory of stress, the pattern of responses exhibited by physiological variables during a single bout of exercise is the direct result of the disruption of homeostasis and neuroendocrine activation. As shown in Table 2.3, homeostasis is disrupted as the neuroendocrine system responds to coordinate all of the physiological processes required to sustain exercise. This is the Shock phase of the Alarm-Reaction. For many physiological processes (respiration, circulation, energy production, and so forth), the initial response is an elevation in function. The degree of elevation and constancy of this elevation depends on the intensity and duration of the exercise. The attainment of the appropriate changes in physiological function begins in the Countershock phase of the Alarm-Reaction and stabilizes in the Stage of Resistance if the same exercise intensity is maintained for at least 1–3 minutes. This is termed a physiological *steady state* or *steady rate*. The Stage of Exhaustion that results from a single bout of exercise, even incremental exercise to maximum, is typically some degree of fatigue or reduced capacity to respond to stimulation, accompanied by a feeling of tiredness. This fatigue is temporary and readily reversed with proper rest and nutrition.

Training programs are made up of a series of acute bouts of exercise organized in such a way as to provide an overload that puts the body into the Alarm-Reaction followed by recovery processes that not only restore homeostasis, but also encourage supercompensation or adaptation (Kenttä and Hassmén, 1998; Kuipers, 1998; O'Toole, 1998). This can be manifested by altered homeostatic levels at rest, dampened homeostatic disruptions to absolute submaximal exercise loads, and/or enhanced maximal performances or physiological responses. When these adaptations occur, the body has achieved a Stage of Resistance. Table 2.3 indicates which of the training principles introduced in Chapter 1 operate in the three stages of Selye's general adaptation syndrome.

Table 2.3
Selye's Theory of Stress Applied to Exercise Physiology

Stage	Exercise Response	Training Principles	Training Adaptation/ Maladaptation

I. Alarm-Reaction
  a. Shock
  b. Countershock
	Neuroendocrine system stimulated
	  a. Homeostasis disrupted
	  b. Begin to attain elevated steady state
		Warm-up/cool-down
		Overload
		
		Reversibility
		Progression[1]
			Dampened response to equal acute exercise stimulus
			Reversible with detraining

II. Stage of Resistance	Elevated homeostatic steady state maintained if exercise intensity is unchanged	Adaptation Maintenance Specificity (SAID) Individualization	Enhanced function Increased maximal exercise capacity depending on individual neuroendocrine physiology and imposed demand Overreaching[2]
III. Stage of Exhaustion	Fatigue, a temporary state, reversed by proper rest and nutrition	Retrogression/plateau/ reversibility	Overreaching Overtraining Maladaptive changes in neuroendocrine systems

1. The cycle of adaptation and progression occurs repeatedly during a training program.

2. If overreaching is planned and recovery is sufficient, positive adaptation results; if overreaching is accompanied by insufficient recovery and additional overload, overtraining will result.

The goal of a training program is to alternate the exerciser between Stages I and II and to avoid Stage III. The primary way in which this proceeds is by the cyclical interaction (shown by the arrows in Table 2.3) between adaptation (changes that occur in response to an overload) and progression (change in overload in response to adaptation). Each progression of the overload should allow for adaptation. However, this is not always accomplished.

Training Adaptation and Maladaptation

Training and its relationship to fitness goals and athletic performance exist on a continuum that is best described as an inverted U (Figure 2.15) (Fry, et al., 1991; Kuipers, 1998; Rowbottom, et al., 1998). At one end of the continuum are individuals who are undertrained and whose fitness level and performance abilities are dictated by genetics, diseases, and nonexercise lifestyle choices. Individuals whose training programs lack sufficient volume, intensity, or progression for either improvement or maintenance of fitness or performance are undertrained. The goal of optimal training is the attainment of peak fitness and/or performance. However, if the training overload is too much or improperly applied, then maladaptation is possible. The first step toward maladaptation is *overreaching,* a short-term decrement in performance capacity that is easily recovered from and generally lasts only a few days to 2 weeks. Overreaching can either result from planned shock microcycles, as described in the periodization section in Chapter 1, or result inadvertently from too much stress and too little planned recovery (especially insufficient metabolic recovery) (Fry, et al., 1991; Fry and Kraemer, 1997; Kuipers, 1998). If overreaching is planned and recovery is sufficient, positive adaptation and improved

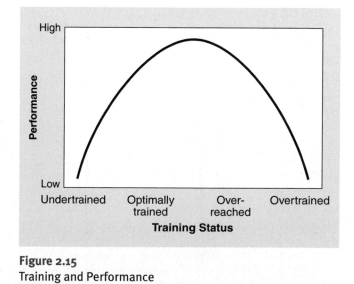

Figure 2.15
Training and Performance

Focus on Application

✳ Ratings of Perceived Exertion and Recovery

Researchers have begun to suggest that the adequacy of recovery from training be monitored through the use of rating scales. One system (Kenttä and Hassmén, 1998) proposes that recovery from training be assessed using two total quality recovery (TQR) scales. The TQR perceived (TQRper) scale is a subjective rating by the individual to the query "How do you rate your overall recovery for the previous 24 hours?" The TQR action scale (TQRact) allows the athlete to accumulate "recovery points" based on his or her activities in the previous 24 hours. Up to 10 points can be awarded for nutrition and hydration; up to 4 points for sleep and rest; up to 3 points for relaxation and emotional support; and up to 3 points for stretching and active rest. Because the point values for the action items are not set in stone, but rather are determined by the athlete and his or her coach/trainer, they should be established before implementing this scale. Based on this system, recovery is adequate if both the TQRper and TQRact are at or above the training stress as measured by the Borg Rating of Perceived Exertion Scale for the workout preceding the recovery.

Foster (1998) bases his technique on Borg's category ratio scale (CR-10) and the duration of each day's workout (multiplying the two together) to obtain a training session load. Each week the mean and standard deviation of the training load is computed as an index of training variability. The monotony of the weekly training load is described by dividing the daily mean load by the standard deviation (SD). A small SD and a high quotient indicate little day-to-day variation, that is, high monotony. The strain of the weekly load is determined by multiplying the daily load by 7 days per week and the monotony factor. Both consistent high training monotony and high training strain appear to be related to training maladaptation. Such analyses may lead to early recognition of inappropriate loading and thus allow the coach to modify training before the athlete shows overreaching or overtraining decrements in performance.

The example on the facing page shows how simply substituting one rest day for a long cycling ride reduces the training monotony and strain. Many elite athletes work at a training load of 4000 units per week; thus, even for an elite athlete, the 7-day-a-week program would be considered excessive. This biathlete could substitute the long bike ride for the long run on alternate weeks.

Borg's CR-10 scale	Borg's RPE scale	TQR per scale		Borg's CR-10 scale	Borg's RPE scale	TQR per scale
0.0	6	6		4.5	14	14
0.0 nothing	7 very, very light	7 very, very poor		5.0 heavy/strong		
				5.5	15 hard	15 good
0.5 just noticeable	8	8		6.5	16	16
1.0 very weak	9 very light	9 very poor		7.0 very strong		
1.5	10	10		7.5	17 very hard	17 very good
2.0 light/weak	11 fairly light	11 poor		9.0	18	18
3.0 moderate	12	12		10.0 extremely strong	19 very, very hard	19 very, very good
3.5	13 somewhat hard	13 reasonable		10.0+ (~12) highest possible	20	20
4.0 somewhat strong						

performance, not maladaptation, result. If, however, overreaching is left unchecked or the individual or coach interprets the decrement in performance as an indication that more work must be done, overreaching develops into overtraining. Overtraining, more properly called the **overtraining syndrome (OTS)** (or *staleness*) is a state of chronic decrement in performance and ability to train, in which restoration may take several weeks, months, or even years (Fry, et al., 1991; Fry and Kraemer, 1997; USOC/ACSM, 1999).

Overtraining Syndrome (OTS) A state of chronic decrement in performance and ability to train, in which restoration may take several weeks, months, or even years.

Current Training Program

Day	Training Session	Duration (min)	Perceived Exertion CR-10	Load (units)
Monday	Weight lifting	90	4	360
Tuesday	Running (8 km)	45	3	135
Wednesday	Cycling (48 km)	120	4	480
Thursday	Weight lifting	90	4	360
Friday	Cycling (80 km)	200	6	1200
Saturday	Track intervals	75	7	525
Sunday	Long run (29 km)	180	6	1080

Daily mean load	591
Standard deviation (SD) of daily load	396
Monotony (daily load ÷ SD)	1.49
Weekly load (daily load × 7)	4137
Strain (weekly load × monotony)	6164

Proposed Modifications to Reduce Training Stress

Day	Training Session	Duration (min)	Perceived Exertion CR-10	Load (units)
Monday	Weight lifting	90	4	360
Tuesday	Running (8 km)	45	3	135
Wednesday	Cycling (48 km)	120	4	480
Thursday	Rest day	0	0	0
Friday	Weight lifting	90	4	360
Saturday	Track intervals	75	7	525
Sunday	Long run (29 km)	180	6	1080

Daily mean load	420
Standard deviation (SD) of daily load	345
Monotony (daily load ÷ SD)	1.21
Weekly load (daily load × 7)	2940
Strain (weekly load × monotony)	3557

Sources:
Foster (1998); Kenttä & Hassmén (1998)

Signs and Symptoms of Overreaching and the Overtraining Syndrome

Note that the primary characteristic of both overreaching and the OTS is a drop in performance that is unexpected and unexplainable by injury, illness, or other factors. This drop in performance may be preceded by a period in which performance is maintained but at greater physiological effort. Familiarity with additional signs and symptoms that may be exhibited can help the trainer recognize overreaching or OTS in the athlete.

Overtraining can range from mild to severe. It is most likely to occur in individuals who are highly motivated, in instances where large increases in training occur abruptly, and in situations where the periodization training program includes insufficient rest and recovery. The sooner overtraining is recognized and dealt with, the faster recovery can be expected. The recognition of overtraining necessitates a familiarity with its signs and symptoms. A list of such signs and symptoms is given in Table 2.4. These are outward manifestations of neuroendocrine imbalances, immune system suppression, or a reversal of normal physiological training adaptations (Fry, et al., 1991; Kuipers, 1998; Morris, 1984). This list is by no means all-inclusive, and no single indicator other than a decrement in performance is likely to be common to all individuals who are overtrained. Only those signs and symptoms that require minimal testing or that can be detected by astute observation have been included. Above all, this list should point to the importance of monitoring and interacting with those entrusted to your guidance.

Behavioral and Physiological Causes of OTS

Simply stated, the overtraining syndrome results when the total stress internalized by an individual exceeds his or her capacity to cope, primarily because of insufficient rest or recovery. It is most likely to occur in individuals who are highly motivated and in instances where large increases in training occur abruptly and/or are sustained in heavy training known as *monotonous training*. Because stress is additive, other stressors may compound the stress of training, including frequent competition, preexisting medical conditions, poor nutrition (especially an inadequate intake of carbohydrates and fluid), environmental conditions, and psychosocial factors.

The inability to cope with the total amount of stress imposed on the individual is mediated through the hypothalamus and hence the neural and hormonal systems (Keiser, 1998; Kuipers, 1998; Urhausen and Kindermann, 2000). Two forms of the OTS probably exist: a sympathetic form and a parasympathetic form (Flynn, 1998; Fry and Kraemer, 1997; Kenttä and Hassmén, 1998; Lehmann, Foster, et al., 1998; Lehmann, Netzer, et al., 1998; Urhausen and Kindermann, 2000; Witlert, 2000). The *sympathetic form* is characterized by an increased sympathetic neural tone at rest and during exercise and down regulation of β receptors. Restlessness and hyperexcitability dominate. For example, an elevated resting heart rate, slower heart rate recovery postexercise, decreased appetite and unintentional loss of body mass, excessive sweating, and disturbed sleep patterns are symptomatic of sympathetic overtraining (Fry, et al., 1991). This form is generally considered to be an early indication of overtraining. It appears to be most closely related to high-intensity anaerobic activities (Fry and Kraemer, 1997). The *parasympathetic*

Table 2.4
Signs and Symptoms of Overtraining

Performance-Related

Consistent decrement in performance

Persistent fatigue and sluggishness that leads to several days of poor training

Prolonged recovery from training sessions or competitive events

Reappearance of already corrected errors

Physiological

Decreased maximal work capacities and markers

Increased disruption of homeostasis at submaximal workloads

Headaches or stomachaches out of proportion to life events

Insomnia

Persistent low-grade stiffness and soreness of the muscles and joints

Frequent sore throats, colds, and/or cold sores

Constipation or diarrhea

Loss of appetite; loss of body weight and/or muscle mass when no conscious attempt is being made to diet or when weight loss is undesirable

An elevation of approximately 10% in the morning heart rate taken immediately upon awakening

Amenorrhea

Psychological/Behavioral

Feelings of depression

General apathy, especially toward previously enjoyed activities

Decreased self-esteem

Emotional instability or mood changes

Difficulty concentrating

Loss of competitive drive or desire

Perceived insufficient recovery

form is characterized by sympathetic neural insufficiency, a decreased sensitivity to the pituitary and adrenal hormones, and an increased parasympathetic tone at rest and during exercise. The symptoms of parasympathetic overtraining are less obvious and in isolation may be difficult to distinguish from positive training adaptations (Fry, et al., 1991). For example, resting pulse rates may be low and heart rate recovery from exercise rapid; however, this is typically associated with early fatigue and impaired maximal work capacity markers, such as heart rate and lactate. Apathy, digestive disturbances, and altered immune and reproductive function are common. Parasympathetic overtraining syndrome is the more advanced form. It appears to be most frequently associated with excessive volume training in both aerobic endurance activity and dynamic resistance exercise (Fry and Kraemer, 1997). Individual differences in the nervous system may predispose any given individual to either up regulation (sympathetic) or down regulation (parasympathetic) of the neuroendocrine homeostasis, but either way the overtraining syndrome clearly represents neuroendocrine dysfunction or imbalance. Additionally, some researchers propose that chemicals released from immune cells interact with the sympathetic nervous system and the endocrine system to mediate the body's response in the OTS (Smith, 2000). This theory is discussed in greater detail in Chapter 17. Unfortunately, at this point in time, there is no single or simple hormonal (or immunological) change that can be monitored as an early warning for the OTS, despite the fact that neuroendocrine disorders probably precede the symptoms of the OTS (Urhausen and Kindermann, 2000).

Prevention and Treatment of OTS

The key to preventing the overtraining syndrome is careful periodization of training. The delicate balance between overload/progression and rest/recovery must be attained for each individual. The main protection against OTS is the inclusion of sufficient recovery after heavy physical training. Sufficient recovery may be accomplished by the inclusion of easy days, days of active cross-training, rest days emphasizing stretching and relaxation techniques, or days of complete rest. Adequate sleep, caloric intake (emphasizing carbohydrates for glycogen replenishment), and fluid intake are also necessary to optimize training and avoid OTS (Kenttä and Hassmén, 1998).

Monitoring training is another important factor in preventing OTS. One of the most helpful things that the exerciser can do is to keep a training log, including heart rates, body weight, other physical or mental feelings, and planned versus achieved workouts. With this information and periodic testing in all cycles of the training program, the coach can make adjustments to reverse or, even better, prevent overtraining. Unfortunately, as stated previously, there is no single specific marker that can be used as an index of overtraining (Flynn, 1998; Urhausen, et al., 1995). Instead, the coach should conduct periodic physiological and performance testing during the annual training cycle. These tests must be conducted after a recovery or regeneration cycle when adaptation can accurately be evaluated (Rowbottom, et al., 1998). The Focus on Application box (on pages 46 and 47) presents two techniques, based in part on perceived exertion, that have been shown to be useful in addi-

tion to periodic testing (Foster, 1998; Kenttä and Hassmén, 1998). Perceived exertion scales are described and discussed more completely in Chapter 14. With proper monitoring, adjustments can be made to the periodization plan to lessen the likelihood of progression to OTS.

If training adjustments are insufficient and OTS develops, treatment is required. Treatment requires a medical examination to rule out possible illnesses or injuries as the underlying cause of the decrement in performance. Once illness or injury has been ruled out, the individual must be guided through a recovery program. This must be done carefully, because active—and especially competitive—individuals often resist recommendations to cut down or cease training. As with recovery, rest need not mean total inactivity. Resumption of training must be gradual (USOC/ACSM, 1999). From the standpoint of stress theory, physical fitness may be defined as achieved adaptation to the stress imposed by muscular exercise. Physical fitness resulting from a properly applied training program is usually exhibited in response to an acute exercise task and implies avoidance of overtraining.

Summary

1. The nervous system and the endocrine system both function to help maintain homeostasis and to respond to the stress of exercise. Furthermore, the two systems interact and overlap in multiple ways. Both systems communicate with target cells by chemical messengers.

2. A target cell is activated when the chemical message from the nervous system (neurotransmitter) or endocrine system (hormone) binds to receptors on or in the target cell. Receptor activation can cause one or more of the following: change in the electrical state of the cell, change in enzyme activity, change in secretory activity of the cell, muscle contraction, or protein synthesis.

3. The nervous system can be divided into the central nervous system (CNS), consisting of the brain and spinal cord, and the peripheral nervous system (PNS), consisting of everything outside the CNS. The PNS is divided into afferent and efferent divisions. The afferent division carries information from the periphery to the CNS. The efferent division carries signals from the CNS to effector organs in the periphery. The efferent division is further subdivided into the somatic and autonomic nervous systems. The somatic system sends signals from the CNS to skeletal muscle to initiate muscle contraction.

4. The autonomic nervous system (ANS) carries information from the CNS to cardiac muscle, smooth muscle, and endocrine glands. The ANS has two branches, the sympathetic and parasympathetic nervous system, which work in opposition to each other.

5. The neuron, or nerve cell, is the functional unit of the nervous system. A typical neuron contains dendrites (highly branched extensions of the neuron); a cell body, which acts as the control center of the cell; and an axon, which conducts the action potentials and secretes neurotransmitters.

IP *Nervous I–Anatomy Review* (pages 1–9); *Nervous I–The Membrane Potential* (pages 1–16); *Nervous I–The Action Potential* (pages 1–13)*

6. The somatic nervous system is responsible for initiating muscle contraction. An efferent neuron (called an α motor neuron) releases a neurotransmitter at the site of the junction between the neuron and the muscle. The neurotransmitter causes the cell membrane of the muscle cell to become excited. The excitation of the muscle cell membrane ultimately leads to contraction of the muscle cell.

IP *Muscular–The Neuromuscular Junction* (pages 1–11) (end of last paragraph): *Nervous II–Anatomy Review* (pages 1–9); *Nervous II–Synaptic Transmission* (pages 1–16)

7. The exercise response is mediated primarily through the sympathetic branch of the autonomic nervous system. The primary functions of the sympathetic branch of the ANS during exercise are to enhance cardiorespiratory function, regulate blood flow and maintain blood pressure, maintain thermal balance, and increase fuel mobilization for the production of energy.

8. During exercise, several metabolic hormones (glucagon, insulin, growth hormone, epinephrine [E], norepinephrine [NE]) function together to mobilize fuel for the production of adenosine triphosphate (ATP) and to maintain blood glucose levels.

9. During exercise, several hormones help to enhance cardiac function (E, NE), distribute blood to active tissue (E, NE), and maintain fluid and electrolyte balance (antidiuretic hormone [ADH], renin, aldosterone).

IP *Cardiovascular–Blood Pressure Regulation* (pages 15–29)*

10. Applying Selye's theory of stress to exercise, exercise is a stressor that causes a disruption of the body's homeostasis. During an acute bout of exercise the body may progress from the Alarm-Reaction Stage to the Stages of Resistance and (occa-sionally) Exhaustion. Training programs should be designed to provide an overload that allows adaptation and gradual progression, but avoids the Stage of Exhaustion.

11. The physiological responses to stress are mediated through the hypothalamus by way of the hypothalamic-pituitary-adrenal axis and the brain stem (locus ceruleus)–sympathetic nervous system pathway.

12. Overreaching may be defined as a short-term decrement in performance capacity that is easily recovered from and generally lasts only a few days to 2 weeks. Overtraining (or overtraining syndrome [OTS]) is a state of chronic decrement in performance and in ability to train in which restoration may take several weeks to years.

This topic is available on the InterActive Physiology® Sampler CD that comes with the purchase of a new copy of this book.

Review Questions

1. Define homeostasis, and identify the role of the two systems involved in maintaining homeostasis.

2. Describe receptor activation, and list five changes that may occur in a target cell as a result of receptor activation.

3. Provide a schematic of the structure of the nervous system.

4. Identify three regions of a neuron, and indicate the primary role of each region.

5. What is the role of the somatic nervous system in initiating movement?

6. What is the role of the autonomic nervous system in regulating the exercise response?

7. Create a table that indicates the hormones involved in regulating metabolism and fluid balance and how they respond to exercise.

8. How does the hormonal system adapt as a result of exercise training?

9. What relationship does Selye's theory of stress have with exercise and training?

10. What's the difference between overreaching and overtraining?

11. Identify the behavioral and physiological causes of OTS. What can be done to prevent OTS? What is the most effective way to treat OTS?

12. Prepare a line chart of the neurohormonal physiological basis of the exercise and exercise training stress response.

13. Identify the performance-related, physiological, and behavioral signs and symptoms of overtraining that can be evaluated with little if any laboratory testing.

For further review and additional study tools, go to The Physiology Place (www.physiologyplace.com) and the Student Study Guide for Exercise Phyiology for Health, Fitness, and Performance *by Sharon A. Plowman and Denise L. Smith.*

Passport to the Internet

Visit the following Internet sites to explore further topics and issues related to neurohormonal regulation. To visit an organization's web site, go to www.physiologyplace.com and click on "Passport to the Internet."

The Endocrine Society Home page for the professional endocrinology organization. Visit the "News & Facts" area to read of the latest studies in the field.

Frontiers in Neuroendocrinology Opens to the official journal of the International Society for Neuroendocrinology.

Society for Endocrinology: Online Endocrinology Journals Access a number of the leading journals in the field of endocrinology.

SportsMed Web: The Overtraining Syndrome Affiliated with Rice University, this site provides information that appeals to athletes of all levels. Search through the site and read more about overtraining syndrome.

References

Berent, V. J., & L. Wartofsky: Thyroid function and exercise. In M. P. Warren & N. W. Constantini (eds.), *Sports Endocrinology.* Totawa, NJ: Humana Press, 97–118 (2000).

Borg, G.: *Borg's Perceived Exertion and Pain Scales.* Champaign, IL: Human Kinetics (1998).

Bunt, J. C.: Hormonal alterations due to exercise. *Sports Medicine.* 3:331–345 (1986).

Chilibeck, P. D.: Hormonal regulations of the effects of exercise on bone: Positive and negative effects. In M. P. Warren & N. W. Constantini (eds.), *Sports Endocrinology.* Totawa, NJ: Humana Press, 239–252 (2000).

Chrousos, G. P., & P. W. Gold: The concepts of stress and stress system disorders. *Journal of the American Medical Association.* 267(4):1244–1252 (1992).

Coggan, A. R., & B. D. Williams: Metabolic adaptations to endurance training: Substrate metabolism during exercise. In M. Hargraves (ed.), *Exercise Metabolism.* Champaign, IL: Human Kinetics, 177–210 (1995).

Cumming, D. C.: The male reproductive system, exercise, and training. In M. P. Warren & N. W. Constantini (eds.), *Sports Endocrinology.* Totawa, NJ: Humana Press, 119–132 (2000).

Deschenes, M. R., J. Cocault, W. J. Kraemer, & C. M. Maresh: The neuromuscular junction: Muscle fiber type differences, plasticity and adaptability to increased and decreased activity. *Sports Medicine.* 17(6):358–372 (1994).

Eliakim, A., J. A. Brasel, & D. M. Cooper: Exercise and the growth hormone–insulin-like growth factor-I axis. In M. P. Warren & N. W. Constantini (eds.), *Sports Endocrinology.* Totawa, NJ: Humana Press, 77–96 (2000).

Flynn, M. G.: Future research needs and directions. In R. B. Kreider, A. C. Fry, & M. L. O'Toole (eds.), *Overtraining in Sport.* Champaign, IL: Human Kinetics, 373–383 (1998).

Foster, C.: Monitoring training in athletes with reference to overtraining syndrome. *Medicine and Science in Sports and Exercise.* 30(7):1164–1168 (1998).

Fry, R. W., A. R. Morton, & D. Keast: Overtraining in athletes: An update. *Sports Medicine.* 12(1):32–65 (1991).

Fry, A. C., & W. J. Kraemer: Resistance exercise overtraining and overreaching: Neuroendocrine responses. *Sports Medicine.* 23:106–129 (1997).

Galbo, H.: *Hormonal and Metabolic Adaptation to Exercise.* New York: Thieme-Stratton (1983).

Gleim, G. W., & B. W. Glace: Energy balance and weight control: Endocrine considerations. In M. P. Warren & N. W. Constantini (eds.), *Sports Endocrinology.* Totawa, NJ: Humana Press, 189–206 (2000).

Guyton, A. C.: *Textbook of Medical Physiology* (9th ed.). Philadelphia: W. B. Saunders (1996).

Kapit, W., R. I. Macey, & E. Meisami: *The Physiology Coloring Book* (2nd ed.). San Francisco, CA: Addison Wesley Longman, (2000).

Keiser, H. A.: Neuroendocrine aspects of overtraining. In R. B. Kreider, A. C. Fry, & M. L. O'Toole (eds.), *Overtraining in Sport.* Champaign, IL: Human Kinetics, 145–167 (1998).

Kenttä, G., & P. Hassmén: Overtraining and recovery: A conceptual model. *Sports Medicine.* 26:1–16 (1998).

Kjaer, M., & K. Lange: Adrenergic regulation of energy metabolism. In M. P. Warren & N. W. Constantini (eds.), *Sports Endocrinology.* Totawa, NJ: Humana Press, 181–188 (2000).

Kraemer, W. J.: Endocrine responses and adaptations to strength training. In P. V. Komi (ed.), *Strength and Power in Sport.* London: Blackwell Scientific Publications, 291–304 (1992a).

Kraemer, W. J.: Endocrine responses to resistance exercise. *Medicine and Science in Sports and Exercise.* 20(5) Supplement: S152–S157 (1988).

Kraemer, W. J.: Hormonal mechanisms related to the expression of muscular strength and power. In P. V. Komi (ed.), *Strength and Power in Sport.* London: Blackwell Scientific Publications, 64–76 (1992b).

Kuipers, H.: Training and overtraining: An introduction. *Medicine and Science in Sports and Exercise.* 30(7): 1137–1139 (1998).

Lehmann, M., C. Foster, H.-H. Dickhuth, & U. Gastmann: Autonomic imbalance hypothesis and overtraining syndrome. *Medicine and Science in Sports and Exercise.* 30(7): 1140–1145 (1998).

Lehmann, M., N. Netzer, J. M. Steinacker, A. Opitz-Gress, & U. Gastmann: Physiological responses to short- and long-term overtraining in endurance athletes. In R. B. Kreider, A. C. Fry, & M. L. O'Toole (eds.), *Overtraining in Sport.* Champaign, IL: Human Kinetics, 19–46 (1998).

Marieb, E. N.: *Human Anatomy and Physiology* (5th edition). San Francisco, CA: Benjamin/Cummings (2001).

McComas, A. J.: *Skeletal Muscle: Form and Function.* Champaign, IL: Human Kinetics (1996).

Morris, A. F.: *Sports Medicine: Prevention of Athletic Injuries.* Dubuque, IA: Wm. C. Brown (1984).

O'Toole, M. L.: Overreaching and overtraining in endurance athletes. In R. B. Kreider, A. C. Fry, & M. L. O'Toole (eds.), *Overtraining in Sport.* Champaign, IL: Human Kinetics, 3–17 (1998).

Robergs, R. A., & S. O. Roberts: *Exercise Physiology: Exercise, Performance and Clinical Applications.* St. Louis, MO: Mosby-Year Book (1997).

Rowbottom, D. G., D. Keast, & A. R. Morton: Monitoring and preventing of overreaching and overtraining in endurance athletes. In R. B. Kreider, A. C. Fry, & M. L. O'Toole (eds.), *Overtraining in Sport.* Champaign, IL: Human Kinetics, 47–66 (1998).

Sale, D. G.: Neural adaptations to strength training. In P. V. Komi, (ed.), *Strength and Power in Sport.* London: Blackwell Scientific Publications, 249–265 (1992).

Selye, H.: *The Stress of Life.* New York: McGraw-Hill (1956).

Smith, L. L.: Cytokine hypothesis of overtraining: A physiological adaptation to excessive stress? *Medicine and Science in Sports and Exercise.* 32(2):317–331 (2000).

Sutton, J. R., P. A. Farrell, & V. J. Harber: Hormonal adaptations to physical activity. In C. Bouchard, R. J. Shephard, T. Stephens, J. R. Sutton, & B. D. McPherson (eds.), *Exercise, Fitness, and Health.* Champaign, IL: Human Kinetics, 217–257 (1990).

Urhausen, A., H. Gabriel, & W. Kindermann: Blood hormones as markers of training stress and overtraining. *Sports Medicine.* 20(4):251–276 (1995).

Urhausen, A., & W. Kindermann: The endocrine system in overtraining. In M. P. Warren & N. W. Constantini (eds.), *Sports Endocrinology.* Totowa, NJ: Humana Press, 347–370 (2000).

USOC/ACSM: The Overtraining syndrome in athletes: Identification, prevention and treatment [on-line]. Available *http://www.acsm.org* (1999).

Vallbo, A. B., T. E. Hagbarth, H. E. Torebjork, & B. G. Wallin: Somatosensory, proprioceptive, and sympathetic activity in human peripheral nerves. *Physiological Reviews.* 59:919–957 (1997).

Van de Graaff, K. M., & S. I. Fox: *Concepts of Human Anatomy and Physiology* (2nd edition). Dubuque, IA: Wm. C. Brown (1989).

Vander, A. J., J. Sherman, & D. Luciano: *Human Physiology: The Mechanisms of Body Function.* Boston: McGraw Hill (2001).

Wade, C. E.: Hormonal regulation of fluid homeostasis during and following exercise. In M. P. Warren & N. W. Constantini (eds.), *Sports Endocrinology.* Totowa, NJ: Humana Press, 207–226 (2000).

Witlert, G.: The effects of exercise on the hypothalamo-pituitary-adrenal axis. In M. P. Warren & N. W. Constantini (eds.), *Sports Endocrinology.* Totowa, NJ: Humana Press, 43–56 (2000).

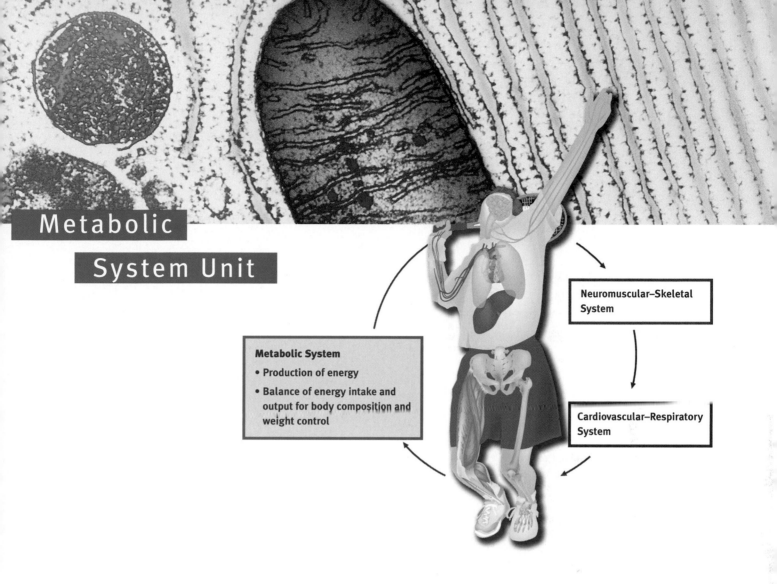

Metabolic System Unit

Metabolic System
- Production of energy
- Balance of energy intake and output for body composition and weight control

Neuromuscular–Skeletal System

Cardiovascular–Respiratory System

Metabolism refers to the sum of all chemical processes within the body. From the exercise physiology standpoint, the most important metabolic process is how muscle cells convert foodstuffs and oxygen to chemical energy (in the form of adenosine triphosphate) to support physical activity. Without the production of adenosine triphosphate through metabolic processes, there could be no movement by the neuromuscular system; indeed, there could be no life. Because most energy production requires the presence of oxygen, metabolism largely depends on the functioning of the cardiorespiratory system.

Chapter 3

Energy

Production

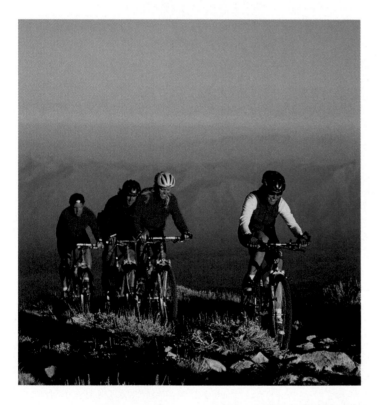

After studying the chapter, you should be able to

- Describe the role of ATP.

- Summarize the processes of cellular respiration for the production of ATP from carbohydrate, fat, and protein fuel substrates.

- Calculate the production of ATP from glucose or glycogen, fatty acid, and amino acid precursors.

- Describe the goals of metabolic regulation during exercise.

- Explain how the production of energy is regulated by intracellular and extracellular factors.

- Compare the relative use of carbohydrate, fat, and protein fuel substrates on the basis of intensity and duration of exercise.

Introduction

Most individuals eat at least three meals a day. Aside from the wide variation in content of those meals and the societal or psychological attributes that might be attached to them, eating is physiologically necessary to provide the energy that is essential for all cellular—and hence bodily—activity. To provide this energy, food must be transformed into chemical energy.

The total of all energy transformations that occur in the body is called **metabolism.** If the energy is *used* to build tissues—as when amino acids are combined to form proteins that make up muscle—the process is called *anabolism.* If the energy is *produced* from the breakdown of foodstuffs and stored so that it is available to do work, the process is called *catabolism.*

It is catabolism that is of primary importance in exercise metabolism. Here the interest is in providing energy to support muscle activity, whether a little or a lot of muscle mass is involved or the exercise is light or heavy, submaximal or maximal. In providing this needed energy, the human body follows the *first law of thermodynamics,* which states that energy is neither created nor destroyed, but only changed in form. Figure 3.1 is a schematic representation of this law and the changes in form representing catabolism. Potential chemical energy—or fuel—is ingested as food. Carbohydrates, fats, and protein can all be used as fuels, although they are not used equally by the body in that capacity. The chemical energy produced from the food fuel is stored as **adenosine triphosphate (ATP).** The ATP then transfers its energy to energy-requiring physiological functions, such as muscle contraction during exercise, where part appears as work done and part as heat. Thus, ATP is stored chemical energy that links the energy-yielding and the energy-requiring functions within all cells. The aim of this chapter is to fully explain ATP and how it is produced from carbohydrate, fat, and protein food sources.

Structurally, ATP is composed of a carbon-nitrogen base called adenine, a 5-carbon sugar called ribose, and three phosphates, symbolized by P_i (inorganic phosphate). Each phosphate group is linked by a chemical bond. When one phosphate is removed, the remaining compound is *adenosine diphosphate* (ADP). When two phosphates are removed, the remaining compound is *adenosine monophosphate* (AMP).

The ATP energy reaction is reversible. When ATP is synthesized from ADP by adding P_i, energy is required. The addition of P_i is known as **phosphorylation.**

$$ADP + P_i + energy \rightarrow ATP$$

When ATP is broken down, energy is released. **Hydrolysis** is a chemical process in which a substance

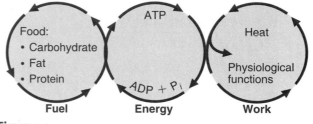

Figure 3.1

Generalized Scheme of Catabolic Energy Transformation in the Human Body

Energy is the capacity to do work. Energy exists in six forms: chemical, mechanical, heat, light, electrical, and nuclear. Movement of the human body (work) represents mechanical energy that is supported by the chemical energy derived from food fuels.

is split into simpler compounds by the addition of water. ATP is split by hydrolysis.

$$ATP \rightarrow ADP + P_i + energy\ for\ work + heat$$

The energy-requiring and energy-releasing reactions involving ATP are **coupled reactions.** Coupled reactions are linked chemical processes in which a change in one substance is accompanied by a change in another; that is, one of these reactions does not occur without the other. As the chemical agent that links the energy-yielding and energy-requiring functions in the cell, ATP is also a universal agent, being the immediate source of energy for virtually all reactions requiring energy in all cells.

ATP is often referred to as cellular energy. Actually, ATP is a high-energy molecule. The term *high energy* means that the probability is high that when a phosphate is removed, energy will be transferred (Brooks, et al., 1999). To better understand how the breakdown of ATP releases energy, consider an analogy. Think

---

Metabolism The total of all energy transformations that occur in the body.

Adenosine Triphosphate (ATP) Stored chemical energy that links the energy-yielding and energy-requiring functions within all cells.

Phosphorylation The addition of a phosphate (P_i).

Hydrolysis A chemical process in which a substance is split into simpler compounds by the addition of water.

Coupled Reactions Linked chemical processes in which a change in one substance is accompanied by a change in another.

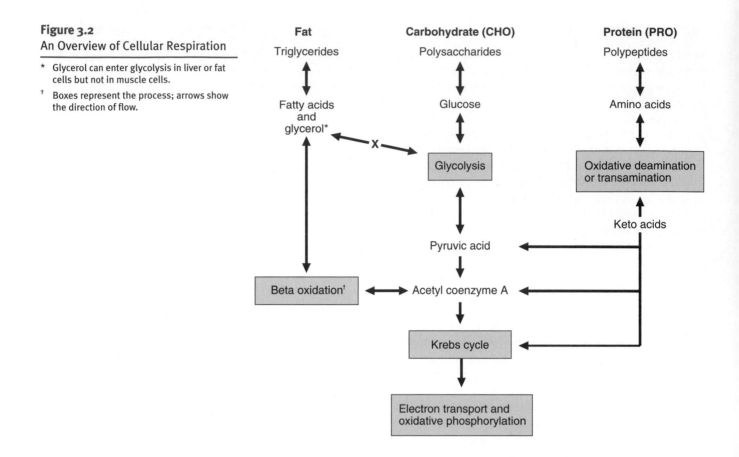

Figure 3.2

An Overview of Cellular Respiration

* Glycerol can enter glycolysis in liver or fat cells but not in muscle cells.

† Boxes represent the process; arrows show the direction of flow.

for a moment about a spring-loaded dart gun. The dart can be considered analogous to P_i. It takes a small amount of energy to "spring-load" the dart; this energy corresponds to the energy involved in the energy-requiring reaction:

$$ADP + P_i + energy \rightarrow ATP$$

Once the dart is loaded, the spring houses potential energy, which is released when the gun is fired. Firing corresponds to the energy-releasing reaction:

$$ATP \rightarrow ADP + P_i + energy$$

The energy available to do work in the intact cell is 12 kcal·mol^{-1} of ATP, although this energy may vary in different cells and under different conditions (Lehninger, 1971).

ATP can be regenerated from ADP in three ways:

1. By interaction of ADP with CP (*creatine phosphate,* which is sometimes designated as PC, or *phosphocreatine*).

2. By anaerobic respiration in the cell cytoplasm.

3. By aerobic respiration in the cell mitochondria.

Phosphocreatine is another high-energy compound stored in muscles. It transfers its phosphate—

and, hence, its potential energy—to ADP to form ATP, leaving creatine:

$$ADP + PC \rightarrow C + ATP$$

PC stores are sacrificed to regenerate ATP and in a working muscle will be depleted in less than 15 sec. The rest of this chapter will concentrate on the more substantial production of ATP by the second and third techniques listed, namely, anaerobic and aerobic cellular respiration.

Cellular Respiration

The process by which cells transfer energy from food to ATP in a stepwise series of reactions is called **cellular respiration.** It is called cellular respiration because the cells rely heavily upon the oxygen that the respiratory system provides for them in order to produce energy. In addition, the by-product of energy production, carbon dioxide, is exhaled through the

Cellular Respiration The process by which cells transfer energy from food to ATP in a stepwise series of reactions; relies heavily on the use of oxygen.

respiratory system. Cellular respiration can be either **anaerobic,** meaning it occurs in the absence of, does not require, nor use oxygen, or **aerobic,** meaning it occurs in the presence of, requires, or uses oxygen. Brain cells cannot produce energy anaerobically, and cardiac muscle cells have only a minimal capacity for anaerobic energy production. Skeletal muscle cells, however, are able to produce energy aerobically and/ or anaerobically as the situation demands it.

Figure 3.2 presents a basic outline of the products and processes of cellular respiration. A detailed discussion of these processes will follow. At this time, however, you need only note the following points.

1. All three major food nutrients, fats (FAT), carbohydrates (CHO), and proteins (PRO), can serve as fuel or **substrates**—the substances acted upon by enzymes—for the production of ATP.

2. The most important immediate forms of the substrates utilized are glucose (GLU), free fatty acids (FFA), and amino acids (AA). Both FFA and glycerol are derived from the breakdown of triglycerides. Some cells can use glycerol directly in glycolysis, but muscle cells cannot.

3. *Acetyl coenzyme A* (acetyl CoA) is the central converting substance (usually called the universal or common intermediate) in the metabolism of FAT, CHO, and PRO. Although the process of glycolysis will provide a small amount of ATP as well as acetyl CoA, both beta oxidation and oxidative deamination or transamination are simply preparatory steps by which FFA and AA are converted to acetyl CoA. That is, beta oxidation and oxidative deamination or transamination are simply processes for converting FFA and AA, respectively, to a common substrate that allows the metabolic pathway to continue. The end result is that the primary metabolic pathways of the Krebs cycle, electron transport system (ETS), and oxidative phosphorylation (OP) are the same no matter what the food precursor. This is certainly more efficient than having totally separate pathways for each food nutrient.

4. Each of the energy-producing processes (glycolysis, Krebs cycle, ETS/OP) consists of a series of steps. This is both good news and bad news for you as a student. It is good news because it allows energy to be released gradually. If all of the energy contained in the food nutrients were released at one time, it would be predominantly released as heat and would destroy tissue. It is bad news because it is easy to be intimidated by or uninterested in so many steps, each with its own chemical structure, enzyme, and long, strange name. There is a logic to these steps, however, and it is on the logic and understanding (rather than the chemical structures) that this discussion will concentrate.

Carbohydrate Metabolism

The discussion of ATP production will begin with carbohydrate metabolism for several reasons. First, many of the energy requirements of the human body are met by carbohydrate metabolism. Second, carbohydrate is the only food nutrient that can be used to create energy anaerobically. Energy for both rest and exercise is provided primarily by aerobic metabolism. However, exercise can often require anaerobic energy production. In that situation carbohydrate is essential. Third, carbohydrate is the preferred fuel of the body because carbohydrate requires less oxygen in order to be metabolized than fat does. And finally, if you understand carbohydrate metabolism, it is relatively simple to understand how fats and proteins are metabolized.

Carbohydrates are composed of carbon, oxygen, and hydrogen. The complete metabolism of carbohydrate requires oxygen, which is supplied by the respiratory system and is transported by the circulatory systems to the muscle cells. The metabolism of carbohydrate also produces carbon dioxide, which is removed via the circulatory and respiratory systems, and water.

The form of carbohydrate that is exclusively metabolized is *glucose,* a 6-carbon sugar arranged in a hexagonal formation and symbolized as $C_6H_{12}O_6$. Thus, all carbohydrate must be broken down into glucose before it can continue through the metabolic pathways. In its most simplistic form the oxidation of carbohydrate can be represented by the equation

$$C_6H_{12}O_6 + 6O_2 \rightarrow 6H_2O + 6CO_2$$

or

$$glucose + oxygen \rightarrow water + carbon\ dioxide$$

In the skeletal muscle, cell oxidation is tightly coupled with phosphorylation to produce energy in the form of ATP, and the equation becomes

$$C_6H_{12}O_6 + 6O_2 + 36(ADP + P_i) \rightarrow$$
$$6CO_2 + 36ATP + 42H_2O$$

or

glucose + oxygen + (adenosine diphosphate + inorganic phosphate) → carbon dioxide + adenosine triphosphate + water

---

Anaerobic In the absence of, not requiring, nor utilizing oxygen.

Aerobic In the presence of, requiring, or utilizing oxygen.

Substrate A substance acted upon by an enzyme.

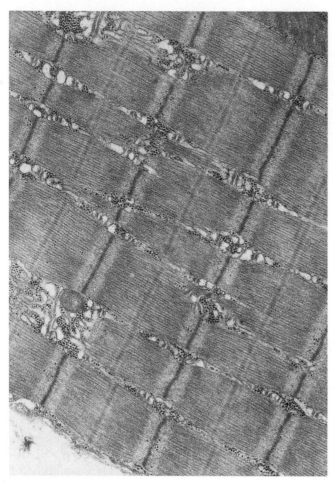

Figure 3.3
Glycogen Storage in Skeletal Muscle

In this electron micrograph of skeletal muscle (EM:25,000×), stored glycogen is visible as the small round black dots.

Source: Photo courtesy of Dian Molsen, Northern Illinois University Electron Microscope Laboratory.

Glycogen Stored form of carbohydrate composed of chains of glucose molecules chemically linked together.

Glycogenolysis The process by which stored glycogen is broken down (hydrolyzed) to provide glucose.

Metabolic Pathway A sequence of enzyme-mediated chemical reactions resulting in a specified product.

Glycolysis The energy pathway responsible for the initial catabolism of glucose in a 10- or 11-step process that begins with glucose or glycogen and ends with the production of pyruvate (aerobic glycolysis) or lactate (anaerobic glycolysis).

When an excess of glucose is available to the cell, it can be stored as **glycogen,** which is a chain of glucose molecules chemically linked together, or converted to and stored as fat. The formation of glycogen from glucose is called *glycogenesis.* Glycogen is stored predominantly in the liver and muscle cells, as shown in the electron micrograph in Figure 3.3. When additional glucose is needed, stored glycogen is broken down (hydrolyzed) to provide glucose, a process called **glycogenolysis.** Because glycogen must first be broken down into glucose, the production of energy from glucose or glycogen is identical after that initial step. The complete breakdown of glucose and glycogen follows the four-stage approach outlined in Figure 3.4 and detailed in later figures.

To keep the concepts *stages* and *steps* clear, think of the four stages as the four quarters of a football game. Each quarter is composed of several series of plays in which the offensive team has four downs to make 10 yards and run more plays or score. In metabolism each stage is like a quarter. Each individual step is analogous to a single football play. When steps are put together as in a series of plays in a drive, a **metabolic pathway** or sequence of enzyme-mediated chemical reactions resulting in a specific product is created. Although the quarters of a game and the stages of metabolism always follow the given numerical succession, there are two major differences. First, football plays should follow no particular order, or it wouldn't be much of a contest. Steps in a metabolic pathway, on the other hand, occur in an absolute, unvarying sequence. Second, one never knows exactly what the score of a football game will be, or even if there will be any scoring, until the game is over. The end result of metabolism, however—the production of ATP energy—is a given, and the amount is precisely known for each fuel utilized.

Stage I: Glycolysis Overview

Much of the importance of glycolysis is simply that it prepares glucose to enter the next stage of metabolism (see Figure 3.4) by converting glucose to pyruvate. Also very important is that ATP is produced during glycolysis. This process is the only way that we can produce ATP in the absence of oxygen (anaerobically).

Glycolysis, which literally means the breakdown or dissolution of sugar, is the energy pathway responsible for the initial catabolism of glucose in a 10- or 11-step process. Glycolysis begins with either glucose or glycogen and ends with the production of either pyruvate (pyruvic acid) by aerobic glycolysis or lactate (lactic acid) by anaerobic glycolysis (Frisell, 1982; Lehninger, 1971; Marieb, 2001; Newsholme and Leech,

1983; Van de Graaff and Fox, 1989). (Note that names ending in -*ate* technically indicate the salts of their respective acids, that is, lactate is the salt of lactic acid. However, the salt and acid forms are often used interchangeably in descriptions of the metabolic pathways.)

Each step is catalyzed by a specific enzyme. An **enzyme** is a protein that accelerates the speed of a chemical reaction without itself being changed by the reaction. It does not cause a reaction that would not otherwise occur; it simply speeds up one that would occur anyway. Metabolic enzymes are easy to identify since their names end in the suffix -*ase*. Generally, their names are also related to the reaction they are catalyzing.

The activity of enzymes is affected by the concentrations of the substrate acted upon and of the enzyme itself, temperature, pH, and the presence or absence of poisons or medications. The discussions that follow assume that the enzymes are acting in a normal physiological environment. Only a few selected enzymes that are especially important or function in regulatory or rate-limiting roles will be named. *Regulatory or rate-limiting enzymes* are the enzymes that are critical in controlling the rate and direction of energy production along a metabolic pathway—just as a traffic light regulates the flow of vehicles along a highway.

As a metabolic pathway, glycolysis begins with the absorption of glucose into the bloodstream from the small intestines or with the release of glucose into the bloodstream from the liver. These steps supply the fuel. Glucose must then be transported into the muscle cell. Transport occurs across the cell membrane via facilitated diffusion, utilizing a protein carrier and occurring down a concentration gradient. Transport is a passive process that does not require the expenditure of energy.

Human muscle and adipose cells contain both GLUT-1 (non–insulin-regulated) and GLUT-4 (insulin-regulated) transporters, or protein carriers, of glucose. However, GLUT-4 transporters represent the primary protein carrier in human skeletal and cardiac muscles. GLUT-1 transporters are located in the sarcolemma or cell membrane. In resting muscles when blood glucose levels are relative stable, most glucose enters by GLUT-1 transport (Brooks, et al., 1999). When glucose and insulin levels are high (for example, following a meal) or during exercise, most glucose enters by GLUT-4 transport. The GLUT-4 transporters are thus activated both by insulin, through a second

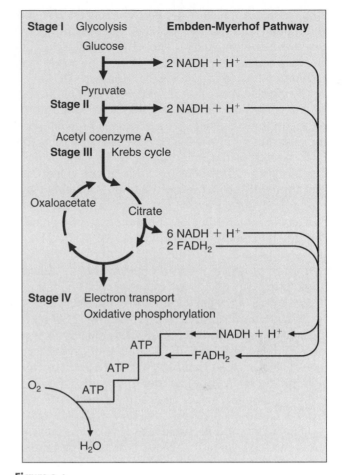

Figure 3.4
The Four Stages of Carbohydrate Cellular Respiration

messenger system, and by muscle contraction. Calcium is probably one of the second messengers (Brooks, et al., 1999; MacLean, et al., 2000). Within skeletal muscle, the number of GLUT-4 transporters is highest in fast-twitch oxidative glycolytic (FOG, Type IIA) fibers, followed by slow-twitch oxidative (SO, Type I) fibers, and is lowest in fast-twitch glycolytic (FG, Type IIB) fibers (Sato, et al., 1996).

GLUT-4 transporters exist intracellularly in small sacs or vesicles within the cytoplasm. When activated, they literally move to the cell surface (translocate) and serve as portals through which glucose enters the cell. The maximal rate of muscle glucose transport is determined both by the total number of GLUT-4 molecules and the proportion that are translocated to the cell membrane (Houston, 1995; Sato, et al., 1996). The dual stimulation of GLUT-4 translocation by insulin and contraction is important because, as you know from Chapter 2 and will examine in greater detail in this chapter, insulin secretion is

---

Enzyme A protein that accelerates the speed of a chemical reaction without itself being changed by the reaction.

suppressed during exercise. Thus, during exercise the predominant activator of GLUT-4 transporters is the muscle contraction itself. The effect of muscle contraction persists into the early recovery period to help rebuild depleted glycogen stores (Houston, 1995).

Glycolysis takes place in the cytoplasm of the cell. The enzymes that catalyze each step are simply free floating in the cytoplasm. The transfer of the intermediary substances between enzymes takes place by *diffusion,* which is the tendency of molecules to move from a region of high concentration to one of low concentration. All of the intermediates (everything but glucose and the pyruvate or lactate) are *phosphorylated compounds*—that is, they contain phosphates. All of the phosphate intermediates, ADP, and ATP are unable to pass through the cell membrane. The cell membrane, however, is freely permeable to glucose and lactate.

Glycolysis, as depicted in Figure 3.5, involves both the utilization and production of ATP. One ATP molecule is used in the first step if the initial fuel is glucose. One ATP is used in step 3 whether the initial fuel is glucose or glycogen. Thus, 1 ATP is used for activation if the initial fuel is glycogen, but 2 ATP are used if the initial fuel is glucose. ATP is produced from ADP + P_i at steps 7 and 10 by a process known as substrate-level phosphorylation. **Substrate-level phosphorylation** is the transfer of P_i directly from the phosphorylated intermediates or substrates to ADP without any oxidation occurring. A net total of 3 ATP are gained if glycogen is the initial fuel, but only 2 ATP are gained if glucose is the initial fuel.

Exactly how glycolysis is accomplished is explained in the following step-by-step analysis. Clarification of the terms *oxidation* and *reduction* and a description of the role of nicotinamide adenine dinucleotide (NAD)

Substrate-Level Phosphorylation The transfer of P_i directly from a phosphorylated intermediate or substrates to ADP without any oxidation occurring.

Oxidation A gain of oxygen, a loss of hydrogen, or the direct loss of electrons by an atom or substance.

Reduction A loss of oxygen, a gain of electrons, or a gain of hydrogen by an atom or substance.

Nicotinamide Adenine Dinucleotide (NAD) A hydrogen carrier in cellular respiration.

Flavin Adenine Dinucleotide (FAD) A hydrogen carrier in cellular respiration.

---

and flavin adenine dinucleotide (FAD) are necessary before proceeding to these steps, however.

Oxidation-Reduction There are three kinds of **oxidation:** a gain of oxygen (hence the name), a loss of hydrogen, or the direct loss of electrons by an atom or substance.

The name of the process whereby an atom or substance gains electrons is called **reduction.** A good way to remember which is which is to put the two words with *e*'s together: reduction = + e^-. Reduction can also mean a loss of oxygen or a gain of hydrogen by an atom or a substance. Electron donors are known as reducing agents and electron acceptors as oxidizing agents. The major electron donors are organic fuels, such as glucose. Oxygen is the final electron acceptor or oxidizing agent in cellular respiration.

When one substance is oxidized, another is simultaneously reduced. The substance that is oxidized also loses energy; the substance that is reduced also gains energy.

Oxidation in the form of hydrogen removal occurs in several of the intermediary steps in catabolism. When hydrogen atoms are removed, they must be transported elsewhere. The two most important hydrogen carriers in cellular respiration are **nicotinamide adenine dinucleotide (NAD)** and **flavin adenine dinucleotide (FAD).** Both NAD and FAD can accept two electrons and two protons from two hydrogen atoms. Each does so in a slightly different manner, however. FAD (the oxidized form is FAD_{ox}) actually binds both protons and is written as $FADH_2$ (or FAD reduced, written FAD_{red}). NAD actually exists as NAD^+ (or NAD oxidized, written NAD_{ox}); when bonded to hydrogen, it is written as $NADH + H^+$ (or NAD reduced, written as NAD_{red}). The symbols NAD^+ and FAD will be used to indicate the oxidized form, and $NADH + H^+$ and $FADH_2$ will be used to indicate the reduced form of these carriers in this text, so it is clear where the hydrogen atoms are. NAD^+ is by far the more important hydrogen carrier in human metabolism.

A helpful analogy of the roles of FAD and NAD is a taxi cab. The purpose of NAD and FAD is to transport (serve as taxis for) the hydrogen. NAD and FAD must pick up hydrogen passengers (be reduced) and they must drop them off (be oxidized) at another point without either the carrier (taxi) or the hydrogen (passengers) being permanently changed.

The Steps of Stage I Refer to Figure 3.5 as each step is explained in the text (Frisell, 1982; Lehninger, 1971; Marieb, 2001; Newsholme and Leech, 1983; Van de Graaff and Fox, 1989).

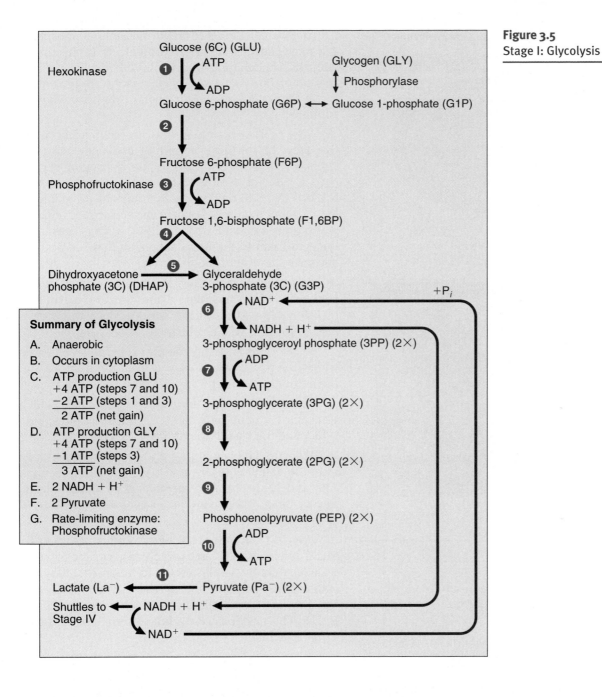

Figure 3.5
Stage I: Glycolysis

Step 1. The glucose molecule is phosphorylated (has a phosphate attached) through the transfer of one phosphate group from ATP to the location of the sixth carbon on the glucose hexagon, producing glucose 6-phosphate. *Hexokinase* is the enzyme that catalyzes this process. This phosphorylation effectively traps the glucose in that particular cell, because the electrical charge of the phosphate group prohibits glucose from crossing the membrane, and the enzyme that can break this phosphate bond is not present in muscle cells.

The same is true for the glycogen in the cells; that is, it is trapped in the muscle where it is stored. On the other hand, the liver possesses enzymes to break down glycogen and release glucose into the bloodstream.

These facts are important because during high-intensity long-term exercise, glycogen stored in specific muscles must be used there. Furthermore, glycogen stored in muscles not used in that activity (for example, the upper body for a running event) cannot be removed as such from the inactive muscles and be transported to the active ones. Therefore, high levels of glycogen need to be stored in the muscles that will be used.

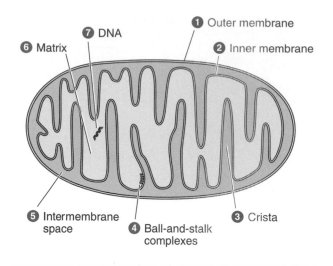

① Outer membrane
⑦ DNA
② Inner membrane
⑥ Matrix
⑤ Intermembrane space
④ Ball-and-stalk complexes
③ Crista

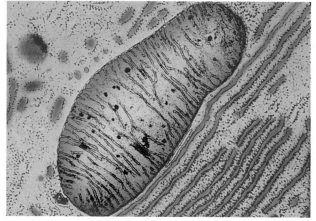

Figure 3.6
Mitochondrion

Step 2. The atoms that make up the glucose 6-phosphate are simply rearranged to form fructose 6-phosphate.

Step 3. Another molecule of ATP is broken down and the phosphate added at the first carbon. This addition places a phosphate group at each end of the molecule and results in the product fructose 1,6-di- or bisphosphate. The prefixes *di-* and *bis-* mean "two." In this case two phosphates are now part of the molecule. This step is catalyzed by the enzyme *phosphofructokinase* (PFK), which is the most important regulatory enzyme in glycolysis.

Step 4. This is the step from which glycolysis, meaning sugar breaking or splitting, gets its name, for here the 6-carbon sugar is split into two 3-carbon sugars. The two sugars are identical in terms of their component atoms but have different names (dihydroxyacetone phosphate, or DHAP, and glyceraldehyde 3-phosphate, or G3P) because the component atoms are arranged differently.

Step 5. The atoms of dihydroxyacetone phosphate are rearranged to form glyceraldehyde 3-phosphate, with the phosphate group at the third carbon. From this point on, each step occurs twice (indicated by 2× in Figure 3.5), once for each of the three carbon subunits.

Step 6. Two reactions that are coupled occur in this step. In the first, a pair of hydrogen atoms is transferred from the G3P to the hydrogen carrier NAD^+, reducing this to $NADH + H^+$. The fate of this $NADH + H^+$ will be dealt with later. This reaction releases enough energy to perform the second reaction, which adds a phosphate from the P_i always present in the cytoplasm to the first carbon, so that the product becomes 1,3-diphosphoglycerate.

Step 7. ATP is finally produced from ADP in this step when the phosphate from the first carbon is transferred to ADP, storing energy. Since this step is also doubled, 2 ATP are formed.

Step 8. This is simply another rearrangement step where the phosphate is moved from the number 3 to the number 2 carbon.

Step 9. A water molecule is removed, which weakens the bond between the remaining phosphate group and the rest of the atoms.

Step 10. The remaining phosphate is transferred from phosphoenolpyruvate (PEP) to ADP, forming ATP and pyruvate. The enzyme is pyruvate kinase. Again, since the reaction happens twice, 2 ATP are produced.

Step 11. If the hydrogen atoms carried by NAD^+ as $NADH + H^+$ are unable to enter the electron transport chain (as described in Stage IV), they are transferred instead to pyruvic acid (pyruvate), forming lactic acid (lactate), which regenerates the NAD^+. The enzyme catalyzing this reaction is *lactic dehydrogenase*.

Note that the formula for the two pyruvic acid molecules formed is $2C_3H_4O_3$ while that of the original glucose was $C_6H_{12}O_6$. Both the number of carbon atoms and the number of oxygen atoms are the same, however, there are four fewer hydrogen atoms in pyruvic acid than in glucose. These are the hydrogen atoms that are carried by the NAD^+. If the endpoint of glycolysis is lactic acid ($2C_3H_6O_3$), all of the hydrogen atoms are accounted for.

When the end product of glycolysis is pyruvic acid, the process is called aerobic glycolysis (or slow glycolysis). When the end product of glycolysis is lactic acid, the process is called anaerobic glycolysis (or fast glycolysis). Glucose predominates as the fuel for slow glycolysis, and glycogen predominates as the fuel for fast glycolysis.

Mitochondria Mitochondria (which is the plural form; the singular is *mitochondrion*) are subcellular organelles that are often called the powerhouses of the cell. The formation of acetyl CoA, Krebs cycle, electron transport, and oxidative phosphorylation all take place in the mitochondria.

Figure 3.6 presents a diagram and an electron micrograph of a mitochondrion: a three-dimensional, discretely encapsulated, bean-shaped structure. In actual living tissue mitochondria exist in many different shapes—and, indeed, they constantly change shapes.

As shown in Figure 3.6, mitochondria have five distinct components. The first component is the outer membrane (labeled as (1) in the figure). As is usual, this membrane serves as a barrier; however, it contains many channels through which solutes can pass and so is permeable to many ions and molecules. The second component (2) is an inner membrane. The inner mitochondrial membrane is impermeable to most ions and molecules unless each has a specific carrier. It is, however, permeable to water and oxygen. The inner membrane is parallel to the outer membrane in spots, but it also consists of a series of folds or convolutions called *crista* (3) (the plural is *cristae*). Protruding across and from the inner membrane is a series of protein-enzyme complexes called ball-and-stalk complexes (4) that have the appearance of a golf ball on a tee. Although the inner membrane has transport functions, the crista portion and especially the ball-and-stalk apparatus are specialized as the locations where ATP synthesis actually takes place.

The area between the two membranes is known simply as the intermembrane space (5). The center portion of the mitochondria is known as the *matrix* (6). The matrix is filled with a gel-like substance composed of water and proteins. Metabolic enzymes and DNA (7) for organelle replication are stored here.

The fact that mitochondria contain their own DNA means that they are self-replicating. When a need for more ATP arises, mitochondria simply split in half and then grow to their former size. This property, discussed later, has specific implications for how an individual adapts to exercise training. It also explains why some cells have only a few mitochondria but others have thousands. Red blood cells are unique in that they contain no mitochondria.

Mitochondria tend to be located where they are needed. Within muscle cells they lie directly beneath

> **Mitochondria** Cell organelles in which the Krebs cycle, electron transport, and oxidative phosphorylation take place.

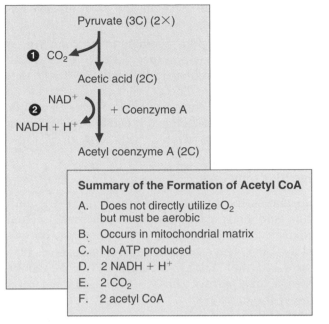

Figure 3.7
Stage II: The Formation of Acetyl Coenzyme A

the cell membrane (and are called *sarcolemmal mitochondria*) and among the contractile elements (which are called *interfibrillar mitochondria*).

Stage II: Formation of Acetyl Coenzyme A

Stage II (Figure 3.7) is a very short metabolic pathway consisting solely of the conversion of pyruvate to acetyl coenzyme A (Frisell, 1982; Lehninger, 1961; Marieb, 2001; Newsholme and Leech, 1983; Van de Graaff and Fox, 1983). No ATP is either used or produced directly. However, a pair of hydrogen atoms (two, because all reactions still happen twice) are removed and picked up by NAD^+ to be transferred to the electron transport chain.

The conversion of pyruvate to acetyl CoA takes place within the mitochondrial matrix (Figure 3.6). This conversion requires that the pyruvate be transported across the mitochondrial membranes via a specific carrier. No oxygen is used directly in this stage, but these steps will only occur in the presence of oxygen. As usual, enzymes catalyze each reaction.

The Steps of Stage II Refer to the diagram in Figure 3.7 for the two steps of Stage II (Frisell, 1982; Lehninger, 1971; Marieb, 2001; Newsholme and Leech, 1983; Van de Graaff and Fox, 1989).

Step 1. Pyruvate is converted to acetic acid. In the process, one molecule of CO_2 is removed. This CO_2, as well as the CO_2 that will be formed in Stage III, diffuses into the bloodstream and is ultimately exhaled via the lungs.

Step 2. Acetic acid is combined with coenzyme A to form acetyl coenzyme A (acetyl CoA). A **coenzyme** is a nonprotein substance derived from a vitamin that activates an enzyme. The conversion of pyruvate to acetyl CoA commits the pyruvate to Stages III and IV since there is no biochemical means of reconverting acetyl CoA back to pyruvate.

Stage III: Krebs Cycle

What makes the **Krebs cycle** a cycle is that it both begins and ends with the same substance, called *oxaloacetate* (or oxaloacetic acid, which is abbreviated as OAA). The cycle is an eight-step process (see Figure 3.8) that actually comprises two metabolic pathways: one pathway for steps 1–3 and the second pathway for steps 4–8.

No ATP is used in the Krebs cycle, and only one step (5) results in the substrate-level phosphorylation production of ATP. However, four steps (3, 4, 6, and 8) result in the removal of hydrogen atoms, which are picked up by either NAD^+ or FAD. This result is critically important, because these are the hydrogen atoms that will provide the electrons for the electron transport system. Carbon dioxide is produced at steps 3 and 4. As with every step since the 6-carbon glucose molecule was split into two 3-carbon units in Stage I (step 4, Figure 3.5), every reaction and product is doubled.

All of the enzymes and hence all of the reactions for the Krebs cycle occur within the mitochondrial matrix, with one exception. The exception is that the

---

Coenzyme A nonprotein substance derived from a vitamin that activates an enzyme.

Krebs Cycle A series of eight chemical reactions that begins and ends with the same substance; energy is liberated for direct substrate phosphorylation of ATP from ADP and P_i; carbon dioxide is formed and hydrogen atoms removed and carried by NAD and FAD to the electron transport system; does not directly utilize oxygen but requires its presence.

Electron Transport System (ETS) The final metabolic pathway; it proceeds as a series of chemical reactions in the mitochondria that transfer electrons from the hydrogen atom carriers NAD and FAD to oxygen; water is formed as a by-product; the electrochemical energy released by the hydrogen ions is coupled to the formation of ATP from ADP and P_i.

---

enzyme succinate dehydrogenase that catalyzes step 6 is located in the inner mitochondrial membrane.

The intermediate molecules as well as the preliminary molecules pyruvic acid and acetyl CoA are keto acids. Although no oxygen is used directly, this stage requires the presence of oxygen.

The Steps of Stage III   The steps for the Krebs cycle (Frisell, 1982; Lehninger, 1971; Marieb, 2001; Newsholme and Leech, 1983; Van de Graaff and Fox, 1989) are presented in Figure 3.8, which you should refer to while reading the discussion.

Step 1. The 2-carbon acetyl CoA combines with the 4-carbon molecule oxaloacetate (OAA) to form citrate or citric acid. It is because of this first product that the cycle is also known as the citric acid cycle. In the reaction the coenzyme A (CoA-SH) is removed from acetyl CoA and is free to convert more pyruvate to acetyl CoA or to be used later in the cycle.

Step 2. The atoms of citric acid (citrate) are rearranged to become isocitrate.

Step 3. Two reactions occur. In the first hydrogen atoms are removed and accepted by the carrier NAD^+, forming $NADH + H^+$. In the second reaction a CO_2 is removed, leaving the 5-carbon α-ketoglutarate.

Step 4. Step 4 is basically a repetition of step 3 in that a pair of hydrogen atoms are removed and picked up by NAD^+ and a CO_2 is also removed. In addition, the remaining structure is attached to coenzyme A (CoA-SH). The resultant succinyl CoA has only four carbons, which will remain intact throughout the rest of the cycle.

Step 5. In this step coenzyme A is displaced by a phosphate group, which, in turn, is transferred, via a substance called guanosine triphosphate (GTP), to ADP to form ATP. This is the only step in the Krebs cycle that produces and stores energy directly. As in glycolysis, this ATP is produced by substrate-level phosphorylation.

Step 6. More hydrogen atoms are removed, but this time the carrier substance is FAD, forming $FADH_2$.

Step 7. Water is added, converting fumarate to malate.

Step 8. A pair of hydrogen atoms is removed and accepted by NAD^+. The remaining atoms once more make up oxaloacetate, and the cycle is ready to begin again.

The ATP produced in Stages I and III can be used immediately to provide energy for the cell. The CO_2 diffuses into the bloodstream, is transported to the

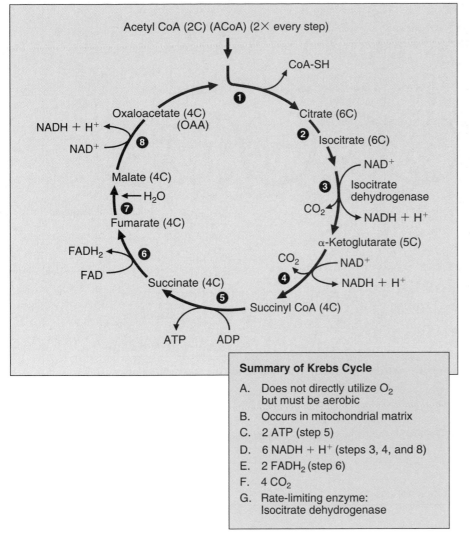

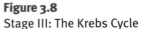
Figure 3.8
Stage III: The Krebs Cycle

Acetyl CoA (2C) (ACoA) (2× every step)

CoA-SH

❶

Oxaloacetate (4C) (OAA)

Citrate (6C)

❷

Isocitrate (6C)

NADH + H⁺

NAD⁺

❽

NAD⁺

❸ Isocitrate dehydrogenase

Malate (4C)

CO_2

NADH + H⁺

H₂O

❼

Fumarate (4C)

α-Ketoglutarate (5C)

FADH₂

CO_2 NAD⁺

❻

❹

NADH + H⁺

FAD

Succinate (4C)

❺

Succinyl CoA (4C)

ATP   ADP

Summary of Krebs Cycle

A.   Does not directly utilize O_2 but must be aerobic
B.   Occurs in mitochondrial matrix
C.   2 ATP (step 5)
D.   6 NADH + H⁺ (steps 3, 4, and 8)
E.   2 FADH₂ (step 6)
F.   4 CO_2
G.   Rate-limiting enzyme: Isocitrate dehydrogenase

lungs, and is exhaled. Now we must determine what happens to all of the hydrogen atoms that are carried as NADH + H⁺ and FADH₂.

Stage IV: Electron Transport and Oxidative Phosphorylation

The **electron transport system (ETS)** or respiratory chain is the final metabolic pathway; it proceeds as a series of chemical reactions in the mitochondria that transfer electrons from the hydrogen atom carriers NAD and FAD to oxygen; water is formed as a by-product and the electrochemical energy released by the hydrogen ions is coupled to the formation of ATP from ADP and P_i (Frisell, 1982; Lehninger, 1971; Marieb, 2001; Newsholme and Leech, 1983; Van de Graaff and Fox, 1989). The chain itself consists of a series of electron (e⁻) carriers and proton pumps embedded in the inner membrane of the mitochon-

dria. Most carriers are proteins or a combination of metal ions (such as iron, Fe) and proteins. The major carriers are indicated in Figure 3.9. These carriers are flavoprotein 1 and 2, the coenzyme Q, and five cytochromes: b, c_1, c, a, and a_3. Coenzyme Q and cytochrome c are mobile and literally move the electrons between the other carriers.

The H⁺ and e⁻ come from the breakdown of the hydrogen atoms released in Stages I, II, and III and transported by NAD⁺ and FAD:

$$2H = 2H^+ + 2e^-$$

The H⁺ are deposited via the proton pumps into the intermembrane space. The e⁻ are shuttled along from one electron acceptor to the next (see Figure 3.9). The e⁻ move along in a series of oxidation-reduction reactions, because each successive carrier has a greater affinity (force of chemical attraction) for them than the preceding one in the sequence. Oxygen has the

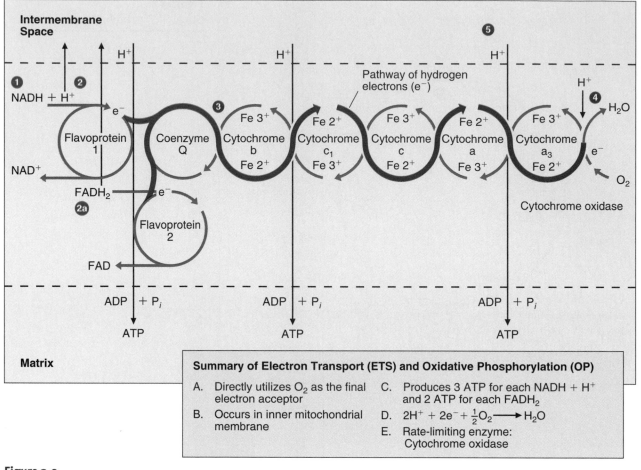

Figure 3.9
Stage IV: Electron Transport and Oxidative Phosphorylation

greatest affinity of all for e⁻ and acts as the final e⁻ acceptor. The additional electrons on the oxygen give it a negative charge and attract the positively charged H^+, thus forming water (Figure 3.10). The H^+ move from the intermembrane space to the matrix through the ball-and-stalk apparatus. This movement of the H^+ activates ATP synthetase, which phosphorylates ADP to ATP.

Thus, the formation of ATP from ADP and P_i is coupled to the movement of H^+ and e⁻ through and along the electron transport chain. The movement of those ions releases energy that is harnessed when ADP is phosphorylated to ATP. Because phosphate is added (phosphorylation) and the NADH + H^+ and

$FADH_2$ are oxidized (electrons removed), the term **oxidative phosphorylation (OP)** is used to denote this formation of ATP. Thus oxidative phosphorylation is the process in which NADH + H^+ and $FADH_2$ are oxidized in the electron transport system and the energy released is used to synthesize ATP from ADP and P_i. Remember that the process of producing ATP directly in glycolysis and the Krebs cycle was called substrate-level phosphorylation because the P_i was transferred directly from phosphorylated intermediates to ADP without any oxidation occurring.

The Steps of Stage IV Again, the series of steps (Frisell, 1982; Lehninger, 1971; Marieb, 2001; Newsholme and Leech, 1983; Van de Graaff and Fox, 1989) presented in Figure 3.9 are necessary so that the energy may be preserved and not released all at once and lost as heat, which would destroy tissue.

Step 1. NADH + H^+ arrives at flavoprotein 1 and transfers the electrons (e⁻) and protons (H^+) from the hydrogen across the inner membrane.

Oxidative Phosphorylation (OP) The process in which NADH + H^+ and $FADH_2$ are oxidized in the electron transport system and the energy released is used to synthesize ATP from ADP and P_i.

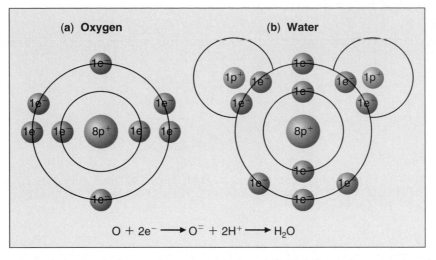

$$O + 2e^- \longrightarrow O^= + 2H^+ \longrightarrow H_2O$$

Figure 3.10
Oxygen as the Final Electron Acceptor

(a) The outer shell of oxygen has room for eight electrons but contains only six. Thus it can accept two electrons at the end of electron transport. (b) When oxygen accepts these two electrons, it then has a double negative charge ($O^=$). Two hydrogen ions (H^+) are thus attracted, and water (H_2O) is formed.

Step 2. The H^+ are released and deposited into the intermembrane space.

Step 2a. This step is really a variation and not a sequential step. If the original hydrogen carrier was FAD instead of NAD^+, the transfer of electrons and protons occurs at flavoprotein 2 instead of flavoprotein 1.

Step 3. The electrons shuttle down the cytochromes, alternately causing the cytochromes to gain (become reduced) and lose (become oxidized) the electrons. In this process they also move across the width of the inner membrane shuttling H^+ from the matrix to the inner membrane space. This shuttling is repeated three times if the carrier is NADH + H^+ and twice if the carrier is $FADH_2$.

Step 4. Oxygen accepts the electrons. This increase in negative charge attracts hydrogen ions and causes the formation of water. Figure 3.10 depicts this step graphically.

Step 5. The H^+ that have been transported into the intermembrane space create an electrochemical gradient. Since the drive is to equalize that gradient, the H^+ leak back into the mitochondrial matrix through the ball-and-stalk complexes which are the enzyme ATP synthase. The movement of H^+ creates an electrical current, and this electrical energy, along with the enzyme action, is somehow used to synthesize ATP from ADP + P_i, both of which are present in the matrix. Each NADH + H^+ is responsible for producing 3 ATP, but each $FADH_2$ produces only 2 ATP.

Step 6. In the final step (depicted in Figure 3.11), the ATP moves out of the mitochondria in exchange for the inward movement of ADP needed for the continual production of energy.

Figure 3.11 summarizes the process of cellular respiration just discussed and shows the interrelationships in a cell. As you study the figure, refer to the individual stage explanations as needed.

ATP Production from Carbohydrate

The number of ATP produced directly by substrate-level phosphorylation and the number of hydrogen atoms being carried by NAD and FAD were pointed out for each stage. These numbers are summarized in Table 3.1 (page 69). From this summary we can compute the total yield of ATP from one molecule of glucose or glycogen.

Stage I (glycolysis) yields a gross production of 4 ATP but uses 2 ATP, yielding a net gain of 2 ATP from direct substrate-level phosphorylation, if the substrate is glucose. If the substrate is glycogen, only 1 ATP is used and the net gain is 3 ATP.

Two NADH + H^+ are also produced. These hydrogen atoms are transported from the cytoplasm, where glycolysis has taken place, into the mitochondria, if the level of pyruvate is not too high and if there is enough oxygen to accept the electrons at the end of the ETS. However, the inner mitochondrial membrane is impermeable to NADH + H^+, meaning that the

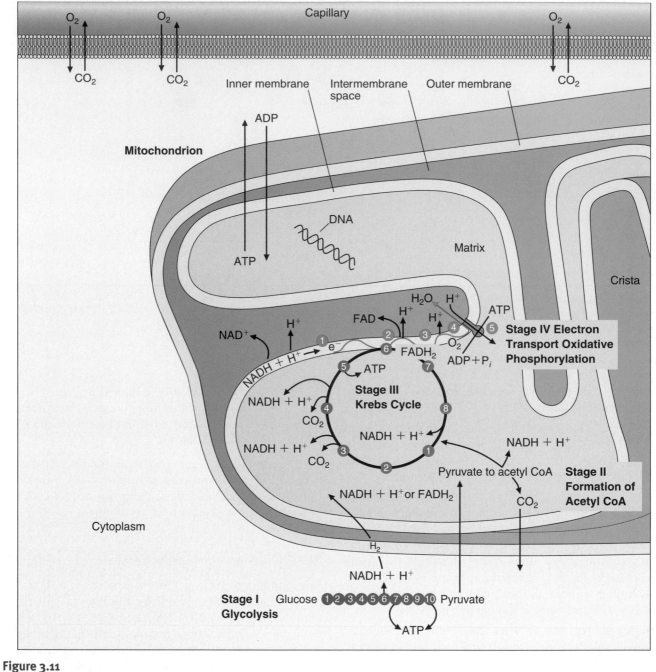

Figure 3.11
Cellular Respiration

membrane does not allow it to pass through. Therefore, a shuttle system must be employed.

Actually, two shuttle systems appear to operate—one for cardiac muscle and the other for skeletal muscle. The cardiac-muscle shuttle system is called the *malate-aspartate shuttle*. It operates by the NADH + H$^+$ in the cytoplasm giving up the hydrogens to malate, which carries them across the inner mitochondrial membrane. Here, mitochondrial NAD$^+$ picks up the H$^+$ and enters the ETS (Newsholme and Leech, 1983).

The skeletal-muscle shuttle system is called the *glycerol-phosphate shuttle*. It operates by the NADH + H$^+$ in the cytoplasm giving up the hydrogens to glycerol phosphate, which carries them into the inner mitochondrial membrane. Here, FAD picks the H$^+$ up and enters the ETS. This shuttle predominates in skeletal muscle (Frisell, 1982; Lehninger, 1971; Marieb, 2001; Newsholme and Leech, 1983; Van de Graaff and Fox, 1989) although there is some evidence that the malate-aspartate shuttle may operate

Table 3.1
ATP Production from Carbohydrate

Metabolic Process Stage	ATP				Hydrogen Atoms and Carrier	
	Heart Muscle		Skeletal Muscle		Heart Muscle	Skeletal Muscle
I. Glycolysis	$+4$ $\underline{-2}$ 2	$+4$ $\underline{-1}^*$	$+4$ $\underline{-2}$ 2	$+4$ $\underline{-1}^*$	2 NADH + H[1]	2 NADH + H[++] $\rightarrow$ 2 FADH$_2$
Glucose						
*Glycogen		3		3		
II. Pyruvate $\rightarrow$ acetyl CoA	0	0	0	0	2 NADH + H$^+$	2 NADH + H$^+$
III. Krebs cycle	2	2	2	2	6 NADH + H$^+$ 2 FADH$_2$	6 NADH + H$^+$ 2 FADH$_2$
IV. ETS/OP: Hydrogen atoms from						
Stage I	6	6	$^\dagger 4$	$^\dagger 4$		
Stage II	6	6	6	6		
Stage III	22	22	22	22		
Total	——	——	——	——		
Glucose	38		36			
Glycogen		39		37		

* If glycogen, not glucose, is fuel.

† Owing to shuttle differences in crossing into mitochondrial membrane, these hydrogen atoms are actually carried by FAD in the mitochondria, reducing the ATP production.

in Type I slow-twitch oxidative skeletal muscle (Houston, 1995). It is the carrier within the mitochondrion that determines how many ATP are produced.

Therefore, in heart muscle the yield from the glycolytic hydrogens is 6 ATP (2 NADH + H$^+$ × 3 = 6 ATP). That of skeletal muscle is only 4 ATP (2 FADH$_2$ × 2 = 4 ATP). No differences exist in the ATP production count for any of the remaining stages between cardiac and skeletal muscle.

Stage II (the conversion of pyruvate to acetyl CoA) yields no substrate-level ATP, but it does produce 2 NADH + H$^+$. Since these molecules are already in the mitochondria, they directly enter the ETS: 2 NADH + H$^+$ × 3 = 6 ATP.

Stage III (the Krebs cycle) produces 2 ATP directly by substrate-level phosphorylation, NADH + H$^+$ at three steps, and FADH$_2$ at one step. Thus, (3 NADH + H$^+$ × 3 = 9 ATP) + (1 FADH$_2$ × 2 = 2 ATP). Since each step occurs twice for each 6-carbon glucose molecule, this yield must be doubled: 9 ATP + 2 ATP = 11 ATP × 2 = 22 ATP.

If we add all of these results for skeletal muscle when glucose is the fuel, we get:

2 ATP	(substrate-level phosphorylation, glycolysis)
4 ATP	(NADH + H$^+$ → FADH$_2$, glycolysis)
6 ATP	(NADH + H$^+$, Stage II)
2 ATP	(substrate-level phosphorylation, Krebs cycle)
22 ATP	(FADH$_2$ + NADH + H$^+$, Krebs cycle ETS/OP)
or 36 ATP	for the aerobic oxidation of one molecule of glucose by skeletal muscle.

Complete the Question of Understanding box.

A Question of Understanding

To understand the calculation, determine the total ATP produced when the aerobic oxidation takes place in heart muscle and the initial fuel is glucose. Check your answer against the value given in Table 3.1. Next, do the same computations assuming that glycogen, not glucose, is the energy substrate. Again, check your answer against the value given in Table 3.1 or in Appendix D.

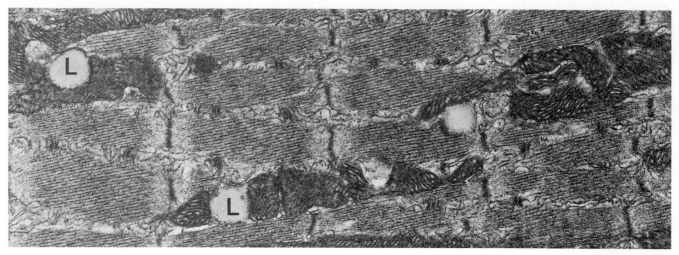

Figure 3.12
Lipid Droplets in Skeletal Muscle

In this electron micrograph of skeletal muscle (EM: 27,200×) lipid droplets are visible in the light round circles, some of which have been labeled "L."

Source: *Cell and Tissue Ultrastructure* by Cross and Mercer. Copyright © 1993 by W. H. Freeman and Company. Used with permission.

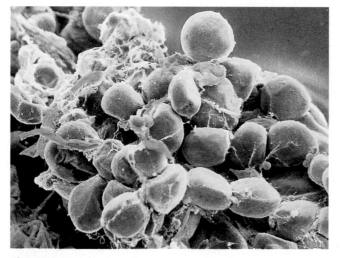

Figure 3.13
Triglyceride Stored in Adipose Tissue

Fat Metabolism

Although the body may prefer to use carbohydrate as fuel from the standpoint of oxygen cost, the importance of fat as an energy source should not be underestimated. Fat is found in many common foods. Fat, in the form of *triglyceride* (sometimes known as triacylglycerol), is the major storage form of energy in humans. Some triglyceride is stored within muscle cells (Figure 3.12), but the vast majority is deposited in adipose cells (Figure 3.13) and comprises approximately

10–15% of the body weight of young males and 20–25% of the body weight of young females (Malina and Bouchard, 1991). Roughly half of this adipocyte storage occurs subcutaneously (under the skin). The remaining stores surround the major organs of the abdomino-thoracic cavity as support and protection. Triglycerides are turned over constantly in the body. In fact, your body fat is turned over completely about every 3–4 weeks, so you are definitely not carrying any of your "baby fat" with you today (Marieb, 2001).

Fat is an excellent storage fuel for several reasons. First, fat is an energy-dense fuel yielding 9.13 kcal per gram; both carbohydrate and protein yield slightly less than 4 kcal per gram. The reason for these figures is related to the chemical structure of the substrates—specifically, the amount of oxidizable carbon and hydrogen. It is easy to appreciate the difference by looking at the chemical composition of the free fatty acid palmitate, which is $C_{16}H_{32}O_2$. This fatty acid has almost three times the amount of C and H, but only a third the amount of O as glucose ($C_6H_{12}O_6$). Remember that it is H that donates the electrons used during oxidative phosphorylation.

Second, carbohydrate, in the form of glycogen, is stored in the muscles with a large amount of water: 2.7 g of water per gram of dried glycogen. Triglyceride is stored dry. Thus, the energy content of fat is not diluted, and hard as it may be to believe, bulk is less than would otherwise be necessary. If humans had to store the comparable energy amount as carbohydrates, we would be at least twice as big (Newsholme and Leech, 1983)!

Third, glycogen stores are relatively small in comparison to fat stores. A person can deplete the stored glycogen in as little as 2 hr of heavy exercise or one day of bed rest, whereas fat supplies can last for weeks, even with moderate activity. Although many Americans often seem concerned about having too much body fat, this storage capacity is undoubtedly important for survival of the species when food is not readily available.

The triglycerides stored in adipose tissue must first be broken down into glycerol and free fatty acids before they can be used as fuel (Figure 3.2). One glycerol and three fatty acids make up a triglyceride. Seven fatty acids predominate in the body, but since three fatty acids combine with a glycerol to make up a triglyceride, there are 343 (7 × 7 × 7) different combinations possible (Péronnet, et al., 1987). Some common fatty acids are oleic acid, palmitic acid, stearic acid, linoleic acid, and palmitoleic acid.

Fatty acids may be saturated, unsaturated, or polyunsaturated. A saturated fatty acid has a chemical bonding arrangement that allows it to hold as many hydrogens as possible. Thus, *saturated* means "saturated with hydrogen." Unsaturated fatty acids have a chemical bonding arrangement with a reduced-hydrogen binding potential and therefore are unsaturated with respect to hydrogens. Polyunsaturated means several bonds are without hydrogens.

The breakdown of triglycerides into glycerol and fatty acids is catalyzed by the enzyme hormone-sensitive lipase. The glycerol is soluble in blood, but the free fatty acids (FFA) are not. Glycerol can enter glycolysis in the cytoplasm (as 3-phosphoglycerate, the product of step 7 in Figure 3.5), but it is not typically utilized by muscle cells in this fashion (Newsholme and Leech, 1983; Péronnet, et al., 1987). The direct role of glycerol as a fuel in the muscle cells during exercise is so minor that it need not be considered. However, glycerol can be converted to glucose by the liver.

FFA must be transported in the blood bound to albumin. Specific receptor sites on the muscle cell membrane receive the FFA into the cell. The FFA must then be translocated or transported from the cytoplasm into the mitochondria. Once in the mitochondrial matrix, the FFA undergoes the process of beta oxidation (Figure 3.14).

Beta Oxidation

Beta oxidation is a cyclic series of steps that breaks off successive pairs of carbon atoms from FFA, which are then used to form acetyl CoA. Remember that

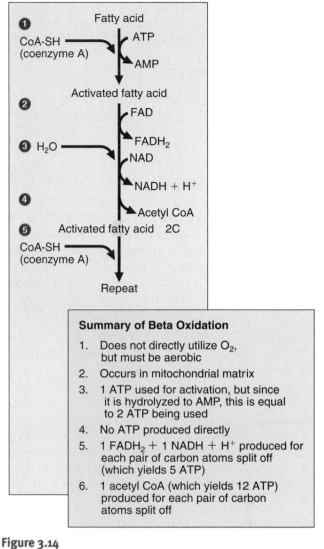

Summary of Beta Oxidation

1. Does not directly utilize O_2, but must be aerobic
2. Occurs in mitochondrial matrix
3. 1 ATP used for activation, but since it is hydrolyzed to AMP, this is equal to 2 ATP being used
4. No ATP produced directly
5. 1 $FADH_2$ + 1 NADH + H^+ produced for each pair of carbon atoms split off (which yields 5 ATP)
6. 1 acetyl CoA (which yields 12 ATP) produced for each pair of carbon atoms split off

Figure 3.14
Beta Oxidation

acetyl CoA is the common intermediate by which all foodstuffs enter the Krebs cycle and electron transport system. The number of cycles depends upon the number of carbons; most fatty acids have 14–24 carbons.

When there is an adequate supply of oxaloacetate to combine with, the fat-derived acetyl CoA enters the Krebs cycle and proceeds through electron transport and oxidative phosphorylation. Figure 3.14 diagrams the steps of beta oxidation, which are explained next.

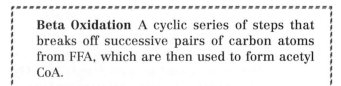

Beta Oxidation A cyclic series of steps that breaks off successive pairs of carbon atoms from FFA, which are then used to form acetyl CoA.

As with glycolysis, ATP is used for activation; but unlike glycolysis, beta oxidation produces no ATP directly, by substrate phosphorylation.

The Steps of Beta Oxidation

Step 1. The fatty acid molecule is activated by the breakdown of 1 ATP to AMP, releasing the energy equivalent of 2 ATP if broken down as it is normally to ADP. Concurrently, coenzyme A is added.

Step 2. FAD is reduced to $FADH_2$. The $FADH_2$ will enter the electron transport chain and produce 2 ATP.

Step 3. A molecule of water is added and NAD^+ is reduced to $NADH + H^+$. The $NADH + H^+$ will enter the electron transport chain and produce 3 ATP. Steps 2 and 3, with the removal of the hydrogen atoms, account for the oxidation portion of the name for this process.

Step 4. The bond between the alpha (α) carbon (C_2) and the beta (β) carbon (C_3) is broken, resulting in the removal of two carbons (C_1 and C_2), which are then used to form acetyl coenzyme A. The cleavage of carbons at the site of the beta carbon explains why the process is called beta oxidation.

Step 5. Steps 1–4 are repeated for each pair of carbons except the last, since the last unit formed is acetyl CoA itself. Therefore, the number of cycles that must be completed to oxidize the fat can be computed using the formula $n/2 - 1$ where n is the number of carbons. The acetyl CoA can enter the Krebs cycle and electron transport system (Figures 3.2, 3.8, and 3.9).

ATP Production from Fatty Acids

The number of ATP produced from the breakdown of fat depends on which fatty acid is utilized. The following example shows a calculation for palmitate.

Example
- - - - - - - - - - - - - - - -

Calculate the number of ATP produced from the breakdown of palmitate (palmitic acid).

The steps in the calculation follow

1. Palmitate is a 16-carbon fatty acid. Therefore, as noted in the previous step 5, it cycles through beta oxidation $n/2 - 1 = 16/2 - 1 = 7$ times.
2. Each cycle produces 1 $FADH_2$ and 1 $NADH + H^+$, as follows:

$FADH_2$	$\rightarrow$ FAD	2 ATP
$NADH + H^+$	$\rightarrow NAD^+$	+ 3 ATP
		5 ATP

This reaction happens 7 times: $7 \times 5 = 35$ ATP.

3. Each cycle (7) plus the last step (1) produces acetyl CoA, for a total of 8. Each acetyl CoA yields 1 ATP, 3 $NADH + H^+$, and 1 $FADH_2$ in the Krebs

cycle. The 3 $NADH + H^+$ will produce 9 ATP, and the $FADH_2$ will produce 2 ATP in the electron transport system. Thus, 12 ATP are produced for each acetyl CoA, for a total of 8 acetyl CoA $\times$ 12 ATP = 96 ATP.

4. Add the results of steps 2 and 3: 96 ATP + 35 ATP = 131 ATP. However, 1 ATP was utilized in step 1 of beta oxidation to activate the fatty acid. Furthermore, this ATP was broken down to AMP, not ADP; hence, the equivalent of 2 ATP were used. Subtracting this result from the total, we get 131 ATP − 2 ATP = 129 ATP from palmitate. ✛

Recall that three acids plus one glycerol make up a triglyceride. These calculations apply to a single specific fatty acid. It has been estimated that for the mixture that comprises human adipose tissue the ATP yield is 138 molecules of ATP per molecule of fatty acid. Complete the Question of Understanding box.

Ketone Bodies and Ketosis

As mentioned earlier, in order for the acetyl CoA produced by beta oxidation to enter the Krebs cycle, a sufficient amount of oxaloacetate is necessary. When carbohydrate supplies are sufficient, this is no problem, and fat is said to burn in the flame of carbohydrate. However, when carbohydrates are inadequate (perhaps as a result of fasting, prolonged exercise, or diabetes mellitus), oxaloacetate is converted to glucose. The production of glucose from noncarbohydrate sources under these conditions is necessary because some tissue, such as the brain and nervous system, rely predominantly on glucose as a fuel (Marieb, 2001).

When oxaloacetate is converted to glucose and is therefore not available to combine with acetyl CoA to form citrate, the liver converts the acetyl CoA derived from the fatty acids into metabolites called *ketones* or *ketone bodies*. Despite the similarity in the names, do not confuse these ketones with keto acids (pyruvic acid and the Krebs cycle intermediates) (Figure 3.8). There are three forms of ketones: acetoacetic acid, beta-hydroxybutyric acid, and acetone. All are strong acids. Acetone gives the breath a very characteristic fruity smell.

The ketone bodies can themselves be used as fuel by muscles, nerves, and the brain. If the

> ### A Question of Understanding
>
> To determine whether you understand the ATP yield from fatty acids, calculate the ATP produced from an 18-carbon fatty acid, such as stearate. Check your answer in Appendix D.

Table 3.2
Transamination and Oxidative Deamination

Transamination	Oxidative Deamination
Generalized	**Generalized**
Amino acid (1) and keto acid (1) $\longrightarrow$ amino acid (2) + keto acid (2).	Amino acid $\longrightarrow$ keto acid + NH_3.
The NH_2 group from amino acid (1) is transferred to keto acid (1), forming a different amino acid (2) and a different keto acid (2).	The NH_2 group is removed from an amino acid, forming a keto acid and ammonia.
Most Common	**Most Common**
Any one of 12 different amino acids + α-ketoglutarate $\longrightarrow$ glutamate + keto acid	Glutamate + H_2O + NAD^+ $\longrightarrow$ NH_3 + α-ketoglutarate + NADH + H^+
Specific Example	**Fate of Products**
Glutamate + pyruvate $\longrightarrow$ alanine + α-ketoglutarate	1. NADH + H^+ enters the electron transport system.
	2. α-ketoglutarate is a Krebs cycle intermediate.
	3. NH_3 (ammonia) is removed in urine. The urea cycle is $2NH_3 + CO_2 \rightarrow NH_2\,CONH_2$ (urea) + H_2O.

ketones are not used but, instead, accumulate, a condition called *ketosis* occurs. The high acidity of ketosis can disrupt normal physiological functioning, especially acid-base balance. Ketosis is more likely to result from an inadequate diet (as in anorexia nervosa) or diabetes than from prolonged exercise, since the muscles will use the ketones as fuel. During exercise aerobically trained individuals can utilize ketones more effectively than untrained individuals.

Protein Metabolism

Proteins are found in many food sources. *Proteins* are large molecules consisting of varying combinations of amino acids linked together. Approximately 20 amino acids occur naturally (Kapit, et al., 1987). Because there are so many ways these amino acids can combine, there is an almost infinite number of possible proteins. Like carbohydrates and fats, amino acids contain atoms of carbon, oxygen, and hydrogen. In addition, they may include sulfur, phosphorus, and iron. All amino acids have in common an amino group containing nitrogen (NH_2).

Proteins are extremely important in the structure and function of the body. Among other things they are components of hemoglobin, contractile elements of the muscle, hormones, fibrin for clotting, tendons, ligaments, and portions of all cell membranes. Because proteins are so important in the body, the constituent amino acids are used predominantly as building blocks, not as a source of energy.

However, amino acids can be, and in certain instances are, used as a fuel source. When amino acids are used as a fuel source, muscles appear to preferentially, but not exclusively, utilize the group of amino acids known as branched-chain amino acids (BCAA): leucine, isoleucine, and valine. In this situation, as with carbohydrate and fat metabolism, the final common pathways of the Krebs cycle, electron transport, and oxidative phosphorylation are utilized. The site of entry into the metabolic pathways varies, as shown in Figure 3.2, with the amino acid (Van de Graaff and Fox, 1989).

Six amino acids can enter metabolism at the level of pyruvic acid, 8 at acetyl CoA, 4 at alpha-ketoglutarate, 4 at succinate, 2 at fumarate, and 2 at oxaloacetate. All of these intermediates except acetyl CoA are, in turn, converted to pyruvate before being utilized to produce energy. The acetyl CoA is used directly in the Krebs cycle and electron transport, as previously described.

Transamination and Oxidative Deamination

Before amino acids can be used as a fuel and enter the pathways at any place, the nitrogen-containing amino group (the NH_2) must be removed. Removal is accomplished by the process of transamination and sometimes oxidative deamination (Frisell, 1982; Lehninger, 1971; Marieb, 2001; Newsholme and Leech, 1983; Van de Graaff and Fox, 1989). These processes are summarized in Table 3.2.

All but two amino acids appear to be able to undergo transamination. **Transamination** involves the

> **Transamination** The transfer of the NH_2 amino group from an amino acid to a keto acid.

transfer of the NH_2 amino group from an amino acid to a keto acid. Remember that keto acids include pyruvic acid, acetyl CoA, and the Krebs cycle intermediates. This process occurs in both the cytoplasm and the mitochondria, predominantly in muscle and liver cells. Transamination results in the formation of a new amino acid and a different keto acid. The most frequent keto acid acceptor of NH_2 is α-ketoglutarate, with glutamate being the amino acid formed (Marieb, 2001; Van de Graaff and Fox, 1989).

Two fates for glutamate are shown in Table 3.2. In the first glutamate is transaminated to alanine, another amino acid. Alanine, in turn, can be converted to glucose in a process called gluconeogenesis (Frisell, 1982; Marieb, 2001). **Gluconeogenesis** is the creation of glucose in the liver from noncarbohydrate sources, particularly glycerol, lactate or pyruvate, and alanine.

In the second process, glutamate undergoes oxidative deamination. In oxidative deamination, the oxidized form of NAD is reduced, and the amino group (NH_2) is removed and becomes NH_3. NH_3 is ammonia, and high concentrations in the body are extremely toxic. The dominant pathway for NH_3 removal is by conversion to urea in the liver (via the urea cycle) and excretion in urine by the kidneys. Oxidative deamination is used much less frequently than transamination.

ATP Production from Amino Acids

Because the amino acid derivatives are ultimately utilized as pyruvate or acetyl CoA, the ATP production count from the amino acids is the same as for glucose from that point on, except that it is not doubled (Péronnet, et al., 1987). Refer to Figure 3.5 to remind yourself why the double count occurred and to Figure 3.2 to see amino acids entering the pathways denoted next.

Pyruvate → acetyl CoA =	$1NADH + H^+$	3 ATP
Krebs cycle		1 ATP
ETS/OP	$3 NADH + H^+$	9 ATP
	$1 FADH_2$	2 ATP
		15 ATP

Acetyl CoA would produce 12 ATP, because the $NADH + H^+$ production from pyruvate to acetyl CoA would be the only step missing.

> **Gluconeogenesis** The creation of glucose in the liver from noncarbohydrate sources, particularly glycerol, lactate or pyruvate, and alanine.

The Regulation of Cellular Respiration and ATP Production

Intracellular

Intracellularly, the production of ATP—and, hence, the flow of substrates through the various metabolic pathways—is regulated predominantly by feedback mechanisms. As has been stated before, each step in each metabolic pathway is catalyzed by a specific enzyme. At least one of these enzymes in each pathway can be acted upon directly by other chemicals in the cell and, as a result, increases or decreases its activity. Such an enzyme is called a *rate-limiting enzyme,* and the other factors that influence it are called *modulators.* When the rate-limiting enzyme is inhibited, every step in the metabolic pathway beyond that point is also inhibited. When the rate-limiting enzyme is stimulated, every step in the metabolic pathway beyond that point is also stimulated.

The primary rate-limiting enzyme in glycolysis is phosphofructokinase (PFK), the enzyme that catalyzes step 3. PFK is stimulated, and subsequently the rate of glycolysis increased, by modulators such as ADP, AMP, P_i, and a rise in pH. ADP, AMP, and P_i modulators are the result of the breakdown of ATP. This is an example of a positive-feedback system in which the by-product of the utilization of a substance stimulates a greater production of that original substance. Conversely, PFK is inhibited, and subsequently the rate of glycolysis decreased, by the modulators ATP, CP, citrate (a Krebs cycle intermediate), FFA, and a drop in pH. Each of these modulators indicates that sufficient substances exist to supply ATP. This is an example of a negative-feedback system in which the formation of a product or other similarly acting product inhibits further production of the product (Newsholme and Leech, 1983).

The primary rate-limiting enzyme in the Krebs cycle is isocitrate dehydrogenase (ICD), which catalyzes step 3. ICD is stimulated by ADP, P_i, and calcium (positive feedback) and is inhibited by ATP (negative feedback) (Newsholme and Leech, 1983).

Cytochrome oxidase—which catalyzes the transfer of electrons to molecular oxygen, resulting in the formation of water—is the rate-limiting enzyme for the electron transport system. It is stimulated by ADP and P_i (positive feedback) and is inhibited by ATP (negative feedback) (Newsholme and Leech, 1983).

A pattern in the modulators is readily evident, with ATP, ADP, and P_i being universally important. When ATP is present in sufficient amounts to satisfy the needs of the cell and to provide some reserve in storage, there is no need to increase its production. Thus, key enzymes in the metabolic pathways are inhibited. However, when muscle activity begins and ATP is broken down into ADP and P_i, these by-products stimulate all

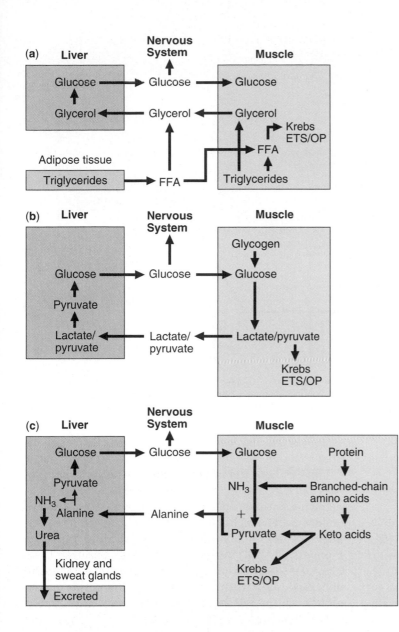

Figure 3.15
Gluconeogenesis

(a) Glycerol-glucose cycle, (b) Cori cycle, (c) Felig cycle.

the metabolic pathways to produce more ATP so that the muscle contractions can continue.

Extracellular

During exercise the metabolic processes must provide ATP for energy and maintain blood glucose levels at near-resting values for the proper functioning of the entire organism. This is because the brain and nervous tissue must have glucose as a fuel. One of the ways of maintaining glucose levels is by the process of gluconeogenesis.

Gluconeogenesis

As defined earlier, gluconeogenesis is the creation (*-genesis*) of new (*-neo*) glucose (*gluco-*) in the liver from noncarbohydrate sources. The primary fuel sources for gluconeogenesis are glycerol, lactate or pyruvate, and alanine. Glycerol is released into the bloodstream when triglycerides are broken down (Figure 3.15a).

Pyruvate is the end product of glycolysis. The majority of the pyruvate is converted to acetyl CoA and enters the Krebs cycle and electron transport system. However, a small portion diffuses out of the muscle cell and into the bloodstream (Péronnet, et al., 1987). Still another portion of the pyruvate (the actual amount depends on the intensity of the activity) is converted to lactate, which also diffuses into the bloodstream. About ten times as much lactate as pyruvate diffuses out of the muscle cells (Figure 3.15b).

Alanine is formed by transamination when the amino group from one amino acid (preferentially, the

Figure 3.16
Extracellular Neurohormonal
Regulation of Metabolism

Notes: TRH is thyroid-releasing hormone; ACTH
is adrenocorticotrophic hormone; GHRH is
growth hormone–releasing hormone; CRH is
corticotrophin-releasing
hormone; TSH is thyroid-stimulating hormone. ↓ decrease, ↑ increase.

Sources: Bunt, 1986; Marieb, 2001; Van de
Graaff & Fox, 1989.

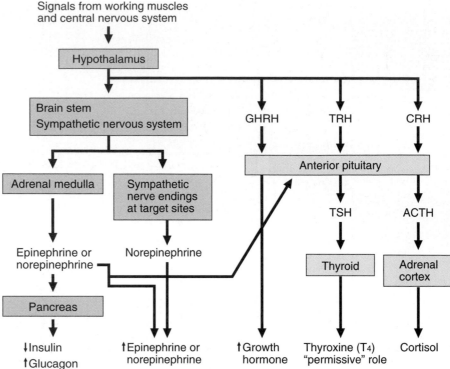

BCAA or an amino acid derived from glutamate) is transferred to pyruvate (Figure 3.15c). Note that in the liver alanine is first reconverted to pyruvate (freeing the NH_3 to enter the urea cycle and be excreted) before being converted to glucose.

In all cases the conversion to glucose takes place in the liver. For each gram of glucose produced 1.02 g of glycerol, 1.43 g of pyruvate, 1.23 g of lactate, or 1.45 g of alanine is utilized (Péronnet, et al., 1987).

The glycerol-glucose cycle has no special name, but the pyruvate/lactate-glucose cycle is known as the *Cori cycle,* and the alanine-glucose cycle is called the *Felig cycle.* The Cori and Felig cycles help maintain normal blood glucose levels so that the brain, nerves, and kidneys as well as the muscles may draw from this supply.

Neurohormonal Coordination

The regulation of blood glucose levels, including gluconeogenesis, is governed jointly by the autonomic nervous system (particularly the sympathetic division) and the endocrine system, which function in a coordinated fashion. Figure 3.16 shows this integration of the two control systems for the regulation of energy production in responding to exercise. Chapter 2 provides a comprehensive explanation of the functioning of the neurohormonal system.

When exercise begins, signals from the working muscles and motor centers in the central nervous

system bring about a neurohormonal response mediated through the hypothalamus. The hypothalamus stimulates both the anterior pituitary and the sympathetic nervous system. The neurotransmitter norepinephrine is released directly from sympathetic nerve endings, and the hormones epinephrine and norepinephrine are released from the adrenal medulla. Epinephrine and norepinephrine both act directly on fuel sites and stimulate the anterior pituitary and pancreas. As a result of the dual stimulation of the anterior pituitary, hormones are released—namely, growth hormone, cortisol, and thyroxine. The release of insulin is inhibited from the pancreas, but glucagon release is stimulated (Bunt, 1986; Galbo, 1983). In general, the result is threefold (see also Table 3.3):

1. An increase in the mobilization and utilization of free fatty acid stores from extramuscular (adipose tissue) and intramuscular stores.

2. An increase in the breakdown of extramuscular (liver) and intramuscular stores of glycogen and the creation of glucose from noncarbohydrate sources (gluconeogenesis) in the liver.

3. A decrease in the uptake of glucose into the nonworking cells.

A two-tier system of hormonal involvement appears to operate on the basis of time of response. The catecholamines (epinephrine and norepinephrine) and glucagon react to an increase in muscular activity

Table 3.3
Hormonal Regulation of Metabolism during Exercise

Effect	Glucagon	Epinephrine and Norepinephrine	Growth Hormone*	Cortisol
Glucose uptake and utilization	↓†		↓†	↓†
Glycogen breakdown (glycogenolysis)	↑	↑	↑	↑
Glycogen formation (glycogenesis)	↓	↓	↑	↑
Gluconeogenesis	↑	↑	↑	↑
FFA storage (lipogenesis)	↓		↓	↓
FFA mobilization (lipolysis)	↑	↑	↑	↑
Amino acid transport and uptake			↑	↑
Protein breakdown				↑

* Heavy exercise.   ↑ = Increases.
† Nonactive cells.   ↓ = Decreases.

in a matter of seconds to minutes. Both assist in all three functions listed. However, epinephrine's influence on fat metabolism is relatively slow (approximately 20 min) and far greater than its effect on glucose metabolism (Guyton, 1986).

The actions of epinephrine, norepinephrine, and glucagon are backed up by growth hormone and cortisol, respectively. The response of growth hormone and cortisol may take hours to become maximal. Thus, these latter two hormones are probably most important for carbohydrate conservation in long-duration activity. This result explains why they can bring about glycogen synthesis, which glucagon and the catecholamines do not (Guyton, 1986).

Insulin secretion is suppressed during exercise. This decrease in insulin and the increase in glucagon, growth hormone, and cortisol cause a decrease in the glucose uptake into cells other than the working muscles. The available glucose is thus spared for the working muscles and the nervous system.

During exercise the working muscles become highly permeable to glucose despite the lack of insulin. As previously noted, the muscle contraction itself stimulates GLUT-4 translocation to the cell surface for the movement of glucose into the working muscle (Houston, 1995; Sato, et al., 1996). The contractile process also helps to break down the intramuscular stores of glycogen and triglycerides (Galbo, 1983; Guyton, 1986).

The increases in protein breakdown and in amino acid transport caused by growth hormone and corti-

sol are important in providing protein precursors for gluconeogenesis. The fact that these hormones are slow responders also explains why protein is not used in significant amounts until long-duration activity.

Because the mobilization of free fatty acids involves the breakdown of triglycerides, glycerol is also released and made available for gluconeogenesis. Note that an accumulation of the other gluconeogenic precursor, lactate, will inhibit free fatty acid release from adipose tissue. Therefore, gluconeogenesis serves a dual purpose in helping to provide glucose and reducing the levels of lactate so that it does not interfere as much with fat utilization.

Thyroxine itself has a number of metabolic functions. However, its role in exercise metabolism appears to be one of potentiation or permissiveness. That is, it helps to create an environment in which the other metabolic hormones can function more effectively, rather than having any major effect itself.

The level of response and reaction to all of these hormones depends on the following:

1. the type, duration, and intensity of the exercise; relative intensity appears to be more important than the absolute workload;

2. the nutritional status, health, training status, and fiber type composition of the exerciser; and

3. the size of the fuel depots, the state of the hormone receptors, and the capacity of the involved enzymes (Galbo, 1983).

Focus on Application

✳ Metabolic Pathways: The Vitamin Connection

Many individuals mistakenly believe that vitamins are a source of energy in the human body. Although this is not true, vitamins do participate in many of the chemical reactions described in this chapter that convert the potential energy of food sources into ATP. You can't light a fire, even if you have plenty of the right kind and size of wood, without a way to produce a spark; neither can your body produce energy without vitamins. However, just as rubbing two sticks (the fuel source) together can produce the needed spark, so does the ingestion of a well balanced diet (the fuel source) provide the needed vitamins. On the other hand, too much wood added to the fire may be counterproductive and wasteful; similarly, the ingestion of excessive amounts of vitamins does not increase the activity of the enzymes for which the vitamins act as coenzymes. Listed below are the six vitamins that are particularly important for energy metabolism, their actions, and selected dietary sources (vanderBeek, 1985).   ✳

Vitamin	Function in Metabolism	Selected Dietary Sources
B₁ (thiamine)	Coenzyme involved in the conversion of pyruvate to acetyl CoA during carbohydrate metabolism	Lean meats, eggs, whole grains, leafy green vegetables, legumes
B₂ (riboflavin)	Basis of coenzyme FAD which serves as hydrogen acceptor in the mitochondria	Milk, eggs, lean meat, green vegetables
Niacin (nicotinamide)	Basis of coenzyme NAD which is the primary hydrogen carrier in both the cytoplasm and mitochondria	Lean meat, fish, legumes, whole grains, peanuts
B₆ (pyridoxine)	Functions as coenzyme in amino acid transamination reactions; required coenzyme for glycogenolysis action of the enzyme phosphorylase	Meat, poultry, fish, white and sweet potatoes, tomatoes, spinach
Pantothenic Acid	Functions as coenzyme A in the formation of acetyl CoA from pyruvate	Meat, legumes, whole grains, eggs
Biotin	Essential as coenzyme for a number of enzymes in the Krebs cycle and gluconeogenesis	Eggs, legumes, nuts

Fuel Utilization at Rest and during Exercise

The preceding discussion explained how each of the major fuel sources—fats, carbohydrates, and proteins—produces ATP energy for the human body. At rest, it has been estimated that fats contribute from 41–67%, carbohydrates from 33–42%, and proteins from just a trace to 17% of the total daily energy requirements of the human body (Lemon and Nagel, 1981).

During exercise various forms of each fuel are utilized to supply the working muscle with the additional ATP energy needed to sustain movement. In order to understand which energy sources are used during exercise, it is first necessary to know approximately how much of each energy substrate is available for use. Table 3.4 shows the tissue fuel stores in an average adult male who weighs 65 kg and has 8.45 kg (13%) body fat and 30 kg of muscle. Protein stores have been omitted because the major tissue storage of protein is in the muscles and complete degradation (breakdown) of muscle to sustain energy metabolism is neither realistic nor desirable under normal circumstances.

Several important points should be noted from Table 3.4. First, triglycerides provide the greatest source of potential energy (77,150 kcal is enough energy to sustain life for approximately 47 days!). Second, comparatively, very little carbohydrate is actually stored. In fact, the human body's stores of carbohydrate are only enough to support life for 1¼ days if all three sources (muscle glycogen, liver glycogen, and circulating glucose) are added together. Thus, carbohydrate replenishment on a regular basis is essential. Third, exercise has a major impact on how long each fuel can supply energy.

Table 3.4 assumes that each fuel is acting independently, which in fact never happens. Tables 3.5 and 3.6 provide more realistic views of what actually happens during exercise. Table 3.5 depicts the relative utilization of each substrate source as influenced by the type, intensity, and duration of the activity. Very short duration, very high-intensity dynamic activity and static contractions are special cases that rely predominantly on energy substrates stored in the muscle fibers—that is, ATP-PC and glycogen (which can quickly be broken down into ATP to provide energy).

Table 3.4
Tissue Fuel Stores in Average Adult Males (body weight = 65 kg, percent body fat = 13)

Tissue Fuel	Total Energy*			Estimated Period Fuel Would Supply Energy[†]		
	g	kJ	Kcal	Basal[‡] (days)	Walk[‡] (days)	Run[‡] (min)
Triglycerides[§] (fatty acids)	8,450	322,789	77,150	47.46	11.25	5223
Liver glycogen[‖]	80	1,275	305	0.19	0.05	20.7
Muscle glycogen (28.25 kg muscle[#])	425	7,384**	1,743**	1.07	0.25	118
Circulating glucose (blood + extracellular)	20	319	76	0.05	0.01	5.2

* Conversion factors utilized: glucose, 3.81 kcal·g^{-1}; fatty acid, 9.13 kcal·g^{-1}; kcal × 4.184 = kJ (Bursztein, et al., 1989; Péronnet, et al., 1987).

[†] Calculations assume that each fuel is the only fuel utilized. In reality, the fuels are utilized with mixtures that depend on the type, intensity, and duration of the activity and the training, fiber type proportions, and nutritional status of the exerciser.

[‡] Kilocalorie cost of exercise: basal 0.174 kcal·kg^{-1}·10 min^{-1} walking at 3.5 mi·hr^{-1} = 0.733 kcal·kg^{-1}·10 min^{-1}; running at 8.7 mi·hr^{-1} (6:54 mile) = 2.273 kcal·10 min^{-1} (Consolazio, et al., 1963).

[§] 65 kg body weight × 0.13 (fraction of body fat) = 8.45 kg fat.

[‖] Liver equals approximately 2.5% body weight. Normal glycogen content is 50 g·kg^{-1}; extracellular glucose includes the portion in liver available to circulation (Péronnet, et al., 1987).

[#] Weight of the muscle is approximately equal to half the lean body mass.

** Muscle fatty acid values would equal this value because 1 kg of muscle contains approximately 13.5 g fatty acid and 1.5 g glycerol. The triglyceride value includes the muscle store (Péronnet, et al., 1987).

Sources: Based on Kapit, et al. (2000); Newsholme & Leech (1983).

Table 3.5
Relative Degree of Fuel Utilization in Muscle for Various Types of Exercise

Fuel	Exercise Condition					
	Rest	Very High-Intensity, Very Short Duration (< 3 min), and Static Contractions	High-Intensity (80–85% max), Short-Duration (< 40 min)	High-Intensity (70–80% max), Moderate-Duration (40–150 min)	Moderate-Intensity (60–70% max), Long-Duration (> 150 min)	Low-Intensity (< 50% max), Long-Duration (> 150 min)
Muscle glycogen	Negligible	High	High	High	Moderate	Low
Liver glycogen/ blood glucose	Moderate	Negligible	High	High	Moderate	Moderate
Free fatty acid (FFA)	Moderate	Negligible	Low	Moderate	High	High
Amino acid	Low	Negligible	Negligible	Low	Low	Low

Sources: Based on Felig & Wahren (1975); Pernow & Saltin (1971).

Focus on Research

Sex Differences in Substrate Utilization

Friedlander, A. L., G. A. Casazza, M. A. Horning, M. J. Huie, M. F. Piacentini, J. K. Trimmer, & G. A. Brooks: Training-induced alterations of carbohydrate metabolism in women: Women respond differently from men. *Journal of Applied Physiology* 85(3):1175–1186 (1998).

The data presented in Tables 3.5 and 3.6 show variations not only in the reliance on carbohydrate, fat, and protein substrates based on exercise intensity, but also among the various components of carbohydrate used as a fuel (glucose, and muscle and liver glycogen). Data from this study by Friedlander, et al., demonstrate that there might also be meaningful variations among fuel substrates between the sexes. Substrate utilization in young adult males and females was determined at rest and at 45% $\dot{V}O_2$peak and 65% $\dot{V}O_2$peak exercise intensities on a cycle ergometer. Although only those comparisons marked with an asterisk (*) in the accompanying graphs attained statistical significance, the overall pattern that can be seen in panel (a) is that carbohydrates provided a higher percentage of the total energy supply for males than for females. Conversely, the pattern in panel (b) shows that the females used relatively more glucose than other carbohydrate sources (presumably glycogen and lactate) than did the males. Both of these trends were true at rest before and after training, at the two submaximal power outputs pretraining (45% UT and 65% UT), at the same absolute power output pretraining and posttraining (65% UT and 65% TR), and at the new relative power output posttraining (65% TR).

The mechanism to explain these differences is unknown. However, the authors speculate that hormonal differences may have been the cause. Factors that may influence these differences include the amount of circulating epinephrine (although these values did not differ between the males and females in this study), receptor availability and affinity for epinephrine (which was not tested), or the interaction of other circulating hormones, especially estrogen and progesterone (higher, of course, in the females) with epinephrine. It is also possible, because many of the differences were significant only after training, that the sympathetic nervous system in males and females may adapt differently to exercise training.

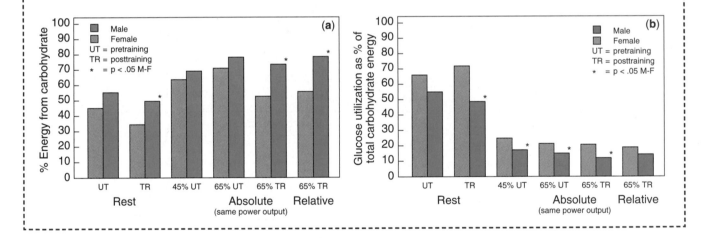

Table 3.6
Fuel Utilization by 70-kg Male Runner at Different Distances and Levels of Performance

	10 km (6.2 mi)		42.2 km (26.2 mi)	
	Fast	Slow	Fast	Slow
Performance	0:30:00	1:00:00	2:21:00	5:12:00
Circulating glucose (g)	9.7	13.4	120.5	217.8
Muscle glycogen (g)	149.0	134.0	403.0	69.0
Liver glycogen (g)	20.1	10.9	73.7	103.9
Fatty acids (g)	7.0	12.0	104.0	229.0
Branched-chain amino acids (g) (BCAA)	0.7	0.9	15.7	48.5

Source: Péronnet, et al. (1987).

The other exercises listed in Table 3.5 are assumed to be predominantly dynamic and to a large extent aerobic (utilizing oxygen). In general, the lower the intensity, the more important fat is as a fuel; the higher the intensity, the more important carbohydrates are as fuel. Duration has a similar effect in that the shorter the duration, the more important carbohydrates are as a fuel, with fat being utilized more and more as the duration lengthens. Fats come into play over the long term because the glycogen stores can and will be depleted. Indeed, long-duration activities often exhibit a three-part sequence in which muscle glycogen, bloodborne glucose (including glucose that has been broken down from liver glycogen and glucose that has been created by gluconeogenesis), and fatty acids successively predominate as the major fuel source. Protein may account for 5–15% of the total energy supply in activities lasting more than an hour (Felig and Wharen, 1975; Lemon and Nagel, 1981; Pernow and Saltin, 1971).

Table 3.6 provides an estimation of how fuel utilization varies by race distance [10 km (6.2 mi) and 42.2 km (26.2 mi), or marathon distance] and performance (a "fast" and a "slow" time for each distance). Compare the muscle glycogen utilization in the fast and the slow conditions. At the short distance (less than 1 hr) there is not much difference, but during the marathon almost six times as much muscle glycogen is used by the faster runner. Conversely, the greatest amount of fat is utilized by the slow marathoner. Circulating glucose use is much higher in marathoners because the longer duration and lower intensity permit the liver to generate (by gluconeogenesis) and release glucose into the bloodstream. The 10-km runner has sufficient muscle glycogen stores and does not need to rely on external glucose production. Very little protein (BCAA) is used by either of the 10-km runners, but a small amount provides some energy for the marathoners.

A complex interaction exists between exercise energy needs and the fuel sources that provide this energy within the human organism.

Summary

1. The process by which ATP is formed from food is called cellular respiration.

2. Carbohydrate metabolism consists of four stages that convert glucose or glycogen into carbon dioxide, water, and ATP energy.

3. Stage I of carbohydrate metabolism is known as glycolysis. Glycolysis consists of a series of 10 or 11 steps; it occurs in the cytoplasm of cells and is anaerobic. It begins with glucose or glycogen and ends with pyruvate (pyruvic acid) or lactate (lactic acid). In the process a net gain of 2 ATP is achieved by substrate-level phosphorylation if the fuel was glucose and 3 ATP if the fuel was glycogen. A pair of NADH + H$^+$ also result.

IP *Muscular–Metabolism* (pages 11–18)

4. Stage II of carbohydrate metabolism has no identifying name, but it results in the formation of acetyl coenzyme A from pyruvate. These two steps occur in the mitochondrial matrix; although no oxygen is used directly, the process must be aerobic. No ATP is produced, but two pairs of hydrogen atoms are released and picked up by NAD$^+$, forming NADH + H$^+$.

IP *Muscular–Muscle Metabolism* (page 19)

5. Stage III of carbohydrate metabolism is the Krebs cycle (sometimes known as the citric acid cycle). This stage consists of eight steps and also occurs in the mitochondrial matrix; again, no oxygen is used directly, but it also must be aerobic. Two ATP are produced by substrate-level phosphorylation and pairs of hydrogen atoms are removed at four separate steps. In three cases the hydrogens are picked up by NAD$^+$ and in the fourth by FAD.

IP *Muscular–Metabolism* (pages 20–22)

6. Stage IV of carbohydrate metabolism is known as electron transport and oxidative phosphorylation. Electron transport takes place in the inner mitochondrial membrane and, as the name implies, consists of relaying electrons from the hydrogen atoms from one protein carrier to another and transporting the remaining hydrogen ions into the intermembrane space. In the process an electrical current is created. This electrical energy is then used to synthesize ATP from ADP by the addition of a phosphate as the H$^+$ move through the ball-and-stalk apparatus into the mitochondrial matrix. For each hydrogen carried to the electron transport system by NAD$^+$, 3 ATP are formed. For each hydrogen carried by FAD to the electron transport chain, 2 ATP are formed.

7. A total of 36 ATP are produced if the fuel substrate is glucose and the muscle is skeletal. A total of 37 ATP are produced if the fuel substrate is glycogen and the muscle is skeletal. A total of 38 ATP are produced if the fuel substrate is glucose and the muscle is cardiac. A total of 39 ATP are produced if the fuel substrate is glycogen and the muscle is cardiac.

8. Triglycerides stored in adipose cells or stored intramuscularly are the major storage form of energy in humans. Triglycerides are composed of fatty acids and glycerol. Muscle cells can only use fatty acids as a fuel.

9. Fatty acid can only be utilized as a fuel source aerobically within the mitochondria. Fatty acids must undergo the process of beta oxidation—which involves the removal of hydrogen atoms (oxidation) and the removal of pairs of carbons (at the beta carbon location) to form acetyl coenzyme A—before entering the Krebs cycle and electron transport.

10. The ATP produced from each fatty acid depends upon the number of carbon pairs. For the mixture that comprises human adipose tissue the ATP yield is 138 molecules of ATP per molecule of fatty acids.

11. When glucose supplies are inadequate and oxaloacetate must be converted to glucose, the acetyl coenzyme A derived from fatty acids is converted into three forms of ketones: acetoacetic acid, beta-hydroxybutyric acid, and acetone. Acetone gives the breath a characteristic fruity smell.

12. Amino acids are used primarily in anabolic processes in human cells, building proteins such as hemoglobin and the contractile elements of muscle. However, amino acids—and especially the branched-chain amino acids (valine, leucine, and isoleucine)—can be used as a fuel source and may contribute as much as 5–15% of the energy supply in long term, dynamic endurance activity.

13. All amino acids contain an amino group (NH_2). Before an amino acid can be used as a fuel, this amino group must be removed. Removal of the amino group is accomplished by two processes: oxidative deamination or transamination (most common). Entry into the Krebs cycle and electron transport then occur at several locations, but ultimately all of the intermediates except acetyl CoA are converted to pyruvate before being used to produce energy.

14. Fifteen ATP are derived from each of the amino acid derivatives utilized as pyruvate, and 12 ATP are produced from each derivative utilized as acetyl CoA.

15. ATP energy production has both intracellular and extracellular regulation. Intracellular regulation operates primarily by the feedback stimulation (by ADP, AMP, P_i, and a rise in pH) or inhibition (by ATP, CP, citrate, and a drop in pH) of the rate-limiting enzyme. Extracellular regulation is achieved by the coordinated action of the sympathetic nervous system (via norepinephrine) and the hormonal system (norepinephrine, epinephrine, glucagon, cortisol, growth hormone, and cortisol).

16. The goal of metabolism during exercise is threefold:
    a. To increase the mobilization and utilization of free fatty acid from adipose tissue and intramuscular stores.
    b. To decrease the uptake of glucose into nonworking muscle cells while at the same time providing glucose for nerve and brain cells.
    c. To increase the breakdown of liver and muscle stores of glycogen and create glucose from noncarbohydrate sources in the liver.

17. The creation of glucose from noncarbohydrate sources is called gluconeogenesis. The primary fuel sources for gluconeogenesis are glycerol, lactate or pyruvate, and alanine.

18. Fatty acids comprise the largest fuel supply. Other fuels, in descending order, are total muscle glycogen, liver glycogen, and circulating glucose.

19. Which energy substrate is utilized and in what amounts depends upon the complex interaction of the type, duration, and intensity of exercise; the proportion of muscle fiber types involved; and the training status, long-term nutritional state, and short-term dietary status of the exerciser.

20. In general, very short duration, high-intensity dynamic activity and static contractions are special cases that rely predominantly on the ATP-PC and glycogen stored in the muscle fibers.

21. In dynamic aerobic activity the higher the intensity, the more important carbohydrates (glucose and glycogen) are as a fuel; the lower the intensity, the more important fats are as a fuel. Likewise, the shorter the duration, the more important carbohydrates are as a fuel; the longer the duration, the more that fat is utilized. In activities lasting more than an hour, protein makes a small but important contribution to the energy supply.

Review Questions

1. Distinguish between anabolism and catabolism. Is cellular respiration anabolic or catabolic?

2. Name and briefly summarize the four steps of carbohydrate metabolism.

3. Explain how a count of 36 ATP is achieved by cellular respiration if the fuel substrate is glucose in skeletal muscle. Why is the ATP count from carbohydrate sometimes 37, 38, or 39 instead of 36?

4. Why is beta oxidation necessary before fat can be used as an energy substrate? Describe what occurs during beta oxidation.

5. State how the calculation is completed to determine the number of ATP produced from fatty acids. Complete an example using a fat having 24 carbons.

6. Name and describe the process that amino acids must undergo before being used as a fuel substrate. Why is this process necessary?

7. Identify the locations in the metabolic pathways where amino acids may enter. How does the ATP count differ between these locations?

8. Why is acetyl coenzyme A called the universal common intermediate?

9. Why would the breath of someone suffering from anorexia nervosa smell sweet?

10. Describe the role of enzymes in the metabolic pathways. Identify the rate-limiting enzymes in Stages I, III, and IV of carbohydrate metabolism. How are enzymes regulated?

11. What are the goals of metabolic regulation during exercise? How are these goals achieved by the interaction of the sympathetic nervous system and the hormonal system?

12. Compare the relative availability and use of carbohydrate, fat, and protein fuel substrates on the basis of intensity and duration of exercise.

For further review and additional study tools, go to The Physiology Place (www.physiologyplace.com) and the Student Study Guide for Exercise Physiology for Health, Fitness, and Performance *by Sharon A. Plowman and Denise L. Smith.*

Passport to the Internet

Visit the following Internet sites to explore further topics and issues related to understanding energy production. To visit an organization's web site, go to www.physiologyplace.com and click on "Passport to the Internet."

Metabolic Pathways of Biochemistry   This site provides graphic representation of all major metabolic pathways. The site serves as a thorough resource for students and researchers alike. Visit to explore many of the concepts discussed in this book.

The Biology Project   Developed by the University of Arizona, the Biology Project is an interactive online resource for studying biology that provides very useful information on energy production. The site contains numerous problem sets designed to provide a basic understanding of the fundamental biological concepts. Enter the "Biochemistry" area and click on "Metabolism," listed under "Energy Reactions." Work your way through each of the problem sets to review your knowledge of metabolism.

References

Brooks, G. A., T. D. Fahey, T. P. White, & K. M. Baldwin: *Exercise Physiology: Human Bioenergetics and Its Applications* (3rd edition). Mountain View, CA: Mayfield (1999).

Bunt, J. C.: Hormonal alterations due to exercise. *Sports Medicine.* 3(5):331–345 (1986).

Bursztein, S., D. H. Elwyn, J. Askanazi, & J. M. Kinney: *Energy Metabolism, Indirect Calorimetry and Nutrition.* Baltimore: Williams & Wilkins (1989).

Consolazio, C. F., R. E. Johnson, & L. J. Pecora: *Physiological Measurements of Metabolic Functions in Man.* New York: McGraw-Hill (1963).

Felig, P., & J. Wahren: Fuel homeostasis in exercise. *New England Journal of Medicine.* 293(4):1078–1084 (1975).

Frisell, W. R.: *Human Biochemistry.* New York: Macmillan (1982).

Galbo, H.: *Hormonal and Metabolic Adaptation to Exercise.* New York: Thieme-Stratton (1983).

Guyton, A. C.: *Textbook of Medical Physiology* (7th edition). Philadelphia: Saunders (1986).

Houston, M. E.: *Biochemistry Primer for Exercise Science.* Champaign, IL: Human Kinetics (1995).

Kapit, W., R. I. Macey, & E. Meisami: *The Physiology Coloring Book.* New York: Harper & Row (1987).

Lehninger, A. L.: *Bioenergetics* (2nd edition). Menlo Park, CA: Benjamin (1971).

Lemon, P. W. R., & F. J. Nagel: Effects of exercise on protein and amino acid metabolism. *Medicine and Science in Sports and Exercise.* 13(3):141–149 (1981).

MacLean, P. S., D. Zheng, & G. L. Dohm: Muscle glucose transporter (GLUT 4) gene expression during exercise. *Exercise and Sport Sciences Reviews.* 28(4): 148–152 (2000).

Malina, R. M., & C. Bouchard: *Growth, Maturation and Physical Activity.* Champaign, IL: Human Kinetics (1991).

Marieb, E. N.: *Human Anatomy and Physiology* (5th edition). San Francisco: Benjamin Cummings (2001).

Newsholme, E. A., & A. R. Leech: *Biochemistry for the Medical Sciences.* New York: John Wiley (1983).

Pernow, B., & B. Saltin (eds.): *Muscle Metabolism During Exercise.* New York: Plenum (1971).

Péronnet, F., G. Thibault, M. Ledoux, & G. Brisson: *Performance in Endurance Events: Energy Balance, Nutrition, and Temperature Regulation in Distance Running.* London, Ontario, Canada: Spodym (1987).

Salway, J. G.: *Metabolism at a Glance.* Oxford, England: Blackwell Science (1994).

Sato, Y., Y. Oshida, I. Ohsawa, N. Nakai, Ohsaki, K. Yamanouchi, J. Sato, Y. Shimomura, & H. Ohno: The role of glucose transport in the regulation of glucose transport by muscle. In R. J. Maughm & S. M. Shirreffs (eds.), *Biochemistry of Exercise IX.* Champaign, IL: Human Kinetics (1996).

vanderBeek, E. J.: Vitamins and endurance training: Food for thought for running, or faddish claims? *Sports Medicine* 2:175–197 (1985).

Van de Graaff, K. M., & S. I. Fox: *Concepts of Human Anatomy and Physiology* (2nd edition). Dubuque, IA: Wm. C. Brown (1989).

Chapter 4

Anaerobic Metabolism
during Exercise

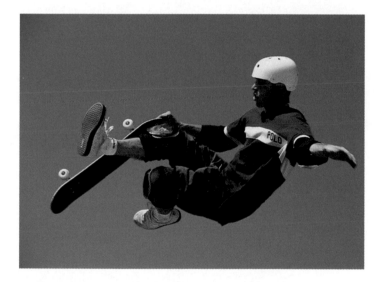

After studying the chapter, you should be able to

- Describe the energy continuum as it relates to varying durations of maximal maintainable exercise.

- Provide examples of sports or events within sports in which the ATP-PC, lactic, or oxygen system predominates.

- List the major variables that are typically measured to describe the anaerobic response to exercise and, where appropriate, the actual exercise test itself.

- Explain the physiological reasons why lactate may accumulate in the blood.

- Distinguish between the power and the capacity of the ATP-PC, lactic, and oxygen systems.

- Identify the oxygen deficit and excess postexercise oxygen consumption, and explain the causes of each.

- Describe the changes in ATP and PC that occur during constant-load, heavy exercise lasting 3 min or less.

- Describe the changes in lactate accumulation that occur during constant-load, high-intensity, anaerobic exercise lasting 3 min or less; short-term, light to moderate, and moderate to heavy submaximal aerobic exercise; long-term moderate to heavy submaximal aerobic exercise, during incremental exercise to maximum, and dynamic resistance exercise.

- Differentiate between the terms *anaerobic threshold, ventilatory threshold,* and *lactate threshold;* and explain why *anaerobic threshold* is a misnomer.

- Discuss why the accumulation of lactate is a physiological and performance problem.

- Explain the fate of lactate during exercise and recovery.

- Compare anaerobic metabolism during exercise for males versus females; children and adolescents versus young and middle-aged adults; and the elderly versus young and middle-aged adults.

- Identify the impact of genetics on anaerobic characteristics.

The Energy Continuum

Chapter 3 explained how ATP, the ultimate energy source for all human work, is produced in the metabolic pathways. The emphasis there was on the energy substrate (carbohydrate, fat, or protein) that was utilized as a fuel. This chapter and the next will look at ATP production and utilization on the basis of the need for oxygen. Anaerobic metabolism does not require oxygen to produce ATP, but aerobic metabolism does. Critical to understanding anaerobic and aerobic exercise metabolism is the fact that these processes are not mutually exclusive; that is, anaerobic metabolism and aerobic metabolism are not either/or situations in terms of how ATP is provided. Both systems can and usually do work concurrently. When describing muscular exercise, the terms *aerobic* or *anaerobic* refer to which system predominates.

Figure 4.1 reviews the three sources of ATP introduced in Chapter 3. Figure 4.1a describes *alactic anaerobic metabolism,* sometimes called the *phosphagen* or *ATP-PC system.* Once ATP has been produced, it is stored in the muscle. This amount is relatively small and can provide energy for only 1–2 sec of maximal effort. However, another high-energy compound, phosphocreatine (PC), also known as creatine phosphate (CP), can be used to resynthesize ATP from ADP instantaneously. The amount of PC in muscle is about three times that of ATP (Gollnick and King, 1969). Muscles differ in the amount of stored PC by fiber type. Muscle fiber types are fully described in Chapter 19, but briefly, fibers that produce energy predominantly by anaerobic glycolysis are called *glycolytic;* those that produce energy predominantly aerobically are called *oxidative.* Glycolytic fibers are also fast twitch; oxidative fibers are primarily slow twitch. Fast-twitch fibers have proportionally more PC than ATP compared to slow-twitch oxidative fibers. Any time the energy demand is increased—whether the activity is simply turning a page of this book, coming out of the blocks for a sprint, or starting out on a long bicycle ride—at least part of the immediate need for energy is supplied by these stored forms, which must ultimately be replenished. These sources are also used preferentially in high-intensity, very short duration activity. Together, the ATP-PC supply can support slightly less than 10 sec of maximal activity. This ATP-PC system neither uses oxygen nor produces lactic acid and is thus said to be *alactic anaerobic.*

Figure 4.1b represents *anaerobic glycolysis,* also called the *lactic acid (LA) system.* When the demands for ATP exceed the capacity of the phosphagen system and the aerobic system (at the initiation of any activity or during high-intensity, short-duration exercise), anaerobic (fast) glycolysis is utilized. This is rather like

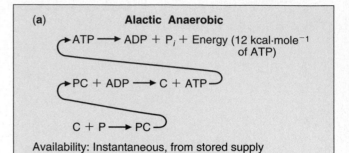

(a) **Alactic Anaerobic**

$$ATP \longrightarrow ADP + P_i + Energy\ (12\ kcal \cdot mole^{-1}$$
$$of\ ATP)$$

$$PC + ADP \longrightarrow C + ATP$$

$$C + P \longrightarrow PC$$

Availability: Instantaneous, from stored supply

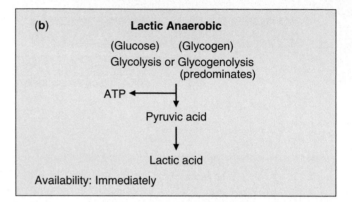

(b) **Lactic Anaerobic**

(Glucose)   (Glycogen)
Glycolysis or Glycogenolysis
(predominates)

ATP ←

Pyruvic acid

↓

Lactic acid

Availability: Immediately

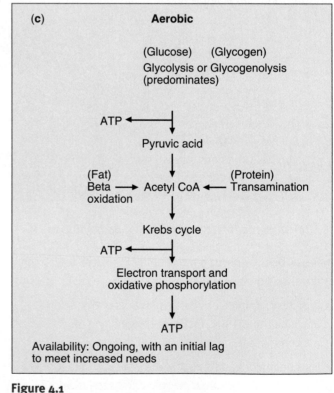

(c) **Aerobic**

(Glucose)   (Glycogen)
Glycolysis or Glycogenolysis
(predominates)

ATP ←

Pyruvic acid

↓

(Fat)   (Protein)
Beta → Acetyl CoA ← Transamination
oxidation

↓

Krebs cycle

ATP ←

Electron transport and
oxidative phosphorylation

↓

ATP

Availability: Ongoing, with an initial lag
to meet increased needs

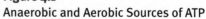

Figure 4.1
Anaerobic and Aerobic Sources of ATP

calling in the reserves, for glycolysis can provide the supplemental energy quickly. This system makes such activities as a 1500-m speed skating event possible.

Focus on Application

✳ Creatine as an Ergogenic Aid

Because of its role in the rephosphorylation of ATP from ADP and the theoretical impact this might have on performance and fatigue resistance, creatine (primarily in the form of creatine monohydrate) has enjoyed unprecedented popularity as an ergogenic aid. It has been established that oral creatine supplementation can increase muscle phosphocreatine (PC) content by approximately 20%, depending on an individual's starting level. There is an upper limit for storage, so if an individual is already at that point ($\sim$160 mmol·kg^{-1} of dry muscle) supplementation will not further increase storage. Excess ingested creatine is excreted in the urine (American College of Sports Medicine [ACSM], 2000; Zoeller, 1998). This can explain why one individual might respond to creatine monohydrate supplementation and another be a "nonresponder."

Despite numerous studies, the effectiveness of creatine supplementation has not been established. An American College of Sports Medicine Roundtable consensus statement concluded that the majority (approximately two-thirds) of the studies reviewed that measured muscular force and/or power output during short bouts of maximal exercise in healthy young (18–35 yr) adults (almost exclusively males) showed an enhancement. The greatest improvement in performance seemed to be found in the later bouts of a repetitive series of exercises in which the high power output lasted only a matter of seconds separated by rest periods of 20–60 sec (ACSM, 2000). These increases have been seen largely in average power outputs, however, not in peak power outputs (Zoeller, 1998). A number of studies have also indicated that creatine supplementation, along with heavy resistance training, enhances the normal training adaptation (ACSM, 2000). However, when a mathematical analysis (called a meta-analysis) was conducted of studies that tested anaerobic performance, creatine supplementation showed no significant improvements for fatigue resistance, power, speed, strength, or total work (Misic, et al., 2000).

As with any supplement, concerns have been expressed regarding the safety of creatine ingestion. Two credible reviews have concluded that although there have been numerous anecdotal reports of gastrointestinal disturbances (nausea/vomiting/diarrhea), liver and kidney dysfunction, cardiovascular/thermal impairment, and muscular damage (cramps/strains), the supporting evidence, with a few notable exceptions, is not definitive. The most notable exceptions involved documented medical case reports of individuals with preexisting kidney problems that were aggravated with creatine supplementation and resolved when the supplementation was stopped. The following precautions are advised (ACSM, 2000; Poortmans and Francaux, 2000):

1. Individuals with preexisting kidney dysfunction or those at high risk for kidney disease (for example, diabetics and individuals with a family history of kidney disease) should either avoid creatine supplementation or undergo regular medical monitoring. Regular check-ups are recommended for everyone taking creatine because any individual may react adversely to any substance, and excess creatine is a burden that must be eliminated by the kidneys.
2. Individuals wishing to maintain or decrease body weight while participating in strenuous exercise should avoid creatine supplementation.
3. High-dose creatine supplementation should be avoided during periods of physical activity under high thermal stress.
4. Adequate fluid and electrolytes should always be ingested.
5. Individuals under the age of 18 should not supplement with creatine.
6. Pregnant or lactating females should not supplement with creatine.
7. The ingestion of creatine during exercise should be avoided. ✳

Sources:

American College of Sports Medicine Roundtable (2000); Misic, et al. (2000); Poortmans & Francaux (2000); Zoeller & Angelopoulos (1998).

That is the benefit. The cost is that the production of lactic acid often exceeds clearance, and lactate accumulates. Because this system does not involve the utilization of oxygen but does result in the production of lactic acid, it is said to be *lactic anaerobic.*

Figure 4.1c shows *aerobic oxidation,* also termed the *O_2 system.* The generation of ATP from aerobic (slow) glycolysis, the Krebs cycle, and electron transport–oxidative phosphorylation is constantly in operation at some level. Under resting conditions this

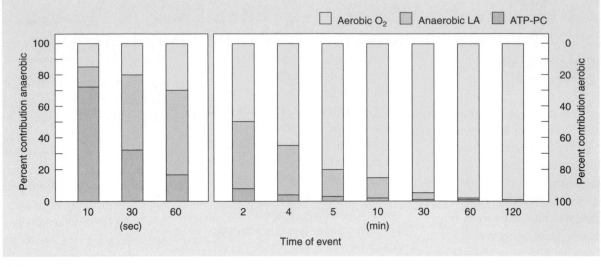

Figure 4.2
Time-Energy System Continuum

Approximate relative contributions of aerobic and anaerobic energy production at maximal maintainable intensity for varying durations.

Note: The graphs assume 100% $\dot{V}O_2$max at 10 min; 95% $\dot{V}O_2$max at 30 min; 85% $\dot{V}O_2$max at 60 min; and 80% $\dot{V}O_2$max at 120 min. ATP-PC ≤ 10 s.

Sources: Åstrand & Rodahl (1977); Gollnick & Hermansen (1973).

system provides basically all of the energy needed. When activity begins or occurs at moderate levels of intensity, oxidation increases quickly and proceeds at a rate that supplies the needed ATP. If the workload is continuously incremented, aerobic oxidation proceeds at a correspondingly higher rate until its maximal limit is reached. The highest amount of oxygen the body can consume during heavy dynamic exercise for the aerobic production of ATP is called *maximal oxygen uptake,* or $\dot{V}O_2$max. Because $\dot{V}O_2$max is primarily an index of cardiorespiratory capacity, it is discussed in depth in that unit. However, because $\dot{V}O_2$max reflects the amount of oxygen available for the aerobic production of ATP, it is also an important metabolic measure. Both aerobic and anaerobic exercises are often described in terms of a given percentage of $\dot{V}O_2$max (either less than or greater than 100% $\dot{V}O_2$max). Anaerobic metabolic processes are important at the onset of all aerobic exercise, contribute significantly at submaximal levels, and increase their contribution as the exercise intensity gets progressively higher. Depending on an individual's fitness level, lactic anaerobic metabolism begins to make a significant contribution to dynamic activity at approximately 40–60% $\dot{V}O_2$max. However, even then the ability to process oxygen is most important. Because the aerobic system does involve the use of oxygen and proceeds completely to oxidative phosphorylation, it is said to be *aerobic* or *oxidative*.

These three sources of ATP—the phosphagen system (ATP-PC), the glycolytic system (LA), and the oxidative system (O_2)—are recruited in a specific sequence called the *time-energy system continuum*. This continuum assumes that the individual is working at a maximal maintainable intensity for a continuous duration. This means that it is assumed that an individual can go all out for 5 min or less or can work at 100% $\dot{V}O_2$max for 10 min, at 95% $\dot{V}O_2$max for 30 min, at 85% $\dot{V}O_2$max for 60 min, and at 80% $\dot{V}O_2$max for 120 min. Of course, there are individual differences, but these assumptions are reasonable in general.

Figure 4.2 indicates the relative contributions of each of the energy systems to the total energy requirement under these conditions. These values are estimates that sometimes overlap but that do provide general trends as well as some specific values (Åstrand and Rodahl, 1977; Gollnick and Hermansen, 1973). For example, during an all-out event that lasts 30 sec, the dominant metabolism is anaerobic (80%), with approximately 33% being provided by the ATP-PC system and 47% by the LA system. Which system predominates during an event which takes 5 min and what are the percentages? If you take time to analyze the graph, you should discover that the breakdown at 5 min is a mirror image of what occurs at 30 sec. Now 80% of the energy is provided by aerobic oxidative metabolism and only 20% by anaerobic metabolism, split 3% ATP-PC and 17% LA.

Four basic patterns can be discerned from this continuum. Understanding these patterns will be helpful later for developing training programs.

1. All three energy systems (ATP-PC, LA, O_2) are involved in providing energy for all durations of exercise.

2. The ATP-PC system predominates in activities lasting 10 sec or less and still contributes at least 8% of the energy supply for maximal activities up to 2 min in length. Since the ATP-PC system is involved primarily at the onset of longer activities, it becomes a smaller portion of the total energy supply as the duration gets longer.

3. Anaerobic metabolism (ATP-PC and LA) predominates in supplying energy for exercises lasting less than 2 min. However, even exercises lasting as long as 10 min utilize at least 15% anaerobic sources. Within the anaerobic component the longer the duration, the greater the relative importance of the lactic acid system is in comparison to the phosphagen system.

4. By 5 min of exercise, the O_2 system is clearly the dominant system. The longer the duration, the more important it becomes.

The rest of this chapter will concentrate on the anaerobic contribution to energy metabolism. Chapter 5 will concentrate on the aerobic contribution to energy metabolism, although again it must be emphasized that the two systems work together, with one or the other predominating based primarily on the duration and intensity of the activity.

Alactic Anaerobic PC Production

As previously described, alactic anaerobic production of ATP involves the use of phosphocreatine (PC), which is simply creatine bound to inorganic phosphate. An adult human has a creatine level of approximately 120–125 mmol·kg^{-1} of dry muscle, although there is considerable individual variation from a low of 90–100 mmol·kg^{-1} to a high of about 150–160 mmol·kg^{-1}. Each day approximately 2 grams of creatine are degraded in a nonreversible reaction to creatinine. This creatinine is ultimately excreted by the kidneys in urine. The individual counterbalances this loss under normal dietary conditions by ingesting about 1 gram of creatine from meat, poultry, and/or fish and synthesizing another gram in the liver from the amino acids arginine, glycine, and methionine. Close to 95% of the creatine in the body is stored in skeletal muscle. Thirty to 40% is stored as free creatine and the rest as phosphocreatine.

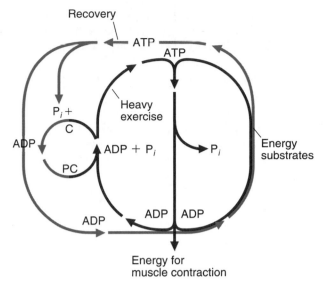

Figure 4.3
Use and Regeneration of ATP-PC

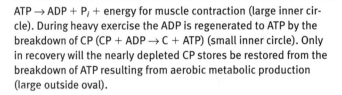

ATP → ADP + P$_i$ + energy for muscle contraction (large inner circle). During heavy exercise the ADP is regenerated to ATP by the breakdown of CP (CP + ADP → C + ATP) (small inner circle). Only in recovery will the nearly depleted CP stores be restored from the breakdown of ATP resulting from aerobic metabolic production (large outside oval).

Figure 4.3 shows the breakdown of ATP and PC during heavy exercise. It also shows the restoration of ATP from energy substrate sources and then restoration of PC from the regenerated ATP. The process continues until both the PC and ATP resting levels are regained. Specifically, when ATP is hydrolyzed by the contractile proteins in muscle (large inner circle), the resulting ADP is rephosphorylated in the cytoplasm by the PC that is available there (small inner circle). In turn, the now free creatine is rephosphorylated at the inner mitochondrial membrane from ATP produced at that site (large outside oval). The remnant ADP is then free, in turn, to be phosphorylated again by oxidative phosphorylation. In addition to providing ATP rapidly, this mechanism, called the creatine phosphate shuttle, is one way in which electron transport and oxidative phosphorylation are regulated (Brooks, et al., 1999).

Lactic Acid/Lactate Production

Lactic acid is produced in muscle cells when the NADH + H$^+$ formed in glycolysis (step 6; see Figure 3.5) is oxidized to NAD$^+$ by a transfer of the hydrogen ions to pyruvic acid which, in turn, is reduced to lactic acid (Brooks, 1985; Newsholme and Leech, 1983). In muscle tissue, lactic acid is produced in amounts that are in equilibrium with pyruvic acid under normal resting conditions. In addition, lactic acid is always produced by red blood cells, portions of the kidneys, and certain tissues within the eye. Both resting and exercise values depend on the balance between lactic acid *production* (*appearance*) and *removal* (*disappearance, or clearance*). This balance of appearance and disappearance is called *turnover*. When production exceeds removal, lactate is said to *accumulate*. The questions, then, especially during exercise are, what conditions result in lactic acid production and what processes lead to lactic acid removal? This section will deal with the first of these two questions.

In general, the relative rates of glycolytic activity (Stage I of carbohydrate metabolism) and oxidative activity (Stages II, III, and IV) determine the production of lactic acid/lactate. Specifically, five factors play important roles: muscle contraction, enzyme activity, muscle fiber type, sympathetic nervous system activation, and insufficient oxygen (anaerobiosis, the onset of anaerobic metabolism).

1. *Muscle contraction.* During exercise, muscle activity obviously increases. The process of muscle contraction requires the release of calcium (Ca^{2+}) from the sarcoplasmic reticulum. In addition to its role in the coupling process of actin and myosin, calcium also causes glycogenolysis by activating the enzyme glycogen phosphorylase. Glycogen is processed by fast glycolysis and results in the production of lactic acid whether oxygen levels are sufficient or not (Brooks, et al., 1999; Fox, 1973).

2. *Enzyme activity.* The conversion of pyruvate and $NADH + H^+$ to lactate and NAD^+ is catalyzed by the enzyme lactic dehydrogenase (LDH), whereas the conversion of pyruvate to acetyl CoA (Stage II) prior to entry into the Krebs cycle is catalyzed by the enzyme pyruvate dehydrogenase (PDH). LDH has the highest rate of functioning of any of the glycolytic enzymes and is much more active than the enzymes that provide alternate pathways for pyruvate metabolism, including PDH and the rate-limiting enzymes in the Krebs cycle. Any increase in pyruvate and $NADH + H^+$ further increases the activity of LDH and results in the production of lactic acid (Spriet, et al., 2000). Therefore, lactic acid production is an inevitable consequence of glycolysis (Brooks, 1986; Gaesser and Brooks, 1975; Spriet, et al., 2000). The more pyruvate provided, the more lactate produced. The shifting of the hydrogen atoms from $NADH + H^+$ to pyruvate forming lactate serves to maintain the *redox potential* of the cell. The redox, or oxidation-reduction, potential is the ratio of $NADH + H^+$ to NAD^+. There is a finite amount of NAD^+ available in the cytoplasm to accept hydrogen atoms in step 6 and keep glycolysis going. To maintain this supply, $NADH + H^+$ must either transfer the hydrogen atoms into the mitochondria to the electron transport chain or give them up to pyruvate.

3. *Muscle fiber type.* During high-intensity, short-duration activities, fast-twitch glycolytic (FG) muscle fibers are preferentially recruited. These fast-contracting glycolytic fibers produce lactic acid when they contract whether oxygen is present in sufficient amounts or not. This response appears to be a function of the specific lactic dehydrogenase enzyme and the low mitochondrial density found in these fibers (Green, 1986).

4. *Sympathetic nervous system activation.* During heavy exercise, activity of the sympathetic nervous system stimulates the release of epinephrine and glucagon (see Figure 3.16). Both of these hormones bring about the breakdown of glycogen, leading ultimately to high levels of glucose-6-phosphate (G6P). (Refresh your memory by referring to Figure 3.5, if necessary, to locate G6P in glycolysis). High levels of G6P increase the rate of glycolysis and, hence, the production of pyruvic acid (Brooks, 1986). As previously described, any increase in pyruvate and $NADH + H^+$ ultimately results in an increase in lactic acid.

5. *Insufficient oxygen (anaerobiosis, onset of anaerobic metabolism).* Finally, during high-intensity, short-duration or near-maximal exercise, the delivery of oxygen to the mitochondria—and hence the availability of oxygen as the final oxygen acceptor at the end of the respiratory chain—can become deficient. Under these circumstances glycolysis proceeds at a rate that produces larger quantities of $NADH + H^+$ than the mitochondria has oxygen to accept. Again, "something" has to be done with the hydrogen atoms so that the NAD^+ can be regenerated. That "something" is the transfer of the hydrogen atoms to pyruvic acid and the formation of lactic acid.

Thus, although lactic acid is associated with high-intensity, short-duration exercise, this is not the only exercise condition that results in the production of lactic acid. Furthermore, although a lack of oxygen can contribute to the production of lactic acid, the presence of lactic acid does not absolutely indicate a lack of oxygen. The presence of lactic acid simply reflects the use of the anaerobic glycolytic pathway for ATP production, and the balance between glycolytic and mitochondrial activity.

Lactate Clearance

Lactate clearance occurs primarily by three processes: oxidation, gluconeogenesis/glyconeogenesis, and transamination. All three processes can involve the movement of lactate.

Once produced, lactate moves readily between cytoplasm and mitochondria, muscle and blood, blood and muscle, active and inactive muscle, glycolytic and oxidative muscle, blood and heart, blood and liver, and blood and skin (Brooks, 2000). Lactate moves between lactate-producing and lactate-consuming sites by means of intracellular and extracellular lactate shuttles. Transport across cellular and mitochondrial membranes occurs by facilitated exchange down concentration and hydrogen ion (pH) gradients utilizing lactate transport proteins known as monocarboxylate transporters (MCTs) (Brooks, 2000).

As of 1998, seven monocarboxylate transporters had been reported in the literature. MCT1 is abundant in oxidative skeletal and cardiac muscle fibers and mitochondrial membranes. MCT4 is most prevalent in the cell membranes of glycolytic skeletal fibers.

The *intracellular lactate shuttle* (Figure 4.4a) involves the movement of lactate by MCT1 transporters between the cytoplasm, where it is produced, and the mitochondria. Once inside the mitochondria, lactate is oxidized to pyruvate and the NAD$^+$ reduced to NADH + H$^+$. The pyruvate proceeds through Stages II, III, and IV of aerobic metabolism, while the NADH + H$^+$ goes directly to Stage IV. This is a very new concept that indicates that muscle cells can both produce and consume lactate at the same time (Brooks, 2000).

Extracellular lactate shuttles act to move lactate between tissues (Figure 4.4b). Muscle cell membrane lactate proteins (MCT1 and MCT4) move the lactate both out of and into tissues. Intermuscularly, most lactate moves out of active fast-twitch glycolytic skeletal muscle cells (FOG, Type IIA and FG, Type IIB) and into active oxidative (slow twitch, SO) skeletal muscle cells. This can occur either by a direct shuttle between the skeletal muscle cells or through the circulation. Once lactate is in the bloodstream, it can also circulate to cardiac cells. During heavy exercise, lactate becomes the preferred fuel of the heart. In this manner glycogenolysis in one cell can supply fuel for another cell. In each of these cases the ultimate fate of the lactate is oxidation to ATP, CO$_2$, and H$_2$O by aerobic metabolism (Brooks, 1986, 2000).

Lactate circulating in the bloodstream can also be transported to the liver where, as described in Chapter 3, it is reconverted by the process of gluconeogenesis into glucose. Indeed, the liver appears to preferentially make glycogen from lactate as

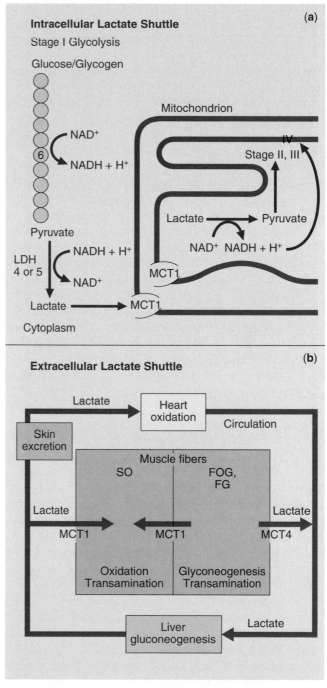

Figure 4.4

Intracellular and Extracellular Lactate Shuttles

(a) The intracellular lactate shuttle transports lactate from the cytoplasm into the mitochondria by MCT1 transporters, where it is reconverted to pyruvate and proceeds through Stages II, III, and IV of metabolism. (b) The extracellular lactate shuttle moves lactate directly between lactic acid–producing fast-twitch glycolytic fibers (FOG and FG) and lactate-consuming slow-twitch oxidative fibers. It also transports lactate through the circulation to the liver, skin, and heart, where it is cleared by oxidation, transamination, gluconeogenesis, or excretion. Most lactate remaining in fast-twitch glycolytic fibers is reconverted to glycogen by glyconeogenesis.

opposed to glucose. In human glycolytic muscle fibers (both fast-twitch oxidative glycolytic and fast-twitch glycolytic), some of the lactate produced during high-intensity exercise is retained, and in the postexercise recovery period it is reconverted to glycogen in that muscle cell. This process is called *glyconeogenesis* (Brooks, et al., 1999; Donovan and Pagliassotti, 2000; Gladden, 2000).

Both oxidative and glycolytic fibers can also clear lactate by transamination. Transamination forms keto acids (Krebs cycle intermediates) and amino acids. The predominant amino acid produced is alanine. In turn, alanine can undergo gluconeogenesis in the liver (Brooks, 1986; Gaesser and Brooks, 1975).

A small amount of lactate in the circulation moves from the blood to the skin and exits the body in sweat. Finally, some lactate will remain as lactate circulating in the blood. This comprises the resting lactate level.

Oxidation is by far the predominant process of lactate clearance both during and after exercise. As stated previously, the accumulation of lactate in the blood depends on the relative rate of appearance (production) and disappearance (clearance), which in turn is directly related to the intensity and duration of the exercise being done.

Measurement of Anaerobic Metabolism

Laboratory Procedures

Unfortunately, there is no generally accepted means by which to directly measure the anaerobic energy contribution to exercise. There are, however, two general approaches to describing the anaerobic exercise response. One approach describes changes in the chemical substances either used in alactic anaerobic metabolism (specifically, ATP and PC levels) or produced as a result of lactic anaerobic metabolism (lactic acid or lactate). The second approach quantifies the amount of work performed or the power generated during short-duration, high-intensity activity. The assumption is that such activity could not be done without anaerobic energy; therefore, measuring such work or power indirectly measures anaerobic energy utilization.

ATP-PC and Lactate

The measurement of ATP, PC, and lactate can be done by chemical analysis of muscle biopsy specimens. Lactate is the most frequently measured variable, in part because it can also be measured from blood samples. The blood sample may be obtained by either venipuncture or finger prick, both of which are less invasive than a muscle biopsy. Another reason for the

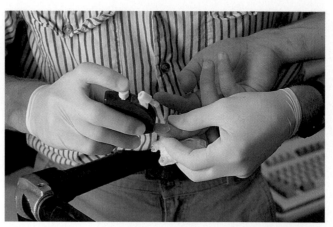

(a)

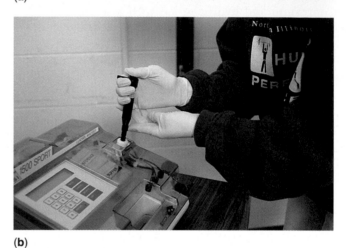

(b)

Figure 4.5
Lactate Analysis

A small sample of blood is obtained by a finger prick (a) and injected into a lactate analyzer (b) for determination of lactate concentration [La⁻].

popularity of lactate analysis is the user-friendly, fast, accurate, and relatively inexpensive analyzers that are available. Figure 4.5 shows an analyzer that requires a minimal blood sample (a 25-μL capillary tube obtained by a finger prick), is portable, and takes less than 5 min for each sample analysis.

At normal pH levels lactic acid will almost completely dissociate into hydrogen ions (H^+) and lactate ($C_3H_5O_3^-$, designated as La^-). Thus, technically, lactic acid is formed, but lactate is what is measured in the bloodstream. Despite this distinction, the terms *lactic acid* and *lactate* are often used synonymously (Brooks, 1985).

Lactate is a small molecule that moves easily from the muscles to the blood and most other fluid compartments. However, much of the lactate that is produced does not get into the bloodstream. It takes time for the portion that does get into the bloodstream to

Table 4.1
Estimated Maximal Power and Capacity in Untrained Males

Energy system	Power		Time	Capacity	
	kcal·min^{-1}	kJ·min^{-1}	hr:min:sec	kcal	kJ
ATP-PC (phosphagen)	72	300	:09–:10	11	45
LA (anaerobic glycolysis)	36	150	1:19.8	48	200
O$_2$ (aerobic glycolysis + Krebs cycle + ETS-OP; fuel = CHO)	7.2–19.1	30–80	2:21:00*	359–1268	1500–5300

*   When all fuels are considered, the time is unlimited.

Sources: Bouchard, Taylor, & Dulac (1991); Bouchard, et al. (1982).

reach an equilibrium between muscle and blood. This equilibrium and the achievement of peak blood values may take as long as 5–10 min. Until equilibrium occurs, muscle lactate values will be higher than blood lactate values. This also means that the highest blood lactate values are typically seen after several minutes of recovery, not during high-intensity work (Gollnick and Hermansen, 1973).

Lactate levels are reported using a variety of units. The two most common are millimoles per liter (mmol·L^{-1}, sometimes designated as mM) or milligrams per 100 milliliters of blood (mg·100 mL^{-1}, sometimes designated as mg% or mg·dL^{-1}). One mmol·L^{-1} is equal to 9 mg·100 mL^{-1}. Resting levels of lactate of 1–2 mmol·L^{-1} or 9–18 mg·100 mL^{-1} are typical. A value of 8 mmol·L^{-1} or 72 mg·100 mL^{-1} is usually taken to indicate that an individual has worked maximally (Åstrand and Rodahl, 1977). Peak values as high as 32 mmol·L^{-1} or 288 mg·100 mL^{-1} have been reported.

Tests of Anaerobic Power and Capacity

Energy system capacity is defined as the total amount of energy that can be produced by an energy system. **Energy system power** is defined as the maximal amount of energy that can be produced per unit of time. Table 4.1 clearly shows that the phosphagen (ATP-PC) system is predominantly a power system with very little capacity. The lactic anaerobic glycolytic system has almost equal power and capacity,

---

Energy System Capacity The total amount of energy that can be produced by an energy system.

Energy System Power The maximal amount of energy that can be produced per unit of time.

---

just slightly favoring capacity. The information on the aerobic (O$_2$) system is included here just to show how truly high in power and low in capacity the anaerobic systems are.

Although the ATP-PC system can put out energy at the rate of 72 kcal·min^{-1}, it can only sustain that value when working maximally for 9–10 sec, for a total output of only 11 kcal (72 kcal·min^{-1} ÷ 60 sec·min^{-1} = 1.2 kcal·sec^{-1}; 11 total kcal ÷ 1.2^{-1} kcal·sec^{-1} = 9.17 sec). The LA system has a lower power (36 kcal·min^{-1}) but can sustain it for almost 1 min and 20 sec (48 kcal ÷ 36 kcal·min^{-1} = 1.33 min = 1:19.8). By comparison, if the O$_2$ system worked at a power output of 9 kcal·min^{-1}, exercise could be sustained for more than 2 hr (1268 kcal ÷ 9 kcal·min^{-1} = 141 min = 2:21) just using carbohydrate fuel sources. In fact, when all fuel supplies are included, the capacity of the aerobic system is, for all intents and purposes, unlimited.

When measuring the anaerobic systems, one would ideally have a test that could distinctly evaluate alactic anaerobic power, alactic anaerobic capacity, lactic anaerobic power, and lactic anaerobic capacity. Because no such tests exist, attempts have been made to get this information indirectly by measuring (1) the total mechanical power generated during high-intensity, short-duration work; (2) the amount of mechanical work done in a specific period of time; or (3) the time required to perform a given amount of presumably anaerobic work (Green, 1995). Two such tests are commonly used in laboratory settings, the Wingate Anaerobic Test (WAT) and the Maragaria-Kalamen Stair Climb (Bouchard, et al., 1982).

The Wingate Anaerobic Test   The Wingate Anaerobic Test depicted in Figure 4.6 is probably the most well known of several bicycle ergometer tests used to measure anaerobic power and capacity. The test is an

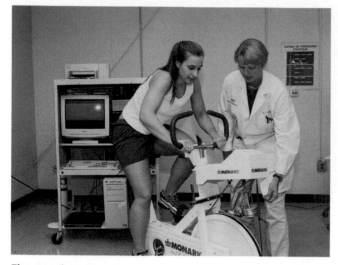

Figure 4.6
Wingate Anaerobic Test

This subject is performing the Wingate Anaerobic Test. Once she is pedaling as fast as she can, the tester releases the weight, providing a resistance based on the subject's body weight. The subject will then continue to pedal as quickly as possible for 30 seconds. Data from sensors attached to the flywheel are relayed to the computer for calculation of peak power, mean power, and fatigue index.

all-out ride for 30 sec against a resistance based on body weight. Resistance values of 0.075 kg·kg^{-1} body weight for children, 0.086 kg·kg^{-1} body weight for adult females, and 0.095 kg·kg^{-1} body weight for adult males appear to be optimal. Athletes may need values as high as 0.10 kg·kg^{-1} of body weight, but the most common value used (as in the example that follows) is 0.075 kg·kg^{-1} body weight (Vandewalle, et al., 1987). The revolutions (rev) of the flywheel are counted per second during the test, and from the available information three variables are determined.

Computer-generated results from a typical test are given in Table 4.2. The subject was a 129-lb female physical education major, but not an athlete. Note that these results are for a leg test; an arm version is also available. Calculations for the resistance

> **Peak Power (PP)** The maximum power (force times distance divided by time) exerted during very short (5 sec or less) duration work.
>
> **Mean Power (MP)** The average power (force times distance divided by time) exerted during short (typically 30 sec) duration work.
>
> **Fatigue Index (FI)** Percentage of peak power drop-off during high-intensity, short-duration work.

she used (4.4 kg) are shown on Table 4.2. The data contained in the table will be used to calculate three variables: peak power, mean power, and fatigue index. **Peak power (PP)** is defined as the maximal power (force times distance divided by time) exerted during very short (5 sec or less) duration work. **Mean power (MP)** is defined as the average power (force times distance divided by time) exerted during short (typically 30 sec) duration work. The **fatigue index (FI)** is the percentage of peak power drop-off during high-intensity, short-duration work. Each of these variables requires the use of different time periods in the calculations.

The first variable computed is *peak power* (PP), the maximum power exerted during the highest 5-sec period. This usually occurs early in the activity and, in the example given, is the time between 2 and 6 sec where 10.25 rev were completed. Peak power can be expressed in absolute terms as kgm·5 sec^{-1} or prorated to a full minute as kgm·min^{-1} or watts (W). Peak power can also be expressed relative to body weight as kgm·5 sec^{-1}·kg^{-1}, kgm·min^{-1}·kg^{-1}, or W·kg^{-1}. The formula for peak power is

4.1 peak power (kgm·5 sec^{-1}) = maximal revolutions in 5 sec × distance that the flywheel travels per revolution (m) × force setting (kg)

or

$$PP = rev(max) \text{ in 5 sec} \times D \cdot rev^{-1} \times F$$

Example

Thus for this example the calculation is

$$PP = 10.25 \text{ rev} \times 6 \text{ m·rev}^{-1} \times 4.4 \text{ kg}$$
$$= 270.6 \text{ kgm·5 sec}^{-1}$$

Prorated to a full minute, PP is

$$PP = 270.6 \text{ kgm·5 sec}^{-1} \times 12$$
$$(60 \text{ sec·min}^{-1} \div 5 \text{ sec} = 12)$$
$$= 3247.2 \text{ kgm·min}^{-1}$$

Relative to body weight PP is

$$PP = 3247.2 \text{ kgm·min}^{-1} \div 58.5 \text{ kg}$$
$$= 55.50 \text{ kgm·min}^{-1}·kg^{-1}$$

When converted to watts (1 W = 6.12 kgm·min^{-1}), the relative value is

$$PP = 55.5 \text{ kgm·min}^{-1} \div 6.12 \text{ kgm·min}^{-1}·W^{-1}$$
$$= 9.07 \text{ W·kg}^{-1}$$ ✛

Originally, peak power was thought to reflect only alactic processes—alactic anaerobic capacity, in particular. However, subsequent research has shown that muscle lactate levels rise to high values as early as 10 sec into such high-intensity work. This result indicates that glycolytic processes are occurring

Table 4.2

Results for the Wingate Leg Test

Weight is 129 lb = 58.50 kg; resistance for legs is 58.50 kg × 0.075 kg·kg^{-1}; body weight = 4.4 kg.

Inclusive Time (sec)	5-sec Total Revolutions	kgm·min^{-1}·kg^{-1}	W·kg^{-1}
1–5	10.00	54.15	8.85
2–6	10.25	55.50	9.07
3–7	9.75	52.80	8.63
4–8	9.50	51.44	8.41
5–9	9.25	50.09	8.18
6–10	9.00	48.74	7.96
7–11	8.25	44.67	7.30
8–12	8.00	43.32	7.08
9–13	7.75	41.97	6.86
10–14	7.50	40.61	6.64
11–15	7.50	40.61	6.64
12–16	7.50	40.61	6.64
13–17	7.25	39.26	6.41
14–18	7.25	39.26	6.41
15–19	7.00	37.91	6.19
16–20	7.00	37.91	6.19
17–21	6.75	36.55	5.97
18–22	6.75	36.55	5.97
19–23	6.50	35.20	5.75
20–24	6.50	35.20	5.75
21–25	6.25	33.84	5.53
22–26	6.25	33.84	5.53
23–27	6.00	32.49	5.31
24–28	6.00	32.49	5.31
25–29	5.75	31.14	5.09
26–30	5.50	29.78	4.87

Total pedal revolutions = 45.25.

Highest 5-sec absolute peak power = 3247.20 kgm·min^{-1}.

Highest 5-sec relative peak power = 55.50 kgm·min^{-1}·kg^{-1}
    = 9.07 W·kg^{-1}.

Mean absolute power = 2389.20 kgm·min^{-1}.

Mean relative power = 40.84 kgm·min^{-1}·kg^{-1} = 6.67 W·kg^{-1}.

Fatigue index = 100 − (lowest 5 sec divided by highest 5 sec) × 100
    = 46.34%.

almost immediately along with ATP-CP breakdown. Therefore, peak power cannot be interpreted as being only alactic (Bar-Or, 1987).

The second variable calculated is *mean power*, and it can also be expressed in both absolute and relative units. Mean power (MP) is the average power sustained throughout the 30-second ride. The formula for mean power is

4.2 mean power (kgm·30 sec^{-1} = total number of revolutions in 30 sec × distance that the flywheel travels per revolution (m) × force setting (kg)

or

MP = rev(total) in 30 sec × D·rev^{-1} × F

Example

Thus for this example the calculation is

$$MP = 45.25 \text{ rev} \times 6 \text{ m·rev}^{-1} \times 4.4 \text{ kg}$$
$$= 1194.6 \text{ kgm·30 sec}$$

Prorated to a full minute, MP is

$$MP = 1194.6 \text{ kgm} \times 2 \quad (60 \text{ sec·min}^{-1} \div 30 \text{ sec} = 2)$$
$$= 2389.2 \text{ kgm·min}^{-1}$$

Related to body weight MP is

$$MP = 2389.2 \text{ kgm·min}^{-1} \div 58.5 \text{ kg}$$
$$= 40.84 \text{ kgm·min}^{-1}·\text{kg}^{-1}$$

When converted to watts MP is

$$MP = 40.84 \text{ kgm·min}^{-1}·\text{kg}^{-1} \div 6.12 \text{ kgm· min}^{-1}·\text{W}^{-1}$$
$$= 6.67 \text{ W·kg}^{-1}$$

Mean power is sometimes said to represent lactic anaerobic capacity, although this has not been substantiated (Bar-Or, 1987).

The third variable that can be computed is the *fatigue index* (FI), or the percentage of peak power drop-off during high-intensity, short-duration work. It is calculated using the highest 5-sec power (PP) and the lowest 5-sec power (LP). Little is known about the relationship of the fatigue index to anaerobic fitness (Bar-Or, 1987).

4.3 fatigue index (%) = [1 − (lowest power kgm· 5 sec^{-1} ÷ (peak power kgm·5 sec^{-1})] × 100

or

$$FI = \left[1 - \left(\frac{LP}{PP} \right) \right] \times 100$$

Example
- - - - - - - - - - - - - - - - - - - -

In our example the highest 5-sec power is 270.6 kgm. Using the peak power formula of Equation 4.1 but with the lowest 5-sec total, we get

LP = 5.50 rev × 6 m·rev^{-1} × 4.4 kg
  = 145.2 kg·5 sec^{-1}

[1 − (145.2 kg·5 sec^{-1} ÷ 270.6 kg·5 sec^{-1})]
                              × 100 = 46.34% ✚

Although the WAT is not a purely anaerobic test (the aerobic component has been measured at between 13% and 29%), it is predominantly anaerobic. It compares well (with correlations generally above 0.75) with other tests of anaerobic power and capacity and is widely used (Bar-Or, 1987; Patton and Duggan, 1987).

The Margaria-Kalamen Stair Climb   To perform the Margaria-Kalamen test, an individual runs for 6 m on the level and then climbs a staircase, taking three steps at a time. Power in kgm·sec^{-1} is calculated by using, respectively, the weight of the subject, the vertical height between the third and ninth steps, and the time between the third and ninth steps (Bouchard, et al., 1982; Vandewalle, et al., 1987). The use of electronic switch mats or photoelectric cells is essential for accuracy. This test is considered to be a test of alactic anaerobic power because of the short time involved—usually less than 5 sec for the entire test and close to 1 sec for the measured time between the third and ninth steps.

Field Tests   There are no field tests available to estimate the ATP-PC used or the lactate produced during exercise. However, performance in high-intensity, short-duration activity can give an indication of anaerobic power and capacity. Two types of activities

are commonly used: vertical jump tests and sprints (sometimes done as shuttles) or middle-distance runs.

In vertical jump tests several different protocols are utilized, including variations in the starting posture, the use or nonuse of arms, and what body part displacement is measured. The one commonality is the end value measured: the height jumped. When the jump is performed on a force platform, actual power values can be calculated, and the test is considered to be a laboratory test. When the jump is performed as a field test on a normal surface, work (force × distance), not power, is estimated. The height of the vertical jump and peak power as determined from force plate data have been shown to be highly correlated (r = 0.92). For these reasons, vertical jump height is seen as an acceptable indicator of anaerobic alactic power (Vandewalle, et al., 1987).

For sprints and middle-distance runs, the involvement of the various energy systems is related to the time of the all-out activity, as shown in Figure 4.2. Therefore, runs whose distance can be covered in a distinct time range (depending somewhat on age, sex, and training status) can be utilized as field tests of anaerobic metabolism (Cheetham, et al., 1986). For example, dashes of 40, 50, or 60 yd or m will take approximately 4–15 sec and can be used as an indication of alactic anaerobic power and/or capacity. Longer runs, probably between 200 and 800 m (or 220 and 880 yd) and lasting 40–120 sec, can be used as an indication of lactic anaerobic power and capacity. Faster speeds in covering a given distance would indicate increased anaerobic power and/or capacity.

The Anaerobic Exercise Response

Oxygen Deficit and Excess Postexercise Oxygen Consumption

When exercise begins, no matter how light or heavy it is, there is an immediate need for additional energy. Thus, the most obvious exercise response is an increase in metabolism. All three energy systems will be involved in this response, with their relative contributions being proportional to the intensity and duration of the activity.

Figure 4.7 shows two scenarios for going from rest to different intensities of exercise. In Figure 4.7a the activity is a moderate submaximal bout. The oxygen requirement for this particular exercise is 1.4 L·min^{-1}. The individual has a $\dot{V}O_2$max of 2.5 L·min^{-1}. Therefore, this individual is working at 56% $\dot{V}O_2$max. The area under the smoothed curve during both exercise and recovery represents oxygen used. Notice, however, that there is an initial lag during which the oxygen supplied and utilized is below the oxygen requirement for providing energy. This difference between the oxygen required during exercise and the oxygen supplied and utilized is called the **oxygen deficit.** Because of this supply and demand discrepancy, anaerobic sources must be involved in providing energy at the onset of all activity.

The O_2 deficit has traditionally been explained as the inability of the circulatory and respiratory systems to respond quickly enough to the increased energy demands. Evidence now, however, indicates that the O_2 deficit is probably due to limited cellular utilization of O_2 as a result of metabolic adjustments (Sahlin, et al., 1988). That is, the increasing levels of ADP, P_i, and NADH + H^+, brought about by the suddenly elevated energy demands, stimulate both aerobic and anaerobic energy processes, not just one or the other. Thus, it is not that the aerobic system cannot supply all of the needed energy but that the regulatory system does not allow it to. Therefore, during the transition from rest to work, energy is supplied by

1. O_2 transport and utilization;

2. utilization of O_2 stores in capillary blood and bound to myoglobin;

3. the splitting of stored ATP-PC; and

4. anaerobic glycolysis, with the concomitant production of lactic acid (Saris, et al., 1985).

Eventually, if the exercise intensity is low enough (as in the example in Figure 4.7a), the aerobic system will predominate and the oxygen supply will equal the oxygen demand. This condition is called steady-state, steady-rate, or steady-level exercise.

Figure 4.7b shows a smoothed plot of O_2 consumption at rest and during and after an exercise bout in which the energy requirement is greater than $\dot{V}O_2$max, sometimes called **supramaximal exercise.** The initial period of lag between O_2 supply and demand is once again evident and, as in the first example, the added energy is provided by stored ATP-PC, anaerobic glycolysis, and stored O_2. However, in this case, when the O_2 consumption plateaus or levels off, it is at $\dot{V}O_2$max, and more energy is still needed if exercise is to continue.

Oxygen Deficit The difference between the oxygen required during exercise and the oxygen supplied and utilized. Occurs at the onset of all activity.

Supramaximal Exercise An exercise bout in which the energy requirement is greater than that which can be supplied aerobically at $\dot{V}O_2$max.

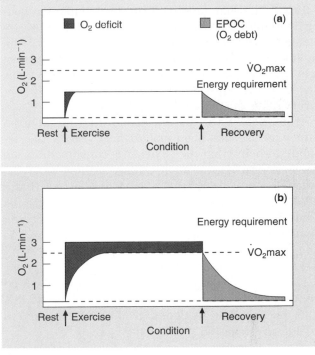

Figure 4.7
Oxygen Deficit and Excess Postexercise Oxygen Consumption (EPOC) during Submaximal Exercise and Supramaximal Exercise

(a) During light to moderate submaximal exercise, both the oxygen deficit, indicated by the convex curve at the start of exercise, and the excess postexercise oxygen consumption, indicated by the concave curve during the recovery time period, are small. (b) During heavy or supramaximal exercise both the O_2 deficit and the EPOC are large. Under both conditions energy is supplied during the O_2 deficit period by using stored ATP-PC, anaerobic glycolysis, and oxygen stores in capillary blood and bound to myoglobin. The heavier the exercise the more the reliance on anaerobic glycolysis. The EPOC is a result of the restoration of ATP-PC, removal of lactate, restoration of O_2 stores, elevated cardiovascular and respiratory function, elevated hormonal levels, and especially, the elevated body temperature.

This plateau is not considered to be a steady state because the energy demands are not being totally met aerobically. The supplemental energy is provided by anaerobic glycolysis. Exactly what the energy demand is in this situation is difficult to determine precisely, because, as stated before, lactic acid levels do not reflect production alone. However, without the anaerobic energy contribution this activity could not continue. The maximal ability to tolerate lactic acid accumulation will determine to a large extent how long the activity can continue.

The recovery from exercise represented by the concave curves following the cessation of exercise in both Figures 4.7a and 4.7b shows that oxygen consumption drops quickly (a fast component lasting 2–3 min) and then tapers off (a slow component lasting 3–60 min). The magnitude and duration of this elevated oxygen consumption will depend primarily on the intensity of the preceding exercise. In the case of light submaximal work (Figure 4.7a) recovery takes place quickly; after heavy exercise (Figure 4.7b) recovery takes much longer.

Historically, this period of elevated metabolism after exercise has been called the *O₂ debt,* the assumption being that the "extra" O₂ consumed during the "debt" period was being utilized to "pay back" the deficit incurred in the early part of exercise (Bahr, 1992; Stainsby and Barclay, 1970). More recently, the terms *O₂ recovery* or **excess postexercise oxygen consumption (EPOC)** have come into favor. EPOC is defined as the oxygen consumption during recovery that is above normal resting values.

A critical question is what causes this elevated metabolism in recovery. Although there is, at this time, no complete explanation of EPOC, six factors have been suggested.

1. *Restoration of ATP-PC stores:* About 10% of the EPOC is utilized to rephosphorylate creatine and ADP to PC and ATP, respectively, thus restoring these substances to resting levels (Bahr, 1992; Gaesser and Brooks, 1975). Approximately 50% of the ATP-PC is restored in 30 sec (Margaria, et al., 1933). This time is called the *half-life restoration* of ATP-PC. Full recovery requires slightly over 2 min (Fox, 1973).

2. *Restoration of O₂ stores:* Although the amount of O₂ stored in the blood (bound to hemoglobin) and muscle (bound to myoglobin) is not large, it does need to be replenished at the cessation of exercise. Replenishment probably occurs completely within 2–3 min (Bahr, 1992; Stainsby and Barclay, 1970).

3. *Elevated cardiovascular-respiratory function:* Both the respiratory system and the cardiovascular system remain elevated postexercise; that is, neither the breathing rate and depth nor heart rate recover instantaneously. Although this circumstance enables the extra amounts of oxygen to be processed, the actual energy cost of these cardiovascular-respiratory processes probably accounts for only 1–2% of the excess oxygen (Bahr, 1992; Stainsby and Barclay, 1970).

4. *Elevated hormonal levels:* During exercise the circulating levels of the catecholamines (epinephrine and norepinephrine), thyroxine, and cortisol are all increased (Figure 3.16 and Table 3.3). In addition to their fuel mobilization and utilization effects, these hormones increase Na^+-K^+ pump activity in muscles and nerves by changing cell membrane permeability to Na^+ and K^+. As an active transport process, the Na^+-K^+ pump requires ATP. The increased need for ATP means an increased need for O_2. Until the hormones are cleared from the bloodstream, the additional O_2 and ATP use is a significant contributor to the EPOC (Bahr, 1992; Gaesser and Brooks, 1975).

5. *Elevated body temperature:* When ATP is broken down to supply the energy for chemical, electrical, or mechanical work, heat is produced as a by-product. During exercise, heat production may exceed heat dissipation, causing a rise in body core temperature. For each degree Celsius that body temperature rises, the metabolic rate increases approximately 13–15% (Kapit, et al., 1987). Thus, in recovery, although the need for high levels of energy to support the exercise has ceased, the influence of the elevated temperature has not, because cooling takes some time to occur. This temperature effect is by far the most important reason for EPOC, accounting for as much as 60–70% of the slow component after exercise at 50–80% $\dot{V}O_2$max (Bahr, 1992; Gaesser and Brooks, 1975).

6. *Lactate removal:* The lactate that has accumulated must be removed. Historically, it was thought that the majority of this lactate was converted to glycogen and that this conversion was the primary cause of the slow component of EPOC. As previously described, the fate of lactic acid is now seen as more complex and its contribution as a causative factor for EPOC is minimal (Gaesser and Brooks, 1975; Stainsby and Barclay, 1970).

Anaerobic Exercise Responses

ATP-PC Changes

Figure 4.8 indicates what happens to ATP and PC levels in both muscle and blood during constant-load, supramaximal exercise (105–110% $\dot{V}O_2$max) lasting 3 min or less. As shown in the figure, the ATP level in the muscle decreases only slightly. In fact, the maximum ATP depletion observed in skeletal muscle after heavy exercise is only about 30–40% in both males and females. Thus, even after exhaustive work 60–70% of the resting amount of ATP is still present (Cheetham, et al., 1986; Gollnick and King, 1969).

Conversely, the level of PC changes dramatically such that it is nearly depleted. The greatest depletion of PC occurs in the initial 20 sec of exercise, with the result that ATP is almost maintained at resting levels during that time span. From 20 to 180 sec the decline

---

Excess Postexercise Oxygen Consumption (EPOC) Oxygen consumption during recovery that is above normal resting values.

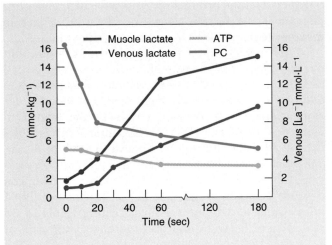

Figure 4.8

Time Course for the Depletion of PC and ATP and the Accumulation of Lactate in Muscle and Veins

Muscle levels of ATP are maintained relatively constant during high-intensity, short-duration exercise at the expense of PC. Muscle lactate levels rise sooner and higher than venous levels owing to the diffusion time lag and dilution.

Source: Modified from P. D. Gollnick & L. Hermansen. Biochemical adaptation to exercise: Anaerobic metabolism. In J. H. Wilmore (ed.), *Exercise and Sport Sciences Reviews*. New York: Academic Press (1973). Reprinted by permission of Williams & Wilkins.

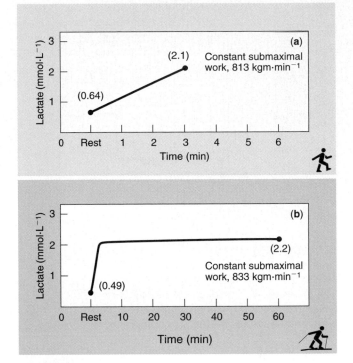

Figure 4.9

Lactate Accumulation during Short- and Long-Term Dynamic Aerobic Constant Submaximal Work

After an initial rise in accumulation during the oxygen deficit period (a), lactate levels off and remains relatively constant during long duration submaximal aerobic work (b).

Source: Based on data from Freund et al. (1990).

in PC and ATP is both gradual and parallel (Gollnick and Hermansen, 1973). Obviously, the ATP level is maintained at the expense of the PC. However, some ATP is also being provided from glycolysis, as indicated by the rise in lactate. Compare the theoretical basis of the Wingate Anaerobic Test with these data.

Lactate Changes

Lactate levels in response to exercise depend primarily on the intensity of the exercise. Acute exercise does not result in any meaningful enhancement of lactate transporters. Instead, transmembrane lactate and hydrogen ion gradients increase. Lactate transport is faster in oxidative fibers than in glycolytic ones. The fast transport of lactate by oxidative fibers may reflect lactate's role as an energy substrate, while the slower transport in glycolytic fibers may contribute to a greater retention of lactate during recovery for reconversion into glycogen (Gladden, 2000).

Short-Term, High-Intensity Supramaximal Exercise

Figure 4.8 includes both muscle and blood lactate response to high-intensity, short-duration (3 min or less), supramaximal exercise. As the figure shows,

muscle lactate levels rise immediately with the onset of such hard work (105–110% $\dot{V}O_2$max) and continue to rise throughout the length of the task. The blood lactate values show a similar pattern, if the lag for diffusion time is taken into account. This lactate response (a rapid and consistent accumulation) is representative of what occurs when the exercise bout is greater than 90% $\dot{V}O_2$max (Gollnick and Hermansen, 1973).

Short- and Long-Term, Low-Intensity Submaximal Aerobic Exercise

Figure 4.9 depicts what occurs in both short-term and long-term low-intensity submaximal aerobic activity. During the first 3 min of such steady-state work the lactate (La^-) level rises (Figure 4.9a). This increase reflects the lactate accumulated during the oxygen deficit (Gollnick and Hermansen, 1973). When a similar workload is continued for 60 min, the lactate level remains unchanged after the initial rise (Figure 4.9b). The reason for this result lies in the balance

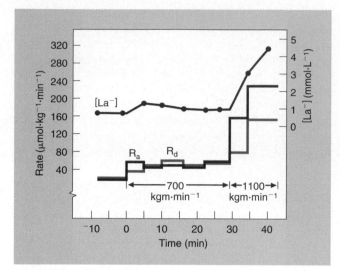

Figure 4.10

The Impact of the Rates of Lactate Appearance and Disappearance on Lactate Accumulation during Light and Heavy Submaximal Aerobic Exercise

During light (700 kgm·min⁻¹ submaximal aerobic exercise, the rate of lactate disappearance (R_d) (left y-axis) lags behind the rate of lactate appearance (R_a) (left y-axis) to a small extent, but then catches up so that the 30-min lactate concentration [La⁻] value (right y-axis) approximates rest. During heavy submaximal exercise (minutes 30–45) the R_d lags behind R_a and [La⁻] increases.

Source: G. A. Brooks. Anaerobic threshold: Review of the concept and directions for further research. *Medicine and Science in Sports and Exercise.* 17(1):22–31 (1985). Reprinted by permission.

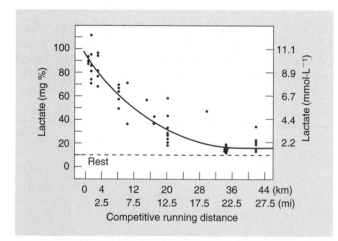

Figure 4.11

Lactate Accumulation Resulting from Increasing Distances of Competitive Running Races

Blood lactate accumulation shows an inverse curvilinear relationship with distance in running races.

Source: D. L. Costill. Metabolic responses during distance running. *Journal of Applied Physiology.* 28(3):251–255 (1970). Reprinted by permission of the American Physiological Society.

between lactate production (the rate of lactate appearance) and lactate clearance (the rate of lactate disappearance).

Figure 4.10 shows the results from a study that directly measured the rate of lactate appearance (R_a) and the rate of lactate disappearance (R_d) by radioactive tracers as well as the blood levels of lactate concentration ([La⁻]) (Brooks, 1985). In the transition from rest to steady-state submaximal exercise, the rate of both lactate appearance and lactate disappearance increased. During the next 30 min of exercise, the turnover rate was higher than at rest. The result was an initial increase in [La⁻], which declined after 5 min of activity to almost resting levels by 30 min. When the workload was increased, the rate of clearance (R_d) was no longer able to keep up with the rate of production (R_a), and the lactate concentration in the blood [La⁻] showed a sharp increase.

Figure 4.11 shows how lactate level varies with competitive distance (and hence duration) in highly trained male runners. At the shorter distances the predominant energy source is anaerobic, and the anticipated high lactate values are seen. As the distance increases and more of the energy is supplied aerobically, the intensity that can be maintained decreases. As a result, lactate also decreases, doing so in a negative exponential curvilinear pattern. By approximately 30 km (18 mi) the lactate levels are no different from what they are at rest.

Long-Term, Moderate to Heavy Submaximal Aerobic Exercise

The importance of the intensity of exercise, even at the marathon distance, is illustrated in Figure 4.12. Two groups of runners were equated according to their V̇O₂max. One group ran a simulated marathon on the treadmill at 73.3% V̇O₂max (in 2 hr 45 min or less); the other group ran the same distance but at 64.5% V̇O₂max (in 3 hr 45 min or slightly less). Within the slow group blood lactate values remained relatively stable and at a level considered to be within normal resting amounts. The blood lactate levels in the fast group were statistically significantly higher throughout the marathon than those of the slow group. As absolutes, however, both sets of values were low, with the slow group being within a normal resting range and the fast group barely above normal resting levels (O'Brien et al., 1993).

In general, during light to moderate work (that is, less than 50–60% of V̇O₂max), the blood lactate level is likely to rise slightly at first. Then it either will remain the same or will decrease slightly, even if the exercise lasts 30–60 min.

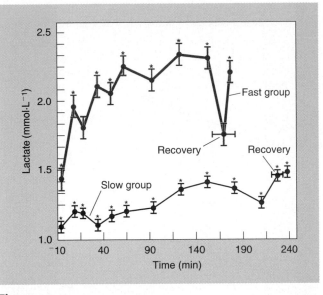

Figure 4.12
Blood Lactate Accumulation
during the Marathon

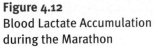

Blood lactate accumulation during a fast marathon (2 hr and 45 min or less) was greater than the accumulation during a slow marathon (3 hr and 45 min or less). The lactate levels for the slow marathoners never exceeded normal resting levels and the lactate levels for the fast marathoners barely exceeded normal resting levels.

Source: M. J. O'Brien, C. A. Viguie, R. S. Mazzeo, & G. A. Brooks. Carbohydrate dependence during marathon running. *Medicine and Science in Sports Exercise.* 25(9):1009–1017 (1993). Reprinted by permission.

At moderate to heavy intensities between 50 and 85% $\dot{V}O_2$max (depending on the genetic characteristics and training status of the individual), lactate levels will elevate rapidly during the first 5–10 min of exercise. If the workload continues for more than 10 min, the lactate level may continue to rise, may stabilize, or may decline, depending on the individual and other conditions.

One of these "other conditions" may be the exercise intensity in relation to the individual's maximal lactate steady state. **Maximal lactate steady state (MLSS)** is the highest workload that can be maintained over time without a continual rise in blood lactate; it indicates an exercise intensity above which lactate production exceeds clearance. MLSS is determined by a series of workloads performed on different days. Each succeeding workload gets progressively harder until the blood lactate accumulation increases more or less steadily throughout the test or increases more than 1 mmol·L^{-1} after the initial rise and establishment of a plateau in the early minutes. Thus, in a 30 min test this means that changes in the first 10 min are ignored and only the last 20 min used to determine if the change is less than or greater than 1 mmol·L^{-1}. When the blood lactate concentration meets the criterion, the previous workload that exhibited a plateau in lactate throughout the duration (after the initial rise) is labeled as the MLSS workload. Often the MLSS workload is compared to the individual's maximal workload and expressed as a percentage known as MLSS intensity (Beneke, et al., 2000). Performances at the MLSS intensity will result in a steady state for lactate; performances below this intensity will show declining lactate values, and performances above this level will exhibit progressively increasing lactate values. Extensive endurance performance cannot be completed above the MLSS, but portions of the event certainly may be.

Incremental Exercise to Maximum

Figure 4.13 depicts the accumulation of lactate during incremental exercise to maximum. The oxygen consumption (Figure 4.13a) increases in a rectilinear pattern to meet the increasing demands for energy, but blood lactate (Figure 4.13b) shows very little initial change and then increases continuously (Hughes, et al., 1982; Hughson, et al., 1987). These particular results are below the 8 mmol·L^{-1} generally considered to indicate a maximal test, however. As depicted, this pattern is best described as a positively accelerating exponential curve. Alternatively, the accumulation of lactate during incremental exercise can be depicted, as in Figure 4.14, as a rectilinear rise with two breakpoints or thresholds.

Since the early 1970s a great deal of attention has been paid to a concept that has been labeled variously as the *anaerobic threshold,* the *ventilatory threshold(s),* or the **lactate threshold(s).** The original concept of an anaerobic threshold is based upon the lactate response to incremental exercise, as depicted in Figure 4.14, and the relationship of the lactate response to minute ventilation (the volume of air breathed each minute).

Maximal Lactate Steady State (MLSS) The highest workload that can be maintained over time without a continual rise in blood lactate; it indicates an exercise intensity above which lactate production exceeds clearance.

Lactate Thresholds Points on the linear-curvilinear continuum of lactate accumulation that appear to indicate sharp rises, often labeled as the first (LT1) and second (LT2) lactate threshold.

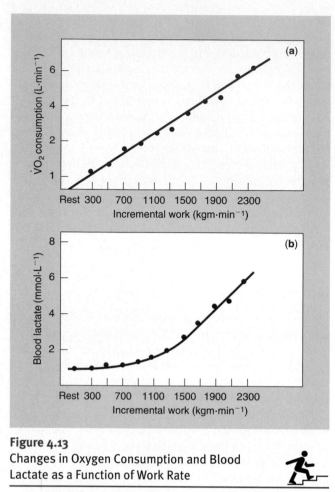

Figure 4.13

Changes in Oxygen Consumption and Blood
Lactate as a Function of Work Rate

The rise in O_2 consumption is directly proportional to the increase
in workload. Blood lactate levels show very little change at low
work rates and then increase continuously in a curvilinear pattern.

Source: Modified from E. F. Hughes, S. C. Turner, & G. A. Brooks. Effects of
glycogen depletion and pedaling speed on anaerobic threshold. *Journal
of Applied Physiology.* 52(6):1598–1607 (1982). Reprinted by permission
of the American Physiological Society.

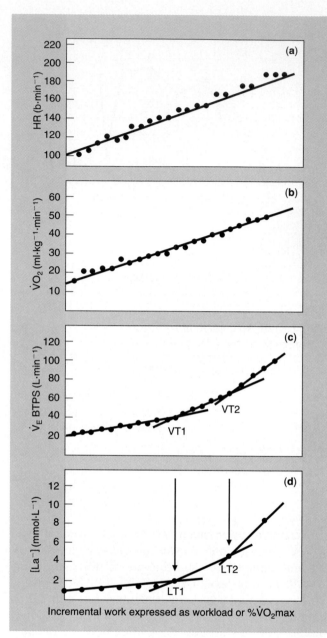

Figure 4.14

Ventilatory and Lactate Thresholds during
Incremental Work to Maximum

Both heart rate (a) and O2 consumption (b) increase in direct rectilinear patterns during an incremental work task whether the work
is expressed in terms of absolute workload or percentage of
$\dot{V}O_2$max. In contrast, both ventilation (c) and lactate (d) appear
to exhibit two distinct breakpoints as they rise. The circumstance
of VT1 occurring at the same time as LT1 and VT2 occurring at the
same time as LT2 is coincidental.

As espoused by Wasserman and his colleagues
(1973), the *anaerobic threshold* is defined as the exercise intensity, usually described as a percentage of
$\dot{V}O_2$max or workload, above which blood lactate levels rise and minute ventilation increases disproportionately in relation to oxygen consumption. The
onset of anaerobic metabolism (or anaerobiosis),
which is assumed to lead to the lactate accumulation,
is attributed to the failure of the cardiovascular system to supply the oxygen required to the muscle tissue. The disproportionate rise in ventilation is attributed to excess carbon dioxide resulting from the
buffering of the lactic acid (Jones and Ehrsam, 1982;
Wasserman and McIlroy, 1964).

Theoretically, these interactions can occur as follows: Lactic acid is a strong acid, and as noted before
in this chapter, it readily dissociates into hydrogen
ions (H^+) and lactate (La^-). Because an excess of hydrogen ions would change the pH (or acid-base balance) of the muscles and blood, the body attempts to
bind these hydrogen ions to a chemical buffer. For

example, sodium bicarbonate (a weak base) may be used as a buffer in the reaction:

$$NaHCO_3 + HLa \leftrightarrow NaLa + H_2CO_3$$

sodium + lactic $\leftrightarrow$ sodium + carbonic
bicarbonate acid lactate acid

Carbonic acid is a much weaker acid than lactic acid and can be further dissociated into water and carbon dioxide:

$$H_2CO_3 \leftrightarrow H_2O + CO_2$$

Carbon dioxide is a potent stimulant for respiration and can easily be removed from the body through respiration, thereby assisting in the maintenance of pH (Pitts, 1974). The carbon dioxide thus formed is said to be *nonmetabolic carbon dioxide,* since it does not result from the immediate breakdown of an energy substrate (carbohydrate, fat, or protein).

Figure 4.14 clearly shows that there are distinct breaks from linearity in respiration (Figure 4.14c) despite a continuous rectilinear rise in heart rate (Figure 4.14a) and oxygen consumption (Figure 4.14b) during incremental work to maximum. These breakpoints (Figure 4.14c) have been labeled as VT1 (the first ventilatory threshold) and VT2 (the second ventilatory threshold). They were originally thought to result from corresponding lactate thresholds (labeled in Figure 4.14d as LT1 and LT2, the first lactate threshold and the second lactate threshold) as a result of the buffering of lactic acid. The original work by Wasserman and others postulated only one anaerobic threshold (which would have been VT1 in Figure 4.14c), but later work identified at least two thresholds, which were given various names (Jacobs, 1986; Reinhard, et al., 1979; Skinner and McLellan, 1980). The designations VT1 and VT2 and LT1 and LT2 are used here for simplicity and because no causal mechanism is implied.

The idea that the point of lactate accumulation can be determined noninvasively by respiratory values typically measured during laboratory exercise testing of oxygen consumption is appealing, since few people truly enjoy having multiple blood samples taken. However, the terminology, determination, and mechanistic explanations are not without controversy (Walsh and Banister, 1988). Four concerns are discussed.

The primary concern is that the presence of lactate does not automatically mean that the oxygen supply is inadequate (Hughes, et al., 1982). This fact was discussed at length earlier in this chapter. Lactate accumulation does not occur at the time of increased production; rather, it occurs when the turnover rate (or balance between production and removal) cannot keep up and appearance exceeds clearance.

Figure 4.15a shows this concept graphically for incremental exercise. That is, as the exercise and

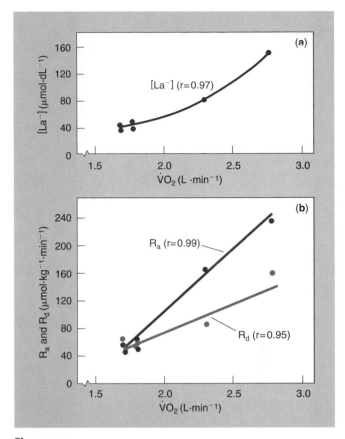

Figure 4.15

The Rate of Appearance (R_a), the Rate of Disappearance (R_d), and the Resultant Accumulation of Lactate as a Consequence of Incremental Exercise

The measured change in lactate concentration [La⁻] (a) is a result of a growing imbalance between the rate of appearance (R_a) and the rate of disappearance (R_d) (b) as exercise intensity increases.

Source: G. A. Brooks. Anaerobic threshold: Review of the concept and directions for future research. *Medicine and Science in Sports and Exercise.* 17(1):22–31 (1985). Reprinted by permission.

oxygen consumption increases, the rate of lactate appearance (R_a) in the muscle does also (Figure 4.15b). At low-intensity exercise the rate of lactate disappearance (R_d) does not differ much from R_a. However, as the intensity increases, the gap between R_a and R_d grows progressively wider. The result is the blood lactate concentration [La⁻] depicted in Figure 4.15a. Thus, it is incorrect to label the appearance of elevated levels of lactic acid in the blood as representing an anaerobic threshold.

A second concern is exactly how to interpret the lactate response to incremental work. Look closely at the lactate patterns in Figures 4.13 and 4.14. Basically, the circles representing individual data points are the same. However, in Figure 4.14 lines are imposed on the data points that clearly indicate two

Focus on Research

The Impact of Dehydration on the Lactate Threshold

Moquin, A., & R. S. Mazzeo: Effect of mild dehydration on the lactate threshold in women. *Medicine and Science in Sports and Exercise.* 32(2):396–402 (2000).

Seven collegiate female rowers participated in two incremental exercise bouts to maximum on a cycle ergometer. One trial (hydrated state) was preceded the night before by a 45-min submaximal ride at a heart rate of 130–150 $b\cdot min^{-1}$ during which the participants were allowed unlimited access to fluid. The other trial (dehydrated state) consisted of the same submaximal exercise, but the participants performed in a full sweat suit and were denied fluid until after the incremental test the next morning. See the table for results.

Despite only a mild dehydration—associated with a net drop of 1.5% in body weight—a statistically significant ($p < .05$) shift did occur in the lactate threshold, defined as the first lactate threshold, or LT1, to a lower percentage of peak oxygen consumption. This was accompanied by a significant decrease in work performance both in terms of power output and time to exhaustion. However, similar values were attained for maximal heart rate, oxygen consumption, and lactate. Thus, it appears that dehydration (or the failure to rehydrate adequately after exercise) alters the relative contributions of aerobic and anaerobic metabolism to an external workload and negatively affects performance. Guidelines for hydration will be presented in Chapter 7. The effects of dehydration on cardiovascular responses to exercise are detailed in Chapter 15.

Variable	Hydrated Trial	Dehydrated Trial
Body weight loss (kg)	0.8 ± 0.2	$1.8 \pm 0.2^*$
Performance time (min)	17.3 ± 0.7	$16.3 \pm 0.7^*$
Power output at max (W)	250.0 ± 7.7	$235.7 \pm 9.21^*$
$\dot{V}O_2$peak ($L\cdot min^{-1}$)	3.1 ± 0.2	3.0 ± 0.1
HRmax ($b\cdot min^{-1}$)	181.6 ± 2.9	180.6 ± 2.4
Lactate max ($mmol\cdot L^{-1}$)	4.65 ± 0.27	5.36 ± 0.83
Lactate threshold —LT1 ($\%\dot{V}O_2$peak)	72.2 ± 1.1	$65.5 \pm 1.8^*$

$^*p < .05$

breaks in the linearity, or two thresholds (Skinner and McLellan, 1980). The same data points are described as an exponential curve in Figure 4.13 (Hughson, et al., 1987). Experimental evidence and mathematical models (Hughson, et al., 1987) support the curvilinear interpretation. Nevertheless, the term *lactate threshold* continues to be used to indicate marked increases in the accumulation of lactate. The ventilatory thresholds are always considered to be true breakpoints.

A third concern involves carbon dioxide. Carbon dioxide is involved in the control of respiration (see Chapter 10). An excess of hydrogen ions from a source such as lactic acid can cause an increase in the amount of carbon dioxide through the bicarbonate buffering system just described. However, the presence of lactic acid is not the only mechanism that can account for an increase in carbon dioxide or the concomitant increase in minute ventilation (Inbar and Bar-Or, 1986). Evidence is particularly strong in McArdle's syndrome patients. McArdle's syndrome patients are deficient in the enzyme glycogen phosphorylase, which is necessary to convert glycogen to lactic acid. Thus, no matter how hard these patients exercise, their lactic acid values remain negligible. On the other hand, their minute ventilation values have the same distinctive breakpoints shown by anyone not deficient in glycogen phosphorylase (Heck, et al., 1985). Thus, something other than the accumulation of lactic acid must be operating to explain the ventilatory response.

Fourth, the lactate thresholds and the ventilatory thresholds do not change to the same extent in the same individuals as a result of training, glycogen depletion, caffeine ingestion, and/or varying pedaling rates (Hughes, et al., 1982; Poole and Gaesser, 1985). If they were causally linked, they should change together.

Current theory, therefore, says that although lactic acid increases and ventilatory breaks or thresholds often occur simultaneously, these responses are due to coincidence, not cause and effect (Brooks, 1985; Walsh and Banister, 1988). Exactly what these various thresholds mean is still unknown.

Despite a lack of complete understanding of the lactate threshold, the amount of work an athlete can do before accumulating large amounts of lactate has a definite bearing on performance. Distance running

Table 4.3
Lactic Anaerobic Exercise Response

Short-Term, Light to Moderate, Submaximal Exercise	Short-Term, Moderate to Heavy, Submaximal Exercise	Long-Term, Moderate to Heavy, Submaximal Exercise	Short-Term, High-Intensity, Supramaximal Exercise	Incremental Exercise to Maximum	Dynamic Resistance Exercise
≤ 2 mmol·L^{-1}	~4–6 mmol·L^{-1}	Depends on relationship to MLSS	Large increase; interval may go to 32 mmol·L^{-1}	Positive exponential curve; LT1 ~2 mmol·L^{-1}, LT2 ~4 mmol·L^{-1}; max = > 8 mmol·L^{-1}	4–21 mmol·L^{-1}; greatest with high volume and circuit type

performance, for example, depends to a large extent on some combination of $\dot{V}O_2$max, the oxygen cost of running at a given submaximal speed (called economy), and the ability to run at a high percentage of $\dot{V}O_2$max without a large accumulation of lactic acid (Costill, et al., 1973; Farrell, et al., 1979; Kinderman, et al., 1979). An indication of the running speed that represents the optimal percentage of $\dot{V}O_2$max can be achieved by determining the lactate thresholds. The first lactate threshold (LT1) generally occurs between 40 and 60% of $\dot{V}O_2$max; the second (LT2) is generally over 80% of $\dot{V}O_2$max and possibly as high as 95% of $\dot{V}O_2$max. LT1 is sometimes equated with a lactate concentration of 2 mmol·L^{-1} and LT2 with a lactate concentration of 4 mmol·L^{-1}. This 4 mmol·L^{-1} level, also called the *onset of blood lactate accumulation* (OBLA), is frequently used to decide both training loads and racing strategies (Hermansen, et al., 1975; Jacobs, 1986). Running at a pace that results in a continual accumulation of lactate has a detrimental effect on endurance time that is directly related to changes brought about by the lactate.

Dynamic Resistance Exercise

Lactate responses to dynamic resistance exercise vary greatly because the possible combination of exercises, repetitions, sets, and rest periods is almost endless. In addition, values are generally not taken repeatedly during the workout; instead, the most frequent reported values are simply postexercise ones. In general, postexercise lactate values have been shown to range from approximately 4–19 mmoL·L^{-1}. The higher values result from high-volume, moderate-load, short rest period sequences and circuit type exercise bouts (Bangsbo, et al., 1994; Burleson, et al., 1998; Keul, et al., 1978; Reynolds, et al., 1997; Tesch, 1992).

Table 4.3 summarizes the anaerobic metabolic exercise responses discussed in this section.

Why Is Lactic Acid a Problem?

It is the hydrogen ions (H$^+$) that dissociate from lactic acid, rather than undissociated lactic acid or lactate (La$^-$), that present the primary problems to the body. This distinction is important, because at normal pH levels lactic acid is almost completely dissociated immediately to H$^+$ and La$^-$ (C$_3$H$_5$O$_3$$^-$) (Brooks, 1985). As long as the amount of free H$^+$ does not exceed the ability of the chemical and physiological mechanisms to buffer them and maintain the pH at a relatively stable level, there are few problems. Most problems arise when the amount of lactic acid—and hence H$^+$—exceeds the body's immediate buffering capacity and pH decreases. The blood has become more acidic. At that point pain is perceived and performance suffers. The mechanisms of these results are described in the following subsections.

Pain Anyone who has raced or run the 400-m distance all out understands the pain caused by lactic acid. Such an event takes between approximately 45 sec and 3 min (depending on the ability of the runner) and relies heavily on the ATP-PC and LA systems to supply the needed energy. The resultant hydrogen ions accumulate and stimulate pain nerve endings located in the muscle (Guyton, 1986).

Performance Decrement The decrement in performance associated with lactic acid is brought about by fatigue that is both metabolic and muscular in origin.

1. Metabolic fatigue is a result of a reduced production of ATP linked to enzyme changes, changes in membrane transport mechanisms, and changes in substrate availability.

Enzymes—in particular, the rate-limiting enzymes in the metabolic pathways—can be inactivated by high hydrogen ion concentrations (low pH). The hydrogen ion attaches to these enzyme molecules and in so doing changes their size, shape, and hence ability to function. Phosphofructokinase (PFK) is thought to be particularly sensitive, although oxidative enzymes can also be affected (Hultman and Salin, 1980).

At the same time, changes occur in membrane transport mechanisms (either to the carriers in the membrane or to the permeability channels). These changes affect the movement of molecules across the cell membrane and between the cytoplasm and organelles such as the mitochondria (Hultman and Salin, 1980).

Energy substrate availability can be inhibited by a high concentration of hydrogen ions. Glycogen breakdown is slowed by the inactivation of the enzyme glycogen phosphorylase. Fatty acid utilization is decreased because lactic acid inhibits mobilization. Thus, a double-jeopardy situation is evident. With fatty acid availability low, a greater reliance is placed on carbohydrate sources at the time when glycogen breakdown is inhibited. At the same time, phosphocreatine (PC) breakdown is accelerated, leading to a faster depletion of substrate for ATP regeneration (Åstrand and Rodahl, 1977; Davis, 1985; Hultman and Salin, 1980).

Thus, both the inactivation of enzymes and the decrement in substrate availability will lead to a reduction in the production of ATP and, ultimately, a decrement in performance.

2. Muscular fatigue is evidenced by reduced force and velocity of muscle contraction. The contraction of skeletal muscle and the influence of lactic acid on muscular fatigue are explained in depth in Chapters 19 and 20, respectively. Suffice it to say here that a lowered pH can have two major effects on muscle contraction. The first is an inhibition of actomyosin ATPase, the enzyme responsible for the breakdown of ATP to provide the immediate energy for muscle contraction. The second is an interference of H^+ with the actions and uptake of calcium (Ca^{2+}) that is necessary for the excitation-contraction coupling and relaxation of the protein cross-bridges within the muscle fiber. High levels of lactate ions (La^-) may also interfere with cross-bridging (Hogan, et al., 1995). The result of these actions is a decrease in both the force a muscle can exert and the velocity of muscle contraction.

Time Frame for Lactate Removal Postexercise

Lactate is removed from the bloodstream relatively rapidly following exercise (Gollnick, et al., 1986). However, removal does not occur at a constant rate. If it did, then higher levels of lactate would take proportionately longer to dissipate than lower levels. For example, if you could do one push-up in 2 sec and you couldn't change that rate or speed, then 10 push-ups would take twice as long to do as 5 push-ups (20 versus 10 sec). On the other hand, if you could change that rate, you might be able to do 10 in the same time as you did 5 (in 10 sec). Many chemical reactions have this ability to change the rate or speed at which they occur. That is, the rate is proportional to the amount of substrate and product present. The more substrate available and the less product, the faster the reaction proceeds, and vice versa. This characteristic is called the *mass action effect.* Lactate appears to be one of those substrates whose utilization and conversion is linked with the amount of substrate present (Bonen, et al., 1979).

Thus, despite wide interindividual differences (which may be related to muscle fiber type), in a resting recovery situation approximately half of the lactate is removed in about 15–25 min no matter what the starting level is. This time is called the *half-life of lactate.* Near-resting levels are achieved in about 30–60 min, regardless of the starting level. Thus, the initial postexercise concentration of lactate is the first factor that influences the rate of removal. The higher the concentration, the faster the rate of removal is (Bonen, et al., 1979; Hermansen and Stensvold, 1972; Hogan, et al., 1995).

Figure 4.16 shows typical resting recovery curves from cycling and running studies. Note that in each case the value close to 50% (shown in parentheses) of the initial postexercise lactate levels occurs between 15 and 25 min of recovery.

The second factor that determines the rate of lactate removal is whether the individual follows a rest (passive) recovery or an exercise (active) recovery regimen. Third, if an exercise recovery is employed, the intensity of the exercise (expressed as a percentage of $\dot{V}O_2max$) will make a difference. Fourth, the modality of the exercise employed in the recovery phase may influence the optimal percentage of $\dot{V}O_2max$ at which removal occurs. And finally, whether the recovery exercise is continuous or intermittent seems to make a difference.

Evidence suggests that lactate removal occurs more quickly when an individual exercises during recovery than when he or she rests by sitting quietly (Bangsbo, et al., 1994). Figure 4.17 shows the results of a study conducted by Bonen and Belcastro (1976). Six trained runners completed a mile run on three different occasions. In randomized order they then performed three different 20-min recoveries: (1) seated rest, (2) continuous jogging at a self-selected pace, and (3) self-selected active recovery. During self-selected active recovery the subjects did calisthenics,

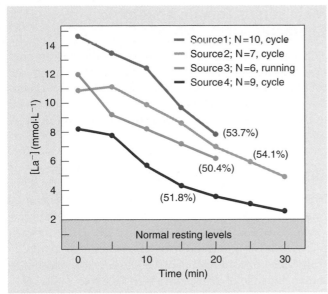

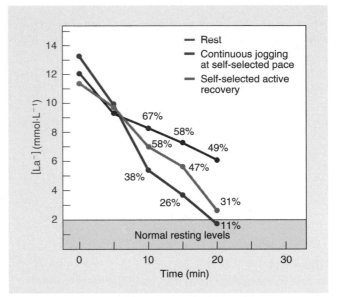

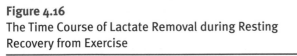

Figure 4.16

The Time Course of Lactate Removal during Resting Recovery from Exercise

During resting recovery from exercise, lactate exhibits a half-life of 15–25 minutes.

Sources: Bonen, et al. (1979); Belcastro & Bonen (1975); Bonen & Belcastro (1976); McGrail, et al. (1978).

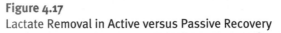

Figure 4.17

Lactate Removal in Active versus Passive Recovery

Lactate removal is faster under active than passive conditions, although the magnitude of the benefit of active recovery depends on the type and intensity of the activity. In this study, continuous jogging at 61.4% $\dot{V}O_2$max was more effective than a mixture of walking, jogging, and calisthenics.

Source: Bonen & Belcastro (1976).

walked, jogged, and rested for variable portions of the total time.

As shown in Figure 4.17, after 5 min there is no appreciable difference in the level of lactate between the different recovery protocols. However, over the next 15 min the level of lactate removal was significantly faster for the jogging recovery than for either the self-selected active recovery or the rest recovery. The self-selected activity (which is what you would typically see athletes doing at a track meet), although not as good as continuous jogging (in part because it was intermittent), was still significantly better than resting recovery.

After 20 min of jogging recovery, the lactate that remained was within the normal resting levels of 1–2 mmol·L^{-1}. The self-selected active recovery had removed 70% of the lactate, but the resting recovery had only removed 50% of the lactate. Thus, full recovery was, and generalizing is, delayed if a seated rest is employed. Because athletes who run the distances from 400–1500 m (or the English equivalents of 440 yd to 1 mi) often double at track meets, such a delay could impair their performances in the second event. On the basis of these results, an athlete competing or training at distances that are likely to cause large accumulations of lactic acid should cool down with an active continuous recovery.

Why does activity increase the rate of lactate removal? The rate of lactate removal by the liver appears to be the same whether an individual is resting or exercising. However, during exercise blood flow is increased, as is the oxidation of lactate by skeletal and cardiac muscles (Bangsbo, et al., 1994; Belcastro and Bonen, 1975; Gollnick and Hermansen, 1973; Hogan, et al., 1995; McGrail, et al., 1978). These changes appear to be primarily responsible for the beneficial effects of an active recovery.

At what intensity should an active recovery be performed? Studies that have attempted to answer this question have found an inverted U-shaped response (Belcastro and Bonen, 1975; Hogan, et al., 1995). That is, up to a point, a higher intensity of exercise (as measured by percentage of $\dot{V}O_2$max) during recovery is better. But after that point, as the intensity continues to rise, the removal rate decreases. This pattern is depicted in Figure 4.18, where the curve is both an inverted U-shape and skewed toward the lower $\dot{V}O_2$max percentage values, with the optimal rate being between 29% and 45% of $\dot{V}O_2$max. These data were collected after cycle ergometer rides. Data collected for track and treadmill exercises show the same type of inverted U-shaped curve response, but in the 55–70% $\dot{V}O_2$max range (Belcastro and Bonen,

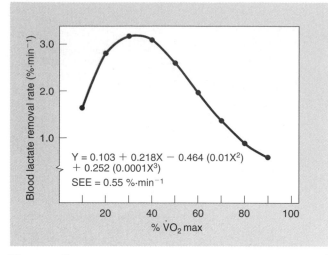

Figure 4.18

Lactate Removal Rate as a Function of the Percentage of $\dot{V}O_2$max in Recovery Exercise for Cycling

Source: A. N. Belcastro & A. Bonen. Lactic acid removal rates during controlled and uncontrolled recovery exercise. *Journal of Applied Physiology.* 39(6):932–936 (1975). Modified and reprinted by permission of the American Physiological Association.

1975; Hogan, et al., 1995.) This difference in optimal intensity may be a function of the modality (there is a higher static component for the cycle ergometer than for running) or of the training status of the subjects tested.

The actual value of these optimal percentages should not be surprising. The first lactate threshold has been shown to occur between 40% and 60% of $\dot{V}O_2$max and may be higher in trained individuals. Thus, it appears that the optimal intensity for recovery would be just below an individual's lactate threshold, where lactate production is minimal but clearance is maximized.

One word of caution: Although an active recovery is best for lactate removal, it can delay glycogen resynthesis by further depleting glycogen stores (Choi, et al., 1994). This has more relevance for an individual attempting to recover from a hard interval-training session than for someone just completing a middle-distance race and preparing for another. Glycogen depletion is likely to be more severe in the former case, and getting rid of the lactate quickly is more of an immediate concern in the latter case. For athletes recovering from an interval training session or competing in heats on successive days, the best procedure may be to combine an initial dynamic active recovery (just to the point of regaining a near-resting heart rate) with stretching and then engage in a passive recovery during which carbohydrates are consumed.

Male versus Female Anaerobic Characteristics

The anaerobic characteristics of females are in general lower than those of males during the young and middle-aged adult years. Much of the difference is undoubtedly related to the smaller overall muscle mass of the average female compared with that of the average male (Wells, 1991).

The Availability and Utilization of ATP-PC

Neither the local resting stores of ATP per kilogram of muscle nor the utilization of ATP-PC during exercise varies between the sexes (Brooks, 1986; Gollnick, et al., 1986). However, in terms of total energy available from these phosphagen sources, males will exceed females because of muscle mass differences.

The Accumulation of Lactate

Resting levels of lactate are the same for males and females. Lactate thresholds, when expressed as a percentage of $\dot{V}O_2$max, are also the same for both sexes, although the absolute workload at which the lactate thresholds occur will be higher for males than for females. Thus, at any given absolute workload that is still submaximal but above LT1 or LT2, females will have a higher lactate value than males. Consequently, the workload is more stressful for females and requires a greater anaerobic contribution. However, at a given relative workload or percentage of $\dot{V}O_2$max above the lactate thresholds, lactate concentrations are equal for both sexes (Wells, 1991).

Lactate values at maximal exercise from ages 16 through 50 are higher by approximately 0.5–2.0 $mmol \cdot L^{-1}$ for males than for females (see Figure 4.19). Once again, females are generally doing less in terms of an absolute workload than males at maximum.

The accumulation of lactate during maximal exercise presents a special dilemma for nursing mothers. A portion of the lactate present in blood diffuses into breast milk and remains present for at least 90 min (Wallace, et al., 1992; Wallace and Rabin, 1991). Infants have fully developed taste buds at birth and can detect sour tastes such as that produced by lactic acid. In fact, it has been reported that some infants will reject postexercise milk if it contains lactic acid (Wallace, et al., 1992). If a nursing mother finds that her infant fusses or refuses to nurse after she has exercised, she can try one of several things. The first option is to feed the baby just prior to exercising or collect the milk at that time and store it for later feeding. The second possibility is to discard postexercise milk and implement supplemental feeding. The third

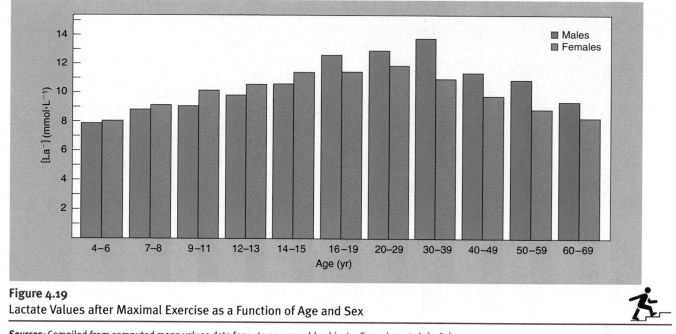

Figure 4.19
Lactate Values after Maximal Exercise as a Function of Age and Sex

Sources: Compiled from computed mean values data for 4- to 20-year-old subjects: Cumming, et al. (1985);
Saris, et al. (1985); Åstrand, et al. (1963); & Eriksson (1972). Computed mean values data for 20- to 60-year-old
subjects: Bouhuys, et al. (1966); Sidney & Shephard (1977); I. Åstrand (1960); Robinson (1938); and
P. Åstrand (1952).

possibility is to experiment with lower-intensity work-outs that may not lead to a substantial lactate accumulation. Indeed, lactating women participating in a moderate submaximal aerobic exercise program (60–70% heart rate reserve, progressing from 20 to 45 $min \cdot d^{-1}$, 5 $d \cdot wk^{-1}$ for 12 weeks) did not report any difficulties nursing after exercise (Dewey, et al, 1994). A later study that investigated maximal exercise and 30-min exercise sessions at LT1 and 20% below LT1 confirmed that the appearance of lactate in breast milk is a function of exercise intensity. Milk lactate levels were significantly higher following maximal and LT1 threshold intensity exercise, but not the LT1-20% intensity session, when compared to nonexercise control values. LT1-20% represents moderate exercise that was performed at a rate of perceived exertion of 12. Infant acceptance of postexercise milk was not directly reported in this study, but the role of lactate in infant rejection of milk in the previously described study was questioned (Quinn and Carey, 1999).

Mechanical Power and Capacity

As previously mentioned, on average males produce higher absolute work output than females. Data available from the Wingate Anaerobic Test show that values for peak power for women are approximately 65% of values for men if expressed in watts, improve to 83% if expressed in watts per kilogram of body weight, and come close to being equal at 94% when expressed in watts per kilogram of lean body mass. The corresponding comparisons for mean power are 68%, 87%, and 98%, respectively. The peak power of women (in watts per kilogram of body weight) is very similar to the mean power of men. The fatigue index does not show a significant sex difference, indicating that both sexes tire at the same rate (Makrides, et al., 1985).

Anaerobic Exercise Characteristics of Children

The anaerobic characteristics of children are not as well-developed as those of adults. Furthermore, children do not tend to be the metabolic specialists that adults are. For example, one would not expect Leroy Burrell (1994 world record holder in the 100-m dash, with a time of 9.85) to do well at the marathon distance, nor Joan Benoit Samuelson (first women's Olympic marathon winner in 1984) to be successful at the sprint distances. Yet watch children at play (Figure 4.20) and, more often than not, the fastest at short distances or strength-type events will also do well at long distances or in aerobic-type games such as soccer. Although much research is still needed to explain the anaerobic differences between children and adults, some patterns are apparent (Bar-Or, 1983).

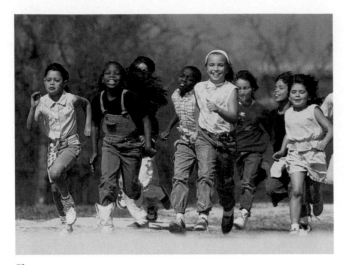

Figure 4.20

Children tend not to be metabolic specialists in their play, but can perform anaerobic short-distance or strength-type activities as well as aerobic long-distance type activities.

The Availability and Utilization of ATP-PC

Local resting stores of ATP per kilogram of wet muscle weight appear to be the same for a child and for an adult. Levels of resting PC per kilogram of wet muscle weight have been reported as slightly lower in children (Bar-Or, 1983; Shephard, 1982) or no different from adult levels (Eriksson, 1972; Shephard, 1982). There is agreement that the rate of utilization of these reserves during exercise does not differ. However, because children are smaller in stature than adults, the total amount of energy that can be generated from this source is lower.

The Accumulation of Lactate

On the average, blood lactate values obtained during submaximal exercise and after maximal exercise are lower in children than in adults (Rowland, 1990; Shephard, 1982). Furthermore, peak lactate values after maximal exercise exhibit a relatively positive rectilinear increase with age until adulthood. Figure 4.19 depicts this relationship. It also shows that there is no meaningful sex difference in children in the ability to accumulate lactate, although the girls' values are slightly higher than the boys' values throughout the growth period.

Several theories have been postulated to explain children's inability to sustain high lactate levels. All of these ideas are based upon two assumptions: that the children tested did indeed put forth a maximal effort, and that there is a physiological cause for the observed differences.

The Muscle Enzyme Theory

Eriksson (1972) and others have shown that phosphofructokinase (PFK) activity in 11- to 13-yr-old boys is 2.5–3 times lower than in trained or sedentary adult men. Since PFK is a rate-limiting enzyme of glycolysis, this lowered activity may be indicative of a decreased ability to produce lactic acid. In addition, the availability and the utilization of glycogen as a substrate are both lower in children than in adults. However, other glycolytic enzymes, such as lactic dehydrogenase (the enzyme involved in the conversion of pyruvic acid to lactic acid), show just the opposite response; that is, the highest level of activity has been seen in 12- to 14-yr-old boys (Berg, et al., 1986). Therefore, no definitive conclusion can be made about the role of the glycolytic enzymes.

In general, the oxidative enzymes show higher activity in young children than in older individuals (Berg, 1986; Williams, et al., 1990). This result, along with higher mitochondrial density and intracellular lipids, means that lipid utilization is greater in the child. Thus, it may be that children have a finer balance between aerobic and anaerobic metabolism than adults. Additional evidence for this observation comes from the fact that children show a lower oxygen deficit and reach a steady state faster than adults (Åstrand, 1952; Reybrouck, 1989; Shephard, 1982).

Sexual Maturation Theory

Limited evidence suggests that the increase in glycolytic capacity (and hence the production of lactate) in children is related to the hormonal changes that occur to bring about sexual maturation (Williams, et al., 1990). In particular, testosterone is thought to have a role.

Neurohormonal Regulation Theory

It has been shown that sympathetic nervous system activity is significantly lower in children than in adults at maximal exercise. One of the results of sympathetic stimulation during exercise is hepatic vasoconstriction. The liver plays a major role in the clearance of lactate. If blood flow to the liver is reduced, not as much lactate is cleared. Thus, because the child maintains a higher liver blood flow, more lactate can be cleared. This implies that children are not deficient in the production of lactate but are, instead, better able to remove or reconvert it than adults (Berg and Keul, 1988; Mácek and Vávra, 1985; Rowland, 1990).

Which of these theories—muscle enzyme, sexual maturation, neurohormonal regulation—or which combination of them is correct remains to be shown.

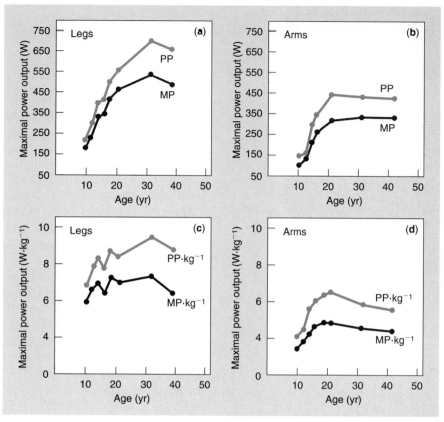

Figure 4.21
The Effect of Age on Anaerobic Performance

Cross-sectional data on 306 males who performed both an arm and a leg Wingate Anaerobic Test. The pattern of increase in values from childhood to young adulthood is similar for leg (a and c) and arm (b and d) cycling whether the unit of measurement is absolute (a and b) or relative (c and d).

Source: O. Inbar & O. Bar-Or. Anaerobic characteristics in male children and adolescents. *Medicine and Science in Sports and Exercise.* 18(3):264–269 (1986). Reprinted by permission.

The Lactate Threshold(s)

The phenomenon of ventilatory breakpoints and lactate accumulation is seen in children as well as in adults (Gaisl and Buchberger, 1979). Because children do not utilize anaerobic metabolism as early in work as adults do, the work level of children at the fixed lactate levels of 4 mmol·L^{-1} will be relatively higher than that of adults (Kanaley and Boileau, 1988; Reybrouck, 1989). Williams et al. (1990) report a value of almost 92% of $\dot{V}O_2$max for 4 mmol·L^{-1} of lactate in 11- to 13-yr-old boys and girls. Values for adults tend to be about 15% below this value. Thus, the child is working relatively harder (at a higher %$\dot{V}O_2$max) than the adult at the same lactate level. Consequently, the assessment of exercise capacity and the monitoring of training by a 4-mmol·L^{-1} value is inappropriate in prepubertal children.

Mechanical Power and Capacity

Peak power and peak power per kilogram of body weight have consistently been shown to be lower in prepubertal boys and girls than in adolescents or young adults when evaluated by the Margaria-Kalamen Stair Climb test. The results are similar to those for the Wingate Anaerobic Test, although there is a lack of information on females of all ages (Figure 4.21). In boys peak power and mean power increase consistently from age 10 to young adulthood. This is true whether the values are expressed in absolute terms (watts) or are corrected for body weight (watts per kilogram). The absolute differences between children and adults, however, are much greater (children can achieve only about 30% of adult values) than the relative differences (children can achieve about 60–85% of the adult values). Peak values seem to occur in the late thirties for the legs and the late twenties for the arms (Bar-Or, 1988; Hughson, et al., 1987).

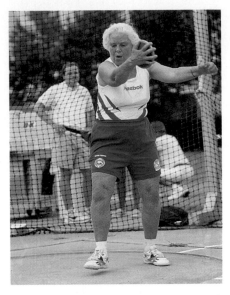

Figure 4.22

Anaerobic metabolic processes function less effectively in the elderly than in younger adults, but participation in anaerobic sports such as throwing the discus can still be enjoyed.

Anaerobic Exercise Characteristics of Older Adults

Evidence detailing anaerobic characteristics in the elderly is scarce. The reason is undoubtedly a combination of caution on the part of researchers and uncertain motivation on the part of subjects when faced with the necessarily high-intensity exercise. What data are available indicate that anaerobic variables show a common aging pattern; that is, there is typically a peak in the second or third decade and then a gradual decline into the sixth decade. Despite this, the elderly can still participate successfully in basically anaerobic activities (Figure 4.22). One must always remember when interpreting aging results, however, that no one knows how much of the reduction is a direct result of aging, how much is the result of detraining that accompanies the reduced acti-vity level of the elderly, and how much is the result of disease.

The Availability and Utilization of ATP-PC

Local resting stores of ATP-PC are reduced and levels of creatine and ADP are elevated in muscles of the elderly (Kanaley and Boileau, 1988; Simoneau, et al., 1986). Results from the Margaria-Kalamen Stair Climb test have shown a reduction in ATP-PC power of as much as 45% and a reduction in ATP-PC capacity of 32% from youth to old age (Shephard, 1982). This means that ATP-PC stores are both reduced and unable to be used as quickly. The result is a decrease in alactic anaerobic power.

The Accumulation of Lactate

On the average, resting levels of blood lactate are remarkably consistent across the entire age span, varying only from 1 to 2 mmol·L^{-1}.

Lactate values during the same absolute submaximal work show a tendency to be higher for individuals over the age of 50 (I. Åstrand, 1960; P.-O. Åstrand, 1952, 1956; Robinson, 1938). However, this generalization is confounded by the fact that at any given absolute load of work, the older individual is working at a higher percentage of his or her maximal aerobic power, which would be expected to involve anaerobic metabolism more (Sidney and Shephard, 1977). When younger and older individuals work at the same relative workload (%$\dot{V}O_2$max), lactate concentrations are lower in older people than in the young, probably because the elderly are using less muscle mass to do less work (Kohrt, et al., 1993). Data are unavailable on the lactate thresholds in the elderly.

Maximal lactate levels reach a peak between 16 and 39 yr of age and then show a gradual decline (see Figure 4.19). Both males and females exhibit the same pattern, with the absolute values of females being considerably lower than those of males.

Physiological factors appear to contribute to the decline in maximal lactate values with age (Shephard, 1982; Smith and Serfass, 1981). First, activity of the enzyme lactate dehydrogenase (which catalyzes the conversion of pyruvic acid to lactic acid) decreases in all muscle fiber types. This decrease effectively slows glycolysis. The reduction in glycolysis may also be related to reduced amounts of glycogen stored in the skeletal muscles of the elderly.

Second, the elderly possess a smaller ratio of muscle mass to blood volume, a smaller ratio of capillary to muscle fiber, and a concomitant slower diffusion of lactic acid out of the active muscle fibers and into the bloodstream (Shephard, 1982). Thus, it may not be that the elderly have a large deficiency in anaerobic capacity at the cellular level; rather, it may simply be that measurements from blood samples are underestimations. Of course, a combination of the first and second factors may also be operating.

Mechanical Power and Capacity

The average peak power value obtained on the Margaria-Kalamen Stair Climb test (Figure 4.23a) declines precipitously over the 20- to 70-yr age range (Bouchard, et al., 1982). Published results are

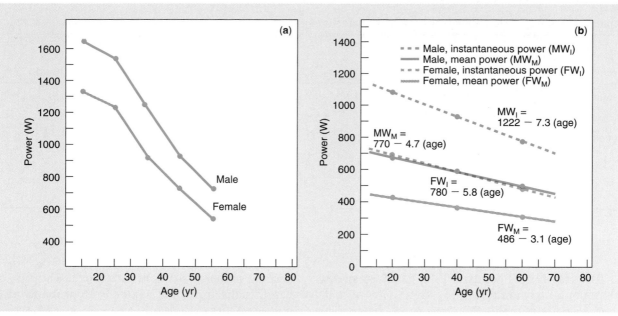

Figure 4.23
Mechanical Power Changes with Age in Males and Females

(a) Average peak power ratings determined from the Margaria-Kalamen Stair Climb are higher for males than females across the age span from adolescence to middle adulthood. Males and females show steady and parallel declines in peak power during the adult years. (b) Instantaneous peak power and mean power measured during a 30-sec cycle ergometer test are higher for males (MW_I and MW_M, respectively) than for females (FW_I and FW_M, respectively) across the age span from late adolescence to older adulthood. Female instantaneous peak power (FW_I) is equal to male mean power (MW_M). Instantaneous peak power and mean power show rectilinear and parallel declines with age in males and females. Each line was calculated from the experimentally determined equation associated with that line on the graph.

Sources: (a) Data from Bouchard et al. (1982). (b) Data from Makrides et al. (1985).

unavailable for the Wingate Anaerobic Test for individuals over the age of 40 and for females except in the 18- to 28-yr range (Maud and Shultz, 1989). However, Makrides et al. (1985) have presented data on 50 male and 50 female subjects from 15 to 70 on a test similar to the WAT (Figure 4.23b). In this case peak power represents an instantaneous value rather than a 5-sec value. Mean power is still the average of 30 sec of pedaling but at a controlled rate of 60 rev·min^{-1}. The results from this study show a decline of approximately 6% for each decade of age for sedentary individuals of both sexes. However, the absolute values for the females are consistently lower than those for the males. Indeed, in the Makrides study the peak power of the females coincides with the mean power of the males. For both sexes lean thigh volume was found to be closely related to peak power and mean power, but it did not account for all the variation in the values or in the decline with age.

Heritability of Anaerobic Characteristics

There is an old saying that "sprinters are born and distance runners are made." Is this statement scientifically defensible? The answer is both yes and no. Since sprinters are the anaerobic athletes, only sprinters will be dealt with here. Very little research has been done on the genetic contribution to differences in alactic and lactic anaerobic power and capacity, which form the basis for successful sprint performances. However, because there is so much interindividual variation in anaerobic values and abilities, genetics is likely to play an important role. Heritability studies ideally compare measures of a given trait for pairs of monozygous (MZ), or identical, twins and dizygous (DZ), or fraternal, twins. The expectation is that the MZ twins will show less variability (that is, be more similar in the trait) than the DZ twins. The studies detailed here comprise what is known at this time.

Table 4.4
Intrapair Correlations of Heritability for Anaerobic Characteristics

Source	Pairs	ATP-PC System $J \cdot kg^{-1}$	$J \cdot kg^{-1}$ FFW^{-1*}	LA System (mmol L^{-1})
Klissouras (1971)	DZ twins (N = 15)			0.76
	MZ twins (N = 10)			0.93
Simoneau, et al. (1986)	Adopted siblings (N = 19)	−0.01	0.06	
	Biological siblings (N = 55)	0.46	0.38	
	DZ twins (N = 31)	0.58	0.44	
	MZ twins (N = 49)	0.80	0.77	

* FFW = fat free body weight.

Klissouras (1971) compared the lactate response to incremental treadmill running in 10 pairs of male DZ and 15 pairs of males MZ twins from 7 to 13. The young age of the subjects was thought to be helpful in controlling for the effect of environment. The lactate responses were more similar for the more closely genetically related MZ twins than for the DZ twins (Table 4.4). The study concluded that the genetic determination for lactate accumulation was 81.4%.

Komi and colleagues provided data on 15 pairs of male and 14 pairs of female twins between the ages of 10 and 14 (1973) and 20 pairs of male and 11 pairs of female twins between the ages of 15 and 24 (1979). The variability in maximal mechanical power as measured by the Margaria-Kalamen Stair Climb was found to be 99.2% genetically determined in the preadolescent boys and 97.8% in the older men. The variability could not be computed for the girls and women.

Simoneau et al. (1986) studied the alactic anaerobic capacity in four groups with increasing genetic communality—that is, adopted siblings, biological siblings, dizygotic twins, and monozygotic twins. Both sexes were included, and the ages ranged from 9 to 33. Alactic anaerobic capacity was determined by the total work output (in joules) on a bicycle ergometer in 10 sec. Table 4.4 shows that the correlations between the work output of the pairs of siblings or twins got steadily higher as the shared genetics increased between the groups. As expected, there was not much difference between the separate-birth biological siblings and dizygotic twins when expressed in joules per kilogram of body weight or joules per kilogram of fat free body weight (FFW). The total genetic effect was estimated to be between 44% and 76%.

On the basis of these data it can only be concluded that there is some degree of genetic influence on anaerobic characteristics but the exact amount is unknown. It can therefore be said that, at least to a certain extent, sprinters are born. On the other hand, as discussed in Chapter 5, so probably are distance runners.

Summary

1. Anaerobic metabolism does not require oxygen to produce adenosine-triphosphate (ATP), but aerobic metabolism does.

2. Anaerobic and aerobic metabolism work together to provide ATP and, hence, energy for exercise. Depending on the duration and intensity of the activity, one or the other predominates.

IP *Muscular–Muscle Metabolism* (pages 3–12; 15–18)

3. The adenosine triphosphate-phosphocreatine (ATP-PC) system predominates in high-intensity exercise that lasts 30 sec or less. The LA system predominates in high-intensity exercise lasting between 30 sec and 1½ min. The aerobic system predominates in exercise lasting from 3–5 min to hours. This sequence is called the time-energy system continuum.

4. There is no generally accepted way to directly measure the anaerobic energy contribution to exercise. One indirect approach is to describe the changes in ATP, PC, and lactate levels. Another is to quantify the amount of work performed or power generated during short-duration, high-intensity activity.

5. Lactic acid/lactate production depends on the use of glycogen as fuel, the formation of pyruvate, and the necessity of preserving the redox potential of the cell. It involves
   a. muscle contraction that in turn depends on calcium release and results in glycogenolysis;

b. the high activity of the enzyme lactate dehydrogenase compared with other glycolytic and oxidative enzymes;

c. recruitment of fast-twitch glycolytic (FG, Type IIA and FOG, Type IIB) muscle fibers;

d. activation of the sympathetic nervous system, which ultimately results in glycogenolysis; and

e. insufficient oxygen, which results in anaerobiosis or the onset of anaerobic metabolism.

6. Lactic acid/lactate clearance utilizes both an intracellular and extracellular shuttle system. MCT1 and MCT4 transporters move lactate by facilitated exchange down concentration and pH gradients.

7. Lactate accumulation results when production (appearance) exceeds clearance (disappearance).

8. The onset of all exercise is characterized by a discrepancy between oxygen demand and oxygen utilization known as the oxygen deficit. This deficit is due not to the cardiovascular-respiratory system's inability to respond but to limited cellular utilization of oxygen as a result of metabolic adjustments. That is, when ATP is broken down into ADP + P_i and elevated levels of NADH + H^+ are present, both aerobic and anaerobic metabolic pathways are stimulated to produce more ATP.

9. During the transition from rest to exercise—the *O₂ debt* period—energy is supplied by:
a. Oxygen transport and utilization.
b. The use of oxygen stores in venous blood and on myoglobin.
c. The splitting of stored ATP-PC.
d. Anaerobic glycolysis with the concomitant production of lactic acid.

10. During recovery from exercise, oxygen consumption remains elevated. The term *excess postexercise oxygen consumption (EPOC)* is used to refer to this phenomenon. The following factors appear to be ongoing during recovery.
a. Restoration of ATPPC stores
b. Restoration of oxygen stores
c. Elevated cardiorespiratory function
d. Elevated hormonal levels
e. Elevated body temperature
f. Lactate removal

11. During exercise, the balance between aerobic and anaerobic metabolism depends on the intensity of the activity in relation to the individual's maximal ability to produce energy using oxygen ($\dot{V}O_2$max).

12. During high-intensity, short-duration (3 min or less) anaerobic exercise ATP levels decrease 30–40%, PC levels decrease 60–70%, and lactate accumulation can increase well over 1000%.

13. The lactate response (increase, decrease, no change after an initial rise) to long-term moderate to heavy submaximal exercise depends to a large extent on the intensity of the exercise in relation to the maximal lactate steady state (MLSS) intensity.

14. During incremental work to maximum lactate accumulates slowly until approximately 40–60% $\dot{V}O_2$max when the continual accumulation is exponentially curvilinear. The term *lactate threshold* (LT) is commonly (although not absolutely accurately) used to describe the point where large increases in lactate accumulation occur.

15. LT1 is typically found between 40 and 60% $\dot{V}O_2$max, and LT2 is found between 80 and 95% $\dot{V}O_2$max. An absolute value of 4 mmol·L^{-1} is termed the *onset of blood lactate accumulation (OBLA)* and is often used as a training and racing guideline.

16. The relationship between the lactate thresholds and ventilatory thresholds appears to be primarily coincidental.

17. The term *anaerobic threshold* is a misnomer and should not be used because the presence of lactate does not automatically mean that the oxygen supply is inadequate.

18. Performance decrements occur with high concentrations of H^+ because of:
a. Pain.
b. Reduced production of ATP through inactivation of enzymes or changes in membrane transport.
c. Inhibition of energy substrate availability because glycogen breakdown is slowed or because fatty acid mobilization is slowed.
d. Reduced force and velocity of muscle contraction.

19. Lactate removal from the bloodstream after exercise follows the law of mass action: The more lactate present, the faster the rate of removal. The half-life of lactate is approximately 15–25 min, with full removal achieved between 30 and 60 min.

20. The time required for lactate removal can be decreased by doing an active recovery at an intensity of approximately 30–45% $\dot{V}O_2$max for cycling and 55–70% $\dot{V}O_2$max for running.

21. The anaerobic characteristics of children are not well developed in comparison with those of adults. The lower amount of ATP-PC available is related to children's small body size.

22. Peak lactate values after incremental exercise to maximum are lower in children than adults and vary directly with age throughout the growth years. There is no meaningful male-female difference in the ability to accumulate lactate during childhood.

23. Mechanical power and capacity are lower for children and adolescents than for adults, whether expressed in absolute terms or corrected for body weight.

24. During the adult years males accumulate higher levels of blood lactate as a result of maximal work than do females, and males exhibit higher mechanical power and capacity even when they are adjusted for body weight.

25. Anaerobic metabolic processes decline from young and middle-aged to older adults. The decline includes lower resting levels of ATP-PC.

26. Peak lactate values after incremental exercise to maximum decline after approximately 40 yr of age. Females exhibit considerably lower peak values than males.

27. The mechanical power and capacity of the elderly decline steadily. The decline is greater in females than in males.

28. The exact degree of genetic influence on anaerobic characteristics is unknown, although estimates range from 44–99%.

Review Questions

1. Describe the energy continuum. For each of the following sports or events, determine the percentage contribution from the ATP-PC, LA, and O_2 systems.

   a. 100-m dash   f. 100-m swim
   b. 800-m run   g. mile run
   c. soccer (not goalie)   h. stealing a base
   d. triathlon   i. wrestling period
   e. volleyball spike

2. List the major variables that are typically measured to describe the anaerobic response to exercise. Where possible, provide an example of an exercise test from which the variable could be determined.

3. Explain the five physiological reasons for the production of lactic acid. What determines whether or not lactate accumulates in the blood? How is lactate cleared?

4. Arrange the ATP-PC, LA, and O_2 systems from highest to lowest in terms of (a) power and (b) capacity. What is the difference between power and capacity?

5. Diagram the oxygen deficit and excess postexercise oxygen consumption for an activity that requires 110% $\dot{V}O_2$max in an individual whose $\dot{V}O_2$max equals 4 $L\cdot min^{-1}$ and whose resting oxygen is 0.25 $L\cdot min^{-1}$. Explain how energy is provided during the oxygen deficit time period and why oxygen remains elevated during recovery.

6. Diagram and explain the changes that take place in ATP, PC, and [La$^-$] during constant-load, heavy exercise lasting 3 min or less.

7. Explain the concept of maximal lactate steady state and why MLSS is important in endurance performance.

8. Diagram the lactate response to incremental work to maximum. The ventilatory and lactate thresholds often occur at approximately the same time. Debate whether this is a result of cause and effect or coincidence. Can either the lactate thresholds or the ventilatory thresholds be accurately described as anaerobic thresholds? Why or why not?

9. What are the physiological effects of lactate accumulation?

10. What is the best way to clear lactate quickly during recovery?

11. What are the effects of sex and age on anaerobic metabolism during exercise?

12. Approximately how much of an individual's anaerobic ability is due to genetic factors? Are sprinters made or born?

For further review and additional study tools, go to The Physiology Place (www.physiologyplace.com) and the Student Study Guide for Exercise Physiology for Health, Fitness, and Performance *by Sharon A. Plowman and Denise L. Smith.*

Passport to the Internet

Visit the following Internet sites to explore further topics and issues related to anaerobic metabolism. To visit an organization's web site, go to www.physiology place.com and click on "Passport to the Internet."

The Nicholas Institut e of Sports Medicine and Ath-letic Trauma (NISMAT) The Nicholas Institute of Sports Medicine and Athletic Trauma (NISMAT) is the first hospital-based facility dedicated to the study of sports medicine in the United States. First explore this complete site. Then go to www.nismat.org/physcor/energy_supply.html for a thorough discussion of muscle energy supply.

Arnot Ogden Medical Center Visit the Arnot Ogden Medical Center for an informative discussion on energy without oxygen.

References

American College of Sports Medicine Roundtable: The physiological and health effects of oral creatine supplementation. *Medicine and Science in Sports and Exercise.* 32(3):706–717 (2000).

Åstrand, I.: Aerobic work capacity in men and women with special reference to age. *Acta Physiologica Scandinavica* (Suppl.). 169:1–92 (1960).

Åstrand, P.-O.: *Experimental Studies of Physical Working Capacity in Relation to Sex and Age.* Copenhagen: Munksgaard (1952).

Åstrand, P.-O.: Human physical fitness with special reference to sex and age. *Physiological Reviews.* 36(3):307–335 (1956).

Åstrand, P.-O., L. Engstrom, B. O. Eriksson, P. Karlberg, I. Nylander, B. Saltin, & C. Thoren: Girl swimmers: With special reference to respiratory and circulatory adaption and gynecological and psychiatric aspects. *Acta Paediatrica* (Suppl.). 147:1–73 (1963).

Åstrand, P.-O., & K. Rodahl: *Textbook of Work Physiology: Physiological Bases of Exercise.* New York: McGraw-Hill (1977).

Bahr, R.: Excess postexercise oxygen consumption—Magnitude, mechanisms and practical implications. *Acta Physiologica Scandinavica* (Suppl.). 605:9–70 (1992).

Bangsbo, J., T. Graham, L. Johansen, & B. Saltin: Muscle lactate metabolism in recovery from intense exhaustive exercise: Impact of light exercise. *Journal of Applied Physiology.* 77(4):1890–1895 (1994).

Bar-Or, O.: *Pediatric Sports Medicine for the Practitioner: From Physiological Principles to Clinical Applications.* New York: Springer-Verlag, 1–65 (1983).

Bar-Or, O.: The prepubescent female. In M. M. Shangold & G. Mirkin (eds.), *Women and Exercise: Physiology and Sports Medicine.* Philadelphia: Davis, 109–119 (1988).

Bar-Or, O.: The Wingate Anaerobic Test: An update on methodology, reliability and validity. *Sports Medicine.* 4:381–394 (1987).

Belcastro, A. N., & A. Bonen: Lactic acid removal rates during controlled and uncontrolled recovery exercise. *Journal of Applied Physiology.* 39(6):932–936 (1975).

Beneke, R.: Anaerobic threshold, individual anaerobic threshold, and maximal lactate steady state in rowing. *Medicine and Science in Sports and Exercise.* 27(6):863–867 (1995).

Beneke, R., M. Hutler, & R. M. Leithauser: Maximal lactate-steady-state independent of performance. *Medicine and Science in Sports and Exercise.* 32(6): 1135-1139 (2000).

Berg, A., & J. Keul: Biochemical changes during exercise in children. In R. M. Malina (ed.), *Young Athletes: Biological, Psychological, and Educational Perspectives.* Champaign, IL: Human Kinetics (1988).

Berg, A., S. S. Kim, & J. Keul: Skeletal muscle enzyme activities in healthy young subjects. *International Journal of Sports Medicine.* 7:236–239 (1986).

Bonen, A.: Lactate transporters (MCT proteins) in heart and skeletal muscles. *Medicine and Science in Sports and Exercise.* 32(4):778–789 (2000).

Bonen, A., & A. N. Belcastro: Comparison of self-selected recovery methods on lactic acid removal rates. *Medicine and Science in Sports.* 8(3):176–178 (1976).

Bonen, A., C. J. Campbell, R. L. Kirby, & A. N. Belcastro: A multiple regression model for blood lactate removal in man. *Pflügers Archives.* 380:205–210 (1979).

Bouchard, C., A. W. Taylor, & S. Dulac: Testing maximal anaerobic power and capacity. In J. D. MacDougall, H. W. Wenger, & H. J. Green (eds.), *Physiological Testing of the High-Performance Athlete* (2nd edition). Champaign, IL: Human Kinetics, 175–221 (1991).

Bouchard, C., A. W. Taylor, J. A. Simoneau, & S. Dulac: Testing anaerobic power and capacity. In J. D. MacDougall, H. A. Wenger, & H. J. Green (eds.), *Physiological Testing of the Elite Athlete.* Hamilton, Ontario: Canadian Association of Sport Sciences Mutual Press Limited, 61–73 (1982).

Bouhuys, A., J. Pool, R. A. Binkhorst, & P. van Leeuwen: Metabolic acidosis of exercise in healthy males. *Journal of Applied Physiology.* 21(3):1040–1046 (1966).

Brooks, G. A.: Anaerobic threshold: Review of the concept and directions for future research. *Medicine and Science in Sports and Exercise.* 17(1):22–31 (1985).

Brooks, G. A.: Intra- and extra-cellular lactate shuttles. *Medicine and Science in Sports and Exercise.* 32(4):790–700 (2000).

Brooks, G. A.: The lactate shuttle during exercise and recovery. *Medicine and Science in Sports and Exercise.* 18(3):360–368 (1986).

Brooks, G. A., T. D. Fahey, T. P. White, & K. M. Baldwin: *Exercise Physiology: Human Bioenergetics and Its Applications* (3rd edition). Mountain View, CA: Mayfield (1999).

Burleson, M. A., Jr., H. S. O'Bryant, M. H. Stone, M. A. Collins, & T. Triplett-McBride: Effect of weight training exercise and treadmill exercise on post-exercise oxygen consumption. *Medicine and Science in Sports and Exercise.* 30(4):518–522 (1998).

Cheetham, M. E., L. H. Boobis, S. Brooks, & C. Williams: Human muscle metabolism during sprint running. *Journal of Applied Physiology.* 61(1):54–60 (1986).

Choi, D., K. J. Cole, B. H. Goodpaster, W. J. Fink, & D. L. Costill: Effect of passive and active recovery on the resynthesis of muscle glycogen. *Medicine and Science in Sports and Exercise.* 26(8):992–996 (1994).

Costill, D. L.: Metabolic responses during distance running. *Journal of Applied Physiology.* 28(3):251–255 (1970).

Costill, D. L., H. Thomason, & E. Roberts: Fractional utilization of the aerobic capacity during distance running. *Medicine and Science in Sports.* 5(4):248–252 (1973).

Cumming, G. R., L. Hastman, & J. McCort: Treadmill endurance times, blood lactate, and exercise blood pressures in normal children. In R. A. Binkhorst, H. C. G. Kemper, & W. H. M. Saris (eds.), *Children and Exercise XI.* Champaign, IL: Human Kinetics 140–150 (1985).

Davis, J. A.: Response to Brooks' manuscript. *Medicine and Science in Sports and Exercise.* 17(1):32–34 (1985).

Dewey, K. G., C. A. Lovelady, L. A. Nommsen-Rivers, M. A. McCrory, & B. Lonnerdal: A randomized study of the effects of aerobic exercise by lactating women on breast-milk volume and composition. *New England Journal of Medicine.* 330(7):449–453 (1994).

Donovan, C. M. & M. J. Pagliassotti: Quantitative assessment of pathways for lactate disposal in skeletal muscle fiber types. *Medicine and Science in Sports and Exercise.* 32(4): 772–777 (2000).

Eriksson, B. O.: Physical training, oxygen supply and muscle metabolism in 11–13 year old boys. *Acta Physiologica Scandinavica* (Suppl.). 384:1–48 (1972).

Farrell, P. A., J. H. Wilmore, E. F. Coyle, J. E. Billing, & D. L. Costill: Plasma lactate accumulation and distance running performance. *Medicine and Science in Sports and Exercise.* 11:338–344 (1979).

Fox, E. L.: Measurement of the maximal lactic (phosphagen) capacity in man. *Medicine and Science in Sports* (abstract). 5:66 (1973).

Freund, H., S. Oyono-Enguéllé, A. Heitz, C. Ott, J. Marbach, M. Gartner, & A. Pape: Comparative lactate kinetics after short and prolonged submaximal exercise. *International Journal of Sports Medicine.* 11(4):284–288 (1990).

Gaesser, G. A., & G. A. Brooks: Muscular efficiency during steady-rate exercise: Effects of speed and work rate. *Journal of Applied Physiology.* 38(6):1132–1139 (1975).

Gaisl, G., & J. Buchberger: Determination of the aerobic and anaerobic thresholds of 10–11 year old boys using blood-gas analysis. In K. Berg & B. O. Eriksson (eds.), *Children and Exercise IX.* Baltimore: University Park Press, International Series of Sport Sciences 93–98 (1979).

Gladden, L. B.: Muscle as a consumer of lactate. *Medicine and Science in Sports and Exercise.* 32(4):764–771 (2000).

Gollnick, P. D., W. M. Bayly, & D. R. Hodgson: Exercise intensity, training, diet, and lactate concentration in muscle and blood. *Medicine and Science in Sports and Exercise.* 18(3):334–340 (1986).

Gollnick, P. D., & L. Hermansen: Biochemical adaptations to exercise: Anaerobic metabolism. In J. H. Wilmore (ed.), *Exercise and Sport Sciences Reviews.* New York: Academic Press (1973).

Gollnick, P. D., & D. W. King: Energy release in the muscle cell. *Medicine and Science in Sports.* 1(1):23–31 (1969).

Green, H. J.: Muscle power: Fiber type recruitment, metabolism and fatigue. In N. L. Jones, M. McCartney, & A. J. McComas (eds.), *Human Muscle Power.* Champaign, IL: Human Kinetics (1986).

Green, S.: Measurement of anaerobic work capacities in humans. *Sports Medicine.* 19(1):32–42 (1995).

Guyton, A. C.: *Textbook of Medical Physiology* (7th edition). Philadelphia: Saunders (1986).

Hagberg, J. M., E. F. Coyle, J. E. Carroll, J. M. Miller, W. H. Martin, & M. H. Brooke: Exercise hyperventilation in patients with McArdle's disease. *Journal of Applied Physiology.* 52:991–994 (1982).

Heck, H., A. Mader, G. Hess, S. Mücke, R. Müller, & W. Hollmann: Justification of the 4-mmol/L lactate threshold. *International Journal of Sports Medicine.* 6:117–130 (1985).

Hermansen, L., S. Maehlum, E. D. R. Pruett, O. Vaage, H. Waldum, & T. Wessel-Aas: Lactate removal at rest and during exercise. In H. Howald & J. R. Poortmans (eds.), *Metabolic Adaptation to Prolonged Exercise.* Basel: Birkhäuser, 101–105 (1975).

Hermansen, L., & I. Stensvold: Production and removal of lactate during exercise in man. *Acta Physiologica Scandinavica.* 86:191–201 (1972).

Hogan, M. C., L. B. Gladden, S. S. Kurdak, & D. C. Poole: Increased [lactate] in working dog muscle reduces tension development independent of pH. *Medicine and Science in Sports and Exercise* 27(3):371–377 (1995).

Hughes, E. F., S. C. Tuner, & G. A. Brooks: Effect of glycogen depletion and pedaling speed on anaerobic threshold. *Journal of Applied Physiology.* 52(6):1598–1607 (1982).

Hughson, R. L., K. H. Weisiger, & G. D. Swanson: Blood lactate concentration increases as a continuous function in progressive exercise. *Journal of Applied Physiology.* 62(5):1975–1981 (1987).

Hultman, E., & K. Sahlin: Acid-base balance during exercise. In R. S. Hutton & D. I. Miller (eds.), *Exercise and Sport Sciences Reviews.* 8:41–128 (1980).

Inbar, O., & O. Bar-Or: Anaerobic characteristics in male children and adolescents. *Medicine and Science in Sports and Exercise.* 18(3):264–269 (1986).

Jacobs, I. Blood lactate: Implications for training and sports performance. *Sports Medicine.* 3:10–25 (1986).

Jones, N. L., & R. E. Ehrsam: The anaerobic threshold. In R. L. Terjung (ed.), *Exercise and Sport Sciences Reviews.* 10:49–83 (1982).

Kanaley, J. A., & R. A. Boileau: The onset of the anaerobic threshold at three stages of physical maturity. *Journal of Sports Medicine and Physical Fitness.* 28(4):367–374 (1988).

Kapit, W., R. I. Macey, & E. Meisami: *The Physiology Coloring Book* (2nd edition). San Francisco: Addison Wesley Longman (2000).

Kenney, R. A. *Physiology of Aging: A Synopsis.* Chicago: Year Book Medical (1982).

Keul, J., G. Haralambie, M. Bruder, & H.-J. Gottstein: The effect of weight lifting exercise on heart rate and metabolism in experienced weight lifters. *Medicine and Science in Sports.* 10(1):13–15 (1978).

Kinderman, W., G. Simon, & J. Keul: The significance of the aerobic-anaerobic transition for the determination of workload intensities during endurance training. *European Journal of Applied Physiology.* 42:25–34 (1979).

Klissouras, V.: Heritability of adaptive variation. *Journal of Applied Physiology.* 31(3):338–344 (1971).

Kohrt, W. M., R. J. Spina, A. A. Ehsani, P. E. Cryer, & J. O. Holloszy: Effects of age, adiposity, and fitness level on plasma catecholamine responses to standing and exercise. *Journal of Applied Physiology.* 75(4):1828–1835 (1993).

Komi, P. V., & J. Karlsson: Physical performance, skeletal muscle enzyme activities, and fibre types in monozygous and dizygous twins of both sexes. *Acta Physiologica Scandinavica* (Suppl.). 462:5–28 (1979).

Komi, P. V., V. Klissouras, & E. Karvinen: Genetic variation in neuromuscular performance. *Internationale Zeitschrift für Angewandte Physiologie.* 31:289–304 (1973).

Kraemer, W. J., L. J. Marchitelli, D. McCurry, S. J. Fleck, J. E. Dziados, E. Harman, A. L. Vela, & P. Frykman: Lactate responses to different resistance exercise protocols: Impact of different variables. *National Strength Conditioning Association Journal.* 8(4):72 (abstract) (1986).

Mácek, M., & J. Vávra: Anaerobic threshold in children. In R. A. Binkhorst, H. C. G. Kemper, & W. H. M. Saris (eds.), *Children and Exercise XI.* Champaign, IL: Human Kinetics Publishers, 110–113 (1985).

Makrides, L., G. J. F. Heigenhauser, N. McCartney, & N. L. Jones: Maximal short term exercise capacity in healthy subjects aged 15–70 years. *Clinical Science.* 69:197–205 (1985).

Margaria, R., M. T. Edwards, & D. B. Dill: The possible mechanisms of contracting and paying the oxygen debt and the role of lactic acid in muscular contraction. *American Journal of Physiology.* 106:689–715 (1933).

Maud, P. J., & B. B. Shultz: Norms for the Wingate Anaerobic Test with comparison to another similar test. *Research Quarterly for Exercise and Sport.* 60(2):144–151 (1989).

McGrail, J. C., A. Bonen, & A. N. Belcastro: Dependence of lactate removal on muscle metabolism in man. *European Journal of Applied Physiology.* 39:87–97 (1978).

Misic, M. M., G. A. Kelley, S. A. Plowman, & G. A. Schlabach: The effects of creatine supplementation on anaerobic performance: Preliminary meta-analytic results. *Medicine and Science in Sports and Exercise.* 32(5) Supplement: S137 (abstract) (2000).

Newsholme, E. A., & A. R. Leech: *Biochemistry for the Medical Sciences.* New York: Wiley (1983).

Noble, B. J., W. J. Kraemer, M. J. Clark, & B. W. Culver: Stress response to high intensity circuit weight training in experienced weight trainers. *Medicine and Science in Sports and Exercise.* 16(2):146 (abstract) (1984).

O'Brien, M. J., C. A. Viguie, R. S. Mazzeo, & G. A. Brooks: Carbohydrate dependence during marathon running. *Medicine and Science in Sports and Exercise.* 25(9):1009–1017 (1993).

Patton, J. F., & A. Duggan: An evaluation of tests of anaerobic power. *Aviation and Space Environmental Medicine.* 58:237–242 (1987).

Pitts, R. F.: *Physiology of the Kidney and Body Fluids* (3rd edition). Chicago: Year Book Medical (1974).

Poole, D. C., & G. A. Gaesser: Response of ventilatory and lactate threshold to continuous and interval training. *Journal of Applied Physiology.* 58(4):1115–1121 (1985).

Poortmans, J. R., & M. Francaux: Adverse effects of creatine supplementation: Fact or fiction? *SportsMedicine.* 30(3): 155–170 (2000).

Quinn, T. J. & G. B. Carey: Does exercise intensity or diet influence lactic acid accumulation in breast milk? *Medicine and Science in Sports and Exercise.* 31(1):105–110 (1999).

Reinhard, V., P. H. Muller, & R. M. Schmulling: Determination of anaerobic threshold by the ventilation equivalent in normal individuals. *Respiration.* 38:36–42 (1979).

Reybrouck, T. M.: The use of the anaerobic threshold in pediatric exercise testing. In O. Bar-Or (ed.), *Advances in Pediatric Sport Sciences.* Champaign, IL: Human Kinetics Publishers, 131–150 (1989).

Reynolds, T. H., IV, P. A. Frye, & G. A. Sforzo: Resistance training and the blood lactate response to resistance exercise in women. *Journal of Strength and Conditioning Research.* 11(2):77–81 (1997).

Robinson, S.: Experimental studies of physical fitness in relation to age. *Arbeitsphysiologie.* 10:251–323 (1938).

Rowland, T. W.: *Exercise and Children's Health.* Champaign, IL: Human Kinetics Publishers (1990).

Sahlin, K., J. M. Ren, & S. Broberg: Oxygen deficit at the onset of submaximal exercise is not due to a delayed oxygen transport. *Acta Physiologica Scandinavica.* 134:175–180 (1988).

Saris, W. H. M., A. M. Noordeloos, B. E. M. Ringnalda, M. A. Van't Hof, & R. A. Binkhorst: Reference values for aerobic power of healthy 4 to 18 year old Dutch children: Preliminary results. In R. A. Binkhorst, H. C. G. Kemper, & W. H. M. Saris (eds.), *Children and Exercise XI.* Champaign, IL: Human Kinetics Publishers, 151–160 (1985).

Shephard, R. J.: *Physical Activity and Growth.* Chicago: Year Book Medical (1982).

Sidney, K. H., & R. J. Shephard: Maximum and submaximum exercise tests in men and women in the seventh, eighth, and ninth decade of life. *Journal of Applied Physiology: Respiratory, Environmental and Exercise Physiology.* 43(2):280–287 (1977).

Simoneau, J. A., G. Lortie, C. Leblanc, & C. Bouchard: Anaerobic alactacid work capacity in adopted and biological siblings. In R. M. Malina & C. Bouchard (eds.), *Sport and Human Genetics.* Champaign, IL: Human Kinetics Publishers, 165–171 (1986).

Skinner, J. S., & T. H. McLellan: The transition from aerobic to anaerobic metabolism. *Research Quarterly for Exercise and Sport.* 51(1):234–248 (1980).

Smith, E. L., & R. C. Serfass (eds.): *Exercise and Aging: The Scientific Basis.* Hillside, NJ: Enslow Publishers (1981).

Spriet, L. L., R. A. Howlett, & G. J. F. Heigenhauser: An enzymatic approach to lactate production in human skeletal muscle during exercise. *Medicine and Science in Sports and Exercise.* 32(4):756–763 (2000).

Stainsby, W. N., & J. K. Barclay: Exercise metabolism: O_2 deficit, steady level O_2 uptake and O_2 uptake for recovery. *Medicine and Science in Sports.* 2(4):177–181 (1970).

Tesch, P. A.: Short- and long-term histochemical and biochemical adaptations in muscle. In P. V. Komi (ed.), *Strength and Power in Sports.* Oxford, England: Blackwell Scientific, 239–248 (1992).

Vandewalle, H., G. Pérès, & H. Monod: Standard anaerobic exercise tests. *Sports Medicine.* 4:268–289 (1987).

Volek, J. S.: Creatine supplementation and its possible role in improving physical performance. *ACSM's Health & Fitness Journal.* 1(4):23–29 (1997).

Wallace, J. P., G. Inbar, & K. Ernsthausen: Infant acceptance of postexercise breast milk. *Pediatrics.* 89(6):1245–1247 (1992).

Wallace, J. P., & J. Rabin: The concentration of lactic acid in breast milk following maximal exercise. *International Journal of Sports Medicine.* 12(3):328–331 (1991).

Walsh, M. L., & E. W. Banister: Possible mechanisms of the anaerobic threshold: A review. *Sports Medicine.* 5:269–302 (1988).

Wasserman, K., & M. B. McIlroy: Detecting the threshold of anaerobic metabolism in cardiac patients during exercise. *American Journal of Cardiology.* 14:844–852 (1964).

Wasserman, K., B. J. Whipp, S. N. Koyal, & W. L. Beaver: Anaerobic threshold and respiratory gas exchange during exercise. *Journal of Applied Physiology.* 35:236–243 (1973).

Wells, C. L.: *Women, Sport and Performance: A Physiological Perspective* (2nd edition). Champaign, IL: Human Kinetics Publishers (1991).

Williams, J. R., N. Armstrong, & B. J. Kirby: The 4mM blood lactate level as an index of exercise performance in 11–13 year old children. *Journal of Sport Sciences.* 8:139–147 (1990).

Zoeller, R. F., & T. J. Angelopoulous: Creatine supplementation and exercise performance. *ACSM's Certified News.* 8(2):1–4 (1998).

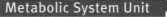
Chapter 5

Aerobic Metabolism during Exercise

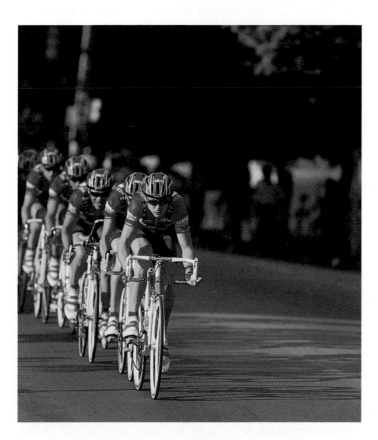

After studying the chapter, you should be able to

- List and explain the major variables used to describe the aerobic metabolic response to exercise.

- Explain the laboratory and field assessment techniques used to obtain information on aerobic metabolism during exercise.

- Compare and contrast oxygen consumption during aerobic (a) short-term, light- to moderate-intensity exercise; (b) long-term, moderate to heavy sub-maximal exercise; (c) incremental aerobic exercise to maximum; (d) static; and (e) dynamic resistance exercise.

- Describe how the oxygen cost of breathing changes during exercise.

- Calculate the respiratory exchange ratio and interpret what it means in terms of energy substrate utilization.

- Calculate the metabolic cost of activity in both kilocalories and metabolic equivalents, and explain how each can be applied.

- Differentiate between gross efficiency, net efficiency, delta efficiency; differentiate between the efficiency and the economy of movement.

- List the ways in which an exercising individual can increase his or her efficiency.

- Compare the walking and running economy between children and young or middle-aged adults, and discuss the possible reasons for the differences.

- Explain why efficiency and economy are important to exercise performance.

- State the impact of genetics on aerobic metabolism during exercise.

Introduction

Chapter 4 concentrated on anaerobic exercise responses; that is, it examined situations in which energy was provided predominantly by the stored ATP-PC or by the production of ATP through anaerobic glycolysis. Chapter 4 also described anaerobic participation in exercises of lower intensity, longer duration, and incremental exercise to maximum. This chapter will concentrate on the aerobic responses to the different intensities, durations, and types of exercise. Keep in mind throughout this chapter that aerobic metabolism predominates in activity lasting 3–5 min or longer but that the onset of all activity involves some amount of anaerobic metabolism during the oxygen deficit period. Excess postexercise oxygen consumption (EPOC) occurs following submaximal as well as maximal exercise and aerobic as well as dynamic resistance exercise.

Laboratory Measurement of Aerobic Metabolism

The primary goal of measuring aerobic metabolism is to quantify how much energy is necessary to complete a given activity. There are a couple of ways to approach this goal. To understand these approaches, consider two known aspects of aerobic metabolism: First, it requires oxygen; and second, it produces heat as a by-product. Therefore, aerobic metabolism can be assessed by measuring oxygen consumption or heat production. Oxygen consumption is measured by indirect open-circuit spirometry, and heat production is measured by calorimetry, as summarized in Figure 5.1.

Calorimetry

The term *calorimetry* is derived from the word *calorie,* the basic unit of heat energy. **Calorimetry** is the measurement of heat energy liberated or absorbed in metabolic processes. *Direct calorimetry* actually measures

---

Calorimetry The measurement of heat energy liberated or absorbed in metabolic processes.

Spirometry An indirect calorimetry method for estimating heat production or calorimetry in which expired air is measured and analyzed for the amount of oxygen consumed and carbon dioxide produced.

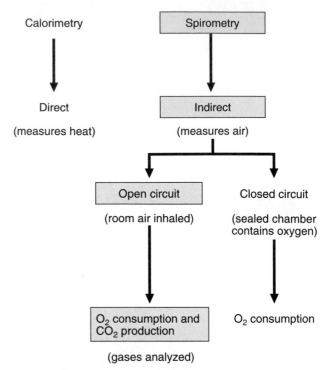

Figure 5.1
Measurement of Aerobic Metabolism

Aerobic metabolism can be measured by direct calorimetry or indirect spirometry. In exercise physiology, open-circuit indirect spirometry, in which expired gases are analyzed for O_2 consumed and CO_2 produced, are typically used.

Note: Boxes indicate processes typically utilized in exercise physiology.

---

heat production. This measurement requires the use of specially constructed chambers in which the heat produced by a subject increases the temperature of the air or water surrounding the walls and is thereby measured.

Accurate exercise data are difficult to obtain because exercise equipment, even if it fits into the usually small quarters, can also emit heat. In addition, the body may store heat (as evidenced by a rise in body temperature) and/or sweat (which must be accounted for). Despite these drawbacks, the direct measurement of heat is the most precise use of the term *calorimetry.*

Spirometry

Spirometry is an indirect calorimetry method for estimating heat production in which expired air is measured and analyzed for the amount of oxygen consumed and carbon dioxide produced. This method is based on the fact that oxygen consumption at rest or during submaximal exercise, when expressed as calories, is equal to the heat produced by the body as measured by direct calorimetry. However, since heat is not measured directly, spirometry is an indirect measure. The oxygen consumption is also directly proportional to the aerobic production of ATP. The measurement of oxygen consumed is based on the amount of air breathed. Spirometry is the measurement of air breathed.

In a *closed system* the subject breathes from a sealed container filled with gas of a designated composition (often 99.9% O_2). Expired CO_2 is usually absorbed by a chemical such as soda lime. The rate of utilization of the available O_2 is then determined. This system has a large error and is rarely used. It is mentioned here so that the terminology of an open circuit can be understood.

In *open-circuit spirometry* the subject inhales room or outdoor air from his or her surroundings and exhales into the same surroundings. The oxygen content of the inhaled air is normally 20.93%; the carbon dioxide does not need to be absorbed but is simply exhaled into the surrounding atmosphere. A sample of the expired air is analyzed for oxygen and carbon dioxide content.

Putting these factors together results in the descriptor *open-circuit indirect spirometry*. The term *open-circuit indirect calorimetry* should be reserved for use when calories are calculated from oxygen consumption, but in fact it is often used interchangeably with *open-circuit indirect spirometry*.

Measuring O_2 consumption by open-circuit indirect spirometry is a valid way to assess aerobic metabolism during resting and steady-state submaximal exercise, conditions when the relationship between O_2 consumption and ATP production remains linear. However, in situations when anaerobic energy production is also involved, the actual energy cost of the exercise will be underestimated, because the linear relationship no longer exists and there is no way to account for the anaerobic portion.

Open-circuit indirect spirometry can be used to measure oxygen consumption during any physical activity. However, the size, sensitivity, and lack of portability of the equipment have, until recently, limited its use to modalities that can be performed in a laboratory or a special swimming pool setup. By far the most popular exercise-testing modalities in the laboratory are the motor-driven treadmill and the cycle ergometer. Measurement can be done at rest, during submaximal exercise, or at maximal levels of exertion. The following section will describe in detail how this measurement is accomplished and, in so doing, will discuss the aerobic response to varying patterns of exercise.

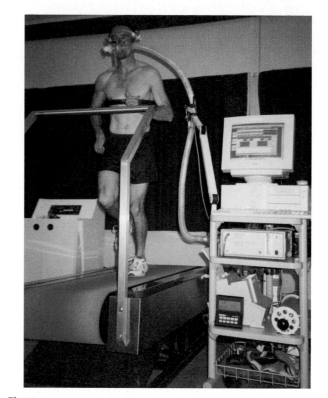

Figure 5.2
Subject Undergoing Assessment of Aerobic Metabolism during Exercise

Aerobic Exercise Responses

Figure 5.2 shows an individual attached to an analysis system for open-circuit indirect spirometry. The individual interacts with the system through the breathing valve, which permits air to flow in only one direction at a time—in from room air and out toward the sampling chamber. The use of the nose-clip ensures that all breathing is done through the mouth.

Oxygen Consumption and Carbon Dioxide Production

Figure 5.3 shows schematic configurations of an open-circuit system in which either the volume of inspired air (Figure 5.3a) or expired air (Figure 5.3b) is measured and the expired air is analyzed for the percentage of oxygen and carbon dioxide. Although oxygen consumption is the variable of primary interest, because of its direct relationship with ATP, determining the amount of carbon dioxide produced is also important, because that measure will enable us to determine information about fuel utilization and caloric expenditure.

Figure 5.3
Open-Circuit Indirect Spirometry with
Online Computer Analysis

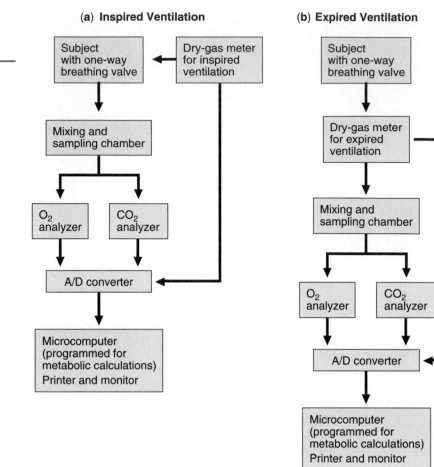

(a) Inspired Ventilation

Subject with one-way breathing valve ← Dry-gas meter for inspired ventilation

Mixing and sampling chamber

O_2 analyzer CO_2 analyzer

A/D converter

Microcomputer (programmed for metabolic calculations) Printer and monitor

(b) Expired Ventilation

Subject with one-way breathing valve

Dry-gas meter for expired ventilation

Mixing and sampling chamber

O_2 analyzer CO_2 analyzer

A/D converter

Microcomputer (programmed for metabolic calculations) Printer and monitor

Oxygen consumption ($\dot{V}O_2$) is the amount of oxygen taken up, transported, and used at the cellular level. It equals the amount of oxygen inspired minus the amount of oxygen expired. **Carbon dioxide produced ($\dot{V}CO_2$)** is the amount of carbon dioxide generated during metabolism, primarily from aerobic cellular respiration. It equals the amount of carbon dioxide expired minus the amount of carbon dioxide inspired. The amount of a gas equals the volume of air (either inhaled or exhaled) times the percentage of the gas. Therefore, to determine these amounts, we need to measure the volume of air either inhaled or exhaled and the percentages of oxygen and carbon dioxide in exhaled air. The percentages of oxygen and carbon dioxide in inhaled air are known to be 20.93% and

---

Oxygen Consumption ($\dot{V}O_2$) The amount of oxygen taken up, transported, and used at the cellular level.

Carbon Dioxide Produced ($\dot{V}CO_2$) The amount of carbon dioxide generated during metabolism.

0.03%, respectively. The mathematical relationships just described can be formulated as follows:

5.1 oxygen consumption ($L \cdot min^{-1}$) = [volume of air inspired ($L \cdot min^{-1}$) × percentage of oxygen in inspired air] − [volume of air expired ($L \cdot min^{-1}$) × percentage of oxygen in expired air]

or

$$\dot{V}O_2 \text{ cons} = (\dot{V}_I \times \%O_2 \text{ insp}) - (\dot{V}_E \times \%O_2 \text{ expir})$$

5.2 carbon dioxide produced ($L \cdot min^{-1}$) = [volume of air expired ($L \cdot min^{-1}$) × percentage of carbon dioxide in expired air] − [volume of air inspired × percentage of carbon dioxide in inspired air]

or

$$\dot{V}CO_2 \text{ prod} = (\dot{V}_E \times \%CO_2 \text{ expir}) \\ - (\dot{V}_I \times \%CO_2 \text{ insp})$$

Because the volume of air inhaled does not usually equal the volume of air exhaled, knowing either the value of air inhaled or exhaled and the gas percentages

Table 5.1
Aerobic Metabolic Responses at Rest and during Submaximal Exercise

Sex = Female	Ambient Temperature = 18°C
Age = 22 yr	Barometric Pressure = 752 mmHg
Weight = 53.4 kg	Relative Humidity = 5%

Time (min)	$\dot{V}_E$ STPD (L·min^{-1})	O$_2$%	CO$_2$%	$\dot{V}O_2$ (L·min^{-1})	$\dot{V}CO_2$ (L·min^{-1})	$\dot{V}O_2$ (mL·kg^{-1}·min^{-1})	RER	HR (b·min^{-1})
Rest (standing)								
1	7.57	17.11	3.26	0.30	0.23	5.61	0.81	75
2	7.58	17.21	3.20	0.29	0.23	5.43	0.82	75
3	8.64	16.95	3.37	0.34	0.28	6.55	0.80	75
$\overline{X}$	7.93	17.09	3.28	0.31	0.25	5.86	0.81	75
3.5 mi·hr^{-1} walking (steady state); 7% grade								
1	21.96	15.85	4.34	1.14	0.93	21.53	0.81	120
2	24.20	15.85	4.60	1.25	1.10	23.59	0.87	136
3	23.46	15.73	4.76	1.25	1.10	23.40	0.88	136
4	26.07	16.02	4.66	1.29	1.20	24.15	0.93	136
5	25.71	15.95	4.73	1.29	1.20	24.34	0.92	136
6	27.53	16.03	4.68	1.35	1.27	25.46	0.93	136
7	25.71	15.91	4.79	1.29	1.22	24.34	0.93	136
8	28.64	16.06	4.68	1.39	1.33	26.21	0.94	136
$\overline{X}$	25.41	15.93	4.66	1.28	1.17	24.13	0.90	136
3.5 mi·hr^{-1} walking (oxygen drift); 7% grade								
33	28.64	16.26	4.56	1.33	1.29	25.09	0.96	140
34	31.21	16.33	4.55	1.43	1.41	26.96	0.98	144
35	31.21	16.32	4.54	1.43	1.39	26.96	0.97	144
36	30.84	16.16	4.67	1.47	1.43	27.71	0.96	146
37	32.31	16.19	4.68	1.52	1.50	28.65	0.97	150

This individual had a $\dot{V}O_2$max of 47.64 mL·kg^{-1}·min^{-1}, or 2.54 L·min^{-1}.

allows us to calculate the other air volume. These calculations are fully described in Appendix B.

Most laboratories use a computer programmed with software to solve Eqs. 5.1 and 5.2. Table 5.1 gives the results of such a computer program for a metabolic test. The first 3 min represent resting values. The next 8 min were determined during treadmill walking at 3.5 mi·hr^{-1} (94 m·min^{-1}, or 5.6 km·hr^{-1}) at 7% grade. Ignore for the time being minutes 33 through 37 as well as the missing minutes. Locate in Figure 5.3, the pieces of equipment referred to as you follow the discussion of these variables. The dot above the volume symbol ($\dot{V}$) indicates per unit of time, which is usually 1 min.

The volume of air inspired ($\dot{V}_I$) or expired ($\dot{V}_E$) is measured by a pneumoscan or flowmeter (labeled as the dry-gas meter in Figure 5.3). Typically, all ventilation values are reported as expired values that have been adjusted to standard temperature (0°C), stan-dard pressure (760 mmHg), and dry (without water vapor) conditions, known as STPD. The process and rationale for standardizing ventilatory volumes are discussed fully in Chapter 10. Standardization permits comparisons between data collected under different conditions. Two things should be noted about the $\dot{V}_E$ STPD values. First, the values for exercise (Ex) are higher than those at rest (R) ($\overline{X}$R = 7.93 L·min^{-1} $\overline{X}$Ex = 25.41). Second, within each condition the values are very stable.

The air the subject exhales is sampled from a mixing chamber and analyzed by electronic gas analyzers that have been previously calibrated by gases of known composition. Information regarding the percentage of expired oxygen (O$_2$% in Table 5.1) and carbon dioxide (CO$_2$% in Table 5.1) is relayed from the gas analyzers along with the ventilation values through an analog-to-digital (A/D) converter, which gets the electronic signals in proper form to a microcomputer.

Focus on Research

Ambient Temperature and Muscle Metabolism

Parkin, J.M., et al. Effect of ambient temperature on human skeletal muscle metabolism during fatiguing submaximal exercise. *Journal of Applied Physiology.* 86(3):902–908 (1999).

It is known that prolonged submaximal exercise to fatigue in comfortable ambient temperature results in glycogen depletion. In fact, it is thought that muscle glycogen depletion causes fatigue. In this study, Parkin and colleagues investigated the effects of ambient temperature on muscle metabolism. Participants in this study exercised at 70% of their peak oxygen consumption on three occasions: once in a cool environment (3°C), once in a thermoneutral environment (20°C), and once in a hot environment (40°C). The graphs present the time to exhaustion and muscle glycogen content at rest and at fatigue in the three conditions.

These data reveal two important points:

1. As expected, the participants could cycle longer before the onset of fatigue in the cooler conditions. In fact, they exercised for almost an hour longer in the cool condition than in the hot condition.
2. Glycogen content in the muscle was significantly greater at fatigue in the hot condition compared to the thermoneutral and cool conditions. This means that muscle glycogen depletion was not the cause of fatigue during exercise to exhaustion in the hot condition.

This study challenges the idea that fatigue during long-duration submaximal exercise is primarily the result of glycogen depletion.

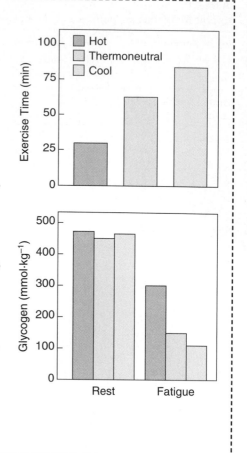

Remember that room air is composed of 20.93% O_2, 0.03% CO_2, 79.04% N_2, and other trace elements such as argon and krypton. The N_2 component is considered to be inert in human metabolism. However, as we have seen in the metabolic pathways, O_2 is consumed when ATP is created aerobically and CO_2 is produced. Therefore, in general, the O_2% will decrease from values in ambient air and range somewhere around 15–16% during moderate exercise. The CO_2 values will be greater than those in room air, increasing to somewhere around 4–6% during moderate exercise. Note these values in Table 5.1. During rest not much oxygen is used, so the percentage exhaled is relatively high ($\overline{X}R = 17.09\%$). The accompanying CO_2% is, as would be expected, relatively low ($\overline{X}R = 3.28\%$). During the exercise portion more O_2 is being used to produce energy; therefore, there is a lower percentage of O_2 exhaled ($\overline{X}E = 15.93\%$). The use of more O_2 to produce more energy also results in the production of more CO_2 ($\overline{X}Ex = 4.66\%$).

The computer uses a software program of metabolic formulas to correct ventilation for temperature (room temperature if V_I is measured; expired air temperature if V_E is measured), relative humidity (if V_I is measured), and barometric pressure. Then using the expired percentage values of O_2 and CO_2, it calculates values for the volume of O_2 consumed ($\dot{V}O_2$ $L \cdot min^{-1}$ and $\dot{V}O_2$ in $mL \cdot kg^{-1} \cdot min^{-1}$), CO_2 produced ($\dot{V}CO_2$ in $L \cdot min^{-1}$), and the ratio of the volume of CO_2 produced divided by the volume of O_2 consumed, known as the respiratory exchange ratio (RER). Sometimes this relationship is designated simply as R, but we will use RER throughout this textbook. The $\dot{V}O_2$ and $\dot{V}CO_2$ values are actual volumes of the gases that are used and produced by the body, respectively. The $L \cdot min^{-1}$ unit represents the absolute amount of gas on a per-minute basis. The $mL \cdot kg^{-1} \cdot min^{-1}$ unit takes into account body size [the body weight (BW) is given at the top of the table], and hence is considered to be a relative value; that is, it describes how many milliliters of gas are consumed (or produced) for each kilogram of body weight each minute.

The absolute unit is highly influenced by body size, with large individuals showing the highest values. Therefore, it is most useful when comparing an individual to himself or herself under different conditions, such as before and after a training program, to determine whether an improvement in fitness has occurred. Use of the absolute unit is particularly important if individuals have lost weight, because the $mL \cdot kg^{-1} \cdot min^{-1}$ value will go up as the weight goes down whether or not actual fitness has improved. The $mL \cdot kg^{-1} \cdot min^{-1}$ value, to an extent, equates individuals by factoring out the influence of body size. It is typically used for comparisons between individuals.

Another unit that can be used to express O_2 consumed and CO_2 produced on a relative basis is $mL \cdot kg$ $FFB^{-1} \cdot min^{-1}$ or $mL \cdot kg$ $LBM^{-1} \cdot min^{-1}$, where FFB stands for fat-free body and LBM stands for lean body mass. To calculate these units, percentage of body fat must be known and used to determine what portion of the total body weight is fat-free or lean. This unit is often used in comparisons between the sexes. However, it is not a very practical measure because no one has yet figured how to avoid carrying one's fat during exercise.

At rest the subject in the example in Table 5.1 is using about 0.31 $L \cdot min^{-1}$, or 310 $mL \cdot min^{-1}$, of oxygen and producing about 0.25 $L \cdot min^{-1}$ of carbon dioxide. During exercise she is using 1.28 $L \cdot min^{-1}$ of oxygen and producing 1.17 $L \cdot min^{-1}$ of carbon dioxide.

Short-Term, Light- to Moderate-Intensity Submaximal Exercise

Look at minutes 1–8 in Table 5.1. During this light exercise there is very little minute-to-minute variation in any of the variables after the first minute of adjustment. A comparison of the mean oxygen cost of these 8 min (24.13 $mL \cdot kg^{-1} \cdot min^{-1}$) with her $\dot{V}O_2$max (47.64 $mL \cdot kg^{-1} \cdot min^{-1}$) shows that the subject is working at approximately 50% $\dot{V}O_2$max. When the exercise performed is at less than 70% $\dot{V}O_2$max and the duration is from 5 to 10 min, the oxygen consumption should level off and remain relatively constant for the duration of the work after the initial rise (Figure 5.4a). This condition is known as steady state or steady-rate exercise. The time to achieve steady state varies from 1 to 3 min in youths and young adults at low and moderate levels of intensity, but it will increase with higher-intensity exercise (Morgan, Martin, et al., 1989). The time to achieve steady state increases in the elderly.

Oxygen Drift A situation that occurs in submaximal activity of long duration, or above 70% $\dot{V}O_2$max, or in hot and humid conditions where the oxygen consumption increases, despite the fact that the oxygen requirement of the activity has not changed.

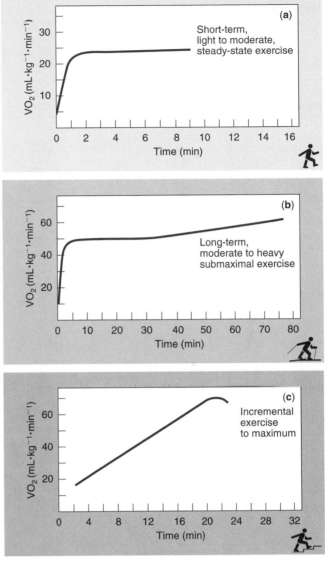

Figure 5.4
Oxygen Consumption Responses to Various Exercises

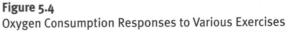

(a) Short-term, light to moderate, submaximal aerobic exercise.
(b) Long-term, moderate to heavy, submaximal dynamic aerobic exercise. (c) Incremental aerobic exercise to maximum.

Long-Term, Moderate to Heavy Submaximal Exercise

Now look carefully at minutes 33 through 37 in Table 5.1. Pay particular attention to the $\dot{V}O_2$ $L \cdot min^{-1}$ and $mL \cdot kg^{-1} \cdot min^{-1}$ values. Despite the fact that the workload has not changed, a gradual increase is seen in these variables. When exercise is performed at a level greater than 70% $\dot{V}O_2$max; or when exercise is performed at a lower percentage of $\dot{V}O_2$max, as in this case, but for a long duration; or if the conditions are hot and humid, a phenomenon known as **oxygen drift**

Table 5.2

Aerobic Metabolic Responses during an Incremental Treadmill Test (Modified Balke Protocol)

Sex = Male   Ambient Temperature = 23°C
Age = 22 yr   Barometric Pressure = 739 mmHg
Weight = 66 kg   Relative Humidity = 13%

Time (min)	$\dot{V}_E$ STPD	O_2%	CO_2%	$\dot{V}O_2$ (L·min^{-1})	$\dot{V}O_2$ (mL·kg^{-1}·min^{-1})	$\dot{V}CO_2$ (L·min^{-1})	RER	HR (b·min^{-1})
2	25.21	16.47	4.45	1.12	16.96	1.10	0.99	82
3	27.31	16.36	4.54	1.25	18.93	1.22	0.98	84
4	29.06	16.30	4.62	1.33	20.30	1.30	0.98	100
5	29.75	16.18	4.71	1.41	21.36	1.39	0.98	98
6	33.62	16.09	4.84	1.62	24.54	1.60	0.99	108
7	30.17	16.08	4.99	1.45	21.96	1.49	1.03	105
8	34.37	15.99	5.03	1.68	25.45	1.72	1.01	120
9	37.92	16.09	5.03	1.81	27.42	1.89	1.04	117
10	37.17	16.07	4.96	1.79	27.12	1.83	1.02	115
11	38.84	15.89	5.00	1.95	29.69	1.93	0.98	123
12	39.56	15.82	5.10	2.01	30.60	2.00	0.99	122
13	39.84	15.57	5.23	2.15	32.57	2.07	0.96	124
14	43.37	15.51	5.30	2.36	35.75	2.28	0.96	132
15	46.64	15.62	5.41	2.45	37.27	2.50	1.01	144
16	47.37	15.68	5.42	2.45	37.27	2.54	1.03	138
17	50.87	15.85	5.21	2.55	38.78	2.62	1.02	143
18	51.53	15.52	5.48	2.78	42.12	2.80	1.01	146
19	55.12	15.73	5.38	2.83	42.87	2.95	1.03	155
20	56.84	15.74	5.32	2.91	44.24	3.00	1.02	158
21	58.54	15.63	5.38	3.08	46.81	3.12	1.01	162
22	59.95	15.58	5.43	3.19	48.33	3.23	1.01	167
23	68.06	15.59	5.47	3.61	54.69	3.70	1.02	180
24	78.06	15.69	5.55	4.01	60.90	4.30	1.07	181
25	85.18	15.70	5.62	4.36	66.21	4.75	1.08	188
26	94.94	15.78	5.75	4.68	71.06	5.39	1.14	192
27	112.96	16.29	5.51	4.98	75.45	6.18	1.24	196
28	139.04	16.97	4.94	5.11	77.52	6.83	1.34	200

occurs. In oxygen drift the oxygen consumption increases despite the fact that the oxygen requirement of the activity has not changed. A schematic representation of oxygen drift is presented in Figure 5.4b.

The oxygen consumption increases (drifts upward) because of rising blood levels of catecholamines (epinephrine and norepinephrine), lactate accumulation (if the % $\dot{V}O_2$ is high enough), shifting substrate utilization (to greater carbohydrate), increased cost of ventilation, and increased body temperature. Thus, although any given level of exercise typically requires a specific amount of oxygen, this amount will show some individual and circumstantial variation (Daniels, 1985).

Incremental Aerobic Exercise to Maximum

Table 5.2 provides the results of a computer program for an incremental treadmill test to maximum. In this case the subject was a very fit male senior exercise science major who regularly and successfully competed in long-distance running, cycling, and duathlon events. In an incremental exercise test such as this the subject is asked to continue to the point of volitional fatigue—that is, until he is too tired to go on any longer. Throughout the test the speed and/or grade is systematically raised so that the exercise becomes progressively harder. The protocol used for this particular test is called the modified Balke. For this test the speed was kept constant at 3.5 mi·hr^{-1} (94 m·min^{-1}). The grade was 0% for the first minute and 2% for the second minute; it increased 1% per minute thereafter. At the treadmill limit of 25% grade, speed was then increased 13.4 m·min^{-1} each minute. Because the increments are small, the individual should be able to adjust to the load in just 1 min for most of the submaximal portion. This subject was able to continue for 28 min.

Because the work is different, the ventilation, $\dot{V}O_2$, and $\dot{V}CO_2$ responses are also different from those of the submaximal steady-state exercise in Table 5.1. In the incremental task ventilation ($\dot{V}O_E$), $\dot{V}O_2$, and $\dot{V}CO_2$ values all increase as a result of the increasing demands for and production of energy. For this particular subject the volume of expired air ($\dot{V}_E$ STPD) rose from 25.21 L·min^{-1} at minute 2 to 139.04 L·min^{-1} at minute 28. This result demonstrates the reserve capacity in the ventilatory system. Oxygen consumption increased from slightly over 1 L·min^{-1} (or almost 17 mL·kg^{-1}·min^{-1}) to just over 5 L·min^{-1} at maximum. At this point the subject was producing as much ATP as he could aerobically. The highest amount of oxygen an individual can take in, transport, and utilize to produce ATP aerobically while breathing air during heavy exercise is **maximal oxygen consumption ($\dot{V}O_2$max)**.

The exercise tester has to decide whether any given test truly is a maximal effort before labeling the highest $\dot{V}O_2$ value as maximal. Several physiological criteria can be used to decide if test results represent a maximal test. These are (a) a lactate value greater than 8 mmol·L^{-1} (Åstrand, 1956; Åstrand and Rodahl, 1977); (b) a heart rate $\pm$ 12 b·min^{-1} of predicted maximal heart rate (220 minus age) (Durstine and Pate, 1988); (c) a respiratory exchange ratio (RER, which is described fully later in this chapter) of 1.0 or 1.1, primarily depending on the age of the subject (Holly, 1988; MacDougall, et al., 1982); and (d) a plateau in oxygen consumption. The classic definition of a plateau is a rise of 2.1 mL·kg^{-1}·min^{-1} or less, or a rise of 0.15 L·min^{-1} or less, in oxygen consumption ($\dot{V}O_2$) with an increase in workload that represents a change in grade of 2.5% while running at 7 mi·hr^{-1} (11.2 km·hr^{-1}) with 3-min stages (Taylor, et al., 1955). Using this criterion for all protocols has been questioned (Howley, et al., 1995). One alternative is defining a plateau as an increase of less than half the expected theoretical rise based on the change in speed,

grade, or speed and grade (Plowman and Liu, 1999). The expected increase can be calculated using the American College of Sports Medicine (2000) equations provided in Appendix B. In this case, the expected difference in oxygen consumption between the last two minutes (27 and 28) is 5.8 mL·kg^{-1}·min^{-1}. Occasionally, an RPE (rating of perceived exertion) of equal to or greater than 17 is used as a psychophysiological criterion (Howley, et al., 1995). Complete the Question of Understanding box to apply these criteria.

The rectilinear increase in $\dot{V}O_2$ can be generalized to all healthy individuals whether they are male or female, young or old, high or low in terms of fitness. This pattern is schematically represented in Figure 5.4c. However, the plateau is not always evident in children and the elderly. In these cases the term *peak oxygen consumption* ($\dot{V}O_2$peak) to describe the highest value attained is more accurate than the term *maximal oxygen consumption* ($\dot{V}O_2$max).

As a result of the increasing ATP production, the amount of CO_2 produced also increases. Note in Table 5.2 that the amount of CO_2 produced ($\dot{V}CO_2$) is generally not equal to the amount of O_2 consumed ($\dot{V}O_2$). Note also that despite the incremental nature of this test, the O_2% and CO_2% do not vary much. There is a slight decline in O_2% and a parallel rise in CO_2% after the first 10 min and then relatively steady values until the last 2 min, when the O_2% goes back up and the CO_2% goes back down just a little. Frequently, as a subject nears maximal exertion, the O_2% may rise to 17% and the CO_2% may drop to 3%. These small percentage changes, especially when they occur in the last couple of minutes, are compensated for by the increasingly larger volumes of air being ventilated.

Static and Dynamic Resistance Exercise

Physiological responses to static exercise are generally described in relation to the percentage of maximal voluntary contraction (MVC) at which they take place. Depending on the muscle group involved, static contractions below 15–25% MVC do not fully occlude blood flow, and so oxygen can be delivered to working muscles. At such loads, however, little extra energy above resting level is required, and oxygen consumption increases minimally, perhaps as little as 50 mL·min^{-1}, but for as long as half an hour (Asmussen, 1981; Shepard et al., 1981).

Maximal Oxygen Consumption ($\dot{V}O_2$max) The highest amount of oxygen an individual can take in and utilize to produce ATP aerobically while breathing air during heavy exercise.

A Question of Understanding

Did this subject meet the HR and $\dot{V}O_2$ criteria for a true maximal test? Check the answers in Appendix D.

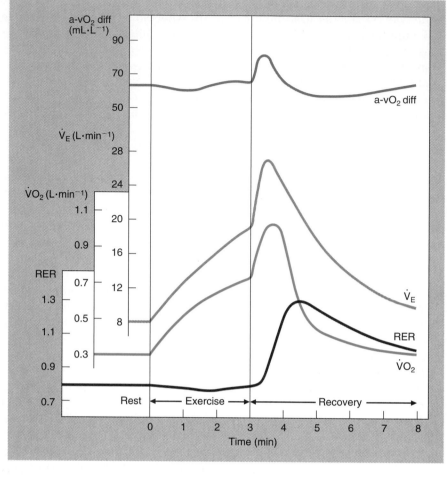

Figure 5.5
Respiratory and Metabolic Responses to Heavy Static Exercise

Heavy static exercise causes small respiratory (a-vO$_2$ diff and $\dot{V}_E$) and metabolic ($\dot{V}O_2$ and RER) responses during the actual contraction. However, each of these variables exhibits an increased rebound effect immediately upon cessation of the exercise before slowly returning to preexercise values.

Source: E. Asmussen. Similarities and dissimilarities between static and dynamic exercise. *Circulation Research* (Suppl.). 48(6):I-3–I-10 (1981). Copyright 1981 by the American Heart Association. Reprinted by permission.

The higher the % MVC of the static contraction, the greater the intramuscular pressure is, the more likely it is that the blood flow will be completely arrested or occluded, and the shorter the time that the contraction can be maintained. If, despite an MVC of 30% or greater, occlusion of blood flow is not complete, an increase in oxygen consumption occurs. This increased oxygen consumption is higher than the amount at lower percentages of MVC but still far below the rise in values that occurs during the aerobic endurance exercises previously described.

In addition to a lower oxygen consumption, there is one other major difference between static and dynamic endurance exercise. At the cessation of static exercise, when blood flow is fully restored, a sudden increase in oxygen consumption is seen (Figure 5.5)

before the slow, gradual decline of the typical EPOC curve begins (Asmussen, 1981; Shepard et al., 1981).

The primary source of energy for dynamic-resistance activity such as weight lifting or wrestling is anaerobic (Fleck and Kraemer, 1987; Fox and Mathews, 1974). In part, anaerobic energy is used because dynamic resistance exercise has a static component to it. In part, anaerobic energy is used due to the high intensity and short duration of the exercise. Despite the predominance of anaerobic energy sources, there is an aerobic component to dynamic resistance activity as well. As mentioned in the previous chapter, even the most widely used anaerobic test, the Wingate Anaerobic Test, has an aerobic energy contribution of almost 30% (Bar-Or, 1987). The more the repetitions and the longer the duration of

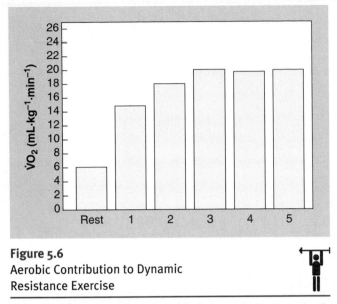

Figure 5.6
Aerobic Contribution to Dynamic
Resistance Exercise

Oxygen consumption was measured before and during five sets of
6–12 repetitions of supine leg presses. The values represent the
combined results of two groups: one performed only the concentric
(lifting) phase, and the other performed both the concentric and
eccentric (lowering) phases. The addition of the eccentric phase
represented such a low additional energy cost above just the concentric energy expenditure that it was not separated out.

Source: Based on Tesch, et al. (1990).

the sets in a weight-lifting workout, the greater will be
the aerobic contribution. Actual values are not available for different routines because such activities are
intended for anaerobic, not aerobic, benefits. However, an example of the oxygen contribution to five
sets of 6–12 repetitions per set of supine leg press exercise can be seen in Figure 5.6 (Tesch, et al., 1990).
For this group of untrained males, a gradual rise in
oxygen consumption can be seen over the first three
sets, at which point the oxygen consumption basically
stabilizes for the remaining two sets. The oxygen cost
represents approximately 33–47% of the average
maximal oxygen consumption for these subjects.
Thus, the aerobic contribution during weight-lifting
exercise can be expected to be somewhat less than
the oxygen costs of most aerobic endurance activities
but higher than the cost of purely static exercise
(Tesch, et al., 1990).

The Oxygen Cost of Breathing

Part of the oxygen used both at rest and during exercise goes to support the respiratory muscles. This
value does not remain constant but varies with the
intensity of activity. During rest the respiratory
system uses about 1–2% of the total body oxygen
consumption, or 2.5 mL·min^{-1} of oxygen. The oxygen

cost of ventilation is higher in children than in adults
and the elderly (Bar-Or, 1983; Pardy, et al., 1984).

During light to moderate submaximal dynamic
aerobic exercise, where $\dot{V}_E$ is less than 60 L·min^{-1},
the respiratory oxygen cost changes to, at most, about
25–100$_E$ mL·min^{-1}. At heavy submaximal exercise,
where $\dot{V}_E$ is anywhere from 60 to 120 L·min^{-1}, respiratory oxygen use may rise from 50 to 400 mL·min^{-1}.
During incremental exercise to maximum, the initial
$\dot{V}_E$ during the lower exercise stages shows a very
gradual curvilinear rise, reflecting the submaximal
changes described previously. At workloads above
those requiring a $\dot{V}_E$ greater than 120 L·min^{-1}, a dramatic exponential curve occurs. In this curve, by the
time a $\dot{V}_E$ of 180 L·min^{-1} is achieved in a very fit individual, 1000–1300 mL·min^{-1} of oxygen is used simply
to support respiration (Pardy, et al., 1984).

There may be a theoretical maximal level of ventilation above which any further increase in oxygen
consumption would be used entirely by the ventilatory
musculature (Bye, et al., 1983; Otis, 1954; Pardy, et
al., 1984). Precisely where this critical level of ventilation occurs is unknown. However, even if there is no
such thing as a critical ventilation level, respiration
does utilize a significant portion, 3–13%, of the $\dot{V}O_2$
during heavy exercise (Bye, et al., 1983; Shephard,
1966). Smoking increases the oxygen cost of respiration during exercise. However, even an abstinence of
just one day can substantially reduce this effect of cigarette smoking (Rode and Shephard, 1971; Shepard,
et al., 1981). In old age the oxygen cost of breathing
may be a significant factor in limiting exercise performance (Shepard, et al., 1981).

Respiratory Quotient/Respiratory
Exchange Ratio

Once the $\dot{V}O_2$ consumed and $\dot{V}CO_2$ produced during
exercise are known, a great deal of useful information
can be derived. One such derived variable—**RER, or
respiratory exchange ratio**—is given in both Table
5.1 and Table 5.2.

The RER reflects on a total body level what is happening at the cellular level. The ratio of the amount of
carbon dioxide (CO_2) produced to the amount of oxygen consumed (O_2) at the cellular level is termed the
respiratory quotient (RQ). The formula is

Respiratory Quotient (RQ) Ratio of the amount
of carbon dioxide produced divided by the
amount of oxygen consumed at cellular level.

Respiratory Exchange Ratio (RER) Ratio of
the volume of CO_2 produced divided by the volume of O_2 consumed on a total body level.

Table 5.3

Energy Production from Carbohydrate, Fat, and Protein

	Carbohydrate		Protein		Fat
Primary utilization in exercise	High-intensity, short-duration exercise		Ultradistance exercise and glucose precursor		Low-intensity, long-duration exercise and glucose precursor
Form in which utilized by muscles	Glucose	Glycogen	*	Branched-chain amino acids	Fatty Acids
Oxygen needed to utilize per gram $(L \cdot g^{-1})$	$0.75 \ L \cdot g^{-1}$	$0.83 \ L \cdot g^{-1}$	$0.965 \ L \cdot g^{-1}$	$1.24 \ L \cdot g^{-1}$	$2.02 \ L \cdot g^{-1}$
Energy produced per gram $(kcal \cdot g^{-1})$	$3.75 \ kcal \cdot g^{-1}$ $15.68 \ kJ \cdot g^{-1}$	$4.17 \ kcal \cdot g^{-1}$ $17.43 \ kJ \cdot g^{-1}$	$4.3 \ kcal \cdot g^{-1}$ $17.97 \ kJ \cdot g^{-1}$	$3.76 \ kcal \cdot g^{-1}$ $18.09 \ kJ \cdot g^{-1}$	$9.3 \ kcal \cdot g^{-1}$ $38.87 \ kj \cdot g^{-1}$
Energy produced per liter of oxygen[†] $(kcal \cdot L \ O_2^{-1})$	$5.03 \ kcal \cdot L \ O_2^{-1}$ $21.03 \ kJ \cdot L \ O_2^{-1}$	$5.03 \ kcal \cdot L \ O_2^{-1}$ $21.03 \ kJ \cdot L \ O_2^{-1}$	$4.46 \ kcal \cdot L \ O_2^{-1}$ $18.64 \ kJ \cdot L \ O_2^{-1}$	$3.03 \ kcal \cdot L \ O_2^{-1}$ $12.67 \ kJ \cdot L \ O_2^{-1}$	$4.61 \ kcal \cdot L \ O_2^{-1}$ $19.27 \ kj \cdot L \ O_2^{-1}$
Carbon dioxide produced $(L \cdot g^{-1})$	$0.75 \ L \cdot g^{-1}$	$0.83 \ L \cdot g^{-1}$	$0.781 \ L \cdot g^{-1}$	$0.92 \ L \cdot g^{-1}$	$1.43 \ L \cdot g^{-1}$

* Values for protein are given. However, the BCAA values are more realistic for muscle activity per 1 g PRO = 1.17 g AA (Morgan, Martin, et al., 1989; Péronnet, et al., 1987).

† Energy produced per liter of oxygen equals the caloric equivalent.

5.3 respiratory quotient = carbon dioxide produced (molecules) ÷ oxygen consumed (molecules)

or

$$RQ = \frac{CO_2}{O_2}$$

This formula may also be computed using liters per gram in place of molecules.

The values of carbon dioxide produced and oxygen consumed are known for the oxidation of carbohydrate, fat, and protein, both on a chemical or molecular level and in absolute amounts $(L \cdot g^{-1})$. The latter values are presented in Table 5.3. The amount of oxygen consumed and the amount of carbon dioxide produced vary between the major fuel sources because of differences in the chemical composition of the fuels. The examples that follow compute the cellular level RQ for each major fuel source both per mole of a specific substrate (the carbohydrate, glucose, $C_6H_{12}O_6$; the fat, palmitic acid, $C_{16}H_{32}O_2$; and the protein, albumin, $C_{72}H_{112}N_2O_{22}S$), and per gram of carbohydrate (glucose), fat (fatty acid) as well as total protein and branched chain amino acids. In each case the oxygen used (left side of the equation) and carbon dioxide produced (right side of the equation) are inserted into Eq. 5.3 to determine RQ.

Example

For carbohydrates:
Glucose (per mole)

$$C_6H_{12}O_6 + 6O_2 \rightarrow 6CO_2 + 6H_2O + energy$$

$$RQ = \frac{6CO_2}{6O_2} = 1.0$$

Glucose (per gram, from Table 5.3):

1 g glucose + 0.75 L O_2 → 0.75 L CO_2 + H_2O
+ 3.75 kcal

$$RQ = \frac{0.75 \ L \ CO_2}{0.75 \ L \ O_2} = 1.0$$

For fat:
Palmitic acid (per mole)

$$C_{16}H_{32}O_2 + 23O_2 \rightarrow 16CO_2 + 15H_2O + energy$$

$$RQ = \frac{16 \ CO_2}{23 \ O_2} = 0.7$$

Fatty acids (per gram, from Table 5.3)

1 g fatty acid + 2.02 L O_2 → 1.43 L CO_2 + H_2O
+ 9.3 kcal

$$RQ = \frac{1.43 \ L \ CO_2}{2.02 \ L \ O_2} = 0.71$$

For protein:
Albumin (per mole)

$$C_{72}H_{112}N_2O_{22}S + 77O_2 \rightarrow 63CO_2 + 38H_2O + SO_3 \\ + 9CO(NH_2) \text{ (urea)}$$

$$RQ = \frac{63CO_2}{77O_2} = 0.82$$

Protein (per gram, from Table 5.3)

$$1 \text{ g protein} + 0.965 \text{ L } O_2 \rightarrow 0.781 \text{ L } CO_2 + H_2O \\ + 4.3 \text{ kcal}$$

$$RQ = \frac{0.781 \text{ L } CO_2}{0.965 \text{ L } O_2} = 0.81$$

Note that if the branched-chain amino acids are used, the RQ would be lower:

$$1 \text{ g BCAA} + 1.24 \text{ L } O_2 \rightarrow 0.92 \text{ L } CO_2 + H_2O + 3.76 \text{ kcal}$$

$$RQ = \frac{0.92 \text{ L } CO_2}{1.24 \text{ } O_2} = 0.74$$

The values of 1.0 for carbohydrate, 0.7 for fat, and 0.81 for protein are the classic accepted values for RQ. ✛

Because these values for RQ have been derived from the cellular oxidation of specific foodstuffs, knowing the RQ allows one to estimate the fuels utilized. However, individuals do not often use only one fuel; thus, the "classic values" are rarely seen. Therefore, in a resting individual an RQ of 0.93 indicates a high reliance on carbohydrate, and an RQ of 0.75 indicates a high reliance on fat. An RQ of 0.82 indicates either a fasting individual burning protein (usually from muscle mass, if in a starvation situation) or more likely, an individual using a normal mixed diet of all three fuels. Remember that protein is not normally used as a major fuel source, especially at rest.

Although these interpretations are acceptable in the resting individual, there are several difficulties with the RQ and its meaning during exercise. In the first place, the O_2 and CO_2 values measured in open-circuit indirect spirometry are ventilatory measures that are indicative of total body gas exchange and not just working muscle. Second, anything that causes hyperventilation will cause an excess of CO_2 to be exhaled, thus falsely elevating the ratio. This result is often seen in stress situations in anticipation of an exercise test or in early recovery from maximal work. Third, if exercise is of a high enough intensity to involve anaerobic metabolism, causing an increase in acidity (a decrease in pH) and a concomitant rise in nonmetabolic CO_2 release, RQ no longer represents just fuel utilization. Values during exercise, especially as an individual approaches maximal effort, usually

exceed 1.0. In this case the assumption is that the fuel source is carbohydrate and the excess CO_2 is a result of anaerobic metabolism. Conversely, after an initial increase during recovery, CO_2 is retained, causing low values (Newsholme and Leech, 1983). For these reasons the term respiratory exchange ratio (RER) is a more accurate one than RQ to describe the ratio of $\dot{V}CO_2$ produced to $\dot{V}O_2$ consumed when determined by open-circuit spirometry.

This involvement of anaerobic metabolism that results in RER values greater than 1.0 allows for the RER as criterion to determine whether an exercise test was truly maximal. The criterion for a true maximal test is an RER greater than 1.1 or at least 1.0, with the lower value predominating for children/ adolescents and the elderly (Holly, 1988; MacDougall, et al., 1982).

Although changing the name from RQ to RER is a more accurate description, RER values still do not distinguish between different forms of a fuel, such as glucose or glycogen, fatty acids, or ketone bodies. Also, when only ventilatory CO_2 and O_2 are measured, there is no indication of protein utilization. To measure protein utilization, the amount of nitrogen excreted (in urine and sweat) must be measured. This task is, at best, a cumbersome one and, at worst, almost impossible to do in exercise situations (Bursztein, et al., 1989; Consolazio et al., 1963). Thus, the RER that is measured by the $\dot{V}CO_2 \text{ L·min}^{-1} \div \dot{V}O_2 \cdot \text{L·min}^{-1}$ during exercise is a nonprotein RER. Again, because protein is not thought to be utilized as a fuel until long-duration activity is in progress, this simplification is not deemed to materially affect the relative percentage of carbohydrate and fat utilization in most situations.

Table 5.4 presents the relative percentages of calories used from carbohydrate and fat for all RER values between 0.7 and 1.0 (Carpenter, 1964). Referring to Table 5.1, we see that during rest the individual in the example had an RER of 0.81. From Table 5.4 this value means that 35.4% of her fuel was carbohydrate and 64.6% fat at that time. During her

---

A Question of Understanding

Look at Table 5.2. Determine the approximate percentages of carbohydrate and fat used at minutes 2, 14, and 28. Check your answer in Appendix D to see whether you are correct. The early minute RER values are higher than expected for the workload, probably from hyperventilation in anticipation of the maximal effort to come in the exercise test. The last three RER values listed in Table 5.2 are greater than 1.1 and indicate the involvement of anaerobic metabolism.

Table 5.4

Percentage of Calories from Carbohydrate (CHO) and Fat and the Caloric Equivalents for Nonprotein RER Values for Each Liter of Oxygen Used

RER	CHO%	Fat%	Caloric Equivalent (kcal·L O_2^{-1})	RER	CHO%	Fat%	Caloric Equivalent (kcal·L O_2^{-1})
0.70	0.0	100.0	4.686	0.86	52.4	47.6	4.875
0.71	1.4	98.6	4.690	0.87	55.8	44.2	4.887
0.72	4.8	95.2	4.702	0.88	59.2	40.8	4.899
0.73	8.2	91.8	4.714	0.89	62.6	37.4	4.911
0.74	11.6	88.4	4.727	0.90	66.0	34.0	4.924
0.75	15.0	85.0	4.739	0.91	69.4	30.6	4.936
0.76	18.4	81.6	4.751	0.92	72.8	27.2	4.948
0.77	21.8	78.2	4.764	0.93	76.2	23.8	4.961
0.78	25.2	74.8	4.776	0.94	79.6	20.4	4.973
0.79	28.6	71.4	4.788	0.95	83.0	17.0	4.985
0.80	32.0	68.0	4.801	0.96	86.4	13.6	4.998
0.81	35.4	64.6	4.813	0.97	89.8	10.2	5.010
0.82	38.8	61.2	4.825	0.98	93.2	6.8	5.022
0.83	42.2	57.8	4.838	0.99	96.6	3.4	5.035
0.84	45.6	54.4	4.850	1.00	100.0	0.0	5.047
0.85	49.0	51.0	4.862				

Source: Modified from T. M. Carpenter. *Tables, Factors, and Formulas for Computing Respiratory Exchange and Biological Transformations of Energy* (4th ed.). Washington, D.C.: Carnegie Institution of Washington, Publication 303C (1964). Reprinted by permission.

8 min of steady-state work the RER averaged 0.90, indicating a major shift in fuel supply. At that RER, 66% of the fuel was carbohydrate and 34% fat.

During the last 5-min interval (minutes 33–37 in Table 5.1), we see an even greater reliance on carbohydrate with approximately 90% of the energy used being supplied by carbohydrate sources. If submaximal exercise were to continue for another 2 hr or more, the RER values would drop back down, indicating a depletion of available carbohydrate fuel stores. How low the RER values would go depends on the amount of carbohydrate originally stored, as well as the exact intensity and duration of the activity. For this reason, athletes often try to carbohydrate load prior to endurance events so that carbohydrate stores are initially high and will last longer. Carbohydrate loading is fully discussed in Chapter 7. Table 5.5 summarizes the oxygen consumption, RER/energy substrate responses to the varying categories of exercise. Check your knowledge by completing the Question of Understanding box on page 133.

Estimation of Caloric Expenditure

Table 5.3 not only shows the oxygen consumed and carbon dioxide produced when each of the energy substrates is utilized, but also indicates the potential energy in terms of kilocalories per gram (kcal·g^{-1}) or kilocalories per liter of oxygen (kcal·L O_2^{-1}) for each substrate. The kcal·L O_2^{-1} figures show that carbohydrates are most efficient in the use of oxygen to provide energy, followed by fat, and finally by protein. However, there really is not a great deal of variation among the substrates.

The potential energy for carbohydrate and for protein depends on whether the form is glucose (3.75 kcal·g^{-1}) or glycogen (4.17 kcal·g^{-1}), all amino acids (4.3 kcal·g^{-1}) or just the branched-chain amino acids (3.76 kcal·g^{-1}). When food is ingested, these distinctions cannot be made; and the net average energy values are rounded to the whole numbers of 4 kcal·g^{-1} for carbohydrate and protein and 9 kcal·g^{-1} for fat. These values are called *Atwater factors* and are used to represent the energy potential of food. From the known values of $\dot{V}O_2$ L·min^{-1} and RER it is possible to compute the kilocalorie (or kilojoule) energy expenditure.

Table 5.4 includes the **caloric equivalent**—the number of kilocalories produced per liter of oxygen consumed—for all values of RER between 0.7 and 1.0. The kilocalories produced per liter of oxygen (kcal·L O_2^{-1}) varies from 4.686 at an RER of 0.7 to

Table 5.5
Aerobic Exercise Responses

		O_2 Consumption	RER/Energy Substrate
Short-term, light to moderate submaximal exercise		Initial rise; plateau at appropriate steady state	.85 to .90 / mixed fat & CHO to predominantly CHO
Short-term, moderate to heavy submaximal exercise		Initial rise; plateau at appropriate steady state	.85 to .90 to 1.0+ / mixed fat & CHO to CHO
Long-term, moderate to heavy submaximal exercise		Initial rise; plateau at steady state; positive drift	.85 to .90 to 1.0+ to .90 to .85 / mixed fat & CHO to CHO; if duration is long enough RER will decrease as CHO supplies are depleted
Short-term, high-intensity, supramaximal exercise		Small increase; provides approximately 30% or less of energy cost	.90 to 1.0+ / predominantly CHO to all CHO
Incremental exercise to maximum		Rectilinear rise; plateau at maximum	.85 to ≥ 1.0 / mixed fat & CHO to glycogen
Static exercise		Small gradual rise during exercise; rebound rise in recovery	.80 to 1.1+ / mixed fat & CHO during exercise with rebound rise in recovery/glycogen
Dynamic resistance exercise		Small gradual rise during exercise; the lighter the load and the higher the reps, the greater the contribution	.90 to 1.0+ / glycogen

5.047 at an RER of 1.0. If the amount of oxygen consumed and the caloric equivalent are known, the caloric cost of an activity can be computed.

To compute the kcal·min^{-1} cost, one must first find the caloric equivalent for the RER in Table 5.4. The rest of the computation is simply a matter of multiplying the oxygen cost by the caloric equivalent. The formula is

5.4 caloric cost of an activity (kcal·min^{-1})
= oxygen consumed (L·min^{-1}) × caloric equivalent (kcal·L O_2^{-1})

Example

Assume that an individual had an RER of 0.91 during exercise that used 2.15 L O_2·min^{-1}. The caloric equivalent for an RER of 0.91 is 4.936 kcal·LO_2^{-1} so the calculation becomes

Caloric Equivalent The number of kilocalories produced per liter of oxygen consumed.

Caloric Cost Energy expenditure of an activity performed for a specified period of time. It may be expressed as total calories (kcal), calories or kjoules per minute (kcal·min^{-1} or kJ·min^{-1}) or relative to body weight (kcal·kg^{-1}·min^{-1} or kJ·kg^{-1}·min^{-1}).

$$2.15\ O_2\ L\cdot min^{-1} \times 4.936\ kcal\cdot L\ O_2^{-1}$$
$$= 10.61\ kcal\cdot min^{-1}\quad \textbf{+}$$

Complete the Question of Understanding boxes below and on page 137.

This **caloric cost** represents the energy expenditure of the activity. It may be expressed as calories or joules per minute (kcal·min^{-1} or kJ·min^{-1}) or relative to body weight (kcal·kg^{-1}·min^{-1} or kJ·kg^{-1}·min^{-1}) or as total calories if the calories per minute is multiplied by the total number of minutes of participation.

If you know the oxygen consumed during any activity, but you do not know the RER, you can estimate the caloric value of that activity by multiplying by 5.0 kcal·L O_2^{-1}. The 5 kcal·L O_2^{-1} value is very close to the average caloric equivalent and is easy to remember. Since one kilocalorie equals 4.18 kilojoules, to convert kcal·min^{-1} to kJ·min^{-1}, multiply by 4.18. For the example we are discussing, we get

$$10.61\ kcal\cdot min^{-1} \times 4.18\ kJ\cdot kcal^{-1} = 44.36\ kJ\cdot min^{-1}$$

A Question of Understanding

Determine the caloric cost (in kilocalories and kilojoules) for minute 14 of Table 5.2. Check your answer in Appendix D.

Focus on Application

✳ Caloric Cost and Exercise Machines

You have been studying exercise physiology for hours, and to take a break you go to the campus recreation center to exercise. Your goal is to burn 300 kcal, so you hop on your favorite piece of exercise equipment, punch in your body weight, select manual protocol and begin. When the console reads 300 kcal you stop—proud of having attained your goal. But did you really?

The answer to that question depends on a number of factors. The console number for kcal is derived mathematically from a prediction equation that typically takes into account your body weight and one or more measures of workload, such as stride rate, stride length, belt speed, elevation, and resistance or power output, depending on whether the equipment is a stair-stepping machine, treadmill, elliptical strider, rowing machine, or cycle ergometer. In general, re-

search studies have shown that under identical conditions, the calorie cost estimations are very consistent (reliable). However, the same cannot be said for the accuracy (validity) of the caloric cost values. For example, in one study Swain et al. (1999) found that an elliptical motion machine significantly overestimated caloric cost (from 39% to 79%), with the larger overestimations occurring at the higher exercise intensities. In another study on an elliptical striding machine, Heselton and colleagues (2000) found that although the mean caloric cost values at two of three workloads were not significantly different, the estimated values were systematically overestimated at levels above 300 kcal per 30-minute workout, and the percentage of individuals whose measured caloric cost fell within 30 kcal of their estimated caloric cost was only 60%, averaged over two trials. Similar overestimations have been found for stair-stepping machines (Riddle and Orringer,

1990; Ryan, et al., 1998), and several studies have reported that holding on to the point where part of the body weight is supported results in a significant overestimation of caloric expenditure for both stair-steppers and the treadmill (Åstrand, 1984; Butts, et al., 1993; Howley, et al., 1992). The manufacturers of these pieces of equipment are trying to provide accurate information to the exerciser, but errors are part of predictions, and the mathematical program cannot adjust if you "cheat" by holding on. So, the answer to our question of whether you burned 300 kcal is "probably not." It is best to interpret the console values for caloric expenditure as an approximation rather than an absolute and to accept that the approximation is probably high.   ✳

Sources:

Åstrand (1984); Butts, et al. (1993); Heselton, et al. (2000); Howley, et al. (1992); Riddle & Orringer (1990); Ryan, et al. (1998); Swain, et al. (1999).

Remember that this caloric cost is an estimate of the aerobic portion only. If we attempt to calculate the caloric cost of all 28 min of the incremental task, the resulting number will be an underestimation, because we cannot calculate the anaerobic energy expenditure. Furthermore, these values include what an individual would expend if he or she were resting quietly. The term used when resting energy expenditure is included is *gross energy expenditure*. If resting energy expenditure is subtracted from gross energy expenditure, net energy expenditure—or the energy expended to do the exercise itself—is the result.

Knowledge of the caloric cost of an activity is helpful in prescribing exercise.

The Metabolic Equivalent (MET)

Although most people are used to seeing energy cost expressed as kilocalories, exercise physiologists and physicians often use MET values. MET is an acronym derived from the term *Metabolic EquivalenT*. One MET represents the average, seated, resting energy cost of an adult and is set at 3.5 mL·kg^{-1}·min of oxygen, or 1 kcal·kg^{-1}·hr^{-1}.

In reality, resting metabolic rate varies among individuals. If an individual's resting, seated energy expenditure is known, this value can be substituted for the 3.5 mL·kg^{-1}·min^{-1} average, but in practice, variations from the average value are not considered to be substantial enough to invalidate its use. Multiples of the 1-MET resting baseline represent the **MET** level or multiples of the resting rate of oxygen consumption of any given activity. Thus, an activity performed at the level of 5 METs would require five times as much energy as is expended at rest.

To calculate MET levels, divide the amount of oxygen utilized (in mL·kg^{-1}·min^{-1}) by 3.5. Hence, if an individual expends 29 mL·kg^{-1}·min^{-1} of O_2 on a task, the MET level is 29 mL·kg^{-1}·min^{-1} ÷ 3.5 mL·kg^{-1}·min^{-1} = 8.3 METs.

To convert from MET to kcal·min^{-1}, it is necessary to know the individual's body weight and use the relationship 1 kcal·kg^{-1}·hr^{-1} = 1 MET (American College of Sports Medicine [ACSM], 1995). For example, if the 8.3-MET activity was done by a female of average weight (68 kg), the calculation is

$$8.3 \text{ METs} = \frac{(8.3 \text{ kcal} \times 68 \text{ kg})}{60 \text{ min·hr}^{-1}} = 9.4 \text{ kcal·min}^{-1}$$

Table 5.6 presents a list of common activities in both METs and kcal·kg^{-1}·min^{-1} for adults. These values can be used for exercise prescriptions. Table 5.7 provides a classification of work intensities for sedentary individuals based on oxygen consumption (L·min^{-1}) and caloric cost (kcal·min^{-1} and kcal·kg^{-1}·min^{-1}). These values can be used as a rough guide for determining how long work can be sustained at each intensity. For example, hiking at a level of 0.05–0.12 kcal·kg^{-1}·min^{-1} (from Table 5.6) can be sustained at least 8 hr a day for several weeks (from Table 5.7), as many individuals who have traveled the length of the Appalachian Trail from Georgia to Maine will attest. Conversely, running at 6 min·mi^{-1} (10 mph) is such heavy work (0.27 kcal·kg^{-1}·min^{-1} from Table 5.6) that it would easily exhaust the untrained individ-

ual in just a few minutes (Table 5.7). Trained individuals would be able to sustain heavy levels of work for longer periods of time. Complete the Question of Understanding box on page 138.

Field Estimates of Energy Expenditure during Exercise

Metabolic Calculations Based on Mechanical Work or Standard Energy Use

In situations where an accurate assessment of mechanical work is possible, energy expenditure, expressed as oxygen consumption (mL·min^{-1}, mL·kg^{-1}·min^{-1}, or METs) can be estimated by a series of calculations. The equations used for the calculations are based on known oxygen costs for steady-state horizontal walking (0.1 mL·kg^{-1}·min^{-1} for each m·min^{-1}), horizontal running (0.2 mL·kg^{-1}·min^{-1} for each m·min^{-1}), vertical rise (1.8 mL·kg^{-1}·min^{-1} for each m·min^{-1} of walking or 0.9 mL·kg^{-1}·min^{-1} for each m·min^{-1} of running), leg ergometer work against resistance (2 mL·kgm^{-1}), and arm ergometer work against resistance (3 mL·kgm^{-1}) (ACSM, 2000). These values do not include the resting metabolic rate of 1 MET or 3.5 mL·kg^{-1}·min^{-1} of oxygen.

Example

If an individual were walking on a track at a 20 min·mi^{-1} pace (3 mi·hr^{-1}), which is a velocity of 80.4 m·min^{-1} (3 mi·hr^{-1} × 26.8 m·min^{-1}·mi·hr^{-1}), the calculation would be as follows:

$$\text{walking oxygen consumption} = 80.4 \text{ m·min}^{-1} \times \left(\frac{0.1 \text{ mL·kg}^{-1}·\text{min}^{-1}}{\text{m·min}^{-1}}\right)$$
$$+ 3.5 \text{ mL·kg}^{-1}·\text{min}^{-1} = 11.54 \text{ mL·kg}^{-1}·\text{min}^{-1}$$

This value can easily be converted to METs as previously described by dividing by 3.5 mL·kg^{-1}·min^{-1}. At the 20 min·mi^{-1} pace, this is 3.3 METs. If you check Table 5.6, you will see that 3.3 is the MET value given for walking at 3 mi·hr^{-1}. ✛

In addition to this equation for horizontal walking, other equations are available and are presented in Appendix B for uphill walking, horizontal and uphill running, bench stepping, leg cycle ergometry, and arm cycle ergometry (ACSM, 2000).

A Question of Understanding

A reasonable and beneficial level of exercise for fat loss is 300 kcal per session (Åstrand, 1952). The oxygen cost of riding a bicycle ergometer at 2 Kp (600 kgm·min^{-1}, or 100 W) at 60 rev·min^{-1} is 1200 mL O_2·min^{-1} above resting metabolism. At this rate, how long should an individual ride in order to burn an excess of 300 kcal? Ignore the cost involved in a warm-up or cool-down. Check your answer in Appendix D.

MET A unit that represents the metabolic equivalent in multiples of the resting rate of oxygen consumption of any given activity.

Table 5.6
MET and Caloric Values for Various Physical Activities

Physical Activity	MET Range	kcal·kg^{-1}·min^{-1}	Physical Activity	MET Range	kcal·kg^{-1}·min^{-1}
Archery	3–4	0.05–0.07	Running (*continued*)		
Backpacking	5–11	0.08–0.18	11 min·mi^{-1}	9.4	0.16
Badminton	4–9	0.07–0.15	10 min·mi^{-1}	10.2	0.17
Basketball			9 min·mi^{-1}	11.2	0.19
Nongame	3–9	0.05–0.15	8 min·mi^{-1}	12.5	0.21
Game play	7–12	0.12–0.20	7 min·mi^{-1}	14.1	0.24
Bed exercise (cardiac)	1–2	0.02–0.03	6 min·mi^{-1}	16.3	0.27
Bicycling, 10 mph	7	0.12	Sailing	2–5	0.03–0.08
Bowling	2–4	0.03–0.07	Scuba diving	5–10	0.08–0.17
Calisthenics	3–8	0.05–0.13	Skating, ice and roller	5–8	0.08–0.13
Canoeing, rowing, kayaking	3–8	0.05–0.13	Skiing,		
			Downhill	5–8	0.08–0.13
Dancing			Cross-country	6–12	0.10–0.20
Social and square	3–7	0.05–0.12	Water	5–7	0.08–0.12
Aerobic	6–9	0.10–0.15	Soccer	5–12	0.08–0.20
Football (touch)	6–10	0.10–0.17	Squash	8–12	0.13–0.20
Golf			Stair climbing	4–8	0.07–0.13
Power cart	2–3	0.03–0.05	Swimming	4–8	0.07–0.13
Walking, carrying bag	4–7	0.07–0.12	Table tennis	3–5	0.05–0.08
Handball	8–12	0.13–0.20	Tennis	4–9	0.07–0.15
Hiking, cross-country	3–7	0.05–0.12	Volleyball	3–6	0.05–0.10
Horseback riding	3–8	0.05–0.13	Walking		
Paddleball, racquetball	8–12	0.13–0.20	1.7 mi·hr^{-1}	2.3	0.04
Rope jumping	8–12	0.13–0.20	2.0 mi·hr^{-1}	2.4	0.04
Running			2.5 mi·hr^{-1}	2.9	0.05
12 min·mi^{-1}	8.7	0.15	3.0 mi·hr^{-1}	3.3	0.06
			3.4 mi·hr^{-1}	3.6	0.06

Note: 1 MET = 1 kcal·kg^{-1}·hr^{-1}; 1 kcal·kg^{-1}·hr^{-1} ÷ 60 min·hr^{-1} = .017 kcal·kg^{-1}·min^{-1}.

Source: Modified from American College of Sports Medicine (2000).

These equations are useful for exercise prescription purposes in a school, health club, or clinical setting where it is not possible to directly measure energy expenditure. Physicians, as mentioned before, often prescribe exercise by MET level and assume that the exercise leader will be able to determine the proper pace for walking or running, resistance on a cycle ergometer, or height and rate for step aerobics. The equations enable the exercise leader to do just that. However, it must always be remembered that the resultant values are just estimates for any given individual in any specific setting. Therefore, workloads should be fine-tuned by using heart rate or rate of perceived exertion (RPE) responses as described in Chapter 13.

Motion Sensors and Accelerometers

Attempts have been made to determine energy cost in the field by measuring movement, assuming that more movement means that more calories have been expended. Probably the most familiar type of motion sensor is the pedometer. After it is set with an individual's stride length, a *pedometer* can be used to record the distance an individual travels by foot. Thus, it is an indication of the quantity of movement. Electronic motion sensors that measure both frequency (or quantity) of movement and intensity of movement are called *accelerometers* (Laporte, et al., 1985). The most popular accelerometer is the Caltrac. Figure 5.7 shows an individual wearing a Caltrac while walking.

A Question of Understanding

How many METs is the subject in Table 5.2 exercising at in minute 14? The answer is in Appendix D.

Table 5.7
Work Classifications Based on Metabolic Cost of Sedentary Individuals

Classification	$\dot{V}O_2$ (L·min^{-1})	kcal·min^{-1}	kcal·kg^{-1}·min^{-1}*	Time Work Can Be Sustained
Light				
Mild	< 0.75	< 4	< 0.06	Indefinitely
Moderate	0.76–1.50	4.1–7.5	0.07–0.11	8 hr daily
Heavy				
Optimal	1.51–2.00	7.6–10	0.12–0.15	8 hr daily for a few weeks only
Strenuous	2.01–2.50	10.1–12.5	0.16–0.18	4 hr 2–3 times per week for a few weeks consecutively
Severe				
Maximal	2.51–3.00	12.51–15.00	0.19–0.22	1–2 hr occasionally
Exhausting	> 3.00	> 15.0	> 0.22	Few minutes, rarely

*   Assume 150 lb or 68 kg, which is the average American weight for a 64.5-in. female. The actual values will vary for different body weights.

Source: Modified from Wells, Balke, & Van Fossan (1957).

Both activity counts and estimated caloric values are displayed directly by Caltrac and require no additional calculations by the user. However, the accuracy of Caltrac for individual assessment of caloric cost has not been definitively determined (Bray, et al., 1992; Haskell, et al., 1993; Haymes and Byrnes, 1993; Maliszewski, et al., 1991; Pambianco, et al., 1990).

Activity Recalls and Questionnaires

The least complex system for estimating energy expenditure, at least from the standpoint of technology, is some form of self- or observer activity report (Laporte, et al., 1985). To determine the caloric cost of a particular exercise session, we must first know the activity that was performed and its intensity and duration. Then the caloric cost of that activity is determined from a chart like the one presented in Table 5.6. Finally, we must know the body weight of the individual exercising. The information is then substituted into the following formula:

5.5 total caloric cost of the activity (kcal) = caloric cost per kilogram of body weight per minute (kcal·kg^{-1}·min^{-1}) × body weight (kg) × exercise time (min)

Example

If a 65-yr-old, 84-kg female walks 3 mi in 1:15, how many kilocalories does she expend?

In order to use Table 5.6, we must first convert 3 mi in 1 hr and 15 min to mi per hour.

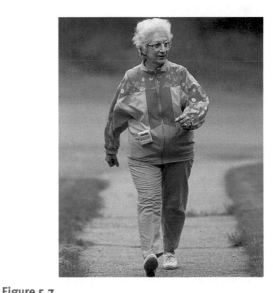

Figure 5.7
A Caltrac Accelerometer

This woman is wearing a Caltrac accelerometer that senses the frequency of her movement as she walks. The results provide an estimate of energy expended.

$$3 \text{ mi} \div \left(\frac{75 \text{ min}}{60 \text{ min}} \right) = 2.4 \text{ mi·hr}^{-1}$$

Looking at Table 5.6, we see that 2.5 mi·hr^{-1} is the closest we can get. Thus, an individual walking at 2.5 mi·hr^{-1} expends 0.05 kcal·kg^{-1}·min^{-1}. Substituting into this formula, we get

0.05 kcal·kg^{-1}·min^{-1} × 84 kg × 75 min = 315 kcal

Therefore, this individual has expended 315 kcal in her walk, which is a good fitness workout.

If an assessment of total daily energy expenditure or even weekly average expenditure is desired, the process becomes more tedious and, as a result, is probably less exact. Even the most willing individuals have only so much time to spend writing down everything they do; and if it is recorded after the fact, some things will be forgotten. Nevertheless, keeping a diary both of approximate energy expended and ingested can provide valuable information for individuals.

Efficiency and Economy

Efficiency

Walk into an appliance store to buy a furnace, hot water heater, washer, dryer, air conditioner, or refrigerator and each of the choices will have a label proclaiming its efficiency rating. Brand X uses only such and such an amount of electricity (for just pennies a day!) to heat 40 gallons of water, wash a load of clothes, and so on. Down the street the car dealer is shouting the praises of the latest midsized economy car. Plenty of leg room, holds five adults comfortably, and gets 35 mi per gallon of gas! In each case the concept is the same. We want to get the most output (in heating, cooling, or miles) for the least input and expense (electrical power, gas, or money). The same holds true when we consider physical labor or exercise output: We want to get the most output (work) for the least input (ATP, kilocalories, or fuel used).

The human body conforms to the first law of thermodynamics, which is also called the law of conservation of energy. Simply put, this law states that energy can neither be created nor destroyed but can only be changed in form. When an individual exercises or performs other external work, the actual work achieved represents only a portion of the total energy utilized. The rest of the energy appears as heat, which must be dissipated or the body temperature will rise. The percentage of energy input that appears as useful external work is called the **mechanical efficiency**, or simply the efficiency of that task.

Efficiency can be calculated in at least three ways. The simplest calculation of efficiency is as *gross efficiency*.

$$\boxed{5.6}\quad \text{gross efficiency} = \frac{\text{work output}}{\text{energy expended}} \times 100$$

Mechanical Efficiency The percentage of energy input that appears as useful external work.

Example

Calculate the gross efficiency for a 22-yr-old female whose body weight (BW) is 65.5 kg. She has ridden a Monark cycle ergometer (flywheel distance = 6 meters) at 50 rev·min^{-1} with a load of 2.5 kp for 15 min.

The external output is calculated as work equals force times distance ($W = F \times D$).

$$W = 2.5 \text{ kp} \times (50 \text{ rev·min}^{-1} \times 6 \text{ m}) \times 15 \text{ min}$$
$$= 11250 \text{ kgm}$$

It takes 426.8 kgm of work to equal one kilocalorie. Therefore,

$$11250 \text{ kgm} \div 426.8 \text{ kcal·kgm}^{-1} = 26.36 \text{ kcal}$$

of work output.

The amount of energy expended is calculated by using Eq. 5.4 and multiplying by the total time of the exercise. The average oxygen consumption for the ride was 1.73 L·min^{-1} and the RER was 0.91. At an RER of 0.91 the caloric equivalent (Table 5.4) is 4.936 kcal·L O_2^{-1}. Substituting into Eq. 5.4 we get

$$1.73 \text{ L } O_2\text{·min}^{-1} \times 4.936 \text{ kcal·L } O_2^{-1}$$
$$= 29.95 \text{ kcal·min}^{-1} \times 15 \text{ min} = 128.09 \text{ kcal}$$

of energy expended.

Eq. 5.6 can now be used to determine gross efficiency.

$$\text{gross efficiency} = \frac{26.36 \text{ kcal}}{128.09 \text{ kcal}} \times 100 = 20.58\% \text{ ✢}$$

A slightly more complex method uses *net efficiency*. In net efficiency the energy expended is corrected for resting metabolic rate.

$$\boxed{5.7}$$

$$\text{net efficiency} = \frac{\text{work output}}{\text{energy expended} - \text{resting}\atop\text{metabolic rate for the}\atop\text{same time period}} \times 100$$

Example

This means in the example used for gross efficiency that the individual's resting metabolic rate (measured to be 1.11 kcal·min^{-1} or 16.6 kcal for the 15 min) must be subtracted from the total energy expenditure of 128.09 kcal before computing for efficiency. Thus, substituting in Eq. 5.7 we get

$$\text{net efficiency} = \frac{26.36 \text{ kcal}}{128.09 \text{ kcal} - 16.6 \text{ kcal}} \times 100$$
$$= 23.64\% \qquad \text{✢}$$

The third technique for reporting efficiency requires the use of at least two workloads and is based on the difference between the two loads. It is called *delta efficiency*.

5.8

$$\text{delta efficiency} = \frac{\text{difference in work output between two loads}}{\text{difference in energy expenditure between the same two loads}} \times 100$$

Example

Calculate the delta efficiency for the 22-yr-old female in the last two examples whose body weight is 65.5 kg. This time she has performed two exercise stages on a treadmill, the first at 0% grade and the second at 10% grade. The speed was a constant 94 m·min^{-1} (3.5 mi·hr^{-1}). The difference in work output is therefore primarily determined by the difference in percent grade, in this case a 10% difference. Treadmill delta efficiency calculations are usually done on a per minute basis. Therefore, instead of calculating the change in work (W = F × D) as in the first two examples, the change (Δ) in work rate or power (P), which is work divided by time, is used (Adams, 1990; Gaesser and Brooks, 1975):

$$\Delta P \text{ kgm·min}^{-1} = BW \text{ (kg)} \times \text{speed (m·min}^{-1}) \times (\% \text{ slope}/100)$$

Substituting, we get

$$\Delta P = 65.5 \text{ kg} \times 94 \text{ m·min}^{-1} \times (10/100)$$
$$= 615.7 \text{ kgm·min}^{-1}$$

Using the conversion of 426.8 kgm of work is equal to 1 kcal, we then divide 615.7 kgm·min^{-1} by 426.8 kgm for a difference in work output of 1.44 kcal·min^{-1}.

As before, energy expenditure is calculated by using Eq. 5.4. The average oxygen consumption at 0% grade is 0.91 L·min^{-1} with an RER of 0.73. The caloric equivalent (Table 5.4) of the 0.73 RER is 4.714 kcal·L O$_2^{-1}$. Substituting into Eq. 5.4 this becomes

$$0.91 \text{ L O}_2\text{·min}^{-1} \times 4.714 \text{ kcal·L O}_2^{-1} = 4.29 \text{ kcal·min}^{-1}$$

The average oxygen consumption at 10% grade was 1.75 L O$_2^{-1}$ and the RER was 0.86. The caloric equivalent of an RER of 0.86 is 4.875 kcal·L O$_2^{-1}$. Substituting these values into Eq. 5.4 we have

$$1.75 \text{ L O}_2\text{·min}^{-1} \times 4.875 \text{ kcal·L O}_2^{-1} = 8.53 \text{ kcal·min}^{-1}$$

To obtain the difference in energy expended at the two workloads, we simply subtract

$$8.53 \text{ kcal·min}^{-1} - 4.29 \text{ kcal·min}^{-1} = 4.24 \text{ kcal·min}^{-1}$$

Eq. 5.8 can now be used to solve for delta efficiency:

$$\text{delta efficiency} = \frac{1.44 \text{ kcal·min}^{-1}}{4.25 \text{ kcal·min}^{-1}} \times 100 = 33.9\% \quad +$$

When used on the same exercise modality, the different methods of calculating efficiency will yield very different results. For example, Gaesser and Brooks (1975) calculated gross efficiencies of 7.5–20.4%, net efficiencies of 9.8–24.1%, and delta efficiencies of 24.4–34% on the bicycle ergometer under the same controlled experimental conditions. Despite these differences, each technique is best suited for particular uses.

Gross efficiency is most useful when values for specific workloads, speeds, or the like, are of interest. For example, it answers the question: What is the efficiency of cycling into a 15 mi·hr^{-1} (24 km·hr^{-1}) head wind, and how might that change with body position? Gross efficiency is also important for applications in nutritional studies where gross energy expenditure is a matter of concern for adequate replenishment, such as during the Tour de France, when replacement is essential if a cyclist is to continue hard riding day after day. Gross efficiency also is the measure that has been reported most frequently, and so it is important for comparison purposes (Donovan and Brooks, 1977).

Because the energy expended during rest really is not used to do external work, net efficiency is actually a better indication of the efficiency of work per se. At the same time, it is not a particularly realistic value, since an individual performing any external work is still expending resting energy.

The most accurate means for determining the effect of speed or work rate on efficiency is the use of delta efficiency. It gives an indication of the relative energy cost of performing an additional increment of work. Delta efficiency is also the technique of choice when calculating efficiency on a treadmill. Its use is necessary because technically no work (calculated as force × distance) is done when the treadmill is horizontal (0% grade), despite the fact that energy is used.

All efficiency calculations assume a submaximal steady-state or steady-rate condition and require that both work output and energy expenditure be expressed in the same units, typically kilocalories. The calculations may be done for the total time, as in the 15-min bicycle ergometer ride used in the example for gross efficiency, or per unit of time, as in the per-minute calculations for the treadmill of delta efficiency. However, time can be a factor, since efficiency is generally high when a large amount of work is performed in a short period of time and low when a small amount of work is performed over a long period of time (Stegeman, 1981).

Because the same amount of physical work in the same or a different exercise modality does not cause the same metabolic effect, it is the energy cost (V̇O$_2$ consumption) that is the deciding factor in determining efficiency (Stegeman, 1981). Figure 5.8 shows this basic relationship. As the energy cost (V̇O$_2$ mL·kg^{-1}·min^{-1} on the left y-axis) increases, efficiency (% efficiency on the right y-axis) decreases, and vice versa.

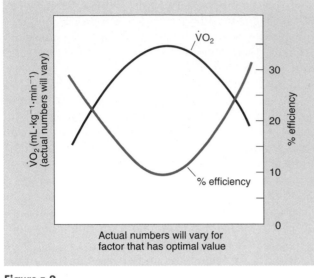

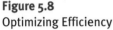

Figure 5.8
Optimizing Efficiency

Note: Optimization means minimizing energy expenditure and maximizing work output.
Source: Cavanaugh & Kram (1985).

Certain factors have been shown to change efficiency and thus can be manipulated by an individual in order to optimize efficiency. For example, the optimal seat height on a bicycle at any given power output has been found to be approximately 109% of leg length. Optimal pedaling frequency at any given power output has been shown to be between 40 and 60 rev·min^{-1} for trained and untrained individuals, despite the fact that trained cyclists self-select a rate closer to 90 rev·min^{-1}. The higher revolutions per minute used by the trained cyclist may optimize muscular forces and lower limb stresses but not metabolic efficiency (Widrick, et al., 1992). When the revolutions per minute are kept constant on a cycle ergometer, efficiency tends to increase from low to high workloads (Cavanagh and Kram, 1985; Hagberg, et al., 1981; Stegeman, 1981). The optimal speed for walking when distance is held constant is between 60 and 100 m·min^{-1} (about 2.25 and 3.75 mi·hr^{-1}, or 16–27 min·mi^{-1}). The optimal grade when speed is held constant is approximately 5% downhill (−5%). The optimal stride length when speed is held constant varies considerably among individuals. Most runners, however, intuitively select a stride length that is very close to optimal for themselves. Therefore, coaches who attempt to alter stride length may be harming efficiency.

Exercise efficiency values are most frequently reported in the 20–25% range. These values may be slightly higher (20–45%) if they are calculated as delta efficiencies and slightly lower (5–20%) if the activity involves air or wind resistance. Overcoming air resistance requires additional energy at all speeds of running and velocities of wind (including no wind). Hence, in a running or cycling race participants often draft off of (or tuck in behind) the front runner. The first athlete must work harder than the athlete tucked behind, who does less work, hoping to save sufficient energy to put on a surge at the end and pass the more fatigued front runner.

The extra energy cost due to air resistance is proportional to the velocity at which the runner is moving raised to the second power, or m·sec^2. Assuming there is no head wind, this amounts to approximately 2% extra energy expenditure for the marathon distance, 4–8% for middle-distance events, and 8–16% for sprints at world-class speeds. Although these percentages may not sound like much, they can be the equivalent of 5 min for the marathoner. At high levels of competition this is a tremendous amount of time and would make a considerable difference in the results (Åstrand, 1952; Davies, 1980; Donavan and Brooks, 1977; Gaesser and Brooks, 1975; Pendergast, et al., 1977; Pugh, 1970). Although a head wind can require additional energy, and thus decrease efficiency, the reverse is not true. A tailwind never assists the runner by decreasing the energy cost proportionally.

The mechanical efficiency of cycling, whether calculated as net efficiency or delta efficiency, appears to be similar in prepubertal children, postpubertal adolescents, and adults (Klausen, et al., 1985; Rowland, 1990). It may be slightly reduced in the elderly. These similarities are true whether the calculations are based on relative (% $\dot{V}O_2$max) or on absolute (kgm·min^{-1} or W) workloads. The similarities also hold for males and females alike (Bal, et al., 1953; Girandola, et al., 1981; Sidney and Shephard, 1977; Taylor, et al., 1950). Because of the constancy of efficiency, cycling is a good family activity.

Economy of Walking and Running

As has been shown, the calculation of efficiency is a ratio of work output to energy expenditure input. However, measuring external work output may be impossible in many activities such as horizontal walking and running during which the reciprocal movements of the arms and legs cancel each other and no vertical gain is attained. Consequently, the energy expended or oxygen cost is often used alone for walking and running as a measure of economy, not efficiency.

Economy is the oxygen cost of walking or running at varying speeds. The most basic generalization

---

Economy The oxygen cost of walking or running at varying speeds.

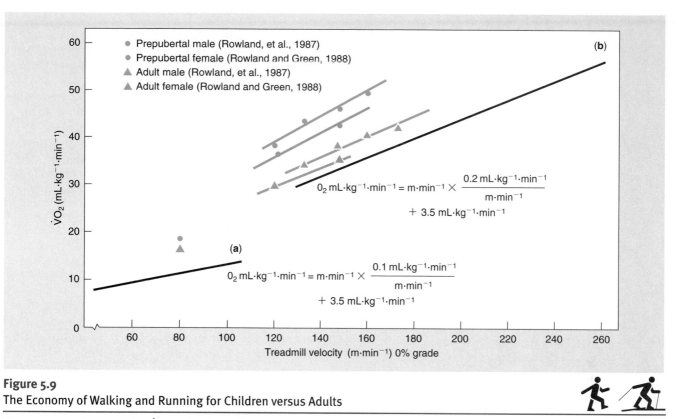

Figure 5.9
The Economy of Walking and Running for Children versus Adults

The oxygen cost (expressed as $\dot{V}O_2$ mL·kg^{-1} min^{-1}) of walking (a) and running (b) increases rectilinearly as velocity increases. However, the slope of the two lines is different, and they do not form a continuous line from slow walking to fast running. Prepubertal males and prepubertal females are less economical than adult males and females as indicated by the higher oxygen cost at each and every velocity.

Sources: American College of Sports Medicine (2000); Rowland, et al. (1987); Rowland & Green (1988).

about economy is that, over a wide range of velocities, the energy cost (in mL·kg^{-1}·min^{-1} of O_2) is rectilinearly related to the speed (in m·min^{-1}). This generalization is true at least at 0% grade on a treadmill when the speed can be accomplished at a submaximal steady-state level (Costill, 1986). Figure 5.9 shows this fundamental relationship. The black lines were computed from the equations recommended by the American College of Sports Medicine (2000). These equations in turn were based on a compilation of research. Note that the relationship between speed and oxygen consumption is not a continuous straight line encompassing both walking (Figure 5.9a) and running (Figure 5.9b). For walking speeds between approximately 50 and 100 m·min^{-1} each m·min^{-1} adds 0.1 mL·kg^{-1}·min^{-1} above resting to the cost of the walk; for running speeds above 134 m·min^{-1} the increment is 0.2 mL·kg^{-1}·min^{-1}. Speeds between 100 and 134 m·min^{-1} represent an awkward area for most people; where it is too fast to walk but too slow to run. Additionally, outdoor running over ground is probably more demanding in terms of oxygen cost

than indoor running on the treadmill at any given velocity, although overground inclined running equals the oxygen cost of treadmill-grade running (ACSM, 2000; Daniels, 1985; Morgan, Baldini, et al., 1989).

For any given individual, running economy appears to be relatively stable if environmental, equipment, and testing factors (such as body temperature, air resistance, footwear, time of day, and training status) are controlled (Morgan, Martin, et al., 1989). Day-to-day variations between 1.6–11% have been reported in the literature for well-trained and elite male runners. On the other hand, differences among individuals in terms of running economy are often extensive, ranging from 20–30%, in subjects of equal training and performance status. The reason for these observations has not been determined (Conley and Krahenbuhl, 1980; Daniels, 1985).

The Influence of Sex on Economy

The influence of sex on the interindividual variation in economy is unclear. Studies report that males

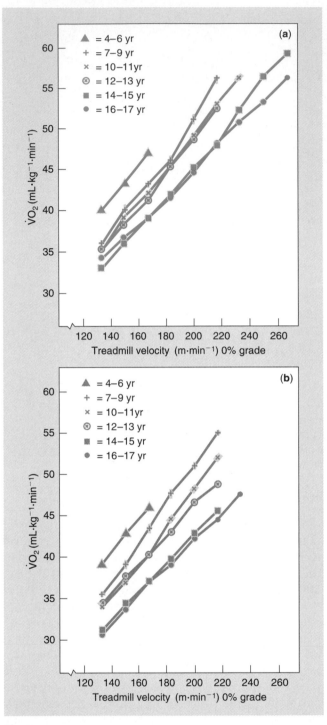

Figure 5.10

Running Economy of Children and Adolescents

Running economy improves as both male (a) and female (b) children age. This can be seen by the almost parallel and successively lower $\dot{V}O_2$ mL·kg^{-1}·min^{-1} values across the tested velocities of running.

Source: P.-O. Åstrand. *Experimental Studies of Physical Working Capacity in Relation to Sex and Age.* Copenhagen: Munksgaard (1952). Modified and printed by permission.

expend more energy (Figure 5.9, green lines), less energy, or the same amount of energy in walking and running as do females (Figure 5.9, gold lines) when values are expressed relative to body mass (per kilogram of body weight). What is clear is that even if the oxygen cost is equal at any given speed, the female, who typically has a lower $\dot{V}O_2$max, will be working at a higher % $\dot{V}O_2$max than the male (Åstrand, 1956; Bhambhani and Singh, 1985; Bransford and Howley, 1977; Bunc and Heller, 1989; Cunningham, 1990; Daniels, 1985; Morgan, Martin, et al., 1989). This fact has implications for the pace at which long distance events can be run.

The Influence of Age on Economy

Age has a clear-cut effect on economy. Ample evidence exists to show that children and adolescents are less economical than adults when running over a wide range of speeds. There is scant evidence to indicate that the elderly may be less economical than young and middle-aged adults. Further research is needed in this area (Adams, et al., 1972; Asmussen, 1981; Daniels, 1985; Girandola, et al., 1981; Larish, et al., 1987; Morgan, Martin, et al., 1989; Robinson, et al., 1976; Rowland and Green, 1988; Rowland, et al., 1987; Rowland, et al., 1988).

Figures 5.9a and 5.9b show the results of two studies conducted in the same laboratory in which male prepubertal children (9–13 yr) were compared with adult males (23–33 yr) (Rowland, et al., 1987) and female prepubertal children (8–12 yr) were compared with adult females (22–35 yr) (Rowland, et al., 1988) and how the four groups compared to the theoretical computed oxygen consumption values. In both sexes the energy cost at all speeds of running was higher for the children than the adults when expressed relative to body mass. No values for walking were available for the males, but at 80 m·min^{-1} there was no apparent age difference for the females. The differences at the running speeds held true whether expressed as an absolute load (m·min^{-1}) or relative load (% $\dot{V}O_2$max). The adult values were much closer to the calculated values than the children's, indicating that the equations should not be used for children.

Figures 5.10a and 5.10b show that children and adolescents differ not only from adults in terms of economy of running but also from each other (Åstrand, 1952). Indeed, there is a progressive decline in oxygen cost (progressive increase in economy) from the youngest (4–6 yr) to the oldest (16–17 yr) age groups in both the boys and girls. A compilation of studies shows the decline in oxygen cost to be about 2% per year from 8 to 18 yr when the same work is performed (Morgan, Martin, et al., 1989). Similar data are available for walking at 80–100 m·min⁻¹ at increasing grades for both boys and girls. These changes are evident from cross-sectional studies in which different individuals are tested at each age, and in longitudinal studies of the same individuals at different ages (Bar-Or, 1983; Costill, 1986; Daniels, et al., 1978).

Much speculation has surrounded the cause of this low economy in children. Five factors are known to be affected by growth and may offer at least a partial explanation.

1. *High basal metabolic rate.* The basal metabolic rate (BMR) is the minimum level of energy required to sustain the body's vital functions in the waking state as measured by oxygen consumption. BMR is highest in young children and progressively declines to adulthood, where it stabilizes until it again declines in old age (Rowland, 1990). (See Figures 5.11 and 9.2.) Hence, gross exercise oxygen consumption values may be higher in children than in adults because resting metabolic rates are higher. Bar-Or (1983) has pointed out that this difference in resting metabolism is only 1–2 mL·kg⁻¹·min⁻¹ and, although this value represents a 25–35% greater BMR in children than in adults, it is unlikely to account for all of the difference in submaximal exercise values. Indeed, when Åstrand (1952) utilized net oxygen values instead of gross (by subtracting the BMRs), the differences between the age groups was reduced but not eliminated.

2. *Large surface area/mass ratio.* A phenomenon exists in the animal kingdom in which smaller animals (such as mice, squirrels, rabbits, or the young of any species) exhibit higher resting metabolic rates per unit of body mass than larger animals (dogs, horses, elephants, or the adults of any species). However, when the unit of comparison is not body mass (that is, per kilogram) but body surface area (that is, per square meter), metabolic rates are similar. This is called the surface law. The surface law appears to be important in the maintenance of normal core temperatures. Body heat loss is directly related to surface area. The larger the surface area, the greater the heat loss is. Relatively speaking, small and/or young adults have greater surface areas per unit of mass than large and/or adult animals. Hence, a higher resting metabolic rate is necessary to maintain body temperature. This phenomenon may be the reason for the elevated BMR in the young (Rowland, 1990; Rowland and Green, 1988; Rowland, et al., 1987). When Rowland and his colleagues (1988, 1987) changed the unit of comparison from mL·kg⁻¹·min⁻¹ to mL·m²·min⁻¹, the differences between the prepubertal and adult subjects of both sexes were no longer significant and were almost eliminated.

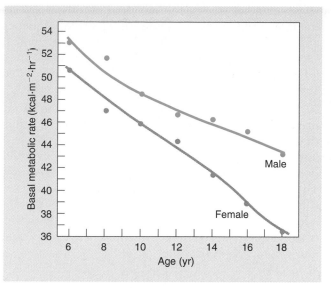

Figure 5.11
Changes in Basal Metabolic Rate with Age

Source: From *Exercise and Children's Health* (pp. 56, 57) by Thomas W. Rowland, Champaign, IL: Human Kinetics. Copyright 1990 by Thomas Rowland. Reprinted by permission.

3. *Immature running mechanics.* Anyone watching a young child and an adult run together can easily see the differences in motor skill (Rowland, 1990; Rowland, et al., 1987). The young child appears to take numerous small, choppy steps involving lots of extraneous movements. Technically, the child has a higher stride frequency; a shorter stride length (although it is proportional to his or her height); a greater vertical displacement; increased ankle, knee, and hip extension at takeoff; a longer nonsupport phase; and a shorter placement of the support foot in front of the center of gravity. The only one of these variables that seems to have any direct effect on the oxygen cost of running is stride frequency. Each stride requires energy to accelerate and brake the body's mass. When only one stride is considered, the oxygen cost does not differ between children and adults. However, at any given pace the child has a greater frequency of strides simply because he or she is anatomically smaller. Thus, more oxygen is utilized to provide the greater energy need (Rowland, et al., 1987).

Support for the importance of stride frequency is also evident from cycling. Cycling is independent of weight (the body weight is supported by the seat) and can be independent of pedaling frequency (analogous to stride frequency), when it is controlled by setting the rev·min⁻¹ with a consistent wheel size. In this situation, as stated previously, no difference in efficiency is apparent between children and adults.

Remember that each individual intuitively selects the most economical combination of stride frequency and length for running. It is best not to attempt to "make" children more economical by training them to lengthen their strides. Stride frequency decreases and stride length increases naturally as the child grows.

4. *Less efficient ventilation.* The volume of air breathed in order to consume 1 L of oxygen is called the *ventilatory equivalent* (VE). Children have a higher VE than adults. The processing of this additional air requires an added expenditure of energy. This increased metabolic cost of respiration may account for part of the increased oxygen costs at submaximal work in children, although not all research evidence is in agreement (Rowland, 1990; Rowland and Green, 1988; Rowland, et al., 1987; Rowland, et al., 1988).

5. *Decreased anaerobic capacity.* As discussed in the preceding chapter, children are less able to generate ATP anaerobically than adults. The measurement of economy by oxygen consumption evaluates only the aerobic energy contribution. It is possible that at higher, but still submaximal, workloads, adults provide a greater amount of the required energy anaerobically and thus exhibit an artificially low oxygen cost value (Rowland, 1990; Rowland, et al., 1987). Evidence from RER values supports this contention. Children typically show lower RERs during submaximal exercise than do adults. Direct measurement of free fatty acid and glycerol levels show, however, that the lower RERs are not the result of an increased utilization of fat as a fuel as might be expected. Instead, it is postulated that the lower RERs result from lower amounts of nonmetabolic "excess CO_2," that is, the CO_2 generated from the buffering of lactic acid.

Why Do Economy and Efficiency Matter?

Economy or efficiency probably matter little in high-intensity, short-term activities such as maximal weight lifts and sprints or in skilled movements such as golf. However, economy or efficiency is extremely important in endurance events. Among those factors critical for success in endurance performances are a high $\dot{V}O_2$max, the ability to work at a high % $\dot{V}O_2$max aerobically, and a high economy measured as a low submaximal oxygen cost at high velocities (Conley and Krahenbuhl, 1980; Costill, 1986; Costill, et al., 1973; Cunningham, 1990; Morgan, Martin, et al., 1989).

Although a high $\dot{V}O_2$max is considered to be a prerequisite for success in distance or endurance events, it generally does not determine performance if participants are relatively homogeneous in that trait. For example, Costill (1986) presents data from two runners (Ted Corbitt and Jim McDonagh) who had similar $\dot{V}O_2$max values (64 and 65 mL·kg^{-1}·min^{-1}). Over a period of two years they competed against each other in 15 major races and the same runner (McDonagh) won each and every time! Obviously, the physiological explanation did not lie in $\dot{V}O_2$max.

The importance of % $\dot{V}O_2$max that can be sustained for long periods is exemplified by the success of such runners as Grete Waitz, Frank Shorter, and Derek Clayton (Costill, 1986). These world-class runners were estimated to use between 85% and 90% $\dot{V}O_2$max when they competed in marathons, whereas less successful marathoners average about 75–80% $\dot{V}O_2$max. Typically, such a high percentage (85–90%) could only be maintained for the shorter (10 mi or less) distance. By being able to continue at that rate for over twice as long as normal, these individuals gained a competitive edge.

A Question of Understanding

The Fitt family plans to run the Cornfest 10-km (6.2 miles) race together. Dr. Phyllis Fitt (the mother) is an exercise physiologist and recently tested everyone in her lab. Given the following information, what is the fastest time they can run with a reasonable chance of everyone finishing in good shape together?

	Daughter	Son	Mother	Father	Grandmother
Age (yr)	12	8	37	45	57
$\dot{V}O_2$max (mL·kg^{-1}·min^{-1})	48	50	50	52	40
$\dot{V}O_2$ (mL·kg^{-1}·min^{-1})					
10 min·mi^{-1}	37	39	30	32	33
9 min·mi^{-1}	40	43	32	34	36
8 min·mi^{-1}	45	48	38	41	40
7 min·mi^{-1}	48	50	43	46	

Hint: Competitive runners typically average 80–90% $\dot{V}O_2$max during distance races of 5–10 mi; fun runners might be expected to be at the lower end of this value.

Table 5.8

Information for Predicted Velocity at $\dot{V}O_2$max for Subjects A and B (Figure 5.12)

Subject	$\dot{V}O_2$ mL·kg^{-1}·min-1 at indicated speed (m·min^{-1})					$\dot{V}O_2$max (mL·kg^{-1}·min^{-1})	v$\dot{V}O_2$max (m·min^{-1})	10-km Run Time	%v$\dot{V}O_2$max for 10 km
	196	215	230	248	268				
A	38.03	40.58	44.30	45.10	—	54.68	304.56	38:21	83.2
B	—	46.13	48.28	50.54	54.88	60.88	306.50	38:09	83.1

Source: Based on Bird (1991).

Additionally, if two runners of widely varying $\dot{V}O_2$max (runner A = 65 mL·kg^{-1}·min^{-1}; runner B = 50 mL·kg^{-1}·min^{-1}) but similar economy attempt to train together, say at an 8-min pace ($\dot{V}O_2$ cost = 40 mL·kg^{-1}·min^{-1}), runner B will be working much harder (80% $\dot{V}O_2$max) than runner A (62% $\dot{V}O_2$max). This variation in effort often occurs when females (average lower $\dot{V}O_2$max, equal economy) run with males.

Differences in economy have a similar effect on performance. If, for example, runner A and runner B had the same $\dot{V}O_2$max (65 mL·kg^{-1}·min^{-1}) but widely varying economies at an 8-min pace (runner A = 55 mL·kg^{-1}·min^{-1}; runner B = 40 mL·kg^{-1}·min^{-1}), then runner A would be working much harder (85% $\dot{V}O_2$max) than runner B (62% $\dot{V}O_2$max). This difference is probably why McDonagh (mentioned earlier) continually beat Corbitt in their races. At all velocities faster than 8 min·mi^{-1} Corbitt used significantly more oxygen than McDonagh (Costill, 1986). He had to be able to make up this difference by running at a higher % $\dot{V}O_2$max or he would lose. Obviously, it was the latter that occurred.

This scenario also occurs when a child (on average equal in $\dot{V}O_2$max to an adult but lower in economy) runs with an adult. At any given speed the child (unless there is a great disparity in his or her favor for $\dot{V}O_2$max) will be working harder than the adult. Although it is important for parents and teachers to encourage children to be active and for adults to do activities with children, the fact that the child will be working proportionally harder at any given running pace must be taken into account. The parent or teacher should match the pace of the child or encourage just a slightly faster pace—not make the child keep up with what feels comfortable to the adult. As a consequence, the adult will have to do his or her hard training without the child along, but the child will enjoy the experience much more. Since there appears to be no difference in efficiency in cycling as a function of either sex or age, as long as the wheel sizes (and hence revolutions per minute) are equal, cycling

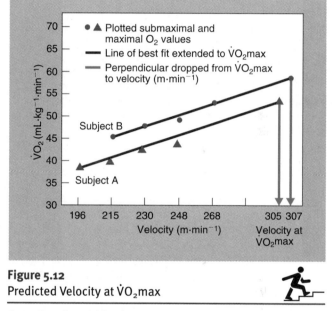

Figure 5.12
Predicted Velocity at $\dot{V}O_2$max

Source: Based on Bird (1991).

may be a better family activity than running. Work through the Question of Understanding box on page 146. Check your answer in Appendix D.

What may matter most to a competitive runner is a combination of economy and $\dot{V}O_2$max known as velocity at $\dot{V}O_2$max (v$\dot{V}O_2$max). The **velocity at $\dot{V}O_2$max** is the speed at which an individual can run when working at his or her maximal oxygen consumption based both on submaximal running economy and $\dot{V}O_2$max. Table 5.8 and Figure 5.12 show how this value is calculated and what it means. To calculate v$\dot{V}O_2$max, $\dot{V}O_2$ values (y-axis) are plotted at several

Velocity at $\dot{V}O_2$max The speed at which an individual can run when working at his or her maximal oxygen consumption; based both on submaximal running economy and $\dot{V}O_2$max.

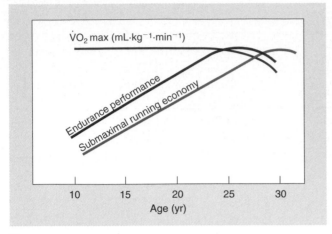

Figure 5.13

The Relationship between Maximal Oxygen Consumption, Endurance Performance, and Submaximal Running Economy from Childhood to Early Adulthood

As children age endurance performance typically improves often despite no improvement in $\dot{V}O_2$ mL·kg^{-1}·min^{-1}. One possible explanation is the parallel improvement in submaximal running economy. In early adulthood all three measures begin to decline.

Source: From *Exercise and Children's Health* (pp. 56, 57) by Thomas W. Rowland, Champaign, IL: Human Kinetics. Copyright 1990 by Thomas Rowland. Reprinted by permission.

submaximal speeds (x-axis) for each individual, and a regression line—a line that best fits the $\dot{V}O_2$ values—is established. The line is extended to include the individual's measured $\dot{V}O_2$max. The speed (or velocity) at which the $\dot{V}O_2$max occurs is then determined by dropping a perpendicular line from the extended line to the x-axis. This velocity is taken as the velocity at $\dot{V}O_2$max (v$\dot{V}O_2$max). As the figure shows, it is possible to achieve the same v$\dot{V}O_2$max with a high economy (that is, a low energy cost at submaximal speeds) and a low $\dot{V}O_2$max (subject A) or with a low economy (that is, a high energy cost at submaximal speeds) and a high $\dot{V}O_2$max (subject B). Individuals such as these two with a similar v$\dot{V}O_2$max would be expected to have similar performances in endurance running events (Bird, 1991; Morgan, Baldini, et al., 1989). All other factors (such as % $\dot{V}O_2$max) being relatively equal, an individual with a high v$\dot{V}O_2$max would be expected to perform better than an individual with a low v$\dot{V}O_2$max.

The low economy of children may be important in explaining another phenomenon. Typically, endurance performance as measured by treadmill time to fatigue, 12-min-run distance, mile-run time, and so on, improves in children with age despite a constant $\dot{V}O_2$max (Figure 5.13). Furthermore, although young athletes generally exhibit $\dot{V}O_2$max values that are higher than

those of nonathletes, when training programs are followed, endurance performance often improves exclusively—or at least more than does $\dot{V}O_2$max. It is possible that improvements in submaximal running economy (through improved skill in the short term) and age improvements in qualitative changes in oxygen delivery (not indicated by $\dot{V}O_2$max) and/or the improvement of anaerobic strength and speed components in the long term account for the enhanced endurance performances regardless of what occurs with $\dot{V}O_2$max. Indeed, submaximal running economy has been found to be statistically related to and to account for a considerable portion of the variance in endurance performance in children and adolescents in most (but not all) studies on this topic. Since $\dot{V}O_2$max remains relatively stable and the O_2 cost of any given speed decreases, the child is progressively working at a lower % $\dot{V}O_2$max as he or she ages. Hence, the individual would be expected to be able to perform (endure) at the same speed for a longer period of time, cover more ground in the same time span, and/or increase the speed at which any given distance is covered (Bar-Or, 1983; Burkett, et al., 1985; Daniels and Oldridge, 1971; Daniels, et al., 1978; Krahenbuhl, et al., 1989; Mayers and Gutin, 1979; McCormack, et al., 1991; Roland, 1990; Roland, et al., 1988).

Finally, for all the reasons cited in the discussion so far, one cannot use adult prediction equations based on $\dot{V}O_2$/speed relationships to predict $\dot{V}O_2$max in children.

Heritability of Aerobic Characteristics

Very little information is available on the impact of genetics on submaximal aerobic metabolism or its determinant characteristics. Bouchard et al (1989) studied the energy cost of incremental, submaximal, cycle ergometer work on 22 pairs of sedentary male dizygous (DZ) twins and 31 pairs of sedentary male monozygous (MZ) twins (16–29 yr old). As anticipated, the MZ twins were more similar in oxygen utilization than the DZ twins. However, the heritability estimate (degree of genetic influence) declined from 90% when exercise was performed at 50 W, to 78% when exercise was performed at 75 W, to 46% when exercise was performed at 100 W. Variability due to heritability was nonsignificant at workloads of 125 W and 150 W. Thus, a significant genetic effect was suggested for low work intensities but not for high ones. Energy substrate utilization (as determined by RER) did not exhibit a consistently greater similarity in the MZ twins than in the DZ twins. These results do little to clarify the possibility of a genetic influence on aerobic characteristics.

Endurance performance—defined as maximal aerobic capacity and measured as total work output in 90 min of pedaling on a bicycle ergometer—was found to be more highly correlated in MZ twins than in DZ twins but had a heritability estimate of only 32% (Bouchard, 1986). On the subcellular level no gene-associated variation has been found in mitochondrial density or metabolic enzyme activity (Bouchard, 1986; Bouchard and Lortie, 1984).

Despite these meager results, a strong genetic potential is deemed important for successful performance and absolutely essential for elite-level competition.

Summary

1. Aerobic metabolism can be measured directly by calorimetry (the measurement of heat production) or indirectly by spirometry (the measurement of air breathed and the analysis of oxygen and carbon dioxide gases). Typically, open-circuit indirect calorimetry is used.

2. During aerobic exercise the amount of oxygen consumed and carbon dioxide produced increases. If the exercise is a short-term submaximal activity, the metabolic costs level off where the energy requirements are met. This activity is called steady-state or steady-rate submaximal exercise.

3. If a submaximal exercise lasts for a long time, is above approximately 70% $\dot{V}O_2$max, or takes place under hot and humid conditions, oxygen drift occurs. The oxygen consumption drifts upward owing to rising levels of catecholamines, lactate, and body temperature as well as an increasing cost of ventilation and a shift in substrate utilization.

4. During incremental exercise to maximum the oxygen consumed rises in a rectilinear pattern proportional to the workload increments until the individual can increase oxygen utilization no more and a plateau occurs. The highest amount of oxygen an individual can take in, transport, and utilize during heavy exercise is called maximal oxygen consumption ($\dot{V}O_2$max).

5. Both static and dynamic resistance activity are predominantly anaerobic activities. The oxygen contribution to the energy cost rarely exceeds one-third to one-half the total energy cost.

6. On the cellular level the ratio of carbon dioxide produced to oxygen consumed is termed the respiratory quotient (RQ); as analyzed from expired air, it is termed the respiratory exchange ratio (RER). Nonprotein RER is used most frequently in determining energy substrate utilization, with 0.7 being interpreted as fat, 1.0 as carbohydrate, and 0.85 as an approximate 50-50 mixture of both.

7. During exercise the higher the intensity, the higher the RER value is. During long-duration submaximal exercise RER may decrease as the carbohydrate stores are depleted. During incremental exercise to maximum RER may increase above 1.0, reflecting carbon dioxide increases from nonmetabolic sources. RERs for high-intensity, static exercise and dynamic resistance exercise are between 0.8 and 1.0^+, reflecting a mixed fuel supply during the static activity followed by hyperventilation and a reliance on glycogen during the dynamic resistance activity.

8. Knowledge of the amount of oxygen consumed, the RER during the same time span, and the caloric equivalent permit the calculation of caloric expenditure ($kcal \cdot min^{-1}$) and metabolic equivalents (METs).

9. Estimates of energy expenditure in nonlaboratory (field) settings can be done by using a series of metabolic formulas, by using motion sensors, or by using activity recall questionnaires and previously established caloric cost charts.

10. Mechanical efficiency, either gross, net, or delta, is some ratio of work output to energy expended. Economy is simply a measure of the energy expended (oxygen consumed); it is used when measuring the work output is difficult. Because the energy cost of walking and running is rectilinear over a wide range of speed, it is possible to estimate oxygen cost or MET values when the speed is known.

11. Individual variation in running economy is high between individuals but is low within the same individual. No clear-cut distinction in running economy has been shown between females and males. Children and adolescents are less economical than adults when running over a wide range of speeds. The elderly may also be less economical than young and middle-aged adults.

12. The exact reason why children are less economical than adults is unknown. However, the following factors have been considered possibilities:
    a. A high basal metabolic rate
    b. A large surface area/mass ratio
    c. Immature running mechanics
    d. Less efficient ventilation
    e. Decreased anaerobic capacity

13. A high economy (that is, a low oxygen cost) at any given velocity of running is beneficial to performance, especially if it is combined with a high $\dot{V}O_2$max and the ability to work consistently at a high %$\dot{V}O_2$max. The higher the velocity at $\dot{V}O_2$max and the greater percentage of v$\dot{V}O_2$max an individual can maintain, the better his or her performance will be. The improvement in running economy may explain why, as they grow and/or train, children typically improve in endurance run performance (such as the mile run) but do not show any significant improvement in $\dot{V}O_2$max.

14. The genetic influence on aerobic metabolic components is unclear. A heritability estimate of about 32% has been found for endurance performance.

Review Questions

1. List the variables used to describe the aerobic metabolic response to exercise. Describe how each one is obtained from laboratory or field tests. Explain what each variable means.

2. Diagram the oxygen consumption response during (a) short-term, light- to moderate-intensity submaximal aerobic exercise; (b) long-term, moderate to heavy submaximal aerobic exercise; (c) incremental aerobic exercise to maximum; (d) static exercise; and (e) dynamic resistance exercise.

3. Describe the relationship between the oxygen cost of breathing and exercise intensity.

4. Explain the respiratory quotient and the respiratory exchange ratio. Relate them to the determination of energy substrate utilization, theoretically and numerically according to exercise intensity, duration, and type.

5. Explain the similarities and differences in describing activity by kilocalories and MET levels. How can both be practically applied?

6. Differentiate, in terms of definition, calculation, and application, between gross efficiency, net efficiency, and delta efficiency. How can a cyclist maximize his or her efficiency?

7. Compare running economy by sex and age. Discuss possible reasons for any observed differences. Give three situations where any observed differences could have significant practical meaning.

8. Show how efficiency or economy can have an impact an exercise performance.

9. Describe the impact of genetics on aerobic metabolism during exercise.

For further review and additional study tools, go to The Physiology Place (www.physiologyplace.com) and the Student Study Guide for Exercise Physiology for Health, Fitness, and Performance *by Sharon A. Plowman and Denise L. Smith.*

Passport to the Internet

Visit the following Internet site to explore further topics and issues related to aerobic metabolism. To visit an organization's web site, go to www.physiology place.com and click on "Passport to the Internet."

The Nicholas Institute of Sports Medicine and Athletic Trauma (NISMAT) The Nicholas Institute of Sports Medicine and Athletic Trauma (NISMAT) is the first hospital-based facility dedicated to the study of sports medicine in the country. Conduct a search for "Aerobic Metabolism," and review the online literature on this subject. In particular, take a look at the "Maximal Oxygen Consumption Primer."

References

Adams, W. C., M. M. McHenry, & E. M. Bernauer: Multistage treadmill walking performance and associated cardiorespiratory responses of middle-aged men. *Clinical Science.* 42:355–370 (1972).

American College of Sports Medicine: *Guidelines for Exercise Testing and Prescription* (6th edition). Baltimore: Williams & Wilkins (2000).

Asmussen, E.: Similarities and dissimilarities between static and dynamic exercise. *Circulation Research* (Suppl. I). 48(6):I-3–I-10 (1981).

Åstrand, P.-O.: *Experimental Studies of Physical Working Capacity in Relation to Sex and Age.* Copenhagen: Munksgaard (1952).

Åstrand, P.-O.: Human physical fitness with special reference to sex and age. *Physiological Reviews.* 36(3):307–335 (1956).

Åstrand, P. O.: Principles of ergometry and their implications in sport practice. *International Journal of Sports Medicine.* 5:102–105 (1984).

Åstrand, P.-O., & K. Rodahl: *Textbook of Work Physiology: Physiological Bases of Exercise.* New York: McGraw-Hill (1977).

Bal, M. E., E. M. Thompson, E. M. McIntosh, C. M. Taylor, & C. MacLeod: Mechanical efficiency in cycling of girls six to fourteen years of age. *Journal of Applied Physiology.* 6:185–188 (1953).

Bar-Or, O.: *Pediatric Sports Medicine for the Practitioner: From Physiological Principles to Clinical Applications.* New York: Springer-Verlag, 1–65 (1983).

Bar-Or, O.: The Wingate Anaerobic Test: An update on methodology, reliability and validity. *Sports Medicine.* 4:381–394 (1987).

Bhambhani, Y., & M. Singh: Metabolic and cinematographic analysis of walking and running in men and women. *Medicine and Science in Sports and Exercise.* 17(1):131–137 (1985).

Bird, J.: The contribution of selected physiological variables to 10 kilometer run time in trained, heterogeneous adult male runners. Unpublished master's thesis, Northern Illinois University, DeKalb, IL, 31 (1991).

Bouchard, C.: Genetics of aerobic power and capacity. In R. M. Malina & C. Bouchard (eds.), *Sports and Human Genetics.* Champaign, IL: Human Kinetics, 59–88 (1986).

Bouchard, C., & B. Lortie: Heredity and endurance performance. *Sports Medicine.* 1(1):38–64 (1984).

Bouchard, C., A. Tremblay, A. Nadeau, J. P. Despres, G. Thériault, M. R. Boulay, G. Lortie, C. Leblanc, & G. Fournier: Genetic effect in resting and exercise metabolic rates. *Metabolism.* 38(4):364–370 (1989).

Bransford, D. R., & E. T. Howley: Oxygen costs of running in trained and untrained men and women. *Medicine and Science in Sports.* 9(1):41–44 (1977).

Bray, M. S., J. R. Morrow, J. M. Pivarnik, & J. T. Bricker: Caltrac validity for estimating caloric expenditure with children. *Pediatric Exercise Science.* 4:166–179 (1992).

Bunc, V., & J. Heller: Energy cost of running in similarly trained men and women. *European Journal of Applied Physiology.* 59:178–183 (1989).

Burkett, L. N., B. Fernhall, & S. C. Walter: Physiological effects of distance run training on teenage females. *Research Quarterly for Exercise and Sport.* 56(3):215–220 (1985).

Bursztein, S., D. H. Elwyn, J. Askanazi, & J. M. Kinney: *Energy Metabolism, Indirect Calorimetry and Nutrition.* Baltimore: Williams & Wilkins (1989).

Butts, N. K., C. Dodge, & M. McAlpine: Effect of stepping rate on energy costs during StairMaster exercise. *Medicine and Science in Sports and Exercise.* 25(3):378–382 (1993).

Bye, P. T. P., G. A. Farkas, & C. Roussos: Respiratory factors limiting exercise. *Annual Review of Physiology.* 45:439–451 (1983).

Carpenter, T. M.: *Tables, Factors, and Formulas for Computing Respiratory Exchange and Biological Transformations of Energy* (4th edition). Washington, D.C.: Carnegie Institution of Washington, Publication 303C (1964).

Cavanagh, P. R., & R. Kram: Mechanical and muscular factors affecting the efficiency of human movement. *Medicine and Science in Sports and Exercise.* 17(3):326–331 (1985).

Conley, D. L., & G. S. Krahenbuhl: Running economy and distance running performance of highly trained athletes. *Medicine and Science in Sports and Exercise.* 12(5):357–360 (1980).

Consolazio, C. F., R. E. Johnson, & L. J. Pecora: *Physiological Measurements of Metabolic Functions in Man.* New York: McGraw-Hill (1963).

Costill, D. L.: *Inside Running: Basics of Sport Physiology.* Indianapolis: Benchmark Press (1986).

Costill, D. L., H. Thomason, & E. Roberts: Fractional utilization of the aerobic capacity during distance running. *Medicine and Science in Sports.* 5(4):248–252 (1973).

Cunningham, L. N.: Relationship of running economy, ventilatory threshold, and maximal oxygen consumption to running performance in high school females. *Research Quarterly for Exercise and Sport.* 61(4):369–374 (1990).

Daniels, J. T.: A physiologist's view of running economy. *Medicine and Science in Sports and Exercise.* 17(3):332–338 (1985).

Daniels, J., & N. Oldridge: Changes in oxygen consumption of young boys during growth and running training. *Medicine and Science in Sports.* 3(4):161–165 (1971).

Daniels, J., N. Oldridge, F. Nagle, & B. White: Differences and changes in $\dot{V}O_2$ among young runners 10 to 18 years of age. *Medicine and Science in Sports and Exercise.* 10(3):200–203 (1978).

Davies, C. T. M.: Effects of wind assistance and resistance on the forward motion of a runner. *Journal of Applied Physiology: Respiratory, Environmental and Exercise Physiology.* 48(4):702–709 (1980).

Donavan, C. M., & G. A. Brooks: I. Muscular efficiency during steady-rate exercise. II. Effects of walking speed and work rate. *Journal of Applied Physiology: Respiratory, Environmental and Exercise Physiology.* 43(3):431–439 (1977).

Durstine, J. L., & R. R. Pate: Cardiorespiratory responses to acute exercise. In S. N. Blair, P. Palmer, R. R. Pate, L. K. Smith, & C. B. Taylor (eds.). *Resource Manual for Guidelines for Exercise Testing and Prescription.* Philadelphia: Lea & Febiger, 38–54 (1988).

Fleck, S. J., & W. J. Kraemer: *Designing Resistance Training Programs.* Champaign, IL: Human Kinetics (1987).

Fox, E. L., & D. K. Mathews: *Interval Training: Conditioning for Sports and General Fitness.* Philadelphia: Saunders (1974).

Gaesser, G. A., & G. A. Brooks: Muscular efficiency during steady-rate exercise: Effects of speed and work rate. *Journal of Applied Physiology.* 38(6):1132–1139 (1975).

Girandola, R. N., R. A. Wiswell, F. Frisch, & K. Wood: Metabolic differences during exercise in pre- and post-pubescent girls. *Medicine and Science in Sports and Exercise* (abstract). 13(2):110 (1981).

Hagberg, J. M., J. P. Mullin, M. D. Giese, & E. Spitznagel: Effect of pedaling rate on submaximal exercise responses of competitive cyclists. *Journal of Applied Physiology: Respiratory, Environmental and Exercise Physiology.* 51(2):447–451 (1981).

Haskell, W. L., M. C. Yee, A. Evans, & P. J. Irby: Simultaneous measurement of heart rate and body motion to quantitate physical activity. *Medicine and Science in Sports and Exercise.* 25(1):109–115 (1993).

Haymes, E. M., & W. C. Byrnes: Walking and running energy expenditure estimated by Caltrac and indirect calorimetry. *Medicine and Science in Sports and Exercise.* 25(12): 1365–1369 (1993).

Heselton, R., S. A. Plowman, N. S. Hannibal, L. Schuler, K. Jensen, & K. Harkness: The reliability and validity of the caloric expenditure values from an elliptical striding system. *Medicine and Science in Sports and Exercise.* Abstract 32(5) Supplement: S301 (2000).

Holly, R. G.: Measurement of the maximal rate of oxygen uptake. In S. N. Blair, P. Palmer, R. R. Pate, L. K. Smith, & C. B. Taylor (eds.). *Resource Manual for Guidelines for Exercise Testing and Prescription.* Philadelphia: Lea & Febiger, 171–177 (1988).

Howley, E. T., D. R. Bassett, Jr., & H. G. Welch: Criteria for maximal oxygen uptake: Review and commentary. *Medicine and Science in Sports and Exercise.* 27(9):1292–1301 (1955).

Howley, E. T., D. L. Colacino, & T. C. Swensen: Factors affecting the oxygen cost of stepping on an electronic stepping ergometer. *Medicine and Science in Sports and Exercise.* 24(9):1055–1058 (1992).

Klausen, K., B. Rasmussen, L. K. Glensgaard, & O. V. Jensen: Work efficiency of children during submaximal bicycle exercise. In R. A. Binkhorst, H. C. G. Kemper, & M. Saris (eds.), *Children and Exercise XI.* Champaign, IL: Human Kinetics, 210–217 (1985).

Krahenbuhl, G. S., D. W. Morgan, & R. P. Pangrazi: Longitudinal changes in distance-running performance of young males. *International Journal of Sports Medicine.* 10(2): 92–96 (1989).

Laporte, R. E., H. J. Montoye, & C. J. Caspersen: Assessment of physical activity in epidemiologic research: Problems and prospects. *Public Health Reports.* 100(2):131–146 (1985).

Larish, D. D., P. E. Martin, & M. Mungiole: Characteristic patterns of gait in the healthy old. *Annals of the New York Academy of Sciences.* 515:18–32 (1987).

MacDougall, J. D., H. A. Wenger, & H. J. Green (eds.): *Physiological Testing of the Elite Athlete* (first edition). Hamilton, Ontario Canadian Association of Sport Sciences: Mutual Press Limited (1982).

Maliszewski, A. F., P. S. Freedson, C. J. Ebbeling, J. Crussemeyer, & K. B. Kastango: Validity of the Caltrac accelerometer in estimating energy expenditure and activity in children and adults. *Pediatric Exercise Science.* 3(2):141–151 (1991).

Mayers, N., & B. Gutin: Physiological characteristics of elite prepubertal cross-country runners. *Medicine and Science in Sports.* 11(2):172–176 (1979).

McCormack, W. P., K. J. Cureton, T. A. Bullock, & P. G. Weyand: Metabolic determinants of 1-mile run/walk

performance in children. *Medicine and Science in Sports and Exercise.* 23(5):611–617 (1991).

Morgan, D., F. Baldini, P. Martin, & W. Kohrt: Ten km performance and predicted velocity of $\dot{V}O_2$max among well-trained male runners. *Medicine and Science in Sports and Exercise.* 21:78–83 (1989).

Morgan, D. W., P. E. Martin, & G. S. Krahenbuhl: Factors affecting running economy. *Sports Medicine.* 7:310–330 (1989).

Newsholme, E. A., & A. R. Leech: *Biochemistry for the Medical Sciences.* New York: Wiley (1983).

Otis, A. B.: The work of breathing. *Physiological Reviews.* 34:449–458 (1954).

Pambianco, G., R. R. Wing, & R. Robertson: Accuracy and reliability of the Caltrac accelerometer for estimating energy expenditure. *Medicine and Science in Sports and Exercise.* 22(6):858–862 (1990).

Pardy, R. L., S. N. A. Hussain, & P. T. Macklem: The ventilatory pump in exercise. *Clinics in Chest Medicine.* 5(1): 35–49 (1984).

Pendergast, D. R., P. E. de Prampero, A. B. Craig, D. R. Wilson, & D. W. Rennie: Quantitative analysis of the front crawl in men and women. *Journal of Applied Physiology: Respiratory, Environmental and Exercise Physiology.* 43(3): 475–479 (1977).

Péronnet, F., G. Thibault, M. Ledoux, & G. Brisson: *Performance in Endurance Events: Energy Balance, Nutrition, and Temperature Regulation in Distance Running.* London, Ontario: Spodym (1987).

Plowman, S. A., & N. Y.-S. Liu: Norm-referenced and criterion-referenced validity of the one-mile run and PACER in college age individuals. *Measurement in Physical Education and Exercise Science.* 3(2):63–84 (1999).

Pugh, L. G. C. E.: Oxygen intake in track and treadmill running with observations on the effect of air resistance. *Journal of Physiology.* 207:823–835 (1970).

Riddle, S. J., & C. E. Orringer: Measurement of oxygen consumption and cardiovascular response during exercise on the StairMaster 4000PT versus the treadmill. *Medicine and Science in Sports and Exercise.* Abstract 22(2)Supplement: S65 (1990).

Robinson, S., D. B. Dill, R. D. Robinson, S. P. Tzankoff, & J. A. Wagner: Physiological aging of champion runners. *Journal of Applied Physiology.* 41(1):46–51 (1976).

Rode, A., & R. J. Shephard: The influence of cigarette smoking upon the oxygen cost of breathing in near-maximal exercise. *Medicine and Science in Sports.* 3(2):51–55 (1971).

Rowland, T. W.: *Exercise and Children's Health.* Champaign, IL: Human Kinetics (1990).

Rowland, T. W., & G. M. Green: Physiological responses to treadmill exercise in females: Adult-child differences. *Medicine and Science in Sports and Exercise.* 20(5):474–478 (1988).

Rowland, T. W., J. A. Auchinachie, T. J. Keenan, & G. M. Green: Physiologic responses to treadmill running in adult and prepubertal males. *International Journal of Sports Medicine.* 8(4):292–297 (1987).

Rowland, T. W., J. A. Auchinachie, T. J. Keenan, & G. M. Green: Submaximal aerobic running economy and treadmill performance in prepubertal boys. *International Journal of Sports Medicine.* 9(3):201–204 (1988).

Ryan, N. D., J. R. Morrow, Jr., & J. M. Pivarnik: Reliability and validity characteristics of cardiorespiratory responses on the StairMaster 4000PT®. *Measurement in Physical Education and Exercise Science.* 2(2):115–126 (1998).

Shepard, J. T., C. G. Blomquist, A. R. Lind, J. H. Mitchell, & B. Saltin: Static (isometric) exercise: Retrospection and introspection. *Circulation Research* (Suppl. I). 48(6):I-179–I-188 (1981).

Shephard, R. J.: The oxygen cost of breathing during vigorous exercise. *Quarterly Journal of Experimental Physiology.* 51:336–350 (1966).

Sidney, K. H., & R. J. Shepard: Maximum and submaximum exercise tests in men and women in the seventh, eighth, and ninth decade of life. *Journal of Applied Physiology: Respiratory, Environmental and Exercise Physiology.* 43(2): 280–287 (1977).

Stegeman, J.: *Exercise Physiology: Physiological Bases of Work and Sport.* Chicago: Year Book Medical Publishers (1981).

Swain, D. P., N. McClain, K. Davidson, A. Moseley, & N. Reed. Energy expenditure during elliptical motion exercise and comparison to treadmill walking. Abstract. *Medicine and Science in Sports and Exercise.* 31(5) Supplement: S153 (1999).

Taylor, C. M., M. E. Bal, M. W. Lamb, & G. MacLeod: Mechanical efficiency in cycling of boys seven to fifteen years of age. *Journal of Applied Physiology,* 2:563–570 (1950).

Taylor, H. L., E. Buskirk, & A. Henschel: Maximal oxygen intake as an objective measure of cardiorespiratory performance. *Journal of Applied Physiology.* 8:73–80 (1955).

Tesch, P. A., P. Buchanan, & G. A. Dudley: An approach to counteracting long-term microgravity-induced muscle atrophy. *The Physiologist.* 33(1) Supplement: S-77–S-79 (1990).

Wells, J. G., B. Balke, & D. D. VanFossan: Lactic acid accumulation during work. A suggested standardization of work classification. *Journal of Applied Physiology.* 10(1):51–55 (1957).

Widrick, J. J., P. S. Freedson, & J. Hamill: Effect of internal work on the calculation of optimal pedaling rates. *Medicine and Science in Sports and Exercise.* 24(3):376–382 (1992).

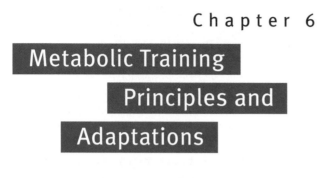

Chapter 6

Metabolic Training Principles and Adaptations

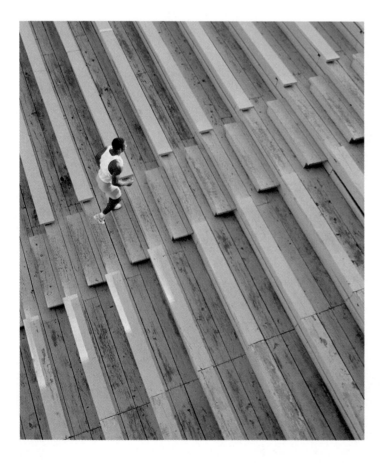

After studying the chapter, you should be able to

- Name and apply the training principles for metabolic enhancement.

- Describe and explain the metabolic adaptations that normally occur as a result of a well-designed and carefully followed training program.

- Discuss the impact of genetics on metabolic train-ability, and derive a practical application from that discussion.

Introduction

To provide a training program that meets an individual's metabolic goals it is necessary to systematically apply the training principles. The way in which these principles are applied will determine the extent to which the aerobic and/or anaerobic systems of energy production are emphasized, which, in turn, will determine the training adaptations that occur.

Application of the Training Principles for Metabolic Enhancement

A general description of the training principles was included in Chapter 1. Each training principle has a special meaning in relation to the metabolic production of energy to support exercise.

Specificity

Any training program must begin with a determination of the goal (Fox and Mathews, 1974; McCafferty and Horvath, 1977). For example, a 50-yr-old male enrolled in a fitness program who wants to break 60 min at a local 10-km race will have a very different training program from a 16-yr-old high school student competing at the 400- and 800-m distances.

Once the goal is established, it is possible to determine an estimate of the relative contributions of the major energy systems by use of a graph such as the one shown in Figure 4.2. For the 50-yr-old male just mentioned, approximately 98% of the energy for his 60-min, 10-km run is derived from the O_2 system, with the remaining 2% coming from the ATP-PC and LA systems. These percentages vary little even if an individual's time is considerably slower or even somewhat faster than 60 min. Thus, the O_2 system should be emphasized in this individual's training regimen.

The high school middle-distance runner is a different story. To plan her training program, it is necessary to know her typical times at those distances. In general, she would be expected to be in the 1:00–3:00 range for both distances. (The American National 2000 record for a high school female was 0:50.74 for the 400-m run and 2:00.07 for the 800-m run.) Events in this range stress all three energy systems with a heavier reliance on the ATP-PC and LA anaerobic systems as her performance speed increases. Because a faster time is the goal, she should emphasize and work on the anaerobic systems.

In general, only by stressing the primary energy system (or systems) used during the performance of the activity can improvement be expected. The one exception to this rule appears to be the development of an *aerobic base* through long-distance endurance work in the general preparatory phase (off-season) for athletes in just about any sport (see Figure 1.5). This base can be viewed as preparation for more intense and specific training for anaerobic sports. The most specific training for metabolic improvement should occur in the specific preparatory phase (preseason) (see Figure 1.5) (McCafferty and Horvath, 1977). Refresh your knowledge of time, distance, and energy systems by answering A Question of Understanding offered in the box below.

For those sports where time is not the measuring stick for performance (such as basketball, football, softball, tennis, and volleyball), it is important to carefully analyze the separate components of the sport and determine which energy system supports each. For example, many people don't realize (until they think about it) that the average football play lasts between 4 and 7 sec and that the total action in a 60-min game, although spread over 3 hr, may be only 12 min. Thus, football training must emphasize the ATP-PC system (the 4–7-sec range), not the O_2 system (the 60-min time). Drills or circuits can be devised that stress the energy systems determined by the sport analysis to be the most important.

Specificity also applies to the major muscle groups and exercise modality involved. Most of the biochemical training adaptations that occur do so only in the muscles that have been trained repeatedly in the way in which they will be used. Thus, the would-be triathlete who emphasizes bicycling and running in his or her program and spends little time on swimming should be more successful (in terms of individual potential) if he or she competed in duathlons instead.

Overload

Overload of the metabolic systems is typically achieved in one of two ways: first, by manipulating time and distance; and second, by monitoring lactic acid levels. Maximal oxygen uptake, although a

---

A Question of Understanding

The American National records in the 1500-m metric mile for girls progress from 7:39 (under 10 yr), to 7:04 (age 11–12 yr), to 4:37.32 (age 13–14 yr), to 4:25.57 (age 15–16 yr) (Athletics Congress of the USA, 1989). How does the energy system contribution vary with these times? Explain this variation on the basis of what you know about the development of the aerobic and anaerobic systems as a child matures. Compare your answer with the answer in Appendix D.

measure of aerobic power and a means of quantifying training load, is more a cardiovascular than a metabolic variable. Factors contributing to the improvement of $\dot{V}O_2$max and the use of % $\dot{V}O_2$max reserve as an overload technique are therefore primarily discussed in the section on application of the training principles in the cardiovascular unit (see Chapter 14).

The Time or Distance Technique

The *time or distance technique* involves some version of continuous and/or interval training. As the name implies, *continuous training* occurs when an individual selects a distance or a time to be active and continues uninterrupted to the end. Typically, a steady pace is maintained throughout the duration of the activity. Thus, the runner who completes an 8-mi training run at a 7:30-min·mi^{-1} pace has done a continuous workout. Sometimes, if such a continuous steady-state aerobic training session is maintained for an extended period of time or distance, it is called a **long slow distance (LSD)** workout. If several periods of increased speed are randomly interspersed into a continuous aerobic workout, the term *fartlek* is used. Thus, a **fartlek workout,** named from the Swedish word meaning "speed play," combines the aerobic demands of a continuous run with the anaerobic demands of sporadic speed intervals. The distance, pace, and frequency of the speed intervals can vary depending on what the individual wishes to accomplish that day.

Interval training is an aerobic and/or anaerobic workout that consists of three elements: a selected work interval (usually a distance), a target time for that distance, and a predetermined recovery or relief period before the next repetition of the work interval

---

Long Slow Distance (LSD) Workout A continuous aerobic training session performed at a steady-state pace for an extended period of time or distance.

Fartlek Workout A type of training session, named from the Swedish word meaning "speed play," that combines the aerobic demands of a continuous run with the anaerobic demands of sporadic speed intervals.

Interval Training An aerobic and/or anaerobic workout that consists of three elements: a selected work interval (usually a distance), a target time for that distance, and a predetermined recovery period before the next repetition of the work interval.

(Fox and Mathews, 1974). The energy system stressed is determined on the basis of the length of time of the work interval. Thus, a work time of less than 30 sec stresses the ATP-PC system; one between 30 sec and 3 min stresses the LA system. Anything over 3–5 min emphasizes the O_2 system. The target time is based on each individual's ability at the selected distance. The length and type of recovery period employed depends on the energy system stressed; but the length is typically between 30 sec and 6 min, and the type may be rest-relief (which can include light aerobic activity and flexibility exercises) or work-relief (which means moderate aerobic activity.) Examples for an ATP-PC, LA, and O_2 interval set are presented in Table 6.1. Note that the three sets are not intended to be combined.

ATP-PC System In the ATP-PC set, the runner is doing 100-m sprints. Each repetition is to be run at 3 sec slower than her best time. A total of eight repetitions are to be completed with 0:54 of rest recovery between each repetition.

The amount of time required to restore half of the ATP-PC that has been used—that is, the half-life restoration period for ATP-PC—is approximately 30 sec, with full restoration occurring by 2 min (Fox and Mathews, 1974). Thus, this individual will restore over half her ATP-PC.

During the same recovery time myoglobin O_2 replenishment is also taking place. The amounts replenished and restored are influenced by the activity of the participant during the recovery phase, with the greatest restoration occurring with rest or light activity such as stretching and walking.

Because the ATP-PC stores recover so quickly, they can be called upon repeatedly to provide energy. Repeatedly stimulating the ATP-PC system should bring about an increase in the capacity of that system. Any major involvement of the LA system is avoided by keeping the work intervals short so that little lactate accumulation occurs.

LA System To stress the lactic acid system requires work durations of 30 sec to 3 min. In this example, the runner is asked to perform five repetitions of 400 m in 1:20, with a work-relief recovery of 2:40 between repetitions. Lactic acid is produced in excess of clearance amounts during heavy work of this duration, resulting in an accumulation of lactate in the blood. Because lactate has a half-life clearance time of 15–25 min, with full clearance taking almost an hour, it is neither practical nor beneficial to allow for even half-life clearance of lactate between repetitions.

Tolerance to lactic acid is increased by incomplete recovery periods of 1 min 30 sec to 3 min. This

Table 6.1
Examples of Time-Distance Interval Training for Runners[*]

Energy System	Competitive Distance	Best Time	Training Distance	Training Time	Repetitions	Recovery Time	Recovery Type
ATP-PC	100 m	:15	100 m	0:18	8	(1:3) 0:54	Rest
LA	1500 m	5:16	400 m	1:20[†]	5	(1:2) 2:40	Work
O$_2$	1500 m	5:16	1200 m	4:24[‡]	3	(1:1/2) 2:12	Rest

[*] This is not intended to be one workout, although the 100-m and 400-m training sets could constitute one work-out and the 1200-m repeats another. Each would then total approximately 2 miles of intervals.

[†] Based on 1–4 sec faster than average 400 m during 1500-m–1600-m race.

[‡] Based on 1–4 sec slower than average 400 m during 1500-m–1600-m race.

amount of rest allows for the replenishment of ATP-PC and myoglobin O$_2$, and it allows the high-intensity work in the next work interval to be partially supplied by the ATP-PC energy system before stressing the LA system again (Fox, et al., 1969). It is intensity (from among the three overload factors of frequency, intensity, and duration) that is most important in improving the capacity of the LA system. Work-relief recovery is typically utilized at these work times, since active recovery does speed up lactate clearance.

O$_2$ System Long work bouts, which are still only a portion of the competitive event (that is, 0.5–1-mi [800–1600 m] repeats for a 10-km runner), can be done to stress the O$_2$ system. The pace is typically close to average pace during competition and may exceed it. The smaller the proportion of the distance, the faster the pace is and the more repetitions there are. However, the intent is that the intervals be done aerobically. The example in Table 6.1 is for 1200 m. Note that the time is longer than simply triple the 400-m time and that the recovery time is proportionally very short. The 2:12 recovery allows for full ATP-PC restoration prior to the start of the next repetition. Because this pace is already relatively low intensity work, a rest or walking recovery is best.

The distance for an interval workout (excluding warm-up and cool-down) should rarely exceed 2–5 mi (3.2–8 km) with a frequency of 1–3 days per week (Costill, 1986). High-intensity interval training taxes the muscles and joints and care must be taken to avoid injury or overtraining. Refer to Chapter 2 for a review of the signs and symptoms of overtraining, if necessary. Continuous work at lower intensities allows for greater frequency and longer durations, both of which lead to a greater volume of training. A higher training volume is particularly important to endurance athletes.

The Lactate Monitoring Technique

Assessing blood lactate concentration ([La$^-$]) is the second common technique for monitoring overload. Ideally, this technique involves the direct measurement of blood lactate levels resulting from a given workout. Currently there is no general agreement about the best way to use blood lactate values to design and monitor training programs. Nomenclature also varies greatly. Generally, however, six categories of workouts or training zones are useful (see Table 6.2). These training zones are based on the identification of the lactate thresholds (LT1 and LT2) obtained during incremental exercise. There is considerable overlap among the zones. The three lower zones (recovery, extensive aerobic, and intensive aerobic) involve predominantly low- to moderate-intensity aerobic activity, whereas each of the three higher zones (threshold, $\dot{V}O_2max$, and anaerobic) represent the transition from aerobic to anaerobic energy supply at progressively higher intensity until both aerobic and anaerobic energy production is maximized (Anderson, 1998; Bourdon, 2000).

Direct measurement of La$^-$ during training is not very practical, however, because of the necessity for special equipment and the cost of taking multiple blood samples. Several studies conducted by Weltman and his colleagues (1995) have demonstrated a reasonably stable relationship between blood lactate values and Borg's rating of perceived exertion (RPE) 6–20 scale. Borg's RPE scale was introduced in Chapter 2 and is presented and described fully in Chapter 14. The range of RPE values corresponding approximately to lactate values for each training zone are presented in Table 6.2.

A better method to individualize the use of RPE is to test the individual in a laboratory and record both RPE and lactate values at each progressive workrate. Figure 6.1 presents such results. This individual reached his LT1 at 220 m·min^{-1}. At that speed

Table 6.2

Training Zones Based on Lactate Thresholds and Values

	Recovery	Extensive Aerobic	Intensive Aerobic	Threshold	$\dot{V}O_2$max	Anaerobic
Relation to LT1 and LT2	< LT1	LT1 to halfway to LT2	> LT1 but < LT2	LT2	> LT2	Maximal
Lactate values mmol·L^{-1}	< 2.0	1.0–3.0	1.5–4.0	2.5–5.5	> 5.0	> 7.0
RPE	< 11–12	11–15	12–15	14–17	17–20	17–20
Workout example	Low-intensity aerobic; e.g., 20–30 min continuous	Long slow distance; e.g., 30 min to 2 hr continuous	Tempo runs; e.g., 10–12 sec slower than 10-km race pace	Fartlek; e.g., 1-min bursts	High-intensity intervals; e.g., 6–8 reps 0:30–3:00	Interval repetitions at maximum; e.g., 2–4 reps 0:45–1:30

Source: Based on information from Anderson (1998) and Bourdon (2000).

he reported an RPE of 12. He reached LT2 at a speed of 260 m·min^{-1} with an RPE of 14. Combining these results with the guidelines from Table 6.2, we can see that his recovery workouts should be performed at an RPE of 9–12; extensive aerobic workouts at 12 or 13; intensive aerobic at 13–14; threshold workouts at 14 and $\dot{V}O_2$max at an RPE of at least 15. The test results presented in Figure 6.1 do not represent a maximal test for this individual. Maximal workouts should

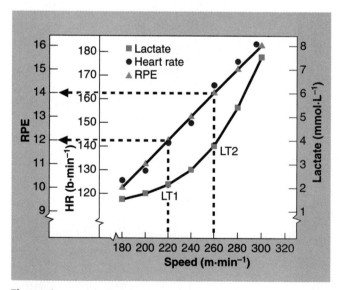

Figure 6.1

Heart Rate, Lactate, and Perceived Exertion Responses to Incremental Exercise as a Basis for Exercise Prescription

LT1 occurred at 220 m·min^{-1}, and LT2 at 260 m·min^{-1} for the individual whose data are plotted. See text for the explanation of how these points are used to prepare an exercise prescription.

elicit an RPE of at least 17 for everyone. Thus, the individual can be given a workout and an RPE value and adjust his or her intensity accordingly. Another alternative method, if an individual has access to laboratory testing facilities, is to determine the relationship between [La$^-$] and HR values. Then HR can be used to estimate the [La$^-$] level during training sessions and the intensity modified accordingly (Dwyer and Bybee, 1983; Gilman and Wells, 1993).

In our example, now reading the rectilinear plot as heart rate, the individual would perform recovery activity between approximately 110 and 140 b·min^{-1}; extensive aerobic exercise bouts between 110 and 155 b·min^{-1}; intensive aerobic exercise between 120 and 165 b·min^{-1}; threshold workouts between 157 and 173 b·min^{-1}; $\dot{V}O_2$max workouts close to 170 b·min^{-1}; and maximal activity at least at 185 b·min^{-1}.

Heart rate primarily reflects the functioning of the cardiovascular system, but lactate levels reflect the metabolic energy system. Fox, Bowers, and Foss (1988) estimate that if the HR-[La$^-$] relationship is not individually determined to ensure that 100% of the individuals are working at or above their "anaerobic threshold," heart rate would have to be greater than 90% of the maximal heart rate or equal to or greater than 85% of the heart rate reserve. Experimental data reported by Weltman (1995) confirm that techniques for exercise prescription involving percentages of heart rate maximum or heart rate reserve do not reflect specific blood lactate concentrations.

Whichever system is used to prescribe an individual's training session, it is important to provide a mixture of workout types to maximize the possibility for improvement and prevent boredom.

Rest/Recovery/Adaptation

Adaptation is evident when a given distance or workload can be covered in a faster time with an equal or lower perception of fatigue or exertion and/or in the same time span with less physiological disruption (lower [La⁻] values) and faster recovery. The key to adaption for energy production in muscles appears to be allowing for sufficient recovery time between hard-intensity workouts. Cyclic training programs that alternately stress the desired specific energy system (hard day) and allow it to recover (easy day) induce optimal adaptation (McCafferty and Horvath, 1977; Weltman, et al., 1978). Too many successive hard days working the same muscles and same energy system can lead to a lack of adaptation because of overtraining, and too many successive easy days can lead to a lack of adaptation because of undertraining.

Progression

Once adaptation occurs, the workload should be progressed if further improvement is desired. Progression can be done by increasing the distance or workload, decreasing the time, increasing the number of repetitions or sessions, decreasing the length of the relief interval, or changing the frequency of the various types of workouts per week. The key to successful progression is an increase in intensity and total training volume. The progression should be gradual. A general rule of thumb is that the increment in **training volume**—which is the total amount of work done, usually expressed as mileage or load—should not exceed more than 10% per week. For example, if an individual is currently cycling 60 mi per week, the distance should not be increased by more than 6 mi the following week. Steploading, as described in Chapter 1, should be used.

Often in fitness work the challenge is to prevent an individual from doing too much too soon. The 50-yr-old man remembers when he was a high school star athlete and wants to regain that feeling and physique *now*! The fitness leader must gently be more realistic and err, if at all, on the side of caution in exercise prescription and progression.

The limit of metabolic adaptation appears to be achieved in approximately 10 days to 3 weeks if training is not progressed (Hickson, et al., 1981). The ultimate limit may be set by genetics.

> **Training Volume** The total amount of work done, usually expressed as mileage or load.

Individualization

The first step in individualizing training is, as mentioned earlier, to match the sport, event, or fitness goal of the participant with the specific mix of energy system demands. The second step is to evaluate each individual. The third step is to develop a periodization sequence for general preparation, specific preparation, competitive, and transition phases. The fourth step is to develop a format, that is, the number of days devoted per week for each type of training or energy system stressed. The fifth step is to determine the training load (distance, workload, repetitions, or the like) on the basis of the individual's evaluation and modified by how he or she responds and adapts to the program. Interpreting and adjusting to an individual's response is the art of being a coach or fitness leader.

Maintenance

Once a specific level of endurance adaptation has been achieved, it appears that this level can be maintained by the same or by a reduced volume of work. However, the way that the volume is reduced is critical. If the training intensity is maintained, reductions of one-third to two-thirds in frequency and duration have been shown to maintain aerobic power ($\dot{V}O_2$max), endurance performance (at a given absolute or relative submaximal workload), and lactate accumulation levels at submaximal loads. This maintenance may last for at least several months. One day per week may be sufficient for short periods of time (say during a one-week vacation) if intensity is maintained (Chaloupka and Fox, 1975; Neufer, 1989; Weltman, 1995). Conversely, a reduction in intensity brings about a reduction in training adaptation.

It also seems to be important that the mode of exercise is consistent or closely simulated, because, as mentioned previously, many of the training adaptations that occur are specific to the muscles involved. Thus, *cross training*—the utilization of different modalities to reduce localized stress but increase overall training volume—is likely to be more beneficial for the cardiovascular system than for the metabolic system.

The level of maintenance training necessary for the anaerobic energy systems to operate at maximal levels is unknown. However, sprint performances deteriorate less quickly in response to a decrease in training than do endurance performances (Wilmore and Costill, 1988).

Many fitness participants are primarily in a maintenance mode after the initial several months or first year of participation. The appropriate level for maintenance should be determined by individual goals.

Maintenance should occur primarily during the competitive training cycle of an athlete.

A special kind of maintenance called tapering is often used by athletes in individual sports such as swimming, cycling, and running. A **training taper** is a reduction in training volume prior to important competitions that is intended to allow the athlete to recover from previous hard training, maintain physiological conditioning, and improve performance. Athletes often fear that if they taper for more than just a few days, their competitive fitness and performance will suffer. However, studies consistently show that if intensity is maintained while training volume is reduced, physiological adaptations are retained and performance is either equaled or improved after a taper of 7 to 21 days (Costill, et al., 1985; Houmard, et al., 1990; Johns, et al., 1992; Shepley, et al., 1992).

The one group of individuals who probably do not respond to these maintenance and taper guidelines with joy are those who are injured. Maintaining a high level of intensity in the training modality is one of the most difficult tasks for an injured individual. Research continues in an attempt to solve this problem, such as trying to determine whether work in the water can be substituted for land-based work. In the meantime, the injured individual who cannot continue to train at his or her preinjury level should probably accept the fact that he or she will experience a loss of adaptation.

Retrogression/Plateau/Reversibility

The training principle of retrogression, plateau, and reversibility is not one that a coach or fitness leader applies as much as anticipates and reacts to. At one or more points in the process of training, an individual will fail to improve with progression and will either stay at the same level (*plateau*) or show a performance or physiological decrement (*retrogression*). When a pattern of nonimprovement occurs, it is important to check for other signs of overtraining. A shift in training emphasis or the inclusion of more easy days may be warranted. Remember that a reduction in training does not necessarily lead to detraining. Of course, not all plateaus can be explained as overtraining; sometimes there is no explanation.

If an individual ceases training completely, for whatever reason, detraining will occur. This *reversibility* of training adaptations in skeletal and

> **Training Taper** A reduction in training prior to important competitions that is intended to allow the athlete to recover from previous hard training, maintain physiological conditioning, and improve performance.

metabolic potential occurs within days to weeks after training ceases. A reduction in both maximal and submaximal performance ultimately follows. It should come as no surprise that those metabolic factors that show the greatest improvement with training—that is, those involved with aerobic energy production (see training adaptations later in this chapter)—also show the greatest reversal. Within 3 to 6 weeks after the cessation of activity, pretraining levels are typically reached again, especially if the training program was of short duration. Individuals with a long and established training history, however, tend to show an initial rapid decline in some aerobic variables but then level off at higher-than-pretraining levels. Anaerobic metabolic variables show less incremental increase with training and less loss with detraining. This fact may explain why sprint performance is more resistant to inactivity than endurance performance. Complete bed rest or immobilization accelerates detraining (Coyle, et al., 1984; Neufer, 1989; Ready and Quinney, 1982; Wilmore and Costill, 1988).

Retraining does not occur as rapidly as detraining and is not easier or more rapid than initial training (Wilmore and Costill, 1988). Although direct experimental evidence is scanty, the consequences of detraining and retraining appear to be similar for adults, children, and adolescents (Bar-Or, 1983).

Warm-Up and Cool-Down

The information about warm-up is sparse in relation to the effects on metabolic function, but several generalizations seem to be warranted. An elevated body temperature—and more specifically, an elevated muscle temperature—increases the rate at which the metabolic processes in the cells can proceed. This rate increase occurs in large part because enzyme activity is temperature-dependent, exhibiting a steady rise from 0°C to approximately 40°C before plateauing and ultimately declining. At the same time, oxygen is more readily released from red blood cells and transported into the mitochondria at elevated temperatures (Van de Graaff and Fox, 1989). One consequence of increased body temperature is a decreased oxygen deficit at the initiation of exercise (Gutin et al., 1976). Another consequence is a greater availability of oxygen to the muscles during work. When more oxygen is available sooner, less reliance is placed on anaerobic metabolism, and less lactate accumulates at any given heavy workload. At lighter endurance workloads a greater utilization of fats for the production of energy is possible earlier in the activity. This early use of fats serves to spare carbohydrate and extend the time a given high-intensity effort can be continued. These beneficial metabolic effects of a warm-up appear to exist for children and adolescents as well as adults (Bar-Or, 1983).

In devising a warm-up to achieve these metabolic benefits, several considerations need to be taken into account (Franks, 1983).

1. The activity should involve large muscle groups that will elevate the body temperature from 37° to 38° or 39°C. This temperature elevation generally occurs simultaneously with the onset of sweating.

2. The activity should last approximately 5–20 min and end no longer than 15 min before the hard phase of the workout or competitive performance. The harder the planned workout, the longer the warm-up phase should be. The less time elapsing between the warm-up and the performance, the better it is for an athlete.

3. The intensity of the warm-up should be such that it does not fatigue the participant. Highly fit individuals can utilize longer, more intense warm-ups than low fit individuals. Generally speaking, the warm-up for endurance activities can occur at a lower intensity (25–30% $\dot{V}O_2$max or less than 35% HRmax) than for sprinting or anaerobic activities (45–50% $\dot{V}O_2$max or 50–60% HRmax). Higher values in the range of 60–80% $\dot{V}O_2$max (70–85% HRmax) may be needed by highly conditioned athletes to elevate core temperature. In any case, it is probably best to stay below the lactate threshold.

4. The warm-up may be built into an endurance workout if the participant begins at a low intensity and progresses nonstop into higher levels of work.

5. Identical warm-ups of explosive tasks (such as long or high jumping) at full speed should be used sparingly. The action can be patterned at lower levels.

6. An intermittent or interval type warm-up has been found to be more beneficial for children than a continuous warm-up (Bar-Or, 1983).

The primary metabolic value of a cool-down lies in the fact that lactate is dissipated faster during an active recovery. As described in Chapter 4, the lactate removal rate is maximized if the cool-down activity is of moderate intensity (a little higher than the individual tends to self-select) and continues for approximately 20 min.

In general, all of the training principles appear to apply to both sexes and, except where noted, to all ages. At the very least, there is insufficient evidence for modifying any of the general concepts on the basis of age or sex, although individual differences should always be kept in mind.

Metabolic Adaptations to Exercise Training

When the training principles just discussed are systematically applied and rigorously followed, a number of adaptations occur relative to the production and utilization of energy. The extent to which the adaptations occur depends on the initial fitness level of the individual and his or her genetic potential. Figure 6.2 is an expanded version of Figure 3.4 showing the metabolic pathways you studied earlier. Numbers have been inserted following the naming of some factors to indicate sites where these adaptations occur. The following discussion will follow that numerical sequence. Refer to Figure 6.2 as you read.

Substrate or Fuel Supply

Regulatory Hormones

Primary among the metabolic adaptations to a training program are changes that occur in the hormones responsible for the regulation of metabolism (see Chapters 2 and 3, Figure 3.16, and Table 3.3). Although little is known about the impact of training on the hypothalamic-releasing factors and adrenocorticotrophic hormone (ACTH), a definite pattern is seen for the five hormones directly involved in carbohydrate, fat, and protein substrate regulation. That pattern is one of a blunted response in which the amount of hormone secreted during submaximal activity is reduced. This pattern occurs whether the load is absolute or relative and in both the fast-responding and slow-responding hormones. Thus, the rise in glucagon is lower and the suppression of insulin less; the rise in norepinephrine and epinephrine is less; the rise in growth hormone is less; and the rise in cortisol is less during submaximal exercise in trained individuals than in untrained individuals (Galbo, 1983). Because of these smaller disruptions at submaximal levels, more work can be done before maximum is reached.

Carbohydrate (1)

The rate-limiting step for glucose utilization in muscles is glucose transport, and glucose transport is primarily a function of GLUT-4 transporters. Exercise training increases GLUT-4 number and concentration in skeletal muscle (Sato, et al., 1996). This results in a greater uptake of glucose under the influence of insulin. Thus, at any resting insulin level, whole body glucose clearance is enhanced. This occurs in both young and elderly healthy individuals as well as in individuals with non–insulin-dependent diabetes (Dela, 1996). Despite this increase in the number of

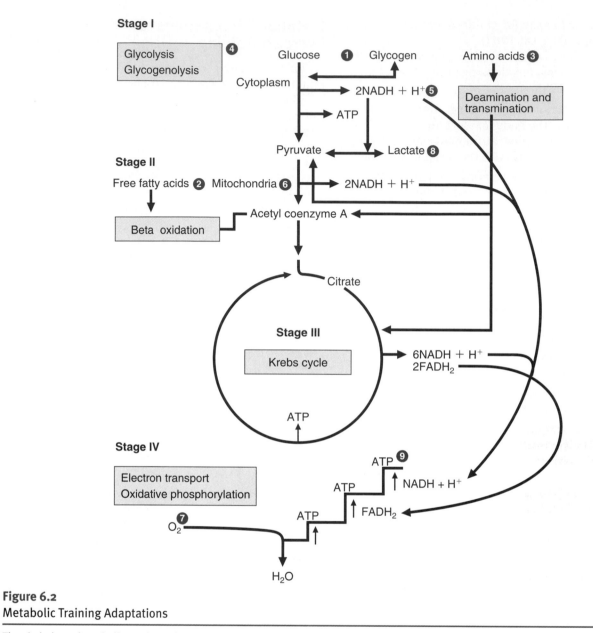

Figure 6.2
Metabolic Training Adaptations

The circled numbers indicate sites where training changes occur. The boxes indicate processes.

GLUT-4 transporters, endurance exercise training reduces glucose utilization during both absolute and relative, moderate-intensity submaximal exercise. The precise mechanisms for this apparent paradox are unknown at this point in time (Coggan, 1996).

Both endurance and sprint training bring about an increase of muscle and liver glycogen reserves. In addition, at the same absolute submaximal workload (that is, the same rate of oxygen consumption) muscle and liver glycogen depletion occurs at a slower rate in the trained individual than in the untrained individual (Abernethy, et al., 1990; Gollnick, et al., 1973; Holloszy, 1973; Holloszy and Coyle, 1984;

Karlsson, et al., 1972). Thus, the trained individual uses less total carbohydrate in his or her fuel mixture. These changes are seen in lower RER values (Figure 6.3a on page 165). Because glycogen is the primary source of fuel for high-intensity work, a larger supply of glycogen used less quickly enables an individual to participate in fairly intense activities at submaximal levels for longer periods of time before fatigue occurs. On the other hand, sprint training can also increase the rate of glycogenolysis at higher levels of work, giving the exerciser a fast supply of energy when needed for short bursts of maximal or supramaximal activity.

Fat (2)

The trained individual is able to use his or her carbohydrate stores more slowly than the untrained individual because of the changes that occur in fat metabolism. Both trained and untrained individuals have more than adequate stores of fat. However, the rate of free fatty acid oxidation is determined not by the storage amount but by the concentration of free fatty acids in the bloodstream and the capacity of the tissues to oxidize the fat. Training brings about several adaptations in fat metabolism, including the following:

1. an increased mobilization or release of free fatty acids from the adipose tissue;

2. an increased level of plasma free fatty acids during submaximal exercise;

3. an increase in fat storage adjacent to the mitochondria within the muscles; and

4. an increased capacity to utilize fat at any given plasma concentration.

The increased reliance on fat as a fuel is said to have a *glycogen-sparing effect* and is responsible for lowered RER values (Figure 6.3a) at the same absolute and same relative (% $\dot{V}O_2$max) work intensities. Because glycogen supplies last longer, there is a delay in fatigue and greater endurance at submaximal work levels. Both endurance and sprint training have glycogen-sparing effects (Abernethy, et al., 1990; Gollnick, et al., 1973; Holloszy, 1973; Holloszy and Coyle, 1984).

Protein (3)

Despite the fact that proteins are the least important energy substrate, changes do occur as a result of endurance training, which enhance their role. Adaptations in protein metabolism include an increased ability to utilize the branched chain amino acid leucine and an increased capacity to form alanine and release it from muscle cells. This increased production of alanine is accompanied by decreased levels in the plasma, probably indicating an accelerated removal for gluconeogenesis. In ultraendurance events, this increased gluconeogenesis effect would be beneficial in maintaining blood glucose levels (Abernethy, et al., 1990; Holloszy and Coyle, 1984; Hood and Terjung, 1990).

Enzyme Activity

The key to increasing the production of ATP is enzyme activity. Since every step in each metabolic pathway is catalyzed by a separate enzyme, the potential for this training adaptation to influence energy production is great. However, it appears that not all enzymes respond to the same training stimulus nor change to the same extent.

Glycolytic Enzymes (4)

The results of studies investigating the activity of the glycolytic enzymes have been contradictory, with most showing little (if any) change but some showing increased activity. Glycolysis is involved in both the aerobic and anaerobic production of energy, and it may be that high-intensity training is required for some glycolytic enzymes to adapt but that others respond better to endurance training. Three key enzymes have shown significant training changes: glycogen phosphorylase, phosphofructokinase, and lactic dehydrogenase.

Glycogen Phosphorylase   Glycogen phosphorylase catalyzes the breakdown of glycogen stored in the muscle cells so that it may be used as fuel in glycolysis. An increase in this enzyme's activity has been found with high-intensity sprint training. The ability to break down glycogen quickly is important in near-maximal, maximal, and supramaximal exercise.

Phosphofructokinase (PFK)   PFK is the main rate-limiting enzyme of glycolysis. Results from both endurance and sprint training studies are inconsistent but tend to suggest an increase in activity with adequate levels of training. Increased PFK activity leads to a faster and greater quantity of ATP being produced glycolytically.

Lactic Dehydrogenase (LDH)   LDH catalyzes the conversion of pyruvate into lactate. It exists in several discrete forms, including a cardiac muscle form that has a low affinity for pyruvate (thus making the formation of lactate less likely) and a skeletal muscle form that has a high affinity for pyruvate (thus making the formation of lactic acid more likely). Endurance training tends to have two effects on LDH. It lowers the overall activity of LDH, and it causes a shift from the skeletal muscle to the cardiac muscle form. Thus, lactate is less likely to be produced in skeletal muscle, and pyruvate is more likely to enter the mitochondria for use as an aerobic fuel. Both of these changes are beneficial to endurance performance (Abernethy, et al., 1990; Gollnick and Hermansen, 1973; Holloszy and Coyle, 1984; Sjödin, et al., 1982).

Shuttles (5)

You will recall that the hydrogen ions removed in glycolysis must be transported across the mitochondrial membrane by a shuttle since that membrane is impermeable to NADH + H$^+$. No training changes have been found to occur in the glycerol-phosphate shuttle enzymes that predominate in skeletal muscle. Conversely, large increases in the enzymes of the cardiac muscle's malate-aspartate shuttle both in the cytoplasm and mitochondria have been found, thus increasing shuttle activity. This increase enhances aerobic metabolism in the heart (Holloszy and Coyle, 1984).

Mitochondrial Enzymes (6)

Changes in the mitochondrial enzymes of the Krebs cycle, electron transport, and oxidative phosphorylation are coupled with changes in the mitochondria themselves. Both the size and the number of the mitochondria increase with training. Thus, mitochondria occupy a proportionally larger share of the muscle fiber space. The sarcolemmal mitochondria are affected to a greater degree than the interfibrillar mitochondria. The stimulus for these increases appears to be contractile activity itself, rather than any external stimulus such as hormonal changes, since only those muscles directly involved in the exercise training show these changes. For example, a runner would exhibit an increase in mitochondrial size and number only in the legs, whereas a cross-country skier would show mitochondrial increases in both arms and legs.

Within limits, the extent of the augmentation in the mitochondria seems to be a function of the total amount of contractile activity. That is, the more contractions there are, the greater is the change in the mitochondria. It does not seem to matter whether the increase in contractile activity is achieved by completing more contractions per unit of time (speed work) or by keeping the rate of contractions steady but increasing the duration (endurance training). Resistance training does not appear to enhance mitochondria.

With larger mitochondria more transport sites are available for the movement of pyruvate into the mitochondria. The enzymatic activity per unit of mitochondria appears to be the same for trained and untrained individuals; however, the greater mitochondrial protein content means an overall greater enzyme activity to utilize the pyruvate. Interestingly, although most mitochondrial enzymes increase in activity, not all do; nor is the rate of change the same for all. The overall effect of the increased enzyme activity

and the increased availability of pyruvate is an enhanced capacity to generate ATP by oxidative phosphorylation. This augmented capacity is more important in supplying energy for submaximal exercise than for maximal exercise (Abernethy, et al., 1990; Gollnick, et al., 1986; Holloszy, 1973; Holloszy and Coyle, 1984).

Oxygen Utilization (7)

Maximal Oxygen Uptake

Maximal oxygen uptake ($\dot{V}O_2$max) increases with training (Figure 6.3b). Even though this is a measure of the amount of oxygen utilized at the muscle level, $\dot{V}O_2$max is determined more by the cardiovascular system's ability to deliver oxygen than by the muscle's ability to use it. Evidence for the subsidiary role of muscle in determining $\dot{V}O_2$max includes the fact that individuals can have essentially the same mitochondrial content but very different $\dot{V}O_2$max values. Conversely, individuals with equivalent $\dot{V}O_2$max values can have quite different mitochondrial enzyme levels. Additionally, small training changes can occur in one (mitochondrial activity or $\dot{V}O_2$max) without concomitant changes in the other—although, typically, both will increase. These differences probably explain why some runners are more economical (use less oxygen at a given pace than others do) and others possess a greater aerobic power (have a higher $\dot{V}O_2$max) (Holloszy and Coyle, 1984).

Submaximal Oxygen Cost

The oxygen cost ($\dot{V}O_2$ in mL·min^{-1} or mL·kg^{-1}·min^{-1}) of any given absolute submaximal workload is the same before and after training, assuming that no skill is involved where efficiency would change (Gollnick, et al., 1986; Holloszy and Coyle, 1984) (Figure 6.3b). For example, if an individual has a smooth, coordinated front crawl stroke but has not participated in lap swimming, the oxygen cost of covering any given distance at a set pace will remain the same as this person trains. However, for an individual who is just learning the front crawl stroke, the oxygen cost would actually go down. It would decrease not because of a change in the exercise oxygen requirements but because extraneous inefficient movements that add to the oxygen cost are eliminated as skill is improved (Daniels, et al., 1978; Ekblom, 1968; Gardner, et al., 1989).

Running economy depends both on the energy needed to move at a particular speed (*external energy*) and on the energy used to produce that energy (*internal energy*). Specifically, internal energy is associated with oxygen delivery (ventilation and heart rate in particular), thermoregulation, and substrate metabolism (remember that it takes more oxygen to utilize fat as a fuel than to burn carbohydrate). Theoretically, internal energy demand can be lowered by decreasing ventilation and heart rate costs and by increasing the percentage of carbohydrate. The first two changes do typically occur with training, but the last one does not. Indeed, the trained individual utilizes a higher percentage of fat at any given submaximal load than does an untrained individual. The primary possibility for improving external energy demand is stride length. However, studies have shown that experienced runners freely select the optimal stride length, so additional improvements in training status do little to change stride length. High-intensity interval training has produced improvements in running economy, but the evidence is not strong (Bailey and Pak, 1991; Conley, et al., 1981; Sjödin, et al., 1982). Decreased efficiency or economy, on the other hand, can occur. If so, it should be interpreted as a symptom of overtraining (Fry, et al., 1991).

If an individual increases his or her $\dot{V}O_2$max yet the oxygen cost of any given (absolute) workload remains the same, then the % $\dot{V}O_2$max at which that individual is doing the given workload will go down. The task will be relatively easier for the individual, and endurance performance will be greatly enhanced. This improvement is a consequence of the biochemical adaptations in the muscle rather than changes in oxygen delivery.

The myoglobin concentration in muscles increases with endurance training in the muscles directly involved in the activity. As a consequence, the rate of oxygen diffusion through the cytoplasm into the mitochondria increases, making more oxygen available quickly.

Oxygen Deficit and Drift

The oxygen deficit at the onset of activity is smaller, but is not eliminated, in a trained individual. The primary reason for this reduction is that oxidative phosphorylation is activated sooner owing to the increased number of mitochondria that are sensitive to low levels of ADP and P_i. This result is advantageous to the exerciser, because less lactic acid will be produced and less creatine phosphate will be depleted (Holloszy, 1973; Holloszy and Coyle, 1984).

The magnitude of oxygen drift will also be less after training. This change may be caused by concomitant reductions in epinephrine, norepinephrine, lactate, and body temperature rise during any given submaximal workload (Casaburi, et al., 1987; Hagberg, et al., 1978).

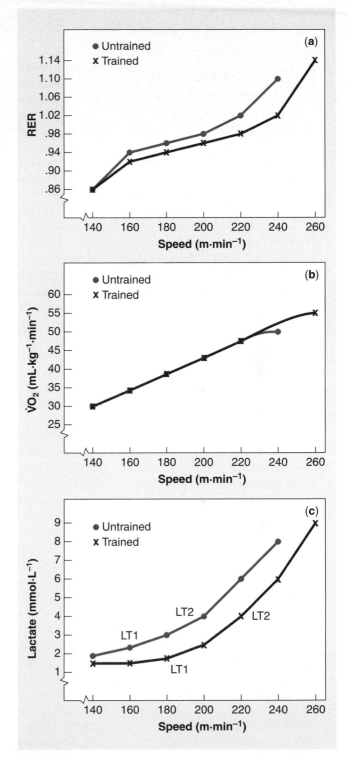

Figure 6.3

Metabolic Responses of Endurance Trained versus Untrained Individuals to Incremental Exercise to Maximum

Focus on Application

✳ Oxygen Free Radicals, Exercise Intensity, and Exercise Training Adaptations

Cancer, atherosclerosis, cataracts, Alzheimer's disease, diabetes, loss of memory, and aging may all, in part, be caused by free radical damage (Keith, 1999). What are free radicals? How can they cause so many different problems? What is the link between oxygen free radicals, exercise, and exercise training adaptations?

Under normal conditions, electrons orbiting in the shells of a molecule are in pairs. If a single electron is added or removed, instability is created. The resultant structure is called a free radical. Free radicals have a drive to return to a balanced stable state and attempt to do so by either taking an electron from, giving an electron to, or sharing an electron with another atom. Often a chain reaction is set up that results in damage (oxidative stress) to lipids (especially the lipid bilayer of cell membranes), proteins (in enzymes, immune cells, joints, and muscles), and DNA (breaking stands or shifting bases, thus influencing the genetic code). These are the changes that ultimately can lead to the disease conditions listed earlier (Alessio and Blasi, 1997; Jenkins, 1993; Keith, 1999).

Free radicals can be produced from sources that originate outside the body, such as x-rays, UV rays from sunlight, air pollutants (ozone, nitric oxide from car exhaust),

cigarette smoke, toxic chemicals (some pesticides), and physical injury (from contact sports or concussions). They may also be produced from sources that originate within the body, specifically as part of normal immune function and as a normal by-product of the production of energy (Keith, 1999).

Acute exercise is involved in several ways. During the aerobic production of ATP, single electrons leak from electron transport in Stage IV in the mitochondria. The principal location of this continuous electron leak is at coenzyme Q. The higher the rate of metabolism (as in moving from rest to submaximal to maximal exercise), the more free radicals are produced. Possibly as much as 4–5% of the oxygen consumed is converted to free radicals. Anaerobic energy production provides an abundance of hydrogen ions that can react with an oxygen free radical to form a reactive oxygen species, such as hydrogen peroxide, H_2O_2. Hypoxia leads to a freeing of metals (Fe, Cu, Mg) that are needed to catalyze free radical production. Exercise-induced hyperthermia may trigger free radical proliferation. Any damage to muscle fibers leads to increased immune response.

Despite the increased production of free radicals resulting from exercise, it is unlikely that exercise results in substantial damages to the normal healthy individual. The body has a number of natural defenses, and antioxidants ingested from food provide additional defenses. Each cell contains a variety of antioxidant

scavenger enzymes, predominantly superoxide dismutase (SOD), catalase (CAT), and glutathione peroxidase (GPX). Antioxidant vitamins, minerals, and phytochemicals include vitamin E, vitamin C, beta carotene (precursor of vitamin A), selenium, and flavonoids.

Acute exercise has been shown to selectively enhance the antioxidant enzymes. In addition, most exercise training studies have shown increased antioxidant levels following exercise, although tolerance does appear to be better following moderate-intensity rather than maximal-intensity exercise. This applies to both aerobic endurance exercise and dynamic resistance exercise. Part of the training adaptation may be due to increases in the cytochromes in electron transport, which reduces electron leakage (Alessio and Blasi, 1997).

All individuals, but especially those doing high-intensity training, should make sure that their diets contain large amounts of antioxidant-rich foods, primarily fruits and vegetables. Prunes, raisins, blueberries, strawberries, oranges, spinach, broccoli, beets, onions, corn, eggplant, nuts, and whole grains are particularly beneficial. Supplementation with 100–400 IU of vitamin E may be warranted (Jenkins, 1993; Keith, 1999).   ✳

Sources:

Alessio & Blasi (1997); Jenkins (1993); Keith (1999).

Lactate Accumulation (8)

Lactic acid is produced when the hydrogen atoms carried on $NADH + H^+$ are transferred to pyruvic acid in a reaction catalyzed by lactic dehydrogenase. Lactate accumulates when the rate of production exceeds the rate of clearance. It is a matter of some debate whether the rate of production decreases or the rate of clearance increases more as a result of training.

Factors that lead to a decrease in lactate production include

1. fuel shifts;

2. enzyme activity changes; and

3. blunted neurohomormonal responses.

Pyruvate is the end product of carbohydrate metabolism (glycolysis). Less carbohydrate is utilized at an absolute submaximal workload after training; therefore, less pyruvate is available for conversion into lactate. Pyruvate dehydrogenase activity increases, converting more pyruvate to acetyl CoA. LDH enzyme shifts from the skeletal muscle form, which favors lactic acid production, to the cardiac muscle form, which has a lower affinity for pyruvate. In addition, glycolysis is inhibited following training by several factors, two of which are related to the increased utilization of fat during submaximal exercise. The first is a high concentration of free fatty acid in the cytoplasm, and the second is a high level of citrate (the first product in the Krebs cycle). Both factors cause the rate-limiting enzyme PFK to slow down glycolysis and, hence, decrease the possible production of lactic acid. Finally, a smaller increase in the concentration of epinephrine and norepinephrine has been found at the same absolute and relative workloads in trained individuals. This decreased sympathetic stimulation may also decrease the activation of glycogenolysis and the potential production of lactic acid (Gollnick, et al., 1986; Holloszy and Coyle, 1984).

There are also several changes that lead to higher rates of clearance. These can be classified into two main factors:

1. enhanced lactate transport; and

2. enhanced lactate oxidation.

Lactate transport is enhanced by a combination of increased substrate affinity, increased intrinsic activity, and increased density of the mitochondrial membrane and cell membrane MCT1 lactate transporters. At the same time, mitochondrial size, number, and enzyme concentrations are elevated. Taken together, these enable muscle cells to increase both the extracellular and intracellular lactate shuttle mechanisms. There is an overall uptake of lactate by muscles, and, consequently, more lactate can be oxidized more rapidly during exercise. Concomitantly, blood flow to the liver is enhanced, which aids in lactate removal overall (Bonen, 2000; Brooks, 2000; Brooks, et al., 1999; Gladden, 2000; Pilegaard, et al., 1994). These adaptations mean that the change in the rate of clearance probably is more important than the change in the rate of production (Brooks, 1991; Donovan and Brooks, 1983; Mazzeo, et al., 1986). The result is a decreased concentration of lactate in the muscles and blood at the same relative workload (% $\dot{V}O_2max$) after training.

As a consequence of the change in the ratio of lactate clearance to production, a higher workload (both in absolute and relative terms) is required to achieve lactate levels in the 2- to 4-$mmol \cdot L^{-1}$ range (Figure 6.3c). This means that an individual can improve performance by exercising at a higher relative intensity for a given period of time and yet delay the onset of fatigue since the lactate thresholds (LT1 and LT2) have been raised (Allen, et al., 1985; Henritze, et al., 1985; Holloszy and Coyle, 1984; Skinner and Morgan, 1985; Williams, et al., 1967; Yoshida, et al., 1982).

At maximal aerobic/anaerobic endurance exercise, the level of lactic acid accumulation is higher as a result of training. The higher level probably results from the greater glycogen stores and increased activity of some of the glycolytic enzymes other than LDH (Abernethy, et al., 1990; Gollnick, et al., 1986). It may also be a result that is more psychological than physiological, in that the trained individual is more motivated and is better able to tolerate the pain caused by lactic acid (Galbo, 1983) and is working at a higher absolute load.

Resistance training has been shown to affect lactate response to both weight-lifting exercise and dynamic aerobic exercise. For example, after 10 weeks of strength training (3 sets of 7 exercises at 8–12 repetitions with 60–90 seconds of rest between sets, 3 days per week), college females significantly improved their squat 1-RM. When blood lactate values were compared before and after training at the same absolute load (70% and 50% of pretraining 1-RM), there was a significant reduction from 8 $mmol \cdot L^{-1}$ to 6 $mmol \cdot L^{-1}$. When the same relative load was compared (70% and 50% of pretraining 1-RM versus 70% and 50% of posttraining 1-RM), there was no significant difference in lactate levels (8 $mmol \cdot L^{-1}$ versus 7.5 $mmol \cdot L^{-1}$). These results indicate that more work could be done before the same accumulation of lactate was obtained after training than before training. Interestingly, the heart rate responses did not vary among the three testing conditions (before, after absolute loads, and after relative loads), but RPE responses paralleled the changes in blood lactate (Reynolds, et al., 1997).

Table 6.3

Estimated Maximal Power and Capacity for Untrained (UT) and Trained (TR) Males

System	Power				Capacity			
	kcal·min^{-1}		kJ·min^{-1}		kcal·min^{-1}		kJ·min^{-1}	
	UT	TR	UT	TR	UT	TR	UT	TR
Phosphagens (ATP-PC)	72	96	300	400	11	13	45	55
Anaerobic glycolysis (LA)	36	60	150	250	48	72	200	300
Aerobic glycolysis plus Krebs cycle plus ETS/OP (O$_2$)	7–19	32–37	30–80	135–155	360–1270	10,770–19,140	1500–5300	45,000–80,000

Source: Modified from Bouchard, Taylor, & Dulac (1991); Bouchard, et al. (1982).

In a 12-week study young adult males trained using a circuit of 10 exercises 3 times per session, doing 8–10 repetitions with 30 seconds of rest between exercises, 3 days per week. As anticipated, the experimental group significantly improved in both 1-RM upper and lower body strength and leg peak torque, while the controls did not. Neither group changed their treadmill $\dot{V}O_2$max nor cycle ergometer $\dot{V}O_2$peak. However, the experimental subjects cycled 33% longer at 75% $\dot{V}O_2$peak after training, and blood lactate concentrations were significantly reduced at all submaximal intensities tested. Lactate threshold (defined as an absolute value of 3.3 mmol·L^{-1}) increased by 12%. These results support the generalization that a higher intensity of endurance exercise can be accomplished before reaching the same level of blood lactate concentration, whether the training modality is dynamic aerobic endurance or dynamic resistance activity (Marcinik, et al., 1991).

ATP Production, Storage, and Turnover

ATP-PC (9)

Although exercise training increases the potential for the production of larger quantities of ATP by oxidative phosphorylation, it does not change the efficiency of converting fuel to ATP or ATP to work. Thirty-six ATP are still produced from glucose in skeletal muscle, and the potential energy per mole of ATP is still between 7 and 12 kcal (Abernethy, et al., 1990; Gollnick, et al., 1986; Gollnick and Hermansen, 1973; Holloszy, 1973; Karlsson, et al., 1972; Skinner and Morgan, 1985).

However, the amount of ATP and PC stored in the resting muscle is higher in the trained than in the untrained individual, especially if muscle mass increases. Whether this amount is large enough to markedly increase anaerobic capacity is questionable. At the same absolute workload there is less depletion of the PC and degradation of ATP levels after training. At the same

relative workload PC depletion and ATP degradation do not change with training. However, the activity of the enzymes responsible for the breakdown of ATP to ADP and the regeneration of ADP and ATP increase. Hence, the rate of turnover of ATP and PC increases. Taken together, the ATP-PC-LA changes indicate an increased anaerobic power and capacity with sprint type training (Medbø and Burgers, 1990). Values for the ATP-PC, LA, and O$_2$ systems are presented in Table 6.3 contrasting the trained and untrained male. It can be seen that the LA system changes much more with training than does the ATP-PC system, but that the greatest change is in the O$_2$ system (Bouchard et al., 1991, 1982).

Work Output

Work output—measured as watts or kilocalories per kilogram of body weight on a bicycle test such as the 10-sec or 30-sec Wingate Anaerobic Test and/or a 90-sec test—shows improvements with training. This result is evidenced by higher scores of athletes when compared to nonathletes and by higher posttraining than pretraining scores in all populations. Furthermore, sprint or power type athletes typically show higher anaerobic values and greater adaptations than endurance athletes. Elite sprinters and power athletes score higher than do less successful competitors (Bar-Or, 1987; Beld, et al., 1989; Horswill, et al., 1989; Patton and Dugan, 1987).

Aerobically, a trained individual can continue any given submaximal workload for a longer period of time than an untrained individual. The trained individual can also accomplish more total work to a higher absolute workload before achieving his or her maximum than an untrained individual can. Overall, the trained individual has a metabolic system capable of supporting enhanced performance, both at submaximal and at maximal levels. These changes, summarized in Table 6.4, are specific to the training employed.

Table 6.4
Metabolic Training Adaptations

1. **Fuel Supply**
   a. Carbohydrate
      (1) ↑ GLUT-4 transporter number and concentration.
      (2) ↓ glucose utilization.
      (3) ↑ Muscle and liver glycogen reserves.
      (4) ↓ Rate of muscle and liver glycogen depletion at absolute submaximal loads, that is, glycogen-sparing.
      (5) ↑ Velocity of glycogenolysis at maximal work.

   b. Fat
      (1) ↑ Mobilization, transportation, and beta oxidation of free fatty acids.
      (2) ↑ Fat storage adjacent to mitochondria.
      (3) ↑ Utilization of fat as fuel at same absolute and same relative workloads.

   c. Protein
      (1) ↑ Ability to utilize the BCAA leucine as fuel.
      (2) ↑ Gluconeogenesis from alanine.

2. **Enzyme Activity**
   a. ↑ Selected glycolytic enzyme activity: glycogen phosphorylase and probably phosphofructokinase.
   b. ↓ LDH activity with some conversion from the skeletal muscle to cardiac muscle form.
   c. ↑ Activity of the malate-aspartate shuttle enzymes but not the glycerol-phosphate shuttle enzymes.
   d. ↑ Number and size of mitochondria.
   e. ↑ Activity of most, but not all, of the enzymes of the Krebs cycle, electron transport, and oxidative phosphorylation due to greater mitochondrial protein amount.

3. **O_2 Utilization**
   a. ↑ $\dot{V}O_2$max with aerobic endurance training but not dynamic resistance training.
   b. = $\dot{V}O_2$ cost at absolute submaximal workload.
   c. ↑ Myoglobin concentration.
   d. ↓ Oxygen deficit.
   e. ↓ Oxygen drift.

4. **Lactic Acid Accumulation**
   a. ↑ MCT1 lactate transporters.
   b. ↑ Intracellular and extracellular lactate shuttle activity.
   c. ↓ La^- accumulation at same absolute workload and % $\dot{V}O_2$max relative intensity for endurance activity.
   d. ↓ La^- accumulation at same absolute load but = La^- accumulation at same relative intensity for resistance exercise.
   e. ↑ Workload to achieve lactate thresholds.
   f. ↑ $[La^-]$ at maximum.

5. **ATP Productions, Storage, and Turnover**
   a. = ATP from gram of precursor fuel substrate.
   b. ↑ ATP-PC storage.
   c. ↓ Depletion of PC and degradation of ATP at same absolute workload.
   d. = Depletion of PC and degradation of ATP at same relative workload.
   e. ↑ ATP-PC turnover.

↑, increase; ↓, decrease; =, no change.

Focus on Research

Substrate Training Adaptations in Children

Duncan, G. E., & E. I. Howley: Metabolic and perceptual responses to short-term cycle training in children. *Pediatric Exercise Science* 10:110–122 (1998).

As has been described in the text, it has been clearly established in adults that the primary substrate utilized to fuel exercise depends on the modality, intensity, and duration of the activity as well as the training status of the exerciser. The "crossover" concept states that at some point, as the intensity increases during incremental exercise, the predominant fuel source will shift from fat to carbohydrate. The crossover point is the power output at which this occurs.

This study by Duncan and Howley shows that the same processes occur in children. Twenty-three boys and girls (ages 7–12) volunteered and were divided into a training group (N = 10) and a control group (N = 13). All were tested for $\dot{V}O_2$peak on a cycle ergometer and then at five power outputs designed to elicit approximately 35%, 45%, 55%, 65%, and 75% of $\dot{V}O_2$ peak. RER values were determined by open circuit spirometry for the five-stage submaximal test before and after 4 weeks of training. Training consisted of three 10-min work bouts separated by 1–2 min of rest at roughly 50% $\dot{V}O_2$peak, three times per week.

The results, presented in the accompanying graph, clearly show that as the intensity of the submaximal exercise increased, so did the percentage of carbohydrate utilized as fuel, both before and after the training. Furthermore, the crossover point was delayed or shifted to the right in the training group (data for the control group are not shown). This means that the trained children could work harder while using fat as the predominant fuel. Training apparently has the same carbohydrate-sparing benefit for children as for adults.

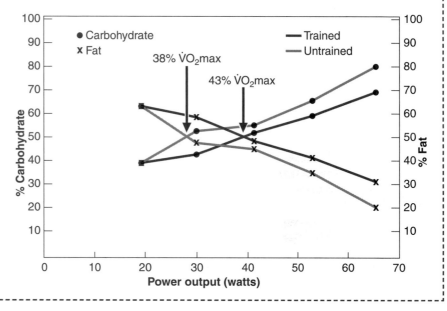

The Influence of Age and Sex on Metabolic Training Adaptations

With the exception of $\dot{V}O_2$max (which is discussed in the cardiovascular-respiratory unit), there is a scarcity of research data on most of the metabolic variables across the age spectrum. What scattered evidence is available indicates that training and detraining changes in children, adolescents, and the elderly are similar to changes for adults in the 20- to 50-yr range. This is especially true if the changes are considered relative to baseline values (that is, as a percentage of change) and not as absolutes (Adeniran and Toriola, 1988; Bar-Or, 1983; Clarke, 1977; Eriksson, 1972; Gaisl and Wiesspeiner, 1986; Massicotte and MacNab, 1974; Rotstein, et al., 1986; Rowland, 1990).

Data concerning metabolic adaptations in females of all ages are also minimal, again with the exception of $\dot{V}O_2$max (Shepard, 1978; Tlusty, 1969; Wells, 1991). Studies have shown the following adaptations in females as a result of appropriate specific training:

1. Fuel utilization shifts in favor of fat.
2. Lactic acid levels decrease during submaximal work and increase at maximal effort.
3. Enzyme levels change.
4. Submaximal $\dot{V}O_2$ consumption remains stable or decreases slightly.
5. Anaerobic power and capacity increase (Wells, 1991; Weltman, et al., 1978).

In short, both males and females respond to the same training with the same adaptations. This is not to say that sex differences are obliterated in equally trained males and females in the metabolic variables—just that both sexes are trainable and probably to the same extent.

Detraining also appears to operate in the same way and to the same extent for males and females.

The Impact of Genetics on Metabolic Trainability

Genetics impacts human physiological variables two ways. The first impact is directly on the expression of that variable. For example, at least 50% of an individual's endurance capacity, as measured by the maximal amount of work done on a cycle ergometer in 90 min, can be accounted for by heritability (Bouchard, 1986). Other examples have been discussed for both anaerobic and aerobic metabolism in previous chapters.

The second way in which genetics impacts physiology is on the adaptation to training of any variable. Research in which multiple pairs of monozygous (MZ) twins have been trained under laboratory conditions has shown that for many of the variables examined the impact of genetics on trainability is stronger than the heritability of the trait itself in sedentary individuals. Furthermore, the influence of genetics is sometimes stronger the closer the individual is to achieving his or her maximal potential.

Although many of the energy system variables whose training adaptations have just been described have not been investigated to date, specific information is available on several (Bouchard, 1986).

Submaximal Substrate or Fuel Utilization

Adaptations in substrate availability and utilization that occur as a result of aerobic endurance training are largely genetically based. In particular, data show that the change in epinephrine-stimulated lipolysis or breakdown of fat from isolated adipose cells that results from training is genetically dependent. The genetic influence on the training-induced ability to mobilize fat is also reflected in the ability to utilize fat during light submaximal exercise. Forty-four percent of the variance in the training adaptation of the respiratory exchange ratio can be attributed to genetics. Likewise, 42% of the variance of submaximal oxygen cost at the same absolute load depends on genetics (Bouchard, et al., 1992).

Maximal Work Output and Oxygen Consumption

Approximately 70% of the variance in the training increase in work output in 90 sec (primarily lactic anaerobic metabolism) can be accounted for by genetics. For training changes in $\dot{V}O_2$max and 90-min maximal work capacity, the amount of variance accounted for by genetics is approximately 75% and 80%, respectively. Both the training adaptations and the percentage of that work increase that can be accounted for by genetics are smaller for a 10-sec (alactic anaerobic) task: only about 30%. Maximal aerobic endurance capacity is about 60% more trainable than $\dot{V}O_2$max. Males show higher trainability in maximal aerobic endurance capacity than females (Bouchard, 1986). Genetically dependent training changes in both glycolytic and oxidative muscle enzyme activity underlie these changes (Bouchard, 1986; Hamel, et al., 1986).

Genetic Variability

One of the most interesting aspects of the genetic impact on trainability is the wide range of adaptation. For example, following a 20-week endurance training program in which the mean improvement in endurance performance was about 50% of the pretraining work output, the range of improvement was from 16 to 97% (Bouchard, et al., 1992). Similarly wide ranges have been shown for other variables, suggesting that most of the individual differences in responding to the same training program are genetically determined (Bouchard, 1993; Bouchard, et al., 1988). Thus, it appears that there are both low and high responders. And there may be as much as a threefold to tenfold variation between high and low responders. Indeed, some people (probably less than 5% of the population) may be nonresponders. In addition, there are also early and late responders. Early responders show metabolic adaptations very quickly, within the first 5–7 weeks of a training program. Late responders may show little initial progress but after 8 weeks or so appear to make a major breakthrough. These variations, of course, are the basis for the individualization training principle (Bouchard, et al., 1988; Hamel, et al., 1986).

Unfortunately, there is no way at the present time to determine an individual's genetic training potential for either the aerobic or the anaerobic system. Thus, the physical educator, coach, or fitness leader must be alert for these variations and counsel those under their tutelage accordingly (Bouchard, 1993).

Summary

1. The most important considerations in applying each training principle to achieve metabolic adaptations are as follows:
   a. For specificity, match the energy system of the activity.
   b. For overload, manipulate time and distance or lactate level.
   c. For adaptation, alternate hard and easy days.
   d. For progression, reoverload if additional improvement is desired.
   e. For individualization, evaluate the individual according to the demands of the activity and develop a periodization training sequence, system, and load on the basis of your evaluation.
   f. For maintenance, emphasize intensity.
   g. For retrogression, plateau, and detraining, evaluate the training adaptations and modify as indicated.
   h. For warm-up and cool-down, include activities that will actually elevate or reduce body temperature, respectively.

2. Properly prescribed training programs bring about adaptations in fuel supply, enzyme activity, oxygen utilization, lactate accumulation, and ATP production, storage, and turnover.

3. Most of the variation between individuals in metabolic training adaptation is genetically based. Long-term, lactic anaerobic, and aerobic metabolic training adaptations are influenced more by genetics than are short-term, alactic anaerobic adaptations.

Review Questions

1. Name and briefly describe the eight training principles. Select a sport or fitness activity and show how each of the training principles can be specifically applied to that activity.

2. Describe and explain the metabolic adaptations to exercise training for each of the following factors:
   a. Substrate or fuel supply
   b. Enzyme activity
   c. Oxygen utilization
   d. Lactate accumulation
   e. ATP production, storage, and turnover

3. Discuss the impact of genetics on the metabolic adaptations to exercise training in terms of the following factors:
   a. Submaximal substrate or fuel utilization

b. Maximal work output and oxygen consumption
c. Variability of response

4. Derive a practical application from this discussion, and provide a realistic example.

For further review and additional study tools, go to The Physiology Place (www.physiologyplace.com) and the Student Study Guide for Exercise Physiology for Health, Fitness, and Performance *by Sharon A. Plowman and Denise L. Smith.*

Passport to the Internet

Visit the following Internet sites to explore further topics and issues related to training principles and adaptations. To visit an organization's web site, go to www.physiologyplace.com and click on "Passport to the Internet."

Runners World Online *Runners World* is one of the leading magazines for dedicated runners. This online resource provides training advice and general information about running.

President's Council on Physical Fitness and Sports The President's Council on Physical Fitness and Sports (PCPFS) serves as a catalyst to promote, encourage, and motivate Americans of all ages to become physically active and participate in sports. Surf this site for hands-on information as well as the latest research on these efforts.

References

Abernethy, P. J., R. Thayer, & A. W. Taylor: Acute and chronic responses of skeletal muscle to endurance and sprint exercise: A review. *Sports Medicine.* 10(6):365–389 (1990).

Adeniran, S. A., & A. L. Toriola: Effects of continuous and interval running programmes on aerobic and anaerobic capacities in schoolgirls aged 13 to 17 years. *Journal of Sports Medicine and Physical Fitness.* 28:260–266 (1988).

Alessio, H., & E. R. Blasi: Physical activity as a natural antioxidant booster and its effect on a healthy life span. *Research Quarterly for Exercise and Sport.* 68(4):292–302 (1997).

Allen, W. K., D. R. Seals, B. F. Hurley, A. A. Ehsani, & J. M. Hagberg: Lactate threshold and distance-running performance in young and older endurance athletes. *Journal of Applied Physiology.* 58(4):1281–1284 (1985).

Anderson, O.: The rise and fall of tempo training. *Running Research.* 14(8):1, 4–5 (1998).

Athletics Congress of the USA: *1989–1990 Competition Rules for Athletics: World and American Records.* Indianapolis: Author (1989).

Bailey, S. P., & R. R. Pate: Feasibility of improving running economy. *Sports Medicine.* 12(4):228–246 (1991).

Bar-Or, O.: *Pediatric Sports Medicine for the Practitioner: From Physiological Principles to Clinical Applications.* New York: Springer-Verlag, 1–65 (1983).

Bar-Or, O.: The Wingate Anaerobic Test: An update on the methodology, reliability and validity. *Sports Medicine* 4:381–394 (1987).

Beld, K., J. Skinner, & Z. Tran: Load optimization for peak and mean power output on the Wingate Anaerobic Test. *Medicine and Science in Sports and Exercise* (Suppl. 164). 21(2):S28 (1989).

Bonen, A.: Lactate transporters (MCT proteins) in heart and skeletal muscles. *Medicine and Science in Sports and Exercise.* 32(4):778–789 (2000).

Bouchard, C.: Genetics of aerobic power and capacity. In R. M. Malina & C. Bouchard (eds.), *Sport and Human Genetics.* 1984 Olympic Scientific Congress Proceedings, Vol. 4. Champaign, IL: Human Kinetics, 59–88 (1986).

Bouchard, C.: Heredity and Health-Related Fitness. *Physical Activity and Fitness Research Digest.* Washington, DC: President's Council on Physical Fitness and Sports, 1(4) (1993).

Bouchard, C., M. R. Boulay, J. A. Simoneau, G. Lortie, & L. Pérusse: Heredity and trainability of aerobic and anaerobic performances: An update. *Sports Medicine.* 5:69–73 (1988).

Bouchard, C., F. T. Dionne, J.-A. Simoneau, & M. R. Boulay: Genetics of aerobic and anaerobic performance. In J. O. Holloszy (ed.), *Exercise and Sport Sciences Reviews.* Baltimore: Williams & Wilkins, 20 (1992).

Bouchard, C., A. W. Taylor, & S. Dulac: Testing maximal anaerobic power and capacity. In J. D. MacDougall, H. W. Wenger, & H. J. Green (eds.), *Physiological Testing of the High-Performance Athlete* (2nd edition). Champaign, IL: Human Kinetics, 175–221 (1991).

Bouchard, C., A. W. Taylor, J. A. Simoneau, & S. Dulac: Testing anaerobic power and capacity. In J. D. MacDougall, H. A. Wenger, & H. J. Green (eds.), *Physiological Testing of the Elite Athlete* (1st edition). Hamilton, Ontario: Canadian Association of Sport Sciences Mutual Press Limited, 61–73 (1982).

Bourdon, P.: Blood lactate transition thresholds: Concepts and controversies. In C. J. Gore (ed.), *Physiological Tests for Elite Athletes.* Champaign, IL: Human Kinetics, 50–65 (2000).

Brooks, G. A.: Current concepts in lactate exchange. *Medicine and Science in Sports and Exercise.* 23(8):895–906 (1991).

Brooks, G. A.: Intra- and extra-cellular lactate shuttles. *Medicine and Science in Sports and Exercise.* 32(4):790–799 (2000).

Brooks, G. A., T. D. Fahey, T. P. White, & K. M. Baldwin: *Exercise Physiology: Human Bioenergetics and Its Applications.* (3rd edition). Mountain View, CA: Mayfield (1999).

Casaburi, R., T. W. Storer, I. Ben-Dov, & K. Wasserman: Effect of endurance training on possible determinants of $\dot{V}O_2$ during heavy exercise. *Journal of Applied Physiology.* 62(1):199–207 (1987).

Chaloupka, E. C., & E. L. Fox: Physiological effects of two maintenance programs following eight weeks of interval training. *Federation Proceedings* (abstract). 34(3):443 (1975).

Clarke, H. H. (ed.): Exercise and aging. *Physical Fitness Research Digest.* Washington, DC: President's Council on Physical Fitness and Sports, 7(2) (1977).

Coggan, A. R.: Effect of endurance training on glucose metabolism during exercise: Stable isotope studies. In R. J. Maughan & S. M. Shirreffs (eds.), *Biochemistry of Exercise IX.* Champaign, IL: Human Kinetics, 27–35(1996).

Conley, D., G. Krahenbuhl, & L. Burkett: Training for aerobic capacity and running economy. *Physician and Sportsmedicine.* 9(4):107–115 (1981).

Costill, D. L.: *Inside Running: Basics of Sport Physiology.* Indianapolis: Benchmark Press (1986).

Costill, D. L., D. S. King, R. Thomas, & M. Hargreaves: Effects of reduced training on muscular power in swimmers. *Physician and Sportsmedicine.* 13:94–101 (1985).

Coyle, E. F., W. H. Martin, D. R. Sinacore, M. J. Joyner, J. M. Hagberg, & J. O. Holloszy: Time course of loss of adaptations after stopping prolonged intense endurance training. *Journal of Applied Physiology: Respiratory, Environmental and Exercise Physiology.* 57(6):1857–1864 (1984).

Daniels, J., N. Oldridge, F. Nagle, & B. White: Differences and changes in $\dot{V}O_2$ among young runners 10 to 18 years of age. *Medicine and Science in Sports and Exercise.* 10(3):200–203 (1978).

Dela, F.: Carbohydrate metabolism in human muscle studied with the glycemic clamp technique: The influence of physical training. In R. J. Maughan & S. M. Shirreffs (eds.), *Biochemistry of Exercise IX.* Champaign, IL: Human Kinetics, 13–26 (1996).

Donovan, C. M., & G. A. Brooks: Endurance training affects lactate clearance, not lactate production. *American Journal of Physiology.* 244:E83–E92 (1983).

Dwyer, J., & R. Bybee: Heart rate indices of the anaerobic threshold. *Medicine and Science in Sports and Exercise.* 15(1):72–76 (1983).

Ekblom, B., P.-O. Åstrand, B. Saltin, J. Stenberg, & B. Wallström: Effect of training on circulatory response to exercise. *Journal of Applied Physiology.* 24(4):518–528 (1968).

Eriksson, B. O.: Physical training, oxygen supply and muscle metabolism in 11–13 year old boys. *Acta Physiologica Scandinavica.* Suppl. 384:1–48 (1972).

Fox, E. L., R. W. Bowers, & M. L. Foss: *The Physiological Basis of Physical Education and Athletics* (4th edition). Philadelphia: Saunders College (1988).

Fox, E. L., & D. K. Mathews: *Interval Training: Conditioning for Sports and General Fitness.* Philadelphia: W. B. Saunders (1974).

Fox, E. L., S. Robinson, & D. L. Wiegman: Metabolic energy sources during continuous and interval running. *Journal of Applied Physiology.* 27(2):174–178 (1969).

Franks, B. D.: Physical warm-up. In M. H. Williams (ed.), *Ergogenic Aids in Sport.* Champaign, IL: Human Kinetics, 340–375 (1983).

Fry, R. W., A. R. Morton, & D. Keast: Overtraining in athletics: An update. *Sports Medicine*. 12(1):32–65 (1991).

Gaisl, G., & G. Wiesspeiner: Training prescriptions for 9- to 17-year-old figure skaters based on lactate assessment in the laboratory and on the ice. In J. Rutenfranz, R. Mocellin, & F. Klimt (eds.), *Children and Exercise XII*. Champaign, IL: Human Kinetics, 17:59–65 (1986).

Galbo, H.: *Hormonal and Metabolic Adaptation to Exercise*. New York: Thieme-Stratton, Inc. (1983).

Gardner, A. W., E. T. Poehlman, & D. L. Corrigan: Effect of endurance training on gross energy expenditure during exercise. *Human Biology*. 61(4):559–569 (1989).

Gilman, M. B., & C. L. Wells: The use of heart rates to monitor exercise intensity in relation to metabolic variables. *International Journal of Sports Medicine*. 14(6):3334–3339 (1993).

Gladden, L. B.: Muscle as a consumer of lactate. *Medicine and Science in Sports and Exercise*. 32(4): 764–771 (2000).

Gollnick, P. D., W. M. Bayly, & D. R. Hodgson: Exercise intensity, training, diet, and lactate concentration in muscle and blood. *Medicine and Science in Sports and Exercise*. 18(3):334–340 (1986).

Gollnick, P. D., & L. Hermansen: Biochemical adaptations in exercise: Anaerobic metabolism. In J. H. Wilmore (ed.), *Exercise and Sport Sciences Reviews*. New York: Academic Press (1973).

Gutin, B., K. Stewart, S. Lewis, & J. Kruper: Oxygen consumption in the first stages of strenuous work as a function of prior exercise. *Journal of Sports Medicine and Physical Fitness*. 16(1):60–65 (1976).

Hagberg, J. M., J. P. Mullin, & F. J. Nagle: Oxygen consumption during constant-load exercise. *Journal of Applied Physiology: Respiratory, Environmental and Exercise Physiology*. 45(3):381–384 (1978).

Hamel, P., J.-A. Simoneau, G. Lortie, M. R. Boulay, & C. Bouchard: Heredity and muscle adaptation to endurance training. *Medicine and Science in Sports and Exercise*. 18(6):690–696 (1986).

Henritze, J., A. Weltman, R. L. Schurrer, & K. Barlow: Effects of training at and above the lactate threshold on the lactate threshold and maximal oxygen uptake. *European Journal of Applied Physiology*. 54:84–88 (1985).

Hickson, R. C., J. M. Hagberg, A. A. Ehsani, & J. O. Holloszy: Time course of the adaptive response of aerobic power and heart rate to training. *Medicine and Science in Sports and Exercise*. 13(1):17–20 (1981).

Holloszy, J. O.: Biochemical adaptations to exercise: Aerobic metabolism. In J. H. Wilmore (ed.), *Exercise and Sport Sciences Reviews*. New York: Academic Press, 1:45–71 (1973).

Holloszy, J. O., & E. F. Coyle: Adaptations of skeletal muscle to endurance exercise and their metabolic consequences. *Journal of Applied Physiology: Respiratory, Environmental and Exercise Physiology*. 56:831–838 (1984).

Hood, D. A., & R. L. Terjung: Amino acid metabolism during exercise and following endurance training. *Sports Medicine*. 9(1):23–35 (1990).

Horswill, C. A., J. R. Scott, & P. Galea: Comparison of maximum aerobic power, maximum anaerobic power, and skinfold thickness of elite and nonelite junior wrestlers. *International Journal of Sports Medicine*. 10:165–168 (1989).

Houmard, J. A., D. L. Costill, J. B. Mitchell, S. H. Park, R. C. Hickner, & J. M. Roemmich: Reduced training maintains performance in distance runners. *International Journal of Sports Medicine*. 11:46–52 (1990).

Jenkins, R. R.: Exercise, oxidative stress, and antioxidants: A review. *International Journal of Sport Nutrition*. 3:356–375 (1993).

Johns, R. A., J. A. Houmard, R. W. Kobe, T. Hortobagyi, N. J. Bruno, J. M. Wells, & M. H. Shinebarger: Effects of taper on swim power, stroke distance, and performance. *Medicine and Science in Sports and Exercise*. 24(10): 1141–1146 (1992).

Karlsson, J., L.-O. Nordesjö, L. Jorfeldt, & B. Saltin: Muscle lactate, ATP, and CP levels during exercise after physical training in man. *Journal of Applied Physiology*. 33(2): 199–203 (1972).

Keith, R. E.: Antioxidants and Health. *Alabama Cooperative Extension System*. HE-778 (1999).

Londeree, B. R.: Effect of training on lactate/ventilatory thresholds: A meta-analysis. *Medicine and Science in Sports and Exercise*. 29(6):837–843 (1997).

Marcinik, E. J., J. Potts, G. Schlabach, S. Will, P. Dawson, & B. F. Hurley: Effects of strength training on lactate threshold and endurance performance. *Medicine and Science in Sports and Exercise*. 23(6):739–743 (1991).

Massicotte, D. R., & R. B. J. MacNab: Cardiorespiratory adaptations to training at specified intensities in children. *Medicine and Science in Sports*. 6(4):242–246 (1974).

Mazzeo, R. S., G. A. Brooks, D. A. Schoeller, & T. F. Budinger: Disposal of blood $[1^{-13}C]$ lactate in humans during rest and exercise. *Journal of Applied Physiology*. 60(1):232–241 (1986).

McCafferty, W. B., & S. M. Horvath: Specificity of exercise and specificity of training: A subcellular review. *Research Quarterly*. 48(2):358–371 (1977).

Medbø, J. I., & S. Burgers: Effect of training on the anaerobic capacity. *Medicine and Science in Sports and Exercise*. 22(4):501–507 (1990).

Neufer, P. D.: The effect of detraining and reduced training on the physiological adaptations to aerobic exercise training. *Sports Medicine*. 8(5):302–321 (1989).

Pilegaard, H., J. Bango, E. A. Richter, & C. Juel: Lactate transport studied in sarcolemmal giant vesicles from human muscle biopsies: Relation to training status. *Journal of Applied Physiology*. 77(4):1858–1862 (1994).

Patton, J. F., & A. Duggan: An evaluation of tests of anaerobic power. *Aviation and Space Environmental Medicine*. 58:237–242 (1987).

Ready, A. E., & H. A. Quinney: Alternations in anaerobic threshold as the result of endurance training and detraining. *Medicine in Sports and Exercise*. 14(4):292–296 (1982).

Reynolds, T. H., P. A. Frye, & G. A. Sforzo: Resistance training and the blood lactate response to resistance exercise in women. *Journal of Strength and Conditioning Research.* 11(2):77–81 (1997).

Rotstein, A., R. Dotan, O. Bar-Or, & G. Tenenbaum: Effect of training on anaerobic threshold, maximal aerobic power and anaerobic performance of preadolescent boys. *International Journal of Sports Medicine.* 7(5):281–286 (1986).

Rowland, T. W.: *Exercise and Children's Health.* Champaign, IL: Human Kinetics (1990).

Sato, Y., Y. Oshida, I. Ohsawa, N. Nakai, N. Ohsaki, K. Yamanouchi, J. Sato, Y. Shimomura, & H. Ohno: The role of glucose transport in the regulation of glucose utilization by muscle. In R. J. Maughan & S. M. Shirreffs (eds.), *Biochemistry of Exercise IX.* Champaign, IL: Human Kinetics (1996).

Shepard, R. J.: *Physical Activity and Aging.* Chicago: Year Book Medical Publishers (1978).

Shepley, B., J. D. MacDougall, N. Cipriano, J. R. Sutton, G. Coates, & M. Tarnopolsky: Physiological effects of tapering in highly trained athletes. *Journal of Applied Physiology.* 72:706–711 (1992).

Sjödin, B., I. Jacobs, & J. Svedenhag: Changes in onset of blood lactate accumulation (OBLA) and muscle enzymes after training at OBLA. *European Journal of Applied Physiology.* 49:45–57 (1982).

Skinner, J. S., & D. W. Morgan: Aspects of anaerobic performance. In D. H. Clarke & H. M. Eckert (eds.), *Limits of Human Performance.* Champaign, IL: Human Kinetics, 131–144 (1985).

Tlusty, L.: Physical fitness in old age. II. Anaerobic capacity, anaerobic work in graded exercise, recovery after maximum work performance in elderly individuals. *Respiration.* 26:287–299 (1969).

Van de Graaff, K. M., & S. I. Fox: *Concepts of Human Anatomy and Physiology* (2nd edition). Dubuque, IA: Brown (1989).

Wells, C. L.: *Women, Sport and Performance: A Physiological Perspective* (2nd edition). Champaign, IL: Human Kinetics (1991).

Weltman, A.: *The Blood Lactate Response to Exercise.* Champaign, IL: Human Kinetics (1995).

Weltman, A., R. J. Moffatt, & B. A. Stamford: Supramaximal training in females: Effects on anaerobic power output, anaerobic capacity, and aerobic power. *Journal of Sports Medicine and Physical Fitness.* 18(3):237–244 (1978).

Williams, C. G., C. H. Wyndham, R. Kok, & M. J. E. von Rahden: Effect of training on maximal oxygen intake and on anaerobic metabolism in man. *Internationale Zeitschrift fuer Angewandte Physiologie Einschliesslich Arbeitsphysiologie.* 24:18–23 (1967).

Wilmore, J. H., & D. L. Costill: *Training for Sport and Activity: The Physiological Basis of the Conditioning Process* (3rd edition). Dubuque, IA: Brown (1988).

Yoshida, T., S. Yoshihiro, & N. Takeuchi: Endurance training regimen based upon arterial blood lactate: Effects on anaerobic threshold. *European Journal of Applied Physiology.* 49:223–230 (1982).

Chapter 7

Nutrition for Fitness and Athletics

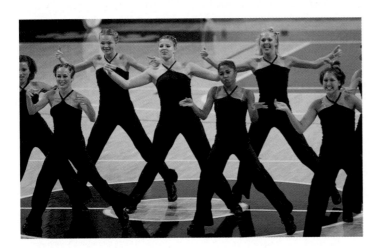

After studying the chapter, you should be able to

- List the goals for nutrition during training and for nutrition during competition, and explain why they are different.

- Compare a balanced diet for sedentary individuals with a balanced diet for active individuals in terms of caloric intake; carbohydrate, fat, and protein intake; and vitamin, mineral, and fluid requirements.

- Discuss the positive and negative aspects of a high-carbohydrate diet.

- Interpret the glycemic index; identify common high-, moderate-, and low-glycemic foods; and explain the best use of each classification.

- Discuss the situations where an increase in protein ingestion above the RDA is advisable and when it is not advisable.

- Describe a training situation when fat intake can be too low.

- Compare the theory of carbohydrate loading for endurance athletes to its use for bodybuilders.

- Compare the classic versus the modified techniques of carbohydrate loading in terms of diet and exercise for endurance event competitors.

- Develop a pre-event meal plan for athletic competition.

- Develop a plan for feeding during an endurance event and defend it.

- Describe optimal fluid ingestion during and after exercise.

- Judge the value of commercially available sport drinks.

- Differentiate among the eating disorders anorexia nervosa, bulimia nervosa, and anorexia athletica by definition and characteristics.

- Identify the risk factors for developing an eating disorder.

- Construct a list of guidelines to help prevent or deal with eating disorders in exercise settings.

Introduction

Proper nutrition and exercise are natural partners for health, fitness, and athletic performances. Consequently, many fitness enthusiasts pursue healthy diets, and athletes try to optimize athletic performance by identifying appropriate diets. Although these trends are very positive, they also have the potential to be taken to an extreme—an extreme that may simply involve spending money needlessly on "nutritional supplements" or that may actually be harmful, such as eating disorders. It is the responsibility of all fitness professionals to understand what constitutes optimal nutrition for fitness and athletics.

Nutrition education should be a part of physical fitness classes, community adult fitness and rehabilitation programs, and athletic training. Most individuals who are training regularly want to eat right, but they may confuse advertisements and media hype with factual information.

The issue of optimal nutrition for fitness and athletics must be considered for two different situations. The first is training, and the second competition, whether on the "fun run" or elite level. With the possible exception of youth sports, individuals typically spend more total time training than competing. Therefore, daily nutritional practices are the more critical. No amount of dietary manipulation the day of and/or the day before a competition can make up for otherwise poor nutritional habits (Burke and Read, 1989).

Nutrition and Training

Individuals involved in exercise training need to match their training regimen with an appropriate diet. This attempt often involves consultation with a fitness professional, a complete diet analysis, and, many times, a trial-and-error technique to find what works best for a given individual.

The goals of an optimal training diet are

1. to provide caloric and nutrient requirements;
2. to incorporate nutritional practices that promote good health;
3. to achieve and maintain optimal body composition and competition weight;
4. to promote recovery from training sessions and physiological adaptations; and
5. to try variations of precompetition and competition fuel and fluid intake to determine the body's responses (Burke and Read, 1989).

There is almost universal agreement that poor nutritional status impairs work performance. There is also considerable, although not universal, agreement that good general nutrition (the balanced diet recommended for just about everyone; see Table 7.1) is adequate and probably even optimal for most active individuals as well as sedentary individuals.

Unfortunately, the typical American does not eat the recommended healthy balanced diet. Many still

Table 7.1
Balanced Diets

For Sedentary Individuals	For Active Individuals
Calorie balance of intake and expenditure to maintain acceptable body composition and weight	Adequate caloric intake to balance caloric expenditure of training and competition in excess of normal living while maintaining optimal body composition and playing weight
12–15% protein (1.2 g·kg^{-1}·day^{-1}, 7–10 yr; 1.0 g·kg^{-1}·day^{-1}, 11–14 yr; 0.9 g·kg^{-1}·day^{-1}, 15–18 yr; 0.8 g·kg^{-1}·day^{-1}, 19 + yr)	12–15% protein (1.2–2 g·kg^{-1}·day^{-1})
30% fat (⅓ saturated, ⅓ unsaturated, ⅓ polyunsaturated); 65 g (< 20 g saturated)/2000 kcal or 80 g (< 25 g saturated)/2500 kcal)	20–30% fat (⅓ saturated, ⅓ unsaturated, ⅓ polyunsaturated)
55–58% carbohydrate (4.5 g·kg^{-1}·day^{-1})	58–68% carbohydrate (8–10 g·kg^{-1}·day^{-1})
RDA/DRI for vitamins and minerals	RDA/DRI for vitamins and minerals
Fluid intake monitored by thirst; 1880–2350 mL·day^{-1} (64–80 oz·day^{-1})	Fluids adequate to prevent dehydration: 2350–2825 mL·day^{-1} (80–96 oz·day^{-1}) plus 400–600 mL preexercise, 200–400 mL every 15–20 min during exercise, 700 mL postexercise

Sources: Based on information from Brotherhood (1984); Haymes (1983); U.S. Department of Agriculture, Dietary Guidelines Advisory Committee (1995).

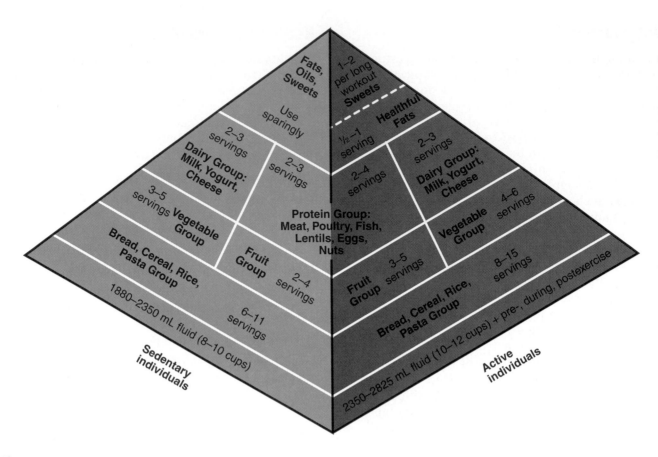

Figure 7.1
Food Guide Pyramid for Sedentary and Active Individuals

The United States Department of Agriculture food pyramid (left side) provides a suggested number of servings to be consumed daily from each food group. The smaller numbers are intended for individuals consuming approximately 1600 kcal per day, whereas the higher numbers assume a caloric intake of approximately 2800 kcal. The modified food pyramid (right side) illustrates how active individuals should spread their additional caloric intake among the food groups.

Sources: Applegate (2000); United States Department of Agriculture, Dietary Guidelines Advisory Committee (1995).

consume too much fat (37–42%) and too little carbohydrate (43–48%). If the recommended percentages (not more than 30% fat and 55–58% carbohydrate) are consumed, the vast majority of youth sport, middle and secondary school, and college athletes, as well as fitness participants of all ages, will not need any modification in their diet. For those athletes or fitness participants training very long, hard, and often and/or competing at an elite level, a few modifications may be beneficial (Allen, et al., 1979; American Dietetic Association, 1987; Belko, 1987; Brotherhood, 1984; Burke and Read, 1989; Lemon and Nagle, 1981; Nieman, 1990). Table 7.1 summarizes these recommendations, which are discussed in the following sections. Figure 7.1 illustrates these through the food pyramid daily recommendations. Recommended Daily Allowances (RDA) are in the process of being converted to Dietary Reference Intakes (DRI).

Kilocalories

The most obvious distinction between active and inactive individuals is the number of calories required per day. Everyone needs sufficient calories to support daily needs, and children need adequate calories for growth. In addition, an active individual can expend several hundred to several thousand kilocalories more per day than a sedentary individual. The actual amount depends on the size of the individual and the intensity, duration, and frequency of the workouts. Big football players doing two-a-days and smaller endurance athletes expend large amounts of energy, but golfers or softball and baseball players of any size expend much smaller amounts. Some athletes may actually increase their daily energy expenditure by 25–50% during the season (American Dietetic Association, 1987; Brotherhood, 1984; Burke and Read,

1989; Leaf and Frisa, 1989). Costill (1988) cites figures of 900–2400 kcal·day^{-1} expended for elite distance runners, 6000 kcal·day^{-1} for cyclists, and 1250–3750 kcal·day^{-1} for swimmers during training. These calories must be replaced.

Published reports indicate that male basketball and football players may consume as many as 9000–11,000 kcal·day^{-1}, triathletes 3500–6400 kcal·day^{-1} (female and male), cross-country skiers 4000–5500 kcal·day^{-1} (female and male), and track and field athletes (male) 3500–4700 kcal·day^{-1}, depending on the event. It is highly likely that these athletes are adequately resupplying their energy needs (Burke and Read, 1989).

However, competitors in other sports (long-distance running, gymnastics, wrestling, and dance) often attempt to maintain extremely low and, in some cases, "unnatural" body fat and body weight. Intake values as low as 600 kcal·day^{-1} for male gymnasts and 900 kcal·day^{-1} for female ballet dancers have been reported. It is equally likely that these athletes are *not* adequately resupplying their energy needs (Burke and Read, 1989).

If the relative proportion of nutrients remained the same as the calories increased to support training, the active individual would have an acceptable diet. However, some subtle shifting of percentages and/or amounts can be of benefit in certain situations. Chief among them is an increased percentage of carbohydrate ingestion for endurance athletes.

Carbohydrate

The earlier discussion of carbohydrate metabolism (Chapter 3) pointed out several important facts about carbohydrates as a fuel for exercise (American Dietetic Association, 1987; Burke and Read, 1989; Costill, 1988; Nieman, 1990):

1. The higher the intensity of exercise (whether continuous or intermittent; aerobic, anaerobic, or aerobic-anaerobic), the more important glycogen is as a fuel.
2. The body can only store limited amounts of carbohydrates. Training increases the ability to store carbohydrate and to spare carbohydrate. However, 60–90 min of heavy endurance work seriously depletes glycogen stores, and depletion can be complete in 120 min. Muscle glycogen can also be depleted by 15–30 min of near-maximal or supramaximal-intensity interval work.
3. Fat metabolism is linked to carbohydrate metabolism. Fatigue, "hitting the wall," and exhaustion are tied to glycogen depletion during high-intensity, long-duration activity. Thus, having an adequate supply of muscle glycogen is necessary if one is to avoid fatigue. Whatever glycogen is utilized, in training or competition, must be replenished before more heavy work can be done.

The storage of carbohydrate in liver and muscles depends on the level of activity (that is, the severity of glycogen depletion), the extent of muscle trauma, and the amount of dietary carbohydrate. Muscle glycogen resynthesis is highest when the muscle has been depleted, but not necessarily exhausted, and the diet is high in carbohydrate. Muscle fiber damage associated with exhaustive eccentric exercise (in which a contracting muscle is forcibly lengthened), such as running a marathon, may delay resynthesis for as long as 7–10 days despite elevated dietary carbohydrate (Burke and Read, 1989; Costill, 1988).

Given optimal amounts of carbohydrate, muscle glycogen resynthesis is higher (per muscle mass per hour) after short-term, high-intensity exercise than long-term, submaximal endurance exercise. Rates of muscle glycogen resynthesis following dynamic resistance exercise are lower than after short-term, high-intensity exercise but may be less than, equal to, or slightly higher than resynthesis following prolonged endurance exercise. The rate at which glycogen resynthesis occurs depends, to a large part, on the blood lactate concentration (higher levels result in higher rates of synthesis) and eccentric loading (higher levels result in slower rates of resynthesis) (Pascoe and Gladden, 1996).

How much carbohydrate should be included in the diet? The normal recommended intake of carbohydrate is 4.5 g·kg^{-1}·day^{-1}. For an individual utilizing high amounts of carbohydrate in training, 8–10 g·kg^{-1}·day^{-1} are recommended. In some cases this may increase the percentage of carbohydrate to 70–80% of the dietary intake.

Particularly important is the intake of carbohydrate during recovery from exercise when the glycogen that has been used needs to be replenished. Carbohydrate ingestion (50–100 g) should begin as soon after the workout or competition as is practical (15–30 min) and continue at the rate of 50 g every 2 hr until a larger meal of solid food (150–250 g of carbohydrate) is desired and possible (Coyle and Coyle, 1993). Does it matter which carbohydrates are ingested or if carbohydrates only are ingested? The answer to both questions is yes and no.

Liquid carbohydrate sources are as effective as solid carbohydrate sources (Figure 7.2). In fact, liquids may be even more useful, because many individuals are not hungry after an intense bout of exercise and fluid replacement is also important (Costill, 1988; Coyle, 1991). Table 7.2 provides a comparison of some

Table 7.2
Composition of Selected Sports Drinks (per 8 oz or 240 mL)

Name	Type of CHO*	Energy kcal	CHO (g)	CHO† Concentration (%)	Na (mg)	K (mg)	Other
All Sport	F, G	70	20	8.3	55	50	Ca, Cl, P, vitamin C, and 5 B vitamins
Body Fuel 450	GP, F	40	10	4		20	—
Exceed	GP, F	68	17	7	50	45	Ca, Mg, P, Cl
Gatorade	G, S	56	14	6	110	25	Cl, P
Gatorlode	G, GP	280	47	20	95	0	Vitamins
Gator Pro		360	58	24	180	630	Fat, protein, vitamins, minerals
Nutrament	F	240	34	14			Fat, protein
Power Ade	F, GP	70	19	8	55	30	Cl, vitamin C
Propel	S	10	3	0.4	35	40	Vitamins C, E, niacin, B-6, B-12, pantothenic acid
Water		0	0	0	Low	Low	Depends on source

* F = fructose, G = glucose, GP = glucose polymer, and S = sucrose.

† % concentration = [CHO (g)] ÷ [volume (mL)] × 100, rounded to nearest whole percentage.

Sources: Compiled from Applegate (1991); Murray (1987); Nieman (1990); Quaker Oats Company (1990); and from brand labels.

currently available liquid commercial products containing readily available carbohydrates. Table 7.3 provides the macronutrient breakdown for selected nutrition bars and a Snickers® candy bar for comparison purposes (Applegate, 1998; Manore, 2000). Nutrition bars provide a readily available source of

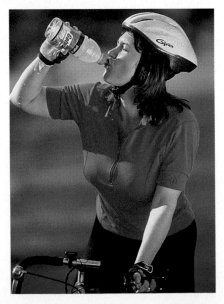

Figure 7.2

Replenishment of carbohydrate during and after exercise training sessions can easily be accomplished by drinking specially formulated sports drinks. Such drinks provide both fuel and fluid.

carbohydrate and fall into two generic categories: high carbohydrate (> 60% of total calories) with minimal fat and protein; and minimal to moderate carbohydrate (20–55% of total calories) with balanced fat and protein (approximately 30% of each). Those which are high in carbohydrate are best for ingestion before, during, and after exercise. Fat consumed during exercise is not readily available for energy; moreover, fat slows digestion and can lead to stomach upset. Bars with 4 g or less of fat (per 230 kcal serving size) are fine for workouts, but bars with higher fat content are best utilized as dietary supplements or snacks. Before or during exercise it is best to select energy bars with no more than 8–10 g of protein because higher protein amounts also slow digestion. Likewise, energy bars that contain more than 5 g of fiber should not be ingested prior to or during exercise because fiber also slows digestion. However, for a snack food, high-fiber bars can be good choices because fiber delays hunger pangs. If a bar is to be used as a meal replacement, one with a higher protein content should be selected. The amount of vitamins and minerals included in many energy bars is probably too small to provide much benefit but may be enough to cause gastrointestinal upset. Whenever an energy bar is eaten, it is important to drink at least 350–475 mL (12–16 ounces) of water to aid in digestion. Energy bars can serve as a convenient, effective fuel source, but they are engineered food and should not replace the groupings in the food pyramid.

Table 7.3

Composition of Selected Energy Bars

Name	Energy (kcal)	Carbohydrate (g)	Carbohydrate (%)	Fat (g)	Fat (%)	Protein (g)	Protein (%)	Fiber (g)	Vitamins/ Minerals
Balance Bar™ (almond brownie)	200	22	43	6	27	15	30	1	25; 25–210% DV*
Clif Bar (peanut butter)	250	45	72	4	14	10	16	4	15
Clif Luna (chocolate pecan pie)	180	24	53	5	25	10	22 (soy)	1	22
EAS Myoplex Delux (chocolate)	340	43	51	7	19	24	28	2	26
Met-Rx Bar (fudge brownie)	320	48	60	2.5	7	27	43	2	22+ L-glutamine
Power Bar (chocolate)	225	42	75	2	8	10	18	3	20; 35–100% DV
Power Bar Essentials™ (chocolate)	180	20	62	4	20	10	22	3	21
Power Bar Protein Plus™	290	15	21	8	25	32	44	1	21
PR-Bar® (bavarian mint)	190	21	44	6	28	13	27	1	23; 35–200% DV
Snickers Bar®	280	35	50	14	45	4	6	1	0
Tiger Sport Bar™	230	43	75	2	8	10	17	3	19; 35–100% DV

*DV = Daily value

Sources: Based on Applegate (1998) and Manore (2000).

Table 7.4

Composition of Selected Sports Gels

Name	Energy (kcal)	Carbohydrate (g)	Carbohydrate (%)	Fat (g)	Fat (%)	Protein (g)	Protein (%)	Fortification
Clif Shot	96	24	100	0	0	0	0	Caffeine (some flavors)
Gu	100	25	100	0	0	0	0	Caffeine
Power Gel	112	28	100	0	0	0	0	Ginseng, Kola nut, caffeine (some flavors)
Squeezy	80	20	100	0	0	0	0	

Another type of prepackaged food for active individuals is an energy gel. Energy gels are products with a consistency of syrup or pudding that come in 0.75 to 1.4 ounce plastic or foil packets. They contain between 20 and 28 g (80–110 kcal) of carbohydrates per serving. Some gels contain electrolytes (especially potassium) and/or caffeine, but none contain fat or protein (Table 7.4). As with energy bars, it is important to ingest sufficient water (approximately 4–8 ounces per ounce of gel) and to try a variety of gels during training to determine individual reactions before ingesting any during competition.

Some forms of simple sugars appear to have different effects on glycogen resynthesis. Glucose and sucrose promote muscle glycogen resynthesis, whereas fructose promotes liver glycogen resynthesis. Fructose alone is not recommended, because it must first be converted to glucose in the liver before muscles can store it as glycogen (Blom, et al., 1987; Costill, 1988; Coyle, 1991). This conversion delays the process of replenishing muscle glycogen stores.

Ingesting protein along with the carbohydrates in the 4-hr time span after exercise has been shown to significantly increase the rate of glycogen storage (Zawadzki, et al., 1992). Some of the liquid supplements listed in Table 7.2 and many of the solid nutrition bars (Table 7.3) include both carbohydrate and proteins.

Perhaps the most important criterion for selecting postexercise carbohydrates is the glycemic index (Coyle, 1991; Coyle and Coyle, 1993; Singh, et al., 1994). The **glycemic index** compares the elevation in blood glucose caused by the ingestion of 50 g of any carbohydrate food with the elevation caused by 50 g of white bread (Wolever, 1990). The glycemic index cannot be predicted by knowing the chemical

> **Glycemic Index** A measure that compares the elevation in blood glucose caused by the ingestion of 50 g of any carbohydrate food with the elevation caused by the ingestion of 50 g of white bread.

Table 7.5
Glycemic Index of Selected Foods

High–Glycemic Food (85 or greater)	Moderate–Glycemic Food (60–85)	Low–Glycemic Food (Under 60)
Sugars, Syrups, and Jellies		
White table sugar		Fructose
Maple syrup		
Honey		
Sports drinks		
(6–20% CHO concentration)		
Cereal Products		
Bagel	Rice	
Bread (white, wheat)	Pasta (spaghetti, macaroni)	Barley
Corn flakes	Bread (whole grain, rye)	All-Bran cereal
Shredded wheat		
Oatmeal		
Puffed wheat and rice		
Fruits		
Raisins	Grapes	Apples
Watermelons	Orange juice	Cherries
	Bananas	Dried apricots
		Peaches
		Pears
		Plums
		Grapefruits
Vegetables		
Potatoes (baked, microwaved, mashed)	Yams	Tomato soup
Carrots	Sweet corn	
Parsnips	Potato chips	
Legumes		
	Baked beans	Beans (butter, green, kidney, navy; dried)
	Beans (kidney, pinto; canned)	Lentils (green, red; dried)
	Peas (chick, green; canned or frozen)	
	Lentils (red, green; canned)	
Dairy Products		
	Ice cream	Milk (skim, whole)
		Yogurt
		Custard

Sources: Compiled from Coyle & Coyle (1993); Jenkins, et al. (1981); Singh, et al. (1994); Wolever (1990); Walton & Rhodes (1997).

composition of the food, including whether it is a simple or a complex carbohydrate. Instead, the glycemic index depends on the speed at which foods are digested and absorbed (Wolever, 1990). White bread has been assigned a glycemic index of 100. High–glycemic foods have a rating of 85 or greater; moderate–glycemic foods rate from 60 to 85; low–glycemic foods have a rating less than 60. Values greater than 100 are possible.

Foods with a high glycemic index cause a fast, high elevation in glucose and insulin; foods with lower indices cause a slower rise in both glucose and insulin. Table 7.5 gives examples of high–, moderate–, and low–glycemic foods. In general, sugars and sports drinks; syrups and jellies; and grain, pasta, and cereal products have high– or moderate–glycemic indices. Most fruits, legumes, and dairy products have low glycemic indices. The glycemic index of energy bars is, unfortunately, unknown. Significantly greater glycogen resynthesis and storage results from the ingestion of high–glycemic foods over a 24-hr period than from the intake of low–glycemic foods (Burke, et al., 1993). Moderate–glycemic foods appear to promote glycogen resynthesis just about as effectively as high–glycemic foods (Coyle and Coyle, 1993). Glycogen resynthesis occurs at about 5–6% per hour under optimal dietary conditions, thus even then requiring approximately 17–20 hr for complete recovery (Coyle, 1991; Coyle and Coyle, 1993).

Focus on Research

Carbohydrate Ingestion and the Inflammatory Response to Strenuous Exercise

Nehlsen-Cannarella, S. L., O. R. Fagoaga, D. C. Nieman, D. A. Henson, D. E. Butterworth, R. L. Schmitt, E. M. Bailey, B. J. Warren, A. Utter, & J. M. Davis. Carbohydrate and the cytokine response to 2.5 h of running. *Journal of Applied Physiology.* 82(5):1662–1667 (1997).

Strenuous exercise results in muscle soreness and injury and evokes an inflammatory response by the immune system. The relationship between muscle damage and overtraining was mentioned in Chapter 2 (the cytokine hypothesis of overtraining), and Chapter 17 discusses the sequence of events by which muscle exertion and subsequent muscle injury activate the inflammatory response. In brief, the inflammatory response and immune response to strenuous exercise are thought to be mediated, to a large extent, by the release of chemicals from immune cells. These chemicals are collectively known as cytokines. Cytokines may be proinflammatory (i.e., IL-6) or anti-inflammatory (i.e., L-1-ra). Because it is possible that carbohydrate ingestion may alter the inflammatory response to strenuous exercise, it is appropriate to consider these events as they relate to metabolism. Nehlsen-Cannarella and colleagues investigated the influence of carbohydrate ingestion on the cytokine response to 2.5 hr of intense running (76.7% $\dot{V}O_2$max). The figures below present the response of IL-6 and IL-1-ra to the exercise bout.

1. There was a greater increase in the proinflammatory cytokine (IL-6) in the placebo group versus the group that ingested carbohydrate immediately postrun and 1.5 hr postrun.
2. There was a greater increase in the anti-inflammatory cytokine (IL-1-ra) in the placebo group versus the group that ingested carbohydrate at 1.5 hr postrun.

These data indicate that carbohydrate ingestion reduces cytokine levels in the inflammatory response. Rather than being a definitive study that suggests that carbohydrate ingestion dampens the inflammatory response, this study begins the exploration of the relationship between nutrient intake and the complex inflammatory and immune response to strenuous exercise.

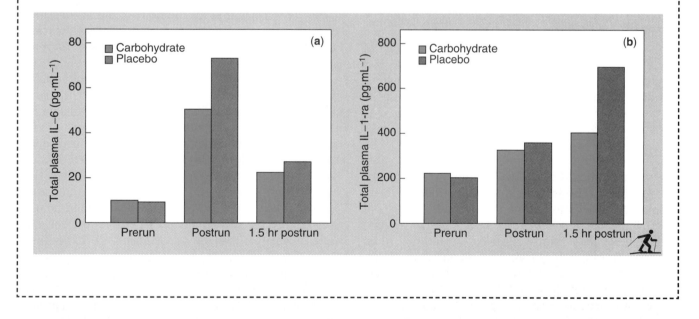

If carbohydrates are not replenished between training bouts, local muscle fatigue will result, and work output during succeeding training sessions will decline (Costill, 1988; Coyle, 1991). Severe depletion followed by a nonoptimal diet will require more than one day of rest, which is one reason to alternate body parts and hard-easy exercise days. If the aim of carbohydrate ingestion is not quick glycogen replenishment but a slower sustained presentation of glucose into the system, as would be the case during a marathon or long hike, then low–glycemic foods are preferable (Coyle and Coyle, 1993).

Although most individuals would benefit from increasing the percentage of carbohydrate ingested, levels as high as 70–80% are recommended only for athletes or fitness participants who are actually using high amounts of carbohydrate in their training regimens. Such individuals include long-distance runners, swimmers, cyclists, and soccer, hockey, or lacrosse players (Costill, 1988; Coyle, 1991).

There is little advantage, and possibly some risk, for a nonendurance athlete such as a golfer, a softball or baseball player, or a fitness walker to ingest 70–80% carbohydrates, especially if much of this food has a high–glycemic index. As mentioned earlier, absorption of a large dose of high–glycemic carbohydrates results in temporary hyperglycemia and an increased insulin response. Glycogen storage is limited in sedentary and nonendurance-trained individuals, and the glycolytic pathway is overloaded. The result is a greater-than-normal reliance on a side pathway that converts the glucose to free fatty acids (and then triglycerides) and cholesterol (Costill, 1988; Newsholme and Leech, 1983). Absorption of the same amount of low–glycemic carbohydrates results in a smaller blood glucose and insulin rise and hence less lipid formation. High blood levels of triglycerides and, more definitively, cholesterol are frequently associated with an increased risk of cardiovascular disease.

Endurance-trained individuals demonstrate less hyperglycemia and a lower insulin response in relation to a given glucose load than do untrained individuals. Thus, endurance-trained individuals appear to be able to convert high dietary levels of carbohydrate, especially high–glycemic foods, into glycogen storage without an elevation of blood lipids. Carbohydrate should be the highest energy substrate in terms of percentage for all individuals, but an additional 10–20% above the normal 55–58% is not recommended for sedentary individuals nor for low-intensity nonendurance athletes (Costill, 1988).

Protein

The optimal amount of dietary protein for individuals engaged in exercise training and competition has been debated practically forever, and it remains an area of controversy. The *recommended daily allowance* (RDA) of protein varies among countries for adults (United States: 0.8 g·kg^{-1} for male and female; Australia: 1.0 g·kg^{-1} for male and female; and Netherlands: 1.0 g·kg^{-1} for female and 1.2 g·kg^{-1} for male) and within countries for various ages. For example, the U.S. RDA decreases from 1.2 g·kg^{-1} for 7- to 10-yr-olds to 1.0 g·kg^{-1} for 11- to 14-yr-olds to 0.9 g·kg^{-1} for 15- to 18-yr-olds. Pregnant or lactating females are encouraged to ingest higher levels of protein, but only the Netherlands officially recommends an increased intake (1.5 g·kg^{-1}·day^{-1}) for physically active individuals (Lemon, 1991, 1989a).

The reluctance of nutritional experts to advocate increased protein intake relative to body weight is based on several factors (Lemon and Nagle, 1981).

First, because of the complexities of metabolism and the inaccuracies of measurement, the RDA for most nutrients, including protein, has not been precisely determined. Second, the estimated recommendations for protein just given are thought to include a considerable safety margin (about 78%). Finally, this safety margin is generally assumed to be sufficient to cover any additional exercise-induced increase in protein requirement. However, in several situations this assumption is questionable.

The first situation in which a higher protein intake might be beneficial is training in which the primary goal is a large increase in muscle mass (Kreider, et al., 1993; Lemon, 1989a, 1989b; Lemon and Nagle, 1981). Individuals involved in resistance training—such as weight lifters, power lifters, bodybuilders, football players, sprinters, and wrestlers—strive for increased muscular strength and/or hypertrophy. Training of this type typically increases protein in the muscle fibers (see Chapter 21). This increased muscle protein probably results from a decrease in the endogenous protein breakdown (which would decrease the need for dietary protein) and an increased protein synthesis from amino acids (which would increase the need for dietary protein). This balance between demand and supply, unfortunately, is generally not precise. In fact, there is evidence that for the body to maintain a positive nitrogen balance—and, hence, maintain the availability of indispensable amino acids—an increase above the RDA is needed. Conversely, there is minimal scientific evidence that amino acid supplementation in excess of the additional amount needed to maintain a positive nitrogen balance will enhance muscle hypertrophy or strength attainment. On the other hand, additional protein may be beneficial to ensure repair of any damaged muscle fiber (Lemon, 1991, 1989a). The consensus of current evidence suggests that strength and speed athletes may need to consume 1.2–2.0 g·kg^{-1}·day^{-1} of protein, which should be possible within the recommended 15% of total caloric intake (American Dietetic Association, 1987; Brotherhood, 1984; Haymes, 1983; Lemon, 1991, 1989a, 1989b; Tarnopolsky, et al., 1988).

The second situation in which increased protein might be beneficial is endurance training. Surprising though it may be, both the need and the evidence for an increased protein intake are stronger here than for resistance and power athletes (Kreider, et al., 1993). When an individual begins a training program, a situation called **sports anemia,** a transient decrease in

---

Sports Anemia A transient decrease in red blood cells and hemoglobin levels (grams per deciliter of blood).

red blood cells and hemoglobin level (grams per deciliter), may develop. During the initial two to three weeks of a training program, blood proteins, including erythrocytes (red blood cells, RBC), may be utilized to increase the myoglobin concentration, mitochondrial mass, and enzymes that are part of the training adaptation. An increased intake of dietary protein may minimize the destruction of red blood cells, promote their regeneration, and provide the protein needed for the other training adaptations to occur. However, there is an alternative explanation for sports anemia that involves plasma volume rather than protein (RBC) degradation. If plasma volume increases but hemoglobin and red blood cells do not (or they do not increase proportionally), a dilution effect may occur, resulting in decreased hemoglobin and red blood cell concentrations. Research supports blood volume changes. However, the two phenomena, increased dilution and protein degradation, are not mutually exclusive. Furthermore, research evidence suggests that experienced and not just novice endurance athletes may also suffer sports anemia (American Dietetic Association, 1987; Haymes, 1983; Lemon, 1989b; Tarnopolsky, et al., 1988).

In addition, high-intensity, long-duration training and competition result in increased amino acid oxidation as fuel, ranging from 5–15% of the total calories used, especially if the individual is depleted of carbohydrates (Brotherhood, 1984). Cool-temperature training (5–20°C, or 40–68°F) also utilizes more protein than warm-weather (30°C, or 86°F) training. Females utilize more protein during exercise in the mid-luteal phase of the menstrual cycle (approximately days 14–21) than during the follicular phase (approximately days 1–7) (Phillips, 1999).

For these reasons, a small increase in the intake of dietary protein to $1.2–1.4$ $g \cdot kg^{-1} \cdot day^{-1}$ is recommended for high-intensity, long-duration aerobic endurance training. Individuals training at less than 50% $\dot{V}O_2max$ for 20–60 $min \cdot day^{-1}$ do not need to increase their protein intake above the RDA.

Several high-energy sport bars (Table 7.3) are formulated to include 30% protein. This high protein percentage, eaten 30 min prior to a workout, is said to stimulate the release of glucagon and inhibit the release of insulin so that more fat is mobilized from adipose sites and used as fuel during exercise. Because glucagon does stimulate utilization of fat and insulin does inhibit fat burning in favor of fat storage, this is theoretically possible. However, research results from controlled studies are not available to support this claim.

While these high-protein energy bars are intended for the immediate preexercise time frame, in the last several years a dietary plan known as the Zone diet has been advocated both for weight loss and as a training diet for enhanced endurance athletic performance (Sears, 1995). This diet, also known as the 40/30/30 diet, recommends a consistent macronutrient intake of 40% carbohydrate, 30% fat, and 30% protein or 1.8 to 2.2 g of protein per kg of fat-free mass (total body mass minus fat mass) per day. Proponents of this diet claim that the diet will alter the hormonal balance between insulin and glucagon. They go another step, claiming that the altered hormonal balance will result in the production of specific substances called *eicosanoids* (Sears, 1995). Eicosanoids are hormonelike derivatives of essential fatty acids. These eicosanoids, it is theorized, produce vasodilation to active muscle, thus allowing greater oxygen delivery. It is theoretically possible to vasodilate arterioles by changing eicosanoid production. However, there is no scientific evidence at this time that the key eicosanoid responsible for improved muscle oxygenation either is found in skeletal muscle or contributes significantly to active muscle vasodilation (Cheuvront, 1999). Overall, a 40/30/30 diet does not provide balanced nutrition for optimal health and performance (Cheuvront, 1999) and cannot be recommended.

What is recommended, in terms of protein intake, is an increased amount of protein per kilogram of body weight, without increasing the percentage above the recommended 12–15% of the total calories ingested (Lemon, 1989a; Paul, 1989). Consider, for example, a 56-kg (123-lb) female triathlete. If her caloric intake goes from 1500 $kcal \cdot day^{-1}$ (12% protein) when sedentary to 2240 $kcal \cdot day^{-1}$ during heavy training while maintaining 12% protein ingestion, this increase now provides her with 1.2 $g \cdot kg^{-1}$ instead of 0.8 $g \cdot kg^{-1}$ of protein. At 15% of these calories, 1.5 $g \cdot kg^{-1}$ of protein would be provided daily. The key point is that the *total* caloric intake must be increased. If the total energy intake is insufficient, then the percentages allotted to protein may be inadequate. For example, if the athlete increased her caloric intake to only 1900 $kcal \cdot day^{-1}$ at 12% protein intake, this increase would amount to only 1 $g \cdot kg^{-1} \cdot day^{-1}$. Also, if the athlete increased her carbohydrate intake to 70%, she would need to carefully select the remaining 30% of her foodstuffs to get an adequate protein intake.

The problem of ingesting too few calories and thus ingesting inadequate protein is especially evident where the athlete is concerned with percentage of body fat or making weight. The problem is compounded if the individual is a child or adolescent. As previously mentioned, individuals in this age range need more protein than adults. Inadequate protein intake at this age might adversely affect not only exercise performance but also growth (Lemon, 1991;

Steen, 1994). Of course, if the extra protein ingested is also excess calories, weight and fat will be gained, and that also is not desirable. For the elderly, the interaction of protein need and exercise is unknown at the current time.

Before deciding to increase dietary protein, the individual's diet should undergo a complete nutritional analysis. It should not be assumed that because an individual falls in one of the categories of strength or endurance athlete, he or she needs additional dietary protein or a protein supplement (Lemon, 1991).

Can too much protein in the diet be harmful to the fitness participant or competitive athlete? In individuals with preexisting liver or kidney abnormalities, a high-protein diet can lead to further deterioration of function (American Dietetic Association, 1987; Lemon, 1989b). There is no evidence, though, that individuals with normal kidneys and livers are harmed from high-protein intake.

Two factors, however, require attention. The first is that the metabolism of protein requires more water than the metabolism of carbohydrate or fat does. Therefore, a concomitant increase in water intake is important for the individual to avoid dehydration if protein intake is increased. The second factor relates to calcium balance. There is evidence in sedentary individuals that increasing dietary protein levels leads to increased calcium excretion, suggesting a loss in bone calcium (Allen, et al., 1979; Lemon and Nagle, 1981). If dietary protein intake is excessive, the result could be an accelerated loss of bone density (see Chapter 18). Many female endurance athletes already exhibit a profile of low bone mineral density (and the possible causative factors of low estrogen and low dietary calcium intake) (Drinkwater, 1986). Whether exercise combined with a high-protein diet would exaggerate or protect against additional calcium loss has not been demonstrated experimentally. Until it is, the female endurance athlete should not conclude that if a high protein diet (12–15% as recommended) is good, then an even higher protein diet (greater than 15%) would be better.

Fat

As discussed earlier (Chapters 3 and 5), fat is a major fuel for exercises of low or moderate intensity, and it is readily available in more-than-adequate storage amounts in most individuals. In addition, studies have documented (Chapter 6) that with endurance training, more fat can be used as a fuel, hence sparing carbohydrate stores; and fat can be used at higher absolute levels of work intensity. The carbohydrate-loading studies described later in the section "Nutrition for Competition" have also shown that following

glycogen depletion a high-fat, low-carbohydrate diet results in a decrement in exercise performance (Bergstrom, et al., 1967).

In direct contrast to this last statement, however, are results from two types of studies. The first type has shown that both untrained obese individuals and well-trained athletes can adapt to a high-fat, low-carbohydrate diet and perform moderately intense (approximately 65% $\dot{V}O_2max$) exercise to exhaustion on a high-fat diet as well as they can when they ingest a normal amount of carbohydrates (Phinney, et al., 1983, 1980). This adaptation occurs within approximately 4 to 5 weeks and could be beneficial for continuous multiday ultraendurance events, such as the cycling Race Across America competition. However, even endurance athletes following this regimen show elevated cholesterol levels. Such a diet is neither prudent nor healthy. High-cholesterol levels are a risk factor for coronary artery disease.

The second type of study has shown that too little fat can cause a decrement in physiological and performance variables. Muoio, et al. (1994) studied six collegiate distance runners under three dietary conditions: their self-selected normal diet, which consisted of 61% CHO, 24% FAT, and 14% PRO; a high-fat diet of 50% CHO, 38% FAT, and 12% PRO; and a high-carbohydrate diet of 73% CHO, 15% FAT, and 12% PRO. Both $\dot{V}O_2max$ and running time to exhaustion were significantly higher following seven days on the high-fat diet than on either the high-carbohydrate or normal diets.

The explanation for these results is theoretically linked to intramuscular stores of triglycerides. Muscle triglycerides are significantly depleted during relatively high intensity submaximal exercise. If low concentrations of intramuscular triglycerides are present at the onset of such activity, there is a reduced availability of free fatty acid substrate for oxidative metabolism. To compensate for this an increased uptake of plasma free fatty acids would be necessary. The rate of exogenous free fatty acid delivery to the working muscle may not be sufficient to supply the needed substrate. Thus, just as glycogen can be depleted from muscle cells and bloodborne glucose not be sufficient to offset this depletion, so possibly can intramuscular free fatty acid depletion not be compensated for by bloodborne free fatty acid.

A low-fat, high-carbohydrate diet results in a reduced supply of intramuscular free fatty acid. However, because a diet that includes 38% fat, as in the study just cited, could represent a health hazard, this level is not recommended. Fat loading at the expense of carbohydrates should not be advised, but neither should any attempt be made to totally remove fat from the diet (Sherman and Leenders, 1995). The recommendation of between 20 and 30% fat for sedentary and moderately active individuals remains the best advice, but it may be that well-trained athletes doing endurance training should not drop below the 30% fat level in their diets. No more than 10% of the ingested fat should be saturated, regardless of activity level (Burke and Read, 1989; Leaf and Frisa, 1989). There is no gram per kilogram per day recommended daily allowance for fat for either sedentary or active individuals of any age or either sex, but, as indicated on Table 7.1, between 65 and 80 g per day are reasonable levels for a total caloric input of 2000–2500 kcal·day^{-1} (U.S. Dept. of Agriculture, Dietary Guidelines Advisory Committee, 1995).

Vitamins

Thirteen compounds are now considered to be vitamins. **Vitamins** are organic substances of plant or animal origin that are essential for normal growth, development, metabolic processes, and energy transformations. For example, vitamin B_6 is important in amino acid metabolism and the breakdown of glycogen to glucose; thiamin (B_1) is important in carbohydrate metabolism. Riboflavin (B_2) and niacin are important as the hydrogen carriers FAD and NAD, respectively. Ascorbic acid (vitamin C) is necessary for the formation of connective tissues and the catecholamines (important in the stress response) and maintenance of capillary walls. Vitamin E influences the flow of electrons within the mitochondrial respiratory chain (Belko, 1987; vander Beek, 1985, 1991).

There is some evidence to suggest that exercise training may cause an increased need for vitamin C (especially in hot climates), B complex vitamins (particularly B_6 and B_2, also especially in hot climates), and vitamin E at high altitudes and as antioxidant defense against free radicals (Belko, 1987; Blom, et al., 1987; vander Beek, 1985, 1991). These increased needs, as with the other nutrients, should be adequately covered if the exerciser concomitantly increases his or her total caloric intake with a balanced diet. The increased needs also mean that athletes who are concerned with restricting body weight or body fat or making weight (gymnasts, dancers, figure skaters, divers, wrestlers, boxers, jockeys) and hence restrict caloric intake could be at risk for an inadequate intake of vitamins. For these individuals a generic, one-a-day vitamin and mineral tablet might be appropriate to ensure adequate intake (Belko, 1987).

After almost 50 years of research there is no evidence that vitamin supplementation, in an adequately nourished individual, improves exercise or athletic performance, speeds up recovery, or decreases injuries (Belko, 1987; Haymes, 1983). Where deficiencies are present, supplementation to normal physiological levels can improve performance. This is another reason for a complete nutritional analysis for anyone training or competing. However, megadoses of vitamins are neither substitutes for vigorous training nor necessary for training adaptations (vander Beek, 1985, 1991). Furthermore, extremely large doses of vitamins (both water- and fat-soluble ones) can be toxic, can impair performance, and, more important, can cause health problems. Once again, if some is good, more is not necessarily better. For example, high doses of vitamin C have been linked with the formation of kidney stones and the breakdown of red blood cells, which causes a loss of hemoglobin. Megadoses of niacin inhibit fatty acid mobilization and utilization during exercise, thereby increasing the rate of glycogen usage (Nieman, 1990).

Minerals

Minerals are elements not of animal or plant origin that are essential constituents of all cells and of many functions in the body. Minerals are classified as microminerals (trace elements) or macrominerals on the basis of the amount contained in the body. Minerals are important in bone density, energy metabolism enzyme function, muscle contraction, oxygen transport, insulin regulation, and ATP composition, to name just a few functions.

Microminerals

Of the 14 essential microminerals, only five (zinc, chromium, copper, selenium, and iron) have been implicated as being affected by or potentially beneficial in enhancing exercise training and/or performance.

Exercise can cause a sizable loss of zinc in sweat and urine, and as a result, training may produce a zinc deficiency. However, excess zinc intake above the RDA (15 mg·day^{-1} for adult males, 12 mg·day^{-1} for adult females) can result in an impaired immune response and decreased iron and copper absorption. There is insufficient evidence to conclude that zinc status or zinc supplementation has any impact on exercise performance

---

Vitamins Organic substances of plant or animal origin that are essential for normal growth, development, metabolic processes, and energy transformations.

Minerals Elements not of animal or plant origin that are essential constituents of all cells and of many functions in the body.

(Campbell and Anderson, 1987; Clarkson, 1991b; Lemon, 1991, 1989b; McDonald and Keen, 1988).

There is speculation, but little evidence, that exercise and training may increase the requirements for chromium (50–200 μg·day^{-1}). Speculation that chromium can increase muscle mass and decrease the percentage of body fat in conjunction with resistance training remains just that—speculation (Lefavi, et al., 1992). Chromium supplementation (as chromium picolinate) has been shown in two studies to enhance lean body mass and in one study to decrease the percentage of body fat with weight training (Campbell and Anderson, 1987; Clarkson 1991a). A fourth study (Hasten, et al., 1992) using male and female college lifters, equally divided into two groups (those supplemented with chromium picolinate and those not), found the only treatment effect to be a greater gain in body weight in the female supplemented group without any concurrent gain in strength. Clearly, more research is needed in this area, including the safety of long-term chromium supplementation (Lefavi, et al., 1992).

There is no evidence that either selenium or copper has an impact on acute or chronic exercise responses, although copper may be lost in sweat. Neither of these trace minerals should be supplemented above the RDA (50–70 μg·day^{-1} for male adolescents and adults, 50–55 μg·day^{-1} for female adolescents and adults, for selenium; 1.5–3.0 mg for copper for everyone) (Campbell and Anderson, 1987; Clarkson, 1991b).

Iron deficiency can be a problem for the exercising or training individual, especially menstruating females. Iron deficiency exists in three stages: (1) iron depletion, or low-storage levels of iron; (2) iron deficiency erythropoiesis, which is an impairment of the ability to produce red blood cells; and (3) iron deficiency anemia, or low-hemoglobin levels (less than 12 g·dL^{-1} for females and less than 13 g·dL^{-1} for males). Iron depletion is not associated with a decrement in performance, and the impact of iron deficiency erythropoiesis is marginal. However, iron deficiency anemia definitely impairs performance. Lower-hemoglobin levels mean lower oxygen transport, lower–blood iron levels due to a low iron absorption, and increased iron excretion (some in sweat). An inadequate dietary intake of iron can compound the problem. Moderate levels of exercise do not appear to affect iron status.

Iron supplementation given to individuals with iron deficiency anemia consistently improves iron status and exercise performance. Iron supplementation given to individuals with iron depletion or iron deficiency erythropoiesis shows variable but primarily nonsignificant changes in performance. Excessive iron intake can inhibit zinc and copper absorption. The iron status of an individual should be ascertained before supplementation exceeding the RDA (18 mg for everyone over the age of 4 yr) is undertaken (American Dietetic Association, 1987; Clarkson, 1990; Haymes, 1983; McDonald and Keen, 1988).

Macrominerals

Macrominerals include calcium, chlorine, magnesium, phosphorus, potassium, sodium, and sulfur. As macromineral electrolytes, chlorine, magnesium, potassium, and sodium are discussed in the section "Fluid Ingestion During Exercise." Sulfur has no direct importance for exercise.

The function of calcium in bone health is directly related to exercise training and is fully described in Chapter 18. Beyond its role in bone health, the relationship between exercise, training, and calcium level and supplementation is largely unknown (Clarkson, 1991a).

Magnesium is lost in sweat and has been linked with aerobic capacity and with aldosterone and cortisol function during exercise. However, there is no evidence that supplemental magnesium increases performance. At the same time, levels above the RDA (400–350 mg·day^{-1} for adolescent and adult males, 300–280 mg·day^{-1} for adolescent and adult females) do not appear to be harmful (McDonald and Keen, 1988).

Several studies have shown that *phosphate loading*—increasing phosphate ingestion for several days prior to an event—may improve performance by delaying the onset of anaerobic metabolism; other studies have shown no beneficial effects. Because phosphorus supplementation over an extended period of time can result in lowered blood calcium levels, it is not recommended. The RDA for phosphorus is 1200 mg·day^{-1} for adolescent males and the DRI is 700 mg·day^{-1} for adult males and females (Clarkson, 1991a).

In summary, the pattern here is the same as the one for vitamins. The primary concern is that the exerciser ingest the RDA/DRI and, unless some deficiency has been diagnosed, only the RDA/DRI. For those who are strictly limiting their caloric intake, the combined generic, vitamin-and-mineral, one-a-day pill can be recommended.

Nutrition for Competition

The goals of an optimal competitive diet are

1. to ensure adequate fuel supplies in the pre-event time span;

2. to ensure adequate fuel supplies during the event, no matter what the duration;

3. to facilitate temperature regulation by preventing dehydration;

Table 7.6
Carbohydrate Loading

	Days Prior to Competition							Day of Competition
	−7	−6	−5	−4	−3	−2	−1	
Classic Technique								
Diet	Mixed diet 50% CHO	< 5% CHO or < 2 g CHO·kg^{-1}·day^{-1}	Continue from previous day	Continue from previous day	80–90% CHO > 10–12 g CHO·kg^{-1}·day^{-1}	Continue from previous day	Continue from previous day	High CHO pre-event meal Possible during-event CHO feeding
Exercise	Exercise to exhaustion	90–120 min 65–85% V̇O$_2$max	Continue from previous day	Continue from previous day or exercise to exhaustion	Rest	Rest	Rest	Continuous endurance event lasting 60–90 min, 65–85% V̇O$_2$max
Modified Technique								
Diet	50% CHO or 4.5 g CHO·kg^{-1}·day^{-1}	Continue from previous day	Continue from previous day	Continue from previous day	70% CHO or 8–10 g CHO·kg^{-1}·day^{-1}	Continue from previous day	Continue from previous day	High CHO pre-event meal Possible during-event CHO feeding
Exercise	90 min 75% V̇O$_2$max	Continue from previous day	40 min 75% V̇O$_2$max	Continue from previous day	20 min 75% V̇O$_2$max or 30–60 min 50–70% V̇O$_2$max	Continue from previous day	Rest	Continuous endurance event lasting 60–90 min, 65–85% V̇O$_2$max

4. to achieve desired weight classifications while maintaining fuel and water supplies; and

5. to avoid gastrointestinal discomfort during competition.

Depending on the event, precompetition dietary adjustment may be a matter of hours or days. Most manipulation centers around carbohydrate consumption (Burke and Read, 1989).

Carbohydrate Loading (Glycogen Supercompensation)

For individuals competing in continuous endurance events lasting at least 90 min at 65 to 85% V̇O$_2$max, **carbohydrate loading,** sometimes called **glycogen supercompensation,** may be utilized (American Dietetic Association, 1987; Brotherhood, 1984; Hawley, et al., 1997). Carbohydrate loading is a process of nutritional modification that results in an additional storage of glycogen in muscle fibers that can be approximately three to four times the normal level. As mentioned previously, the time to exhaustion in long-

duration relatively high intensity activities is linked to initial levels of muscle glycogen. Although a high starting level of muscle glycogen will not enable an athlete to perform at a higher intensity (run faster per mile), it will allow him or her to maintain a given pace for a longer period of time.

Table 7.6 presents two carbohydrate loading techniques. The first, labeled as the classic technique, is based on studies by Swedish investigators in the 1960s (Bergstrom, et al., 1967). This technique involves hard exercise to deplete muscle glycogen stores one week prior to the competitive event, followed by 3 days of hard training and 3 days of rest. During the first 3 days after the depletion run, the individual is supposed to eat almost no carbohydrates;

> **Carbohydrate Loading (Glycogen Supercompensation)** A process of nutritional modification that results in an additional storage of glycogen in muscle fiber that can be approximately three to four times the normal levels.

then for the next 3 days he or she eats almost exclusively carbohydrates.

This technique is effective but is not without its problems. The high-fat, high-protein ingestion after the exercise depletion phase is one problem. A diet with so little carbohydrate (less than 5%) means that an individual is ingesting high levels of fat, which is not healthy. Thus, this technique can cause high blood lipid levels. In addition, the ingested fat is incompletely metabolized, and high levels of ketones appear in the blood (ketosis) (Costill, 1988; Newsholme and Leech, 1983). Hypoglycemia (abnormally low blood glucose levels) can also occur, leading to fatigue, restlessness, mental disturbances, irritability, and weakness. At the very least, it is difficult, if not impossible, to maintain the hard training recommended during this phase. At the same time, the 80–90% carbohydrate diet for the 3 days prior to competition can leave the athlete feeling stiff and heavy owing to water retention. Since approximately 2.7 g of water are stored with each gram of glycogen, water retention can add approximately 1–2 kg to the body weight. It has been theorized that this water could be important in delaying or preventing dehydration, but it has not been shown to have any beneficial effect on body temperature regulation or dehydration. Thus an athlete who had trained for months for an event such as a marathon could find himself/herself down both psychologically and physiologically in the week prior to competition.

Subsequent research has shown that neither the exhaustive glycogen depletion exercise nor the 3 days of high-protein, high-fat diet are necessary to maximize muscle glycogen storage (Sherman, 1983, 1989). So, the modified carbohydrate-loading technique presented in Table 7.6 emphasizes a slow downward taper in duration and/or intensity of the training regimen. This taper is accompanied by an always average, but increasing, percentage of carbohydrates in the diet. An athlete already modifying his or her training diet to include high levels of carbohydrate will have very few changes to make.

The practice of carbohydrate loading does not appear in any way to adversely affect the normal healthy individual (American Dietetic Association, 1987; Goss and Karam, 1987; Sherman, 1983, 1989). Obviously, individuals with diabetes should consult with a physician before attempting carbohydrate loading. There is no evidence to support the suggestion that carbohydrate loading is effective only if not done more than once or twice a year. Supercompensation may actually be occurring daily in an athlete undergoing strenuous training and eating 70% carbohydrate.

While carbohydrate loading was and is intended for the endurance athlete, bodybuilders often follow a version of the modified carbohydrate-loading tech-

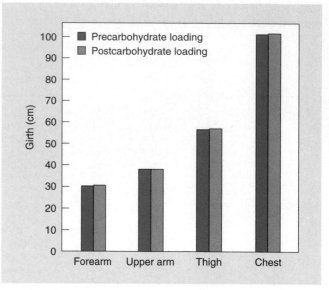

Figure 7.3

Girth Measurements in Bodybuilders with and without Carbohydrate Loading

Source: Based on data from Balon, et al. (1992).

nique (Kroculick, 1988). The primary difference is a restriction of water intake during the high carbohydrate ingestion phase. This water restriction has nothing to do with energy requirements during competition; it is based on the belief that water will then be sucked from beneath the skin for storage with glycogen and lead to an increase in muscle size and definition for competition. In addition, stored glycogen is said to result in a harder muscle. Evidence in support of this consequence is primarily anecdotal.

Results from the only available scientific study are presented in Figure 7.3. Nine male bodybuilders had girth measurements taken after a normal dietary routine (55% CHO, 15% PRO, and 30% FAT) and after a traditional carbohydrate loading regimen (3 days of 10% CHO, 33% PRO, and 57% FAT, followed by 3 days of 80% CHO, 15% PRO, and 5% FAT). Identical weight-lifting workouts were followed during both dietary manipulations and prior to girth measurement. The trials were randomized. No measurement of muscle definition was made, but as the figure shows, diet prior to testing had no effect on muscle girth measurements (Balon, et al., 1992).

Pre-Event Meal

Most road races and other endurance events, unless scheduled for the convenience of the television audience such as during the Olympics, take place in the morning. Competing after an overnight fast is probably not a good idea for an athlete in any sport, but

Focus on Application

✳ The Glycemic Index of Pre-Event Meals

The glycemic index of food ingested 30–60 min prior to exercise may impact the ensuing performance. A group of cyclists consumed (in random order) either a high–glycemic index meal (corn flakes, low-fat milk, banana), a low–glycemic index meal (All-Bran, low-fat yogurt, apple), or water 30 min prior to cycling 2 hr at 70% $\dot{V}O_2$max followed by cycling to exhaustion at 100% $\dot{V}O_2$max. Compared with the high–glycemic index meal, the low–glycemic index meal resulted in significantly lower plasma insulin levels during the first 20 min of exercise; significantly lower RER and RPE during the 2 hrs of cycling; and significantly higher plasma glucose levels at the end of the 2 hr of cycling. Time to exhaustion was 59% longer in the low–glycemic index trial than the high–glycemic index one, and 72% longer than the control ride (DeMarco, et al., 1999). Thus, recommending low– glycemic index pre-event meals, especially if the event is an endurance one that might require near maximal performance toward the end (such as sprinting or finishing uphill during a mountain bike race) would seem prudent. As always, individuals might respond differently to any given meal, so an athlete should experiment with any food combination before ingesting it prior to competition. ✳

Source:

DeMarco, et al., (1999).

it is most detrimental for the endurance athlete. Liver glycogen is the primary endogenous source of blood glucose, and an overnight fast reduces the liver's supply of glycogen. For this reason, approximately 50–100 g of carbohydrate should be included in the pre-event meal, with only enough fat and protein to ward off hunger pangs. A major question is the timing of this meal.

The ingestion of carbohydrate within one hour prior to exercise remains controversial. Theoretically, such a regimen should be detrimental to performance, for the following reasons. The ingestion of carbohydrate causes an increase in blood glucose. The increase of blood glucose causes a concomitant increase in insulin. Insulin favors the removal of blood glucose from the bloodstream, inhibits the release of glucose from the liver, and inhibits the mobilization of free fatty acids, which are used, along with carbohydrate, as fuel for exercise. These actions can cause hypoglycemia and may cause a greater dependency on muscle glycogen stores, depleting them at a faster rate.

Despite the popular acceptance of this reasoning, the research literature is far from conclusive (Burke and Read, 1989; Coyle, 1991). Eight studies conducted between 1979 and 1989 examined endurance performance following carbohydrate ingestion 1 hr or less (usually 30–45 min) before the exercise. One study reported a negative effect; four studies reported no significant effect, either positive or negative; and the other three reported improved performance. These results can be interpreted either as one against and three for or five against (one negative and four no difference) and three for carbohydrate feeding during this time frame. Other studies have shown that if the carbohydrate-feeding time is reduced to 5 min or less before the exercise, performance is improved.

The glucose or glycogen status of the individual prior to the feeding may be important in determining whether or not the response is beneficial (Clarkson, 1991b). Fasted individuals may be more sensitive to glucose ingestion within this time span than those who have been recently fed and had followed a carbohydrate-loading regimen. Alternatively, the glycemic index might be the key to unraveling the confusion. The Focus on Application box above provides evidence in support of the idea that a low–glycemic index, but not a high–moderate–glycemic index carbohydrate meal can be beneficial if ingested 30–60 min prior to exercise.

A much more substantial case can be made in favor of a pre-event meal 3–4 hr prior to competition (Burke and Read, 1989; Costill, 1988; Coyle, 1991). For example, when Neufer et al. (1987) fed subjects 200 g of cereal, bread, and fruit 4 hr prior to riding a cycle ergometer, an 11% increase in power performance occurred. When the same protocol was followed with the addition of a candy bar 5 min before the exercise, the improvement was 22%. On the basis of this study and others, a light meal of 200–500 kcal, including 50–100 g of carbohydrate and plenty of fluid, is recommended 3–4 hr prior to an endurance event, with the option of a last-minute snack. Table 7.7 summarizes this information. It is important that this meal consist of foods that the individual likes and tolerates well. The absence or presence of gastrointestinal distress can be the difference between a PR (personal record) or a DNF (did not finish). High levels of fructose ingestion as the sole carbohydrate source prior to exercise have been associated with gastrointestinal distress and thus should be avoided.

Table 7.7
Recommended Eating on Game Day

Sport	−3 to −4 hr	−2 hr	−5–0 min	Event Begins	+15–30 min Repeated for Duration of Event	Recovery (+15–30 min past)
Nonendurance	Light balanced meal of high % CHO Fluid ingestion	Fluid ingestion 400–600 mL	—	—	Water as desired	Fluid ingestion
Endurance	200–500-kcal meal with 50–100 g CHO Fluid ingestion	Fluid ingestion 400–600 mL	CHO approximately 50 g (optional)		Fluid ingestion CHO (optional): 200–400 mL 30–60 g·hr^{-1} Some Na	Fluid ingestion 50–100 g CHO Some Na

Feeding during Exercise

When exercise begins, insulin release is suppressed, and catecholamine secretion is increased. Thus, the potentially detrimental changes associated with carbohydrate ingestion are no longer of concern. Indeed, both theoretically and experimentally, there is support for the ingestion of carbohydrates once the activity begins. Even small amounts of carbohydrates (about 25 g·hr^{-1}) taken at 15–30 min intervals have been found to prevent a decline in blood glucose and delay fatigue during the latter portion of an endurance event longer than 1 hr. Note that fatigue can be caused by many factors, and carbohydrate feeding merely delays but does not prevent fatigue.

Carbohydrate feedings during intermittent exercise such as soccer or basketball have also been shown to be beneficial (Burke and Read, 1989; Costill, 1988; Coyle, 1991). Oranges at half time may thus be more than a simple tradition, although modern-day carbohydrate beverages are probably more convenient. In addition, carbohydrates move through the stomach rapidly and are less likely than other nutrients to cause gastrointestinal and abdominal disturbances (Burke and Read, 1989; Coyle, 1991). The recommendation is to take in approximately 30–60 g of carbohydrates each hour, beginning early in the exercise. As noted, this can be accomplished at the same time as fluid replenishment.

No differences have been found when glucose, fructose, sucrose, or glucose polymer solutions (maltodextrins) have been compared in terms of rate of gastric emptying or impact on performance. Glucose, sucrose, and glucose polymers stimulate fluid absorption in the stomach, but fructose does not (Coleman, 1988). As for preexercise conditions, fructose ingestion (as the only carbohydrate source) during exercise

has been associated with gastrointestinal distress and is not associated with performance improvement.

Research supports the position that beverages containing 2.5–10% carbohydrate are absorbed by the body as rapidly as water. A concentration of 4–8% is thought to be optimal (American College of Sports Medicine [ACSM], 1996). Drinks containing less than 5% carbohydrate do not provide enough energy to enhance performance, and drinks that exceed 10% carbohydrate (such as soda pop) are often detrimental since they tend to cause abdominal cramps, nausea, and diarrhea (Coleman, 1988).

In general, high–glycemic index foods should be ingested during exercise. They are rapidly digested and absorbed and are thus likely to maintain blood glucose levels. Low–glycemic index carbohydrates are digested more slowly and thus may both cause gastric distress and fail to maintain blood glucose levels (Walton and Rhodes, 1997). One high-carbohydrate energy bar, 24 ounces of sports drink, and two packets of gel are equivalent. Any of these can provide the 30–60 g of carbohydrate recommended per hour of endurance exercise.

Fluid Ingestion during and after Exercise

As previously discussed (Chapter 5) the human body is only about 20–45% efficient, depending on how efficiency is calculated. The energy output that is not utilized as work appears as heat. Normal resting body temperature is in the range of 36.1–37.8°C. Thermal balance in this range is maintained by summing the factors of metabolic heat production, radiant heat exchange, conductive heat exchange, convective heat exchange, and evaporation (Chapter 15) (Haymes and Wells, 1986).

In cool, dry weather heat generated by moderate exercise can be dissipated by radiation and convection. In moderately warm, dry weather, radiation and convection decrease, and sweating must be utilized. In hot weather, when the skin and environmental temperatures are nearly the same, radiation and convection cannot contribute to heat loss (and, indeed, may contribute to heat gain if the ambient temperature is higher), so evaporation alone can dissipate heat. The evaporative heat loss depends on environmental conditions (percentage of relative humidity and air movement), the rate of sweat secretion, and the electrolyte concentration of the sweat. The evaporation of 1 g of water from the skin surface removes slightly less than 0.6 kcal of heat (Nadel, 1988).

During heavy exercise, metabolic heat production can increase in active muscles 100 times that of inactive muscle. If this heat is not dissipated, the internal temperature will rise 1°C every 5–8 min, resulting in overheating (hyperthermia) and collapse of the individual within 15–20 min. Thus, sweating under these conditions is absolutely essential (Nadel, 1988). However, sweating does not occur without a price, and that price is the removal of fluid from the body (Maughan, 1991). A 70-kg, 2:30 marathoner can lose 5 L of body water, or 1–2 $L \cdot hr^{-1}$. Sweat, of course, is not pure water; it includes the electrolytes sodium (Na^+), chloride (Cl^-), and potassium (K^+) and traces of amino acids, bicarbonate (HCO_3^-), carbon dioxide (CO_2), copper, glucose, hormones, iron, lactic acid, magnesium (Mg^+), nitrogen (N), phosphates (PO_4^{-2}), urea, vitamins, and zinc (Murray, 1987). The exact proportion of these elements in sweat varies among individuals and within the same individual under different conditions (Haymes and Wells, 1986).

Although shifting occurs in the internal water compartments to provide the liquid portion of sweat, ultimately much of the water lost through sweating comes from blood plasma. If this water is not replaced, the individual may perform poorly and suffer from heat injuries (Chapter 15).

To avoid dehydration, adequate, and often forced, fluid intake is necessary (American Dietetic Association, 1987; Nieman, 1990). Thirst is an inadequate guide to the amount of water needed. Whether to supplement with plain water or a carbohydrate and/or electrolyte beverage (sports drink) is a matter of much debate. For the vast majority of sports or fitness workouts, plain water is the beverage of choice. Again, however, endurance events may be the exception (American Dietetic Association, 1987).

The rate at which an ingested fluid actually enters the body's water supply depends upon the rate at which it leaves the stomach (called *gastric emptying*) and the rate at which it is absorbed across the intestinal membrane (*intestinal absorption*). Both gastric emptying and intestinal absorption are influenced by the composition of the ingested fluid.

Three factors need to be considered for gastric emptying. First, the gastric-emptying rate decreases as the caloric content of the ingested fluid increases. However, the differences in the gastric-emptying rate of solutions between 2.5 and 10% carbohydrate are negligible between each other and compared to plain water (Coleman, 1988; Maughan, 1991). Second, the rate of gastric emptying is exponentially related to the volume of fluid in the stomach (Maughan, 1991; Murray, 1987). That is, the amount of beverage emptied from the stomach is relatively large in the first minutes and then the rate slows down. Therefore, frequent ingestion of small amounts of fluid is preferable to the reverse. Thus, 200–400 mL of fluid should be ingested every 15–30 min, because approximately 400 mL can be cleared in 15 min (American Dietetic Association, 1987; Nieman, 1990). Third, the temperature of the fluid may be important. It has typically been suggested that any sports drink that is ingested should be cold to enhance gastric emptying. Recent evidence suggests, though, that the gastric-emptying rates of hot and cold beverages are the same (Maughan, 1991). The real advantage of a cold drink may simply be that it tastes better to a hot, sweaty athlete, thereby encouraging more drinking. Of course, a cold fluid also does not add heat to the body, which a hot fluid would. Fluid temperatures between 15 to 22°C (59–72°F) are recommended (ACSM, 1996).

Intestinal absorption is not influenced by as many factors as gastric emptying is. However, research has shown that the presence of glucose and sodium greatly increases intestinal fluid absorption over plain water. Thus, small percentages of glucose do not inhibit gastric emptying and will enhance intestinal absorption if accompanied by sodium.

In those situations where fluid replacement is more important than energy substrate supplementation (such as in a relatively short endurance event of 1–2 hr or an activity in high heat and humidity), the carbohydrate concentration should be low (2.5–8%) and the sodium content moderately high (30–110 mg). Although this may sound like a lot, it is not. An 8-oz glass of 2% milk or tomato juice contains over 100 mg of sodium. The sodium is generally in the form of sodium chloride (common table salt). Conversely, in those situations where substrate provision is more important than fluid replacement (a long endurance event of over 2 hr in temperate environmental conditions), a more concentrated carbohydrate solution (6–10%) with sodium should be ingested (Maughan, 1991; Murray, 1987).

If large quantities of plain water are ingested in events lasting longer than 4 hr, hyponatremia (low sodium, sometimes called "water intoxication") may occur. Hyponatremia is a serious condition that not only affects performance but also can lead to brain damage and death. Thus, in ultraendurance events athletes are urged to drink electrolyte beverages. Conversely, there is no advantage to drinking beverages of any composition but water in activities lasting less than 30 min (Brouns, 1991; Maughan, 1991; Murray, 1987).

Although it has been claimed that electrolytes make sports drinks more palatable and hence encourage drinking, the available evidence indicates that sodium, as mentioned earlier, is the only electrolyte that is physiologically beneficial when consumed during exercise (Maughan, 1991; Murray, 1987). Evidence does not indicate that matching the content of sweat—even if this were possible, considering its extreme variability—is necessary (Haymes and Wells, 1986). Despite the great amount of attention given to it, potassium loss in sweat is low and of little consequence during exercise. The general consensus is that electrolyte losses will be replaced through normal food intake after exercise. An exception again may be sodium. Sodium appears to be important in postexercise beverages for reasons other than intestinal absorption. In the postexercise period, if drinks with little or no sodium are ingested, the plasma becomes diluted, stimulating urine production and fluid excretion. This also shuts off the thirst drive and rehydration is delayed (ACSM, 1996; Maughan, 1991; Nose, et al., 1988). Once again, however, if some is good, more is not better. Salt tablets should never be ingested (Steen, 1994). Such highly concentrated amounts of salt can lead to gastrointestinal discomfort, dehydration, and electrolyte loss (Steen, 1994).

Because most commercially available sports drinks (Table 7.2) do contain varying amounts of electrolytes other than sodium, it must be asked whether

---

Anorexia Nervosa An eating disorder characterized by marked self-induced weight loss accompanied by reproductive hormonal changes and an intense fear of fatness.

Bulimia Nervosa An eating disorder marked by an unrealistic appraisal of body weight and/or shape that is manifested by alternating bingeing and purging behavior.

Anorexia Athletica An eating disorder occurring primarily in young, female athletes that is characterized by a food intake less than that required to support the training regimen and by body weight no more than 95% of normal.

A Question of Understanding

On the basis of the composition of the selected sports drinks given in Table 7.2 and from the text discussion, group the sports drinks into the indicated categories for a serious, but not world-class, marathoner (2:45–3:45). Support your groupings scientifically. Check your classifications against the answer in Appendix D.

1. Training replenishment and carbohydrate loading

   Drink   *Support*

2. Pre-event meal

   Drink   *Support*

3. During training runs and competition

   Drink   *Support*

---

these inclusions are harmful. A qualified no is the answer. There have been no cases of problems arising from the ingestion of commercial sports drinks reported in the literature (Nose, et al., 1988). One can only assume, given the ongoing debate about such products, that such occurrences would have been publicized had they occurred.

Do the problem outlined in the Question of Understanding box above to put together a package of fluids for ingestion by the indicated athlete.

Eating Disorders

Whereas most individuals participating in fitness programs or athletics see nutrition as a partner with exercise to help them achieve their goals of health or successful competition, a few have a distorted view of food and develop eating disorders. Of course, eating disorders are not limited to physically active individuals, but symptoms of eating disorders are more prevalent among athletes than nonathletes, and there is also cause for concern about fitness instructors, including personal trainers (Thompson and Sherman, 1993). The problem occurs much more frequently in females than males, and typically has its onset after menarche but prior to age 30. Males are likely to have actually been overweight or obese before their eating disorder, whereas females simply perceived themselves as such (Sundgot-Borgen, 1994a, 1993b; Thompson and Sherman, 1993).

Three types of eating disorders are of greatest concern for individuals working with active individuals: anorexia nervosa (AN), bulimia nervosa (BN), and anorexia athletica (AA). **Anorexia nervosa,** often referred to as the *self-starvation syndrome,* is

Table 7.8
Diagnostic Criteria for Selected Eating Disorders

Anorexia Nervosa	Bulimia Nervosa	Anorexia Athletica
Refusal to maintain body weight above that considered normal for height and age; marked self-induced weight loss	Recurrent episodes of binge eating (rapid consumption of large quantities of calorie-dense food, often secretly)	Weight loss (> 5% below normal for age and height)*
Intense fear of weight gain or becoming fat despite being underweight	Purging or compensating for bingeing by self-induced vomiting, use of diuretics or laxatives, vigorous exercise, and strict food restriction or fasting	Absence of medical disorder to explain weight loss*
Endocrine changes manifested by amenorrhea (for at least three consecutive cycles) in females and loss of sexual interest and potency in males	Exhibiting bingeing or inappropriate compensatory behavior at least twice a week for three months	Excess fear of becoming fat*
	Unrealistic appraisal of body weight and shape	Food intake < 1200 kcal·day^{-1}
		Delayed puberty
		Primary or secondary amenorrhea or oligomenorrhea
		Binge eating that is not high in calories
		Purging
		Gastrointestinal complaints
		Distorted body image
		Compulsive exercise in addition to normal needed training

* Absolute criteria; others may or may not be present.

Sources: Based on American Psychiatric Association (1994); Sundgot-Borgen (1994a, 1994b).

characterized by marked self-induced weight loss accompanied by reproductive hormonal changes and an intense fear of fatness. **Bulimia nervosa** is marked by an unrealistic appraisal of body weight and/or shape and is manifested by alternating bingeing and purging behavior. **Anorexia athletica,** occurring primarily in young female athletes, is characterized by a food intake that is less than that required to support the training regimen and body weight at least 5% below normal. The precise criteria for each are included in Table 7.8. Both anorexia nervosa and bulimia nervosa are among the eating disorders recognized by the American Psychiatric Association (1994). Anorexia athletica is characterized by elements of both of the other two disorders, and individuals suffering from anorexia athletica may exhibit a variety of symptoms (Sundgot-Borgen, 1994a, 1994b).

The specific causes of eating disorders are unknown (Sundgot-Borgen, 1994a, 1994b). Psychological, genetic-biological, and sociocultural factors have been implicated but not proven. Individuals who are conscientious and achievement-oriented, who seek perfection, but who, at the same time, have a low self-esteem and a high need for approval seem to have a psychological predisposition for an eating disorder. Eating disorders also appear to run in families and are more strongly associated in identical than fraternal twins. By the same token, our cultural obsession with thinness may be considered a social predisposi-

tion, although why some young girls succumb to the pressure but most don't is unknown (Leon, 1991; Sundgot-Borgen, 1994a). The sport/fitness environment emphasizes performance and often demands, in fact or perception, an ideal body size, shape, weight, or composition, both as a means to achieving high performance and, in the aesthetic sports, as a major part of the performance itself (Thompson and Sherman, 1993). Once an individual with a substantial predisposition begins a very restrictive diet, a cycling, self-perpetuating, self-reinforcing process begins; and the individual develops an eating disorder.

Sundgot-Borgen (1994b) identified a series of risk factors or trigger conditions for eating disorders. These results were obtained from a study that tested 522 elite female Norwegian athletes (out of a possible 603 in the entire country). Ninety-two athletes (17%) were found to have AN (N = 7), BN (N = 43), or AA (N = 42). The six risk factors included:

1. *Dieting at an early age.* Dieting is a risk factor, especially if recommended by a coach who indicates that losing weight or fat would enable the athlete to improve her performance. Thus, the fact that athletes in weight-dependent sports (judo, karate) and aesthetic sports (gymnastics, diving, figure skating, dancing) have the highest incidence of eating disorders is not unexpected (Sundgot-Borgen, 1993a).

2. *Unsupervised dieting.* Athletes are rarely given guidance by someone trained in nutrition and knowledgeable about their sports' requirements. Those who are given such assistance often don't follow the good advice.

3. *Lack of acceptance of pubertal changes.* Young female athletes are often distressed at the bodily changes that occur as they mature—particularly menarche and the increasing levels of body fat. Many young athletes are also aware that a delayed menarche is often associated with athletic success (see Chapter 20).

4. *Early sport-specific training.* An individual's somatotype (body type) has a great influence on which sports she can successfully compete in. If this influence is disregarded, a young child may select a sport she enjoys (such as gymnastics) only to find that her body outgrows it. Being a generalist as a child allows more options later—although realistically, that becomes harder to do if one wishes to compete on the international level.

5. *A large increase in training volume accompanied by a significant weight loss.* Athletes do not always spontaneously increase energy intake when the energy expenditure increases. The weight loss is viewed as being good, and there is no incentive to eat more. Thus, the vicious cycle is in place.

6. *Traumatic events.* A traumatic event can be anything, but it is often associated with an illness or injury that prevents training (and increases the fear of gaining weight) and/or the loss of a coach who the athlete often sees as being vital to her career.

The consequences of an eating disorder can be dire. At the very least, the individual's nutritional status is compromised. Figure 7.4 shows a representative sample of nutrient intake in the Norwegian study of elite women athletes previously mentioned (Sundgot-Borgen, 1993a). The control group (labeled C) consisted of 30 athletes not classified as being at risk for developing an eating disorder. However, 27% of those athletes were on a diet. Except for the bulimic group, all other groups had a lower total energy intake than recommended. The bulimic group also had a diet that differed in composition from that of the other groups. They ate more fat (30% versus 20%) and less protein (10% versus 20%) than the other groups but an equal amount of carbohydrates as the other groups. Despite the equality of percentage of carbohydrates, only the bulimic group was taking in sufficient amounts of carbohydrates in grams per kilogram per day. Those with anorexia nervosa showed the greatest nutritional disturbance. They were simply not ingesting enough of anything.

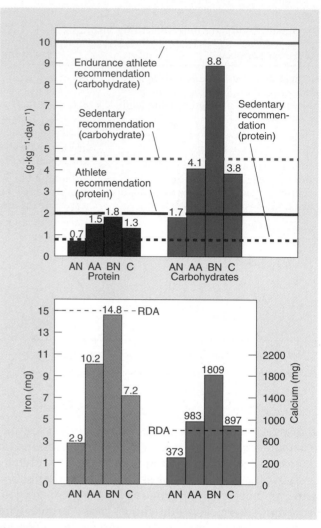

Figure 7.4
Nutrient Intake in Elite Norwegian Female Athletes

AN = anorexia nervosa (N = 7); AA = anorexia athletica (N = 43); BN = bulimia nervosa (N = 92); C = control (N = 30).

Source: Based on data from Sundgot-Borgen (1993a).

Although the bulimic group appears to be getting sufficient nutrients in terms of carbohydrates, protein, calcium, and iron, note that these values are pre-purging intakes. The majority of the bulimia nervosa group and one-third of the anorexia athletica group vomited within 15 min of eating on a regular basis. Thus, the nutrients were ingested, but they were not absorbed. Individuals who purge by the use of diuretics or laxatives, in contrast, have minimal caloric loss; but they do lose electrolytes and can become dehydrated.

The loss of electrolytes, especially potassium, can have serious cardiac implications, whereas lack of fluid impacts blood pressure levels. Extensive hormonal changes, gastrointestinal complications, skin and hair problems, anemia, disordered thermoregulation, and dental abnormalities are just a few of the other medical problems associated with eating disorders. At times, these medical complications are severe enough to cause death (Brownell, et al., 1992).

As a coach, physical educator, or exercise leader, your role is to be part of the solution, not part of the problem. To this end it is important to adhere to the following:

1. Encourage youngsters to try a variety of sports. As much as possible, try to guide them into more than one sport experience where they can potentially be successful.

2. Identify realistic, healthy weight goals appropriate for each youngster's stage of maturation. If weight goals are called for at all, provide target weight ranges that allow for growth and development. Allow for individual differences. Male coaches, in particular, must accept that females naturally have a higher percentage of body fat than males, even when both sexes train equally (Thompson and Sherman, 1993).

3. Monitor weight and body composition privately to avoid competition and possible embarrassment. Do not post weights. Avoid all derogatory or teasing remarks about body size, shape, or weight. Coaches should not be directly involved in any decision regarding weight or in actually weighing athletes (Thompson and Sherman, 1993).

4. Monitor weight and body composition to detect continued and unwarranted weight losses, or weight and fat fluctuations, without always equating weight loss as a positive outcome.

5. Provide proper nutritional guidance—if need be, in conjunction with a nutritionist—and emphasize nutrition for performance, not weight and fat control.

6. Provide a realistic, progressive training program to which the student, athlete, or fitness participant can gradually adjust both in terms of energy input and energy output.

7. Provide a realistic, progressive training program to avoid overtraining, illnesses, and injuries.

8. Monitor the relationship between any weight loss and performance. In the early stages of an eating disorder, performance may improve, which, in turn, can spur the individual on to greater weight loss. However, sooner or later performance will decline owing to malnutrition, depletion of glycogen stores, associated health problems, and the loss of fluid and muscle mass with concomitant decreases in muscular endurance, strength, speed, and coordination.

9. Provide an atmosphere that is supportive of pubertal changes and accept them so that young participants will see them in a positive light.

10. Provide an atmosphere that values the individual and his or her health and well-being above athletic performance or appearance.

11. Be aware of symptoms of eating disorders. However, do not assume that merely educating individuals about eating disorders will be enough to prevent or cure them. Precisely the opposite can occur (Thompson and Sherman, 1993).

12. Seek professional help in dealing with any individual you suspect of having an eating disorder. The first response to being questioned is often denial. Do not delay. The sooner treatment is started, the better the chances are for a full recovery (Steen, 1994).

13. Never allow treatment to become secondary to an individual's participation in sports or fitness activities.

Summary

1. There are five goals in an optimal training diet:
   a. to provide caloric and nutrient requirements;
   b. to incorporate nutritional practices that promote good health;
   c. to achieve and maintain optimal body composition and playing weight;
   d. to promote recovery from training sessions and for physiological adaptations; and
   e. to try variations of precompetition and competition fuel and fluid intake to determine bodily responses.

2. A balanced nutritional diet composed of sufficient calories to maintain acceptable body weight and composition, with 12–15% protein, 30% fat, 55–58% carbohydrate, the RDA for vitamins and minerals, and sufficient fluid for hydration, is adequate and probably optimal for all but hard-training elite, competitive athletes.

3. Active individuals who are satisfied with their body weight and composition must ingest sufficient calories to balance those expended. This should proportionally increase nutrient intake.

4. For an individual utilizing high levels of carbohydrates in training, $8–10 \text{ g·kg}^{-1}\text{·day}^{-1}$ are recommended. This value may increase the intake to 70–80% carbohydrate.

5. Carbohydrate ingestion should begin as soon after activity as possible to restore glycogen storage

in the muscle. It should consist primarily of high– and moderate–glycemic index foods. Low–glycemic index foods do not induce adequate muscle glycogen resynthesis.

6. Excessive carbohydrate intake in individuals not training heavily in endurance activity can lead to elevated levels of blood lipids.

7. Strength, speed, and ultraendurance athletes may need to consume 1.2–2 $g \cdot kg^{-1} \cdot day^{-1}$ of protein, up from the RDA of 0.8 $g \cdot kg^{-1} \cdot day^{-1}$ for sedentary adults. This increased intake should not exceed 15% of the total caloric intake.

8. Excessive protein intake leads to calcium excretion, which may in turn lead to accelerated problems of osteoporosis in young amenorrheic female athletes.

9. Although endurance athletes can adapt to burning high amounts of fat as fuel, high levels of cholesterol also result from a high-fat diet. Therefore, fats should be maintained at no more than 30% of the calories ingested.

10. Vitamins are important in the production of energy. However, there is no evidence that vitamin supplementation in an adequately nourished individual improves performance, speeds up recovery, or reduces injuries. Where deficiencies are present, supplementation to normal physiological levels can improve performance.

11. Excessive levels of vitamins can be toxic.

12. There is insufficient evidence to conclude that supplementation of zinc, chromium, selenium, copper, iron, or any other micronutrient above normal levels has any impact on exercise performance. Iron supplementation given to individuals with iron deficiency anemia consistently improves performance, but supplementation should not be done unless needed clinically.

13. Excessive, unnecessary iron intake can inhibit zinc and copper absorption.

14. There is no evidence that supplementation of the macrominerals calcium and magnesium increases exercise performance. Phosphate loading may delay the onset of anaerobic metabolism effects.

15. Phosphate supplementation over an extended period of time can result in lowered blood calcium levels.

16. Nutritional analysis should always precede any supplementation to determine need and safety.

17. There are five goals of an optimal competitive diet:
   a. to ensure adequate fuel supplies in the pre-event time span;
   b. to ensure adequate supplies during the event;
   c. to facilitate temperature regulation by prevention of dehydration;
   d. to achieve desired weight classifications while maintaining fuel and water supplies; and
   e. to avoid gastrointestinal discomfort during competition.

18. Carbohydrate loading is beneficial only for individuals competing in endurance events of at least 60–90 min at 65–85% $\dot{V}O_2$max.

19. The modified carbohydrate-loading technique in which an individual increases the percentage of carbohydrate ingested from 50 to 70% while gradually tapering training the week before competition is the recommended procedure.

20. A light meal composed primarily of carbohydrate and accompanied by fluids is recommended 3–4 hr prior to competition. Fluid should continue to be ingested right up to the time of the event. Carbohydrate ingested 30–60 min before an event should consist of low–glycemic index foods.

21. Carbohydrate beverages ingested in small amounts (200–400 mL) at 15–30-min intervals during endurance activity can prevent a decline in glucose and delay fatigue. Beverages containing 4 to 8% carbohydrate are recommended for optimal benefit. All carbohydrates ingested during an event should be high–glycemic index foods.

22. Thirst is not an adequate guide to the amount of fluid needed during activity. Plain water may be sufficient except in endurance events (over 4 hr), where a sport beverage is recommended.

23. Electrolyte losses are usually replaced through normal food intake after exercise. However, sodium in a postexercise beverage may help with fluid retention.

24. Three types of eating disorders are of great concern for personnel working with active individuals: anorexia nervosa, bulimia nervosa, and anorexia athletica. Although there are technical differences among the three disorders, all involve a restriction of food intake or a purging of food ingested in a binge, a desire for more and more weight loss, and a denial of having a problem.

25. The exact cause of eating disorders is unknown. More athletes than nonathletes suffer from eating

disorders, and most cases occur in weight-dependent or aesthetic sports. Far more females than males have eating disorders.

26. Personnel working with active individuals between the ages of 10 and 25 should be aware of and try to avoid situations that might trigger an eating disorder.

Review Questions

1. List the goals for nutrition during training and the goals for nutrition during competition. Explain why they are different.

2. Prepare a table comparing a balanced diet for a sedentary individual and one for an active individual. Include caloric intake, percentages, and grams per kilogram per day recommendations for the major nutrients, as well as similarities or differences in vitamin, mineral, and fluid ingestion.

3. Discuss the positive and negative aspects of a high-carbohydrate diet.

4. Define the glycemic index, and describe how foods are divided into high, moderate, and low categories. Using the glycemic index, develop a post-Century bike ride (100 mi) snack to be eaten approximately 30 min after the ride, and develop a snack to be eaten during a day of hiking on the Appalachian Trail. Explain your choices.

5. Discuss the situations in which an increase in protein above the RDA is advisable and situations in which such an increase is not advisable.

6. Describe a training situation and the theory behind when fat intake can be too low.

7. Compare the theory behind the use of carbohydrate loading for endurance athletes with the theory behind the use of carbohydrate loading for bodybuilders.

8. Compare the classic and the modified techniques of carbohydrate loading in terms of diet and exercise for endurance athletes. Explain the reasons for the modifications.

9. Prepare a table of a comprehensive fluid and nutrient intake for pre-event, during-the-event, and postevent diets for a football player and a triathlete.

10. Define and list the characteristics of anorexia nervosa, bulimia nervosa, and anorexia athletica.

11. Identify the risk factors for developing an eating disorder. Prepare a set of guidelines that

might be useful in counteracting these risk factors or dealing with the disorder early in its progression.

For further review and additional study tools, go to The Physiology Place (www.physiologyplace.com) and the Student Study Guide for Exercise Physiology for Health, Fitness, and Performance *by Sharon A. Plowman and Denise L. Smith.*

Passport to the Internet

Visit the following Internet sites to explore further topics and issues related to nutrition and exercise. To visit an organization's web site, go to www.physiologyplace.com, and click on "Passport to the Internet."

U.S. Department of Agriculture Food and Nutrition Information Center   The Food and Nutrition Information Center (FNIC) is one of several information centers available from the Department of Agriculture's Research Services. The site contains a depth of information about nutrition, including a special section on dietary supplements.

National Women's Health Information Center   The National Women's Health Information Center (NWHIC) is a service of the Office of Women's Health in the Department of Health and Human Services. This special site provides a vast array of information on women's health issues. Go to www.4women.gov/owh/pub/eatingdis.htm to read a detailed report on eating disorders and their complications for females and males.

Gatorade Sports Science Institute   Check out the Gatorade Sports Science Institute, a research and educational facility established to share current information and expand knowledge on sports nutrition and exercise science to enhance the performance and well-being of athletes.

References

Allen, L. H., E. A. Oddoye, & S. Margen: Protein-induced hypercalciuria: A longer term study. *American Journal of Clinical Nutrition.* (32):741–749 (1979).

American College of Sports Medicine: Position stand: Exercise and fluid replacement. *Medicine and Science in Sports and Exercise.* 28(1):i–vii (1996).

American Dietetic Association: Nutrition for physical fitness and athletic performance for adults: Technical support paper. *Journal of the American Dietetic Association.* 87(7):934–939 (1987).

American Psychiatric Association: *Diagnostic and Statistical Manual of Mental Disorders* (4th edition). Washington, DC: American Psychiatric Association (1994).

Applegate, L.: Drinks to your health. *Runner's World.* 26(7):24–26 (1991).

Applegate, L.: Taking the bar. *Runner's World.* 33(10):24–28 (1998).

Applegate, L.: The pyramid plan. *Runner's World.* 35(3):20 (2000).

Balon, T. W., J. F. Horowitz, & K. M. Fitzsimmons: Effects of carbohydrate loading and weight-lifting on muscle girth. *International Journal of Sports Nutrition.* 2(4):328–334 (1992).

Belko, A. Z.: Vitamins and exercise—an update. *Medicine and Science in Sports and Exercise.* (Suppl.). 19(5): S191–S196 (1987).

Bergstrom, J., L. Hermansen, E. Hultman, & B. Saltin: Diet, muscle glycogen and physical performance. *Acta Physiologica Scandinavica.* 7:140–150 (1967).

Blom, P. C. S., A. T. Hostmark, O. Vaage, K. R. Kardel, & S. Maehlum: Effects of different post-exercise sugar diets on the rate of muscle glycogen synthesis. *Medicine and Science in Sports and Exercise.* 19(5):491–496 (1987).

Brotherhood, J. R.: Nutrition and sports performance. *Sports Medicine.* 1:350–389 (1984).

Brouns, F.: Heat-sweat-dehydration-rehydration: A praxis oriented approach. *Journal of Sports Sciences.* 9:143–152 (1991).

Brownell, K. D., J. Rodin, & J. H. Wilmore: *Eating, Body Weight and Performance in Athletics: Disorders of Modern Society.* Philadelphia: Lea & Febiger (1992).

Burke, L. M., & R. S. D. Read: Sport nutrition: Approaching the nineties. *Sports Medicine.* 8(2):80–100 (1989).

Burke, L. M., G. R. Collier, & M. Hargreaves: Muscle glycogen storage after prolonged exercise: Effect of the glycemic index of carbohydrate feedings. *Journal of Applied Physiology.* 75(2):1019–1023 (1993).

Campbell, W. W., & R. A. Anderson: Effects of aerobic exercise and training on the trace minerals chromium, zinc and copper. *Sports Medicine.* 4:9–18 (1987).

Cheuvront, S. N.: The Zone diet and athletic performance. *Sports Medicine.* 27(4):213–228 (1999).

Clarkson, P. M.: Minerals: Exercise performance and supplementation in athletes. *Journal of Sports Sciences.* 9:91–116 (1991a).

Clarkson, P. M.: *Tired Blood: Iron Deficiency in Athletes and Effects of Iron Supplementation.* Sports Science Exchange, vol. 3, no. 28. Chicago: Gatorade Sports Science Institute (1990).

Clarkson, P. M.: *Trace Mineral Requirements for Athletes: To Supplement or Not to Supplement.* Sports Science Exchange, vol. 4, no. 33. Chicago: Gatorade Sports Science Institute (1991b).

Coleman, E.: *Sports Drink Update.* Sports Science Exchange, vol. 1, no. 5. Chicago: Gatorade Sports Science Institute (1988).

Coombes, J. S., & K. L. Hamilton: The effectiveness of commercially available sports drinks. *Sports Medicine.* 29(3): 181–209 (2000).

Costill, D. L.: Carbohydrates for exercise: Dietary demands for optimal performance. *International Journal of Sports Medicine.* 9(1):1–18 (1988).

Coyle, E. F.: Timing and method of increased carbohydrate intake to cope with heavy training, competition and recovery. *Journal of Sport Sciences.* (9):29–52 (1991).

Coyle, E. F., & E. Coyle: Carbohydrates that speed recovery from training. *The Physician and Sportsmedicine.* 21(2):111–123 (1993).

DeMarco, H. D., K. P. Sucher, C. J. Cisar, & G. E. Butterfield: Pre-exercise carbohydrate meals: Application of the glycemic index. *Medicine and Science in Exercise and Sports.* 31(1): 164–170 (1999).

Drinkwater, B. L.: Relationship between altered reproductive function and osteoporosis. In J. L. Pohl & C. H. Brown (eds.), *The Menstrual Cycle and Physical Activity.* Champaign, IL: Human Kinetics, 117–127 (1986).

Goss, F. L., & C. Karam: The effects of glycogen supercompensation on the electrocardiographic response during exercise. *Research Quarterly for Exercise and Sport.* 58(1): 68–71 (1987).

Hasten, D. L., E. P. Rome, B. D. Franks, & M. Hegsted: Effects of chromium picolinate on beginning weight training students. *International Journal of Sport Nutrition.* 2(4): 343–350 (1992).

Hawley, J. A., E. J. Schabort, T. D. Noakes, & S. C. Dennis. Carbohydrate-loading and exercise performance. *Sports Medicine.* 24(2): 73–81 (1997).

Haymes, E. M.: Protein, vitamins, and iron. In M. H. Williams (ed.), *Ergogenic Aids in Sports.* Champaign, IL: Human Kinetics, 27–55 (1983).

Haymes, E. M., & C. L. Wells: *Environment and Human Performance.* Champaign, IL: Human Kinetics (1986).

Jenkins, D. J. A., D. M. Thomas, M. S. Wolever, R. H. Taylor, H. Barker, H. Fielden, J. M. Baldwin, A. C. Bowling, H. C. Newman, A. L. Jenkins, & D. V. Goff: Glycemic index of foods: A physiological basis for carbohydrate exchange. *American Journal of Clinical Nutrition.* 34:362–366 (1981).

Kreider, R. B., V. Miriel, & E. Bertun: Amino acid supplementation and exercise performance: An analysis of the proposed ergogenic value. *Sports Medicine.* 16(3):190–209 (1993).

Kroculick, S. T.: Carb loading: How to look full and ripped on contest day. *Ironman.* December: 152–153 (1988).

Leaf, A., & K. B. Frisa: Eating for health or for athletic performance? *American Journal of Clinical Nutrition.* 49:1066–1069 (1989).

Lefavi, R. G., R. A. Anderson, R. E. Keith, G. D. Wilson, J. L. McMillan, & M. H. Stone: Efficacy of chromium supplementation in athletes: Emphasis on anabolism. *International Journal of Sports Nutrition.* 2(2):111–122 (1992).

Lemon, P. W. R.: Effects of exercise on protein requirements. *Journal of Sports Sciences.* 9:53–70 (1991).

Lemon, P. W. R.: *Influence of Dietary Protein and Total Energy Intake on Strength Improvement.* Sports Science Exchange, vol. 2, no. 14. Chicago: Gatorade Sports Science Institute (1989a).

Lemon, P. W. R.: Nutrition for muscular development of young athletes. In C. V. Gisolfi & D. R. Lamb (eds.), *Perspectives in Exercise Science and Sports Medicine.* Indianapolis: Benchmark Press, 369–400 (1989b).

Lemon, P. W. R., & F. J. Nagle: Effects of exercise on protein and amino acid metabolism. *Medicine and Science in Sports and Exercise.* 13(3):141–149 (1981).

Leon, G. R.: Eating disorders in female athletes. *Sports Medicine.* 12(4):219–227 (1991).

Manore, M. M.: Energy bars: Picking the right one for you. *ACSM's Health & Fitness Journal.* 4 (5):33–35 (2000).

Maughan, R. J.: Fluid and electrolyte loss and replacement in exercise. *Journal of Sports Sciences.* 9:117–142 (1991).

McDonald, R., & C. L. Keen: Iron, zinc and magnesium nutrition and athletic performance. *Sports Medicine.* 5:171–184 (1988).

Muoio, D. M., J. J. Leddy, P. J. Horvath, A. B. Awad, & D. R. Pendergast: Effect of dietary fat on metabolic adjustments to maximal $\dot{V}O_2$ and endurance in runners. *Medicine and Science in Sports and Exercise.* 26(1):81–88 (1994).

Murray, R.: The effects of consuming carbohydrate-electrolyte beverages on gastric emptying and fluid absorption during and following exercise. *Sports Medicine.* 4:322–351 (1987).

Nadel, E. R.: *New Ideas for Rehydration During and After Exercise in Hot Weather.* Sports Science Exchange, vol. 1, no. 3. Chicago: Gatorade Sports Science Institute (1988).

Neufer, P. D., D. L. Costill, M. G. Flynn, J. P. Kirwan, J. B. Mitchell, & J. Houmard: Improvements in exercise performance: Effects of carbohydrate feedings and diet. *Journal of Applied Physiology.* 62(3):983–988 (1987).

Newsholme, E. A., & A. R. Leech: *Biochemistry for the Medical Sciences.* New York: John Wiley & Sons (1983).

Nieman, D. C.: *Fitness and Sports Medicine: An Introduction.* Palo Alto, CA: Bull Publishing (1990).

Nose, H. M., G. W. Mack, X. Shi, & E. R. Nadel: Involvement of sodium retention hormones during rehydration in humans. *Journal of Applied Physiology.* 65(1):332–336 (1988).

Pascoe, D. D., & L. B. Gladden: Muscle glycogen resynthesis after short-term, high intensity exercise and resistance exercise. *Sports Medicine.* 21(2):98–118 (1996).

Paul, G. L.: Dietary protein requirements of physically active individuals. *Sports Medicine.* 8(3):154–176 (1989).

Phillips, S. M.: Protein metabolism and exercise: Potential sex-based differences. In M. Tarnopolsky (ed.), *Gender Differences in Metabolism: Practical and Nutritional Implications.* Boca Raton: CRC Press, 155–178 (1999).

Phinney, S. D., B. R. Bistrian, W. J. Evans, E. Gervion, & G. L. Blackburn: The human metabolic response to chronic ketosis without caloric restriction: Preservation of submaximal exercise capability with reduced carbohydrate oxidation. *Metabolism.* 32:769–776 (1983).

Phinney, S. D., E. S. Horton, E. A. H. Sims, J. S. Hanson, E. Danforth, & B. M. LaGrange: Capacity for moderate exercise in obese subjects after adaptation to a hypocaloric diet. *Journal of Clinical Investigations.* 66:1152–1161 (1980).

Quaker Oats Company: *The Science of Gatorade.* Barrington, IL: Author (1990).

Sears, B.: *Enter the Zone: A Dietary Road Map to Lose Weight Permanently, Reset Your Genetic Code, Prevent Disease, Achieve Maximal Physical Performance, Enhance Mental Productivity.* New York: Harper Collins (1995).

Sherman, W. M.: Carbohydrates, muscle glycogen, and muscle glycogen supercompensation. In M. H. Williams (ed.), *Ergogenic Aids in Sport.* Champaign, IL: Human Kinetics, 3–26 (1983).

Sherman, W. M.: *Muscle Glycogen Supercompensation During the Week Before Athletic Competition.* Sports Science Exchange, vol. 2, no. 16. Chicago: Gatorade Sports Science Institute (1989).

Sherman, W. M., & N. Leenders: Fat loading: The next magic bullet? *International Journal of Sport Nutrition.* 5:S1–S12 (1995).

Singh, A., P. A. Pelletier, & P. A. Deuster: Dietary requirements for ultraendurance exercise. *Sports Medicine.* 18(5): 301–308 (1994).

Steen, S. N.: Nutrition for young athletes: Special considerations. *Sports Medicine.* 17(3):152–162 (1994).

Sundgot-Borgen, J.: Eating disorders in female athletes. *Sports Medicine.* 17(3):176–188 (1994a).

Sundgot-Borgen, J.: Nutrient intake of female elite athletes suffering from eating disorders. *International Journal of Sport Nutrition.* 3(4):431–442 (1993a).

Sundgot-Borgen, J.: Prevalence of eating disorders in elite female athletes. *International Journal of Sport Nutrition.* 3(1):29–40 (1993b).

Sundgot-Borgen, J.: Risk and trigger factors for the development of eating disorders in female elite athletes. *Medicine and Science in Sports and Exercise.* 26(4):414–419 (1994b).

Tarnopolsky, M. A., J. D. MacDougall, & S. A. Atkinson: Influence of protein intake and training status on nitrogen balance and lean body mass. *Journal of Applied Physiology.* 64(1):187–193 (1988).

Thompson, R. A., & R. T. Sherman: *Helping Athletes with Eating Disorders.* Champaign, IL: Human Kinetics (1993).

U.S. Department of Agriculture, Agriculture Research Service, Dietary Guidelines Advisory Committee: Report of the Dietary Guidelines Advisory Committee on the Dietary Guidelines for Americans, 1995, to the Secretary of Health and Human Services and the Secretary of Agriculture, 58pp. (1995).

vander Beek, E. J.: Vitamins and endurance training: Food for running or faddish claims? *Sports Medicine* 2:175–197 (1985).

vander Beek, E. J.: Vitamin supplementation and physical exercise performance. *Journal of Sports Sciences.* 9:77–89 (1991).

Walton, P., & E. C. Rhodes: Glycaemic index and optimal performance. *Sports Medicine.* 23(3):164–172 (1997).

Wolever, T. M. S.: The glycemic index. In G. H. Bourne (ed.), Aspects of some vitamins, minerals and enzymes in health and disease. *World Review of Nutrition and Dietetics.* 62:120–185 (1990).

Zawadzki, K. M., B. B. Yaspelkis III, & J. L. Ivy: Carbohydrate-protein complex increases the rate of muscle glycogen storage after exercise. *Journal of Applied Physiology.* 72(5):1854–1859 (1992).

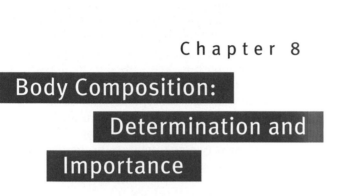

Chapter 8

Body Composition: Determination and Importance

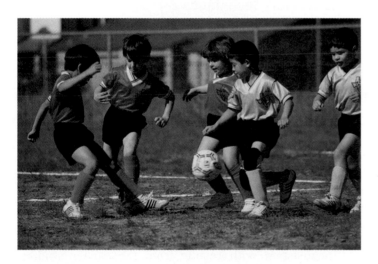

After studying the chapter, you should be able to

- Describe the technique of hydrostatic weighing (densitometry) and explain its theoretical basis.

- Calculate body density and percent body fat.

- Discuss variations in the basic assumptions of densitometry apparent in children, adolescents, and the elderly; and show how these variations have practical meaning.

- List and identify the strengths and weaknesses of the field estimates of body composition.

- Compare the percent body fat estimated by skinfolds and bioelectrical impedance with the percent body fat determined by hydrostatic weighing.

- Contrast the percent body fat and the patterns of fat distribution in an average adult male and in an average adult female.

- Differentiate between overweight and obesity.

- Describe what happens to adipose cells in obesity.

- List and discuss the health risks of being overweight or obese and the impact of physical fitness on these risks.

- Debate the importance of heredity in body composition.

Introduction

Answer the following questions to yourself. Is your body weight just right, a little high, very high, a little low, or very low? Is your percent body fat just right, a little high, very high, a little low, or very low? Do you like the way you look in a bathing suit? What mental images did you use as you answered the questions?

If you are a female, chances are that no matter what the reality of your body weight, composition, or shape, you feel that your values are too high and you are dissatisfied with your shape. You are probably incorrect in your assessment, but you are certainly not alone. For example, one study (Lutter, 1994) presented active women with five figures that represented individuals who were 20% underweight, 10% underweight, average weight and size, 10% overweight, and 20% overweight. The subjects were asked to select the figure they would like to look like. Only 14% wanted the average shape; 44% wanted to be 10% underweight, and 38% wanted to be 20% underweight!

These feelings are, of course, a result of cultural expectations. There have been times in Western civilization (for example, in the seventeenth century) when plumpness was the norm for feminine attractiveness. Within our own century, great changes have occurred in the idealization of the female body. An analysis of *Playboy* centerfolds and Miss America Pageant contestants from 1960 to 1980 showed that the percentage of average weight (average weight being based on mean population values) for these individuals declined steadily from approximately 90% to almost 80%. At the same time, average hip and bust values for these icons of beauty declined, while waist and height values increased. Thus, the ideal shape changed from the hourglass curve to a more tubular profile (Garner, 1980).

In another study, young and middle-aged males and females were asked to select a body silhouette that reflected their current one, the ideal they would like to look like, and the one considered the most attractive to the opposite sex. Both the young (59%) and the middle-aged (65%) females rated their current figures as being significantly larger than the ideal or attractive shape. However, neither the young nor the middle-aged men reported any significant differences between current, ideal, and most attractive silhouettes. Only 25% of the young and 29% of the middle-aged men expressed a desire to be smaller (Tiggemann, 1992). Thus if you are a male, chances are that no matter what the reality of your body weight, composition, or shape, you are not concerned with your body weight per se. You might like larger muscles and greater muscle definition, which would imply a lower percent body fat and a more triangular shape. Data on Mr. America or Mr. Universe contestants are not available to substantiate this impression, but just look at the muscle magazines at any newsstand. What did you compare yourself with mentally? Hopefully you called to mind standards that are consistent with good health, but most likely, you compared yourself to some image presented by the media.

Whether you are female or male, if you have a positive self-image and are content with your body, are eating right, and are exercising regularly, congratulations and keep up the good work. Unfortunately, as a physical education exercise specialist, you will be dealing with a public that has more questions and concerns about body composition and weight control than just about anything else we deal with. These next two chapters are designed to present you with an understanding of these crucial areas.

Body Composition Assessment

Laboratory Techniques

Although it is unpleasant to think about, the only way to directly assess body composition is by dissection of human cadavers. Not only are few bodies available for such studies, but the technique is also difficult and not without problems. From 1945 to 1984 (the time from the earliest to the latest reported studies) body composition analysis has been performed on only 40 cadavers. While the study of these bodies provided a great deal of information, particularly regarding the densities of body tissues, they were not used to determine the accuracy (validity) of the more commonly used laboratory techniques. Theoretically, direct cadaver analysis should be the most accurate technique; however, the newer cadaver studies have often been inconsistent with results from the earlier studies. Thus, when dealing with body composition analysis, keep in mind that some techniques are better than others, and none is likely to be 100% accurate (Behnke and Wilmore, 1974; Brodie, 1988a).

Many methods are currently available for the laboratory assessment of body composition and could possibly serve as criterion measures. Techniques such as computed tomography, dual-energy X-ray absorptiometry, excretion of muscle metabolites, isotope dilution, magnetic resonance imaging, neutron activation, ultrasound, whole-body counting of potassium 40, total body electrical conductivity (TOBEC), and air plethysmography (Bod Pod system) are very accurate (Brodie, 1988a, 1988b). Unfortunately, at this time they are also often expensive, cumbersome, and/or time-consuming, requiring sensitive instrumentation run by highly trained technicians.

A	Total body weight (mass) (TBW)					
B	Fat-free weight 55–96% of TBW					Fat 4–45% of TBW
C	Muscle 48%	Bone 16%	Skin 14%	Blood 9%	Organs 13%	Storage + essential fat
D	Water 72–74%		Protein 19–21%		Bone mineral 7%	Fat

Figure 8.1
Models of Body Composition

Source: Lohman (1986).

The dual-energy X-ray absorptiometry (DXA) technique is pictured and described in Chapter 18 because this equipment is considered to be the "gold standard," or criterion measure, for the assessment of bone mineral density. However, DXA also allows the simultaneous measurement of fat and lean soft tissue for the determination of body composition. It is possible that in the near future, DXA may become the criterion standard for body composition assessment as well. However, pending more research, the label of criterion measurement for body composition (Behnke and Wilmore, 1974; Goldman and Buskirk, 1961) still belongs to hydrostatic or underwater weighing.

Hydrostatic (Underwater) Weighing: Densitometry

Hydrostatic, or underwater, **weighing** determines body composition through the calculation of body density (Behnke and Wilmore, 1974; Goldman and Buskirk, 1961). We have Archimedes, a Greek mathematician who lived in the second century B.C., to thank for this technique. When King Hieron of Syracuse commissioned a new crown, he suspected that the jeweler substituted silver for pure gold inside the crown. The king asked Archimedes to determine the composition of the crown without harming it in any way. Legend has it that as Archimedes was pondering this issue at the public baths, he solved the problem and went running through the streets naked, shouting, "Eureka!" ("I have found it!").

What Archimedes observed was that an amount of water was displaced from the bath equal to the volume of the body entering the bath. Archimedes also reasoned that the body (or any other object floating or submerged) is buoyed up by a counterforce equal to the weight of the water displaced. Thus **Archimedes' principle** states that a partially or fully submerged object experiences an upward buoyant force equal to the weight or the volume of fluid displaced by the object. Based on this principle, the volume of any object, including the human body, can be measured by determining the weight lost by complete submersion underwater. When Archimedes compared the amount of

water displaced by a mass of pure gold and a mass of pure silver equal to the mass of the king's crown, he found that the crown displaced more water than the gold, but less than the silver. He confirmed this result by weighing, underwater, weights of gold and silver equal to the weight of the crown in air, and found the crown to have an intermediate value. Thus, the crown was not pure gold (only about 75%), and we can only speculate as to the fate of the jeweler (Behnke and Wilmore, 1974).

Even if you have never been weighed underwater, you probably have a basic understanding of the principle just described. Think back to a swimming class. Could you float easily, or were you a sinker who could walk on the bottom of the pool? How would you describe those who were either floaters or sinkers in terms of being lean or fat? Whether you floated or sank depended on your body density, and *body density* (mass per unit volume) is determined to a large extent by the amount of body fat that is carried. The density of bone and muscle tissue is greater than the density of fat tissue; hence, the leaner, more muscular individual will weigh more underwater (and tend to sink) than an individual with a large amount of fat (who tends to float).

Whole-body **densitometry,** which is the measurement of mass per unit volume, is the foundation of hydrostatic weighing. It is based on dividing the body into two compartments: fat and fat-free weight. In Figure 8.1, rows A and B indicate this division. Row C

Hydrostatic Weighing Criterion measure for determining body composition through the calculation of body density.

Archimedes' Principle The principle that a partially or fully submerged object will experience an upward buoyant force equal to the weight or the volume of fluid displaced by the object.

Densitometry The measurement of mass per unit volume.

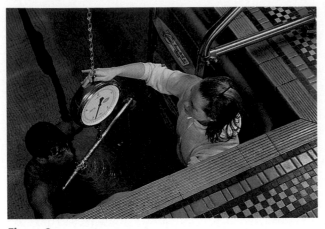

Figure 8.2
Hydrostatic Weighing

The technique for determining body density by hydrostatic (underwater) weighing is based on Archimedes' principle.

lists the component parts of the **fat-free weight** (all of the tissues of the body minus the extractable fat) as muscle, bone, skin, blood, and organs and represents a second model. The fat compartment includes both storage and essential fats. *Storage fat* is the fat in the subcutaneous adipose tissues and the fat surrounding the various internal organs (visceral fat). *Essential fat* includes the fat in bone marrow, central nervous system, cell membranes, heart, lungs, liver, spleen, kidneys, intestines, and muscles.

Note that although the terms *lean body mass* (LBM) and *fat-free weight* (FFW; sometimes called the fat-free body, FFB, or fat-free mass, FFM) are used interchangeably, they are slightly different. Technically, LBM includes the essential fat, but FFW does not. Chemically, FFW is composed of water, proteins, and bone mineral (Figure 8.1, row D), and this represents a third model of compartmentalization or composition (Lohman, 1986). Although each of these models (B, C, and D) describes the composition of the body, when the term *body composition* is used in exercise physiology, it generally refers to model B. That is, **body composition** is defined as the partitioning of body mass into fat-free mass (weight or percentage) and fat mass (weight or percentage).

Compartmentalizing the body into only fat and fat-free weight (not water, mineral, protein, and fat)

Fat-Free Weight The weight of body tissue excluding extractable fat.

Body Composition The partitioning of body mass into fat-free mass (weight or percentage) and fat mass (weight or percentage).

---

and using this two-compartment model to determine percent body fat (%BF) depends upon the following assumptions:

1. The densities of the fat and fat-free weight are known and additive.

2. The densities of water, bone mineral, and protein that make up the fat-free weight are known and relatively constant from individual to individual.

3. The percentage of each fat-free component is relatively stable from individual to individual.

4. The individual being evaluated differs from the assumptions of the equation being used only in the amount of storage fat.

Hydrostatic weighing determines body density (D_B), defined as mass (M) or weight (WT) divided by volume (V) according to the following formula (Behnke and Wilmore, 1974):

8.1 body density ($g \cdot cc^{-1}$) = mass in air (g) ÷ {{[mass in air (g) − mass in water (g)] ÷ [density of water ($g \cdot cc^{-1}$)]} − [residual volume (L) + volume of gastrointestinal air (0.1 L)]}

or

$$D_B = \frac{M_A}{\dfrac{(M_A - M_W)}{D_W} - (RV + V_G)}$$

The mass of an individual in air (M_A) can be obtained either by weighing that individual nude on a sensitive, calibrated scale or by weighing the subject's bathing suit and then subtracting the weight of the suit from the weight of the subject wearing the suit. The volume of the human body is obtained by applying Archimedes' principle. In practice, the individual being weighed is submerged in water, attached in some way to a scale or strain gauge instrumentation (Figure 8.2). The subject then exhales as much air as possible and sits quietly for 3–7 sec while the weight is recorded. Multiple trials are usually necessary. The highest consistent weight is selected from the trials, and the weight of the apparatus, called the tare weight, is then subtracted from the scale weight. The resultant weight is the underwater weight (M_W). Body weight may be measured in lb or kg, but calculations are typically done in metric units, so conversion may be necessary. Not all air can be expelled from the body, and air makes the body buoyant (hence lighter in weight). Therefore, the underwater weight must be corrected for residual volume (the volume of air remaining in the lungs following maximal expiration) and for gastrointestinal gases, the assumed constant equal to 100 mL, or 0.1 L in Equation 8.1. The underwater weight must also be corrected for the density of the water, D_W, which in turn is temperature-dependent.

Example

For example, the following measurements were obtained from a football player:

M_A = 225 lb (102.3 kg)   Water Temperature = 34°C

M_W = 6.07 kg   Water Density at 34°C = 0.9944

RV = 1.583 L

Substituting into Eq. 8.1 we get

$$D_B \frac{102.3 \text{ kg}}{\left(\dfrac{102.3 \text{ kg} - 6.07 \text{ kg}}{0.9944}\right) - (1.583 \text{ L} + 0.1 \text{ L})}$$

Remember that the numerator in this equation represents mass and the denominator represents volume. In the metric system 1 L of water (a volume measure) weighs 1 kg (a mass measure), and conversely 1 kg of mass occupies 1 L of volume (Appendix A). Therefore, the equation can be solved as written.

$$D_B = \frac{102.3 \text{ kg}}{96.77 - 1.683 \text{ L}}$$

$$= \frac{102.3 \text{ kg}}{95.089 \text{ L}} = 1.0758 \text{ kg·L}^{-1}$$

Although kg·L^{-1} is an accurate unit, the D_B is usually reported in g·cc^{-1} units. Dividing the kg·L^{-1} unit by 1000 yields g·mL^{-1}. Then, because 1 mL equals 1 cc (cubic centimeter) the cc designation can easily be substituted for the mL and typically is. ✛

Once body density has been obtained, percent body fat (%BF) can be calculated. The two most widely used formulas for converting body density to %BF were developed by Siri and by Brozek. They have been derived differently but, within the density units of 1.09 and 1.03 g·cc^{-1}, agree within 1% on the %BF values calculated. At lower densities the Siri formula gives increasingly higher %BF values than the Brozek formula (Lohman, 1981).

8.2 Brozek: %BF = $\left[\left(\dfrac{4.570}{D_B}\right) - 4.142\right] \times 100$

8.3 Siri: %BF = $\left[\left(\dfrac{4.950}{D_B}\right) - 4.5\right] \times 100$

Brozek's formula assumes that the individual has neither lost nor gained substantial amounts of body weight recently.

Example

If we use the body density results from the football player in the preceding example in Equation 8.2 and Equation 8.3 we get

Brozek: %BF = $\left[\left(\dfrac{4.570}{1.0758}\right)\right] - 4.142 \times 100 = 10.6\%$

Siri: %BF = $\left[\left(\dfrac{4.950}{1.0758}\right)\right] - 4.50 \times 100 = 10.1\%$

As expected, the %BF values are within 1% of each other with an actual difference of only 0.5% (10.6% − 10.1% = 0.5%). ✛

Once %BF has been determined, body weight at any selected fat percentage can be calculated using the following sequence of formulas. The first formula simply determines the amount of fat-free weight (FFW) an individual currently has (WT$_1$).

8.4 fat-free weight = current body weight (lb or kg) $\times \left(\dfrac{100\% - \text{percent body fat}}{100}\right)$

or

$$FFW = WT_1 \times \left(\frac{100\% - \%BF}{100}\right)$$

The second formula calculates the desired weight (WT$_2$).

8.5 body weight at the selected percent of body fat (lb or kg) = [100 × fat-free weight (lb or kg)] ÷ (100% − selected percent body fat)

or

$$WT_2 = \frac{100 \times FFW}{100\% - \%BF}$$

The third formula calculates the amount of weight to be gained or lost.

8.6 weight to gain or lose (lb or kg) = body weight at selected percent body fat − current body weight

or

$$\Delta WT = WT_2 - WT_1$$

Example

For example, an individual who currently weighs 150 lb at a body fat of 25% wishes to reduce her body fat to 17%. Equation 8.4 is used to calculate her current fat-free weight.

$$FFW = 150 \text{ lb} \times \left(\frac{100\% - 25\%}{100}\right) = 112.50 \text{ lb}$$

Her current fat-free weight and selected %BF are then substituted into Equation 8.5 to obtain her weight goal.

$$WT_2 = \frac{100 \times 112.50 \text{ lb}}{100\% - 17\%} = 135.54 \text{ lb}$$

Comparing her current weight to her goal weight in Equation 8.6 we get

$$\Delta WT = 135.5 \text{ lb} - 150 \text{ lb} = -14.5 \text{ lb}$$

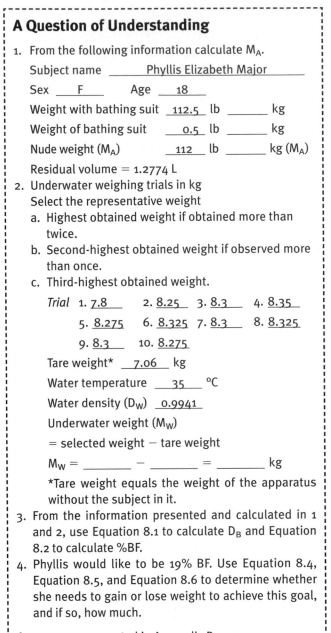

A Question of Understanding

1. From the following information calculate M_A.

   Subject name _____Phyllis Elizabeth Major_____

   Sex __F__   Age __18__

   Weight with bathing suit __112.5__ lb _____ kg

   Weight of bathing suit __0.5__ lb _____ kg

   Nude weight (M_A)   __112__ lb _____ kg (M_A)

   Residual volume = 1.2774 L

2. Underwater weighing trials in kg
   Select the representative weight
   a. Highest obtained weight if obtained more than twice.
   b. Second-highest obtained weight if observed more than once.
   c. Third-highest obtained weight.

   Trial 1. __7.8__   2. __8.25__   3. __8.3__   4. __8.35__

   5. __8.275__   6. __8.325__ 7. __8.3__   8. __8.325__

   9. __8.3__   10. __8.275__

   Tare weight* __7.06__ kg

   Water temperature __35__ °C

   Water density (D_W) __0.9941__

   Underwater weight (M_W)

   = selected weight − tare weight

   M_W = _____ − _____ = _____ kg

   *Tare weight equals the weight of the apparatus without the subject in it.

3. From the information presented and calculated in 1 and 2, use Equation 8.1 to calculate D_B and Equation 8.2 to calculate %BF.

4. Phyllis would like to be 19% BF. Use Equation 8.4, Equation 8.5, and Equation 8.6 to determine whether she needs to gain or lose weight to achieve this goal, and if so, how much.

Answers are presented in Appendix D.

This means that if this individual wishes to be 17% BF she must reduce her current weight by 14.5 lb. Of course, these calculations assume that in the process of losing weight muscle mass is maintained. This assumption is not always true. ✛

Now read the Question of Understanding box above and complete the problems given. The data are presented as they would be recorded during an actual experiment. You will need to do some conversions and analysis to select the correct M_A and M_W. As you do each calculation, mentally review why each step needs to be done to assure yourself that you understand the underlying principles.

When the measuring technique is properly conducted, the error of %BF determined by densitometry is approximately 2.7% for adults. This error is primarily due to variations in the composition of the fat-free mass (Lohman, 1981). The error is always lowest if the equation utilized closely matches the individual being tested with the sample on which the equation was developed (Heyward and Stolarczyk, 1996).

Densitometry: Children and Adolescents, and the Elderly

The previous section outlined the basic assumptions underlying hydrostatic weighing (densitometry). Research has cast doubt upon all of these assumptions with regard to children and adolescents (Lohman et al., 1984).

The values for the FFW or FFB components for adults (males and females) are assumed to be approximately 73% for water and 7% for mineral content, with an overall density of FFW of 1.100 $g\cdot cc^{-1}$ (Figure 8.3, dashed lines) (Boileau, et al., 1984; Lohman, 1986). Protein, not shown on the graph, makes up about 20% of the FFW of adults.

Boileau et al. (1984) have shown that the percentage of water in FFW decreases (Figure 8.3b) from 77–78% at ages 7–9 yr to 73% at approximately age 20 in a steady but slightly curvilinear fashion. Across the age span females have a slightly higher percentage of water in FFW than males. Conversely, the percentage of mineral content in FFW (Figure 8.3c) increases from approximately 5% at ages 7–9 to the 7% at age 20. This change is also slightly curvilinear, and the female values are consistently lower than the male values. The protein change is minimal (and therefore not presented in Figure 8.3), varying only about 1% (from 19 to 20%) over the age span. The result of these changes is that body density also increases in a curvilinear fashion from approximately 1.08 to 1.10 $g\cdot cc^{-1}$ for adult males and to 1.095 $g\cdot cc^{-1}$ for adult females. This means adult females never meet the 1.10-$g\cdot cc^{-1}$ assumed value (Figure 8.3a) (Lohman, 1986).

Because the components are constantly changing as children mature, no single formula can be used for children of different ages. Neither can one formula be used for boys and for girls. Table 8.1 shows the array of age and sex formulas needed.

The use of equations developed with the assumption of the composition of adult components will

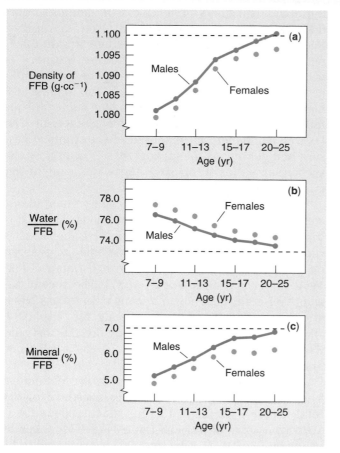

Figure 8.3

Estimated Changes in Fat-Free Body Composition as a Function of Age

The density of the fat-free body, also known as the fat-free weight, is much lower in both male and female children than in adults. FFB density increases as the child matures, but the female density is lower at each age than the male density and never reaches the assumed adult values of 1.1.

The percentage of the FFB that is composed of water is higher in both male and female children than in adults. As the child matures, the percentage of water in the FFB declines, but the female percentage is always higher than the male even after adulthood is reached.

The percentage of FFB that is composed of minerals is lower in both male and female children than in adults. As the child matures, the percentage of minerals in the FFB increases, but the female percentage is always lower than the male percentage even after adulthood is reached.

Source: T. G. Lohman. Applicability of body composition techniques and constants for children and youth. In K. B. Pandolf (ed.), *Exercise and Sport Science Reviews,* New York: Macmillan, 14:325–327 (1986). Reprinted by permission of Williams & Wilkins.

overestimate the %BF of the child or adolescent. This can be illustrated as follows. If the D_B of a 9-yr-old girl is determined to be 1.065 g·cc^{-1} by hydrostatic

Table 8.1

Formulas for Converting Body Density to Percent Body Fat in Children and Adolescents, by Sex

Age (Yr)	Male	Female
7–9	$\left(\dfrac{5.38}{D_B} - 4.97\right) \times 100$	$\left(\dfrac{5.43}{D_B} - 5.03\right) \times 100$
9–11	$\left(\dfrac{5.30}{D_B} - 4.89\right) \times 100$	$\left(\dfrac{5.35}{D_B} - 4.95\right) \times 100$
11–13	$\left(\dfrac{5.23}{D_B} - 4.81\right) \times 100$	$\left(\dfrac{5.25}{D_B} - 4.84\right) \times 100$
13–15	$\left(\dfrac{5.07}{D_B} - 4.64\right) \times 100$	$\left(\dfrac{5.12}{D_B} - 4.69\right) \times 100$
15–17	$\left(\dfrac{5.03}{D_B} - 4.59\right) \times 100$	$\left(\dfrac{5.07}{D_B} - 4.64\right) \times 100$
17–20	$\left(\dfrac{4.98}{D_B} - 4.53\right) \times 100$	$\left(\dfrac{5.05}{D_B} - 4.62\right) \times 100$

Calculated from the density FFW constant (D_1) reported by Lohman (1986), and a density of fat constant (D_2) of 0.9 g·cc^{-1} according to the formula

$$\%BF = \frac{1}{D_B}\left[\left(\frac{D_1 D_2}{D_1 - D_2}\right) - \left(\frac{D_2}{(D_1 - D_2)}\right)\right] \times 100$$

weighing, the %BF calculated by the Brozek formula (Equation 8.2) is

$$\left(\frac{4.570}{1.065}\right) - 4.142 \times 100 = 14.9\%$$

The Lohman (1986) age- and sex-specific formula yields

$$\left(\frac{5.35}{1.065}\right) - 4.95 \times 100 = 7.3\% \quad \text{(see Table 8.1)}$$

The majority of research published to date for children and adolescents has been on normally active nonathletes. Further work is in progress to determine the effects of physical activity and/or athletic participation on bone mineral, hydration, and body density values throughout the growth years. Percent body fat values of young athletes, even if the appropriate age and sex formulas are used, must be interpreted cautiously. Although the pediatric formulas are better than adult formulas, even the pediatric formulas may need to be revised for young athletes. In addition, research in the area of body composition, on both sedentary and active youths, should directly measure water (W) and bone mineral content (M) of the FFW as well as body density in

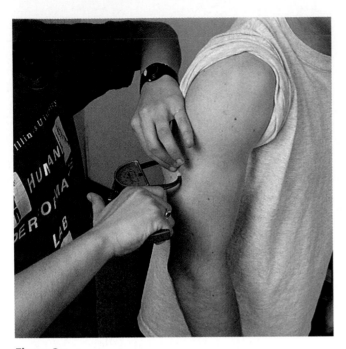

Figure 8.4
Measurement of Triceps Skinfold Using a Calibrated
Skinfold Caliper

order to more accurately account for all body compartments. These variables should be used in a more complex formula such as

$$\boxed{8.7} \; \%BF = \left(\frac{2.747}{D_B}\right) - 0.714(W) + 1.146(M) - 2.0503$$

At the other end of the age continuum, the elderly, consideration needs to be given to the effect of the loss of bone mineral density (termed osteopenia) on the determination of %BF. Theoretically, a loss of bone mineral density would cause a decrease in body density and, thus, an overestimation of %BF if it were not accounted for (Ballor, et al., 1988; Brodie, 1988a; Lohman, 1986).

Field Tests of Body Composition

Skinfolds

The most widely used anthropometric estimation of body size or composition involves the measurement of skinfolds at selected sites. **Skinfolds** (or fatfolds) are

> **Skinfolds** The double thickness of skin plus the adipose tissue between the parallel layers of skin.

the double thickness of skin plus the adipose tissue between the parallel layers of skin (see Figure 8.4). Because there are only slight variations in skin thickness among individuals, the resulting measure is taken as an indication of the thickness of the subcutaneous fat (Behnke and Wilmore, 1974). Technically, however, adipose tissue (and hence the subcutaneous fatfold) has both a fat and a fat-free component. The fat-free component is composed of water, blood vessels, and nerves. As the fat content of the adipose tissue increases (as in obesity), the water content decreases (Roche, 1987).

The use of skinfold thicknesses to estimate body composition is based on two assumptions. The first is that the total subcutaneous adipose tissue mass is represented by the selected skinfold sites. In general, evidence supports this assumption (Lohman, 1981; McArdle, et al., 1991; Roche, 1987). The second assumption is that the subcutaneous tissue mass has a known relationship with total body fat. Table 8.2 shows the distribution of total body fat and the relative percentages of each storage site for a reference male and a reference female 20–24 yr old.

Most of the values in Table 8.2 are estimates. They indicate that approximately one-third of the total fat for both males (3.1 kg subcutaneous fat ÷ 10.3–10.5 kg total fat) and females (5.1 kg subcutaneous fat ÷ 13.4–17.2 kg total fat) is estimated to be subcutaneous. Other estimates put this value as high as 70% and as low as 20%. With advancing age a proportionally smaller amount of fat is stored subcutaneously. Thus, any given skinfold would then represent a smaller percentage of total body fat. It may also be that lean individuals and fat individuals store their fat in proportionally different ways. Additionally, females may store more or less fat subcutaneously than males (Lohman, 1981; McArdle, et al., 1991). There is little disagreement regarding the differences between essential fat amounts for males and females. The higher essential fat values in females are generally attributed to the energy requirements of pregnancy and lactation.

These variations in the estimation of subcutaneous fat percentage mean that the second assumption is not as firmly based as the first (Brodie, 1988a). One way of dealing with this problem is to make sure that the equations that are used are age-adjusted or generalized for sedentary individuals and population-specific for various athletic groups.

When skinfolds are taken by trained professionals and the appropriate equations are used, the accuracy of skinfold prediction of percent body fat is within 3–5% compared with underwater weighing. Improper techniques can result in large prediction

Table 8.2

Percentage of Fat Distribution in a Reference Male and a Reference Female

Distribution Site	70-kg Male Fat Kg	%	56.8-kg Female Fat Kg	%
Total body	10.5	15	15.3	27
Essential	2.1	3	4.9–6.8	9–12
Storage	8.2–8.4	12	8.5–10.4	15–18
Subcutaneous	3.1	4	5.1	9
Intermuscular	3.3	5	3.5	6
Intramuscular	0.8	1	0.6	1
Abdominothoracic cavity	1.0	1	1.2	2

Source: Modified from Behnke & Wilmore (1974); Lohman (1981).

Table 8.3

Calculation of %BF from Skinfolds

Group	Equation
Adult males	$\%BF = 0.39287(X_1) = 0.00105(X_1)^2 + 0.15772(X_2) - 5.18845$, where X_1 = sum of abdominal, suprailiac, and triceps skinfolds and X_2 = age
Adult females	$\%BF = 0.41563(X_1) - 0.00112(X_1)^2 + 0.03661(X_2) + 4.03653$, where X_1 = sum of abdominal, suprailiac, and triceps skinfolds and X_2 = age
Male children and adolescents (8–18 yr)	$\% BF = 0.735(X_1) + 1.0$, where X_1 = sum of triceps and calf skinfolds
Female children and adolescents (8–18 yr)	$\% BF = 0.610(X_1) + 5.1$, where X_1 = sum of triceps and calf skinfolds

Note: The last two equations were developed taking into account body density, percentage of water in FFW, and bone mineral content variations by age.

Source: Based on information in Golding, et al. (1989); Jackson & Pollock (1985); Slaughter, et al. (1988).

errors. The greatest source of error arises from an improper location of the skinfold site to be tested. Therefore, anyone wishing to use this method to predict percent body fat should locate the site precisely and practice the technique repeatedly before using it. Table 8.3 presents equations that can be used to predict percent body fat from two to three skinfold sites. These equations are specific for sex and for age.

Skinfold or fatfold thickness values may be used in ways other than to predict percent body fat. First, the millimeter values of several sites (usually 5–7 from anatomically diverse locations) can be added to form a sum of skinfolds. Such a sum is an indication of the relative degree of fatness between individuals. Or it can be used to detect changes within a given individual, if measurements are taken repeatedly over time. Second, fatfolds may be used to determine the pattern of distribution of subcutaneous fat. Such a pattern has emerged as an important predictor of the health hazards of obesity (Harrison, et al., 1988; McArdle, et al., 1991; Roche, 1987; Van Itallie, 1988).

Bioelectrical Impedance (Impedance Plethysmography)

The determination of body composition by *bioelectrical impedance analysis* (BIA) has gained a great deal of acceptance in fitness facilities due primarily to the ease with which the procedure can be conducted. In BIA four electrodes are attached to a quietly resting supine subject's hands and feet (two per limb either ipsilaterally or contralaterally) (Figure 8.5). A harmless, sensationless, low-amperage (80 µA), radio frequency (50 kHz) electrical current is passed between

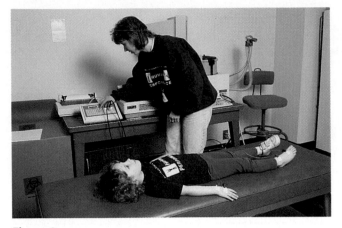

Figure 8.5
Determination of Body Composition by Bioelectrical Impedance

the electrodes; and the resistance to the current is recorded. A reading of resistance (in ohms) is obtained. It is assumed that the body volume is defined as a cylinder of constant cross-sectional area and uniform density distribution. Body volume is more often defined as height squared divided by resistance ($HT^2 \div R$) (Baumgartner, et al., 1990; Brodie, 1988b; Van Loan, 1990).

The ability to conduct the electrical current is directly related to the amount of water and electrolytes in the various body tissues. The flow of the electrical current is easier in fat-free tissue (hence it offers less resistance) than fat tissue because the fat-free tissue contains a higher percentage of water and electrolytes. Therefore, individuals with large amounts of fat-free weight will show low resistance values, and those with large amounts of fat weight will show high resistance values.

Because the BIA technique is actually measuring total body water (TBW), estimates can be made of body density and fat-free weight on the basis of the obtained TBW and the known percentages of water in the body and in the FFW. Another technique is to derive regression equations from height, resistance, and/or other anthropometric variables (such as weight, age, sex, skinfolds, or circumferences) to directly predict FFW or %BF. In most cases hydrostatic weighing is used as the criterion measure. As with skinfolds, a number of equations have been generated in this manner.

As you might suspect from this discussion, the accuracy of BIA measurement depends highly on the maintenance of a normal level of hydration. Either too much fluid (hyperhydration) or too little fluid

(hypohydration or dehydration) will affect the readings. The exact effect is controversial. Theoretically, an increase in body water should decrease resistance and %BF. There is some experimental evidence supporting this theory; however, other studies have shown the opposite result. That is, dehydration caused by exercise has decreased resistance, and hyperhydration from ingestion of replacement supplements has increased resistance. This variance may be related to whether the electrolyte content changes proportionally to water and to the shift in water between compartments. What is clear is that individuals should be measured 3–4 hr after the ingestion of a meal or after an exercise session and should not be under the influence of anything, such as caffeine, that might act as a diuretic (Baumgartner, et al., 1990; Deurenberg, et al., 1988; Stump, et al., 1988; Van Loan, 1990).

The accuracy of BIA also depends on both ambient and skin temperatures. Resistance is higher under cool temperatures than under warm ones. Thus, if an individual is tested repeatedly over a period of 15–20 min and is in an environment that permits body cooling to occur, the %BF estimate will go up as the skin temperature goes down. Care must therefore be taken that testing is done at a neutral temperature (27–29°C; 80–84°F) when the subject is neither overheated nor chilled (Caton, et al., 1988; Stump, et al., 1988).

A third factor that influences the accuracy of BIA estimates of body composition are the equations used. These equations include those for body geometry, cross-sectional area, and current distribution, as well as those used to convert resistance to TBW, body density, and %BF. Each of the electrical assumptions is violated by the human body but apparently not sufficiently to negate the use of BIA. However, these violations do limit the accuracy for estimating TBW, FFW, and %BF to individuals not at the extremes of leanness or fatness. Furthermore, if the criterion measure upon which the equation was based did not take into account the age-related differences in TBW, the inaccuracies would be confounded (Baumgartner, et al., 1990; Brodie, 1988a; Hodgdon and Fitzgerald, 1987).

BIA values under standard conditions will be consistent, but the accuracy is probably no better than that achieved by skinfolds (Baumgartner, et al., 1990).

Height and Weight

In some situations, such as when large numbers of individuals are being evaluated, the only measures of body size that can easily be obtained are height and weight. These values are often used in conjunction with height and weight charts that include standards such as acceptable body weight (less than 10% over the chart weight), overweight (10–20% over the chart weight) and obese (more than 20% over the chart weight). Such use of height and weight charts is minimally acceptable for large group data but is not recommended as a source of what one "should" weigh for individuals, for the following reasons (Burton, et al., 1985; Himes and Frisamcho, 1988; Nieman, 1990; Powers and Howley, 1990):

1. The most commonly available height and weight charts were compiled from lowest mortality data on individuals who purchased life insurance in nongroup situations. The age range was 25–59 yr. Some people were included more than once when they purchased more than one policy. Thus, the sample was neither randomly drawn, as is necessary statistically, nor truly representative of the total American population, especially the elderly, lower-socioeconomic groups, and specific ethnic groups.

2. Individuals with known heart disease, cancer, and/or diabetes were excluded, but smokers were included. Thus, risk factors, other than body weight, were ignored in determining mortality ratios.

3. Only body weights at the time of purchasing the insurance, not at the time of death, were considered. This omission could greatly affect the values. In addition, in many cases height and weight were self-reported and not measured. The accuracy of self-reported data must be questioned.

4. The determination of frame size is not always defined. Even when it is, frame size is very difficult to defend and interpret in relation to body weight.

5. The 1983 Metropolitan Life Insurance height-weight chart shows higher weight values at a given height and frame size than the comparable 1959 chart, reflecting the trend of a national weight gain. The 1959 table values were listed as desirable weights (that is, weights associated with the lowest mortality), but not so the 1983 table values. If the Metropolitan tables are the only thing available for use, the 1959 (not the 1983) version should be selected, except for the elderly. Some evidence suggests that desirable weights are slightly higher in the elderly. Therefore, the 1983 tables can be used for this population.

6. Weight per se does not provide any information on body composition. What matters is the %BF, not the body weight, because %BF is related to health.

If height and weight are the only variables available, and if height and weight charts should not be used, a reasonable alternative is still available: the body mass index.

Body Mass Index

Body mass index (BMI) is a ratio of total body weight to height. Several ratios have been proposed, but the one used most frequently is weight (in kilograms) divided by height (in meters) squared [WT/HT^2 (kg·m^{-2})]. This ratio is also known as the Quetelet index (Brodie, 1988a; Revicki and Israel, 1986; Satwanti, 1980). Calculated BMI can then be compared against standard values to determine whether the individual has acceptable body weight, is overweight, or is obese (see Table 8.4).

Example

For example, if a female subject (age = 30 yr) weighs 165 lb and is 5 ft 8 in. tall, calculation of her BMI first requires conversion to metric units. Dividing 165 lb by 2.2 kg·lb^{-1} gives a weight of 75 kg. Multiplying 68 in. by 2.54 cm·in^{-1} gives 172.7 cm (1.73 m). Height value squared is 2.98 m^2. Thus, BMI = 75 ÷ 2.98 = 25.2. Check Table 8.4 to see whether this is an acceptable, overweight, or obesity value for this individual.   ✛

Note that the table gives both upper and lower ranges of acceptable values. Being too lean is no more desirable than being too fat in a normal, nonathletic population. Athletes often have body composition values below these standards, but as we discussed in the previous chapter in terms of eating disorders, too lean can be a problem or the sign of one. Body composition for athletes will be discussed later in this chapter.

The selection of BMI values of 27.8 for males and 27.3 for females as the upper limit of acceptable is based on the data graphed in Figure 8.6 on page 215. The figure shows that for adults there is a curvilinear increase in excess mortality (a greater number of deaths than expected in a given population) with an increasing BMI (Bray, 1985). Significant increases in risk begin at a BMI of 27.3 for females and 27.8 for males. Therefore, in 1987, the National Center for Health Statistics defined obesity as a BMI of 27.3 for females and 27.8 for males (Lohman, 1994). These are the key values that were used to determine the standards presented in

Table 8.4
Commonly Used Standards for Acceptable Body Weight, Overweight, and Obesity in Nonathletes

	Acceptable Body Weight		Overweight[*]		Obesity	
	Male	Female	Male	Female	Male	Female
BMI (kg·m^{-2})						
5 yr	14.7–20	16.2–21	> 20	> 21		
6 yr	14.7–20	16.2–21	> 20	> 21		
7 yr	14.9–20	16.2–22	> 20	> 22		
8 yr	15.1–20	16.2–22	> 20	> 22		
9 yr	15.2–20	16.2–23	> 20	> 23		
10 yr	15.3–21	16.6–23.5	> 21	> 23.5		
11 yr	15.8–21	16.9–24	> 21	> 24		
12 yr	16.0–22	16.9–24.5	> 22	> 24.5		
13 yr	16.6–23	17.5–24.5	> 23	> 24.5		
14 yr	17.5–24.5	17.5–25	> 24.5	> 25		
15 yr	18.1–25	17.5–25	> 25	> 25		
16 yr	18.5–26.5	17.5–25	> 26.5	> 25		
17 yr	18.8–27	17.5–26	> 27	> 26		
17+ yr	19–27.8	18–27.3	> 27.8[*]	> 27.3[*]	I = 30–34.9	
					II = 35–39.9	
					III = ≥ 40	
%BF						
5–18 yr	10–20%	14–25%	20–25%	26–31%	≥ 25%	≥ 32%
> 18 yr	12–18%	16–25%	19–24%	26–31%	≥ 25%	≥ 32%
Skinfolds[†]						
5–18 yr	10–25	16–30	25–31	31–36	> 32	> 36
> 18 yr					> 45	> 69

[*] BMI 25–29.9 kg·m^{-2} is sometimes designated as overweight range for adults.

[†] Sum of triceps and calf for children and adolescents; sum of triceps and subscapular for adults.

Source: Based on Bray (1987); Bubb (1992); Lohman (1994, 1987); Nieman (1990); Simoupoulos (1987).

Table 8.4. More recently, international agencies (National Heart, Lung, and Blood Institute, 1998; World Health Organization, 1988) adopted BMI standards of < 18.5 for underweight, 18.5–24.9 for normal weight, 25–29.9 for overweight, and ≥ 30 for obesity. Obesity was further divided into three classes. Class I obesity is indicated by a BMI of 30–34.9, Class II by a BMI of 35–39.9, and Class III by a BMI ≥ 40. All values are in kg·m^{-2}. Values between 25 and 27.3 (females) and 27.8 (males) represent being somewhat overweight, but as indicated previously, with only a slightly elevated risk of developing obesity-related health problems.

BMI has been shown to correlate highly with %BF derived from skinfold measures (r = 0.74) and hydrostatic weighing (r = 0.58–0.85). These correlations indicate a moderate relationship, but they also suggest that there is considerable measurement error in using BMI as an estimate of body adiposity. Thus individuals with a normal BMI can actually have high body fat levels, and individuals with high BMIs (especially those in the 25–27 kg·m^{-2} range) may actually have normal, acceptable body fat levels. Individuals who are obviously active and/or muscular should have percent body fat more directly measured (Gallagher, et al., 1996). In situations where the same group of individuals were evaluated, skinfolds generally predicted %BF better than BMI did. Furthermore, at any given BMI females will have a higher percent body fat than males, and older individuals will have a higher percent body fat than younger individuals (Gallagher, et al., 1996). Nevertheless, BMI is often

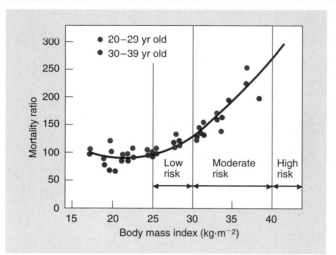

Figure 8.6
The Relationship between Body Mass Index and Mortality

The risk of excess mortality (depicted as a mortality ratio where 100 represents normal mortality) from increasing values for body mass index (BMI) is described by a J-shaped curve. BMI values from 15 to 25 represent no excess mortality risk. BMI values from 25 to 30 represent a low risk, from 30 to 40 a moderate risk, and over 40 a high risk of excess mortality.

Source: G. A. Bray. Complications of obesity. *Annals of Internal Medicine.* 103:1052–1062 (1985). Reprinted by permission of American College of Physicians.

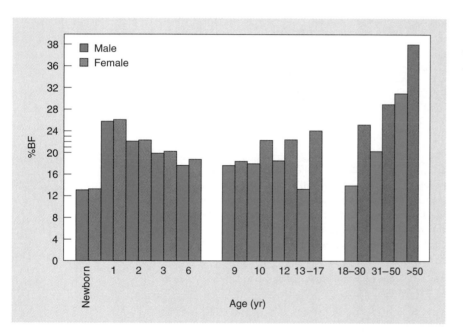

Figure 8.7
Percent Body Fat Changes with Age

Source: Boileau, et al. (1984); Dietz (1987); Fomon, et al. (1982); Friiz-Hansen (1965); Malina, et al. (1982); McArdle, et al. (1991); Plowman, et al. (1991).

used as an indication of overweight or obesity, particularly when mass screening is done.

Overweight and Obesity

Although being overweight is what bothers most people, it is really %BF that should be of concern. Excess weight can be caused by high levels of lean muscle mass, but additional muscle mass is beneficial. Except in rare instances, such as providing protection from the cold water for an English Channel swimmer, excess fat is not beneficial.

Figure 8.7 shows average %BF values for males and females across the age spectrum from infancy to 50 yr. Prior to puberty (which begins at approximately 10 yr for females and 12 yr for males), there is very little sex difference in %BF. The 10–20% range, representing acceptable body weight and composition, is very close to actual measured values during this time span. After puberty male values drop until approximately 30 yr of age and then rise; female values rise slowly and then tend to jump. By age 30 both male and female averages fall in the overweight category, and by age 50 they fall into the obesity category.

The data used to construct Figure 8.7 were not based on a random sampling of the United States population but on available published sources. In contrast, Figure 8.8 presents the results from the 1976–1980 National Health and Nutrition Examination Survey–II (NHANES II), which can be considered

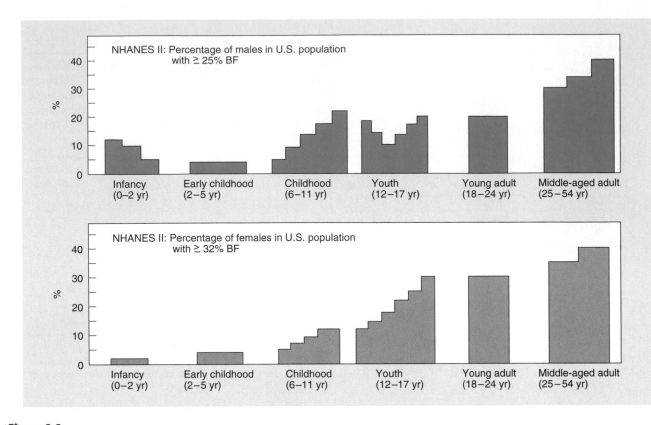

Figure 8.8

Prevalence of Obesity in U.S. Population

Obesity was defined in the National Health and Nutrition Examination Survey–II as 25% BF for males and 32% BF for females. The values were calculated from triceps plus subscapular skinfold measures taken on a representative sample of Americans. The percentage of individuals who are classified as obese shows an inconsistent but definite increasing trend from infancy to adulthood for both males and females. By late middle age (last bar) almost 40% of the American population is estimated to be obese.

Source: "Assessment of body composition in children" by T. G. Lohman, *Pediatric Exercise Science,* (Vol. 1, No. 1), p. 26. Copyright 1989 by Human Kinetics. Reprinted by permission.

representative of the population. In this survey obesity was also defined as 25% BF for males and 32% BF for females. It depicts not average %BF levels but the percentage of obesity across the age spectrum (Lohman, 1989). As shown, the incidence of obesity increases rather steadily as both males and females age, being a problem for females earlier than it is for males. By middle age fully one-third of the U.S. population can be considered obese. Although these data are not shown on the graph, another 25–30% of adults are estimated to be overweight, and the percentage of young people who are overweight doubled between 1980 and 2000. Thus, despite what appears to be a national obsession with thinness, diets, and weight control, large numbers of Americans of all ages are either overweight or obese; and the problem intensifies as the calendar years go by (Williamson, 1993).

What Happens to Adipose Cells in Obesity? The Cellular Basis of Obesity

Adipose tissue is composed of a matrix of connective tissue in which white adipose cells (adipocytes) appear singularly or in small clusters. A typical cell (Figure 8.9) looks something like a signet ring: a metal band with some type of stone or jewel at the top. The nucleus of the cell appears as the stone or jewel of the ring in the cell membrane which forms the band of the ring. The space within the confines of the cell is where the triglyceride droplets are stored (Marieb, 2000). The brown adipose cell in Figure 8.9 will be discussed later.

There are about 30–50 billion fat cells in an adult of acceptable weight. Females have approximately 50% more fat cells than males. Adipocytes can change in size about tenfold if needed to store triglycerides. Apparently, this increase in size (or hypertrophy) is the way in which increasing levels of fat are first stored. Sometimes when the fat cell size is enlarged, the increased size causes a bulging between the fibrous tissue strands, causing a dimply, waffled appearance. These lumpy areas are often labeled as *cellulite*. As can be seen from this discussion, though, cellulite is simply fat (Bjorntop, 1987, 1989).

Once the upper limit of fat storage by hypertrophy is approached (somewhere around 30 kg of fat), fat cell hyperplasia occurs. **Hyperplasia** in general is growth in a tissue or organ through an increase in the number of cells. In fat tissue hyperplasia is the development of new adipocytes from immature precursor cells. Adipocytes themselves do not divide and multiply, but hypertrophy in adipocytes stimulates cell division and maturation in precursor cells (Malina and Bouchard, 1991). Thus, a newly overweight adult is likely to have the same number of fat cells as when he or she was of normal weight, but these adipocytes will be larger than before. An obese individual may have enlarged adipocytes, an increased number of adipocytes, or both. Obese individuals may have as many as 75–80 billion fat cells. Once created, fat cell numbers are not naturally reduced, even if body weight and body fat are lost (Sjöström and Björntorp, 1974). Liposuction—the surgical removal of adipose tissue—is the only way to get rid of adipocytes. The maintenance of large numbers of adipocytes may be one reason why it is so difficult for obese individuals to maintain a weight/fat loss once it occurs.

These facts emphasize the importance of avoiding the maturation of extra fat cells. Overweight or obese infants, children, or adolescents tend to become overweight or obese adults, although adolescent obesity is more predictive of adult obesity than are obesity at birth or in infancy (Charney, et al., 1975; Dietz, 1987; Lohman, 1989).

Figure 8.10 indicates the typical pattern in cell size (Figure 8.10a) and number (Figure 8.10b) that occurs in normal (nonobese) children and adolescents (Malina and Bouchard, 1991). From birth to young adulthood the average cell size doubles or even triples. Most of this increase in size happens during the first year after birth. From 1 yr to the onset of puberty there is no significant increase in size and no sex difference. At puberty, cell size increases in females but remains fairly constant in males. Not all adipose cells are the same size; internal (visceral) fat

White Adipose Cell

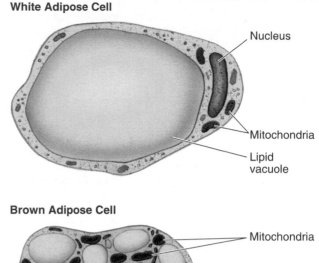

Brown Adipose Cell

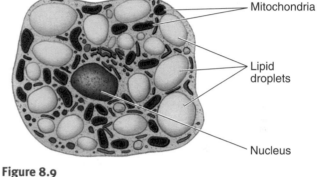

Figure 8.9
Adipose Cells

White and brown adipose cells both store lipid as triglyceride, but do so in slightly different ways. White adipose cells contain one large fat droplet; brown adipose cells contain many small fat droplets. Most of the fat stored in the human body is stored in white adipose cells.

Source: *Growth, Maturation and Physical Activity* (p. 134) by Robert M. Malina and Claude Bouchard. Champaign, IL: Human Kinetics. Copyright 1991 by Robert Malina and Claude Bouchard. Reprinted by permission.

cells are generally smaller than subcutaneous fat cells. Furthermore, not all subcutaneous cells are equal in size. For example, gluteal adipocytes tend to be larger than abdominal adipocytes, which in turn are larger than subscapular cells.

At birth the number of adipocytes is approximately 5 billion. For the number to increase to the average adult value of 30 billion, considerable change must occur. However, little increase in number occurs during the first year after birth when the cell size is changing so drastically (see Figure 8.10b). From 1 yr to the onset of puberty, there is a gradual but steady increase in number, with no difference appearing between the sexes. This gradual increase can double or even triple the number of fat cells. At puberty the cellularity of adipose tissues increases greatly in both males and females, but the female increase far exceeds the male increase. This increase in fat cell

---

Hyperplasia Growth in a tissue or organ through an increase in the number of cells.

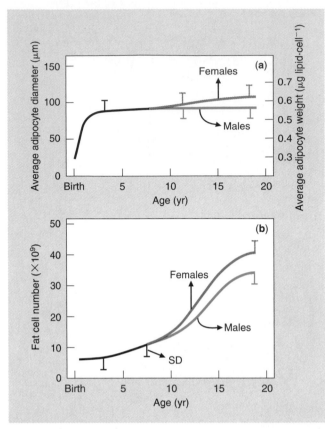

Figure 8.10

Adipose Cell Size and Number Changes with Growth

(a) The greatest change in adipose cell size occurs between birth and 1 year. Until approximately age 10, cell size is similar in males and females. After age 10 the difference between males and females gradually widens, and individual variations (indicated by the vertical lines) become more apparent. (b) The number of adipose cells gradually increases over the childhood years in males and females at a similar rate. At approximately age 10 in both sexes, the rate of increase in fat cell number accelerates, but females far exceed males. Individual differences indicated by vertical bars (labeled SD for standard deviation) increase considerably with age.

Source: Growth, Maturation and Physical Activity (pp. 138, 139) by Robert M. Malina and Claude Bouchard. Champaign, IL: Human Kinetics. Copyright 1991 by Robert Malina and Claude Bouchard. Reprinted by permission.

number plateaus in late adolescence and early adulthood and ideally remains at that level. In reality, however, hyperplasia can and often does occur in adulthood (Malina and Bouchard, 1991). Thus, although there are two critical periods—infancy and adolescence—in the development of adipocytes, this should not be interpreted as meaning that fat cells cannot be added during adulthood.

Some individuals produce more adipocytes than others during growth, and this can amount to billions of cells. During the growth changes males tend to accumulate more subcutaneous fat on the trunk and females on the extremities.

Fat Distribution Patterns

The location of fat storage varies among individuals. In general, humans distribute fat in three basic patterns: android, gynoid, and intermediate patterns (Figure 8.11). The *android pattern,* also known as the abdominal or apple pattern, is predominately found in males. It is characterized by the storage of fat in the nape of the neck, shoulders, and abdomen (upper part of the body). In this pattern the largest quantity of fat is stored internally, not subcutaneously. The result is the classic potbelly shape. Individuals with potbellies often make the claim that they are not fat and occasionally challenge others to hit them in the stomach as hard as possible to prove their superior musculature. In fact, the hardness of the abdominal region is caused by the excess fat in the abdominal cavity pushing against the abdominal muscles and stretching them taut, not by muscle tone or hypertrophy. Once the amount of fat to be stored exceeds the capacity of the abdominal cavity, subcutaneous sites are loaded (Campaigne, 1990; Stamford, 1991).

The *gynoid pattern,* also called the gluteofemoral or pear pattern, is found predominantly among females. It is characterized by the storage of fat in the lower part of the body, specifically, in the thighs and buttocks, with the largest quantity being stored subcutaneously. No pseudohardness is apparent. These sites tend to be soft and to jiggle (Campaigne, 1990; Stamford, 1991).

There is a growing body of evidence that the deposition of fat in the gluteal-femoral region by females is linked to reproductive function. In particular, gluteal-femoral fat may furnish energy for the development of the fetus primarily during the latter states of pregnancy and for the newborn child during lactation. As would be expected, these fat deposits are controlled by the steroid hormones.

The third type of fat pattern is known simply as the *intermediate pattern.* In this pattern, fat is stored in both the upper and the lower parts of the body, giving a somewhat rectangular cubic appearance. Note that all three patterns are found in both males and females, despite the sex-specific predominance associated with android and gynoid shapes (Campaigne, 1990; Stamford, 1991).

Abdominal fat deposits are easily mobilized; therefore it is possible to reduce fat accumulation in this area relatively easily. Conversely, gluteal-femoral fat deposits are not easily mobilized, and so it is not possible to reduce fat accumulation in these areas easily. The potential for reshaping the gluteofemoral

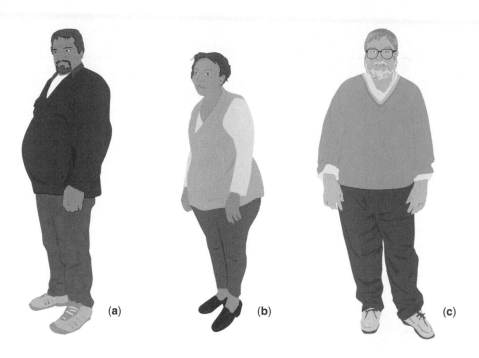

Figure 8.11
Patterns of Fat Distribution

(a) Android; (b) Gynoid; (c) Intermediate.

(a)   (b)   (c)

fat pattern is extremely limited (Campaigne, 1990; Stamford, 1991).

The reason behind the variation in fat deposit mobilization is hormonally based. Two different receptors, alpha and beta, have been identified in fat cells; they vary in their ability to facilitate or inhibit fat incorporation into the cell or fat mobilization out of the cell. Alpha-receptors inhibit fat transfer to and from the adipocytes, and beta-receptors enhance these transfers. Enzyme activity is concomitantly increased or decreased. Alpha-receptors predominate in the lower body and are thus more abundant in the gynoid pattern. Beta-receptors are concentrated in the upper body and are more abundant in the android pattern. Thus, the adipose cells in the abdominal region are more unstable.

Under the influence of epinephrine (released from the adrenal medulla), fat from the abdominal cells is easily mobilized and dumped into the circulatory system. If the free fatty acids and glycerol can be used (directly or indirectly) as fuel to support exercise, there is no problem. However, when epinephrine is released in times of emotional stress, there is no need for the excess fuel; the fatty acids and glycerol are then routed to the liver, where they are primarily converted to low-density lipoproteins (LDLs). LDLs are largely composed of cholesterol and are associated with atherosclerosis and an increased risk of coronary artery disease (CAD). (See Chapter 16 for an in-depth discussion of CAD risk factors.)

In addition, abdominal fat cells tend to be larger than fat cells found in other parts of the body. Larger fat cells are associated with glucose intolerance (the inability to dispose of a glucose load effectively), coupled with insulin resistance and hyperglycemia, and an excess of insulin in the blood (hyperinsulinemia). These conditions are associated with diabetes mellitus (a CAD risk factor) and hypertension (a CAD risk factor). The latter occurs because of the action of insulin in promoting reabsorption of sodium by the kidneys (Brownell, et al., 1987; Campaigne, 1990; Stamford, 1991).

Table 8.5 summarizes the differences between android and gynoid fat patterns.

Waist-to-Hip Ratio

Simply looking in the mirror while naked is probably the best way to determine whether you are android, gynoid, or intermediate in terms of fat distribution. Computation of a waist-to-hip ratio is suggested as a way to estimate the health risk of the pattern of fat distribution. Research has shown that the waist-to-hip ratio (W/H) is a stronger predictor for diabetes, coronary artery disease, and overall death risk than body weight, body mass index, or percent body fat (Brownell, et al., 1987; Folsom, et al., 1993).

Waist circumference is measured with a tape measure, to the nearest centimeter, at the level of the natural indentation or at the navel if no indentation is apparent. Hip circumference is measured at the largest site. Both measures should be taken while the individual is standing and is without clothes. The average value for females ages 17–39 is 0.80, and this value increases with age to above 0.90. Comparable averages for males range from 0.90 to 0.98. Values

Table 8.5
Patterns of Fat Distribution

Factor	Android	Gynoid
Sex it predominates in	Males	Females
Regional fat storage	Upper body (neck, abdomen)	Lower body (thighs, buttocks)
Fat storage site	Internal	Subcutaneous
Characteristic of fat deposit	Hard	Soft
Adipose tissue receptors	Beta	Alpha
Mobilizing hormone	Epinephrine	Reproductive, especially prolactin
Adipose cell size	Large	Small
Fat mobilization	Easy	Difficult
Major risk	Coronary artery disease, glucose intolerance, diabetes, hypertension	Psychological

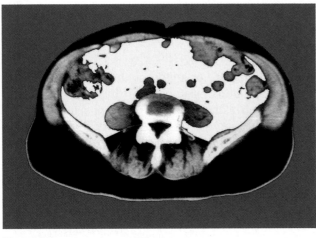

Figure 8.12
Visceral Abdominal Tissue

Computed tomography (CT) scan at the L4–L5 intravertebral space. The abdominal visceral fat depot is in yellow; the subcutaneous fat depot (both outside the muscle wall and below the skin) is in black.

above these averages raise the health risks for individuals of both sexes (Stamford, 1991).

In 1998, the National Heart, Lung, and Blood Institute expert panel on obesity concluded that waist circumference (also known as waist girth) alone was more strongly related to visceral abdominal adipose tissue and more predictive of disease risk than the waist-to-hip ratio. High risk was defined as a waist measure > 102 cm (> 40 inches) for males and > 88 cm (> 35 inches) for females with a BMI between 25 and > 35 $kg \cdot m^{-2}$. Waist circumference has little additional benefit as a predictor of health risk for a BMI >35 because essentially all individuals in this category will have waist measures above the cited cutoff values (National Heart, Lung, and Blood Institute, 1998).

Health Risks of Overweight and Obesity

Individuals who are overweight from an excess of body fat, but are not obese, incur mild to moderate health risks. Individuals who are obese possess an excess of body fat that represents a significant health risk particularly if that excess fat is visceral. Figure 8.12 presents an image of visceral abdominal tissue (VAT). The amount of fat and the distribution of that fat are linked to higher risks of major diseases. These diseases, discussed in the following sections, lead to increased mortality or decreased longevity.

Cardiovascular Disease

Framingham, Massachusetts, has been the site of a longitudinal study investigating the risk factors for heart disease in more than 5000 residents. Data from 26–30 yr of follow-up have shown that overweight or obesity is a significant predictor of cardiovascular disease, independent of age, cholesterol, systolic blood pressure, cigarette smoking, and glucose tolerance. The Framingham investigators have concluded that if everyone were at or within 10% of his or her desirable weight, there would be 25% less coronary heart disease and 35% less congestive heart failure and stroke. The risk is greater for those who become obese early in life rather than in old age (Bray, 1987; Burton, et al., 1985; Pi-Sunyer, 1993; Simopoulos, 1987). And as mentioned in the previous section, the degree of risk is higher for those who store their fat in the android pattern than in the gynoid pattern.

Hypertension (High Blood Pressure)

There is a strong association between elevated blood pressure and excess body weight and fat. The relationship varies directly, and a reduction in blood

Focus on Research

Exercise Training and Visceral Fat in Obese Children

Owen, S., B. Gutin, J. Allison, S. Riggs, & M. Ferguson. Effect of physical training on total and visceral fat in obese children. *Medicine and Science in Sport and Exercise.* 31(1):143–148 (1999).

High levels of total body fat mass and visceral adipose tissue (VAT) place children at greater risk for coronary artery disease and non–insulin-dependent diabetes mellitus. Owen and colleagues conducted this study to determine whether controlled physical training would have a favorable impact on VAT and percent body fat. These authors assigned volunteers to a control group or a physical training group. The physical training group exercised for 40 minutes at an average heart rate of 157 b·min⁻¹, 5 days a week, for 4 months. The graph presents the percentage change in several variables in the training group and in the control group after 4 months.

These data indicate that during an exercise program obese children

1. were capable of participating in a high-intensity exercise training program;
2. experienced a loss in fat mass, percent body fat, and subcutaneous abdominal adipose tissue, (SAAT), whereas the control group experienced a gain in fat mass and SAAT over the same period; and
3. experienced a smaller increase in VAT compared to the control group.

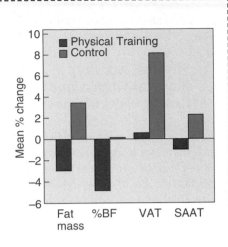

This study indicates that increasing the physical activity of obese children, even without dietary intervention, can improve aspects of body composition that are related to cardiovascular risk factors.

pressure usually follows weight loss (Bray, 1987; Burton, et al., 1985; Pi-Sunyer, 1993). Hypertension is also a very strong and independent risk factor for coronary heart disease.

Gallbladder Disease and Hypercholesterolemia (High Cholesterol)

In the Framingham study mentioned previously individuals who were 20% or more above the average weight for their height were about twice as likely to develop gallbladder disease as those who were 10% less than the average weight. In another study the frequency of gallbladder disease was largely explained by weight, age, and, in females, the number of viable pregnancies (parity). Obese females between age 20 and 30 yr had a 600% greater chance of having gallbladder disease than average-weight females. Within all age groups the frequency of gallbladder disease increased with the level of body weight. The body weight of males with gallstones has also been shown to be significantly more than the body weight of men without gallstones (Bray, 1987; Pi-Sunyer, 1993).

At least part of the explanation for the increased gallbladder disease in overweight or obese individuals can be linked to the effect of increased body weight and fat on cholesterol. There is a significant relationship between fatness and cholesterol level that is direct and positive. Cholesterol production is also related to body weight such that 1 excess kg of body weight increases cholesterol production 20–22 mg·dL⁻¹. Bile is produced in the liver and stored in the gallbladder and always contains some cholesterol. The bile of obese individuals is more saturated with cholesterol than that of nonobese individuals. This increased presence of cholesterol in bile is the likely cause of the increased risk of gallbladder disease (Bray, 1987).

Diabetes Mellitus

Diabetes is a disorder of carbohydrate (glucose) metabolism. Overweight or obesity appears to cause a deterioration in glucose tolerance (leading to high levels of blood glucose) and to aggravate the appearance of diabetes. Weight loss reduces this risk, and Type II diabetes can thus often be controlled by diet and weight loss (Bray, 1987; Burton, et al., 1985; Pi-Sunyer, 1993).

Cancer

The American Cancer Society has published data on 750,000 individuals studied between 1959 and 1972. In these studies, as BMI increased, so did the incidence

Focus on Application

✳ Physical Activity/ Physical Fitness and the Health Risks of Obesity

Epidemiological evidence indicates that there is a relationship between physical activity/physical fitness and the health risks of overweight/obesity. Epidemiology is the science that compares the rates of death (mortality), disease (morbidity), or functional status in one portion of the population exposed to a potential risk factor with another portion of the population not exposed to the potential risk factor. The results are most frequently reported as a relative risk ratio (RR). The relative risk is often adjusted for other factors, such as age, smoking habit, family history, alcohol intake, and so on, to mathematically control for any influence these factors might have (Blair and Brodney, 1999; Welk and Blair, 2000).

The health risks of overweight and obesity have been detailed in this chapter. It is well established that one way to reduce the health risks associated with overweight and

obesity is to lose body weight and, more specifically, body fat. However, it is also well established that this is easier said than done, and the same is true for maintaining any weight loss that might be achieved. So, the question becomes, Can physical activity or physical fitness weaken or blunt the increased risk of morbidity or mortality in overweight/obese individuals who remain overweight or obese?

A compilation of studies that can shed light on this question is presented in the accompanying figure. These studies were conducted at the Institute for Aerobics Research, Cooper Clinic (Dallas, TX), and are based on approximately 22,000 men. Insufficient data are available on female subjects to replicate these studies exactly. The results clearly show that no matter how body composition is measured (BMI, percent body fat, or waist girth), overweight or obese individuals who are fit have a lower risk of all-cause mortality (that is, early death from all causes) than unfit individuals (Blair and Brodney, 1999; Welk and Blair, 2000). Indeed, the fit individuals who were obese

had much less risk of early death than the unfit lean individuals did. This can be seen in the figure by comparing the red bars (fit), which have a RR of approximately 1.0, to the blue bars (unfit), where the relative risk ranges from 1.62 to 4.88. These higher risk ratios mean that the unfit are 62% to approximately 400% more likely to suffer early death than the fit, regardless of body composition level. In addition, the risk of all-cause mortality is similar for fit individuals, no matter what their level of body composition: lean, normal, or obese; that is, the adjusted relative risk for the fit groups deviated only slightly from 1.0 (0.8 to 1.08, which indicates no excessive risk), regardless of body composition (Blair and Brodney, 1999; Welk and Blair, 2000).

It is important to realize that fitness in these studies was determined by a maximal treadmill test, but that only the individuals comprising the bottom 20% (by age-specific distribution) were classified as unfit. In terms of absolute values, this level of fitness is equivalent to a $\dot{V}O_2$max of 28–35 mL·kg^{-1} min^{-1} for 20- to

---

of death from cancer, even independent of cigarette smoking. Overweight males were particularly susceptible to prostate and colorectal cancer; overweight females showed increased rates of breast, cervical, endometrial, uterine, and ovarian cancer. The suspected link, at least for the females, is the level of estrogen. Adipose tissue is a site for estrogen formation in all females and the major site in postmenopausal females. Estrogen formation is increased in overweight and obese individuals owing to the increased number of adipose cells (Bray, 1987; Charney, et al., 1975; Pi-Sunyer, 1993; Simopoulos, 1987).

Miscellaneous Disorders

In addition to the specific diseases just discussed, overweight or obesity has been linked to respiratory dysfunction, joint problems and gout, endocrine

disorder, problems in the administration of anesthetics for surgery, and an impaired physical work capacity (American College of Sports Medicine, 1983; Pi-Sunyer, 1993). The increase in prevalence of these diseases applies to adults, but overweight or obese children also show increased risk factors, though not the actual diseases, compared with normal-weight children (Williams, et al., 1992).

Heredity and Body Composition

There is evidence in humans that both obesity and localized fat deposition are determined solely by genetic transmission in some individuals. Thirteen genetic syndromes have been identified in the medical literature, but all are considered to be pathological disorders and are extremely rare. Even the most common has an incidence rate of only about 1 in 25,000. For

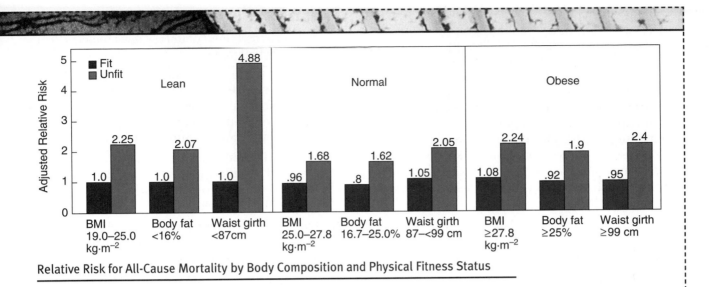

Relative Risk for All-Cause Mortality by Body Composition and Physical Fitness Status

39-yr-old females and males, and 25–33 mL·kg⁻¹ min⁻¹ for 40- to 59-yr-old females and males. These fitness levels can be achieved by as little as 400–1650 kcal of activity per week. This level of energy expenditure is consistent with the recommendation of the Surgeon General: 30 minutes of moderate activity on most, if not all, days of the week (Blair and Brodney, 1999).

The implications for health promotion are clear. There are health risks associated with overweight and obe-sity, and advice to lose weight remains sound. As such, weight loss remains one of the primary reasons individuals join a health club or exercise program. Many overweight/obese individuals, however, become frustrated when the desired weight loss does not happen or does not happen rapidly enough (for whatever reason), and they quickly drop out of the exercise regimen. These individuals should be encouraged to remain or become more active in order to reap the physiological benefits of regular activity. The process of being active, rather than the product of any changes in body weight or percent fat, should be stressed. Stressing the process is more likely to motivate overweight/obese individuals because participation in activity is within each person's control (Welk and Blair, 2000). If the process (regular physical activity) is accomplished, the product (lower health risks) will follow.

Sources:

Blair & Brodag (1999); Welk & Blair (2000).

the vast majority of us the contribution of genetics to our body composition is not nearly so absolute, despite what our experience tells us about familial resemblance (Boileau, et al., 1984).

Studies conducted to determine the contribution of genetics to body composition show the expected pattern of very low relationships between biological siblings, whether born separately or together (dizygotic twins), and moderate relationships between monozygotic twins. Despite these moderate relationships, Bouchard and Perusse (1988) have concluded the following:

1. Only about 5% of the total variation in BMI and skinfold thickness is genetically transferable.

2. About 25–30% of the variance in %BF, FFW, and fat distribution patterning is genetically transferable.

3. About 30% of the transmission of body composition variables is linked to cultural factors, defined as the environment established by the family (such as the role and amount of food consumed, the types of food eaten, and activity patterns).

4. About 45–65% of the variance in body composition is genetically nontransferable.

The first two conclusions may mean that the storage of internal fat is influenced by genetics more than the storage of subcutaneous fat is.

These low to moderate contributions of biological transferability do not mean that heredity does not play a critical role in an individual's body composition. For example, when six pairs of male monozygotic twins were overfed by 1000 kcal·day⁻¹ for 22 days, all responded with significant gains in body weight, skinfold thickness, and fat mass. There were large interpair (between-pair) differences in these gains, but not intrapair (between-twin) differences.

These data indicate that some individuals are genetically programmed for fat gain in response to excess calories, but others are not. A follow-up study lasting for 100 days showed the same response, with some of the pairs exhibiting more of a tendency to gain fat-free mass than fat mass. This tendency to gain fat or fat-free tissue is called *nutrient partitioning*. At the present time there is no way to identify who falls into which category (Bouchard, 1991; Bouchard, et al., 1990). The best advice, therefore, seems to be to avoid consistently ingesting more calories than are utilized—which, of course, is easier said than done for most people.

Summary

1. Hydrostatic, or underwater, weighing is generally considered to be the laboratory criterion measure for the determination of body composition. It is based on densitometry.

2. Densitometry usually divides the body into two components, fat and fat-free weight. Fat-free weight is composed of water, protein, and bone mineral. The components are known and relatively stable in adults but not in children and adolescents. Thus, no single equation, and especially not the adult equations of Brozek or Siri, can be used for children.

3. Skinfolds, bioelectrical impedance, and height and weight indices are frequently used field tests for assessing body composition.

4. Reasonable values for assessing overweight as a risk to health are 26–31% BF or a BMI of > 27.3 kg·m^{-2} for adult females and 19–24% BF or a BMI of > 27.8 kg·m^{-2} for adult males. Comparable standards for obesity are over 32% BF (BMI > 30) for females and over 25% BF (BMI > 30) for males.

5. The size and number of adipocytes increase as a child grows to adulthood. Adult fat gain first involves hypertrophy of the adipocytes and then hyperplasia of precursor cells.

6. The health risks of overweight and obesity include cardiovascular disease, hypertension, gallbladder disease and hypercholesterolemia, diabetes mellitus, and cancer. Physical fitness can blunt these risks in overweight and obese individuals.

7. Heredity influences total percent body fat, fat-free mass, the tendency to gain or lose one or the other, and fat distribution.

Review Questions

1. Define densitometry. Relate densitometry to hydrostatic weighing.

2. Explain the assumptions that must be met in order for hydrostatic weighing to be accurate. What variations in these basic assumptions occur in children, adolescents, and the elderly? State two practical applications of this information.

3. List and identify the strengths and weaknesses of the field estimates of overweight and obesity. Which technique would you select to use in a field setting? Explain why.

4. Compare the accuracy of %BF determined by skinfolds and bioelectrical impedance with %BF determined by hydrostatic weighing.

5. Compare and contrast the %BF, %BF distribution, and patterns of fat distribution between males and females.

6. Differentiate between overweight and obesity.

7. What happens to adipose cells as an individual becomes overweight and then obese?

8. List and briefly discuss the health risks of being overweight or obese.

9. Debate the importance of heredity in body composition.

For further review and additional study tools, go to The Physiology Place (www.physiologyplace.com) and the Student Study Guide for Exercise Physiology for Health, Fitness, and Performance *by Sharon A. Plowman and Denise L. Smith.*

Passport to the Internet

Visit the following Internet sites to explore further topics and issues related to the measurement of body composition. To visit an organization's web site, go to www.physiologyplace.com and click on "Passport to the Internet."

Shape Up America! A nationwide network of over 40 organizations in the fields of medicine, public health, nutrition, and physical activity united to encourage healthy weight and to support increased physical activity. Check out this site and identify the three primary objectives of Shape Up America! What does this organization identify as the key step in reaching these objectives?

Centers for Disease Control and Prevention Visit this government site and look under "Health Topics A to Z" for materials and information on obesity, weight management, and other related topics.

References

American College of Sports Medicine: Proper and improper weight loss programs. *Medicine and Science in Sports and Exercise.* 15:xi–xiii (1983).

Ballor, D. L., V. L. Katch, M. D. Becque, & C. R. Marks: Resistance weight training during caloric restriction enhances lean body weight maintenance. *American Journal of Clinical Nutrition.* 47:19–25 (1988).

Baumgartner, R. N., W. C. Chumlea, & A. F. Roche: Bioelectrical impedance for body composition. In K. B. Pandolf (ed.), *Exercise and Sport Sciences Reviews.* Baltimore: Williams & Wilkins, 18, 193–224 (1990).

Beeson, V., C. Ray, R. A. Coxon, & S. Kreitzman: The myth of the yo-yo: Consistent rate of weight loss with successive dieting by VLCD. *International Journal of Obesity.* 13:135–139 (1989).

Behnke, A. R., & J. H. Wilmore: *Evaluation and Regulation of Body Build and Composition.* Englewood Cliffs, NJ: Prentice-Hall (1974).

Björntorp, P. A.: Fat cell distribution and metabolism. In R. J. Wurtman & J. J. Wurtman (eds.), *Annals of the New York Academy of Science.* New York: New York Academy of Science, 499:66–72 (1987).

Björntorp, P. A.: Sex differences in the regulation of energy balance with exercise. *American Journal of Clinical Nutrition.* 49:958–961 (1989).

Blair, S. N., & S. Brodney: Effects of physical inactivity and obesity on morbidity and mortality: Current evidence and research issues. *Medicine and Science in Sports and Exercise.* 31(11) Supplement: S646–S662 (1999).

Boileau, R. A., T. G. Lohman, M. H. Slaughter, T. E. Ball, S. B. Going, & M. K. Hendrix: Hydration of the fat-free body in children during maturation. *Human Biology.* 56(4):651–666 (1984).

Bouchard, C.: Heredity and the path to overweight and obesity. *Medicine and Science in Sports and Exercise.* 23(3): 285–291 (1991).

Bouchard, C., & L. Perusse: Heredity and body fat. *Annual Review of Nutrition.* 8:259–277 (1988).

Bouchard, C. T., A. Tremblay, A. Nadeau, J. Dussault, J. P. Depres, G. Theriault, P. J. Lupien, O. Serresse, M. R. Boulay, & G. Fournier: Long-term exercise training with constant energy intake. 1. Effect on body composition. *International Journal of Obesity.* 14:57–73 (1990).

Bray, G. A.: Complications of obesity. *Annals of Internal Medicine.* 103(6 pt 2):1052–1062 (1985).

Bray, G. A.: Overweight is risking fate: Definition, classification, prevalence, and risks. *Annals of the New York Academy of Science.* New York: New York Academy of Science, 499: 14–28 (1987).

Brodie, D. A.: Techniques of measurement of body composition: Part I. *Sports Medicine.* 5:11–40 (1988a).

Brodie, D. A.: Techniques of measurement of body composition: Part II. *Sports Medicine.* 5:74–98 (1988b).

Brownell, K. D., S. N. Steen, & J. H. Wilmore: Weight regulation practices in athletes: Analysis of metabolic and health effects. *Medicine and Science in Sports and Exercise.* 19(6):546–556 (1987).

Bubb, W. J.: Relative leanness. In E. T. Howley & B. D. Franks (eds.), *Health Fitness Instructor's Handbook* (2nd edition). Champaign, IL: Human Kinetics (1992).

Burton, B. T., W. R. Foster, J. Hirsch, & T. B. van Itallie: Health implications of obesity: An NIH consensus development conference. *International Journal of Obesity.* 9:155–169 (1985).

Campaigne, B. N.: Body fat distribution in females: Metabolic consequences and implications for weight loss. *Medicine and Science in Sports and Exercise.* 22(3):291–297 (1990).

Caton, J. R., P. A. Mole, W. C. Adams, & D. S. Heustis: Body composition analysis by bioelectrical impedance: Effect of skin temperature. *Medicine and Science in Sports and Exercise.* 20(5):489–491 (1988).

Charney, E., H. C. Goodman, M. McBride, B. Lyon, & R. Pratt: Childhood antecedents of adult obesity. *New England Journal of Medicine.* 295(1):6–9 (1975).

Deurenberg, P. W., I. Paymans, & K. vander Kooy: Factors affecting bioelectrical impedance measurements in humans. *European Journal of Clinical Nutrition.* 42:1017–1022 (1988).

Dietz, W. H.: Childhood obesity. In R. J. Wurtman & J. J. Wurtman (eds.), *Annals of the New York Academy of Science.* New York: New York Academy of Science, 499:47–54 (1987).

Folsom, A. R., S. A. Kaye, T. A. Sellers, C.-P. Hong, J. R. Cerhan, J. D. Potter, & R. J. Prineas: Body fat distribution and 5-year risk of death in older women. *Journal of the American Medical Association.* 269(4):483–487 (1993).

Fomon, S., J. Haschke, E. E. Ziegler, & S. E. Nelson: Body composition of reference children from birth to age 10 years. *American Journal of Clinical Nutrition.* 35: 1169–1175 (1982).

Friiz-Hansen, B.: Hygrometry of growth and aging. In J. E. Brozek (ed.), *Human Body Composition.* Oxford, England: Pergamon Press, 191–209 (1965).

Gallagher, D., M. Visser, D. Sepulveda, R. N. Pierson, T. Harris, & S. B. Heymsfield: How useful is body mass index for comparison of body fatness across age, sex and ethnic groups? *American Journal of Epidemiology.* 146:228–239 (1996).

Garner, D. M., P. E. Garfinkel, D. Schwartz, & M. Thompson: Cultural expectations of thinness in women. *Psychological Reports.* 47:483–491 (1980).

Golding, L. A., C. R. Myers, & W. E. Sinning: *The Y's Way to Physical Fitness* (3rd edition). Champaign, IL: Human Kinetics (1989).

Goldman, R. F., & E. R. Buskirk: Body volume measurement by under water weighing: Description of a method. In J. Brozek & A. Henschel (eds.), *Techniques for Measuring Body Composition.* Washington, DC: National Academy of Sciences—National Research Council, 78–89 (1961).

Harrison, G. G., E. R. Buskirk, J. E. L. Carter, F. E. Johnston, T. G. Lohman, M. L. Pollock, A. F. Roche, & J. Wilmore: Skinfold thickness and measurement technique. In T. G. Lohman, A. F. Roche, & R. Martorell (eds.), *Anthropometric Standardization Reference Manual*. Champaign, IL: Human Kinetics, 55–70 (1988).

Heyward, V. H., & Stolarczyk, L. M.: *Applied Body Composition Assessment*. Champaign, IL: Human Kinetics (1996).

Himes, J. H., & R. A. Frisancho: Estimating frame size. In T. G. Lohman, A. F. Roche, & R. Martorell (eds.), *Anthropometric Standardization Reference Manual*. Champaign, IL: Human Kinetics, 122–124 (1988).

Hodgdon, J. A., & P. I. Fitzgerald: Validity of impedance predictions at various levels of fatness. *Human Biology*. 59(2):281–298 (1987).

Jackson, A. S., & M. L. Pollock: Practical assessment of body composition. *Physician and Sportsmedicine*. 13:76–90 (1985).

Lohman, T. G.: Applicability of body composition techniques and constants for children and youth. In K. B. Pandolf (ed.), *Exercise and Sport Sciences Reviews*. New York: Macmillan, 14:325–357 (1986).

Lohman, T. G.: Assessment of body composition in children. *Pediatric Exercise Science*. 1:19–30 (1989).

Lohman, T. G.: Body composition. In J. R. Morrow, H. B. Falls, & H. W. Kohl (eds.), *FITNESSGRAM Technical Reference Manual*. Dallas: Cooper Institute for Aerobics Research (1994).

Lohman, T. G.: Skinfolds and body density and their relation to body fatness: A review. *Human Biology*. 53(2): 181–225 (1981).

Lohman, T. G.: The use of skinfold to estimate body fatness on children and youth. *Journal of Physical Education, Recreation and Dance*. 58(9):98–102 (1987).

Lohman T. G., R. A. Boileau, & M. H. Slaughter: Body composition in children and youth. In R. A. Boileau (ed.), *Advances in Pediatric Sport Sciences*. Champaign, IL: Human Kinetics, 29–57 (1984).

Lutter, J. M.: Is your attitude weighing you down? *Melpomene Journal*. 13(1):13–16 (1994).

Malina, R. M., & C. Bouchard: *Growth, Maturation and Physical Activity*. Champaign, IL: Human Kinetics (1991).

Malina, R. M., B. W. Meleski, & R. F. Shoup: Anthropometric, body composition, and maturity characteristics of selected school-age athletes. *Pediatric Clinics of North America*. 29(6):1305–1323 (1982).

Marieb, E. N.: *Human Anatomy and Physiology* (5th edition). San Francisco, CA: Benjamin Cummings (2000).

McArdle, W. D., F. I. Katch, & V. L. Katch: *Exercise Physiology: Energy, Nutrition, and Human Performance* (3rd edition). Philadelphia: Lea & Febiger (1991).

National Center for Chronic Disease Prevention and Health Promotion: *Adolescent and School Health*. http://www.cdc.gov/nccdphp/dash/presphyactrpt/summary.ntm (2000).

National Heart, Lung, and Blood Institute: Executive summary of the clinical guidelines on the identification, evaluation, and treatment of overweight and obesity in adults. *Journal of the American Dietetic Association*. 98(10): 1178–1191 (1998).

Nieman, D. C.: *Fitness and Sports Medicine: An Introduction*. Palo Alto, CA: Bull Publishing (1990).

Pi-Sunyer, F. X.: Medical hazards of obesity. *Annals of Internal Medicine*. 119(7 pt 2):655–660 (1993).

Plowman, S. A., N. Y. Liu, & C. L. Wells: Body composition and sexual maturation in premenarcheal athletes and nonathletes. *Medicine and Science in Sports and Exercise*. 23(1):23–29 (1991).

Powers, S. K., & E. T. Howley: *Exercise Physiology: Theory and Application to Fitness and Performance*. Dubuque, IA: Brown (1990).

Revicki, D. A., & R. G. Israel: Relationship between body mass indices and measures of body adiposity. *American Journal of Public Health*. 76:992–994 (1986).

Roche, A. F.: Some aspects of the criterion methods for the measurement of body composition. *Human Biology*. 59(2):209–220 (1987).

Satwanti, B. S., I. P. Singh, & H. Bharadwaj: Body fat from skinfold thicknesses and weight-height indices: A comparison. *Zeitschrift für Morphologie und Anthropologie*. 71(1): 93–100 (1980).

Simopoulos, A. P.: Characteristics of obesity: An overview. In R. J. Wurtman & J. J. Wurtman (eds.), *Annals of the New York Academy of Science*. New York: New York Academy of Science, 499 4–13 (1987).

Sjöström, L., & P. Björntorp: Body composition and adipose tissue cellularity in human obesity. *Acta Medica Scandinavica*. 195:201–211 (1974).

Slaughter, M. H., T. G. Lohman, R. A. Boileau, C. A. Horswill, R. J. Stillman, M. D. Van Loan, & D. A. Bemben: Skinfold equation for estimation of body fatness in children and youth. *Human Biology*. 60(5):709–723 (1988).

Stamford, B.: Apples and pears: Where you "wear" your fat can affect your health. *The Physician and Sportsmedicine*. 19(1):123–124 (1991).

Stump, C. S., L. B. Houtkooper, M. H. Heweitt, S. B. Going, & T. G. Lohman: Bioelectrical impedance variability with dehydration and exercise. *Medicine and Science in Sports and Exercise*. 20(2):S82 (1988).

Tiggemann, M.: Body-size dissatisfaction: Individual differences in age and gender, and relationship with self-esteem. *Personality and Individual Differences*. 13(1):39–43 (1992).

Van Itallie, T. B.: Topography of body fat: Relationship to risk of cardiovascular and other diseases. In T. G. Lohman, A. F. Roche, & R. Martorell (eds.), *Anthropometric Standardization Reference Manual*. Champaign, IL: Human Kinetics, 143–149 (1988).

Van Loan, M. D.: Bioelectrical impedance analysis to determine fat-free mass, total body water and body fat. *Sports Medicine*. 10(4):205–217 (1990).

Welk, G. J., & S. N. Blair; Physical activity protects against the health risk of obesity. *President's Council on Physical Fitness and Sports Research Digest.* Series 3 (12):1–8 (2000).

Williams, D. P., S. B. Going, T. G. Lohman, D. P. Harsha, S. R. Srinivasau, L. S. Webber, & G. S. Beneuson: Body fatness and risk for elevated blood pressure, total cholesterol, and serum lipoprotein ratios in children and adolescents. *American Journal of Public Health.* 82:358–363 (1992).

Williamson, D. F.: Descriptive epidemiology of body weight and weight change in U.S. adults. *Annals of Internal Medicine.* 119(7 pt 2):646–649 (1993).

World Health Organization: Obesity: Preventing and managing the global epidemic. *Report of a WHO Consultation on Obesity.* Geneva: World Health Organization (1998).

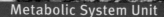
Chapter 9

Body Composition and Weight Control

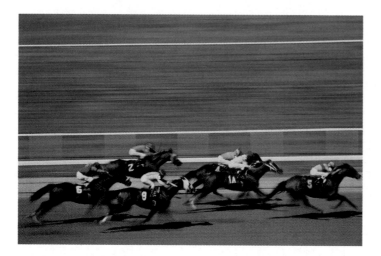

After studying the chapter, you should be able to

- State the caloric balance equation, and define and explain its components.

- Discuss the impact of diet, as caloric restriction, on the components of the caloric balance equation.

- Discuss the impact of an exercise session on the components of the caloric balance equation.

- Discuss the impact of exercise training on the components of the caloric balance equation.

- Compare and contrast the effects of diet alone, exercise alone, and diet plus exercise combined on body weight and composition control.

- Apply the training principles to body weight and composition control.

- Compose guidelines for making weight in a sport.

The Caloric Balance Equation

At its most basic level, weight control follows the first law of thermodynamics. The **first law of thermodynamics,** sometimes called the **law of conservation of energy,** states that energy can neither be created nor destroyed, but only changed in form. This law was described fully in Chapter 3.

When the body converts the potential chemical energy of food into other chemical, mechanical, or heat energy, it follows the law of conservation of energy. Theoretically, if the amount of energy taken in equals the amount of energy expended, the body is in balance and the weight (mass) remains stable. If an excess of energy is ingested, that energy is neither destroyed nor lost; rather, weight (mass) is gained. If insufficient energy is ingested in relation to expenditure, the needed energy cannot be created but must be provided from storage sites, and weight (mass) is reduced.

Energy, in the forms involved in the human body, is most frequently described in terms of kilocalories (kcal) or kilojoules (kJ). One **kilocalorie** is the amount of heat needed to raise the temperature of 1 kg of water 1°C. One kilocalorie is equal to 4.186 kJ. A calorie is equal to 0.001 kcal. The term *calorie* is often used generically, however, as in the statement "Caloric intake should be equal to caloric output," even though the units would be kilocalories. The caloric equivalent of 1 lb of fat is 3500 kcal.

The **caloric balance equation,** the mathematical summation of the caloric intake (+) and energy expenditure (−) from all sources, quantifies the law of conservation of energy. It describes the source of potential energy as food ingested and the various uses of that energy. The input and output can be partitioned into the following elements:

caloric balance = + food ingested (kcal)
  − basal or resting metabolic rate (kcal)
  − thermogenesis (kcal)
  − work or exercise metabolism (kcal)
  − energy excreted in waste products (kcal)

Food intake represents the only positive factor in the caloric balance equation. It is the only way that energy can be added to the system. Energy is expended in three ways. The first is basal or resting metabolic rate, the second is thermogenesis, and the third is work or exercise. These are the negative factors in the caloric balance equation.

Figure 9.1 indicates that the basal or resting metabolic rate accounts for the majority of the total

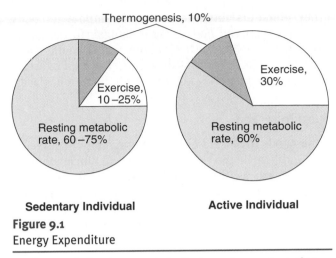

Sedentary Individual **Active Individual**

Figure 9.1
Energy Expenditure

Resting metabolic rate accounts for the largest percentage of energy expended in both inactive and active individuals, although the exact percentage varies between the two groups. The percentage of energy expended during exercise is higher in active than in inactive individuals. Thermogenesis accounts for about 10% of the energy expended in both active and inactive individuals.

Source: Modified from Poehlman (1989).

energy expenditure, varying from approximately 60% to approximately 75% in active and sedentary individuals, respectively. Thermogenesis accounts for a relatively stable 10% in both sedentary and active individuals. The thermic effect of exercise is obviously higher in active individuals, and it depends on the intensity, duration, and frequency of exercise (Poehlman, 1989).

If the amount of energy in the food ingested exceeds the energy expended, the body is in a positive balance, and body weight will increase. If the amount of energy in the food ingested is less than the energy expended, the body is in a negative balance, and body weight will decrease. The amount of energy excreted in waste products is insignificant and rarely measured. It need not be considered here further. The

First Law of Thermodynamics or the **Law of Conservation of Energy** Energy can neither be created nor destroyed but only changed in form.

Kilocalorie The amount of heat needed to raise the temperature of 1 kg of water 1°C.

Caloric Balance Equation The mathematical summation of the caloric intake (+) and energy expenditure (−) from all sources.

other elements have considerable impact on body weight (mass) and body weight control. In the pages that follow, each of these elements will be defined and discussed. The impact of diet, exercise, and exercise training on each of the elements will be emphasized.

Food Ingested

Little needs to be said about food intake per se. We all eat, and lists of the potential energy (calorie) content of foods are readily available. Labels on packaged foods at the grocery store have printed kilocalorie values as well as a nutrient breakdown. Getting into the habit of reading food labels is a good idea and should enable you to make wise food choices in terms of both nutritional and energy content.

Impact of Diet on Food Intake

The term **diet** may mean many things, including the food regularly consumed during the course of normal living. It is also used to mean a restriction of caloric intake. This second meaning is how the term is being used in this chapter. Therefore, "going on a diet" should, by definition, mean a reduction in food intake.

Impact of Exercise and Exercise Training on Food Intake

The relationship between exercise, exercise training, appetite, and energy intake is complex and difficult to discern. Appetite and the amount of food ingested are influenced by physiological, nutritional, behavioral, and psychological factors in humans. It is not just a matter of a physiological drive to balance energy demand and supply (Blundell and King, 1999; Titchenal, 1988; Wilmore, 1983). People eat or don't eat for a variety of reasons. For example, when you are upset, do you cease eating, or do you consume everything in sight?

It is also very difficult to accurately measure food intake. Feeding individuals in a controlled setting where food can be measured may cause changes in eating behavior. Asking individuals to write down everything they eat necessitates a faith that they are neither over- nor (more likely) underreporting. For these reasons conducting studies on the effects of exercise and/or exercise training on appetite in humans is difficult. Despite the difficulties, the following generalizations can be drawn from the studies that are available:

1. Neither a transient reduction nor an increase in energy intake immediately following a single bout of exercise has been clearly established in humans. In one study the subjective rating of appetite was lowered in female subjects following 30 min of exercise at 50% $\dot{V}O_2$max. Despite this decreased subjective rating, food intake at the postexercise meal and for two days after was not affected. A chemical known to have anorectic (loss of appetite) properties in rats is also known to increase in response to exercise in humans; however, it has not been shown to actually decrease the human appetite.

2. Physically active males, females, adults, and children (such as heavy manual laborers and athletes) consume more calories than sedentary individuals. Yet the active individuals generally maintain their body weight and composition at or below normal levels.

3. Energy intake in both males and females generally increases or remains unchanged in response to exercise training. Which response occurs appears to depend on the fitness and body composition status of the individual. Highly trained athletes and lean individuals usually increase their energy intake in response to increased training loads. Untrained and/or obese individuals most often do not change energy intake in response to exercise training.

4. When chronic exercise training ceases, energy intake in humans is spontaneously reduced. Unfortunately, this reduction does not appear to be matched to the reduced energy expenditure. The result is often a positive energy balance, a regain of lost body weight, and a concomitant elevation of body fat.

Resting or Basal Metabolism

Basal energy expenditure, more commonly called **basal metabolic rate (BMR),** is defined as the level of energy required to sustain the body's vital functions in the waking state. Technically, this definition means that the individual is resting quietly in a supine position, has not eaten for 8–18 hr, is at normal body

---

Diet (a) The food regularly consumed during the course of normal living; (b) a restriction of caloric intake.

Basal Metabolic Rate (BMR) The level of energy required to sustain the body's vital functions in the waking state, when the individual is in a fasted condition, at normal body and room temperature, and without psychological stress.

Table 9.1
Surface Area in Square Meters for Different Heights and Weights

Height (cm)	Weight (kg)																
	25	30	35	40	45	50	55	60	65	70	75	80	85	90	95	100	105
200							1.84	1.91	1.97	2.03	2.09	2.15	2.21	2.26	2.31	2.36	2.41
195						1.73	1.80	1.87	1.93	1.99	2.05	2.11	2.17	2.22	2.27	2.32	2.37
190				1.56	1.63	1.70	1.77	1.84	1.90	1.96	2.02	2.08	2.13	2.18	2.23	2.28	2.33
185				1.53	1.60	1.67	1.74	1.80	1.86	1.92	1.98	2.04	2.09	2.14	2.19	2.24	2.29
180				1.49	1.57	1.64	1.71	1.77	1.83	1.89	1.95	2.00	2.05	2.10	2.15	2.20	2.25
175	1.19	1.28	1.36	1.46	1.53	1.60	1.67	1.73	1.79	1.85	1.91	1.96	2.01	2.06	2.11	2.16	2.21
170	1.17	1.26	1.34	1.43	1.50	1.57	1.63	1.69	1.75	1.81	1.86	1.91	1.96	2.01	2.06	2.11	
165	1.14	1.23	1.31	1.40	1.47	1.54	1.60	1.66	1.72	1.78	1.83	1.88	1.93	1.98	2.03	2.07	
160	1.12	1.21	1.29	1.37	1.44	1.50	1.56	1.62	1.68	1.73	1.78	1.83	1.88	1.93	1.98		
155	1.09	1.18	1.26	1.33	1.40	1.46	1.52	1.58	1.64	1.69	1.74	1.79	1.84	1.89			
150	1.06	1.15	1.23	1.30	1.36	1.42	1.48	1.54	1.60	1.65	1.70	1.75	1.80				
145	1.03	1.12	1.20	1.27	1.33	1.39	1.45	1.51	1.56	1.61	1.66	1.71					
140	1.00	1.09	1.17	1.24	1.30	1.36	1.42	1.47	1.52	1.57							
135	0.97	1.06	1.14	1.20	1.26	1.32	1.38	1.43	1.48								
130	0.95	1.04	1.11	1.17	1.23	1.29	1.35	1.40									
125	0.93	1.01	1.08	1.14	1.20	1.26	1.31	1.36									
120	0.91	0.98	1.04	1.10	1.16	1.22	1.27										

Source: D. Dubois & E. F. DuBois. Clinical calorimetry: A formula to estimate the approximate surface area if height and weight be known. *Archives of Internal Medicine.* 17:863–871 (1916). Reprinted by permission of *Archives of Internal Medicine.*

temperature (37°C) and neutral ambient temperature (27–29°C; 80–84°F), and is without feelings of psychological stress. Because of the difficulty of obtaining truly basal conditions in most laboratory settings, the term resting metabolic rate is probably a more accurate descriptor. **Resting metabolic rate (RMR)** is defined as the energy expended while an individual is resting quietly in a supine position. The two terms are often used interchangeably, since the measured differences are small. That practice will be followed here, with the term RMR used primarily but not exclusively (Bursztein, et al., 1989).

A variety of organs and processes are responsible for energy consumption at rest. The liver is the largest consumer of energy at rest (29–32%), followed by the brain (19–21%), muscles (18%), heart (10%), lungs (9%), and kidneys (7%). The muscle energy is primarily for the maintenance of tonus or tension, necessary even in sleep. On the cellular level the energy is used to fuel ion pumps (particularly the sodium–

potassium pump), synthesize and degrade cellular constituents, conduct electrical impulses, and secrete various substances, including hormones (Bogert, et al., 1973; Bursztein, et al., 1989).

Basal or resting metabolism is usually related to body surface area and expressed in $kcal \cdot m^{-2}$. It may also be expressed in $kcal \cdot day^{-1}$ or $\dot{V}O_2$ $mL \cdot min^{-1}$. The choice of measurement unit depends on the intended use of the information. If the interest lies in comparing submaximal or maximal oxygen values, then the choice is $\dot{V}O_2$ $mL \cdot min^{-1}$. In many cases, however, the interest lies in determining caloric needs, and then one of the kilocalorie units is utilized. Tables or graphs are available that allow one to estimate body surface area (BSA, in square meters) from height and weight (Table 9.1) and standard BMR values per BSA (Figure 9.2). From these values BMR ($kcal \cdot day^{-1}$) can be computed.

9.1 basal metabolic rate ($kcal \cdot day^{-1}$) = standard basal metabolic rate ($kcal \cdot m^{-2} \cdot hr^{-1}$) $\times$ body surface area (m^2) $\times$ 24 $hr \cdot day^{-1}$

or

$$BMR = \text{standard BMR} \times BSA \times 24$$

Resting Metabolic Rate (RMR) The energy expended while an individual is resting quietly in a supine position.

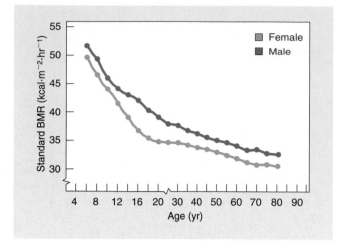

Figure 9.2
Standard Basal Metabolic Rate Across the Age Span

Standard basal metabolic rates decline steeply during childhood and adolescence and then more gradually during the adult years. At every age, male values are higher than female values, despite being prorated to body surface area.

Sources: Calculated from Brownell, et al. (1987); Bursztein, et al. (1989).

Example

A 22-yr-old female is 5 ft 5 in (165 cm) tall and weighs 143 lb (65 kg). According to Table 9.1, her BSA is 1.72 m^2. The number closest to her age on Figure 9.2 is 20 yr. Because this individual is female the lower line is used to estimate a standard BMR of 35.1 kcal·m^{-2}·hr^{-1}. Substituting these values into Equation 9.1 we get

$$BMR \ kcal·day^{-1} = 35.1 \ kcal·m^{-2}·hr^{-1}$$
$$\times 1.72 \ m^2 \times 24 \ hr·day^{-1}$$
$$BMR = 1448 \ kcal·day^{-1}$$

Somewhat less cumbersome is the use of prediction equations such as those presented in Table 9.2. For the individual in the previous example the calculation becomes RMR = 447.593 + (3.098 × 165) + (9.247 × 65) − (4.330 × 22) = 1464.6 kcal·day^{-1}. Although the two techniques do not agree exactly, they are very comparable for practical use.

Eighty-five percent of all normal subjects have estimated RMR values within 10% of measured values. The other 15% of the population have either higher or lower values. The range of variation may exceed 20%. Thus an individual who has a 20% higher RMR than average is able to ingest more calories without gaining weight, but the individual with a 20% lower RMR must ingest less or gain weight (Bursztein, et al., 1989; Guyton, 1986).

Table 9.2
Estimation of Basal (Resting) Metabolic Rate

Males

$$RMR = 88.362 + (4.799 \times HT)$$
$$+ (13.397 \times WT) - (5.677 \times AGE)$$

Females

$$RMR = 447.593 + (3.098 \times HT)$$
$$+ (9.247 \times WT) - (4.330 \times AGE)$$

where HT = height (in centimeters), WT = weight (in kilograms), AGE = age (in years).

Source: Based on Roza & Shizgal (1984).

Two criterion measures are available for RMR. The first is open-circuit indirect calorimetry, which was described in Chapter 5. The second is a blood test for the determination of protein-bound iodine (PBI). The iodine comes from thyroxine (T$_4$), the hormone secreted by the thyroid gland, which has the greatest impact on BMR. This test gives a relative indication of BMR, not a direct kcal·day^{-1} value (Bogert, et al., 1973).

The prediction equations in Table 9.2 give an indication of the primary nonhormonal factors that influence RMR. What are they? If you said body size, age, and sex, you are absolutely correct. RMR relates best to body surface area externally and to cell mass internally. Obese individuals have a larger surface area and a larger cell mass (both fat and fat-free) than average-weight individuals. Hence, not surprisingly, the RMR of obese individuals is higher than that of the normal-weight individuals (Jequier, 1987).

The influence of age and sex can be seen in Figure 9.2. RMR is highest in infants and young children. The drop from age 6 to 18 is approximately 25%, or 2% per year. The decline then slows to about 2–3% per decade after that age. Part of this decline in RMR may be attributed to and be responsible for the increment in %BF that usually occurs as people age.

Figure 9.2 also clearly shows that at all ages average-weight females have lower RMR than do average-weight males. The difference, which is least in young children, is accentuated at puberty and then tends to remain at about 5–6% through middle age and old age. In terms of calories, the RMR of adult males averages between 1500 and 1800 kcal·day^{-1} and the RMR of adult females averages between 1200 and 1450 kcal·day^{-1}. The lower female values are partially because females have smaller internal organs than males and tend to be smaller in terms of total body mass, on average, than males. However, the most obvious explanation is the difference in body cell mass, particularly muscle tissue. Females on average have a higher %BF than do males. At any body weight, for each 1% increase in body fat the RMR decreases 0.6 kcal·hr^{-1} or 14.4 kcal·day^{-1}. If we assume a 10% difference in %BF between the average male and average female, the result can amount to 144 kcal·day^{-1}. When RMR is expressed relative to FFW, the sex differences disappear (Bogert, et al., 1973; Bursztein, et al., 1989).

Another factor that influences resting metabolic rate is body core temperature. For each degree increase in Celsius or Fahrenheit temperature, metabolic rate increases 13% or 7.2%, respectively. Similarly, a decrease in body temperature, at least until the point where shivering is induced, reduces energy expenditure.

A genetic effect has been documented for RMR. Correlations for RMR measured in kilojoules per kilogram of body weight were found to be 0.38 for dizygotic (DZ) twins and 0.78 for monozygotic (MZ) twins of both sexes. The genetic effect (heritability) was deemed to account for approximately 40% of the variance between individuals after adjustments for age, sex, and body composition. By itself, this genetic effect has considerable potential for predisposing an individual to gaining or losing fat over time (Bouchard, 1991; Bouchard, et al., 1989).

The Impact of Diet on Resting Metabolic Rate

The amount and the type of food ingested affect RMR. The effect of caloric restriction on RMR is well documented and clear-cut. Severe caloric restriction decreases RMR (Apfelbaum, et al., 1971; Bray, 1969; Brownell, et al., 1987; Grande, Anderson, et al., 1958; Mole, et al., 1989). Because resting metabolism represents the greatest percentage of daily caloric expenditure in sedentary individuals, the result is a discouraging effect of slowing the weight loss that would be expected from the amount of dietary restriction and negative balance.

Example

One lb (0.45 kg) of body fat contains the energy equivalent of approximately 3500 kcal. In order for a person to lose 1 lb of weight according to the caloric balance equation, the amount of calories expended must exceed the amount ingested by 3500 kcal. If an individual expends 2000 kcal·day^{-1} and ingests 2000 kcal·day^{-1}, weight should be maintained. If that same individual maintains this activity level but reduces his/her caloric intake to just 1000 kcal·day^{-1}, a weight loss of 2 lb per week would be anticipated (2000 kcal·day^{-1} − 1000 kcal·day^{-1} = −1000 kcal·day^{-1}; −1000 kcal·day^{-1} × 7 days·week^{-1} =

−7000 kcal; −7000 kcal ÷ 3500 kcal = −2 lb), assuming that approximately 75% of the 2000 kcal·day^{-1} expenditure or 1500 kcal·day^{-1} is expended by RMR.

However, within 2–3 weeks of such a restricted diet, the RMR will have been reduced by approximately 15% (the range is typically 10–20%) to 1275 kcal·day^{-1}. The difference is now −1775 kcal·day^{-1} expended + 1000 kcal·day^{-1} ingested = −775 kcal·day^{-1}; −775 kcal·day^{-1} × 7 days·week^{-1} = −5425 kcal; −5425 kcal ÷ 3500 kcal·lb^{-1} = −1.5 lb instead of −2 lb per week. As the drop in RMR continues with severe caloric restriction, the weight loss becomes progressively slower (Mole, et al., 1989).

Researchers speculate that this decline in RMR is the body's protective response to energy restriction. Conversely, a short-term excessive ingestion of food and calories results in an elevation of RMR (Apfelbaum, et al., 1971). This elevation has been seen as protection against an increase in the body's "natural" weight (Brownell, et al., 1987; Poehlman, 1989).

The Impact of Exercise on Resting Metabolic Rate

The energy cost of exercise, in oxygen or calorie units, includes a resting component. METs (Chapter 5) express the energy cost of activity in multiples of the resting metabolic rate. Therefore, although metabolism is definitely elevated by exercise, it is not the resting metabolism itself that is elevated. The resting metabolism is assumed to remain constant; the increase in energy consumption is attributed solely to the activity demands and responses.

Immediately after exercise, the metabolic rate remains elevated. This rate is called the excess postexercise oxygen consumption (EPOC) and was discussed in Chapter 5. This recovery oxygen utilization represents additional calories that are expended as a direct result of the response to exercise. These calories are typically not included in the measured caloric cost of the activity. Thus, if an individual expends 250–300 kcal walking or jogging 3 mi, an additional 20–30 kcal may be expended during the hour or two after exercise until complete recovery is achieved. This expenditure, however, also does not mean that the resting metabolic rate itself has been affected.

In order for it to be concluded that the resting metabolism is changed by exercise, the change would have to be evident 24 or 48 hr after exercise. Research evidence for such a change is mixed and difficult to interpret. The inconsistency of the evidence can partially be attributed to the intensity and duration of the exercise involved. Mild to heavy exercise of moderate duration (35–86% $\dot{V}O_2$max for 20–80 min)

Focus on Research

Impact of Body Composition on Resting Metabolic Rate and Submaximal Exercise Oxygen Consumption

McInnis, K. J., & G. J. Balady: Effect of body composition on oxygen uptake during treadmill exercise: Body builders versus weight-matched men. *Research Quarterly for Exercise and Sport.* 70(2):150–156 (1999).

As described in Chapter 5, energy expenditure (expressed as kilocalories per minute) during submaximal weight-bearing exercise is directly related to oxygen consumption during the activity. If the activity is walking or running, the oxygen consumption in turn is related to treadmill speed and grade, and body weight of the exerciser. The purpose of this study was to determine whether there were any differences in oxygen consumption during submaximal treadmill activity between two groups of young adult males who were matched for body weight but who varied in body composition. Percent body fat and fat-free mass were determined from bioelectrical impedance analysis. Oxygen consumption was measured directly by open circuit indirect spirometry. The results are presented in the table below.

These results indicate that gross oxygen consumption was significantly higher for the lean body builders than for the overweight sedentary individuals at all three submaximal workloads despite no difference in total body weight. However, when net oxygen consumption values (exercise $\dot{V}O_2$ minus rest $\dot{V}O_2$) were compared, no statistically significant differences remained, indicating that the difference in resting metabolic rate was probably the reason for the differences seen during exercise. Further analysis showed that when oxygen consumption was expressed as mL·kg FFM^{-1}·min^{-1}, there were no differences at rest or during exercise. This suggests that the difference seen at rest was due to the higher total FFM of the body builders.

Variable	Sedentary Overweight N = 14	Lean Body Builders N = 14
Body weight (kg)	99 ± 9	99 ± 7
BMI (kg·m^{-2})	32 ± 2	31 ± 2
Body fat (%)	24 ± 5	8 ± 3*
Fat-free mass (FFM) (kg)	73 ± 9	91 ± 7*
Resting metabolic rate ($\dot{V}O_2$ mL·kg^{-1}·min^{-1})	4.0 ± 1	5.6 ± 1*
1.7 m·hr^{-1}/10% (gross/net) ($\dot{V}O_2$ mL·kg^{-1}·min^{-1})	$16.1 \pm 2/12.1 \pm 2.6$	18.5 ± 2*/12.8 ± 2.3
2.5 m·hr^{-1}/12% (gross/net) ($\dot{V}O_2$ mL·kg^{-1}·min^{-1})	$23.1 \pm 2/19.1 \pm 3.1$	26.6 ± 3*/20.9 ± 3.0
3.4 m·hr^{-1}/14% (gross/net) ($\dot{V}O_2$ mL·kg^{-1}·min^{-1})	$33.5 \pm 5/29.5 \pm 5.1$	39.3 ± 5*/33.6 ± 5.3

*$p < .05$ = statistically significant difference

has generally been shown to cause no long-term metabolic elevation in RMR, whereas longer, moderate exercise (50–70% $\dot{V}O_2$max; 80–180 min) has.

There is a problem, however, in interpreting metabolic changes 24 or 48 hr after exercise as being caused by the exercise. Studies showing an increase in resting metabolic rate over the long term, even after heavy exercise, have not controlled for the ingestion of food. The elevated metabolism observed was probably due, at least in part, to the thermic effect of the meals taken. (The thermic effect of a meal will be fully explained later in this chapter.) Consequently, it is unlikely that exercise causes any permanent change in resting metabolic rate per se—at least not light or moderate aerobic endurance exercise nor dynamic resistance activity (Bingham, et al., 1989; Horton, 1985; Melby, et al., 1993; Poehlman, 1989).

Exercise Training and Resting Metabolic Rate

The effect of exercise training on RMR is controversial. Some studies have shown that trained individuals exhibit higher RMRs than sedentary individuals or that training programs bring about an increase in RMR, but others have not. An occasional study has even shown a decrease in RMR when exercise training was added to severe caloric restriction (Poehlman, 1989).

Cross-sectional studies have reported higher RMRs (adjusted for body size) in trained individuals or athletes than in untrained individuals. In some cases the difference amounted to 200 kcal·day^{-1}. The difference persisted when the subjects were matched not only on body weight but also on fat-free weight or body fat content. These results suggest that the role of exercise training in the elevation of RMR is separate from its influence in maintaining muscle mass (Poehlman, 1989).

In addition, a significant, direct rectilinear relationship (r = 0.77) has been shown to exist between the level of training or fitness as measured by $\dot{V}O_2$max and RMR. In one study, moderately trained men ($\dot{V}O_2$max $\leq$ 55 mL·kg^{-1}·min^{-1}) and untrained men had similar RMRs, but highly trained men ($\dot{V}O_2$max 55–80 mL·kg^{-1}·min^{-1}) had significantly higher RMRs than both the moderately trained and the untrained individuals (Poehlman, 1989). Thus, one reason why some studies have not revealed differences between trained and untrained individuals may be that the trained individuals were simply not trained enough. In these studies neither the trained nor the untrained individuals were restricted calorically. Therefore, it may be that what is occurring is a last-bout effect by those training at high levels (Melby, et al., 1993). Or it may be that a high-energy flux (heavy training volume with caloric balance) is the cause. Individuals in a high-energy flux condition have shown higher levels of norepinephrine and RMR than when they were in a state of low-energy flux (sedentary, but in caloric balance) (Bullough, et al., 1995)

Longitudinal studies investigating the impact of exercise training on RMR often add the exercise component after several weeks of severe caloric restriction in an attempt to reverse the decline in RMR. Others simply examine the impact of training on RMR during a calorically balanced state. High-intensity programs performed daily have not only brought about a return to baseline in RMR but also, in some instances, caused an elevation of 7–10%. In those studies showing a reversal of the decline in RMR, the change began within just a few days, which is well before any change would be expected in body composition. Thus the conclusion again is that the effect of training on RMR is over and above any change in muscle mass. The increases in RMR above pretraining levels in nondieting individuals could again reflect increased norepinephrine levels (Brownell, et al., 1987; Mole, et al., 1989; Nieman, et al., 1988; Poehlman, 1989; Poehlman and Danforth, 1991).

In those studies that have shown an additional decline in RMR when exercise was added to caloric restriction, the decline is often explained as being part of the body's protective mechanism. If RMR declines when calories are restricted, burning additional calories in activity simply makes matters worse. Therefore, it is logical that the RMR would decrease even further. It has been suggested that this decline occurs in individuals (such as some athletes) who are attempting to maintain body weights below their natural level (Brownell, et al., 1987).

It is important to realize that if diet and/or exercise results in a loss of body weight (mass), then a proportional long-term reduction in RMR should be expected. Despite the claims of many overweight individuals to the contrary, overweight or obese people can have higher RMRs than normal-weight individuals of similar age, sex, and height to begin with. With weight loss this higher RMR should not be expected to be maintained (Garrow, 1987; Wadden, et al., 1990).

Because RMR is highly correlated with or related to fat-free weight (FFW), but not entirely dependent on it, it might be expected that resistance weight training would bring about an increase in RMR. Again, the data are not definitive. Perhaps the most impressive evidence for this idea comes from a study with males 50–65 yr old. After 16 weeks of heavy resistance strength training, these subjects exhibited no change in total body weight but showed a decrease in %BF, an increase in FFW, and an increase in RMR. This increase in RMR remained significant even when expressed per kilogram of FFW. Resting norepinephrine levels also increased. The researchers concluded that the increase in RMR with strength training was only partially due to the increase in FFW and may also have been linked to an increase in basal sympathetic nervous system activity (Pratley, 1994). This conclusion reinforces the idea that RMR is not totally dependent on muscle mass.

A 24-week strength training study resulted in significant increases in RMR in young and old males, but not in females, perhaps reflecting sex differences in sympathetic nervous activity (Lemmer, et al., 2001).

Weight Cycling

A special concern regarding the influence of diet on RMR is weight cycling. **Weight cycling** is defined as repeated bouts of weight loss and regain (Schelkun, 1991). Sometimes this cycling is called the rhythm method of girth control or the yo-yo effect. Most dieters repeatedly lose weight and then gain weight again, despite their best intentions not to. Some athletes (wrestler, jockeys, and the like) (Figure 9.3) lose and gain weight purposely as they make weight for competition and then make up for missed meals by eating large quantities. Dieters may take months or years to complete each cycle; weight class athletes will do the same thing in 2 or 3 days. Furthermore, dieters may lose and gain 20–100 lb or more in each cycle, but athletes generally lose or gain less than 20 lb.

> **Weight Cycling** Repeated bouts of weight loss and regain.

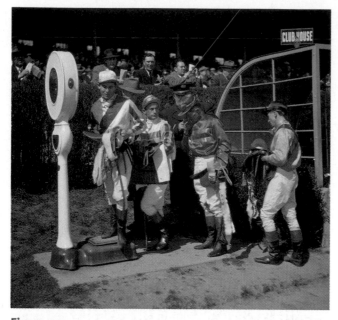

Figure 9.3
Some athletes, such as jockeys, undergo repeated bouts of weight cycling to make weight in their sport.

It has been theorized that weight cycling slows down the RMR, increases the difficulty of subsequent weight loss, and enhances abdominal fat (Blackburn, et al., 1989; Nash, 1987). Despite the theory, experimental evidence from studies testing the influence of weight cycling on RMR has presented inconclusive results. High school wrestlers who weight-cycled exhibited a 15% lower RMR than those who did not (Steen, 1988). However, college wrestlers who weight-cycled had RMRs similar to those of non–weight-cycling wrestlers, and both wrestling groups had higher RMR values than nonwrestling controls (Schmidt, et al., 1993). Perhaps an initially lower RMR necessitated weight cycling in the high school wrestlers and not the reverse. These results cannot be considered conclusive evidence one way or the other.

Studies using dieters, whether initially obese or overweight, are also conflicting, with two of three studies (Beeson, et al., 1989; van Dale and Saris, 1989; Wadden, et al., 1992) finding no evidence that a history of weight cycling affected RMR. One study that has received a great deal of attention did find that prior weight cycling made subsequent weight loss harder (Blackburn, et al., 1989). This study followed two groups (hospital inpatients and outpatients) of obese individuals who exhibited weight cycling over a 9-yr period. During the first attempt at supervised weight loss the outpatients lost an average of 0.19 kg·day^{-1} or 11 kg in 72 days. After regaining 120% of the weight loss these individuals underwent the same regimen again and lost an average of 0.15 kg·day^{-1} or 8 kg in 72 days. Results for the inpatients were even more definitive. During the first weight loss cycle these individuals lost an average of 0.47 kg·day^{-1} in 31 days for a total of 12 kg. They regained 115% of their weight loss. The second time around the weight loss average was only 0.37 kg·day^{-1} for a total loss of 6 kg in 20 days (Blackburn, et al., 1989).

These data suggest a slowing of the rate of weight loss with successive dieting. However, the subjects in this study were also older during the second weight loss cycle, and age does decrease RMR. Furthermore, there was less adherence to the diet during the second weight loss cycle than during the first, which would affect both the rate and the amount of weight loss (Wing, 1992). Finally, three other studies found no relationship between weight loss in one cycle and the subsequent rate or amount of weight loss in later cycles (Beeson, et al., 1989; van Dale and Saris, 1989; Wadden, et al., 1992).

One other study (Rodin, et al., 1990) found that weight cycling was associated with upper-body (abdominal) fat deposition. However, three similar studies found no difference in fat distribution or waist-to-hip ratio as a function of weight-cycling history (Jeffery, et al., 1992; van Dale and Saris, 1989; Wadden, et al., 1992). There is no evidence that weight cycling leads to increased abdominal visceral fat deposition.

Neither body fat distribution nor body composition appears to be adversely affected by a history of weight cycling in humans (National Task Force on the Prevention and Treatment of Obesity, 1994). Remaining overweight or obese is not preferable, from a physiological standpoint, to undergoing repeated attempts at weight loss (National Task Force on the Prevention and Treatment of Obesity, 1994). Taken together, the research does not support any of the theoretical concerns mentioned at the beginning of this discussion (Wing, 1992).

Thermogenesis

Think about this. The temperature is 38°C (100°F) with a relative humidity of 80%. Your apartment air conditioner is not working. You are hungry, but you can't afford to go out to eat. In your food stock are ground beef, red beans and rice, tuna, and the ingredients for both a fruit and a tossed salad. Which do you select?

In all probability you will pick one or both of the salad options, intuitively going for the meal that will not add to your heat load. Actually, though, following ingestion of any meal, energy metabolism is enhanced. This energy increase is due, in part, to the energy-requiring processes of digestion, absorption, assimilation, and synthesis of protein, fat, and carbohydrate.

However, more energy is expended than can be accounted for by these processes. The extra energy expenditure usually peaks in 30–90 min but, depending on the size and content of the meal, may last as long as 4–6 hr. This energy all appears in the form of heat. The production of heat is called **thermogenesis.** For any given meal, the increased heat production as a result of food ingestion is called the **thermic effect of a meal (TEM).** Cumulatively, the energy expenditure associated with the ingestion of all food during a day is called the *thermic effect of feeding* (TEF). TEF is what is depicted as thermogenesis in Figure 9.1 as constituting approximately 10% of daily energy expenditure (Blanchard, 1982; Poehlman, 1989).

There is some evidence for a link between thermogenesis and the control of body weight. TEF is thought to be a survival technique. When stimulated, TEF allows the individual to adapt to a diet low in nutrients by the ingestion of more food without gaining weight. When suppressed, TEF allows the body to maintain its weight during fasting or starvation situations. The stimulus or suppression appears to be mediated through the sympathetic nervous system (Blanchard, 1982).

Precisely how thermogenesis occurs has not been determined, but probably some mechanism for the uncoupling of oxidative phosphorylation is involved. That is, energy substrates are oxidized, but ATP is not produced. Instead, heat is produced. This process may occur at specific steps in the metabolic pathways (known as substrate or futile cycling) or in brown adipose tissue (BAT) (Himms-Hagen, 1984) (see Figure 8.9). Humans, however, have only about 1% of body weight as BAT after early postnatal life. Changes in the sodium-potassium pump activity have also been proposed (Blanchard, 1982). These mechanisms may, in part, be responsible for why some individuals can seemingly eat everything in sight and not gain weight, while others eat much less proportionately and gain weight. Most studies comparing the thermic response of lean and obese individuals to a test meal do indeed show a blunted TEM in the obese (Blanchard, 1982; Jequier, 1987; Newsholme, 1980; Schutz, et al., 1984; Schwartz, 1983; Segal, et al., 1987; Segal, et al., 1985; Segal, et al., 1984; Shetty, et al., 1981).

Thermogenesis The production of heat.

Thermic Effect of a Meal (TEM) The increased heat production as a result of food ingestion.

The Impact of Diet on the Thermic Effect of a Meal

Both the total caloric content and the percent composition of a meal have an impact on the thermic effect of the meal. The greatest thermic effect occurs with protein (15–25%). Carbohydrate and fat show only about half the thermic increase shown by protein, with carbohydrate's increase being slightly higher than fat's. These differences would seem to indicate that a high-protein diet would be valuable for individuals wishing to expend extra calories. However, as mentioned in Chapter 7, high-protein diets can exacerbate kidney and liver problems in individuals with preexisting conditions and may result in excessive losses of calcium. For these reasons, diets exceeding 15% protein are not recommended no matter what the thermic effect (Belko, et al., 1986; Glickman, et al., 1948; Nair, et al., 1983; Swaminathan, et al., 1985).

If the percentages of protein, fat, and carbohydrate are kept constant and close to those values recommended for a healthy diet (55% CHO, 30% FAT, 15% PRO), a direct relationship is found between the caloric content of a meal and TEM; that is, higher-caloric meals cause a higher thermic effect. As a result, an individual on a restricted caloric diet will burn fewer calories through dietary-induced thermogenesis than he or she would when eating larger meals (Belko, et al., 1986; Bursztein, et al., 1989).

The Impact of Exercise on the Thermic Effect of a Meal

Both meal ingestion and exercise stimulate the sympathetic nervous system and thermogenesis. Because many people are interested in maximizing energy expenditure, it was deemed of interest to determine whether a combination of exercise plus a meal in close temporal proximity would potentiate (or increase) the singular effect of either exercise or food. A number of studies have been completed following two basic sequences. After a period of rest the subjects eat a meal and then exercise. Or conversely, after a period of rest the subjects exercise and then eat a meal. In both sequences some studies have shown that TEM was enhanced due to exercise (Belko, et al., 1986; Segal, et al., 1987; Segal, et al., 1985; Segal, et al., 1984; Zahorska-Markiewiez, 1980), while others have shown that TEM was not enhanced due to exercise (Dallasso and James, 1984; Pacy, et al., 1985; Welle, 1984; Willms and Plowman, 1991). The studies have been so diverse in terms of subjects, meal composition and energy value, exercise mode, intensity, and duration that it is not possible to determine a pattern for when the effect appeared to be additive and when it did not.

Figure 9.4
Exercise is an important component of body weight/body composition control.

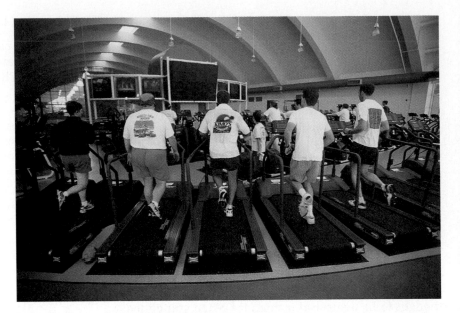

Exercise Training and the Thermic Effect of a Meal

Studies investigating the effects of training, either cross-sectionally or longitudinally, have shown that aerobic-trained individuals have a larger, smaller, or similar TEM response. As in the studies dealing with the acute effects of exercise, there is a wide diversity of subjects (especially in training level), meal composition, and meal energy value. However, a pattern is evident here. The level of fitness or training is the key, and the pattern follows that of an inverted U. Moderate levels of fitness (around 50–55 mL·kg^{-1}·min^{-1} $\dot{V}O_2$max for males; unknown for females) in young nonobese adults appear to enhance TEM above that of unfit subjects. High levels of fitness (greater than 65 mL·kg^{-1}·min^{-1} $\dot{V}O_2$max) appear to decrease TEM.

In both cases the results are probably good news. They mean that the individual beginning a physical fitness program to get in shape and lose a few pounds will benefit from an enhanced thermic effect. By expending more calories in that way, he or she may lose weight slightly faster. The highly trained and active individual, in contrast, is able to preserve energy needed to sustain his or her exercise training. The reduced stimulation of the sympathetic nervous system and catecholamines that accompanies exercise training has been suggested as the reason for a lower TEM in highly trained individuals (Poehlman, 1989). If the intent in highly trained individuals is to preserve energy for activity, it is unclear why they also exhibit an elevated RMR (see "Exercise Training and Resting Metabolic Rate"). For whatever reason, it seems that moderate levels of exercise training, which are probably attainable by large numbers of individuals, may

enhance TEM but not RMR. Conversely, high levels of exercise training decrease TEM, but elevate RMR (Poehlman, 1989).

Only one study has compared the thermic effect of a meal-exercise combination in resistance-trained individuals. In this study the $\dot{V}O_2$max was similar between the resistance-trained (52 mL·kg^{-1}·min^{-1}) and untrained (51.1 mL·kg^{-1}·min^{-1}) subjects and within the range of the moderately fit just cited; but the untrained subjects had a significantly higher TEM (Gilbert, et al., 1991).

Genetics may also play a part in explaining the interaction of TEM and training. For example, when six pairs of male monozygotic twins underwent a 22-day exercise training program, four sets showed a decreased TEM after training, and the remaining two showed an increase. Despite this wide between-pair difference, the intrapair resemblance was high (r = 0.72). Both the degree and the direction of response to TEM following training may in large part be hereditary. Thus, heredity may be one of the factors contributing to individual variations in body composition and weight change (Bouchard, et al., 1990).

The Impact of Diet, Exercise, and Exercise Training on Energy Expenditure

The last element in the caloric balance equation is the amount of energy expended in manual work or exercise. Restricting calories does not change the energy expended in any activity except as it influences body weight. However, individuals on calorically restrictive diets may have insufficient energy and may not be able to do as much physical work or exercise.

Table 9.3

Impact of Diet, Exercise, and Exercise Training on the Caloric Balance Equation

Caloric Balance Factor	Diet	Exercise Response	Training Adaptation
Food ingested (+)	By definition, a reduction occurs	No clearly established effect; appetite does not decrease	Energy intake increases (highly trained and lean individuals) or remains constant (untrained and obese individuals); when training ceases, food intake spontaneously decreases but does not match the decrease in expenditure
BMR and/or RMR (−)	Severe caloric restriction causes a 10–20% decrease; weight cycling does not decrease	Unchanged per se but metabolic rate postexercise remains elevated	No consistent effect is evident
Thermogenesis (TEM) (−)	Decreases because fewer calories are being ingested; dependent on composition of meals	No consistent additive effect in either a sequence of food-exercise or exercise-food	Inverted U response, dependent on fitness level; moderate levels of fitness and training increase TEM; high levels of fitness and training decrease TEM
Work or exercise expenditure (−)	If calories are insufficient, may voluntarily do less exercise; but no direct effect on caloric cost	By definition, an increase occurs	A cumulative increase occurs; relatively constant per kg BW

By definition, exercise will increase energy expenditure and the effects of training will be cumulative. Unless efficiency and/or body weight change, the caloric expenditure of any activity will not change with exercise training.

Table 9.3 summarizes all that has been discussed about the impact of diet, exercise, and exercise training on all of the elements of the caloric balance equation.

The Effect of Diet, Exercise Training, and Diet Plus Exercise Training on Body Composition and Weight

Many people wish to lose weight strictly for aesthetics (to look better) without caring what is lost. The concern from a physiological standpoint, however, is fourfold:

1. to lose body fat;
2. to preserve fat-free weight;
3. to maintain or improve health; and
4. to maintain or improve performance, in the case of athletes.

Many factors influence whether these goals can be and are met. These factors include the following:

1. The initial status of the individual. (Is he or she a few pounds overweight, or is he or she obese? What are his or her genetic predispositions?)

2. The type of diet selected. (Is the caloric restriction minimal, moderate, severe, or maximal? What are the percentages of the basic nutrients included in the diet?)

3. The length of time of the weight-reducing program (24–48 hr, 5–20 weeks, or longer).

4. Whether or not exercise training is included as part of the program, and if so, the amount and type of exercise (dynamic aerobic endurance, weight-bearing or non–weight-bearing, or dynamic resistance training).

Exact responses to all possible combinations of these factors are not available. But some generalizations can be made.

The Effects of Diet on Body Composition and Weight

The vast majority of individuals on a weight-reducing regimen elect to diet. Caloric restriction may be minimal (a deficit of about 250–500 kcal·day^{-1}), moderate (a total intake of 1200–1500 kcal·day^{-1}), severe (a

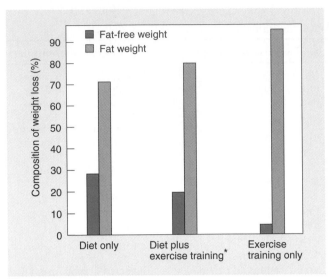

Figure 9.5
Effects of Diet, Exercise, Training, and Diet Plus Exercise on the Composition of Weight Loss

Almost 30% of the weight lost by dietary restriction is fat-free weight. When exercise is added to dietary caloric restriction, the loss of fat-free weight is reduced. The smallest loss of fat-free weight occurs if the caloric deficit is achieved by exercise alone.

* Diets were generally very low calorie or low-calorie (400–1000 kcal·day^{-1}).

Sources: Based on data from Donnelly, et al. (1991); Walberg (1989); Hagan (1988); Heymsfield, et al. (1988); Zuti & Golding (1976); Hagan, et al. (1986); Depres, et al. (1985); Bouchard, et al. (1990); Ballor, et al. (1988).

total intake of 400–800 kcal·day^{-1}, or maximal (fasting, or zero caloric intake). Strictly adhered to, all will bring about a weight loss.

Figure 9.5 shows that in dietary restriction approximately 28% of the lost total body weight is fat-free weight and 72% is fat weight. These values, however, are composites primarily from studies with severe caloric restriction. The percentages will vary on the basis of the caloric content of the diet. Thus, body weight loss from total fasting is split equally between body fat (50%) and fat-free weight (50%); from very low (400–800 kcal·day^{-1}) or low- (800–1200 kcal·day^{-1}) calorie diets the split is approximately 75% body fat and 25% fat-free weight; and from 1200–1500 kcal·day^{-1} diets 90% body-fat and only 10% fat-free weight (Nieman, 1990). Fasting, which is obviously incompatible with life over the long haul, is not recommended as a dietary technique. The use of low-calorie and very low calorie diets should be undertaken only in extreme situations and only under the direct supervision of a physician. This technique is typically reserved for extremely obese individuals and is often conducted on a live-in basis in a metabolic ward of a hospital. The 1200–1500 kcal·day^{-1}

regimen is often recommended, but even that does not totally preserve lean body mass (American College of Sports Medicine [ACSM], 1983).

The importance of the FFW loss may depend on how much excess weight the individual started with. Obese individuals have an excess of both body fat and FFW. That is, their excess body weight is composed of 62–78% fat and 22–38% FFW. The excess of FFW is necessary to support and move the large bulk that accompanies obesity. Therefore, as one loses total body weight, less FFW would be needed; and its loss would therefore not be unexpected. Thus, loss of some FFW in such an individual may not be critical, but its preservation would also not be detrimental from a health standpoint. Therefore, individuals with less weight to lose need to protect their FFW (Brown, et al., 1983; Donnelly, et al., 1991; Jequier, 1987; Pacy, et al., 1986, Pavlou, et al., 1989).

Recall that fat-free weight is composed of water, protein, and bone mineral (Figure 8.1). There is no indication that bone mineral content changes with a loss of body weight. The relative proportions of the loss of water and protein when dieting varies with the time course of the diet. During the first several days of a diet, the majority of any weight loss (55–70%) is water loss. But by the end of the first month this percentage is considerably reduced (to ≈ 40%) and after 7 to 8 months it may be as low as 5%. The protein (primarily the component of muscle tissue) loss is a consistent 5% in a nonexercising dieter (Grande, Anderson, et al., 1958; Heymsfield, et al., 1989). What does this say about the proportion of fat loss? Simply that the percentage of fat loss is a mirror image of the percentage of water loss: little fat is lost at first and then progressively more fat is lost as caloric restriction continues.

Given these facts alone, would you recommend a series of short, very-low calorie diet (VLCD) regimens for quick weight loss or a slow steady approach? Why? Check your thinking in the section on the application of training principles under the subsection "Adaptation."

Strangely enough, restricting water intake while dieting causes a higher proportion of water to be lost, not less, which could lead to dehydration. More total weight is lost if water is restricted, but not more fat. Water intake should not be restricted when dieting (Grande, Taylor, et al., 1958; Heymsfield, et al., 1989).

The Effects of Exercise Training on Body Composition and Weight

On the one hand, few people wishing to lose body weight would set out to do it entirely by exercising.

You will come across some of these people in Y's and health clubs across the country, but they are a minority. On the other hand, there are many individuals who consciously or unconsciously do control their body weight through exercise training. These are, of course, athletes. If we ignore the fact that some athletes also closely watch their caloric intake, indirect evidence of the role of exercise on body composition can be inferred from the %BF values measured on various groups of athletes. Figure 9.6 presents a compilation of available data.

Keeping in mind that the average %BF for a young adult male is 13–15% and that for a young adult female it is 25% (Figure 8.7), several conclusions are discernible from the graph. First, even in the athletic population, the male-female difference in %BF is maintained. Second, athletes in different sports, both male and female, vary considerably in their %BF, from much leaner than average to slightly above average. Third, the %BF values appear to have a direct relationship to the demands of the sport. Athletes in sports where body aesthetics play a part in success (dance, figure skating, body building, gymnastics) tend to have low %BF values. Endurance athletes (cyclists, cross-country skiers, distance runners, triathletes) also tend to have low %BF values. Athletes in predominantly motor skill sports (baseball, golf, volleyball) tend to be just about average. The only athletes consistently at or above average %BF values are the field event participants.

These data tend to support the value of exercise training in maintaining a low %BF, because athletes in activities known to have high caloric costs and engaged in for long periods of time have the lowest %BF values. However, the problem of self-selection arises when dealing with studies of this type; that is, we do not know whether individuals who are genetically programmed for leanness and success in these sports naturally gravitate to them, or whether the training demands of the sport determine the body composition of the performer. Both factors are probably operating.

Although the mean values cited show a definite pattern, a wide range of variability exists among successful athletes in any given event. For example, successful female distance runners have an average measured %BF value of 16.5%. Included in that group, however, is an athlete who won six consecutive international cross-country championships and another who held the 1972 world best time for the marathon; both of these runners had only 6%BF. At the other end of the range, the mid-1970s world record holder for the 50-mi run tested at 35.8%BF (Brownell, et al., 1987). These extremes point out the importance of not establishing a specific %BF value

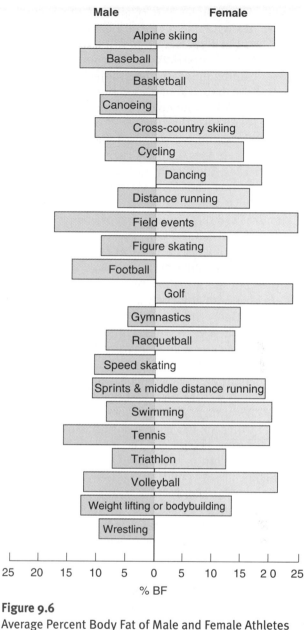

Figure 9.6

Average Percent Body Fat of Male and Female Athletes (17–35 yr) in Selected Sports

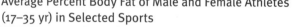

Source: Based on a literature review presented in Wilmore & Costill (1988).

for all athletes in any sport. The average values should not be interpreted as values that all athletes competing in a particular sport should achieve. If %BF values are suggested to athletes, they should be in the form of a range of values. The health and the performance of the athlete need to be monitored within that range, and individual adjustments should be made on the basis of this monitoring. Eating disorders, which are sometimes associated with attempts to control body composition for sport, are discussed fully in Chapter 7.

Figure 9.5 includes the results of three studies that were designed to determine whether weight could be lost but FFW maintained by exercise training without caloric restriction. The column is labeled "exercise training only." In the studies that make up this pool, less than 5% of the weight lost could be attributed to FFW. Indeed, only one study showed any FFW loss. In the other two FFW was gained. Only in those studies where a caloric deficit was achieved did a body weight loss occur. A recent re-view (Wing, 1999) indicates that exercise alone can produce weight loss, but the loss is generally a modest amount.

Wilmore (1983) compiled a list of body weight and body composition changes from 55 training studies whose general purpose was to improve physical fitness. The average body fat change was a decrease of only 1.6%, but at the same time a 1% increase occurred in FFW. No information was provided about the caloric balance in these studies. It must be emphasized that the key to weight and fat loss is not exercise per se but the achievement of a caloric deficit through exercise (Donnelly, et al., 1991; Walberg, 1989). Diet alone can also achieve a caloric deficit; but when weight is lost through dieting alone, it includes a greater percentage of FFW. The evidence discussed earlier is strong for the conclusion that exercise can maintain or even increase FFW, no matter what the caloric balance, but a substantial weight and fat loss will be achieved only when a negative caloric balance is achieved. Dynamic aerobic endurance activity is most helpful in increasing caloric expenditure; dynamic resistance activity (which is low in caloric cost) acts more directly to increase muscle mass.

Recent evidence has shown that overweight individuals (both male and female) benefit from exercise even if they remain overweight. The Focus on Application box in Chapter 8 discussed some of this evidence. Active overweight persons have better risk profiles for the diseases identified earlier and lower rates of morbidity and mortality than their sedentary counterparts. These health gains are related to the beneficial changes in glucose-insulin responses and lipoprotein values. Thus, the value of exercise training for overweight individuals goes far beyond the sometimes minor contribution to weight loss (Bray, 1985).

Children and adolescents appear to be similar to adults in relation to the influence of exercise training on body composition. Comparisons of young athletes with their sedentary counterparts typically show that the athletes, both boys and girls, have a lower percent body fat and higher fat-free weight values. The variation among sports is similar to that for adults. There is also evidence from training studies that a

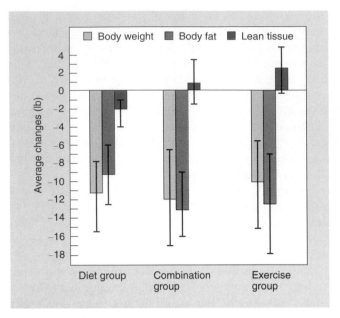

Figure 9.7
Weight Loss Is Similar, but Body Composition Changes Vary Depending on the Means of Achieving a Caloric Deficit

Total weight loss was very similar in three groups of women who achieved their caloric deficit by diet, diet plus exercise, or exercise alone. Both exercise groups not only maintained lean muscle mass tissue but added some.

Source: W. B. Zuti & L. A. Golding. Comparing diet and exercise as weight reducing tools. *The Physician and Sports Medicine.* 4:49–53 (1976). Reprinted by permission of McGraw-Hill Inc.

decrement in percent body fat results from systematically applied exercise programs (Boileau, et al., 1985; Epstein and Goldfield, 1999; Plowman, 1989).

The Effects of Diet Plus Exercise Training on Body Composition and Weight

Studies that have combined diet and exercise seem to suggest that this approach is best for positive, long-term changes. Body weight is not lost faster in combined exercise-plus-diet programs than in diet alone programs, but the loss may be somewhat more than diet alone (Wing, 1999). Furthermore, the desirable maintenance of FFW is achieved. Figure 9.5 shows (from a composite of studies) that when exercise is added to caloric restriction, 20% of the total weight loss is FFW and 80% is fat. This is more FFW loss than when exercise alone is used to achieve the caloric deficit, but less than when diet is used alone. In some cases muscle mass can actually be gained, as shown in Figure 9.7. Note that despite the increase of lean tissue when an exercise component is included, the total weight loss is very similar in all three groups of women in this study (Zuti and Golding, 1976).

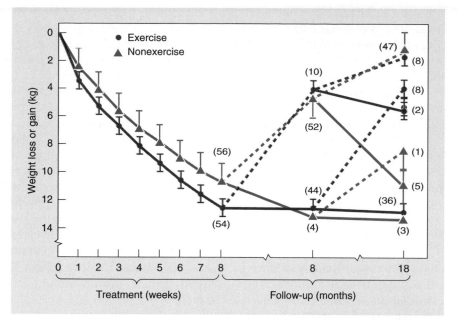

Figure 9.8
The Importance of Exercise in Maintaining Weight Loss

Subjects who exercised and dieted lost only slightly more weight than those who only dieted over an 8-week period. However, only those individuals who continued to exercise were able to maintain or regain their weight loss over a follow-up period of 18 months.

Source: K. N. Pavlou, S. Krey, & W. P. Steffee. Exercise as an adjunct to weight loss and maintenance in moderately obese subjects. *American Journal of Nutrition.* 49:1115–1123 (1989). © *American Journal of Clinical Nutrition.* American Society of Clinical Nutrition. Reprinted by permission.

The key to weight loss while maintaining FFW is probably the total caloric deficit and the nutrient content (PRO and CHO) of the calories ingested (Walberg, 1989). One advantage of adding exercise to a weight loss regimen may simply be that it allows an individual to ingest more kilocalories and still be in a negative caloric balance. Eating a moderately restricted diet allows for adequate nutrition and lifestyle changes that can be tolerated for a lifetime; in contrast, a VLCD can seldom be sustained for a prolonged time.

A study by Pavlou et al. (1989, 1985) illustrates that another benefit of adding exercise to a restricted caloric diet is the ability to maintain a weight loss. In this study (the results are depicted in Figure 9.8), 56 policemen lost an average of 10.1 kg by four preselected, calorically restricted, liquid and solid food diets over an 8-week period. Another 56 policemen lost an average of 12.2 kg when 90 min of supervised walk-jog-run plus calisthenics and relaxation exercises three times per week (for a total of 1500 kcal expenditure per week) were added to the same four diet routines. Subjects were reassessed at 8 and 18 months after the 8-week program.

Follow the lines in Figure 9.8 by the number of subjects at each time point to understand the follow-up

results. At the 8-month follow-up 52 of the 56 dieters had regained all but 3.75 kg (≈63%) of their lost weight. Ten of the diet-plus-exercise group had ceased the exercise program and also regained all but about 3.5 kg (≈71%) of their lost weight. Conversely, the 44 who continued to exercise maintained their entire weight loss, and 4 of the diet group who added exercise lost an additional 3 kg.

At 18 months 47 of the original dieters and 8 of the 10 original diet-plus-exercise group continued to be sedentary and had regained all of their weight loss. The 2 diet-plus-exercise individuals who went back to exercising lost approximately 2 kg again. Their net loss was then approximately 5 kg, the same as 8 individuals who had stopped exercising between the 8th and 18th month.

Five men who had originally been just dieters became exercisers between the 8th and 18th month and reduced their weight to the level of the original loss. One of the 4 individuals from the diet group who began to exercise at the 8th month stopped and regained 5.5 kg. The 36 men in the original diet-plus-exercise group and 3 of the 4 from the diet-only group who began to exercise immediately at the end of the 8-week session maintained their entire weight loss.

Thus, all subjects—no matter how they had originally lost weight—regained the weight lost 1½ yr later if they did not exercise consistently during the intervening time. Conversely, all subjects—no matter how they had originally lost weight—maintained their weight loss after 1½ yr if they did exercise.

Regardless of how successful an initial weight loss diet is, most individuals regain at least a third of the lost weight within a year. Therefore, the contribution of exercise just described is extremely beneficial (Schelkun, 1991). This study used an exercise program that totaled approximately 1500 kcal·week^{-1} in just three sessions. This exercise could just as effectively be divided into five sessions of 300 kcal or six of 250 kcal. The calories expended in exercise are cumulative and the effect is the same no matter how long it takes as long as a deficit is ultimately achieved.

Why is it so hard to keep weight off once it has been lost? There is no definite answer to that question. Interest is currently centered on the enzyme lipoprotein lipase as a possible culprit. Lipoprotein lipase is the enzyme responsible for fat synthesis and storage in adipose tissue. It has been theorized that lipoprotein lipase notifies the brain when fat cells have shrunk, as they would when the body is losing weight. In response, appetite increases and fat cells refill. In other words, starving leads to stuffing. Not only does the appetite increase, but also it appears to be selectively predisposed to disproportionately increase the amount of fat ingested. Fat, of course, is calorically dense. Furthermore, after restrictive dieting the individual can more easily convert other excess food nutrients to fatty acids.

Previously or currently obese individuals seem to be more susceptible to the stimulus and response of lipoprotein lipase. In these individuals lipoprotein lipase activity may be twice as high as in nondieting individuals. That is the bad news. The good news is that when people who are not obese but mildly or moderately overweight diet, the changes in lipoprotein lipase activity are minimal. It may be that a certain amount of weight (approximately 15% of total body weight) must be lost before lipoprotein lipase activity becomes a counterproductive factor (Gershoff, 1991, 1992; Nash, 1987; Schelkun, 1991).

A change in food efficiency may be another factor that complicates the problem of maintaining weight loss. **Food efficiency** is an index of the amount of calories an individual needs to ingest in order to maintain a given weight or percent body fat. Food efficiency increases when the calories needed to sustain a certain weight (or percent fat) decrease. This response could be protective if food were scarce. Food efficiency decreases when the number of calories needed to sustain a certain weight (or percent fat) increases. This is what every dieter would like to have happen, but which does not happen (Brodie, 1988).

Several studies exemplify what appears to happen. In one study a group of obese individuals lost an average of 52 kg (114.4 lb) but remained 60% overweight (39 kg or 85.8 lb, excess) when compared with a normal weight control group. The daily caloric needs (2171 kcal·day^{-1}) of the reduced-weight obese individuals to maintain their weight were found to be 25% lower than the value estimated from their body size and almost 5% lower than the value needed by much lighter normal-weight controls (2280 kcal·day^{-1}).

Another major possibility is a residual reduction in RMR. The impact of RMR is particularly important because it accounts for the highest percentage of daily energy expenditure. When data from 124 formerly obese and 121 control subjects were compared, it was determined that RMR adjusted for fat mass and fat-free mass was 2.9% lower in the formerly obese than the never obese. In addition, a larger percentage (15.3% versus 3.3%) of the formerly obese had a low RMR. When 12 studies were combined in a traditional meta-analysis, relative RMR was 5.1% lower in the formerly obese group than the control group. The authors concluded that the cause of the lower RMR remained unknown; however, the implication was clear. A low RMR is likely to contribute to the formerly obese individual's difficulty in maintaining a weight loss (Astrup, et al., 1999). These and other data suggest an increased food efficiency, an RMR that has remained depressed, or other compensatory changes in energy expenditure that oppose the maintenance of a body weight lower than usual (Leibel and Hirsch, 1984; Leibel, et al., 1995).

Finally, several studies in which dietary and activity analysis were done indicate that some female distance runners ingest only between 1400 and 1990 kcal·day^{-1} while training as much as 65 mi·week^{-1}. These caloric intake values are much lower than those for comparably sized, inactive females of the same age. Again, these results suggest that food efficiency is operating. It may be that food efficiency operates at the two extremes of obesity and excessive thinness when the body reacts to protect against what is perceived as starvation and a wasting away. Food efficiency may not be much of a factor for those losing a moderate amount of weight. More information is needed on this phenomenon (Brownell, et al., 1987).

> **Food Efficiency** An index of the amount of calories an individual needs to ingest in order to maintain a given weight or percent body fat.

Focus on Application

✳ Guidelines for Evaluating a Weight-Loss Diet

Throughout this text you are presented with guidelines for developing, and hence evaluating, exercise programs through the use of the training principles. Because the most effective technique for weight loss and control is a combination of diet and exercise, the following guidelines are presented to assist in the development and evaluation of diets intended for weight loss. An acceptable diet should meet the following standards:

1. Provide a daily energy intake of approximately 500–1000 kcal below normal prediet intake, but not lower than resting metabolic rate (RMR)(approximately 1200 kcal·d^{-1} for females and 1500 kcal·d^{-1} for males) or the total calories halfway between RMR and 30% above RMR.

2. Meet the nutritional requirements of ≥55% carbohydrate, ~15% protein, and ≤30% total fat (8–10% saturated, up to 15% monounsaturated, up to 10% polyunsaturated) and the RDA/DRI for vitamins and minerals.

3. Emphasize a variety of food choices and allow for individual and cultural preferences in terms of acquisition, taste, preparation, and cost.

4. Not be based on some "secret" ingredient or "magic" combination of foods, or require the simultaneous ingestion of "fat burning" or other supplements. The recommendation to take a daily multivitamin may be acceptable.

5. Be backed by credible scientific or medical organizations (for example, the American Dietetic Association or the American Heart Association) and/or well-designed research published in peer-reviewed journals that supports both the effectiveness and safety of the diet. Anyone may write a diet book; the publication of diet books is not regulated by any governmental agency or professional society. If someone is going to make money on the diet, "let the buyer beware."

6. Include at least three meals per day (more frequent smaller meals are also acceptable) and drinking 8–10 8-ounce glasses of water per day. Alcohol intake should be controlled.   ✳

Sources:

American College of Sports Medicine (2000); van Horn, et al. (1998).

The Effects of Diet, Exercise, and Diet Plus Exercise on Abdominal Obesity

Of special concern is the impact of diet, exercise, and diet plus exercise on abdominal fat, both subcutaneous tissue and visceral abdominal tissue, or VAT. The concern relates to the fact that abdominal fat is known to be an independent predictor of the metabolic risk factors that are the antecedents for Type II (non–insulin-dependent) diabetes and various cardiovascular diseases. A review of the studies that investigated the impact of diet alone on VAT found that for every kilogram of weight loss, VAT was reduced 3–4 cm^2, or approximately 2–3% of the total VAT. Furthermore, there appeared to be a preferential reduction in VAT (which is desirable) over subcutaneous fat loss. However, the subjects in these studies were almost exclusively obese females, so whether the results can be generalized to males is unknown (Ross, 1997).

The impact of exercise alone on abdominal obesity has been confounded by what measure was used to evaluate it and whether or not a weight loss was achieved. In general, in the absence of weight loss, abdominal fat levels are not reduced if measured by waist-to-hip ratio or waist circumference. Conversely, physical activity with or without weight loss is associated with reductions in visceral and abdominal subcutaneous fat loss if measured by techniques such as magnetic resonance imaging (MRI) or computerized tomography (CT scan) (Ross and Janssen, 1999).

The few studies that have looked at the impact of diet plus exercise on VAT have shown that the relative reduction in VAT is similar to the response induced by diet alone; that is, the addition of exercise did not provide any preferential benefit for the reduction of VAT (Ross, 1997).

Application of the Training Principles for Weight and Body Composition Loss and/or Control

On the basis of the previous discussion of the impact of diet, exercise training, and diet plus exercise training on body weight and composition, the following guidelines are presented for the application of the training principles to achieve weight and body composition loss, change, and/or control. These guidelines are intended for the mildly or moderately overweight and overfat individuals that the physical educator or fitness leader is likely to encounter; they are not meant for the more severely obese individuals, who require more drastic reductions and medical supervision.

Specificity

The general goals of weight and body composition control should be as stated previously: to maximize the decrease in body weight or body fat while minimizing fat-free weight loss and supplying adequate nutrition. Such a program should become a lifestyle and not be just a temporary test of willpower and discipline.

In order to achieve these goals, a program that combines dietary caloric restriction and both dynamic aerobic endurance exercise and dynamic resistance training exercise is recommended. The combined caloric deficit should bring about a weight loss of no more than 0.5–1 kg (1–2 lb) per week (ACSM, et al., 2000). Evidence suggests that slow weight losses are healthier and easier to maintain than fast weight losses. Because one pound (that is, 0.45 kg) of fat equals 3500 kcal, a deficit of 3500–7000 kcal per week or 500–1000 kcal·day^{-1} is needed to achieve the 0.5–1 kg desired weight loss.

The endurance exercise modality selected (walking, jogging, cycling, swimming, aerobic dancing, stair stepping or stair climbing) should not matter if it is used in conjunction with a weight resistance program. However, for reasons that are neither known nor understood, swim training used by itself does not usually bring about changes in body composition. This is unfortunate, because non–weight-bearing activities such as swimming or cycling may be the least stressful orthopedically for overweight individuals beginning an exercise program. Exercise in water also overcomes other problems often seen when overweight individuals exercise, such as joint immobility, body instability, and heat intolerance. Because of these positive aspects, activity in water (aqua aerobics, walking-jogging, or swimming) may still be the exercise of choice. The addition of dynamic resistance training to water-based training is of even greater importance than it is to land-based exercise modalities (Kieres and Plowman, 1991; Sheldahl, 1985).

Another way to interpret specificity in relation to weight control might be a desire to reduce body fat from a specific location, called *spot reduction*. The idea behind spot reduction is that fat will be selectively mobilized and hence reduced from the area that is exercised. Thus, an individual wishing to reduce his or her abdominal region would concentrate on pelvic tilts, curls, and sit-ups.

Consistent training of specific muscles can increase muscle tone, which may give a slimming appearance (or if hypertrophy occurs, give a more defined appearance). However, there is no experimental evidence that fat (in the form of fatty acids) is mobilized preferentially from adipose cells located near active muscles; that is, spot reducing may be an attractive idea, but in reality, it does not work, either for males or for females. In one study 27 women who performed calisthenics for the abdomen, hips, and thighs were compared with 29 women who performed aerobic activities (Noland and Kearney, 1978). Both groups worked out three times per week for 30 min for 10 weeks. Although %BF did not decrease significantly in either group, several girth and skinfold measures did decrease in both groups. There was no indication of any preferential site reduction in the specifically selected areas, however. Likewise, when 13 men underwent a 27-day training program during which 5004 sit-ups were performed, no significant changes occurred in %BF, skinfold, or girth measurements either as a result of training in the same subjects or in comparison with six nonexercising controls. Adipose biopsy measures did show significant decreases in cell diameters; however, there was no significant difference in these changes between the heavily exercised abdominal site and the nonexercised gluteal and subscapular locations (Katch, et al., 1984).

Fat is mobilized to be used as a fuel by hormonal action. Hormones circulate to all parts of the body via the bloodstream. The distribution of body fat in the android (abdominal), gynoid (gluteofemoral), or intermediate pattern does not appear to affect the amount of weight lost by caloric deficit, nor is the relative distribution of fat altered by the weight loss. That is, the general shape of the individual is preserved despite a reduction in the total amount of fat and despite any attempt at spot reduction. Because spot reduction does not work, any activity that burns enough calories to cause a negative caloric balance can be utilized.

Overload

In the situation where weight loss is the goal, overload really means the attainment of a net deficit. However, the general guidelines for the application of the training principles for dynamic aerobic endurance training outlined in Chapters 6 and 14 also apply here. The one exception is a shift in the importance of intensity and duration. The bottom line is that burning large numbers of calories is what is most important.

Previously sedentary, unfit, and overweight or overfat individuals cannot work at high-intensity levels for even short periods of time, and they should not try to. Instead, low-intensity activities continued for a long duration are recommended. A study by Milesis et al. (1976) exemplifies the importance of duration. Fifty-nine young adult male subjects were divided into four roughly equal groups: a control group whose lifestyle remained unchanged and three exercise groups who engaged in a progressive walk-jog program for 15, 30, or 45 minutes three times per week for 20 weeks. The intensity level was the same for all groups, and no dietary restrictions were involved. Skinfold thickness and percent body fat were significantly reduced in all experimental groups, compared with the controls, but were proportional to the duration of training. Body weight decreased significantly only in the 30- and 45-min exercise groups.

The American College of Sports Medicine (1990) recommends that the threshold level for total body weight and fat weight reduction is an aerobic program 20–60 min in duration with a combination of intensity and duration that will expend at least 300 kcal per session three times per week. If the frequency is raised to four times per week, then a 200-kcal expenditure each session is deemed to be sufficient. Thus, the recommendation for weight loss is any combination of frequency, duration, and intensity of exercise that will burn sufficient calories to obtain a deficit.

This recommendation is contrary to an often mentioned misconception that the way to lose fat is to burn fat doing long-duration, low-intensity exercise. Although it is true that fat is the dominant fuel in long-duration, low-intensity exercise, the important factor in weight loss is to establish a caloric deficit, regardless of the fuel being used. This principle is exemplified in a study by Ballor et al. (1990) on two groups of obese women on equally restricted caloric intakes (1200 kcal·day^{-1}). One group exercised on the cycle ergometer at 51% of their peak $\dot{V}O_2$max for 50 min and the other at 85% of their peak $\dot{V}O_2$max for 25 min. The low-intensity group expended an average of 283 kcal per session at an RER of 0.80, and the high-intensity group expended an average of 260 kcal per session at an RER of 0.92. The estimated fat utilization was 26% for the high-intensity group and 66.6% for the low-intensity group. Although the high-intensity group did improve their cardiovascular fitness more, both groups lost equal amounts of body weight, fat-free mass, fat mass, and percent body fat, and decreased the sum of five skinfold thicknesses.

The advantage of the low-intensity exercise was not an increased loss of fat but a better initial tolerance to the exercise sessions. Individuals who are overweight or obese are also frequently out of shape, and low-intensity work at the initiation of an exercise program is probably more appropriate and less likely to bring about muscle and joint problems than is a high-intensity program. On the other hand, more active or higher fit individuals need not be concerned that in order to reap the weight control benefits of exercise, they need to slow down. The intensity and duration can be manipulated to best suit each individual interested in body weight or composition control.

Increasing caloric expenditure above 300 kcal of exercise and increasing the frequency of the exercise will enhance the fat and weight loss. An individual combining dynamic aerobic endurance and resistance weight training can alternate days (three each) and still have a rest day or can combine sessions on each of 3 or 4 days. The caloric cost of dynamic resistance exercise is less than that of dynamic endurance exercise and this difference needs to be taken into account when designing the exercise program.

In calculations of the energy cost of an activity session the net, not the gross, value should be used. That is, the calories that would have been burned anyway, had the individual been sedentary, should be subtracted from the cost of the exercise (ACSM, 2000; Pacy, et al., 1986). For example, if the energy cost of playing tennis is 7.1 kcal·min^{-1} but the individual would have expended 1.3 kcal·min^{-1} at rest the net cost is 5.8 kcal·min^{-1}. Thus, it would take almost 52 min of tennis to burn 300 excess calories, not 42 min.

Rest/Recovery/Adaptation

The importance of adaptation in caloric deficit lies in the fact that the composition of the weight loss varies the longer the deficit is maintained. Thus, the answer to the question previously posed regarding whether a series of short, very calorically restricted diets or one consistent, moderate-deficit diet is better is definitely the latter. The individual must get past the early water loss stages and into the stage where fat loss is proportionally the greatest. This adaptation will occur in addition to the specific adaptations to the exercise training.

Progression

The greatest progression will be made in the number of calories that can be expended in exercise as the individual adapts to the training. When the calories expended in exercise increase, the amount of food ingested can be kept at the same level, hence increasing the deficit and/or possibly offsetting the decrease in RMR that may occur. Another possibility is to increase the amount of food ingested proportionally to maintain the same relative deficit. Progression should not be interpreted as an attempt to exercise more and more while eating less and less.

Individualization

In order to tailor a weight or fat loss program for an individual, several evaluations and calculations are helpful. The first is the direct measurement or estimation of the RMR. Formulas such as those presented earlier in the chapter (Table 9.2) enable RMR to be estimated fairly easily. The second is a dietary analysis of the nutrient and caloric intake of the individual. Computer programs are available for this analysis. The third is an analysis of the amount of calories normally expended in daily activity. Lists of the caloric cost per kilogram of activities, such as the list presented in Chapter 5, Table 5.6, are available for this calculation.

Once these numbers are available, the relative proportion of the caloric deficit to come from food intake and from energy expenditure can be determined. How much comes from which category should depend on the intake and fitness levels of the individual.

Example

If a sedentary, unfit individual ingests 2000 kcal·day^{-1} and expends 1800 kcal·day^{-1}, 1350 kcal of which is RMR, then an initial 650-kcal decrement makes sense (2000 − 1800 = 200 kcal to get to a caloric balance, and a 450-kcal deficit for a 1.3-lb weight loss per week). If the individual is really unfit, 100 kcal·day^{-1} of exercise may be all he or she is able to do; the other 550 kcal will need to come from the calories ingested. This diet would still allow for a caloric ingestion of 1350 kcal. If, however, the individual is relatively fit, a higher number of calories can be expended in exercise and either a greater intake of food allowed or a greater deficit achieved.   ✛

The caloric ingestion should not fall below the RMR. Although the flat values of 1200 and 1500 kcal·day^{-1} (female and male, respectively) are often suggested as a lower limit of caloric intake (ACSM, 1983), a more individualized system is to calculate a value halfway between RMR and 30% above RMR (Schelkun, 1991).

Retrogression/Plateau/Reversibility

Weight loss tends to be uneven, even if caloric intake and output remain the same. Weight loss is fastest in the early stages of caloric deficit and then tends to level off. This pattern occurs, at least in part, because of the early loss of large amounts of glycogen and water. Later, RMR may decrease, and food efficiency may become a factor (Astrup, et al., 1999; Bray, 1969). Although few who are attempting to lose weight will want to hear about these patterns, they need to be informed in order to get mentally prepared to deal with them. Reverting to old habits of food intake and a sedentary lifestyle (in a sense, detraining) will result in a rapid retrogression or complete reversal, exemplified by regaining lost weight, as was seen in the study described by Pavlou et al. (1989, 1985).

Maintenance

As discussed previously, many more people manage to lose weight than to maintain that weight loss. The key to the maintenance of a weight or fat loss is exercise training (Wing, 1999). Although the amount of food ingested cannot be disregarded, those who continue to exercise are able to eat enough to satisfy their physiological and psychological need for food without creating a positive balance. Those who do not exercise often cannot handle the food deprivation needed; as a result, they overeat for their activity level. The level of food intake and exercise output at the weight the individual wishes to maintain must be continued for life.

Making Weight for Sport

Although athletes in many sports are concerned with maintaining a low body weight and/or a low percent body fat (Brownell, et al., 1987), only a few sports organize the competition around weight classes. The original intention was to make the competitions as fair as possible by matching individuals of approximately the same size. However, in practice, many participants manipulate their body weights and drop down to lower-weight classes under the assumption that they will then have an advantage over their opponents. One wonders what possible advantage there can be when both competitors are following the same strategy (although each athlete will always think he or she can drop down more than his or her opponent) and, more importantly, what the health and performance implications are. Despite the concerns, dropping into a lower-weight class is routinely done, often by individuals in their growth years. Boxers, wrestlers, and jockeys all engage in making weight, but by far the most research attention has been directed toward wrestlers (Figure 9.9).

The American College of Sports Medicine (1996) has published several versions of the "Position Stand on Weight Loss in Wrestlers," the latest in 1996. The techniques typically utilized by wrestlers and the

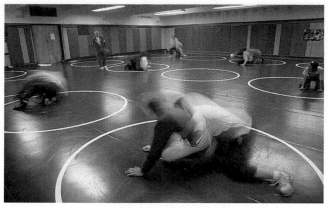

Figure 9.9
Making weight by following sound scientific guidelines should be an important goal for wrestlers at all levels of competition.

physiological consequences were detailed in the 1976 version, as well as a number of suggestions for "making weight" in a healthier manner. Unfortunately, these recommendations appear to have had little impact on the patterns of weight loss and regain in wrestlers.

Over a decade later a study of 63 college and 368 high school wrestlers reported that 44% of the college wrestlers had weight fluctuations between 2.7 and 4.5 kg (6–10 lb) and 41% had fluctuations between 5.0 and 9.1 kg (11–20 lb) per week (Steen, et al., 1988). The majority of the high school wrestlers fluctuated slightly less, with 49% reporting variations of 1.4–2.3 kg (3–5 lb), 23% reporting variations of 2.7–4.5 kg (6–10 lb), and 21% reporting variations of 0–1 kg (0–2 lb). Techniques utilized still included fluid and food restriction (including fasting), vomiting, laxatives, diuretics, time in a sauna, and exercise in a rubber suit. Thirty-five percent of the college sample had lost between 5.0 and 9.1 kg over 100 times in their lives!

Another 1990 study confirmed the detrimental effects of weight loss on physiological parameters (strength, peak aerobic power, anaerobic power, anaerobic capacity, and lactate threshold) (Webster and Weltman, 1990). The wrestlers in this study elected to lose weight by 1–2 hr of exercise in a rubber suit after a 1.5-hr practice session combined with food restriction. The negative work responses were probably the result of dehydration and glycogen depletion. Thus, the conflict between tradition and science continues.

The key to changing the situation appears to be convincing coaches, athletes, trainers, parents, and officials in charge of the sports that a proper weight can and should be determined based on percent body fat, not just body weight at the time of weigh-in. Body fat should be determined in the preseason, and a minimal weight should be determined on the basis of the guideline of not less than 7%BF for male competitors younger than 16 yr and not less than 5%BF for males 16 yr or older. Female wrestlers need a minimum of 12–14%BF. Total body weight loss should not exceed 7%. Body fat should be lost gradually over a period of weeks to achieve the desired wrestling weight. Consideration should be given to allowing the wrestler to compete in a higher-weight class as the season goes on if a substantial increase in height (0.5 in. or more) and/or lean body mass occurs (Tipton, 1990).

It is important that the %BF determinations be accurate. Coaches and/or trainers can learn to take accurate skinfold and other anthropometric measurements and utilize these in sport-specific equations such as the one that follows. This equation is recommended on the basis of studies with wrestlers (Lohman, 1981).

9.2 body density (g·cc^{-1} = 1.0982 − {[0.000815 × sum of triceps + subscapular + abdominal skinfolds (mm)] + [0.0000084 × sum of triceps + subscapular + abdominal skinfolds squared (mm)]}

$$D_B = 1.0982 - (0.000815 \text{ sum of skinfolds} + 0.0000084 \text{ sum of skinfolds}^2)$$
(ACSM, 1983)

Example

If a 17-yr-old wrestler weighed 165 lb and his sum of skinfolds for the selected sites was 46 mm, the calculation would be:

$$D_B = 1.0982 - [0.000815 (46) + 0.0000084(2116)]$$
$$= 1.0429 \text{ g·cc}^{-1}$$

The D_B value is then substituted into the age-appropriate formula presented in Table 8.1 for a male adolescent to determine %BF. For a 17-yr-old this is

$$\%BF = \left(\frac{5.03}{D_B} - 4.59 \right) \times 100 = 23.31$$

Equations 8.4, 8.5, and 8.6 are then used to determine the wrestler's most appropriate competitive weight. Using Equation 8.4

$$FFW = 165 \text{ lb} \times \left(\frac{100\% - 23.3\%}{100} \right) = 126.6 \text{ lb}$$

Using Equation 8.5

$$WT_2 = \frac{100 \times 126.6}{100\% - 16.3\%} = 151.3 \text{ lb}$$

Note: 16% is used here as the desirable %BF, not 5%, which is the lowest recommended %BF for a wrestler of this age. The 16.3% complies with the recommendation that weight loss not exceed 7% of body weight.

A Question of Understanding

Calculate the weight at which the following 14-yr-old wrestler should compete.

Name: Zachary   Triceps skinfold: 8 mm

Weight: 138 lb   Subscapular skinfold: 9 mm

                        Abdominal skinfold: 12 mm

How much weight does Zachary need to gain or lose to achieve this weight?

To get down to 5%BF, this wrestler would need to lose 18.3% of his body weight, and that is too much. Using Equation 8.6

$$151.3 \text{ lb} - 165 \text{ lb} = -13.7 \text{ lb}$$

To achieve his recommended body weight, this wrestler needs to lose 13.7 lb. ✛

Complete the problem in the Question of Understanding box and check your answer in Appendix D.

Specific guidelines for making weight have not been established for other sports, but the principles discussed here can and should be applied.

Summary

1. Weight gain, loss, and stabilization follow the first law of thermodynamics as expressed in the caloric balance equation. The components of this equation are food ingestion (+), resting or basal metabolic rate (−), thermogenesis (−) and exercise (−).

2. Diet, acute exercise, and exercise training can have an impact on the components of the caloric balance equation.

3. The goal of weight or fat control should be to lose body fat, to preserve fat-free weight, to maintain or improve health, and in the case of athletes to maintain or improve performance.

4. Twenty-eight percent of the total weight lost by diet alone is FFW, 72% is fat; 20% of the total weight loss by diet plus exercise is FFW, 80% is fat; only 4.5% of the weight lost by exercise alone is FFW, 95.5% is fat. Thus exercise helps to preserve FFW during times of caloric deficit.

5. A combination of diet plus exercise is the preferred technique for body composition and body weight control both in accomplishing an initial loss and in the maintenance of a weight loss.

6. The exercise training component of weight and fat control should include both an aerobic endurance portion (to burn at least 200–300 kcal per session) and a resistance weight training portion (to maintain and/or build fat-free weight).

7. Proper weight for wrestling should be determined based on %BF. The %BF should not be less than 7% for competitors under the age of 16 yr nor less than 5% for older competitors. Body weight loss should not exceed 7%, and this weight should be maintained throughout the season, except for allowing for more weight if height increases more than 1.25 cm (0.5 in).

Review Questions

1. State the caloric balance equation, and relate it to the first law of thermodynamics. Define and explain the components of the caloric balance equation.

2. Discuss the impact of dietary restriction on the components of the caloric balance equation.

3. Discuss the impact of exercise on the components of the caloric balance equation.

4. Discuss the impact of exercise training on the components of the caloric balance equation.

5. Compare and contrast the effects of diet alone, exercise alone, and diet and exercise combined on body weight and composition control.

6. List the training principles. Explain how each should be specifically applied for body weight or body composition control or maintenance.

7. Defend or refute the following statements, using evidence provided in this chapter.

   a. Weight cycling makes subsequent weight loss physiologically more difficult.

   b. The most important reason to add exercise or exercise training to a weight loss or maintenance program is that exercise decreases appetite.

   c. If food is eaten near the time of exercise (either directly prior to or after), the thermic response is potentiated (made more effective), so that more calories are burned and weight is lost faster.

   d. The maintenance of, increase in, or decrease in resting metabolic rate depends on the maintenance or change in lean body mass.

e. To lose fat, burn fat by doing long-duration, low-intensity exercise.

8. Prepare a set of weight control guidelines for a jockey.

For further review and additional study tools, go to The Physiology Place (www.physiologyplace.com) and the Student Study Guide for Exercise Physiology for Health, Fitness, and Performance by Sharon A. Plowman and Denise L. Smith.

Passport to the Internet

Visit the following Internet sites to explore further topics and issues related to body composition and weight management. To visit an organization's web site, go to www.physiologyplace.com and click on "Passport to the Internet."

University of Illinois Nutritional Analysis Tool The University of Illinois at Urbana-Champaign Food Science and Human Nutrition Department has developed a Nutritional Analysis Tool to promote healthy eating. Although not intended to replace the advice of a physician or health professional, the site does help individuals gain some insight into their dietary patterns and establish a nutrient-dense diet for themselves. Analyze your dietary habits and check out the energy calculator to determine how many calories you expend.

DietWorldOnline.Com An online support center containing comprehensive resources and links to many areas on the Internet that provide information, knowledge, and support needed to help with weight loss. Although not affiliated with a medical or other professional organization, the site provides a great deal of practical information for the layperson.

The Cooper Institute This comprehensive site connects you with the world-renowned Cooper Institute, known for intensive research in the area of fitness and physical health. Visit this site for the latest scientific updates. Visit the Clinical Weight Management Research Center and evaluate your weight management risk level.

References

American College of Sports Medicine: *ACSM's Guidelines for Exercise Testing and Prescription* (6th edition). Philadelphia: Lippincott Williams & Wilkins (2000).

American College of Sports Medicine: Position stand on weight loss in wrestlers. *Medicine and Science in Sports.* 28(2):ix–xii (1996).

American College of Sports Medicine: Proper and improper weight loss programs. *Medicine and Science in Sports and Exercise.* 15:xi–xiii (1983).

American College of Sports Medicine: The recommended quantity and quality of exercise for developing and maintaining cardiorespiratory and muscular fitness in healthy adults. *Medicine and Science in Sports and Exercise.* 22(2):265–274 (1990).

American College of Sports Medicine, American Dietetic Association, & Dietitians of Canada: Joint position statement: Nutrition and athletic performance. *Medicine and Science in Sports and Exercise.* 32(12):2130–2145 (2000).

Apfelbaum, M., J. Bostarron, & D. Lacatis: Effect of caloric restriction and excessive caloric intake on energy expenditure. *American Journal of Clinical Nutrition.* 24:1405–1409 (1971).

Astrup, A., P. C. Gotzsche, K. vandeWerken, C. Ranneries, S. Toubro, A. Raben, & B. Buemann: Meta-analysis of resting metabolic rate in formerly obese subjects. *American Journal of Clinical Nutrition.* 69:1117–1122 (1999).

Ballor, D. L., V. L. Katch, M. D. Becque, & C. R. Marks: Resistance weight training during caloric restriction enhances lean body weight maintenance. *American Journal of Clinical Nutrition.* 47:19–25 (1988).

Ballor, D. L., J. P. McCarthy, & E. J. Wilterdink: Exercise intensity does not affect the composition of diet- and exercise-induced body mass loss. *American Journal of Clinical Nutrition.* 51:142–146 (1990).

Beeson, V., C. Ray, R. A. Coxon, & S. Kreitzman: The myth of the yo-yo: Consistent rate of weight loss with successive dieting by VLCD. *International Journal of Obesity.* 13:135–139 (1989).

Belko, A. Z., T. F. Barbier, & E. C. Wong: Effect of energy and protein intake and exercise intensity on the thermic effect of food. *American Journal of Clinical Nutrition.* 43:863–869 (1986).

Bingham, S. A., G. R. Goldberg, W. A. Coward, A. M. Prentice, & J. H. Cummings: The effect of exercise and improved physical fitness on basal metabolic rate. *British Journal of Nutrition.* 61:155–173 (1989).

Blackburn, G. L., G. T. Wilson, B. S. Kanders, L. J. Stein, P. T. Lavin, J. Adler, & K. D. Brownell: Weight cycling: The experience of human dieters. *American Journal of Clinical Nutrition.* 49:1105–1109 (1989).

Blanchard, M. S.: Thermogenesis and its relationship to obesity and exercise. *Quest.* 34(2):143–153 (1982).

Blundell, J. E., & N. A. King: Physical activity and regulation of food intake: Current evidence. *Medicine and Science in Sports and Exercise.* 31(11)Supplement: S573–S583 (1999).

Bogert, L. J., G. M. Briggs, & D. H. Calloway: *Nutrition and Physical Fitness* (9th edition). Philadelphia: Saunders (1973).

Boileau, R. A., T. G. Lohman, & M. H. Slaughter: Exercise and body composition in children and youth. *Scandinavian Journal of Sport Sciences.* 7:17–27 (1985).

Bouchard, C.: Heredity and the path to overweight and obesity. *Medicine and Science in Sports and Exercise.* 23(3):285–291 (1991).

Bouchard, C. T., A. Tremblay, A. Nadeau, J. P. Despres, G. Theriault, M. R. Goulay, G. Lortie, C. Leblanc, & G. Fournier: Genetic effect in resting and exercise metabolic rates. *Metabolism.* 38(4):364–370 (1989).

Bouchard, C. T., A. Tremblay, A. Nadeau, J. Dussault, J. P. Depres, G. Theriault, P. J. Lupien, O. Serresse, M. R. Boulay, & G. Fournier: Long-term exercise training with constant energy intake. 1. Effect on body composition. *International Journal of Obesity.* 14:57–73 (1990).

Bray, G. A.: Complications of obesity. *Annals of Internal Medicine.* 103(6 pt 2):1052–1062 (1985).

Bray, G. A.: Effect of caloric restriction on energy expenditure in obese patients. *Lancet.* 2:397–398 (1969).

Brodie, D. A.: Techniques of measurement of body composition: Part I. *Sports Medicine.* 5:11–40 (1988).

Brown, M. R., W. J. Klish, J. Hollander, M. A. Campbell, & G. B. Forbes: A high protein, low calorie liquid diet in the treatment of very obese adolescents: Long-term effect on lean body mass. *The American Journal of Clinical Nutrition.* 38:20–31 (1983).

Brownell, K. D., S. N. Steen, & J. H. Wilmore: Weight regulation practices in athletes: Analysis of metabolic and health effects. *Medicine and Science in Sports and Exercise.* 19(6):546–556 (1987).

Bullough, R. C., C. A. Gillette, M. A. Harris, & C. L. Melby: Interaction of acute changes in exercise energy expenditure and energy intake on resting metabolic rate. *American Journal of Clinical Nutrition.* 61:473–481 (1995).

Bursztein, S. E., D. H. Elwyn, J. Askanazi, & J. M. Kinney: *Energy Metabolism, Indirect Calorimetry and Nutrition.* Baltimore: Williams & Wilkins (1989).

Dallasso, H. M., & W. P. James: Whole-body calorimetry studies in adult men. 2. The interaction of exercise and overfeeding on the thermic effect of a meal. *British Journal of Nutrition.* 52:65–72 (1984).

Despres, J. P., C. Bouchard, A. Tremblay, R. Savard, & M. Marcotte: Effects of aerobic training on fat distribution in male subjects. *Medicine and Science in Sports and Exercise.* 17(1):113–118 (1985).

Donnelly, J. E., J. Jakicic, & S. Gunderson: Diet and body composition: Effect of very low calorie diets and exercise. *Sports Medicine.* 12(4):237–249 (1991).

Epstein, L. H., & G. S. Goldfield: Physical activity in the treatment of childhood overweight and obesity: Current evidence and research issues. *Medicine and Science in Sports and Exercise.* 31(11) Supplement: S553–S559 (1999).

Garrow, J. S.: Energy balance in man: An overview. *American Journal of Clinical Nutrition.* 45:1114–1119 (1987).

Gershoff, S. N. (ed.): Ask the experts. *Tufts University Diet & Nutrition Letter.* 9(7):8 (1991).

Gershoff, S. N. (ed.): Ask the experts. *Tufts University Diet & Nutrition Letter.* 9(11):7 (1992).

Gilbert, J. A., J. E. Misner, R. A. Boileau, L. Ji, & M. H. Slaughter: Lower thermic effect of a meal post-exercise in aerobically trained and resistance-trained subjects. *Medicine and Science in Sports and Exercise.* 23(7):825–830 (1991).

Glickman, N. M., H. H. Mitchell, E. H. Lambert, & W. Keeton: The total specific dynamic action of high-protein and high-carbohydrate diets of human subjects. *Journal of Nutrition.* 36:41–57 (1948).

Grande, F. A., J. T. Anderson, & A. Keys: Changes of basal metabolic rate in man in semistarvation and refeeding. *Journal of Applied Physiology.* 12(2):230–238 (1958).

Grande, F. T., H. L. Taylor, J. T. Anderson, E. Buskirk, & A. Keys: Water exchange in men on a restricted water intake and a low calorie carbohydrate diet accompanied by physical work. *Journal of Applied Physiology.* 12(2):202–210 (1958).

Guyton, A. C.: *Textbook of Medical Physiology* (7th edition). Philadelphia: Saunders (1986).

Hagan, R. D.: Benefits of aerobic conditioning and diet for overweight adults. *Sports Medicine.* 5:144–155 (1988).

Hagan, R. D., S. J. Upton, L. Wong, & J. Whittam: The effects of aerobic conditioning and/or calorie restriction in overweight men and women. *Medicine and Science in Sports and Exercise.* 18(1):87–94 (1986).

Heymsfield, S. B., K. Casper, J. Hearn, & D. Guy: Rate of weight loss during underfeeding: Relation to level of physical activity. *Metabolism.* 38(3):215–233 (1989).

Himms-Hagen, J.: Thermogenesis in brown adipose tissue as an energy buffer. *The New England Journal of Medicine.* 311(24):1549–1558 (1984).

Horton, E. S.: Metabolic aspects of exercise and weight reduction. *Medicine and Science in Sports and Exercise.* 18(1):10–18 (1985).

Jeffery, R. W., R. R. Wing, & S. A. French: Weight cycling and cardiovascular risk factors in obese men and women. *American Journal of Clinical Nutrition.* 55:641–644 (1992).

Jequier, E.: Energy, obesity, and body weight standards. *The American Journal of Clinical Nutrition.* 45:1035–1047 (1987).

Katch, F. I., P. M. Clarkson, W. Kroll, T. McBride, & A. Wilcox: Effects of sit-up exercise training on adipose cell size and adiposity. *Research Quarterly for Exercise and Sport.* 55(3):242–247 (1984).

Kieres, J., & S. Plowman: Effects of swimming and land exercises versus swimming and water exercises on body composition of college students. *Journal of Sports Medicine and Physical Fitness.* 31(2):189–195 (1991).

Leibel, R. L., & J. Hirsch: Diminished energy requirements in reduced-obese patients. *Metabolism.* 33(2):164–170 (1984).

Leibel, R. L., M. Rosenbaum, & J. Hirsch: Changes in energy expenditure resulting from altering body weight. *The New England Journal of Medicine.* 332:621–628 (1995).

Lemmer, J. T., F. M. Ivey, A. S. Ryan, G. F. Martel, D. E. Hurlbut, J. E. Metter, J. L. Fozard, J. L. Fleg, & B. F. Hurley: Effect of strength training on resting metabolic rate and physical activity: Age and gender comparisons. *Medicine and Science in Sports and Exercise.* 33(4):532–541 (2001).

Lohman, T. G.: Skinfolds and body density and their relation to body fatness: A review. *Human Biology.* 53(2):181–225 (1981).

Melby, C., C. Scholl, G. Edwards, & R. Bullough: Effect of acute resistance exercise on postexercise energy expenditure and resting metabolic rate. *Journal of Applied Physiology.* 75(4):1847–1853 (1993).

Milesis, C. A., M. L. Pollock, M. D. Bah, J. J. Ayres, A. Ward, & A. C. Linnerod: Effects of different durations of physical training on cardiorespiratory function, body composition, and serum lipids. *Research Quarterly.* 47(4):716–725 (1976).

Mole, P. A., J. S. Stern, C. L. Schultz, E. M. Bernauer, & B. J. Holcomb: Exercise reverses depressed metabolic rate produced by severe caloric restriction. *Medicine and Science in Sports and Exercise.* 21(1):29–33 (1989).

Nair, K. S., D. Halliday, & J. S. Garrow: Thermic response to isoenergetic protein, carbohydrate or fat meals in lean and obese subjects. *Clinical Science.* 66:307–312 (1983).

Nash, J. D.: Eating behavior and body weight: Physiological influences. *American Journal of Health Promotion.* 1(3):5–15 (1987).

National Task Force on the Prevention and Treatment of Obesity: Weight cycling. *Journal of the American Medical Association.* 272(15):1196–1202 (1994).

Newsholme, E. A.: A possible metabolic basis for the control of body weight. *New England Journal of Medicine.* 302(7):400–405 (1980).

Nieman, D. C.: *Fitness and Sports Medicine: An Introduction.* Palo Alto, CA: Bull Publishing (1990).

Nieman, D. C., J. L. Haig, E. D. DeGuis, G. P. Dizon, U. D. Register: Reducing diet and exercise training effects on resting metabolic rates in mildly obese women. *Journal of Sports Medicine and Physical Fitness.* 28(1):79–88 (1988).

Noland, M., & J. T. Kearney: Anthropometric and densitometric responses of women to specific and general exercise. *Research Quarterly.* 49(3):322–328 (1978).

Pacy, P. J., N. Barton, J. D. Webster, & J. Garrow: The energy cost of aerobic exercise in fed and fasted normal subjects. *American Journal of Clinical Nutrition.* 42:764–768 (1985).

Pacy, P. J., J. Webster, & J. S. Garrow: Exercise and obesity. *Sports Medicine.* 3:89–113 (1986).

Pavlou, K. N., S. Krey, & W. P. Steffee: Exercise as an adjunct to weight loss and maintenance in moderately obese subjects. *American Journal of Clinical Nutrition.* 49:1115–1123 (1989).

Pavlou, K. N., W. P. Steffee, R. H. Lerman, & B. A. Burrows: Effects of dieting and exercise on lean body mass, oxygen uptake, and strength. *Medicine and Science in Sports and Exercise.* 17(4):466–471 (1985).

Plowman, S. A.: Maturation and exercise training in children. *Pediatric Exercise Science.* 1:303–312 (1989).

Poehlman, E. T.: A review: Exercise and its influence on resting energy metabolism in man. *Medicine and Science in Sports and Exercise.* 21(5):515–525 (1989).

Poehlman, E. T., & E. Danforth, Jr.: Endurance training increases metabolic rate and norepinephrine appearance rate in older individuals. *American Journal of Physiology.* 261:E233–E239 (1991).

Pratley, R., B. Nicklas, M. Robin, J. Miller, A. Smith, M. Smith, B. Hurley, & A. Goldberg: Strength training increases resting metabolic rate and norepinephrine levels in healthy 50- to 65-yr-old men. *Journal of Applied Physiology.* 76(1):133–137 (1994).

Rodin, J., N. Radke-Sharpe, M. Rebuffe-Scrive, & M. R. C. Greenwood: Weight cycling and fat distribution. *International Journal of Obesity.* 14:303–310 (1990).

Ross, R.: Effects of diet- and exercise-induced weight loss on visceral adipose tissue in men and women. *SportsMedicine.* 24(1):55–64 (1997).

Ross, R., & I. Janssen: Is abdominal fat preferentially reduced in response to exercise-induced weight loss? *Medicine and Science in Sports and Exercise.* 31(11) Supplement: S568–S572 (1999).

Roza, A. M., & H. M. Shizgal: The Harris Benedict equation reevaluated: Resting energy requirements and the body cell mass. *American Journal of Clinical Nutrition.* 40:168–182 (1984).

Schelkun, P. H.: The risks of riding the weight-loss roller coaster. *The Physician and Sportsmedicine.* 19(6):149–156 (1991).

Schmidt, W. D., D. Corrigan, & C. L. Melby: Two seasons of weight cycling does not lower resting metabolic rate in college wrestlers. *Medicine and Science in Sports and Exercise.* 25(5):613–619 (1993).

Schutz, Y. B., T. Bessard, & E. Jequier: Diet-induced thermogenesis measured over a whole day in obese and nonobese women. *American Journal of Clinical Nutrition.* 40:542–552 (1984).

Schwartz, R. S., J. B. Halter, & E. L. Bierman: Reduced thermic effect of feeding in obesity: Role of norepinephrine. *Metabolism.* 32:114–117 (1983).

Segal, K. R., B. Gutin, J. Albu, & F. Pi-Sunyer: Thermic effects of food and exercise in lean and obese men of similar lean body mass. *American Journal of Physiology.* 252:E110–E117 (1987).

Segal, K. R., B. Gutin, A. M. Nyman, & F. X. Pi-Sunyer: Thermic effect of food at rest, during exercise, and after exercise in lean and obese men of similar body weight. *Journal of Clinical Investigation.* 76:1107–1112 (1985).

Segal, K. R., E. Presta, & B. Gutin: Thermic effect of food during graded exercise in normal weight and obese men. *American Journal of Clinical Nutrition.* 40:995–1000 (1984).

Sheldahl, L. M.: Special ergometric techniques and weight reduction. *Medicine and Science in Sports and Exercise.* 18(1):25–30 (1985).

Shetty, P. S., R. T. Jung, W. P. James, M. A. Barrand, & B. A. Callingham: Postprandial thermogenesis in obesity. *Clinical Science.* 60:519–525 (1981).

Steen, S. N., R. A. Oppliger, & K. D. Brownell: Metabolic effects of repeated weight loss and regain in adolescent wrestlers. *Journal of the American Medical Association.* 260(1):47–50 (1988).

Swaminathan, R. K., R. F. King, J. Holmfield, R. A. Siwek, M. Baker, & J. K. Wales: Thermic effect of feeding carbohydrate, fat, protein, and mixed meat in lean and obese subjects. *American Journal of Clinical Nutrition.* 42:177–181 (1985).

Tipton, C. M.: Making and maintaining weight for interscholastic wrestling. *Sports Science Exchange.* 2(22) (1990).

Titchenal, C. A.: Exercise and food intake: What is the relationship? *Sports Medicine.* 6:135–145 (1988).

van Dale, O., & W. H. M. Saris: Repetitive weight loss and weight regain: Effects on weight reduction, resting metabolic rate, and lipolytic activity before and after exercise and/or diet treatment. *American Journal of Clinical Nutrition.* 49:409–416 (1989).

van Horn, L., K. Donato, S. Kumanyika, M. Winston, T. E. Prewitt, & L. Snetselaar: The dietitian's role in developing and implementing the first federal obesity guidelines. *Journal of the American Dietetic Association.* 98(10): 1115–1117 (1998).

Wadden, T. A., S. Bartlett, & K. A. Letizia: Relationship of dieting history to resting metabolic rate, body composition, eating behavior and subsequent weight loss. *American Journal of Clinical Nutrition.* 56:206S–211S (1992).

Wadden, T. A., G. D. Foster, K. A. Letizia, & J. L. Mullen: Long-term effects of dieting on resting metabolic rate in obese outpatients. *Journal of the American Medical Association.* 264(6):707–711 (1990).

Walberg, J. L.: Aerobic exercise and resistance weight-training during weight reduction: Implications for obese persons and athletes. *Sports Medicine.* 47:343–356 (1989).

Webster, S. R., & R. Weltman: Physiological effects of a weight loss regimen practiced by college wrestlers. *Medicine and Science in Sports and Exercise.* 22(2):229–234 (1990).

Welle, S.: Metabolic response to a meal during rest and low intensity exercise. *American Journal of Clinical Nutrition.* 40:990–994 (1984).

Willms, W. L., & S. A. Plowman: The separate and sequential effects of exercise and meal ingestion on energy expenditure. *Annals of Nutrition and Metabolism.* 35(6):347–356 (1991).

Wilmore, J. H.: Appetite and body composition consequent to physical activity. *Research Quarterly for Exercise and Sport.* 54(4):415–425 (1983).

Wilmore, J. H., & D. L. Costill: *Training for Sport and Activity: The Physiological Basis of the Conditioning Process* (3rd edition). Dubuque, IA: Brown (1988).

Wing, R. R.: Weight cycling in humans: A review of the literature. *Annals of Behavioral Medicine.* 14(2):113–119 (1992).

Wing, R. R.: Physical activity in the treatment of the adulthood overweight and obesity: Current evidence and research issues. *Medicine and Science in Sports and Exercise.* 31(11) Supplement: S547–S552 (1999).

Zahorska-Markiewicz, B.: Thermic effect of food and exercise in obesity. *European Journal of Applied Physiology.* 44:231–235 (1980).

Zuti, W. B., & L. A. Golding: Comparing diet and exercise as weight reducing tools. *The Physician and Sportsmedicine.* 4:49–53 (1976).

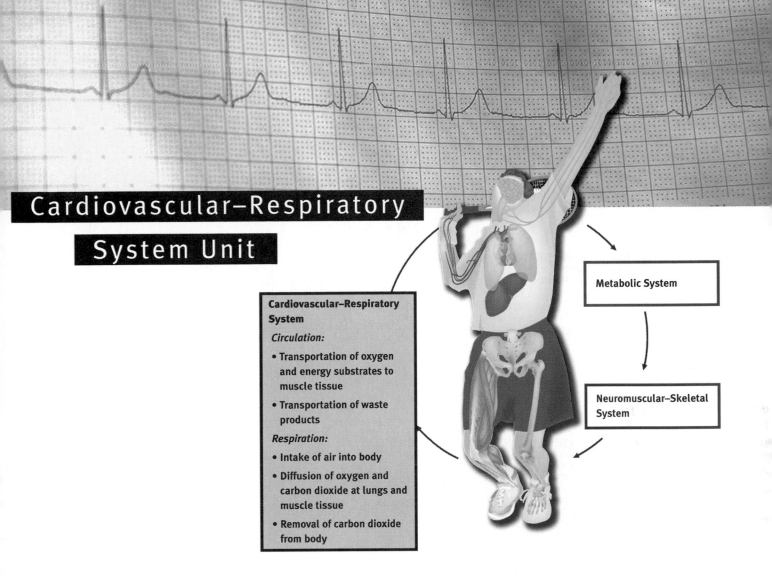

Cardiovascular–Respiratory System Unit

Cardiovascular–Respiratory System

Circulation:
- Transportation of oxygen and energy substrates to muscle tissue
- Transportation of waste products

Respiration:
- Intake of air into body
- Diffusion of oxygen and carbon dioxide at lungs and muscle tissue
- Removal of carbon dioxide from body

Metabolic System

Neuromuscular–Skeletal System

The cardiorespiratory system is responsible for bringing oxygen into the body (respiratory system) and transporting it to the cells (cardiovascular system), which use the oxygen for the production of energy (through the process of cellular respiration). Thus, the respiratory and cardiovascular systems are functionally linked and often referred to collectively as the cardiovascular-respiratory, or cardiorespiratory system. The cardiorespiratory system directly supports metabolism by delivering oxygen to the cells of the body. The metabolic production of ATP from oxygen and foodstuffs then directly supports the neuromuscular system by providing the energy for muscle contraction.

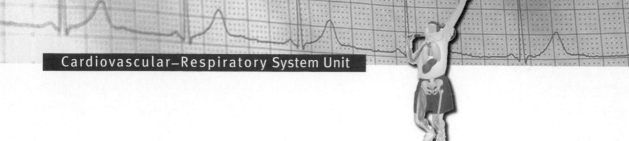
Chapter 10

Respiration

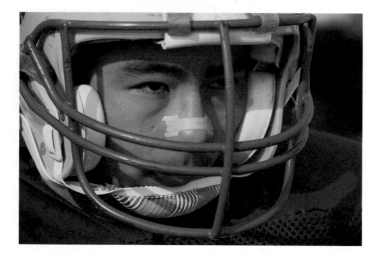

After studying the chapter, you should be able to

- Distinguish between and explain the component variables of pulmonary ventilation, external respiration, and internal respiration.

- Identify the conductive and respiratory zones of the respiratory system and compare the functions of the two zones.

- Explain the mechanics of breathing.

- Differentiate between pulmonary circulation and bronchial circulation.

- Describe static and dynamic lung volumes.

- Distinguish between the conditions under which respiratory measures are collected and reported.

- Calculate minute and alveolar ventilation, the partial pressure of a gas in a mixture, the amount of oxygen carried per deciliter of blood, and the arteriovenous oxygen difference.

- Explain how respiration is regulated at rest and during exercise.

- Explain how oxygen and carbon dioxide are transported in the circulatory system and how oxygen is released to the tissues.

- Explain the role of respiration in acid-base balance.

Introduction

The common denominator for all sports and physical activity is muscle action. For muscles to be able to act, energy must be provided. The first link in the chain of supplying a large portion of this energy is respiration, for it is respiration that provides oxygen to and removes carbon dioxide from the body.

Although it is typical to think of respiration as being synonymous with breathing and/or ventilation, technically it is not. Figure 10.1 presents an overview of respiration. As the figure shows, the volume of air flowing into the lungs from the external environment through either the nose or mouth is called **pulmonary ventilation.** Ventilation is accomplished by breathing, the alternation of inspiration and expiration that causes the air to move. The actual exchange of the gases oxygen (O_2) and carbon dioxide (CO_2) between the lungs and the blood is known as **external respiration.** At the cellular level, oxygen and carbon dioxide gases are again exchanged; this exchange is called **internal respiration. Cellular respiration** is the utilization of oxygen by the cells to produce energy with carbon dioxide as a by-product. Cellular respiration includes both aerobic (with O_2) and anaerobic (without O_2) energy production and is discussed in Chapter 3. This chapter concentrates on pulmonary ventilation, external respiration, and internal respiration.

Structure of the Pulmonary System

The respiratory system consists of two major portions: (1) the conductive zone, which transports the air to the lungs; and (2) the respiratory zone, where gas exchange takes place.

The Conductive Zone

The basic structure of the conductive zone is shown in Figure 10.2. Everything from the nose, or mouth, to the terminal bronchioles comprises the *conductive zone* (Martin, et al., 1979). The primary role of the conductive zone is to transport air. Because no exchange of gases takes place, this zone is also called *anatomical dead space.* As a general guideline, the amount of anatomical dead space can be estimated as 1 mL for each 1 lb of "ideal" body weight (Slonim and Hamilton, 1976). Hence, a 130-lb female who is at her ideal weight has an estimated 130 mL of anatomical dead space. However, if this individual were to gain 20 lb, she would not then also gain anatomical dead space; that estimate would remain at 130 mL. Anatomical dead space is important in determining alveolar ventilation, as discussed later in the chapter.

A second important role of the conductive zone is to warm and humidify the air. By the time the air reaches the lungs, it has been warmed to body temperature (normally ~37°C) and has been 99.5% saturated with water vapor. This protective mechanism maintains core body temperature and protects the

---

Pulmonary Ventilation The process by which air is moved into the lungs.

External Respiration The exchange of gases between the lungs and the blood.

Internal Respiration The exchange of gases at the cellular level.

Cellular Respiration The utilization of oxygen by the cells to produce energy.

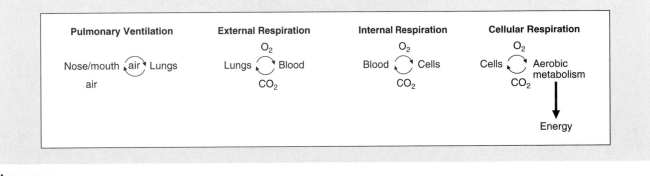

Figure 10.1
Overview of Respiration

Respiration consists of four separate parts. The first is pulmonary ventilation, in which air is moved into and out of the body. The second, external respiration, involves the exchange of oxygen and carbon dioxide between the lungs and the blood. The third is internal respiration, which involves the exchange of oxygen and carbon dioxide at the cellular or tissue level. Finally, cellular respiration is the utilization of oxygen to produce energy, which also produces carbon dioxide as a by-product.

Figure 10.2

Anatomy of the Pulmonary System

The pulmonary system is divided into two zones—the conductive zone transports air to the lungs, and the respiratory zone is where gas exchange takes place.

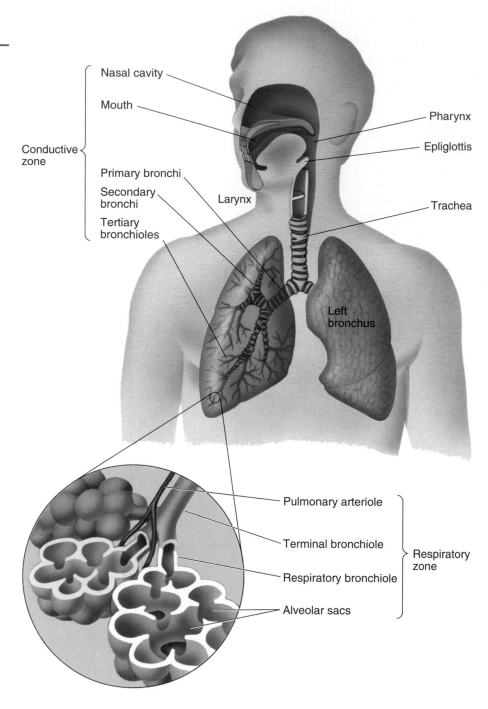

Conductive zone

- Nasal cavity
- Mouth
- Primary bronchi
- Secondary bronchi
- Tertiary bronchioles
- Larynx

- Pharynx
- Epliglottis
- Trachea
- Left bronchus

- Pulmonary arteriole
- Terminal bronchiole
- Respiratory bronchiole
- Alveolar sacs

Respiratory zone

lungs from injury (Slonim and Hamilton, 1976). The warming and humidifying of air is easily accomplished over a wide range of environmental temperatures under resting conditions, when the volume of air transported is small and the air is inhaled through the nose. During heavy exercise, however, large volumes of air are inhaled primarily through the mouth, thus bypassing the warming and moisturizing sites of the nose and nasal cavity. As a result, the mouth and throat may feel dry. If heavy exercise takes place in cold weather (especially at subzero temperatures), dryness increases and actual throat pain may be felt. These uncomfortable feelings are not a symptom of freezing of the lungs; rather they are the result of the drying and cooling of the upper airway. The lower portions of the conductive zone still moisturize and warm the air sufficiently before it reaches the lungs. A scarf worn across the mouth will trap both the moisture and the heat from the exhaled air and decrease or eliminate the uncomfortable sensations.

A third role of the conductive zone is to filter incoming air. The nasal cavity, pharynx, larynx, trachea, and bronchial system are all lined with ciliated mucous membranes (Figure 10.2). These membranes trap impurities and foreign particles (particulates) that are inhaled. Both smoke and environmental air pollutants diminish ciliary activity and can ultimately destroy the cilia.

The Respiratory Zone

The *respiratory zone* consists of the respiratory bronchioles, the alveolar ducts, alveolar sacs (or grapelike clusters), and the alveoli (see Figure 10.2). The *alveoli* are the actual site of gas exchange between the pulmonary system and cardiovascular system. At birth humans possess approximately 24 million alveoli. This number increases to about 300 million by the age of 8 yr and remains constant until 30 yr of age, when it begins a gradual decline. Although each individual alveolus is small, only about 0.2 mm in diameter, collectively the alveoli in a young adult have a total surface area of 70 to 80 m^2 (Slonim and Hamilton, 1976). This area would cover a badminton court or even a tennis court if flattened out. Despite this large surface area, the lungs weigh only about 2.2 lb (1 kg). The membrane between the alveoli and capillaries is actually composed of five very thin layers, two of which are the endothelial cells that comprise the alveoli and capillaries themselves. Despite the number of layers, the thickness is less than the paper this book is printed on, and gas exchange takes place easily (Martin, et al., 1979).

Some alveoli have no capillary blood supply and therefore cannot participate in gas exchange; these alveoli make up a *physiological dead space*. The amount of physiological dead space is minimal in healthy individuals; thus, the total dead space is only slightly larger than the anatomical dead space (Slonim and Hamilton, 1976).

Mechanics of Breathing

The movement of air into the lungs from the atmosphere depends on two factors—pressure gradient (ΔP) and resistance (R). The relationship between these factors is expressed by the equation for *airflow* ($\dot{V}$):

10.1 airflow ($L \cdot min^{-1}$) = $\dfrac{\text{pressure gradient (mmHg)}}{\text{resistance (R unit)}}$

or

$$\dot{V} = \frac{\Delta P}{R}$$

A *pressure gradient* is simply the difference (difference is represented by the Greek capital letter Δ, delta) between two pressures. The larger the differences in pressure, the larger the pressure gradient is. Gases—in this case air, which is a mixture of gases—move from areas of high pressure to areas of low pressure.

Resistance is the sum of the forces opposing the flow of the gases. About 20% of the resistance to airflow is caused by tissue friction as the lungs move during inspiration and expiration. The remaining 80% is due to the friction between the gas molecules and the walls of the airway (airway resistance) and the internal friction between the gas molecules themselves (viscosity). Airway resistance is determined by the size of the airway and the smoothness or turbulence of the airflow.

Equation 10.1 indicates that in order for air to flow, the pressure gradient must be greater than the resistance to the flow. Thus, for inspiration to take place, pressure must be higher in the atmosphere than in the lungs; for expiration, pressure in the alveoli of the lungs must be higher than in the atmosphere. Figure 10.3 shows how the inspiratory pressure gradient is created.

A key to understanding Figure 10.3 is Boyle's law. *Boyle's law* states that the pressure of a gas is inversely related to its volume (or vice versa) under conditions of constant temperature: Low pressure is associated with large volume, and high pressure is associated with small volume.

For pulmonary ventilation, an increase in chest cavity volume is accomplished by muscle contraction for inspiration. This increase in volume leads to an internal lung pressure decrease, according to Boyle's law. As a result, the chest cavity exhibits a negative pressure relative to the atmosphere. Thus, a pressure gradient has been created. Air flows into the chest cavity in an attempt to equalize this pressure difference.

The main inspiratory muscle is the dome-shaped diaphragm. Upon neural stimulation, the diaphragm contracts and moves downward, elongating the chest cavity (see Figure 10.3b). Further enlargement of the chest cavity can come from the action of the external intercostal muscles as well as others (known collectively as the accessory muscles), which elevate the rib cage and bring about expansion both laterally (side to side) and anteroposteriorly (front to back). The extent of accessory muscle activity and the resultant drop in pressure depends on the depth of the inspiration.

The changes in chest cavity volume are transferred to the lungs themselves owing to the presence and function of pleura. *Pleura* is a thin, double-layered membrane that lines both the chest cavity

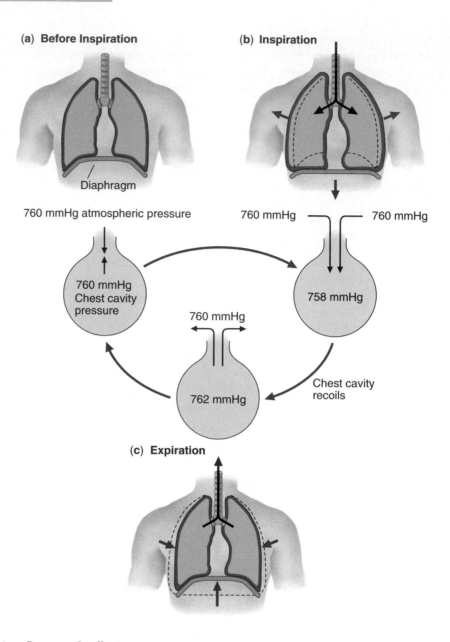

(a) Before Inspiration

Diaphragm

760 mmHg atmospheric pressure

760 mmHg
Chest cavity
pressure

(b) Inspiration

760 mmHg — 760 mmHg

758 mmHg

Chest cavity
recoils

760 mmHg

762 mmHg

(c) Expiration

Figure 10.3

Inspiratory and Expiratory Pressure Gradients

Inspiration and expiration are accomplished by the creation of pressure gradients. (a) The respiratory musculature is relaxed, atmospheric pressure equals chest cavity pressure, and so no air movement occurs. (b) The external intercostals and diaphragm contract, moving the ribs up and out and the diaphragm down, respectively. This muscle action enlarges the chest cavity laterally, anterioposterially, and downward, increasing the volume. As a result, chest cavity pressure is lower than atmospheric pressure, and air flows in. (c) The inspiratory muscles relax, and the chest cavity recoils, creating a pressure higher than atmospheric pressure. Air flows out. The respiratory cycle then begins again.

(the inner surfaces of the thorax, sternum, ribs, vertebrae, and diaphragm) and the external lung surfaces. The portion covering the chest cavity is called *parietal pleura;* the portion covering the external lung surfaces is called the *visceral* or *pulmonary pleura.* A fluid secreted by the pleura fills the space between the pleura (the intrapleural space) and allows the lungs to glide smoothly over the chest cavity walls. It also causes the parietal and pulmonary pleura to adhere to each other in the same way that two pieces of glass are held together by a thin film of water. Because of this adhesion, the lungs themselves move when muscle action causes movement of the chest cavity (Guyton, 1986; Martin, et al., 1979).

Focus on Application

✳ Nasal Dilators

Originally intended as a sleep aid, the Breathe Right Strip™ nasal dilator has been embraced by a broad range of exercisers, including professional athletes from football players to marathoners. The Breathe Right™ has been shown to increase nasal valve area by 25% (Griffin, et al., 1997) and to decrease air resistance in the nasal cavity by approximately 30% (Wetzstein, 1996). The question is whether this larger area and decreased resistance results in a higher tidal volume (V_T), lower frequency of breathing (f), and changes in minute ventilation ($\dot{V}_E$) that might in turn result in better alveolar ventilation ($\dot{V}_A$), external respiration [(A-a)PO_2 diff], arterial oxygenation (PaO_2), or decreases in oxygen consumption ($\dot{V}O_2$) based on a lower energy cost for pulmonary ventilation.

Although one study by Griffin and colleagues showed decreased $\dot{V}_E$ and $\dot{V}O_2$ during submaximal cycling while the exercisers were wearing the nasal dilator, the vast preponderance of available evidence to date has failed to support the use of dilator strips. Studies that have reported pulmonary ventilation responses to short-term (20-min), moderate (55% $\dot{V}O_2$max) cycling (Brown, et al., 1997), incremental exercise to maximum on a cycle ergometer (Huffman, et al., 1996; O'Kroy, 2000) or treadmill (Clapp and Bishop, 1996), and to high-intensity, short-duration activity (the Wingate Anaerobic Test; Young, et al., 1996) have all reported no significant differences for $\dot{V}_E$ L·min^{-1} between an experimental trial using the Breathe Right™ and a control trial in which the exercisers wore nothing on the nose. Nor were any significant differences noted among experimental, control, and placebo trials. In the placebo trial, exercisers wore a fake strip with the same appearance as a Breathe Right™. Furthermore, no significant differences have been found between or among conditions for V_T or f in those studies which reported these variables. Finally, the amount of oxygen consumed during submaximal, maximal, and supramaximal exercise has not been shown to differ by condition.

These experimental results make theoretical sense because arterial saturation is already approximately 97–98% at rest and, as you will learn in Chapter 11, is maintained at close to this level during exercise. Therefore, the use of nasal dilators during exercise does not appear to be warranted.   ✳

Sources:

Brown, et al., 1997; Clapp and Bishop, 1996; Griffin, et al., 1997; Huffman, et al., 1996; O'Kroy, 2000; Wetzstein, 1996; Young, et al., 1996.

During normal resting conditions, expiration occurs simply because the diaphragm and other inspiratory muscles relax. When the muscles are relaxed, both the lungs and the muscles, which are highly elastic, recoil to their original positions. This elastic recoil decreases lung volume and thus creates a pressure inside the chest cavity that is higher than the atmospheric pressure. As the chest cavity decreases in volume, the intrathoracic pressure increases slightly above that of the atmosphere. The result is that air moves out of the lungs into the atmosphere. The pressures equalize again, and the cycle repeats itself with the next inspiration. A complete respiratory cycle includes both inspiration and expiration.

During heavy breathing, as in exercise, expiration is an active process. The primary expiratory muscles are the abdominals and the internal intercostals. The abdominals (rectus abdominus, the obliques, and the transverse abdominus) push the abdominal organs—and hence the diaphragm—upward; the internal intercostals pull the ribs inward and down. This decrease in chest volume increases intrathoracic pressure quicker than passive elastic recoil does, and the air is forced out of the lungs faster.

The pleura also serve a purpose during expiration. Pressure in the intrapleural space fluctuates with breathing in a way that parallels pressure within the lungs. However, the intrapleural pressure is always negative (−4 to −8 mmHg) relative to the intrapulmonary (lung) pressure. This negative pressure protects the lungs from collapsing. If the intrapleural pressure were equal to the atmospheric pressure, the lungs would collapse at the end of expiration because of the elastic recoil.

Because muscle activity is involved during the respiratory cycle of inhalation and exhalation, energy is consumed. During rest, however, this energy consumption (restricted to inspiratory muscles) amounts to only 1–2% of the total energy expenditure in nonsmokers (Pardy, et al., 1984).

Respiratory Circulation

The lung has two different circulatory systems: pulmonary circulation, which serves the external respiratory function, and bronchial circulation, which supplies the internal respiration needs of the lung tissue itself (Figure 10.4).

Figure 10.4
Lung Circulatory Systems

Pulmonary circulation (a) serves
the process of external respiration, picking up oxygen for, and
unloading carbon dioxide from
the body as a whole at the alveoli.
Bronchial circulation (b) serves
the process of internal respiration,
unloading oxygen to, and picking
up carbon dioxide from the lung
tissue.

Source: Modified from W. J. Germann &
C. L. Stanfield, *Principles of Human
Physiology.* San Francisco:
Benjamin Cummings (2002).

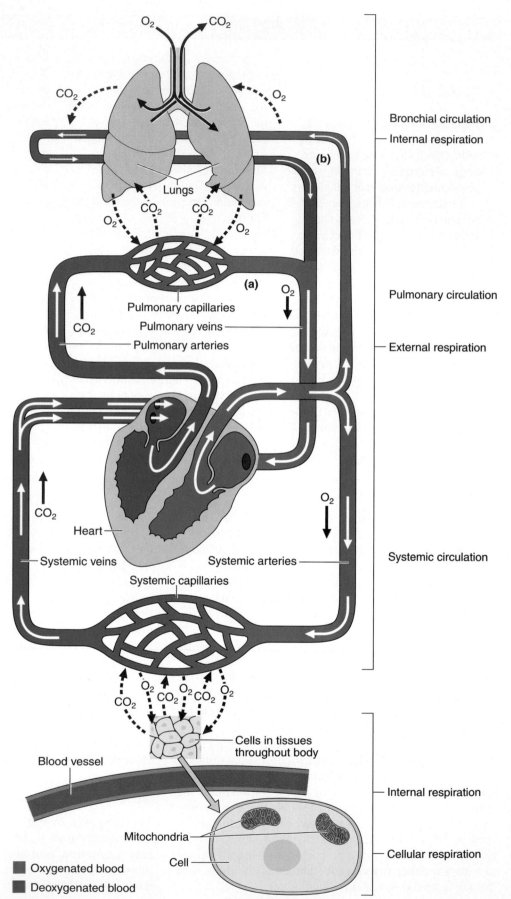

Pulmonary circulation parallels the divisions of the structures in the conductive zone, branching in a treelike manner called arborization. Arborization ends in a dense alveolar capillary network, blanketing most but not all alveoli. **Perfusion of the lung** is the phrase used to describe the capillary blood flow through this network (Guyton, 1986; Martin, et al., 1979).

The pulmonary artery exits from the right ventricle of the heart and gives rise to the capillary network in the lungs (Figure 10.4a). The pulmonary vein arises from this capillary network and enters the heart at the left atrium. As with pulmonary airflow and the rest of the circulatory system, blood flows through this circuit owing to differences in pressure—that is, a pressure gradient that can overcome resistance to the flow. Normal pulmonary artery blood pressure is low, only 25/10 mmHg; but venous pulmonary blood pressure is even lower, only 7 mmHg. Although this pressure gradient between the pulmonary artery and vein is not large, it is sufficient to bring about the blood flow. However, because of these low pressures, gravity affects pulmonary circulation more than the systemic or total body circulation. Thus, whatever portion of the lungs is lowest is perfused best. Whichever portion of the lungs is better perfused with blood is also better ventilated (Guyton, 1986; Leff and Schumacker, 1993; Martin, et al., 1979).

Bronchial circulation (Figure 10.4b) consists of relatively small systemic arteries that originate from the descending portion of the aorta, called the thoracic artery, travel through the lungs, and return as veins that empty into the pulmonary venous system. Thus, not all of the pulmonary venous blood is fully oxygenated (Slonim and Hamilton, 1976).

Minute Ventilation/Alveolar Ventilation

Measurement of pulmonary ventilation as either the amount of air inspired or the amount of air expired in 1 min is known as **minute ventilation** or **minute volume**. The most common units of measurement are liters per minute ($L \cdot min^{-1}$) and milliliters per minute ($mL \cdot min^{-1}$). Inspired minute ventilation is symbolized as $\dot{V}_I$, where V is volume, the "dot" indicates per unit of time, and the subscript I stands for inspired. The symbol for expired ventilation $\dot{V}_E$ merely substitutes a subscripted E, meaning expired, for the I.

Minute ventilation is dependent upon **tidal volume** (V_T), the amount of air inhaled or exhaled per breath and the frequency (f) of breaths per minute. The equation is

10.2   minute ventilation ($mL \cdot min^{-1}$)
= tidal volume ($mL \cdot br^{-1}$) × frequency ($br \cdot min^{-1}$)

or

$$\dot{V} = V_T \times f$$

Milliliters per minute are then commonly converted to liters per minute by dividing by 1000.

At rest a normal young adult will ventilate at a frequency of 12–15 times per minute and have a tidal volume of 400–600 mL. Children ventilate at a much faster rate but with a smaller tidal volume.

Example

Compute $\dot{V}_E$ when f = 15 $br \cdot min^{-1}$ and V_T= 400 mL. You should have set up and solved the equation as follows:

$$\dot{V}_E = (400 \text{ mL} \cdot br^{-1}) \times (15 \text{ br} \cdot min^{-1})$$
$$= 6000 \text{ mL} \cdot min^{-1}$$
$$6000 \text{ mL} \cdot min^{-1} \div 1000 \text{ mL} \cdot L^{-1} = 6.0 \text{ L} \cdot min^{-1}$$

Because minute ventilation represents the total amount of air moved into or out of the lungs per minute, it includes the portion of air that fills the conduction zone. Thus, this is not the amount of air that is available for gas exchange. The amount of air that is available for gas exchange is termed **alveolar ventilation** (or anatomical effective ventilation). Alveolar ventilation ($\dot{V}_A$) takes into account tidal volume (V_T), dead space (V_D), and the frequency (f) of breathing. The equation for calculating $\dot{V}_A$ is

10.3   alveolar ventilation ($mL \cdot min^{-1}$)
= [tidal volume ($mL \cdot br^{-1}$) − dead space ($mL \cdot br^{-1}$)] × frequency ($br \cdot min^{-1}$)

or

$$\dot{V}_A = (V_T - V_D) \times f$$

Perfusion of the Lung Pulmonary circulation, especially capillary blood flow.

Minute Ventilation (Minute Volume) ($\dot{V}_I$ or $\dot{V}_E$) The amount of air inspired or expired each minute; the pulmonary ventilation rate per minute; calculated as tidal volume times frequency of breathing.

Tidal Volume (V_T) The amount of air that is inspired or expired in a normal breath.

Alveolar Ventilation ($\dot{V}_A$) The volume of air available for gas exchange; calculated as tidal volume minus dead space volume times frequency.

Example

Calculate alveolar ventilation using the values of f and V_T given in the previous example, for a female who is at her ideal weight of 130 lb. This problem becomes

$$\dot{V}_A = [(400 \text{ mL·br}^{-1}) - (130 \text{ mL·br}^{-1})] \\ \times (15 \text{ br·min}^{-1}) \\ = 4050 \text{ mL·min}^{-1} \div 1000 \text{ mL·L}^{-1} \\ = 4.05 \text{ L·min}^{-1}$$

Typically, approximately 70% of $\dot{V}_I$ reaches the alveoli for gas exchange. In this example, the percentage is 67.5% [(4050 mL·min^{-1}) ÷ (6000 mL·min^{-1})]. ✦

As with minute ventilation, alveolar ventilation can be calculated from either $\dot{V}_E$ or $\dot{V}_I$. The physiological dead space is so negligible in normal healthy individuals that it does not need to be taken into account in these calculations. To be sure you understand the implications of this concept, complete the problems in the Question of Understanding box. The answer is in Appendix D.

A Question of Understanding

1. Given two breathing patterns, A and B, in the accompanying table, calculate the alveolar ventilation.

| | Breathing Pattern | |
	A	B
$\dot{V}_E$ (L·min^{-1})	6	6
V_T (mL·br^{-1})	600	200
f (br·min^{-1})	10	30
V_D (mL·br^{-1})	150	150
$\dot{V}_A$ (mL·min^{-1})	?	?

On the basis of your calculations, is it better to breathe fast and shallowly or slowly and deeply?

2. Individuals learning the front-crawl swimming stroke are often reluctant to exhale air while their faces are in the water. They then try to inhale more air when their faces are turned to the side or to both exhale and inhale in the short time available during the head turn. Why is this not an effective breathing technique?

3. What is the effect of a snorkel on the dead space? What implication does this effect have for breathing with a snorkel?

Total Lung Capacity (TLC) The greatest amount of air that the lungs can contain.

Residual Volume (RV) The amount of air left in the lungs following a maximal exhalation.

Measurement of Lung Volumes

Lung volumes can be measured either statically or dynamically. Static lung volumes are anatomical measures; since they are independent of time, they do not measure flow. Dynamic lung volumes depend on time and hence measure airflow in addition to air volume.

Static Lung Volumes

Take as deep a breath as you can. At this point your lungs contain the maximum amount of air they can hold. This amount of air is called **total lung capacity** (TLC). Figure 10.5 shows that TLC can be divided into four volumes and three other capacities. The definition of each volume and capacity are included on the table. Note that the four capacities are combinations of two or more volumes. All of these volumes and capacities have clinical significance, but only those important in the study of exercise physiology will be discussed briefly here.

As mentioned previously, tidal volume (V_T) represents the amount of air either inhaled or exhaled in a single breath. A normal V_T inflates the lungs to about half of the TLC in the erect sitting or standing position and only about a third in the supine position (Slonim and Hamilton, 1976). When the demand for energy increases during exercise, V_T increases by expanding into both the inspiratory reserve volume (IRV) and expiratory reserve volume (ERV). Thus, the limits of the vital capacity (VC = IRV + V_T + ERV) represent the absolute limits of tidal volume increase during exercise.

Residual volume (RV) is the amount of air left in the lungs following a maximal exhalation. This leftover air is important because it allows for a continuous gas exchange between the alveoli and the capillaries between breaths. If all of the air were forced out, no gas would be available for exchange. During exercise, when V_T expands, the functional residual capacity (FRC) assists in maintaining a smooth exchange, in the following way. The V_T can and does expand into both the IRV and the ERV, but it expands more into the IRV than the ERV, leaving a relatively large FRC intact. This large FRC dilutes the gas changes (the decrease in oxygen and increase in carbon dioxide) caused by the increased energy production and expenditure of exercise. By reducing fluctuation, the FRC stabilizes and smooths the gas exchange.

Despite its beneficial physiological aspects, residual volume also presents a measurement difficulty. When body composition is determined by hydrostatic (underwater) weighing (see Chapter 8), residual volume must be measured. Residual air makes the body buoyant; if it is not accounted for, it reduces the underwater weight. The less an individual weighs

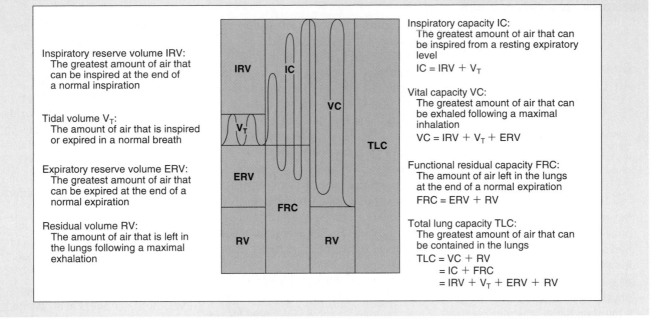

Figure 10.5
Static Lung Volume Spirogram

Total lung capacity (TLC) can be subdivided several ways into four volumes (IRV, V_T, ERV, and RV) and into three other capacities (IC, FRC, and VC). From the normal resting depth of inspiration and expiration (indicated by the wavy line moving up and down, respectively, in the box labeled V_T), both inspiration and expiration can be expanded into the IRV and ERV until all possible air is inhaled and exhaled (VC). The RV remain in the lungs at all times.

underwater, the higher the measured percentage of body fat is. Thus if residual volume is not accounted for, it will be measured as fat. This is the most common reason for determining residual volume in exercise physiology. Sometimes residual volume is estimated from vital capacity (Wilmore, 1969). When it is, residual volume is calculated as 24% of vital capacity for males and 28% of vital capacity for females.

Vital capacity (VC) itself is simply the largest amount of air that can be exhaled following a maximal inhalation. The common way of testing vital capacity is to ask the individual to inhale maximally and then forcefully exhale all of the air as quickly as possible. Because the exhalation is forced, the designation *forced vital capacity,* FVC, is used.

Dynamic Lung Volumes

If volumes are measured at specified time intervals (usually 1 and 3 sec) during a forced vital capacity

test, the name is changed to *forced expiratory volume,* specifically, FEV_1 and FEV_3. This provides information not only on the total volume of air moved but also on the rate of flow of that movement. Normal healthy individuals should be able to exhale at least 80% of their FVC in 1 sec. Because time is now a factor, this measurement is labeled FEV_1. FEV_1 values below 65–70% are indicative of moderate to severe restriction to airflow (Adams, 1994).

The second commonly measured dynamic lung volume is a test of ventilatory capacity called *maximal voluntary ventilation* (MVV). In this test a timed maximal ventilation of either 12 or 15 sec is recorded and then multiplied by 5 (if 12 sec) or 4 (if 15 sec) to extrapolate to the volume that could be ventilated in 1 min. This value is usually higher than what can actually be achieved during exercise in untrained individuals, but it does give a rough estimation of exercise ventilation potential. Low values can reflect not only airway resistance but also poorly conditioned or poorly functioning ventilatory muscles.

Both forced expiratory volume and maximal voluntary ventilation tests are often used as screening tests prior to maximal exercise tests of oxygen consumption.

> **Vital Capacity (VC)** The greatest amount of air that can be exhaled following a maximal inhalation.

Focus on Research

Dynamic Lung Function and All-Cause Mortality

Schunemann, H. J., J. Dorn, B. J. B. Grant, W. Winkelstein, & M. Trevisan: Pulmonary function is a long-term predictor of mortality in the general population: 29-year follow-up of the Buffalo Health Study. *Chest* 118(3): 656–664 (2000).

Beyond the use of residual volume in body composition assessment, the measurement of static and dynamic lung volumes and capacities may appear to be irrelevant to exercise physiology. However, evidence is mounting that at least one measure, forced expiratory volume in one second (FEV$_1$) is related to health.

This epidemiological study extended the link between low values of FEV$_1$ (expressed as a percentage of predicted FEV$_1$ [FEV$_1$%pred]) and mortality (death from all causes). A randomly selected sample of 554 adult men and 641 adult women

were part of a 29-year follow-up. During that time, 302 of the men (54.5%) and 278 (43.4%) of the women died. Only 39 of these deaths (29 male and 10 female) were directly attributed to respiratory disease. Nevertheless, pulmonary function was a significant predictor of all-cause mortality, with each 1% increase in FEV$_1$%pred associated with a 1–1.5% decrease in all-cause mortality. The risk of an early death to individuals scoring in the lowest quintile ($\leq$ 80.2 FEV$_1$%pred for males and $\leq$ 80.5 FEV$_1$%pred for females) was approximately twice as great (2.24 for males, 1.81 for females) when compared to the highest quintile ($\geq$ 108.8 FEV$_1$%pred for males and $\geq$ 113.6 FEV$_1$%pred for females).

The reasons for these results are unknown. It had initially been thought that FEV$_1$%pred was simply a proxy for smoking status, but other research has shown that the association is independent of smoking status and is evident even in individuals

who have never smoked. Possible explanations for the association include the following:

1. Impaired pulmonary function could lead to a decreased tolerance against environmental toxins.
2. Oxidative stress (see the Focus on Application box in Chapter 6 for a discussion of oxidative stress), which is negatively related to FEV$_1$%pred, could adversely affect overall health status; or, conversely, reduced pulmonary function could be an underlying factor responsible for increased oxidative stress.
3. Low FEV$_1$ values may simply adversely affect physical activity patterns. The negative impact of a lack of physical activity has been well documented.

Whatever the reason, at this point in time, forced expiratory volume can be used as a fairly easy health assessment tool. Low values should provide a motivation to begin an exercise training program.

Spirometry

All of the lung volumes and capacities described in the preceding paragraphs—except for total lung capacity, functional residual capacity, and residual volume—can be measured using a spirometer. *Spirometers* typically consist of an inverted container called a bell that fits inside another container usually filled with water. An air tube reaches from the subject's mouth to about the water line. When air is exhaled into the tube, the bell is pushed up; inhalation moves the bell down. A pen connected to the pulley system follows the movements of the bell. In this way, the volumes of air inspired and expired can be measured, and the various volumes, capacities, and flow rates can be calculated. A spirometer that measures air volumes over water is called a *wet spirometer*. Some newer spirometers do not use water and therefore are called *dry spirometers* (Figure 10.6).

Gas Dilution

Total lung capacity, functional residual capacity, and residual volume cannot be measured by simple spirometry because each one includes air that cannot

be exhaled voluntarily from the lungs. Thus, it is necessary to determine the volume of air that remains in the lungs. The most common technique for this measurement is gas dilution. One technique involves the dilution of an inert, insoluble, foreign gas such as helium (He). A second technique involves the dilution of medical grade oxygen and the measurement of nitrogen (N$_2$) and is called the nitrogen washout technique.

Standardization

The respiratory measures detailed above are collected under ambient, or atmospheric, conditions; that is, the temperature measured is the temperature of the room or in the spirometer; the pressure is the barometric pressure of the room; and because the air is exhaled from inside the human body, which is a wet environment, the air is saturated with water vapor. The designation is thus ATPS: ambient (A) temperature (T) and pressure (P), saturated (S). Because ATPS volumes vary from situation to situation, they must be converted to standardized conditions on the basis of the effects of pressure, temperature, and

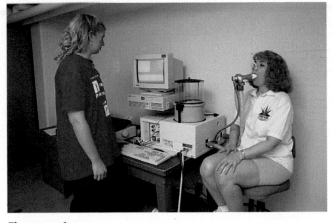

Figure 10.6
A Spirometer

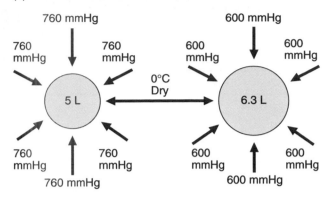

(a) **Effect of Pressure on Volume**

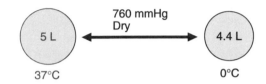

(b) **Effect of Temperature on Volume**

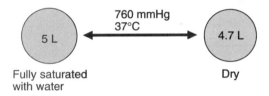

(c) **Effect of Water Vapor on Volume**

Figure 10.7
Effects of Pressure, Temperature, and Water Vapor on Air Volume

(a) The volume of a given quantity of a gas is inversely related to the pressure exerted on it, if the temperature remains constant (Boyle's law). (b) The volume of a given quantity of gas is directly related to the temperature of the gas if the pressure remains constant (Charles's law). (c) The volume of a gas increases as the content of water vapor increases.

water vapor on gas volumes. Figure 10.7 illustrates these three effects, which are described in the following paragraphs.

1. The volume of a given quantity of gas is inversely related to the pressure exerted on it when the temperature remains constant. This effect is Boyle's law and was discussed previously in the explanation of the mechanics of breathing. As shown in Figure 10.7a, when pressure is reduced from 760 to 600 mmHg, 5 L of air expands to 6.3 L. The reverse is also true. If the pressure increases from 600 to 760 mmHg, the volume is reduced, from 6.3 to 5.0 L (Slonim and Hamilton, 1976).

2. The volume of a given quantity of gas is directly related to the temperature of the gas when the pressure remains constant. This effect is described by *Charles's law*. As shown in Figure 10.7b, if the temperature is reduced from 37°C to 0°C, the volume of the gas is also reduced, from 5 to 4.4 L. The reverse is also true. If the temperature rises from 0°C to 37°C, the volume also rises, from 4.4 to 5.0 L.

3. Water molecules evaporate into a gas, such as air, and are responsible for part of the pressure of that gas. The amount of pressure accounted for by the water vapor is related exponentially to temperature. As shown in Figure 10.7c, when a volume of air is converted from saturated to dry air at a constant temperature, the volume is reduced, from 5.0 to 4.7 L. Once again, the reverse is also true. If a gas volume goes from dry to wet at a given temperature, the volume increases (Slonim and Hamilton, 1976).

The numbers representing temperature and pressure in Figure 10.7 were not chosen arbitrarily. They are involved in the two standardized conditions to which

ATPS lung volumes are converted: BTPS and STPD. The abbreviation BTPS means body (B) temperature (T) (37°C), ambient pressure (P), and fully saturated (S) with water vapor. Remember that in its passage through the conduction zone, the air was both warmed and humidified to achieve these values. When converting from ATPS to BTPS, the temperature increases; and the pressure, adjusted for the effects of temperature on water vapor pressure, decreases. From Charles's law (an increase in temperature causes an increase in volume) and Boyle's law (a decrease in pressure causes an increase in volume), the BTPS volume is larger than the originally measured ATPS volume. BTPS is typically used when the anatomical space from which the volume of gas originated is of primary importance. Hence, most lung volumes and capacities are conventionally expressed as BTPS.

Table 10.1

Approximate Gas Partial Pressures in Ambient Air and Selected Ventilatory and Respiratory Sites

Gases	(a) Dry Atmospheric Air, Sea Level			(b) Dry Atmospheric Air, Altitude = (4268 m) 14,000 ft (Pike's Peak)			(c) Alveolar Air, Sea Level		
	%	P_B (mmHg)	P (mmHg)	%	P_B (mmHg)	P (mmHg)	%	P_B (mmHg)	P (mmHg)
O_2	20.93	760	159	20.93	440	92	13.7–14.6	760 − 47 = 713	104–98*
CO_2	0.03	760	0.3	0.03	440	0.1	5.3	760 − 47 = 713	40
N_2	79.04	760	600.7	79.04	440	348	78.7–79.8	760 − 47 = 713	561–569
H_2O	0.00	760	0.0	0.00	440	0.0			47[†]
						440			760

* Owing to minor variations in percentage, the PO_2 in alveolar air is often rounded to 100 mmHg.

[†] Assumes a body temperature of 37°C and PH_2O of 47 mmHg, which must be subtracted from 760 mmHg before determining PO_2, PCO_2, PN_2.

STPD means standard (S) temperature (T) (0°C) and pressure (P) (760 mmHg), dry (D).

Example

Based on the previous discussion, decide whether you think STPD volumes will be greater or smaller than ATPS volumes. Explain your decision. Your reasoning should be as follows. Under typical testing conditions, temperature decreases from ATPS ($\approx$20°C) to STPD (0°C), and by Charles's law, so does volume. Unless the testing is done at sea level, pressure increases from ATPS (variable, but around 735–745 mmHg before considering the influence of water vapor) to STPD (760 mmHg), and according to Boyle's law, volume decreases. Going from wet to dry conditions also decreases the volume. Therefore, the STPD volume is smaller than the originally measured ATPS volume. ✛

STPD volumes are used when it is necessary to know the amount of gas molecules present. Minute ventilation, whether measured as inspired or expired, is typically converted and reported in STPD conditions, although sometimes it may be expressed as BTPS.

Partial Pressure of a Gas: Dalton's Law

Dry, unpolluted atmospheric air is a mixture of gases including oxygen, carbon dioxide, nitrogen, argon, and krypton. Because the latter three are considered to be inert in humans, they are generally linked together and labeled simply as nitrogen, because nitrogen comprises by far the largest amount. Thus, air is said to be composed of 79.04% nitrogen, 20.93% oxygen, and 0.03% carbon dioxide. These percentages are also referred to as fractions of each gas and are then given in a decimal form 0.7904 nitrogen, 0.2093 oxygen, and 0.0003 carbon dioxide. Another way to describe the composition

of a gas mixture such as air is by the partial pressures exerted by each gas (Leff and Schumacker, 1993).

All gases exert pressure. In a mixture of gases the total pressure exerted by the gases is the sum of the pressure of individual gases making up the mixture. Total pressure is standardized to the sea-level barometric pressure of 760 mmHg, but at altitudes above sea level the actual barometric pressure, P_B, must be used. The **partial pressure of a gas (P_G)** is that portion of the total pressure exerted by any single gas within the mixture. The partial pressure of any gas is proportional to its percentage in the total gas mixture. These relationships are known as *Dalton's law of partial pressures.*

The partial pressure of any gas is the product of the total pressure and the fraction of the gas (as a decimal).

10.4 partial pressure of a gas (mmHg) = total pressure (mmHg) × fraction of the gas

or

$$P_G = P_B \times F_G$$

For example, the standardized partial pressure of nitrogen, PN_2, is 760 mmHg × 0.7904 = 600.7 mmHg.

Substituting the appropriate fractions, calculate the PO_2 and PCO_2 of dry atmospheric air. Table 10.1, column a, shows the answers. For extra practice, also calculate the partial pressure of dry atmospheric air at altitude and of alveolar air. Look first at Table 10.1, columns a and b. Notice that the gas percentages are the same at sea level and at altitude, in this case

> **Partial Pressure of a Gas (P_G)** The pressure exerted by an individual gas in a mixture; determined by multiplying the fraction of the gas by the total barometric pressure.

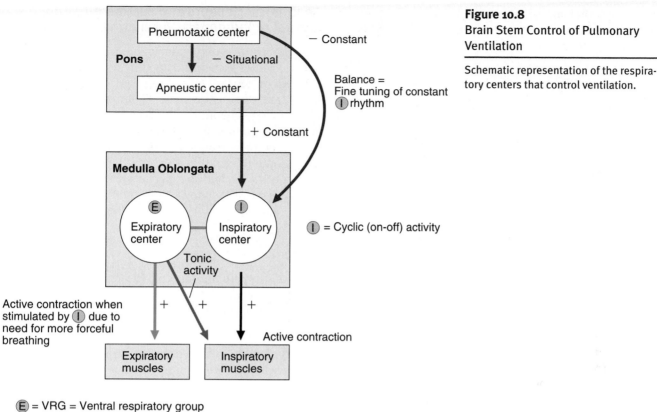

Figure 10.8
Brain Stem Control of Pulmonary
Ventilation

Schematic representation of the respiratory centers that control ventilation.

4268 m (14,000 ft). These percentages would be true
no matter what the selected altitude. Conversely, the
barometric pressure (P_B) is lower at both the selected
altitude and any other altitude in comparison with sea
level. Exactly how much lower than sea level the P_B is
depends on how high the altitude is. At 4268 m
(14,000 ft), P_B is 440 mmHg. As the altitude increases,
the barometric pressure decreases. Now compare
Table 10.1, columns a and c. Notice that now the
barometric pressure values are the same; that is, they
are both standardized to 760 mmHg. However, the
fractions of the gases are different. This variation in
alveolar air from atmospheric air occurs as the percentage of oxygen is diminished by diffusion into the
capillary blood and the percentage of carbon dioxide
is enlarged by diffusion out of the capillary blood. In
addition, water vapor now occupies a percentage of
the total air mixture. At normal body temperature
(37°C), water vapor exerts a pressure of 47 mmHg.
This value must be subtracted from 760 mmHg prior
to multiplying by the fraction of each gas to determine
the partial pressure of each gas.

Knowledge of the partial pressure of gases is important for at least two reasons. The first is that the
partial pressures of oxygen and more definitively

carbon dioxide serve to regulate pulmonary ventilation to bring air into the lungs. The second reason is
that both external and internal respiration depend on
pressure gradients.

Regulation of Pulmonary Ventilation

Breathing, or pulmonary ventilation, is the result of
inspiratory and expiratory muscle contraction and relaxation. The muscle action—and hence the rate,
depth, and rhythm of breathing—is controlled by the
brain and nervous system and is tightly coupled to the
body's overall need for oxygen and the subsequent
production of energy and carbon dioxide. The coordinated control of the respiratory muscles is a very
complex process that is not yet fully understood (Leff
and Schumacker, 1993; Martin, et al., 1979).

The Respiratory Centers

Two respiratory centers, composed of anatomically
distinct neural networks, are located within the
medulla oblongata of the brain stem. These two
centers are schematically diagramed in Figure 10.8.

The more important of the two is the *inspiratory center* (I), also called the *dorsal respiratory group* (DRG). The other center is the *expiratory center* (E), sometimes called the *ventral respiratory group* (VRG). The nerves that make up the inspiratory center depolarize spontaneously in a cyclic, rhythmical on-off pattern. During the "on" portion of the cycle, nerve impulses traveling via motor neurons in the phrenic nerve stimulate the diaphragm and external intercostal inspiratory muscles to contract. Inhalation occurs when the thoracic cavity is enlarged and intrathoracic pressure decreases. During the "off" portion of the cycle the nerve impulses are interrupted, the inspiratory muscles relax, and exhalation occurs. Without outside influence and at rest, the inspiratory center brings about a **respiratory cycle** of approximately 2 sec for inspiration and 3 sec for exhalation (for a rate of 12–15 br·min^{-1}). This normal respiratory rate and oscillating rhythm is known as **eupnea** (Leff and Schumacker, 1993).

The expiratory center appears to have two functions. The first is to maintain inspiratory muscle tone or low-level contraction such that the inspiratory muscles never completely relax. The second is to bring about active contraction of the expiratory muscles (internal intercostals and abdominals) when forceful breathing is required, such as during moderate to heavy exercise. This latter action is instigated by the inspiratory center, which recruits additional accessory muscles at the same time (Leff and Schumacker, 1993; Martin, et al., 1979).

Two neural centers in the pons area of the brain stem also act as respiratory centers and seem to be important for ensuring that the transitions between inhalation and exhalation are smooth. The *pneumotaxic center* constantly transmits inhibitory (indicated on the diagram by a minus sign, −) neural impulses directly to the inspiratory center and situationally to the apneustic center. This limits or, in some cases, shortens inspiration and promotes expiration—thus fine tuning the breathing pattern and preventing lung overinflation. The *apneustic center* continually stimulates (indicated on the diagram by a plus sign, +) the inspiratory center unless inhibited situationally by the pneumotaxic center (Leff and Schumacker, 1993; Martin, et al., 1979).

Respiratory Cycle Inspiration and expiration.

Eupnea Normal respiration rate and rhythm.

Anatomical Sensors and Factors Affecting Control of Pulmonary Ventilation

The inspiratory, expiratory, pneumotaxic, and apneustic centers are influenced by a number of factors through a variety of anatomical sensors that are important during exercise (Dempsey, et al., 1985). Figure 10.9 schematically presents the major factors and where each factor operates. Without outside influences, the rate (frequency) of breathing and tidal volume (depth of breathing) exhibit the greatest changes. A disruption in rhythm rarely occurs except under voluntary control (Guyton, 1986; Leff and Schumacker, 1993; Martin, et al., 1979; Whipp, et al., 1982).

Higher Brain Centers

Both the hypothalamus and the cerebral cortex can influence breathing. The first operates involuntarily and the second voluntarily.

Hypothalamus   The sympathetic nervous system centers in the hypothalamus are activated by pain or strong emotions. They, in turn, send neural messages to the respiratory centers. The reaction can be either stimulatory or inhibitory to breathing. Hyperventilation by an individual who is emotionally upset is an example of hypothalamic stimulation, and having your breath taken away when you jump into very cold water exemplifies hypothalamic inhibition. This hypothalamic control mechanism is also very important in bringing about the increase in respiration upon initiation of movement and sustaining the increase throughout the duration of an activity (Eldridge, 1994).

Cerebral Cortex   Cerebral control of breathing originates in the motor cortex. Such control is important to musicians, singers, and athletes such as swimmers, weight lifters, archers, and shooters, to name just a few. The motor cortex may also operate such that the conscious anticipation of exercise unconsciously increases ventilation. Neural impulses from the motor cortex pass directly to the respiratory muscles, bypassing the control centers in the medulla. Voluntary control is limited, however (Leff and Schumacker, 1993; Martin, et al., 1979). If you doubt this, take a reading break now and jog in place at a fast pace for 3 min. Sit down immediately on stopping, and try holding your breath for 1 min. If you can do that, great; but even if you can, you will probably feel a desire to breathe. More than likely, the automatic drive to breathe will overrule your conscious signal not to; and at some point before the end of the minute, you will gasp for air.

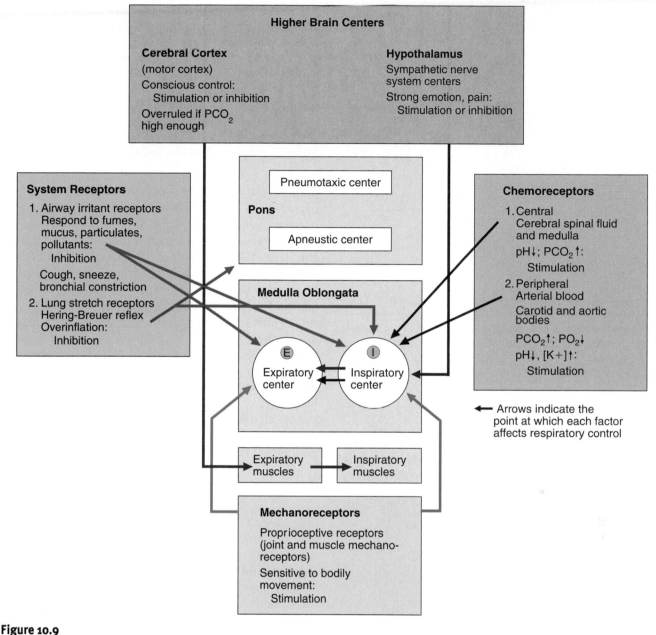

Figure 10.9
Anatomical Sensors and Factors That Influence the Control of Pulmonary Ventilation

Schematic representation of the pathways of action of the factors that influence the brain stem control of ventilation.

Systemic Receptors

The lungs themselves contain several types of receptors that provide sensory information to the respiratory control centers and result in reflex action. Chief among them are irritant receptors and stretch receptors (Leff and Schumacker, 1993; Martin, et al., 1979). Both of these receptors are more important as protective devices than as regulators of normal resting or exercise ventilation.

Irritant Receptors *Irritant receptors* within the conduction zone respond to foreign substances such as chemicals, noxious gases, cold air, mucus, dust, and other pollutant particulates and bring about a reflex response. Depending on the irritating substance and the anatomical location, the response may be a cough, a sneeze, or a bronchial constriction, all of which disrupt the normal breathing pattern (Leff and Schumacker, 1993; Martin, et al., 1979).

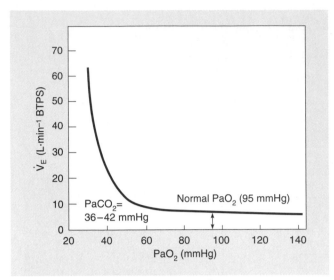

Figure 10.10

The Effect of Arterial PO_2 (PaO_2) on Minute Ventilation

At a normal $PaCO_2$ of 36–42 mmHg, reduced PaO_2 does not stimulate ventilation until the value of PaO_2 is less than 60 mmHg.

Source: A. R. Leff & P. T. Schumacker. *Respiratory Physiology: Basics and Applications.* Philadelphia: W. B. Saunders Company (1993). Reprinted by permission.

Stretch Receptors *Stretch receptors* in the lung respond to deep, fast inflation. Increases in lung volume stimulate the stretch receptors, which send inhibitory impulses to both the apneustic center and the inspiratory center. As a result, inspiration ceases. This reflex is called the *Hering-Breuer reflex.* The threshold for this reflex is quite high. It does not appear to function at rest and plays a minor role in exercise.

Mechanoreceptors

Specific *mechanoreceptors* called proprioceptors exist in skeletal muscles (including respiratory muscles) and joint capsules. These receptors provide information to a variety of sites in the brain about movement and body position in space. Input from these receptors probably plays some minor role in the stimulation of respiration during exercise but are not involved in respiration during rest (Leff and Schumacker, 1993).

Chemoreceptors

Chemoreceptor sensors that respond to fluctuations in chemical substances important to respiration are found in two major anatomical locations. *Central chemoreceptors* are located in the medulla oblongata (but not in the respiratory control centers) and are sensitive to an increased carbon dioxide partial pressure ($\uparrow PCO_2$) and an increased acidity ($\downarrow pH$). *Peripheral chemoreceptors* are located in large arteries, specifically, at the aortic body and the carotid body. In addition to being sensitive to $\uparrow PCO_2$ and $\downarrow pH$, these receptors are also sensitive to a decrease in the partial pressure of oxygen ($\downarrow PO_2$) and an increase in the concentration of potassium ions ($\uparrow [K^+]$). Each of these factors is explained in the following subsections.

Influence of PO_2 The peripheral carotid body chemoreceptors are the main oxygen sensors. Under normal circumstances, a decline in PO_2 has very little impact on minute ventilation other than enhancing sensitivity to $\uparrow PCO_2$ (Leff and Schumacker, 1993).

Figure 10.10 shows that from the normal arterial PO_2 of 95 mmHg (Table 10.1) to a value of about 60 mmHg, minute ventilation does not change if the arterial PCO_2 remains normal (approximately 36–42 mmHg). However, if the arterial PO_2 decreases below 60 mmHg, minute ventilation is stimulated to rise exponentially. This decrease is not a normal physiological event at sea level, even at very heavy levels of exercise, because the arterial PO_2 mmHg is maintained within narrow limits. However, arterial PO_2 may fall below 60 mmHg at altitudes at or above 4268 m (14,000 ft), triggering the graphically depicted increase in minute ventilation (Leff and Schumacker, 1993; Martin, et al., 1979).

Influence of PCO_2 Both the central and the peripheral chemoreceptors are sensitive to an increase in arterial PCO_2. However, the peripheral chemoreceptors respond more directly to PCO_2 than the central chemoreceptors do. The central chemoreceptors respond initially to rising PCO_2 levels but thereafter primarily to the effect these rising PCO_2 levels have on pH. The ventilatory response to PCO_2 is split 40–60% between peripheral and central chemoreceptors, respectively. At rest, the regulation of pH in the cerebrospinal fluid is the primary control mechanism of ventilation.

Figure 10.11 shows the influence of increasing arterial PCO_2 values on minute ventilation. Even a small deviation from the normal value of PCO_2 of approximately 40 mmHg (Table 10.1) causes a large rectilinear increase in minute ventilation when arterial PO_2 is maintained at approximately normal levels ($\approx$95 mmHg). The steepness and the immediacy of this rectilinear increase indicates that the ventilation is much more sensitive to an increase in PCO_2 than to a decrease in PO_2. Hence, PCO_2 is the stronger regulating factor. An increase as small as 5 mmHg in

PCO_2 will almost double ventilation (Leff and Schumacker, 1993).

Holding your breath will cause an increase in arterial PCO_2, called *hypercapnia*. Sometimes an excess of CO_2 in the blood can lead to labored or difficult ventilation, which is termed **dyspnea**. Excess CO_2 is not the only possible cause, and this is not a normal exercise response. A buildup of CO_2 is the reason your conscious control of respiration was overruled when you tried not to breathe after doing the 3-min jog in place. Conversely, **hyperventilation**—defined as increased pulmonary ventilation, especially ventilation that exceeds metabolic requirements, will decrease PCO_2 (called *hypocapnia*) and the drive to breathe. Hyperventilation may be caused by an altitude response to a decreased PO_2, an involuntary response during an anxiety attack, or a conscious attempt to extend breath-holding time.

The decrement in PCO_2 with hyperventilation can have serious consequences. Many people know that hyperventilating will extend breath-holding time, but erroneously believe it does so because more oxygen is taken in. They are unaware that it is CO_2 that is changing (being blown off) and that respiration is more sensitive to PCO_2 changes than to PO_2 changes. Craig (1976) presented a summary of 58 cases of loss of consciousness during underwater swimming and diving following hyperventilation. Of these cases, 40% (23 cases) ended as fatalities, and most of these cases occurred in guarded pools. Because an individual continues patterned motor activity (swimming) after loss of consciousness caused by a lack of oxygen to the brain, these life-threatening cases are difficult for a lifeguard to detect quickly. The beginning swimmer who is frustrated at trying to coordinate arms, legs, and breathing and simply puts his or her head in the water and tries to go as far as possible without breathing is also vulnerable. It is recommended that underwater swimming be limited to one length of a standard 25-yd or 25-m pool.

Influence of pH As with an increase in arterial PCO_2, both the peripheral and central chemoreceptors are sensitive to decreases in pH. The pH level is partially related to CO_2 level. When CO_2 is hydrated, it forms carbonic acid (H_2CO_3) and degrades readily into hydrogen ions (H^+) and bicarbonate (HCO_3^-) according to the following reactions:

$$CO_2 + H_2O \leftrightarrow H_2CO_3 \leftrightarrow H^+ + HCO_3^-$$

carbon dioxide + water $\leftrightarrow$ carbonic acid $\leftrightarrow$ hydrogen ions + bicarbonate

In blood the H^+ can be buffered; but if that capacity is exceeded, any change in arterial pH is detected

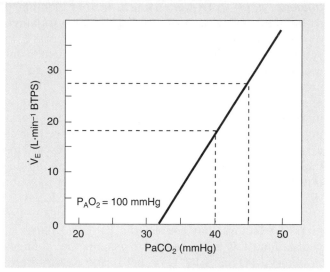

Figure 10.11
The Ventilatory Response to Carbon Dioxide

At a normal P_AO_2 of approximately 100 mmHg, a rise in $PaCO_2$ from the normal value of 40 mmHg to just 45 mmHg almost doubles pulmonary ventilation (from approximately 17 L·min^{-1} to 27 L·min^{-1}, as indicated by the dashed lines intersecting the y-axis) showing how sensitive ventilation is to $PaCO_2$.

Source: Modified from M. Nielsen & H. Smith. Studies on the regulation of respiration in acute hypoxia. *Acta Physiologica Scandinavica.* 4:293–313 (1951). Reprinted by permission.

by the aortic and carotid bodies. The brain and spinal cord are bathed by a protein-free solution known as *cerebrospinal fluid* (CSF). CO_2 easily diffuses across the blood-brain barrier and into the CSF. Because brain cells also produce CO_2 and because CSF has no protein buffers, the pH of CSF is slightly more acidic than that of blood. An excess of H^+ in CSF acts directly on the central chemoreceptors to increase respiration; a decrease in H^+ suppresses respiration.

All changes in pH are, of course, not related to CO_2. For example, during high-intensity exercise large quantities of lactic acid accumulate. If the blood's ability to buffer the resultant H^+ is exceeded, pH will decrease and respiration will increase.

Dyspnea Labored or difficult breathing.

Hyperventilation Increased pulmonary ventilation, especially ventilation that exceeds metabolic requirements; carbon dioxide is blown off, leading to a decrease in its partial pressure in arterial blood.

Influence of [K⁺] Of the chemical factors mentioned so far ($\downarrow PO_2$, $\uparrow PCO_2$, $\downarrow pH$), only $\downarrow pH$ changes enough during exercise to cause the needed increase in ventilation known as **hyperpnea**. Hyperpnea is increased pulmonary ventilation that matches an increased metabolic demand. An increase in [K⁺] may be another factor that changes sufficiently in exercise to increase ventilation. Potassium moves from the working muscles to blood during all intensities of exercise as a result of the establishment of neural impulses. This increased [K⁺], called *hyperkalemia,* directly stimulates the carotid bodies. At rest [K⁺] is not a factor (Eldridge, 1994; Forster and Pau, 1994; Nye, 1994).

Figure 10.9 presented earlier schematically depicts the factors that control the rate and depth of ventilation. It would be logical to assume that changes in arterial PO_2 and PCO_2 occur during exercise and have the primary role in control. However, this is not what happens. Neither PO_2 nor PCO_2 change enough, especially early in exercise or at low to moderate to heavy intensities in untrained individuals to play a major role in ventilatory control during exercise. Exactly which factor is most important is not known precisely, and changes may take place in the sensitivity of the medullary respiratory control centers themselves during exercise. Neural messages from the motor cortex, muscle proprioceptors, and hypothalamic sympathetic nervous system activity as well as increases in the hydrogen ion and potassium ion concentrations all appear to have a role during exercise (Eldridge, 1994; Martin, et al., 1979).

Gas Exchange and Transport

Gas Exchange: Henry's Law

As mentioned previously, knowledge of the partial pressure of gases is important for two reasons. One is that the partial pressures of gases control pulmonary ventilation, as has just been discussed. The second reason is that the movement of O_2 and CO_2 between the alveoli and capillaries (defined as external respiration) and between the capillaries and tissues (defined as internal respiration) occurs by the process of diffusion. **Diffusion** is defined as the tendency of

---

Hyperpnea Increased pulmonary ventilation that matches an increased metabolic demand, such as during exercise.

Diffusion The tendency of gaseous, liquid, or solid molecules to move from areas of high concentration to areas of low concentration by constant random action.

---

gaseous, liquid, or solid molecules to move from areas of high concentration to areas of low concentration by constant random action. Diffusion can only occur if there is a pressure gradient (a difference in the partial pressures of the gas) between the capillary and the tissue. Gases diffuse down a pressure gradient from areas of high pressure to areas of low pressure. The rate of diffusion depends on the magnitude of the pressure gradient (millimeters of mercury at the high end minus millimeters of mercury at the low end), the surface area available for diffusion, the thickness of the barrier between the two locations, and the solubility (ability to be dissolved) of the gas in the barrier liquid. *Henry's law* states that when a mixture of gases is in contact with a liquid, each gas dissolves in the liquid in proportion to its partial pressure and solubility until equilibrium is achieved and the gas partial pressures are equal in both locations (Leff and Schumacker, 1993; Martin, et al., 1979).

External Respiration

External respiration is the movement of gases at the alveolar–pulmonary capillary level. Specifically, oxygen diffuses from the alveoli into the pulmonary capillaries, and carbon dioxide diffuses from the pulmonary capillary to the alveoli. This exchange is diagramed in Figures 10.12a and 10.12d.

Remember that pulmonary circulation originates from the right ventricle of the heart. By definition, an artery is a vessel carrying blood away from the heart. Unlike systemic arteries, the pulmonary artery carries partially deoxygenated blood. The pulmonary arteries quickly branch into capillaries that parallel the alveoli. While they are small, the capillaries do have a definable length.

When the capillary and alveoli first make contact at the arterial end of the capillary, PO_2 in the alveoli (P_AO_2) is high (98–104 mmHg) (see Table 10.1), and PO_2 in the pulmonary capillary is low (40 mmHg). The net diffusion of oxygen is from high to low down the pressure gradient until an equilibrium is reached. Note in Figure 10.12a that this equalization of pressure occurs within the first third of the capillary length. Refer again to Table 10.1 and Figures 10.12a and 10.12b. In Figure 10.12b, notice that PaO_2 is listed as 95 mmHg, not as 98–104 mmHg as given in Table 10.1 and Figure 10.12a. The lower value results because the fully oxygenated blood in the pulmonary vein is diluted with partially oxygenated venous blood ($PvO_2 = 40$ mmHg) from the bronchial vein as blood from both veins flows into the left atrium. Remember that the bronchial artery, the capillaries, and the vein provide blood to and return it from the lungs as part of the systemic circulation and so have the normal

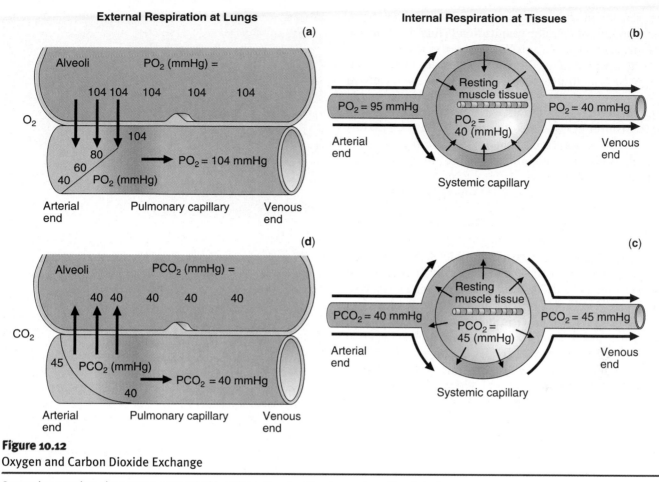

External Respiration at Lungs (a)

Alveoli   PO$_2$ (mmHg) =

104 104   104   104   104

O$_2$

104

80

60

40   PO$_2$ (mmHg)

→ PO$_2$ = 104 mmHg

Arterial end   Pulmonary capillary   Venous end

Internal Respiration at Tissues (b)

PO$_2$ = 95 mmHg

Resting muscle tissue

PO$_2$ = 40 (mmHg)

PO$_2$ = 40 mmHg

Arterial end   Venous end

Systemic capillary

(d)

Alveoli   PCO$_2$ (mmHg) =

40 40   40   40   40

CO$_2$

45   PCO$_2$ (mmHg)

→ PCO$_2$ = 40 mmHg

40

Arterial end   Pulmonary capillary   Venous end

(c)

PCO$_2$ = 40 mmHg

Resting muscle tissue

PCO$_2$ = 45 (mmHg)

PCO$_2$ = 45 mmHg

Arterial end   Venous end

Systemic capillary

Figure 10.12

Oxygen and Carbon Dioxide Exchange

Gas exchange takes place at two anatomical locations: the alveoli-pulmonary capillary interface (called external respiration) and the systemic capillary tissue interface (called internal respiration). (a) External respiration for oxygen, (b) internal respiration for oxygen, (c) internal respiration for carbon dioxide, and (d) external respiration of carbon dioxide.

systemic gas contents and pressures. Although blood from the bronchial vein amounts to only about 2% of the total blood returning to the left atrium, it is sufficient to bring the PaO$_2$ of systemic arterial blood down to approximately 95 mmHg (Guyton, 1986).

At the same time that oxygen is diffusing from the alveoli to the pulmonary capillaries, carbon dioxide is diffusing from the pulmonary capillaries to the alveoli. When any given capillary and alveoli first make contact at the arterial end of the capillary, PCO$_2$ in the capillary is high (about 45 mmHg) and PCO$_2$ in the alveoli is low (40 mmHg) (see Table 10.1). The net diffusion of carbon dioxide is also from high to low pressure down the gradient until an equilibrium is reached. Note in Figure 10.12d that this equalization of pressure occurs within the first third of the capillary length. Note also that the pressure gradient for CO$_2$ is not nearly as steep (5 mmHg) as it is for O$_2$ (64 mmHg). Carbon dioxide simply does not need as great a pressure gradient because it is more soluble.

Again, remember that each gas moves down its own concentration gradient irrespective of the concentration of any other gas.

Internal Respiration

Internal respiration is the movement of gases at the capillary-tissue level. Although the tissue can be any tissue, it is particularly relevant for exercise physiology students to think of the tissue as skeletal muscle tissue. Internal respiration is diagramed in Figures 10.12b and 10.12c. Skeletal muscle fibers are well supplied with capillaries. When blood enters the arterial end of any systemic capillary, PaO$_2$ is high (95 mmHg). Within the tissue, PO$_2$ at rest is low (40 mmHg). The net diffusion of oxygen is once again from high to low pressure until an equilibrium is reached. Blood exiting into the systemic venous system thus has a PvO$_2$ of 40 mmHg, which is maintained until oxygenation occurs again at the alveoli.

Carbon dioxide is produced at the tissue level as a direct result of cellular respiration. Thus, PCO_2 levels are higher (about 45 mmHg) in the tissues than elsewhere in the system. Diffusion occurs as always from the area of high pressure (45 mmHg in the tissue) to the area of low pressure (40 mmHg in the systemic capillary), once again achieving equilibrium. The venous level of PCO_2 is also maintained until it reaches the alveoli, where the carbon dioxide diffuses out of the bloodstream and is exhaled. To make sure that you understand what is happening here, complete the task in the Question of Understanding box below.

Oxygen Transport

Oxygen is carried two ways in the blood. The first way oxygen is transported is in a dissolved form in the liquid portion of the blood. The amount of oxygen transported in this fashion is only about 1.5–3% of the total oxygen transported. However, it is this dissolved component that is responsible for the partial pressure of oxygen in the blood (see Figure 10.12). The dissolved oxygen content is determined by the PO_2 and the solubility of oxygen, which is a constant of 0.00304 mL·dL^{-1}·mmHg at 37°C. The formula is as follows (Guyton, 1986; Leff and Schumacker, 1993; Martin, et al., 1979):

10.5 dissolved O_2 content (mL·dL^{-1}) = PO_2 (mmHg) $\times$ solubility (mL·dL^{-1}·mmHg^{-1})

Example

In normal systemic arterial blood with a PaO_2 of 95 mmHg, the calculation becomes

$$\text{dissolved } O_2 \text{ content} = (95 \text{ mmHg})$$
$$\times (0.00304 \text{ mL·dL}^-\text{·mmHg}^{-1})$$
$$= 0.29 \text{ mL·dL}^{-1}$$

A Question of Understanding

Follow oxygen around the body from the alveoli to the pulmonary capillaries, through the left side of the heart, the systemic arteries, the tissue, the systemic capillaries, the systemic veins, the right side of the heart, and back to the alveoli. Give the PO_2 at each site and any net movement of oxygen. Do the same thing for carbon dioxide, giving PCO_2, but start at the tissue level where carbon dioxide is produced and follow it through the systemic capillaries and veins, the right side of the heart, the pulmonary capillaries and alveoli, the pulmonary vein, the left side of the heart, the systemic arterial system, and back to the systemic capillaries at the tissue level. Check your answer with the one provided in Appendix D.

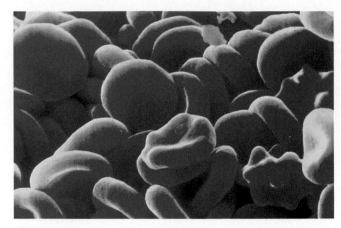

Figure 10.13
Red Blood Cells

An electron micrograph of erythrocytes or red blood cells (RBC) dyed red and showing the biconcave disk shape.

Thus, only 0.29 mL of oxygen is dissolved in a deciliter of arterial blood. You may also see this result expressed in units of milliliters per 100 milliliters (mL·100 mL^{-1}) of blood or as milliliters percent (mL%). All are comparable. ✢

The second way oxygen is transported in the blood is bound to hemoglobin. The vast majority, 97–98.5%, of the oxygen is transported in the bloodstream bound to hemoglobin.

Red Blood Cells and Hemoglobin

Red blood cells (RBC), or erythrocytes, are small, flexible cells shaped like biconcave disks, or miniature doughnuts, with the hole squished in but not pushed out (Figure 10.13). Females typically have a RBC count of 4.3–5.2 million per cubic milliliter of blood; the male count is generally between 5.1 and 5.8 million per cubic milliliter of blood. The total number of red blood cells for the average person is about 35 trillion, with a total surface area of about 2000 times the total body surface area. **Hemoglobin,** which is the protein portion of the RBC that binds with oxygen, constitutes about one-third of a RBC by weight if water is included, but 97% if water is excluded. Normal values for hemoglobin for adult females are 12–16 g·100 mL^{-1} blood, with a mean of 14 g·100 mL^{-1} blood. For adult males the values are

Hemoglobin (Hb) The protein portion of the red blood cell that binds with oxygen, consisting of four iron-containing pigments called hemes and a protein called globin.

14–18 g·100 mL^{-1} blood, with a mean of 16 g·100 mL^{-1} blood. Children have slightly lower values (Martin, et al., 1979).

Hemoglobin consists of four iron-containing pigments called *hemes* and a protein called *globin*. Each iron atom can combine reversibly with one molecule of oxygen. Therefore, each hemoglobin molecule can transport four molecules of oxygen. The chemical symbol for hemoglobin not bound to oxygen, sometimes called deoxyhemoglobin or reduced hemoglobin, is Hb. Hemoglobin bound to oxygen is symbolized HbO$_2$ and is termed oxyhemoglobin. None of the oxygen bound to hemoglobin is used by the RBC.

The Binding of Oxygen with Hb: The Oxygen Dissociation Curve

All four oxygen molecules do not bind with the four heme atoms at the same time. Binding of one oxygen molecule onto a fully deoxygenated hemoglobin molecule changes the shape and increases the binding affinity for the next oxygen molecule. Thus, each succeeding oxygen molecule binds more easily than the preceding one. The result, when graphed, gives the characteristic sigmoid-shaped curve of oxyhemoglobin shown in Figure 10.14. This curve is called the *oxygen dissociation curve,* for reasons that will become clear later.

When all four of its heme groups are bound to oxygen, the hemoglobin molecule is said to be fully saturated. All hemoglobin may not be fully saturated, though. The amount of the oxygen-carrying capacity that is utilized is referred to as **percent saturation of hemoglobin** and is designated as SbO$_2$%. Percent saturation is calculated as

10.6

$$SbO_2\% = \frac{\text{Hb combined with O}_2}{\text{Hb capacity for combining with O}_2} \times 100$$

The symbols SaO$_2$% and SvO$_2$% may be used to distinguish percent saturation of blood in the arteries and veins, respectively, whereas Sb refers nonspecifically to blood.

Percent saturation depends primarily on the partial pressure of oxygen. In arterial blood at a PO$_2$ of

---

Percent Saturation of Hemoglobin (SbO$_2$%)
The ratio of the amount of hemoglobin combined with oxygen to the total hemoglobin capacity for combining with oxygen, expressed as a percentage; indicated generally as SbO$_2$% or specifically as SaO$_2$% for arterial blood or as SvO$_2$% for venous blood.

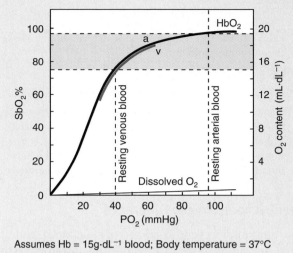

Assumes Hb = 15g·dL^{-1} blood; Body temperature = 37°C
a = arterial blood; PaCO$_2$ = 40 mmHg; pH = 7.4
v = venous blood; PvCO$_2$ = 45 mmHg; pH = 7.38

Figure 10.14
Oxygen Dissociation Curve

Under normal resting conditions approximately 25% of the oxygen being transported in arterial blood is dissociated (released or exchanged by internal respiration) for use by body tissues. The shaded area at the top of the diagram represents this in percentage on the left y-axis and as an absolute amount on the right y-axis. See text for full explanation and calculations.

---

95 mmHg the percent saturation is 97%. Find this value on Figure 10.14 where PO$_2$ is on the x-axis and SbO$_2$% is on the left y-axis. On the same figure determine the SbO$_2$% in normal venous blood. Since the PO$_2$ in normal venous blood is 40 mmHg, you should have determined that the SbO$_2$% was 75%. This value is also shown in Figure 10.14.

The oxygen content of hemoglobin depends upon the hemoglobin level and the physiological oxygen-binding capacity according to the following formula

10.7 oxygen content of hemoglobin (mL·dL^{-1})
= hemoglobin level (gm·dL^{-1}) × oxygen-binding capacity (mL O$_2$·gm Hb^{-1}) × percent saturation (expressed as a decimal fraction)

or

$$HbO_2 = Hb \times 1.34 \times SbO_2\%$$

In this equation the hemoglobin level will, of course, vary from individual to individual. The physiological oxygen-binding capacity is a constant 1.34 mLO$_2$·gmHb^{-1}, and the percent saturation of hemoglobin will vary between arterial and venous blood and resting and exercise conditions.

Example

Using an average hemoglobin level of 15 gm·dL^{-1}, calculate the oxygen content for arterial blood where the percent saturation is 97%.

$$HbO_2 \text{ mL·dL}^{-1} = 15 \text{ gm·dL}^{-1}$$
$$\times 1.34 \text{ mL } O_2 \text{·gm Hb}^{-1} \times .97$$
$$= 19.5 \text{ mL·dL}^{-1}$$

Check Figure 10.14 and look at the right side y-axis. This axis is of O_2 content in mL·dL^{-1} rounded to the nearest whole number. The value for normal arterial blood at 97% saturation is the value just calculated. ✛

Arteriovenous Oxygen Difference

The amount of oxygen released (dissociated) from the blood during one circuit through the systemic system is called the **arteriovenous oxygen difference (a-vO$_2$ diff)**. That is, the a-vO$_2$ diff is the difference between the amount of oxygen returned in venous blood and the amount originally carried in arterial blood. Before we can subtract to obtain the a-vO$_2$ diff, we must calculate the total oxygen in both the arteries and the veins. The amount normally carried in arterial blood has already been determined. It is

$$\begin{aligned} \text{dissolved } O_2 &= 0.29 \text{ mL·dL}^{-1} \\ HbO_2 &= \underline{19.50 \text{ mL·dL}^{-1}} \\ & 19.79 \text{ mL·dL}^{-1} = \text{total } O_2 \text{ content in} \\ &\phantom{= 19.79 \text{ mL·dL}^{-1} =} \text{arterial blood } (aO_2) \end{aligned}$$

Example

Calculate the dissolved O_2 and HbO_2 in venous blood. The calculations are as follows:

$$\begin{aligned} \text{dissolved } O_2 \text{ (venous)} &= 40 \text{ mmHg} \\ &\times 0.00304 \text{ mL } O_2\text{·dL}^{-1}\text{·mmHg} \\ &= 0.12 \text{ mL·dL}^{-1} \\ HbO_2 \text{ (venous)} &= 15 \text{ g·dL}^{-1} \times 1.34 \text{ mL·g}^{-1} \\ &\times 0.75 = 15.08 \text{ mL·dL}^{-1} \end{aligned}$$

Now, add these values.

$$\begin{aligned} \text{dissolved } O_2 &= 0.12 \text{ mL·dL}^{-1} \\ HbO_2 &= \underline{15.08 \text{ mL·dL}^{-1}} \\ & 15.20 \text{ mL·dL}^{-1} \\ &= \text{total } O_2 \text{ content in venous blood } (vO_2) \text{ ✛} \end{aligned}$$

Arteriovenous Oxygen Difference (a-vO$_2$ diff) The difference between the amount of oxygen returned in venous blood and the amount originally carried in arterial blood.

Oxygen Dissociation The separation or release of oxygen from the red blood cells to the tissues.

The a-vO$_2$ diff is calculated by the formula

10.8 a-vO$_2$ diff = O_2 in arterial blood (mL·dL^{-1}) − O_2 in venous blood (mL·dL^{-1})

or

$$\text{a-vO}_2 \text{ diff} = aO_2 - vO_2$$

Hence, the difference, using the values already calculated, is

$$\begin{aligned} \text{a-vO}_2 \text{ diff} &= 19.79 \text{ mL·dL}^{-1} - 15.20 \text{ mL·dL}^{-1} \\ &= 4.59 \text{ mL·dL}^{-1} \end{aligned}$$

Therefore, approximately 5 mL O_2·dL^{-1} are transported to and used by the tissue to support cellular metabolism under normal resting conditions. This means that approximately 25% (4.59 ÷ 19.79 = 0.23 × 100 = 23%) of the oxygen is actually released from the hemoglobin to the tissues and used during rest. And thus, approximately 75% of the oxygen is held in reserve for use during such events as physical exercise. The actual amount of oxygen used, measured as the a-vO$_2$ diff, is called the *coefficient of oxygen utilization*. The normal resting coefficient of oxygen utilization is 4.59 mL·dL^{-1}.

Note that the 75% is also the SbO$_2$% value for venous blood. Refer to Figure 10.14 again. The shaded area at the top—between the SbO$_2$% values of 97 and 75% on the left axis and between the values 19.79 and 15.20 mL·dL^{-1} on the right axis—represents these relative and absolute amounts of O_2 that have been released or dissociated primarily from the RBC cells. On this basis, the curve is called the oxygen dissociation curve. The separation or release of oxygen from the red blood cells to the tissues is called **oxygen dissociation.**

Carbon Dioxide Transport

Carbon dioxide is carried three ways in the blood from muscle or other tissue where it is produced to the lungs, where it is eliminated from the body. As with O_2, the first way it is transported is dissolved in blood plasma. The amount of CO_2 transported in this fashion is only about 5–10% of the total CO_2 transported. However, as with dissolved O_2, it is this dissolved CO_2 component that determines the partial pressure of CO_2 in the blood. Because the exchange of CO_2 in internal and external respiration depends largely upon the PCO$_2$, this is a critical role for dissolved CO_2. The remaining 90–95% of the CO_2 diffuses into the RBCs.

As CO_2 enters the RBC, about 20% combines chemically with the globin portion of the Hb molecule to produce the second form of CO_2 transport—namely, as *carbamino hemoglobin* (HbCO$_2$). Some small quantity may combine with proteins in the plasma as well. Note that when CO_2 combines with Hb, the CO_2 is not competing with oxygen for space on the heme units, because it combines with the globin portion. However, more CO_2 can combine with Hb if it is deoxygenated. That is, the lower the PO_2 and $SbO_2\%$, the greater is the amount of CO_2 that can be carried in the blood. This reaction is known as the *Haldane effect* (Leff and Schumacker, 1993).

At the lung the situation is reversed: As O_2 saturates the Hb, less CO_2 can be combined; so the release of CO_2 is stimulated. Thus, Hb is really a transport vehicle carrying O_2 from the alveoli to the cells and CO_2 from the cells to the alveoli. This task is made easier by the fact that the dissociation (dropping off) of one molecule facilitates the binding (picking up) of the other at both sites.

The third way that CO_2 can be transported is as bicarbonate ions. Approximately 70–75% of the CO_2 is transported in this way. When CO_2 diffuses into the RBCs, it combines with water under the influence of the enzyme carbonic anhydrase and forms carbonic acid (H_2CO_3). Carbonic acid is both weak and unstable and quickly dissociates into hydrogen ions (H^+) and bicarbonate ions (HCO_3^-). The chemical reaction is depicted as

$$\text{carbonic}$$
$$\text{anhydrase}$$
$$CO_2 + H_2O \leftrightarrow H_2CO_3 \leftrightarrow H^+ + HCO_3^-$$

The H^+ binds to Hb ($H^+ + Hb \rightarrow HHb$), thus preventing much change in pH; and the HCO_3^- diffuses into plasma. To counteract this loss of negative charges, chloride ions (Cl^-) move from plasma to the RBC. This ion exchange is called the *chloride shift*. At the lungs, where PCO_2 is relatively low, the reactions are all reversed. The chemical reactions are

$$O_2 + HHb \rightarrow HbO_2 + H^+$$
$$H^+ + HCO_3^- \rightarrow H_2CO_3 \rightarrow CO_2 + H_2O$$

Once back in the form of CO_2, the CO_2 diffuses along its partial pressure gradient from the blood to the alveoli and is exhaled (Guyton, 1986; Leff and Schumacker, 1993; Martin, et al., 1979).

Figure 10.15 summarizes the transport of both oxygen and carbon dioxide in arterial and venous blood. Take time to study that and relate it to the textual information.

The Respiratory System and Acid-Base Balance

The ability of hemoglobin to bind the hydrogen ions (H^+) produced during the transport of carbon dioxide and the ability of pulmonary ventilation both to respond to (Figures 10.9 and 10.11) and to eliminate carbon dioxide are very important in maintaining acid-base balance. These reactions exemplify two of the three lines of defense for regulating acid-base balance, namely, the chemical buffer system and the respiratory system. Furthermore, the partial pressure of carbon dioxide is also directly involved in the third line of defense, renal regulation by the kidneys.

Acid-base balance is defined as a series of mechanisms that attempt to regulate the concentration of hydrogen ions in body fluids. It is vitally important, because virtually all biochemical reactions in the human body require the pH to be maintained within very narrow limits for proper functioning (Martin, et al., 1979; Slonim and Hamilton, 1976). Hydrogen ions originate from a number of sources in the human body, but the majority appear as a result of the production of energy when oxygen is used and carbon dioxide is generated or when lactic acid is accumulated without the use of oxygen.

Chemical buffers are either weak acids or weak bases that respectively release or bind hydrogen ions. They respond instantaneously. Hemoglobin is not the only chemical buffer, but in terms of capacity it is the most important buffer in the blood. Bicarbonate (HCO_3^-) is another important base (Slonim and Hamilton, 1976).

The carbonic acid–bicarbonate system ($H_2CO_3/$ HCO_3^-) not only allows for the temporary buffering of hydrogen ions as they travel through the circulatory system but also provides for the removal from the body of the carbon dioxide formed in the buffering process. The sensitivity of pulmonary ventilation to PCO_2 and pH enables varying amounts of acid production to be dealt with, because increased levels of carbon dioxide can be exhaled as necessary. This respiratory compensation reacts within a matter of 1–3 min (Martin, et al., 1979; Slonim and Hamilton, 1976).

The kidney's role in acid-base balance is twofold: (1) to conserve or eliminate bicarbonate ions, hence stabilizing the amount in the body, and (2) to excrete hydrogen ions. Renal bicarbonate retention or excretion depends on the PCO_2 in arterial blood. The kidneys are the most potent of the acid-base mechanisms. However, they require hours or even days to effectively change pH (Martin, et al., 1979; Slonim and Hamilton, 1976).

In the normal resting condition venous pH is slightly lower than arterial pH (venous = 7.35, arterial = 7.4), but this difference has very little effect on most physiological functions. The key is maintaining arterial pH levels. Thus, not only does the respiratory system deliver oxygen for the production of energy, but it also contributes to the effective functioning of all biochemical reactions through its role in maintaining acid-base balance.

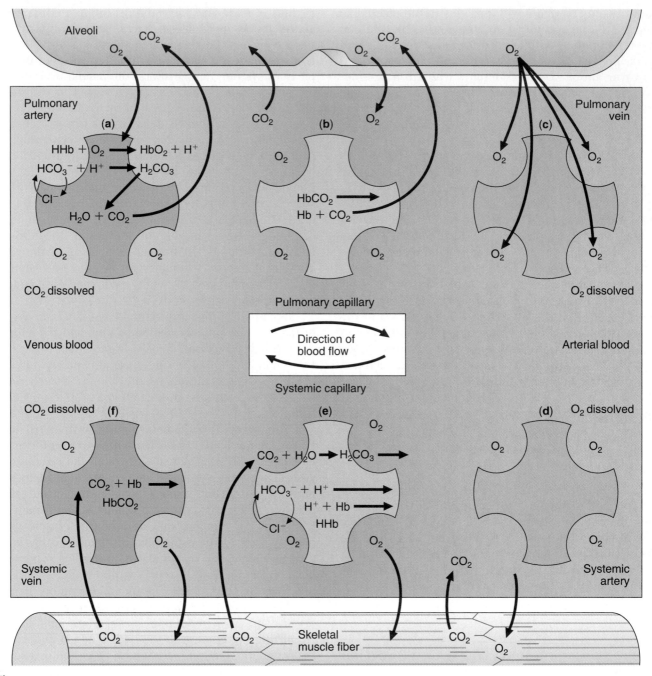

Figure 10.15

Summary of Oxygen and Carbon Dioxide Transport

Oxygen is transported two ways in the circulatory system—dissolved and bound to the heme units of hemoglobin (RBC). Carbon dioxide is transported three ways in the circulatory system—dissolved, bound to the globin portion of hemoglobin, and as bicarbonate. (a) The oxygenation of hemoglobin and diffusion of carbon dioxide from bicarbonate, (b) the diffusion of carbon dioxide from the globin portion of hemoglobin, (c) transport of oxygen on heme portions of hemoglobin, (d) diffusion of oxygen from heme portion of hemoglobin, (e) transport of carbon dioxide as bicarbonate, (f) transport of carbon dioxide on globin portion of hemoglobin.

Summary

1. Respiration consists of pulmonary ventilation and oxygen and carbon dioxide gas exchange at the alveolar (external) and tissue (internal) levels.

2. Structurally, the pulmonary system can be divided into the conductive and respiratory zones. The conductive zone serves to transport air, warm and humidify air, and filter the air. Gas exchange takes place in the respiratory zone.

IP *Respiratory–Anatomy Review* (pages 1–13)*

3. At rest, inspiration is an active process brought about by a pressure gradient that exceeds resistance to the flow of air. Resting expiration is a passive process accomplished primarily by elastic recoil.

IP *Respiratory–Pulmonary Ventilation* (pages 1–19)

4. The conductive zone makes up the anatomical dead space. A physiological dead space occurs when functional alveoli are not supplied with capillaries.

5. Minute ventilation ($\dot{V}_E$ or $\dot{V}_I$) is the respiratory variable most commonly measured in exercise situations. However, alveolar ventilation is the best measure of air available for gas exchange.

6. Residual volume, the amount of air remaining in the lungs after a maximal expiration, must be accounted for when one determines body composition by underwater weighing.

7. Respiratory measures are collected under ambient conditions (ATPS). Most lung volumes and capacities are then converted to body temperature values (BTPS). Minute ventilation may also be converted to standard temperature and pressure, dry (STPD) conditions.

8. Primary control of respiration resides in the medulla oblongata (inspiratory and expiratory centers), with fine tuning provided by the pneumotaxic and apneustic centers in the pons. Factors affecting these centers include:
   a. Conscious thought through the cerebral cortex.
   b. Sympathetic nerve reactions through the hypothalamus.
   c. Irritants or lung inflammation through systemic receptors in the airways and lungs.
   d. PO_2, PCO_2, pH, and K^+ through central and peripheral chemoreceptors.
   e. Movement via proprioceptive stimulation from mechanoreceptors and muscles and joints.

IP *Respiratory–Control of Respiration* (pages 1–16)

9. Gases flow from areas of high pressure to areas of low pressure—that is, always down a pressure gradient. Each gas moves independently. Oxygen moves from the alveoli into arterial blood and red blood cells and then from the red blood cells and capillary blood into the muscle tissues. Carbon dioxide moves from the muscle tissues into capillary blood and red blood cells and then from the venous blood and red blood cells into the alveoli. The P values driving these exchanges are given in Appendix C.

IP *Respiratory–Gas Exchange* (pages 1–17)*

10. Hemoglobin is composed of four iron heme units and one globin (a protein). When fully saturated, each hemoglobin molecule will have oxygen bound to each of its four heme structures. Normal arterial saturation (SaO_2%) is 97%; normal resting venous saturation (SvO_2%) is 75%.

IP *Respiratory–Gas Transport* (pages 1–5)*

11. Oxygen that is released from the red blood cells at the tissue level is said to have been dissociated. At rest the primary drive for this dissociation is the pressure gradient for oxygen.

IP *Respiratory–Gas Transport* (pages 6–10)*

12. At rest only about 25% of circulated oxygen is used; 75% remains saturated in venous blood. These percentages translate into an arteriovenous oxygen difference of approximately 4.6 mL·dL^{-1}.

13. Carbon dioxide is transported from the tissue to the lungs in three ways: dissolved, as carbamino hemoglobin, and as bicarbonate ions. The chemical buffering and removal of carbon dioxide from the body are important in maintaining acid-base balance.

IP *Respiratory–Gas Transport* (pages 11–15)*

*This topic is available on the InterActive Physiology® Sampler CD that comes with the purchase of a new copy of this book.

Review Questions

1. Define *pulmonary ventilation, external respiration,* and *internal respiration.* Define the following variables and classify each as involved in pulmonary ventilation, external respiration, or internal respiration. Some may be classified in more than one way.

(A-a)PO$_2$ diff	V$_T$	PvCO$_2$
a-vO$_2$ diff	$\dot{V}_A$	PvO$_2$
V$_D$	PaO$_2$	SaO$_2$%
f	P$_A$O$_2$	SbO$_2$%
$\dot{V}_E$ and $\dot{V}_I$	PaCO$_2$	SvO$_2$%

2. Diagram the conductive and respiratory zones of the respiratory system. Compare the function of the two zones.

3. Why does air flow into and out of the lungs?

4. What is the functional difference between pulmonary circulation and bronchial circulation? How does bronchial circulation affect the PaO_2?

5. Identify the three capacities and four volumes into which total lung capacity can be divided. Which of them is most responsive during exercise? Which must be accounted for when one determines body composition by hydrostatic (underwater) weighing?

6. Explain the conditions represented by the volume designations ATPS, BTPS, and STPD. Where is each condition most appropriately used? Which volume is typically the largest? Which is the smallest? Name and explain the gas laws that cause these differences.

7. Discuss the primary control of respiration and the factors that affect such control.

8. Describe how oxygen and carbon dioxide are transported in the circulatory system. Note in particular the importance of each transport form and any interaction between the movements of the individual gases.

9. Explain how the transport and removal of carbon dioxide relate to acid-base balance. Why is it important to maintain acid-base balance?

10. Graph a normal resting oxygen dissociation curve. What percentage of the available oxygen is normally dissociated at rest?

For further review and additional study tools, go to The Physiology Place (www.physiologyplace.com) and the Student Study Guide for Exercise Physiology for Health, Fitness, and Performance by Sharon A. Plowman and Denise L. Smith.

Passport to the Internet

Visit the following Internet sites to explore further topics and issues related to respiration. To visit an organization's web site, go to www.physiology place. com, and click on "Passport to the Internet."

National Heart, Lung, and Blood Institute (NHLBI) The web site for this division of the National Institutes of Health presents information and links to resources concerning heart and vascular disease, lung diseases, blood diseases, and sleep disorders.

Ventilation and Ventilatory Control Tests In addition to a thorough discussion on ventilation and venti-latory tests, this site connects to tutorials on a number of subjects. *Note:* Because this site is a personal effort of an individual, its connection may break. If so, conduct your own search for a related site on respiration and ventilation.

Association for Respiratory Technology and Physiology Check out this British professional organization for practitioners working in respiratory physiology and technology. Explore some of the links provided through this web site to numerous other professional organizations in the field.

References

Adams, G. M.: *Exercise Physiology Laboratory Manual* (2nd edition). Dubuque, IA: Brown (1994).

Brown, D. D., D. M. Lawrence, R. A. Steurer, & J. Rogers: The effect of external nasal dilators on submaximal exercise responses. *Medicine and Science in Exercise and Sport.* 29(5)(Supplement): S293 (abstract) (1997).

Clapp, A. J., & P. A. Bishop: Effect of the Breathe Right external nasal dilator during light to moderate exercise. *Medicine and Science in Exercise and Sport.* 28(5)(Supplement): S88 (abstract) (1996).

Craig, A. B.: Summary of 58 cases of loss of consciousness during underwater swimming and diving. *Medicine and Science in Sports.* 8(3):171–175 (1976).

Dempsey, J. A., E. H. Vidruk, & G. S. Mitchell: Pulmonary control systems in exercise: Update. *Federation Proceedings.* 44:2260–2270 (1985).

Eldridge, F. L.: Central integration of mechanisms in exercise hyperpnea. *Medicine and Science in Sports and Exercise.* 26(3):319–327 (1994).

Forster, H. V., & L. G. Pau: The role of the carotid chemoreceptors in the control of breathing during exercise. *Medicine and Science in Sports and Exercise.* 26(3):328–336 (1994).

Griffin, J. W., G. Hunter, D. Ferguson, & M. J. Sillers: Physiologic effects of an external nasal dilator. *Laryngoscope* 107:1235–1238 (1997).

Guyton, A. C.: *Textbook of Medical Physiology* (7th edition). Philadelphia: Saunders (1986).

Huffman, M. S., M. T. Huffman, D. D. Brown, J. C. Quindry, & D. Q. Thomas: Exercise responses using the Breathe Right external nasal dilator. *Medicine and Science in Sports and Exercise.* 28(5)(Supplement): S70 (abstract) (1996).

Leff, A. R., & P. T. Schumacker: *Respiratory Physiology: Basics and Applications.* Philadelphia: Saunders Company (1993).

Martin, B. J., K. E. Sparks, C. W. Zwillich, & J. V. Weil: Low exercise ventilation in endurance athletes. *Medicine and Science in Sports.* 11(2):181–185 (1979).

Nye, P. C. G.: Identification of peripheral chemoreceptor stimuli. *Medicine and Science in Sports and Exercise.* 26(3):311–318 (1994).

O'Kroy, J. A.: Oxygen uptake and ventilatory effects of an external nasal dilator during ergometry. *Medicine and Science in Sports and Exercise.* 32(8):1491–1495 (2000).

Pardy, R. L., S. N. A. Hussain, & P. T. Macklein: The ventilatory pump in exercise. *Clinics in Chest Medicine.* 5(1):35–49 (1984).

Schunemann, H. J., J. Dorn, B. J. B. Grant, W. Winkelstein, & M. Trevisan: Pulmonary function is a long-term predictor of mortality in the general population: 29-year follow-up of the Buffalo Health Study. *Chest* 118 (3); 656–664 (2000).

Slonim, N. B., & L. H. Hamilton: *Respiratory Physiology* (3rd edition). St. Louis: Mosby (1976).

Wetzstein, C.: Breathe Right Strip: How does it affect the nose and how might it benefit exercise? *Research Quarterly for Exercise and Sport.* 67 (Supplement): A-28 (abstract) (1996).

Whipp, B. J., S. A. Ward, N. Lamarra, J. A. Davis, & K. Wasserman: Parameters of ventilatory and gas exchange dynamics during exercise. *Journal of Applied Physiology: Respiratory, Environmental and Exercise Physiology.* 52(6):1506–1513 (1982).

Wilmore, J. H.: The use of actual, predicted, and constant residual volumes in the assessment of body composition by underwater weighing. *Medicine and Science in Sports.* 1:87–90 (1969).

Young, L., J. Sowash, D. Lever, J. Wygand, & R. M. Otto: The effect of Breathrite Aids on acute anaerobic performance and recovery. *Medicine and Science in Sports and Exercise.* 28(5)(Supplement): S17 (abstract) (1996).

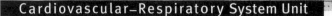
Chapter 11

Respiratory Exercise Response, Training Adaptations, and Special Considerations

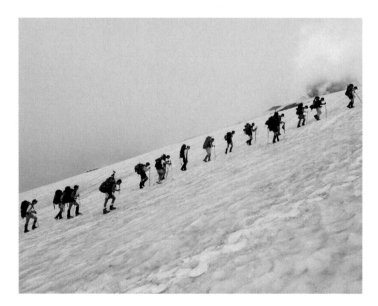

After studying the chapter, you should be able to

- Graph and explain the pattern of response for the major respiratory variables during short-term, light to moderate submaximal aerobic exercise.

- Graph and explain the pattern of response for the major respiratory variables during long-term moderate to heavy submaximal aerobic exercise.

- Graph and explain the pattern of response for the major respiratory variables during incremental aerobic exercise to maximum.

- Graph and explain the pattern of response for the major respiratory variables during static exercise.

- Compare and contrast the pulmonary ventilation, external respiration, and internal respiration responses to short-term, light to moderate submaximal aerobic exercise; long-term, moderate to heavy submaximal aerobic exercise; incremental aerobic exercise to maximum; and static exercise.

- List the exercise training adaptations that consistently occur in the respiratory system.

- Identify variations in resting volumes, exercise responses, and exercise training adaptions among young adults, children and adolescents, and the elderly and between males and females.

- Determine the value of altitude training, hypoxic swim training, and training in polluted conditions.

Response of the Respiratory System to Exercise

During exercise the demand for energy increases, varying, of course, with the type, intensity, and duration of the exercise. In most exercise situations much of the body's ability to respond to the demand for more energy depends on the availability of oxygen. To provide the needed oxygen for aerobic energy production, the respiratory system—including pulmonary ventilation, external respiration, and internal respiration—must respond. Pulmonary ventilation increases to enhance alveolar ventilation; external respiration adjusts in such a way as to maintain the relationship between ventilation and perfusion in most cases; internal respiration responds with the increased extraction of oxygen by the muscles. These changes in respiration not only provide adequate oxygenation for the muscles but also play a major role in maintaining acid-base balance, which is, in turn, closely related to carbon dioxide levels.

In general, all levels of respiratory activity are precisely matched to the rate of work being done. Furthermore, because of this precise control and the large reserve built into the system, respiration in normal, healthy, sedentary, or moderately fit individuals is generally not a limiting factor in activity. This is true despite the perception of feeling out of breath during exercise. Only in the rare situation of some highly trained, elite endurance athletes do the capacities of the cardiovascular and metabolic systems exceed that of the respiratory system such that respiration can be considered a limitation to maximal work.

Of course, changes in pulmonary ventilation would be of little benefit if parallel changes in pulmonary blood volume and flow and total body circulation did not also occur. The specific details of the accompanying cardiovascular responses will be discussed later in this unit.

This section will concentrate on pulmonary ventilation, external respiration, and internal respiration responses to aerobic activity, including short- and long-term, constant-load submaximal activity and incremental exercise to maximum. The most prominent changes in the respiratory system occur within these classifications of activity. A few comments will also be made concerning static exercise responses. However, the response to dynamic resistance activity has not been specifically documented and therefore will not be discussed. When reading this discussion and studying the accompanying graphs, you may wish to refer to the glossary of respiratory symbols summarized in Table 11.1. It should be noted that several variables are involved in more than one process.

Short-Term, Light to Moderate Submaximal Aerobic Exercise

The responses to short-term (meaning 5–10 min), light to moderate submaximal (defined as 30–69% of maximal work capacity) aerobic exercise are diagrammed in Figures 11.1, 11.2 on page 287, and 11.5 on page 290. These responses are discussed in detail in the subsections that follow.

Pulmonary Ventilation

The most obvious response to an increased metabolic demand, such as exercise, is the increase in pulmonary ventilation ($\dot{V}_E$ L·min^{-1}), called *hyperpnea*. What is perhaps a little surprising is the initial immediate reaction. In Figure 11.1a, note that between the

Table 11.1
Respiratory Symbols

Pulmonary Ventilation	External Respiration	Internal Respiration
$\dot{V}_E$ = minute ventilation	$\dot{V}_A$ = alveolar ventilation	a-vO$_2$ diff = amount of oxygen carried in the arteries minus the amount carried in the veins
V_D = dead space	P_AO_2 = partial pressure of oxygen at the alveoli	
V_T = tidal volume		PaO_2 = partial pressure of oxygen dioxide in arterial blood
f = frequency of breathing	PaO_2 = partial pressure of oxygen in arterial blood	
V_D/V_T = ratio of dead space to tidal volume	(A-a)PO$_2$ diff = oxygen or PO$_2$ pressure gradient between the alveoli and arteries	$PaCO_2$ = partial pressure of carbon dioxide in arterial blood
		$PvCO_2$ = partial pressure of carbon dioxide in venous blood
	SaO$_2$% = percent saturation of arterial blood with oxygen	SvO_2% = percent saturation of venous blood with oxygen
	P_ACO_2 = partial pressure of carbon dioxide at the alveoli	PvO_2 = partial pressure of oxygen in venous blood

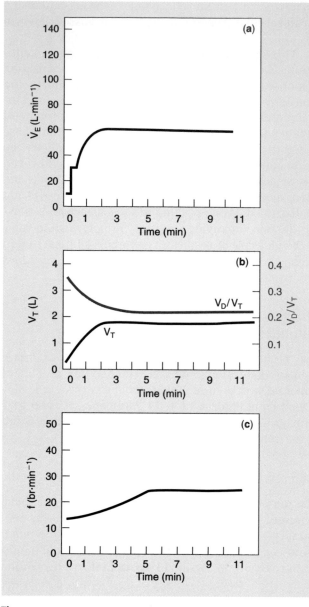

Figure 11.1

Responses of Pulmonary Ventilation Variables to Short-Term, Light to Moderate Submaximal Aerobic Exercise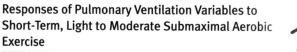

onset of exercise at 0 min and 2 min into the exercise, a triphasic response in $\dot{V}_E$ has occurred. Within the first respiratory cycle at the onset of exercise, there is an initial abrupt increase in $\dot{V}_E$, which is phase 1. It is maintained for approximately 10–20 sec. Phase 2 is the slower exponential rise from the initial elevation to the steady-state leveling off. At the low to moderate workload depicted here, this exponential rise should be completed in 2–3 min. At this point, phase 3, or the new steady state, is achieved. The actual level of the achieved exercise steady state depends on a number of factors, including the workload, the fitness status of

the individual, and the environmental conditions. In the time span depicted, the steady-state level is maintained. The three-phase response at the onset of activity is typically not seen when $\dot{V}_E$ is reported or graphed minute by minute, but it has occurred (Pardy, et al., 1984; Whipp, 1977; Whipp and Ward, 1980; Whipp, et al., 1982).

The initial rise in ventilation occurs primarily because of an increase in tidal volume (Leff and Schumacker, 1993). Theoretically, the potential range of tidal volume is from the resting level to the limits of vital capacity. In reality, rarely is more than 50–65% of vital capacity reached before a plateau occurs. Furthermore, although tidal volume encroaches into both the inspiratory reserve capacity (IRC) and the expiratory reserve capacity (ERC), it encroaches much more into IRC than ERC (Koyal, et al., 1976; Pearce and Milhorn, 1977; Turner, et al., 1968; Younes and Kivinen, 1984).

At light to moderate workloads, the contribution of an increase in breathing frequency to minute ventilation is minimal and gradual. Both tidal volume and frequency level off at a steady state that satisfies the requirements of the short submaximal activity (Figures 11.1b and 11.1c).

Airway resistance decreases owing to bronchodilation as soon as any intensity of exercise begins. Likewise, the ratio of dead space (V_D) to tidal volume (V_T) decreases, and in this case the largest changes are evident at the lowest work rate (Wasserman, et al., 1967; Whipp and Ward, 1980). This result is shown in Figure 11.1b. The depth of the drop in V_D/V_T is moderate at low to moderate exercise intensities. The V_D itself changes minimally with bronchodilation, but with the proportionally larger increase in V_T the ratio declines (Grimby, 1969). This result is important because alveolar ventilation ($\dot{V}_A$) thus increases from about 70% of the total pulmonary ventilation at rest to a higher percentage during exercise. Since $\dot{V}_A$ is the critical ventilation, this reduction in the V_D/V_T ratio means that the appropriate level of $\dot{V}_A$ can be achieved with a smaller rise in $\dot{V}_E$ than would be needed if the ratio did not change (Wasserman and Whipp, 1975).

External Respiration

The $\dot{V}_A$ response to low to moderate exercise is depicted in Figure 11.2a. This curve parallels the change in $\dot{V}_E$, except that the initial adjustments seen in $\dot{V}_E$ are not depicted for $\dot{V}_A$. The rise in $\dot{V}_A$ is sufficient to maintain PO_2 at the alveolar level ($P_{A}O_2$) during short-term submaximal exercise (Figure 11.2b). Maintenance of $P_{A}O_2$ is important because it represents the driving force for oxygen transfer across the alveolar-capillary interface (Powers, et al., 1993; Wasserman, 1978).

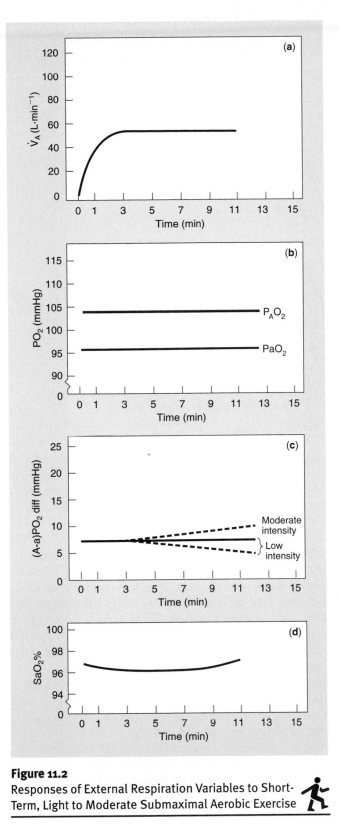

Figure 11.2

Responses of External Respiration Variables to Short-Term, Light to Moderate Submaximal Aerobic Exercise

As explained earlier, under resting conditions there is an inequity in PO_2 between the alveoli (P_AO_2) and systemic arterial blood (PaO_2) owing to the

dilution of the systemic arterial blood with the bronchial venous blood. During short-term, low-intensity submaximal exercise, PaO_2 is maintained and the *alveolar–to–arterial oxygen partial pressure difference,* depicted as (A-a)PO_2 diff in Figure 11.2c, either does not change or decreases slightly (Jones, 1975; Leff and Schumacker, 1993; Wasserman and Whipp, 1975). At moderate workloads a slight increase may be seen. The (A-a)PO_2 diff reflects the efficiency and/or adequacy of oxygen transfer in the lungs during exercise. At the steady-state submaximal levels described here, there is, in essence, no noticeable change in this efficiency.

Gas exchange and blood perfusion in the lungs during low to moderate exercise is sufficient to maintain the saturation of red blood cells with oxygen (SaO_2%) within a narrow range approximating resting levels (Figure 11.2d) (Gurtner, et al., 1975).

Internal Respiration

Recall that internal respiration involves the dissociation of oxygen from the red blood cells so that it may diffuse down the pressure gradient into the muscles and other tissues.

Refer to Figure 11.3 and refamiliarize yourself with the resting relationships described in Chapter 10 and labeled again in this figure. The line for resting arterial blood at 95 mmHg on the x-axis represents the PaO_2. It intersects with the middle curve and indicates a percent saturation of hemoglobin (SbO_2%) of approximately 97% on the left y-axis. The line for resting venous blood at 40 mmHg on the x-axis represents the PvO_2. This line also intersects with the middle curve and indicates a SbO_2 of 75%; that is, at rest 75% of the oxygen remains associated with the red blood cells in venous blood. Thus, a great deal more oxygen could be extracted at the tissue capillary level and normally is during exercise.

Four factors are involved in accomplishing the increased oxygen extraction during exercise:

1. an increased PO_2 gradient;
2. an increased PCO_2;
3. a decreased pH; and
4. an increased temperature.

Each is depicted in the oxygen dissociation curve in Figure 11.3. The way each factor operates is described below.

Increased PO₂ Gradient   Under resting conditions sufficient oxygen remains in the muscle tissue to maintain a PO_2 of 40 mmHg. When exercise increases the demand for energy, the oxygen already in the muscle tissue is used immediately. Since the oxygen is

Figure 11.3
Oxygen Dissociation during Exercise

The center curve represents normal resting values: $PaCO_2$ = 40 mmHg, pH = 7.4, body temperature = 37 °C. During all intensities and types of exercise, the $PaCO_2$ increases, pH decreases (becomes more acidic), and body temperature increases. Each of these conditions causes the curve to shift to the right, with the result that more oxygen is dissociated from red blood cells to be used by the muscles. Consequently, the higher the intensity of exercise, the lower both the oxygen content of the venous blood and the SbO_2% in venous blood, to a minimum of approximately 15%.

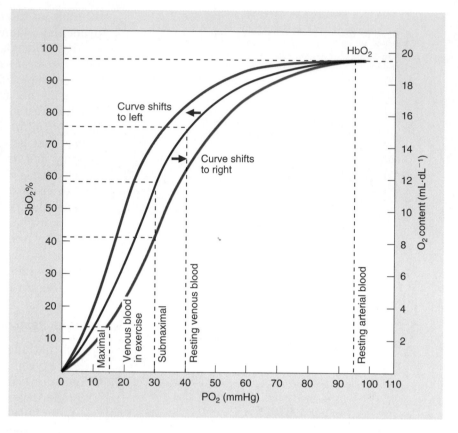

used, the muscle tissue partial pressure is reduced correspondingly. The PO_2 of arterial blood remains unchanged. Therefore, the pressure gradient can be widened from 55 mmHg (95 mmHg at the arterial end of the capillary minus 40 mmHg in the muscle tissue) to possibly 65 mmHg (95 mmHg at the arterial end of the capillary minus 30 mmHg in the muscle tissue) during light submaximal exercise.

Equilibrium is reached between the muscle tissue and the blood by the venous end of the capillary, so the returning venous blood also has the lower PO_2. Refer to Figure 11.3 and find the line labeled submaximal for venous blood in exercise above the x-axis value of 30 mmHg. Assume for the moment that this is the only change that occurs (a false assumption, as will be detailed later, but one which does no harm here). From the figure you can see the effect this increased pressure gradient has on the dissociation of oxygen. By following this submaximal exercise line to where it intersects the solid line middle curve and then to the left y-axis, you can see that the corresponding SbO_2% (actually SvO_2% now) is 60%, not 75%. Thus, instead of 23% of the oxygen being dissociated as it was at rest (97% SaO_2% − 75% SvO_2% = 22%; 22% ÷ 97% = 23%) now 38% (97% SaO_2% − 60 SvO_2% = 37%; 37% ÷ 97% = 38%) has been released from the red blood cells just by changing the pressure gradient. Hence, an additional 15% of the available

oxygen (38% − 23% = 15%) has been dissociated and is used for energy production. Not all submaximal exercise requires the same amount of oxygen, so these numbers are simply illustrative of the effect of a widening pressure gradient.

Increased PCO_2 When oxygen is used to provide energy, carbon dioxide is produced as a by-product. Increasing levels of carbon dioxide mean that PCO_2 increases. An increase in PCO_2 shifts the oxygen dissociation curve to the right. This shift was seen in a minimal way even at rest in the venous curve depicted in Figure 10.14, on page 277. However, during exercise the shift is further to the right. Exactly how far the curve shifts depends on how hard the exercise is and how much carbon dioxide is produced. The shift in the curve to the right means that at any given PO_2 more dissociation occurs, as shown in Figure 11.3. Follow the line for venous blood in exercise from the value of 30 mmHg on the PO_2 x-axis until it intersects the right-hand curve. A horizontal line from this intersection to the left y-axis yields a saturation value of about 41%. Thus, more oxygen is dissociated than would have been if the pressure gradient had been operating alone. Figure 11.4 emphasizes that the actual shift occurs during the red blood cell transit through the capillary before reaching the actual venous blood.

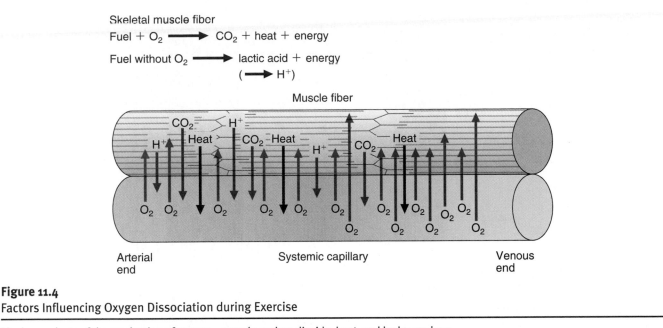

Skeletal muscle fiber

Fuel + O_2 $\longrightarrow$ CO_2 + heat + energy

Fuel without O_2 $\longrightarrow$ lactic acid + energy
($\longrightarrow$ H^+)

Muscle fiber

Arterial end
Systemic capillary
Venous end

Figure 11.4
Factors Influencing Oxygen Dissociation during Exercise

The by-products of the production of energy—namely, carbon dioxide, heat, and hydrogen ions (H^+)—in skeletal muscle fibers stimulate the dissociation of oxygen from red blood cells as they traverse systemic capillaries.

Decreased pH or Increased Hydrogen Ion Concentration
Hydrogen ions (H^+) come from two primary sources during exercise. First, carbon dioxide combines with water to form carbonic acid. The carbonic acid then breaks down into hydrogen ions and bicarbonate. Second, lactic acid breaks down into lactate and hydrogen ions. The presence of increased levels of hydrogen ions lowers the pH to a more acidic level. This more acidic pH shifts the oxygen dissociation curve to the right in the same way that an increased PCO_2 did and with the same results: a greater dissociation of oxygen from red blood cells. How far to the right the curve shifts depends on the amount of hydrogen ions released. As with carbon dioxide, this effect is taking place during the red blood cell's transit through the muscle capillaries (Figure 11.4). The interactive effect of carbon dioxide and pH on the affinity of hemoglobin for oxygen is known as the *Bohr effect* (Guyton, 1986; Kenney, 1982).

Increased Temperature Another by-product of muscle energy production is heat. Heat is also transferred from the muscle tissue (high heat) to the capillary (low heat) (Figure 11.4). The resultant rise in temperature shifts the oxygen dissociation curve to the right. The action is precisely the same as that for the increase in PCO_2 and the decrease in pH, and so it is again depicted by the same shift in Figure 11.3.

Thus, the elevation in the use of oxygen to produce energy during exercise and the by-products of

that energy production operate together to make the reserves of oxygen available: the first (increased oxygen consumption) by widening the pressure gradient, and the other three (increased PCO_2, decreased pH, and increased body temperature) by shifting the oxygen dissociation curve to the right.

The exercise responses for the variables from the oxygen dissociation curve are depicted in Figure 11.5. The best overall indicator of internal respiration is the arteriovenous oxygen difference (a-vO_2 diff) (Gurtner, et al., 1975). Because PaO_2 (Figure 11.5a) and SaO_2% (Figure 11.2d) do not change with short-term, low-intensity exercise, the actual amount of oxygen being carried in the arteries (in milliliters per deciliter) also does not change (Wasserman, et al., 1967). However, because the production of energy uses more oxygen even at these low intensities, the venous oxygen value as well as the PvO_2 (Figure 11.5c) and SvO_2% (Figure 11.5f) will decrease. With an equal arterial oxygen and lower venous oxygen content, the a-vO_2 diff (Figure 11.5e) will increase. Because this is a steady-state submaximal situation, the a-vO_2 diff will level off when sufficient oxygen is being extracted to supply the needs of the cell (Davies, et al., 1972; Dempsey, et al., 1977; Kao, 1974).

Because the production of energy not only uses oxygen but also produces carbon dioxide, it would be anticipated that the PvCO_2 value would increase. As shown in Figure 11.5d, this increase does occur, but it is not particularly large at these low to moderate workloads. The extra carbon dioxide is exhaled easily

Figure 11.5
Responses of Internal Respiration Variables to Short-Term, Light to Moderate Submaximal Aerobic Exercise

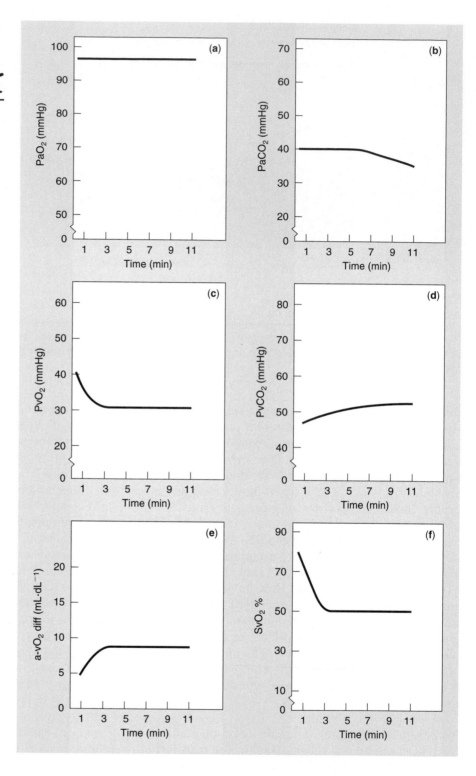

from the lungs and the hyperpnea of exercise may even blow off a little extra carbon dioxide, resulting in a slight decrement in $PaCO_2$ (Figure 11.5b). Regulation of ventilation maintains $PaCO_2$ very close to resting values (Davies, et al., 1972; Dempsey, et al., 1977; Kao, 1974; Wasserman, et al., 1967; Whipp and Ward, 1980).

These combined responses are well within the reserve capacity of the respiratory system for normal, healthy individuals.

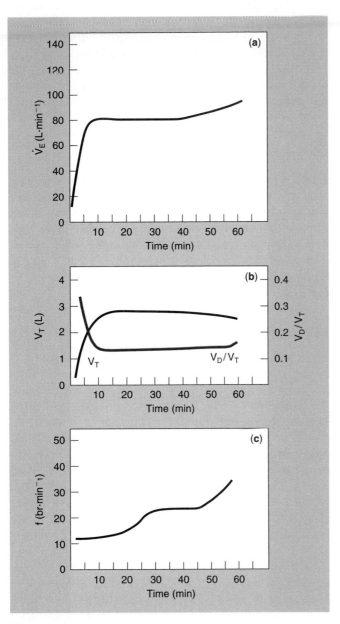

Figure 11.6

Responses of Pulmonary Ventilation Variables to Long-Term, Moderate to Heavy Submaximal Aerobic Exercise

Long-Term, Moderate to Heavy Submaximal Aerobic Exercise

If submaximal aerobic exercise is increased in duration and maintained at high-moderate to heavy intensity (60–75% of maximal working capacity), respiratory responses vary primarily in magnitude when compared with the changes just discussed for short-term, light to moderate submaximal exercise. In addition, several of the variables exhibit a drifting pattern.

Pulmonary Ventilation

Figure 11.6a shows that $\dot{V}_E$ increases to a higher level than during light to moderate submaximal exercise before plateauing at a steady state. The achievement of the steady state may take somewhat longer than at lower work intensities and often is not held throughout the duration of the exercise. Note that after approximately 30 min a gradual rise in $\dot{V}_E$ occurs, despite an unchanging workload, an effect called *ventilatory drift* (Dempsey, et al., 1977; Hanson, et al., 1982; Wasserman, 1978). The precise reason for this drift is unknown (Sawka, et al., 1980), although a rising body temperature is most often speculated as the reason. This drift is both inefficient and advantageous. It is inefficient because it is in excess of the workload demand. It is advantageous to gas exchange because alveolar ventilation parallels the drift and acid-base balance is maintained (Dempsey, et al., 1977; Hanson, et al., 1982).

As for lower-intensity submaximal exercise, the initial change in $\dot{V}_E$ is due primarily to an increase in V_T (Figure 11.6b). However, in the later stages of heavy submaximal work tidal volume may decrease slightly. The drift in $\dot{V}_E$ comes about primarily as a result of increased breathing frequency (Figure 11.6c). The V_D/V_T ratio (Figure 11.6b) still decreases primarily at the onset of activity, but it does so to a greater extent with the heavier workload than at lighter loads. After about an hour of heavy submaximal work, the V_D/V_T ratio may increase very slightly.

External Respiration

As stated earlier, the drift in $\dot{V}_E$ is paralleled by a similar drift in $\dot{V}_A$ (Figure 11.7a). P_AO_2 remains constant (Figure 11.7b), as it did with lower-intensity submaximal work. However, PaO_2 decreases gradually but slightly until about the time when ventilatory drift occurs, forming a shallow U-shaped curve (Dempsey, et al., 1977). It then returns toward baseline values. This variation in PaO_2 while P_AO_2 remains unchanged is reflected in a mirror image relationship in the $(A-a)PO_2$ diff (Figure 11.7c), depicted as a truncated, inverted U-shaped curve. The initial increase in the $(A-a)PO_2$ diff is not a desirable change. It indicates inefficiency in gas exchange. However, the small loss of efficiency seen here has very little practical meaning and does not limit the exercise (Hanson, et al., 1982; Wasserman, et al., 1967).

Internal Respiration

Other than differences in magnitude, all of the internal respiration variables respond in the same way

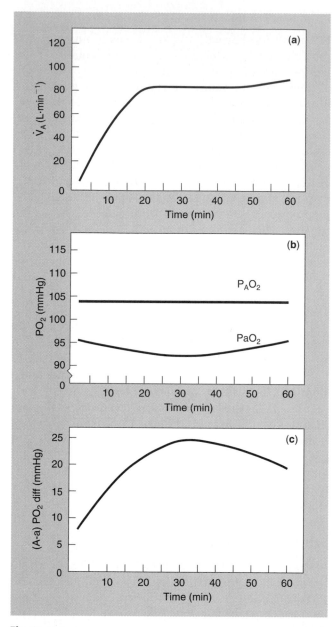

Figure 11.7

Responses of External Respiration Variables to Long-Term, Moderate to Heavy Submaximal Aerobic Exercise

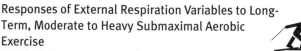

during prolonged, constant, relatively heavy submaximal dynamic exercise as during the shorter, lighter dynamic exercise previously described.

Despite the higher workload and the shallow U-shaped response, PaO_2 is maintained relatively constant (Figure 11.8a). Because of the heavier workload, more oxygen is dissociated and used, and the PvO_2 (Figure 11.8c) and $SvO_2\%$ (Figure 11.8f) decrease to lower levels than in shorter, lighter workloads. The result is a widening of the a-vO_2 diff (Figure 11.8e). The factors responsible for the dissociation of oxygen

are the same as those for lower-intensity exercise. $PaCO_2$ (Figure 11.8b) decreases slightly due to the increased volume of air being exhaled. $PvCO_2$ (Figure 11.8d) increases because the greater use of oxygen to produce energy also results in more carbon dioxide that must be carried in the venous system to the lungs to be exhaled.

Incremental Aerobic Exercise to Maximum

An incremental aerobic exercise bout consists of a series of progressively increasing work intensities, which stop when the individual cannot do any more. The length of each work intensity, often called a *stage,* may vary from 1 to 3 min to allow for the achievement of a steady state, at least until the higher workloads, when a steady state cannot be either attained or maintained.

Pulmonary Ventilation

It might be anticipated that because $\dot{V}_E$ rises and levels off at submaximal workloads, that this rise would be proportional, direct, and rectilinear throughout the entire range, from rest to maximal exercise. However, as shown in Figure 11.9a on page 294, a smooth rise is not completely descriptive of the response. At light to moderate and even heavy intensities, up to approximately 50–75% of maximum workload, $\dot{V}_E$ does increase in a rectilinear fashion. At this point a break in the linearity occurs, and a second, steeper linear rise ensues. This proportional rise continues until approximately 85–95% of maximum workload, when a second break in linearity occurs. The slope of the third linear rise to maximum that follows is even steeper (Koyal, et al., 1976; Powers and Beadle, 1985; Was-serman, 1978). These points where the rectilinear rise in minute ventilation breaks from linearity during incremental exercise to maximum are called **ventilatory thresholds.** The first breakpoint is called the first ventilatory threshold (VT1), and the second breakpoint is called the second ventilatory threshold (VT2).

Precisely what causes these breakpoints is unknown. One theory has linked them with an excess of carbon dioxide resulting from the buffering of lactic acid, and this theory calls the breakpoints anaerobic thresholds. Although carbon dioxide is a known respiratory stimulator, this theory is probably not accurate

Ventilatory Thresholds Points where the rectilinear rise in minute ventilation breaks from linearity during an incremental exercise to maximum.

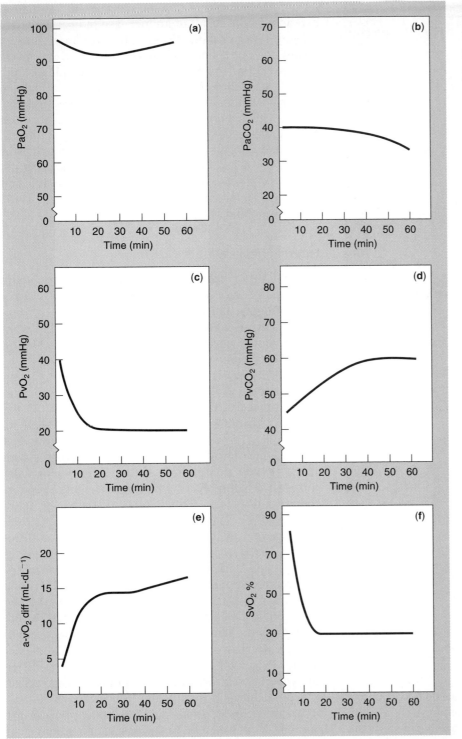

Figure 11.8
Responses of Internal Respiration Variables to Long-Term, Moderate to Heavy Submaximal Aerobic Exercise

(for reasons that are fully discussed in the unit on metabolism). Therefore, the term *ventilatory thresholds* is preferred. Other possible mechanisms—including catecholamine or potassium stimulation of the carotid bodies; limitations in changes in V_T, f, and V_D/V_T to maintain $\dot{V}_A$; increasing body temperatures; and feedback from the skeletal muscle proprioceptors—have

been suggested as causes of the ventilatory thresholds, but their role remains unproven. It is likely that a combination of factors is responsible (Loat and Rhodes, 1993; Skinner and McLellan, 1980; Walsh and Banister, 1988).

Knowledge of the ventilatory thresholds, regardless of why they occur, has some practical benefit. The

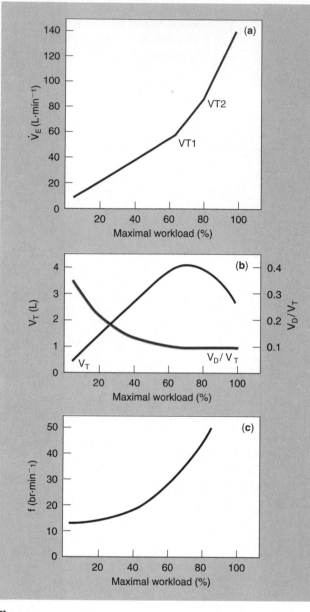

Figure 11.9

Responses of Pulmonary Ventilation Variables to Incremental Aerobic Exercise to Maximum

its highest point, any further increase in ventilation can only be the result of an increase in breathing frequency (Wasserman, 1978). The rise in breathing frequency is exponential at the higher work levels (Figure 11.9c). As with submaximal workloads, the V_D/V_T ratio decreases the most in the initial light to moderate stages of the incremental work (Grimby, 1969). The maximal reduction is reached at about 60% of maximal work, and this value is maintained to maximum. Since the V_D/V_T ratio is reduced to 0.1 (or 10% of V_T), 90% of V_T is available for exchange at the alveoli ($\dot{V}_A$), providing a more efficient ventilation (Grimby, 1969; Jones, 1975; Wasserman, et al., 1967; Wasserman and Whipp, 1975).

External Respiration

Changes in $\dot{V}_A$ parallel the changes in $\dot{V}_E$, including the slope of the rectilinear rises and the two breakpoints (Figure 11.10a). The breakpoints in $\dot{V}_A$, however, occur prior to the breakpoints in $\dot{V}_E$—that is, at slightly lower percentages of maximal work (Jones, 1975; Wasserman, 1978).

The rise in $\dot{V}_A$ is sufficient to maintain P_AO_2 and subsequently PaO_2 through the light to moderate submaximal exercise stages (Figure 11.10b). As the workload becomes higher, P_AO_2 rises exponentially to maximum. This rise provides the driving force that hastens the rate of equilibrium of alveolar gas with mixed venous blood and in so doing maintains PaO_2 and SaO_2% within narrow limits in normal or moderately fit individuals (Figure 11.10d) (Dempsey, 1986; Grimby, 1969; Segal, 1992; Wasserman, et al., 1967; Wasserman and Whipp, 1975). The (A-a)PO_2 diff follows the pattern of the exponential rise in P_AO_2 (Figure 11.10c). The increase of the (A-a)PO_2 diff to approximately 30 mmHg shown in Figure 11.10c is still considered to be a small increase (Jones, 1975).

Refer again to the PaO_2 graph in Figure 11.10b. Note the dotted line, which shows a steep decrease in PaO_2. A decrease of at least 10 mmHg PaO_2 (if persistent) is called **exercise-induced hypoxemia (EIH);** it is a condition in which the amount of oxygen carried in arterial blood is insufficient. Surprisingly, 40–50% of highly trained, healthy, elite male cyclists and runners with $\dot{V}O_2$max in excess of 4.5 L·min^{-1} or 55 mL·kg^{-1}·min^{-1} exhibit this response at work rates from 60% to 90% of maximum. Although most of the

workloads at which the ventilatory thresholds occur are related to endurance exercise performance; that is, the higher the workload where the breaks occur, the greater the intensity of activity that can be sustained (Loat and Rhodes, 1993; Walsh and Banister, 1988).

Once again, the changes in minute ventilation ($\dot{V}_E$) during low to moderate workloads are achieved primarily by an increase in V_T (Figure 11.9b). At very heavy workloads, however, the depth of breathing not only may cease to increase but also may decrease, forming a truncated, inverted U pattern (Dempsey, 1986; Younes and Kivinen, 1984). When V_T reaches

> **Exercise-Induced Hypoxemia (EIH)** A condition found in endurance athletes in which the amount of oxygen carried in arterial blood is severely reduced.

original data centered on these elite adult males, there is now evidence of the occurrence of EIH in females and young and elderly athletes as well (Prefaut, et al., 2000). During EIH the individual's ability to process oxygen and, hence, to perform high-intensity activity is lower than it would be without EIH, although both may be higher than those of untrained or moderately trained individuals. In other words, respiration—more specifically, external respiration—is a limitation to exercise in some highly trained athletes. Furthermore, athletes who exhibit EIH at sea level suffer more severe gas exchange impairments during short-term exposure to higher altitudes than do athletes who do not exhibit EIH at sea level (Powers, et al., 1993).

As shown on the graph in Figures 11.10b and 11.11a, the decline in PaO_2 with EIH can be considerable, ranging from 18 to 38 mmHg below resting values (96 − 18 = 78 mmHg; 96 − 38 = 58 mmHg). At the same time, the $SaO_2\%$ (Figure 11.10d) will be reduced to at least 92–90% and possibly as much as 84% instead of 97% or a decrease of 4% from baseline (Bye, et al., 1983; Powers, et al., 1993).

What causes EIH? There is evidence that a relative hypoventilation induced by endurance training may be involved if the EIH occurs at moderate submaximal exercise intensities (Prefaut, et al. 2000). However, at higher intensities both theoretical and experimental evidence support an inequality between respiratory ventilation and circulatory perfusion as one reason and a limitation in diffusion as another. In turn, the failure to achieve complete diffusion equilibrium may be related to the faster transit time of red blood cells through the capillary bed of athletes with a highly developed cardiovascular system or mild, transient extravascular water accumulation and edema, which lengthens the diffusion distance from the alveolar membrane to the red blood cells (Powers, et al., 1993; Prefaut, et al., 2000; Segal, 1992). In normal sedentary or moderately trained individuals pulmonary capillary blood volume increases with exercise. This increases the surface area for diffusion and slows down the red blood cell transit time sufficiently to allow complete diffusion and equilibration of the gases. In highly trained athletes, pulmonary capillary blood volume reaches its maximum at relatively low workloads (Segal, 1992). Hence, when these elite athletes continue to increase their workloads and total body circulation, pulmonary capillary volume cannot expand anymore. Instead, blood flow velocity increases and red blood cell transit time decreases. As a result, the red blood cell transit time in elite endurance athletes is estimated to be considerably less than that required for gas equilibration (Wagner, 1991). Thus, EIH may be attributed in part to a

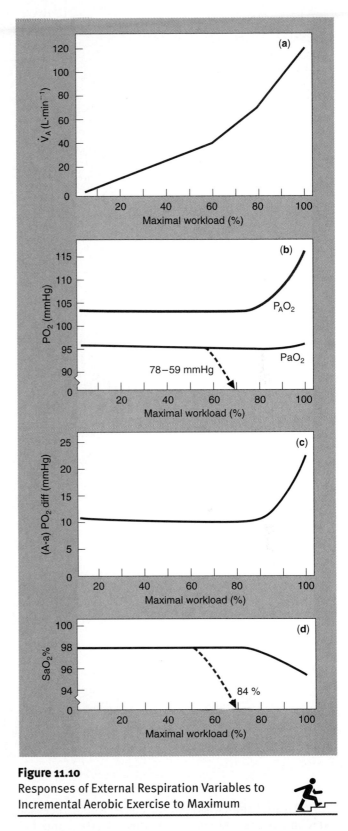

Figure 11.10
Responses of External Respiration Variables to Incremental Aerobic Exercise to Maximum

diffusion limitation as a consequence of this reduced red blood cell transit time. Why EIH occurs in some athletes and not others has not been determined.

Figure 11.11
Responses of Internal Respiration Variables to Incremental Aerobic Exercise to Maximum

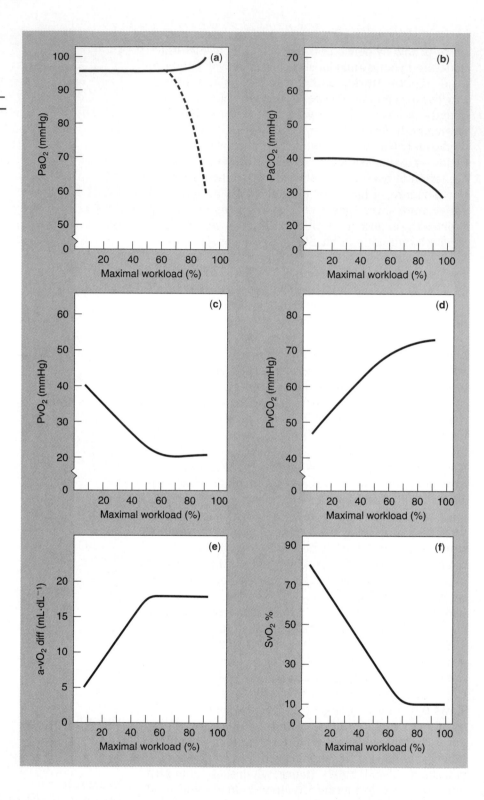

With EIH the (A-a)PO$_2$ diff curve would increase even more than shown in Figure 11.10c, and the SaO$_2$% curve would decline as shown in Figure 11.10d. The (A-a)PO$_2$ diff then becomes a definite indication of lack of efficiency in respiration (Powell, et al., 1964; Shapiro, et al., 1964).

Internal Respiration

The dissociation or release of oxygen reaches its limit during incremental exercise to maximum. At low and moderate workloads, more and more oxygen is released according to the sigmoid-shaped curve in

Figure 11.3. The factors that stimulate the dissociation of oxygen during incremental exercise to maximum are the same as always, but they typically are greater in magnitude; that is, the pressure gradient will be wider, PCO_2 will be higher, pH will be lower, and temperature will be higher as the exercise load increases (Wagner, 1991). It is not possible to extract all the oxygen from the blood perfusing heavily or even maximally exercising muscles. Thus, a muscle PO_2 of 15 mmHg is considered a reasonable lower limit for heavy exercise, with a corresponding maximal pressure gradient of close to 80 mmHg (95 mmHg at the arterial end of the capillary minus 15 mmHg in the muscle tissue). Therefore, some oxygen is always returned in the venous blood. The result is a venous saturation (SvO_2%) of oxygen of approximately 15–35% (Figure 11.11f), which exerts a partial pressure of 15–25 mmHg (Figure 11.11c).

As more oxygen is used to produce more energy, more carbon dioxide is produced. This metabolic carbon dioxide—as well as nonmetabolic carbon dioxide produced in the effort to buffer the lactic acid that accumulates at the higher workloads—brings about the slightly curvilinear rise in $PvCO_2$ shown in Figure 11.11d. Conversely, $PaCO_2$ (Figure 11.11b) is maintained at first and then decreases. This fall in arterial carbon dioxide partial pressure reflects the excess removal of carbon dioxide brought about by alveolar hyperventilation (Dempsey, et al., 1977; Grimby, 1969; Jones, 1975). The a-vO_2 diff (Figure 11.11e) parallels the changes in oxygen dissociation, gradually increasing with the incremental workloads until it can increase no more. It plateaus at approximately 50–60% of the maximal workload (Rowell, 1969; Saltin, 1969).

Thus, even maximal exercise is well within the respiratory reserves for most individuals. Only highly trained endurance athletes whose metabolic and cardiovascular systems have increased greatly exceed their respiratory reserves.

Static Exercise

Static exercise involves the production of force or tension with no mechanical work being done. Therefore, gradations of static exercise are usually expressed relative to an individual's own ability to produce force, called the *maximal voluntary contraction* (MVC), for a given muscle group and held for a specified period of time. This activity is much the same as performing a dynamic exercise at a selected percentage of maximal work, except that in dynamic work the total musculature is generally greater.

In terms of actual energy cost, static exercise is very low in its requirements. However, when static and dynamic exercise require relatively equal amounts of energy, ventilation increases correspondingly. Refer to Figure 5.5. One major difference is apparent, though. At the onset of exercise the initial (0–2 min) three-phase response in $\dot{V}_E$ is absent in static activity. In addition, the a-vO_2 diff either remains the same or decreases slightly during static exercise in contrast to the consistent elevation during dynamic exercise. The maintenance or slight decrease in a-vO_2 diff (Figure 5.5) is undoubtedly related to the occlusion of circulation to the statically contracting muscles. For both $\dot{V}_E$ and a-vO_2 diff, a rebound rise occurs in recovery. In all other aspects the respiratory responses are similar in static exercise and in low-intensity, dynamic endurance exercise. Static exercise does not push the reserve capacity of the respiratory system (Asmussen, 1981).

Table 11.2 summarizes the respiratory responses to exercise that have been discussed in these sections.

Entrainment of Respiration during Exercise

In some, but not all, individuals the performance of rhythmical exercise (such as walking, running, cycling, and rowing) is accompanied by a synchronization of limb movement and breathing frequency called **entrainment** (Bechbache and Duffin, 1977; Caretti, et al., 1992; Clark, et al., 1983; Hill, et al., 1988; Jasinskas, et al., 1980; Kay, et al., 1975; Mahler, et al., 1991). Entrainment means, for example, that an individual always inhales during the recovery phase of rowing and always exhales during the drive portion of the stroke. Or the walker, runner, or cyclist always exhales on the push-off phase of one leg or the other. Unlike swimming, where the coordination of breathing is a function of head placement during any given stroke, and hence a learned response, entrainment occurs without conscious thought.

Subjects who entrain naturally have a lower energy cost during exercise when they entrain but not when they breathe randomly. However, subjects forced to breathe in specific entrainment patterns rather than being allowed to breathe spontaneously do not exhibit any reduction in energy cost nor perceive any decrement in breathing effort with entrained breathing (Maclennan, et al., 1994).

Beginning exercisers often ask how and when they should breathe. The best advice for land activity appears to be to just do whatever comes naturally, be it in a spontaneous or an entrainment pattern. The

> **Entrainment** The synchronization of limb movement and breathing frequency that accompanies rhythmical exercise.

Table 11.2

Respiratory Responses to Exercise*

	Short-Term, Light to Moderate Submaximal Aerobic Exercise	Long-Term, Moderate to Heavy Submaximal Aerobic Exercise[†]	Incremental Aerobic Exercise to Maximum	Static Exercise
Pulmonary Ventilation				
$\dot{V}_E$	Increases rapidly; plateaus	Increases rapidly; plateaus; positive drift	Shows initial rectilinear rise; has two breakpoints	Minor gradual increase; rebound rise in recovery
V_D	Decreases	Decreases	Decreases	All responses the same as for short-term, light to moderate submaximal exercise
V_T	Increases rapidly; plateaus	Increases rapidly; plateaus	Has truncated, inverted U-shaped curve; increases greatly; has incomplete reversal	
f	Slowly increases; plateaus	Increases slowly; plateaus; positive drift	Positive curvilinear rise	
V_D/V_T	Decreases initially; plateaus	Decreases rapidly initially; plateaus	Decreases rapidly initially; levels off at 60% of maximum and is maintained	
External Respiration				
$\dot{V}_A$	Increases rapidly; plateaus	Increases rapidly; plateaus; positive drift	Shows initial rectilinear rise; has two breakpoints	
P_AO_2	Shows no change	Shows no change	Shows no change until approximately 75% of maximum; then positive exponential rise	
PaO_2	Shows no change	Has small U-shaped curve	Shows no change until approximately 75% of maximum; then increases slightly	
$(A-a)PO_2$ diff	Decreases slightly or shows no change (light); increases slightly (moderate)	Has truncated, inverted U-shaped curve; increases rapidly initially; has incomplete reversal	Shows no change until approximately 75% of maximum; then positive exponential rise[‡]	
$SaO_2\%$	Decreases less than 1%; has U-shaped curve	—	—	
Internal Respiration				
$PaCO_2$	Is level; then decreases slightly	Is level; then decreases slightly	Is level; then decreases	
$PvCO_2$	Shows slight linear rise	Shows a gradual linear rise; plateaus	Has sharp rise; levels slightly	
PvO_2	Decreases rapidly; plateaus	Decreases rapidly; plateaus	Decreases sharply; levels off	
$SvO_2\%$	Decreases initially; plateaus	Decreases initially; plateaus	Decreases sharply; never reaches 0	Shows no change or decreases slightly
a-vO_2 diff	Increases rapidly; plateaus	Increases rapidly; plateaus; positive drift	Shows rectilinear rise to 40–60% $\dot{V}O_2$max; plateaus	No change during; rebound rise in recovery

*   Resting values are taken as baseline.

†   The difference between leveling during the short-term, light to moderate and long-term, moderate to heavy submaximal exercise responses is one of magnitude; that is, leveling occurs at a higher value with higher intensities.

‡   Hypoxemia may occur in higher altitudes.

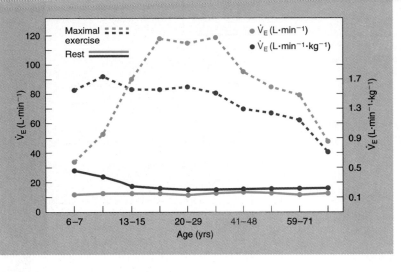

Figure 11.12
Minute Ventilation at Rest and during Maximal Exercise for Males Age 6–76

Source: Based on data from Robinson (1938).

primary exception is weight training. The static component of weight training can cause the **Valsalva maneuver,** a breath-holding action that involves closing of the glottis (which keeps air in the lungs) and contraction of the diaphragm and abdominal musculature. The result is an increase in intra-abdominal pressure and, concomitantly, an abnormal increase in blood pressure. Blood pressures are much lower if breathing is done during the contraction. For this reason it is generally recommended that inhalation occur during the lowering phase of a resistance exercise and exhalation occur during the lifting phase of each repetition (Fleck and Kraemer, 1987).

The Influence of Age and Sex on Respiration at Rest and during Exercise

Children and Adolescents

Lung Volumes and Capacities

In general, the total lung capacity and each of its subdivisions increase in a pattern that deviates only slightly from a straight rectilinear relationship for both males and females as they age from approximately 6 yr to the late teens or early twenties. The forced expiratory volume at one second and maximal voluntary ventilation follow essentially the same in-

cremental pattern in children (P.-O. Åstrand, 1952; P.-O. Åstrand, et al., 1963; Bjure, 1963; Koyal, et al., 1976; Malina and Bouchard, 1991). From birth to approximately age 10, these changes depend largely on the growth and development of the respiratory system. After that, cell proliferation ceases and hypertrophy of existing structures occurs until maturity. Thus, these changes are primarily, but not exclusively, the result of structural enlargement and are strongly related to body height (Bjure, 1963; Johnson and Dempsey, 1991). When the subdivisions of total lung capacity are expressed as a percentage of the total volume, the proportions remain the same from about age 8 to age 20. The anatomical dead space increases in proportion to maturity (Ashley, et al., 1975; Robinson, 1938).

Pulmonary Ventilation

The control of ventilation appears to be similar in children and adults. However, there are some minor differences in minute ventilation and its components across the age span (Zauner, et al., 1989).

Rest The $\dot{V}_E$ at rest is surprisingly consistent regardless of age (Robinson, 1938). Figure 11.12 shows that this value in males varies less than 2 L·min^{-1} from ages 6 to 76. Comparable data are not available for females. When $\dot{V}_E$ is related to body weight, younger boys have a higher $\dot{V}_E$ than older adolescents or adults; but from adolescence to old age there is basically no difference.

Valsalva Maneuver Breath holding that involves closing of the glottis and contraction of the diaphragm and abdominal musculature.

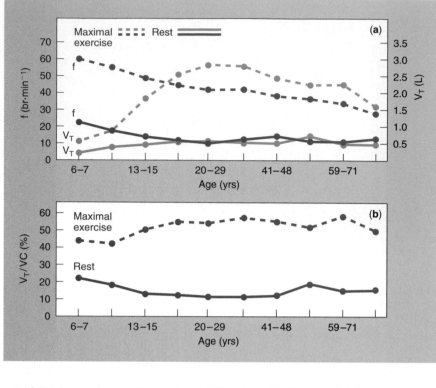

Figure 11.13

Frequency of Breathing, Tidal Volume, and the Percentage of Vital Capacity Used as Tidal Volume at Rest and during Maximal Exercise for Males Age 6–76

Source: Based on data from Robinson (1938).

The remarkably consistent $\dot{V}_E$ is achieved differently by children than by older adolescents and adults. Figure 11.13a shows that breathing frequency is higher and tidal volume lower in youngsters than in older adolescents and adults. From approximately the midteen years until old age, the breathing frequency stabilizes at 10–15 br·min^{-1}, and tidal volume stabilizes at about 500 mL in males (Malina and Bouchard, 1991; Robinson, 1938). Younger children use a higher portion of their vital capacity as a tidal volume than do older adolescents and young adults (Figure 11.13b).

Submaximal Exercise Children's and adolescents' respiratory responses to exercise are quite similar to those of adults, with only some quantitative differences. Thus, $\dot{V}_E$ will rise in response to greater oxygen needs. However, the higher $\dot{V}_E$ in relation to body weight seen at rest is maintained, as is the variation in how $\dot{V}_E$ is obtained; that is, children exhibit a higher breathing frequency and lower tidal volume at any given submaximal load than adults. They also respond with a higher $\dot{V}_E$ in relation to body weight at an equal workload. These differences are considered negative, indicating a wasteful ventilation, and

gradually disappear by late adolescence (Bar-Or, 1983; Robinson, 1938; Rowland, et al., 1987; Rowland and Green, 1988). The differences are exemplified for 11-yr-old girls and boys in comparison to 29-yr-old adults in Figures 11.14a and Figure 11.14b (Rowland, et al., 1987; Rowland and Green, 1988). The speeds are different for the males and females, so direct comparison between the sexes cannot be made. In addition to the differences shown in Figure 11.14, younger children use a marginally lower proportion of their vital capacity during submaximal exercise than do adults.

During prolonged submaximal exercise children and adolescents exhibit the same ventilatory drift as adults. There is nothing in the respiratory response to prolonged exercise that would indicate that children are not suited for such activity (Malina and Bouchard, 1991).

Maximal Exercise In general, children's responses to maximal exercise parallel the differences seen at rest and during submaximal work; that is, the older the child, the higher the $\dot{V}_E$ that can be achieved in absolute terms. The $\dot{V}_E$ in relation to body weight gradually declines from about age 7 until adulthood is

Figure 11.14

Pulmonary Ventilation Responses to Submaximal Exercise in Male and Female Children and Adults

Females: Mean age child = 11.3 yr; adult = 28.7 yr, treadmill speed = 7.3 kph (122 m·min⁻¹).

Males: Mean age child = 11.6 yr; adult = 29.2 yr, treadmill speed = 9.6 kph (160 m·min⁻¹).

Sources: Based on data from (a) Rowland & Green (1988) and (b) Rowland, et al. (1987).

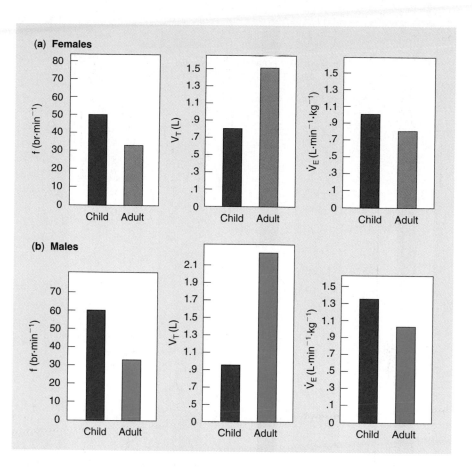

achieved at about 20 years of age, although in 4- to 6-yr-olds this value is comparable to that of young adults (Figure 11.15a) (P.-O. Åstrand, 1952; P.-O. Åstrand, et al., 1963; Fahey, et al., 1979; Krahenbuhl, et al., 1985; Robinson, 1938; Rowland, 1990; Rowland and Green, 1988). Breathing frequency decreases consistently from the youngest children tested to approximately age 20 while tidal volume shows a steady rise over the same time span (Figure 11.15b). The percentage of vital capacity used as tidal volume rises slightly from childhood to young adulthood.

Children exhibit the ventilatory breakpoints during incremental exercise to maximum. However, the breakpoints appear earlier, at lower workloads, than they do for either adolescents or adults. The physiological mechanisms for the ventilatory breakpoints in children are as unclear as they are for adults (Bar-Or, 1983; Rowland and Green, 1988).

External and Internal Respiration

Little is known about the changes in gas exchange and transport that occur during normal growth and maturation. The relatively higher breathing frequency and lower tidal volume of children in relation to adolescents and adults, at rest and during exercise, seem to be offset by their smaller anatomical dead space. Consequently, alveolar ventilation is more than adequate at all values of $\dot{V}_E$ (Bar-Or, 1983; Malina and Bouchard, 1991; Zauner, et al., 1989).

Pulmonary diffusion during exercise does not appear to differ by age. Likewise, there do not appear to be any meaningful aging trends for P_AO_2, PaO_2, or $(A\text{-}a)PO_2$ diff at rest or during exercise. However, PaO_2 decreases slightly and the $(A\text{-}a)PO_2$ diff increases slightly as children mature to adulthood (Bar-Or, 1983; Eriksson, 1972; Robinson, 1938). As a consequence, the percent saturation of arterial blood is also relatively constant across the age span (Robinson, 1938).

The arteriovenous oxygen differences are also very similar at both rest and maximal exercise levels from childhood to maturity. If anything, children may be able to extract about 5% more oxygen during maximal exercise than adults (Eriksson, 1973). Alveolar and arterial oxygen partial pressure levels are slightly lower in young children than in adolescents or adults, possibly reflecting the child's relative hyperventilation (Zauner, et al., 1989).

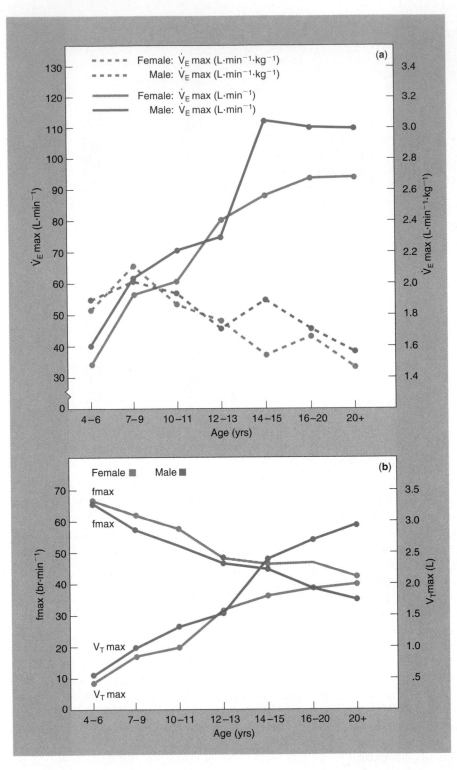

Figure 11.15
Pulmonary Ventilation Responses
to Maximal Treadmill Exercise
as Children Age to Adulthood
for Males and Females

Source: Based on data from P.-O. Åstrand (1952).

The Elderly

Lung Volumes and Capacities

The effect of aging on total lung capacity is controversial. There is evidence that total lung capacity both decreases and stays the same in individuals over the age of 50 (Berglund, et al., 1963; Jain and Gupta, 1974a, 1974b; Johnson and Dempsey, 1991; Kenney, 1982; Stanescu, et al., 1974; Storstein and Voll, 1974). However, research has firmly established that vital capacity and inspiratory capacity decrease with age and that residual volume and functional residual capacity increase, thus changing the percentage of total volume that each occupy (I. Åstrand, 1960;

Focus on Application

✳ Side Stitches

Ever wonder why you sometimes get a stitch in your side when you run, even though you never get that type of side pain swimming or cycling? Two theories have been put forth to explain this phenomenon. Both involve the diaphragm. The first theory posits a change in blood flow as the cause. In this scenario, blood is thought to be shunted away from the diaphragm and other respiratory muscles to the stomach, intestines, and limb muscles. This creates an ischemic pain. The second theory posits mechanical pull as the cause. According to this theory, stitches result from foot impact with the ground: the bouncing of the body causes the peritoneal ligaments from the viscera to pull on the diaphragm, causing pain. This would explain why running, with its pounding movements, is associated with stitches, but not swimming or cycling, in which movement is cushioned.

Experimental evidence has been minimal, but Plunkett and Hopkins (1999) devised a study in which they induced side stitches by having test subjects ingest fluids of varying digestibility. They reasoned that if decreased blood flow were the primary cause, the stitches should develop slowly, with an intensity that related directly to the digestibility of the fluid, and remain despite any maneuvers performed by the subject aimed at reducing the tugging of the peritoneal ligaments. Conversely, if the cause were ligamentous tugging, the stitches should occur rapidly with the ingestion of a large amount of fluid, should remain high with fluids that are not digested, and be alleviated when maneuvers were performed that decreased the pull of the peritoneal ligaments. The results of their study supported the theory that stitches arise when a fluid-engorged stomach tugs on visceral ligaments attached to the diaphragm.

Several practical applications of this research have been suggested. To avoid a side stitch, exercisers should adhere to the following recommendations:

1. Don't exercise immediately after eating a big meal or ingesting a large (close to 1 L) drink. Wait 2–3 hours.
2. When drinking during exercise, take small amounts (200–400 mL) frequently (at 15- to 30-min intervals) rather than a single large drink at a rest stop or aid station.
3. When running downhill, try to keep your breathing regular and your footfalls light.

To deal with a stitch when it occurs:

1. Push in at the location of the pain with your hand, bend forward, and tighten the abdominal muscles.
2. Breathe more deeply to move more air into the lungs at the beginning of each breath, but don't try to force more air out at the end of each breath.
3. Breathe out through pursed lips. This will contract the abdominals.
4. If you experience side stitches frequently, try wearing a light, wide belt around your waist that can be tightened when necessary.   ✳

Source:
Plunkett (1999).

P.-O. Åstrand, 1952; Ericsson and Irnell, 1974; Slonim and Hamilton, 1976; Stanescu, et al., 1974; Turner, et al., 1968). For example, the ratio of residual volume to total lung capacity doubles from about 15–30% in the elderly (Comroe, 1965; Johnson and Dempsey, 1991).

The forced expiratory volume in 1 sec (FEV_1) and maximal voluntary ventilation decline steadily after approximately age 35 in both males and females (Ashley, et al., 1975; Ericsson and Irnell, 1974; Shepard, 1978; Slonim and Hamilton, 1976; Stanescu, et al., 1974). These declines are brought about by a combination of structural and mechanical changes in the respiratory system. These changes include (1) a decrease in the elastic recoil of the lung tissue; (2) a stiffening of the thoracic cage, which decreases chest mobility, necessitating a greater reliance on the diaphragm; (3) a decrease in the intervertebral spaces, which in turn decreases height and changes the shape of the thoracic cavity; (4) losses in respiratory muscle force and velocity of contraction. Of all these changes, the loss of elastic recoil appears to be the most important (Johnson and Dempsey, 1991; Turner, et al., 1968).

Pulmonary Ventilation

Rest Resting $\dot{V}_E$ (Figure 11.12) and its components V_T and f (Figure 11.13a) are remarkably consistent across the entire age span. However, at rest the percentage of vital capacity used as V_T does show a very slight U-shaped curve (Figure 11.13b); that is, both young children and the elderly use slightly more of their vital capacity for V_T at rest than do young adults (Robinson, 1938).

Submaximal Exercise $\dot{V}_E$ rises in the elderly in response to increased energy needs. As for young adults, this increase is accomplished mainly by an increase in V_T at lighter workloads and then by an increased frequency of breathing, if needed. Like children, the elderly seem to have an exaggerated response in $\dot{V}_E$ when compared with younger adults. That is, the absolute $\dot{V}_E$ is higher at any given workload in the elderly than in young adults. Because the vital capacity decreases with age and V_T remains fairly stable, V_T represents a higher percentage of the elderly's vital capacity (I. Åstrand, 1960; P.-O. Åstrand, 1952; Davies, 1972; DeVries and Adams, 1972; Robinson, 1938; Shepard, 1978).

Maximal Exercise With aging both the ability to exercise maximally and the ability to process air decline. The decrement in pulmonary function contributes to the decline in work capacity but probably simply parallels the changes in circulation, metabolism, and muscle function that are also occurring.

The highest $\dot{V}_E$ values are typically seen in young adults, and these may decline by almost half by the seventh decade of life (Figure 11.12). This decline is evident both in absolute values ($\dot{V}_E$ in liters per minute) and in values related to body weight ($\dot{V}_E$ in liters per kilogram per minute). Most of this decline is brought about by a reduction in tidal volume, although maximal breathing frequency does decrease slightly.

The percentage of vital capacity used during maximal work is relatively stable with age from young adulthood on. However, the dead space–to–tidal volume ratio is consistently 15–20% higher in older adults than in younger adults (Robinson, 1938). The ventilatory breakpoints occur at lower absolute and relative workloads in older adults than in younger adults (Shepard, 1978).

External Respiration

Rest The loss of elastic recoil in the lungs not only affects the static and dynamic lung volumes but also influences the distribution of air in the lungs. Thus, ventilation may not be preferentially directed to the base of the lung in the upright posture at rest, although the majority of blood flow is still directed there. Thus, there may be an imbalance between alveolar ventilation and pulmonary perfusion (Johnson and Dempsey, 1991).

In addition, structural changes in the aging lung lead to a decrease in alveolar capillary surface area, which in turn means a decrease in diffusion capacity (Donevan, et al., 1959; Johnson and Dempsey, 1991). Furthermore, pulmonary capillary blood volume decreases owing to a stiffening of both pulmonary arteries and capillaries. The cumulative effects of these changes are a decrease in arterial oxygen partial pressure, but not alveolar, and a widening of the alveolar–to–arterial oxygen difference, although the changes are neither inevitable nor large. The saturation of hemoglobin with oxygen in arterial blood declines about 2–3% from age 10 to age 70 (Robinson, 1938; Shepard, 1978).

Exercise During exercise the increased ventilation that is required results in a more homogeneous distribution of ventilation in the lungs. Although the decreases noted at rest in diffusion surface and pulmonary capillary blood volume remain, the matching of ventilation and perfusion improves during exercise as more of the lung is used. The available reserve is sufficient to meet the demands for oxygen transport even to maximal exercise levels.

Nevertheless, alveolar ventilation is a smaller portion of minute ventilation in older adults than in younger adults. This change does indicate a slightly decreased efficiency of respiration; but general arterial hypoxemia is prevented, and carbon dioxide elimination is adequate. That is, the arterial oxygen and carbon dioxide partial pressures are maintained within narrow limits and are similar to those for younger adults. The alveolar–to–arterial oxygen differences are more variable in the elderly than in younger adults but, on average, are only slightly wider than the usual mean values for younger individuals (Johnson and Dempsey, 1991; Robinson, 1938; Shepard, 1978).

Internal Respiration

At rest and at any given submaximal level of exercise the arteriovenous oxygen difference is greater in older adults than in younger adults. Thus, venous saturation of oxyhemoglobin is lower. Conversely, at maximal exercise the arteriovenous oxygen difference is lower in the elderly than in younger individuals. Maximal values average 14–15 $mL \cdot dL^{-1}$ in older adults but average 15–20 $mL \cdot dL^{-1}$ in younger adults. Some of these changes in the arteriovenous oxygen difference can be attributed to a shift in the oxygen dissociation curve to the left, which makes the release of oxygen to the tissues more difficult (Kenney, 1982; Shepard, 1978). Refer to Figure 11.3 to see this effect.

Male-Female Respiratory Differences

Lung Volumes and Capacities

Values for total lung capacity and each of its subdivisions are lower for females than males across the entire age span, with the possible exception of around 12–13 yr, when girls have had their pubertal growth spurt and boys have not. These differences are carried over into the dynamic measurements of maximal voluntary ventilation and forced expiratory volume in 1 sec. Part of these differences can be attributed in general to the smaller size of the female. However, even prorating values according to height, weight, or surface area does not totally eliminate the difference (P.-O. Åstrand, 1952; Comroe, 1965; Ferris, et al., 1965).

Pulmonary Ventilation

At rest there is no consistent difference in breathing frequency between males and females (Malina and Bouchard, 1991). However, at the same submaximal ventilation females typically display a higher breathing frequency and a lower tidal volume than males. This pattern is maintained at maximal exercise (Saris, et al., 1985). Also, at maximal exercise males exhibit higher minute ventilation at all ages than females, although these differences are narrowed considerably when prorated by body weight (I. Åstrand, 1960; P.-O. Åstrand, 1952). Figures 11.15a and 11.15b show these differences for children and young adults.

External and Internal Respiration

Data to compare males and females are unavailable for most of the external and internal respiratory measures. The arteriovenous oxygen difference has been measured at rest and during submaximal and maximal exercise, but the results show little consistency (Åstrand, et al., 1964; Becklake, et al., 1965; Zwiren, et al., 1983).

Respiratory Training Adaptations

No training principles or guidelines are presented for the respiratory system because training specifically directed toward this system is very rare in nondiseased individuals. What few training adaptations occur do so as a by-product of training for cardiovascular and/or metabolic improvement. Applications of the training principles are presented for these systems in their respective units. The few training adaptations of the respiratory system follow.

Lung Volumes and Capacities

Whether the chronic but intermittent elevations in respiratory demand that occur with physical training actually change the lung itself is unknown. Studies in which the training modality is land based (running, cycling, wrestling, and the like) have found no consistent significant changes in total lung capacity, vital capacity, residual volume, functional residual capacity, or inspiratory capacity in either males or females of any age; nor have they found any differences favoring athletes over nonathletes (Bachman and Horvath, 1968; Cordain, et al., 1990; Dempsey and Fregosi, 1985; Eriksson, 1972; Kaufmann, et al., 1974; Niinimaa and Shepard, 1978; Reuschlein, et al., 1968; Saltin, et al., 1968). Studies where the activities are water based (swimming and scuba diving), however, have shown that swimmers have higher volumes and capacities than both land-based athletes and nonathletes (Cordain, et al., 1990; Leith and Bradley, 1976). In addition, swim training studies have demonstrated increases in total lung capacity and vital capacity in both children and young adults. Similar generalizations can be made for the dynamic measures of forced expiratory volume in 1 sec and maximal voluntary ventilation (Andrew, et al., 1972; Bachman and Horvath, 1968; Clanton, et al., 1987; Vaccaro and Clarke, 1978; Walsh and Banister, 1988).

Precisely why swimmers, and not land-based athletes, show improvements in static and dynamic lung volumes is not known. However, swimmers in all but the backstroke are breathing against the resistance of water in a restricted breathing pattern with repeated expansion of the lungs to total lung capacity. Swimming also takes place with the body in a horizontal position, and this posture is optimal for perfusion of the lung and diffusion of respiratory gases (Cordain and Stager, 1988; Mostyn, et al., 1963).

Pulmonary Ventilation

Changes in $\dot{V}_E$ are the primary and most consistent adaptations seen in the respiratory system as a result of endurance training. Although $\dot{V}_E$ itself does not change at rest, a shift occurs in its components: V_T increases, and f decreases. Not only is this shift maintained during submaximal work, but also the $\dot{V}_E$ is lower as a result of the training. At maximal work $\dot{V}_E$ is higher after training than before, accompanying the ability to do more work. The major component change is an increase in f, but V_T will increase as well (Dempsey, et al., 1977; Mahler, et al., 1991; Rasmussen, et al., 1975; Reid and Thomson, 1985; Whipp, 1977; Wilmore, et al., 1970). In addition, the capacity for sustaining high levels of voluntary ventilation is

Table 11.3
Respiratory Training Adaptations

	Rest	Submaximal Exercise	Maximal Exercise
Lung volumes and capacities	Show no changes from land-based activities; swimming and diving show increases, especially in total lung capacity and vital capacity	—	—
Pulmonary ventilation			
$\dot{V}_E$	Shows no change	Decreases	Increases
V_T	Increases	Increases	Increases
f	Decreases	Decreases	Increases
External respiration, (A-a)PO_2 diff	Shows no change	Decreases	Shows no change
Internal respiration, $PvCO_2$	—	Decreases	—
Oxygen dissociation curve	—	Curve shifts to the right	Curve shifts to the right
a-vO_2 diff	Shows no change in children; increases in young adults	Shows no change in children; inconsistent changes in adults	Shows no change in children; increases in young adults

improved, reflecting an increase in both the strength and the endurance of the respiratory muscles (Krahenbuhl, et al., 1985; Robinson and Kjeldgaard, 1992).

These adaptations are seen within the first 6–10 weeks of a training program and reverse just as quickly upon detraining (Reid and Thomson, 1985). They occur as a result of both land- and water-based activities across the entire age span (Bar-Or, 1983; Fringer and Stull, 1974; Pollock, et al., 1969; Seals, et al., 1984; Zauner and Benson, 1981; Zauner, et al., 1989). The ventilatory thresholds shift to a higher workload as a result of training in children and in adults (Haffor, et al., 1990; Paterson, et al., 1987).

External and Internal Respiration

In a healthy individual of any age and either sex, gas exchange varies little as a result of training (Reid and Thomson, 1985). The diffusion capacity has been reported to be higher in elite swimmers (Comroe, 1965; Magel and Andersen, 1969; Mostyn, et al., 1963; Vaccaro, et al., 1977) and runners (Kaufmann, et al., 1974), but it does not consistently increase at either submaximal or maximal work as a result of training (Saltin, et al., 1968). This observed result may be an example of genetic selection for specific athletes (Comroe, 1965; Dempsey, 1986; Dempsey, et al., 1977; Niinimaa and Shepard, 1978; Reuschlein, et al., 1968; Vaccaro and Clarke, 1978; Wagner, 1991). Even in studies where diffusing capacity has shown an increase, it is most likely due to circulatory changes (an increase in pulmonary capillary volume) and not to any pulmonary membrane change per se.

Arterial values of pH and PCO_2 do not change with training, but venous pH levels increase (become less acidic) and PCO_2 values decrease (Rasmussen, et al., 1975) during the same submaximal exercise. The alveolar–to–arterial oxygen pressure difference decreases at submaximal workloads as a result of training, indicating greater efficiency (Saltin, et al., 1968). Training may also cause the oxygen dissociation curve to shift to the right, facilitating the release of oxygen from the blood into the muscle tissue (Rasmussen, et al., 1975).

In children neither the submaximal nor maximal arteriovenous oxygen difference adapts as a result of training (Bar-Or, 1983; Eriksson, 1973). In young adults the arteriovenous oxygen difference increases at rest (Clausen, 1977; Saltin, et al., 1968) and at maximal exercise as a result of training (Blomqvist and Saltin, 1983; Coyle, et al., 1984; Saltin, et al., 1968). Both increases and decreases in the arteriovenous oxygen difference have been found during submaximal exercise as a result of endurance training (Clausen, 1977; Ekelund, 1967; Ekelund and Holmgren, 1967; Saltin, et al., 1968). Changes in middle-aged and elderly adults are less likely than in younger adults (Green and Crouse, 1993; Saltin, 1969). None of the other partial pressure or saturation variables change significantly and/or consistently with training.

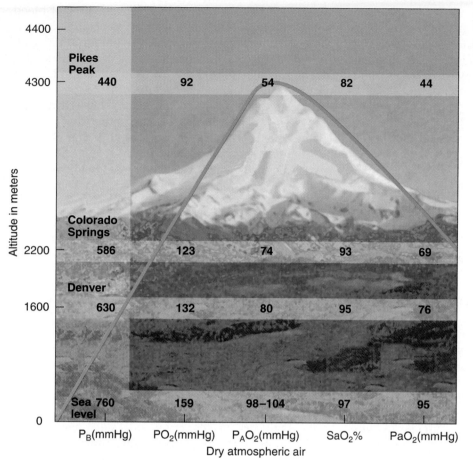

Figure 11.16
The Impact of Altitude on External Respiration

		P_B(mmHg)	PO_2(mmHg)	P_AO_2(mmHg)	SaO_2%	PaO_2(mmHg)
4300	Pikes Peak	440	92	54	82	44
2200	Colorado Springs	586	123	74	93	69
1600	Denver	630	132	80	95	76
0	Sea level	760	159	98–104	97	95

Altitude in meters

Dry atmospheric air

Table 11.3 summarizes the respiratory training adaptations discussed in this section.

Why Are There So Few Respiratory Adaptations to Exercise Training?

The most commonly accepted answer to the question of why there are so few respiratory adaptations to exercise training is that the pulmonary system is endowed with a tremendous reserve capacity that is more than sufficient to meet the demands of even very heavy physical exercise. Thus, when physical training is undertaken, the various components of the respiratory system are not stressed to any significant limits and so do not need to change. At the same time, the cardiovascular and metabolic capacities of muscle are being stressed and do respond by adapting. The adaptations in these systems may ultimately exceed the capability of the respiratory system, as seen in highly trained athletes with exercise-induced hypoxemia. Otherwise, there is no need for great changes in the respiratory system in the normal healthy individual (Dempsey, 1986; Dempsey, et al., 1977).

Special Considerations
The Impact of Altitude on Exercise and Training

The effects of altitude were alluded to several times in Chapter 10. It is time now to deal more directly with the effects of both acute and chronic exposure to altitude and with the issue of whether participation in altitude training can improve athletic performance. Referring back to Table 10.1 and Equation 10.4 may be helpful in comprehending the following discussion.

The percentage of oxygen in air remains constant at 20.93% to an altitude of 100,000 m (328,083 ft) (Clausen, 1977). However, the barometric pressure (P_B) decreases exponentially with an increase in altitude. Thus, air has a lower density (that is, fewer particles per volume) at higher altitudes because the gas has expanded. For instance, at Denver (1600 m, or 5280 ft) P_B is 630 mmHg, and at Colorado Springs (2300 m, or 7590 ft) P_B is 586 mmHg (Figure 11.16). Therefore, the oxygen partial pressure (PO_2) in atmospheric air is reduced. At Denver the PO_2 is 132 mmHg (630 mmHg × 0.2093), and at Colorado Springs it is 123 mmHg (586 mmHg × 0.2093), as

compared to 159 mmHg at sea level (760 mmHg ×
0.2093). Because the partial pressure of the inspired
oxygen decreases with altitude, the alveolar oxygen
partial pressure P_AO_2 also decreases to 80 mmHg and
74 mmHg, respectively, at Denver and Colorado
Springs:

$$[(630 \text{ mmHg}) - (47 \text{ mmHg})] \times (.137 \text{ O}_2) = 80 \text{ mmHg};$$
$$[(586 \text{ mmHg}) - (47 \text{ mmHg})] \times (.137 \text{ O}_2) = 74 \text{ mmHg}$$

This decrease in P_AO_2 reduces the pressure gradient between the returning venous blood (PvO_2) and
the alveoli, resulting in a lower percent saturation
($SaO_2\%$) and arterial partial pressure (PaO_2):

$$80 \text{ mmHg} \times .95 = PaO_2 \text{ of 76 mmHg at Denver};$$
$$74 \text{ mmHg} \times .93 = PaO_2 \text{ of 69 mmHg at}$$
Colorado Springs

This decrement in PaO_2 stimulates an increase in
$\dot{V}_E$ via the aortic and carotid body chemoreceptors, as
compensation to provide more oxygen for alveolar ventilation. The initial increase in $\dot{V}_E$ is *hyperventilation,*
defined as an increase in pulmonary ventilation that
exceeds metabolic requirements, and is achieved
primarily by an increase in respiratory frequency.
Climbers on Mount Everest reportedly averaged
62 br·min^{-1} and a $\dot{V}_E$ of 207 L·min^{-1}, obviously very
high values (Armstrong, 2000). Altitude-induced hyperventilation increases the amount of carbon dioxide
exhaled. In turn, the increased exhalation of carbon
dioxide decreases alveolar and arterial carbon dioxide
partial pressure and increases pH. The decrease in
percent saturation ($SaO_2\%$) and the other resultant
changes at Denver and Colorado Springs are minimal,
perhaps 2–5% because of the flatness of the oxygen dissociation curve (Figure 10.13) in that range. However,
at the top of Pikes Peak (4300 m, or 14,100 ft) $SaO_2\%$ is
82%, and the full effect of altitude is seen (Hannon,
1978; Haymes and Wells, 1986; Ratzin Jackson and
Sharkey, 1988). Table 10.1 and Figure 11.16 show the
external respiration values. The $SaO_2\%$ is approximately 15% less at Pikes Peak than at sea level.

Within the red blood cells a chemical called
2,3-diphosphoglycerate (2,3-DPG) increases at altitude. The effect of the increase in 2,3-DPG is the same
as an increase in carbon dioxide partial pressure, hydrogen ion concentration, and body temperature on
the oxygen dissociation curve (Figure 11.3). That is, it
causes a shift of the oxygen dissociation curve to the
right, thus offsetting the shift to the left (and decreased release of oxygen) that would occur owing to
the decrement in carbon dioxide partial pressure and
increase in pH.

Within two days of altitude exposure hemoglobin
concentration increases, which in turn increases the

amount of oxygen transported per deciliter of blood.
Unfortunately, the hemoglobin concentration increases only because total blood volume initially decreases. That is, the same number of red blood cells
are simply distributed in a smaller volume of blood, a
process called *hemoconcentration.* The blood volume
loss reflects a total body water loss through the kidneys and through increased respiratory evaporation
owing to the compensatory hyperventilation. Such hemoconcentration increases the viscosity of the blood,
which means increased resistance to blood flow. In an
attempt to maintain blood flow, heart rate increases
(Haymes and Wells, 1986; Ratzin Jackson and
Sharkey, 1988).

These changes are compounded during exercise.
The normal exercise increase in diffusion capacity
does not exceed that at sea level, because arterial oxygen partial pressure is decreased and venous oxygen
partial pressure remains the same. As a result, the
normal exercise increase in arteriovenous oxygen difference is not as great at altitude as it is at sea level.

Although the individual probably does not perceive any of the aforementioned changes, except possibly hyperventilation, alterations can also occur in
sensory acuity (vision and hearing), motor skills,
memory, and mood swings to irritability. Dehydration
and weight loss are common, as is sleep disturbance.
In addition, some unpleasant sensations may mark
the onset of altitude sickness. These sensations include the loss of appetite, dizziness, fatigue, nausea,
vomiting, and weakness (Guyton, 1986; Haymes and
Wells, 1986).

The acute effects of altitude are experienced most
directly in terms of the intensity at which an aerobic
endurance activity can be maintained. The higher the
altitude, the greater the impact and the sooner fatigue
is felt. Maximal aerobic power declines, and the intensity at which any endurance event can be performed will be lower, as will the ability to sustain that
activity at higher elevations. This result is true for all
individuals at all age levels, although high-altitude
mountain climbers are impacted the most. Sprints
and other muscular strength, muscular endurance,
and power events do not appear to be disadvantaged
from a physiological standpoint and may even be enhanced because of a reduction in air resistance at
higher elevations (Haymes and Wells, 1986; Ratzin
Jackson and Sharkey, 1988).

Teachers giving fitness tests to students can adjust the cardiovascular endurance items detailed in
Chapter 12 as follows:

1200–2270 m (4000–7500 ft)	7.5%
2300–2730 m (7600–9000 ft)	10.0%
2750–3640 m (9100–12,000 ft)	15.0%

This adjustment would involve either adding time to do the 1-mi run or decreasing the number of laps needed to meet the criterion score for the PACER (Cooper, 1970; Haymes and Wells, 1986). For example, the criterion-referenced standard (minimally acceptable score) for an 11-yr-old boy in the 1-mi run is 11:00. To increase this acceptable time to account for the altitude at Denver (1600 m, or 5280 ft), we can convert the target time to seconds and multiply by 0.075:

$$[(11 \text{ min}) \times (60 \text{ sec·min}^{-1})] \times 0.075$$
$$= 660 \text{ sec} \times 0.075$$
$$= 49.5$$

Thus, an acceptable score might be 11:50 instead of 11:00. Similarly, for the PACER the criterion-referenced standard for a 16-yr-old girl is 32 laps. To account for altitude, we calculate $32 \times 0.075 = 2.4$. Therefore, the criterion target would be 30 laps, not 32 laps.

Athletes who wish to compete at altitude have two choices in attempting to minimize the adverse environmental effects. The first is to arrive at the altitude site 12–18 hr prior to the activity. This is what many collegiate and some professional teams do, even at the moderate altitudes where they compete. Although this strategy does not prevent the effects of altitude, it does minimize the chances that acute altitude sickness will impair performance (Haymes and Wells, 1986; Ratzin Jackson and Sharkey, 1988; Weston, et al., 2001).

The second choice is to train at the same altitude as the eventual competition. During this time the athletes can acclimatize somewhat to the altitude. The minimum amount of time required is 10–20 days, but full acclimatization can take at least a year, and even then the former sea-level resident will not be as physiologically adapted as the individual who was born and has always lived at altitude.

Acclimatization involves subtle but important shifts in the initial attempts of adjusting to the lower oxygen partial pressure. That is, hemoconcentration continues, but the cause shifts from being a decrease in plasma volume with no change in red blood cell count to an increase in both red blood cells under the influence of the hormone erythropoietin (EPO) and blood volume mediated by aldosterone and the antidiuretic hormone (Guyton, 1986). Likewise, hyperventilation is maintained, but instead of an increased frequency of breathing, an increase in tidal volume occurs. Increased tidal volume allows a more effective pulmonary gas exchange. Arterial carbon dioxide partial pressure remains depressed, but arterial oxygen partial pressure increases somewhat as acclimation proceeds (Adams, et al., 1975; Grover, 1978; Guy-

ton, 1986; Hannon, 1978; Haymes and Wells, 1986; Ratzin Jackson and Sharkey, 1988). Females seem to acclimatize to altitude more readily than do males (Grover, 1978).

Unfortunately, these processes of acclimatization do not completely counteract the fundamental hypoxic stress of altitude. Thus, individuals training at altitude cannot train at the same level of intensity for the same period of time as they could at sea level. A reduction of training intensity to 40% of that at sea level may be necessary initially and can usually only be regained up to 75% of sea level intensity (Armstrong, 2000). Highly trained athletes (especially those prone to exercise-induced hypoxemia) are likely to benefit the least from altitude training. Untrained individuals may still be doing more than before, and reap the benefits of the training.

Two patterns have emerged for combining acclimatization and exercise training at altitude. The first pattern or strategy is used primarily by mountaineers and is called "work (climb) high, sleep low." Climbers traditionally establish a series of camp sites, each at a higher altitude than the previous one. During the day, they carry supplies up to the higher camp (camp 2) and work in that vicinity, but then descend at night to camp 1 to sleep. This pattern continues for days or weeks, at which time the climbers reestablish themselves between the old high camp (camp 2) and a new higher location (camp 3) until they are in position for the final ascent of the summit.

The second strategy is to "live high, train low" (Koistinen, et al., 2000; Levine and Stray-Gundersen, 1997). The idea here is to avoid the detrimental effects of altitude (having to train at a greatly reduced exercise intensity with the concomitant detraining effects), while at the same time reaping the benefits of altitude acclimatization, which can improve oxygen-carrying capacity and dissociation. For an example of a study that evaluated this promising, relatively new approach, refer to the Focus on Research box on page 310. As is often the case with any training technique, individual reactions to "living high, training low" can vary widely, and some individuals will not respond at all.

Although living high and training low would seem to simply require a mountain with a nearby accessible valley, such geographical features can be difficult to find and access in practice. One other option that is being used experimentally is a nitrogen house. In this situation, an airtight dwelling is flushed with air diluted with nitrogen. This reduces the oxygen content from 20.93% to approximately 15% and simulates altitude. To train low, the athletes simply leave the house (Koistinen, et al., 2000). A much less costly option that needs further research is to use a nitrogen

Focus on Research

Live High, Train Low

Levine, B. D., & J. Stray-Gundersen: "Living high—training low": Effect of moderate-altitude acclimatization with low-altitude training on performance. *Journal of Applied Physiology.* 83(1): 102–112 (1997).

This study was designed to test the hypothesis that acclimation to living at moderate altitude (2500 m, 8260 ft) combined with training at low altitude (1250 m, 4125 ft) (high-low condition) would improve sea-level (5000 m, 3.1 mi) performance in already well-conditioned athletes more than either both living and training at high altitude (2500–2700 m, 8260–8900 ft), called high-high condition, or sea level, called low-low control condition.

Thirty-nine athletes completed 2 wk of sea-level familiarization and 4 wk of sea-level training prior to being randomized into three groups of 13 athletes (nine males and four females in each group) for 4 wk of high- or low-altitude or sea-level training and living. Training was periodized and tapered before all tests for all groups. As expected, those training at high altitude did so at a slower speed and lower percentage of maximal oxygen uptake than those at sea level. However, the training intensity of the low-altitude training group was reduced by only 6% compared with the sea-level group, whereas that of the high-altitude training group was reduced by 18.5%. Both groups that lived at moderate altitude significantly increased red blood cell mass by 9% and $\dot{V}O_2$max by 5%, while the sea-level group showed neither change. Arteriovenous oxygen difference (a-vO_2 diff) was significantly higher for both altitude groups at velocities near 5000-m run time trial speeds after altitude training. Velocity at $\dot{V}O_2$max increased only for the high-low group. The only group that significantly improved its 5000-m time was the high-low group, by an average of 13.4 ± 10 sec. This improvement persisted for at least 3 wk after the return from altitude when testing was stopped.

These results suggest that an improvement in sea-level performance from altitude training is possible if athletes live at moderate altitude but train at lower levels that permit maintaining a high training intensity.

---

tent. The tent is simply set up on any bed or floor and can be used by the individual for resting and sleeping in his or her own home.

Despite the drawbacks, athletes who train at altitude usually see positive results from that training if the competition is at the same altitude and occurs directly following the training period. The effect of altitude training on later sea-level maximal performance is highly controversial, showing large individual variations. In general, there does not appear to be any advantage to altitude training over that gained from the exercise training itself; that is, the response to the two stressors is not additive (Adams, et al., 1975; Haymes and Wells, 1986).

If an individual chooses to train at moderate altitude, the following guidelines are suggested:

1. Spend a minimum of 2 and a maximum of 4 weeks at altitude at any one time.

2. If both living and training occur at high altitude, maintain the same intensity of exertion that would be used at sea level, but decrease the duration and increase the frequency.

3. Lengthen rest periods.

4. Replace fluids even to the point of hyperhydration (Ratzin Jackson and Sharkey, 1988). Eat a high-calorie, high-carbohydrate diet.

Hypoxic Swim Training

Swimmers have tried their own version of altitude training, called *hypoxic training* or *controlled-frequency breathing.* The general assumption is that if a swimmer inhales once every third, fifth, or seventh arm stroke, instead of every other arm stroke, then the reduced volume of air taken in decreases oxygen partial pressure and creates hypoxia, a decrease in available oxygen. Hypoxia is supposed to bring about the same beneficial effects to the swimmer that running at altitude does for the track athlete.

There are several problems with this idea. First, as you have already learned, altitude training is probably beneficial only for competition at altitude, not at sea level. This restricted benefit is apparent despite the fact that the track athletes often both train and live at altitude for 24 hr a day and do not just experience hypoxia for a few minutes a day. Second, controlled-frequency breathing does not produce hypoxia. What is produced instead is *hypercapnia,* an increase in the partial pressure of carbon dioxide. Third, hypercapnia often causes headaches that last for 30 min or more after the workout ceases. These headaches are painful and may interfere with training.

On the positive side, controlled-frequency breathing may increase buoyancy and improve body position, enabling the swimmer to concentrate on the biomechanics of the stroke. However, it is simply not an effective technique for the training of respiratory, circulatory, metabolic, or neuromuscular functions. At best, controlled-frequency breathing should be used very sparingly and be closely monitored (Dicker, et al., 1980; Holmer and Gullstrand, 1980; Lavoie and Montpetit, 1986; Zempel, 1989).

Exercise Training and Pollution

The impairment of cilia function mentioned in Chapter 10 is not the only respiratory effect of inhaling cigarette smoke and other environmental pollutants. Inhalation of several pollutants [ozone, formed naturally by the action of ultraviolet radiation (UVR) on oxygen as the UVRs enter the earth's atmosphere and by the action of sunlight UVRs on automobile exhaust (Armstrong, 2000); sulfur dioxide from the burning of coal or oil; particulates such as dust or ashes] brings about a reflex bronchioconstriction in the upper airways. If an individual inhales pollutants while exercising, the problem is confounded. As the intensity of exercise increases, both the rate and the depth of breathing also increase. To accommodate this increase, the individual switches from nose to mouth breathing and hence bypasses the cleansing filtration of the nose. As a result, a greater percentage of inhaled pollutants penetrates more deeply into the respiratory tract than would if the individual were at rest. Results may include chest pain (due to the airway constriction), difficulty in breathing, coughing, nose and throat irritation, and decreased performance (Haymes and Wells, 1986; McCafferty, 1981).

If the pollutant is carbon monoxide (CO), it reduces both the ability to carry oxygen and the ability to release oxygen already bound to red blood cells. The affinity of hemoglobin for carbon monoxide is 210–230 times greater than its affinity for oxygen, and carbon monoxide binds at the same site where oxygen would. Thus, when carboxyhemoglobin (COHb) is formed, the arterial percent saturation of oxygen decreases. The release of oxygen from hemoglobin is impaired by a shift in the oxygen dissociation curve to the left (see Figure 11.3). Myoglobin (Mb) and its role in assisting oxygen diffusion through the sarcoplasm to the mitochondria are also affected in two ways. First, the decrement in the release of oxygen from the red blood cells reduces the efficiency of Mb for attracting and holding oxygen within the muscle cells. Second, CO binds directly to Mb with approximately the same affinity as to Hb, thereby reducing myoglobin's ability to combine with whatever oxygen is available. The combined result of the effects of elevated CO levels on Hb and Mb is an earlier and possibly greater dependence on anaerobic metabolism.

This is manifested by a lower exercise intensity at which the lactate thresholds occur, a shorter endurance time at submaximal loads (especially those above the lactate thresholds), a lower maximal exercise performance, and a lower maximal oxygen consumption ($\dot{V}O_2$max) (McDonough and Moffatt, 1999). As little as a 4% carboxyhemoglobin level will have detrimental effects on exercise time and intensity. This level may result if training is done near heavy traffic. If the source of the carbon monoxide is smoking, there will be additional respiratory impact, including increased pulmonary airway resistance, increased oxygen cost of ventilation, and an increased diffusion distance for oxygen and carbon dioxide across the alveolar walls owing to a combination of mucosal swelling and bronchial constriction (McDonough and Moffatt, 1999). Individuals smoking 10 or fewer cigarettes per day average approximately 4% carboxyhemoglobin, and a two-pack-a-day habit almost doubles this value. Nonsmokers riding in a car for 1 hr with a smoker can reach 3% carboxyhemoglobin (Haymes and Wells, 1986).

Athletes are often affected by pollution levels that do not bother spectators. Individuals with cardiovascular and respiratory diseases and children are also particularly vulnerable (McCafferty, 1981). The following recommendations are suggested to minimize the impact of pollutants on an exercise training session or competition.

1. Individuals with health problems making them particularly susceptible to the effects of pollution should not exercise outside when air quality warnings are in effect. Instead, they should seek sites where the air is filtered.

2. Prolonged heavy exercise should be avoided by everyone when hazardous warnings are in effect. Individuals can adapt to breathing pollutants; however, in the long term adaptation is harmful, because it suppresses normal defense mechanisms. Therefore, adaptation should not be attempted.

3. Ozone peaks at around 3 P.M. and is much higher during most of the daylight hours in summer than in winter; carbon monoxide peaks at approximately 7 A.M. and 8 P.M. and is higher in winter than in summer. Thus, heavy outdoor workouts might be best early in the morning and late evening during the summer and around noontime in the winter (Armstrong, 2000). Runners, cyclists, and in-line skaters should seek locations that are lightly traveled by vehicles. Locations upwind with at least 50 ft between motor vehicles and exercisers are best. Trailing close to a pace car or waiting at stoplights behind cars' exhaust pipes should be avoided.

4. At the very least, smoking should be banned from all indoor training and competition sites. Smoking should be discouraged at all times (McCafferty, 1981).

Summary

1. During short-term, light to moderate aerobic exercise, minute ventilation, alveolar ventilation, and the arteriovenous oxygen difference increase rapidly and reach a steady state within approximately 2–3 min. The partial pressure of oxygen at the alveolar and arterial levels does not change, and as a result the alveolar–to–arterial oxygen pressure gradient and percent saturation of arterial hemoglobin with oxygen are maintained. The ratio of dead space to tidal volume, percent saturation of oxygen in venous blood, and the partial pressure of oxygen in venous blood decrease rapidly and reach a steady state within approximately 2–3 min. The partial pressure of carbon dioxide increases in the venous blood as the result of the increased energy production, but the partial pressure of carbon dioxide decreases slightly due to the hyperpnea.

IP *Respiratory–Gas Exchange* (pages 6–14)*

2. During the first 30 min of long-term moderate to heavy aerobic exercise, the only meaningful differences in respiratory responses from short-term light exercise are in magnitude and a slight drop in the arterial partial pressure of oxygen, which, in turn, widens the alveolar to arterial oxygen pressure gradient. After approximately 30 min, minute ventilation, alveolar ventilation, and the arteriovenous oxygen difference exhibit an upward drift. This respiratory drift is associated with a rising body temperature.

IP *Respiratory–Gas Exchange* (pages 15–16)*

3. During incremental aerobic exercise to maximum, both minute ventilation and alveolar ventilation exhibit a rectilinear rise interrupted by two breakpoints that change the slope upward. The arteriovenous oxygen difference rises rectilinearly until approximately 60% of maximal work, where it levels off. The partial pressure of both alveolar and arterial oxygen, and the resultant alveolar to arterial oxygen pressure gradient and percent saturation of arterial blood, remain constant until approximately 75% of maximal work. At this point the first three exhibit a slight exponential rise, and the arterial oxygen saturation percent decreases slightly as a result. The percent saturation of oxygen in venous blood and venous oxygen partial pressure both decrease rectilinearly until approximately 60% of maximal work, where they level off. As the oxygen is extracted and used, carbon dioxide is produced so that the partial pressure of carbon dioxide in venous blood rises sharply at first and then more slowly. The arterial partial pressure of carbon dioxide is maintained initially but then declines as additional carbon dioxide is blown off by the increasing hyperpnea.

IP *Respiratory–Gas Transport* (pages 4–10)*

4. All of the respiratory responses to static exercise are the same as for short-term, light to moderate submaximal aerobic exercise except that oxygen extraction, as denoted by the arteriovenous oxygen difference, either shows no change or decreases slightly and $\dot{V}_E$ and a-vO$_2$ diff exhibit little, if any, change during exercise, with a rebound rise in recovery.

5. During exercise oxygen dissociation is increased by a widening of the O$_2$ pressure gradient, an increase in PCO$_2$, a decrease in pH, and an increase in body temperature. The changes in PCO$_2$, pH, and body temperature increase oxygen release by causing a shift to the right of the oxygen dissociation curve. At altitude the tendency for the decrease in PCO$_2$, caused by the compensatory hyperventilation, to shift the curve to the left and impair oxygen dissociation is counteracted by an increase in 2,3-DPG activity.

6. Individuals should select the breathing pattern, entrainment or spontaneous, that comes most naturally to them when exercising.

7. Many of the differences in respiratory measures when comparing children and adolescents with young adults or males with females are at least partially related to size. Smaller individuals have smaller values.

8. In general, exercise responses are in the same direction but may vary in magnitude across the age span for both males and females.

9. Respiratory training adaptations are minimal in land-based athletes or fitness participants. The most consistent change is in minute ventilation, which goes down during submaximal work and increases at maximum. Swimming and diving show increases in most static and dynamic lung volumes and capacities, particularly in total lung capacity and vital capacity.

10. The relative percentages of oxygen, carbon dioxide, and nitrogen remain the same to an altitude of 100,000 m (328,083 ft). However, because the barometric pressure goes down exponentially as altitude increases, the partial pressures exerted by oxygen and carbon dioxide also decrease with altitude. The result is a decrease in percent saturation of oxygen and a decreased ability to maintain high-intensity aerobic exercise.

11. Individuals who must compete at altitude should arrive at the location either 12–18 hr or 2–4 weeks prior to the event. Acclimatization and training at altitude appear to be beneficial for competing at that same altitude but not for subsequent sea-level competition unless a live high, train low regimen is followed.

12. Hypoxic swim training is a misnomer and is of very little benefit.

13. Exercise in highly polluted air should be avoided. Any adaptation to such conditions is done at the expense of natural defense mechanisms.

This topic is available on the InterActive Physiology® Sampler CD that comes with the purchase of a new copy of this book.

Review Questions

1. List and explain the four factors that increase oxygen dissociation during exercise. What venous percent saturation of oxygen ($SvO_2\%$) remains even under maximal exercise conditions?

2. Compare and contrast the pulmonary ventilation, external respiration, and internal respiration responses to short-term, light to moderate submaximal aerobic exercise; long-term, moderate to heavy submaximal aerobic exercise; incremental aerobic exercise to maximum; and static exercise. Where known, explain the mechanisms for each response.

3. Should fitness participants and athletes be encouraged to practice entrainment as opposed to spontaneous breathing? Why or why not?

4. Explain exercise-induced hypoxemia (EIH), and discuss why it occurs only in highly trained athletes. Relate the factors responsible for EIH to the low incidence of respiratory training adaptations.

5. Prepare a flowchart of the physiological changes that occur as a result of acute exposure to altitude. How are these acute changes modified by acclimatization?

6. Defend or refute this statement: "Hypoxic training, whether achieved by training at altitude or breath holding, is beneficial to an athlete."

For further review and additional study tools, go to The Physiology Place (www.physiologyplace.com) and the Student Study Guide for Exercise Physiology for Health, Fitness, and Performance by Sharon A. Plowman and Denise L. Smith.

Passport to the Internet

Visit the following Internet sites to explore further topics and issues related to respiratory exercise response. To visit an organization's web site, go to www.physiologyplace.com and click on "Passport to the Internet."

American Society of Exercise Physiologists Through this site you can access two professional electronic journals: the *Journal of Exercise Physiology Online*, a professional peer-reviewed Internet-based journal devoted to original research in exercise physiology, and the *Professionalization of Exercise Physiology Online*, which provides ongoing discussions and information on the professionalization of exercise physiology.

Sportscience This online sport science magazine discusses numerous topics related to all areas of exercise response. Go to http://sportsci.org/traintech/altitude/wgh.html for a special report on exercise training at altitude.

American Lung Association Visit the American Lung Association for information on respiratory health promotion, including air pollution issues. Also, check out information available through the Canadian Lung Association. Compare and contrast American and Canadian statistics.

References

Adams, W. C., E. M. Bernauer, D. B. Dill, & J. B. Bomar: Effects of equivalent sea-level and altitude training on $\dot{V}O_{2max}$ and running performance. *Journal of Applied Physiology.* 39(2):262–266 (1975).

Andrew, G. M., M. R. Becklake, J. S. Guleria, & D. V. Bates: Heart and lung functions in swimmers and nonathletes during growth. *Journal of Applied Physiology.* 32(2):245–251 (1972).

Armstrong, L. E.: *Performance in extreme environments.* Champaign, IL: Human Kinetics (2000).

Ashley, F., W. B. Kannel, P. D. Sorlie, & R. Masson: Pulmonary function: Relation to aging, cigarette habit and mortality; the Framingham Study. *Annals of Internal Medicine.* 82:739–745 (1975).

Asmussen, E.: Similarities and dissimilarities between static and dynamic exercise. *Circulation Research* (Suppl. I). 48(6): I-3–I-10 (1981).

Åstrand, I.: Aerobic work capacity in men and women with special reference to age. *Acta Physiologica Scandinavica* (Suppl. 169). 49:1–92 (1960).

Åstrand, P.-O.: *Experimental Studies of Physical Working Capacity in Relation to Sex and Age.* Copenhagen: Munksgaard (1952).

Åstrand, P.-O., T. E. Cuddy, B. Saltin, & J. Stenberg: Cardiac output during submaximal and maximal work. *Journal of Applied Physiology.* 19(2):268–274 (1964).

Åstrand, P.-O., L. Engstrom, B. O. Eriksson, P. Karlberg, I. Nylander, B. Saltin, & C. Thoren: Girl swimmers: With special reference to respiratory and circulatory adaption and gynecological and psychiatric aspects. *Acta Paediatrica* (Suppl.). 147:1–73 (1963).

Bachman, J. C., & S. M. Horvath: Pulmonary function changes which accompany athletic conditioning programs. *Research Quarterly.* 39(2):235–239 (1968).

Bar-Or, O.: *Pediatric Sports Medicine for the Practitioner: From Physiological Principles to Clinical Applications.* New York: Springer-Verlag, 1–65 (1983).

Bechbache, R. R., & J. Duffin: The entrainment of breathing frequency by exercise rhythm. *Journal of Physiology.* 272: 553–561 (1977).

Becklake, M. R., H. Frank, G. R. Dagenais, G. L. Ostiguy, & C. A. Guzman: Influence of age and sex on exercise cardiac output. *Journal of Applied Physiology.* 20(5):938–947 (1965).

Berglund, E., G. Birath, J. Bjure, G. Grimby, I. Kjellmer, L. Sandqvist, & B. Söderholin: Spirometric studies in normal subjects. I. Forced expirograms in subjects between 7 and 70 years of age. *Acta Medica Scandinavica.* 173:185–206 (1963).

Bjure, J.: Spirometric studies in normal subjects. IV. Ventilatory capacities in healthy children 7–17 years of age. *Acta Paediatrica.* 52:232–240 (1963).

Blomqvist, C. G., & B. Saltin: Cardiovascular adaptations to physical training. *Annual Review of Physiology.* 45:169–189 (1983).

Bye, P. T. P., G. A. Farkas, & C. Roussos: Respiratory factors limiting exercise. *Annual Review of Physiology.* 45:439–451 (1983).

Caretti, D. M., P. C. Szlyk, & I. V. Sils: Effects of exercise modality on patterns of ventilation and respiratory timing. *Respiration Physiology.* 90:201–211 (1992).

Clanton, T. L., G. F. Dixon, J. Drake, & J. E. Gadek: Effects of swim training on lung and inspiratory muscle conditioning. *Journal of Applied Physiology.* 62(1):39–46 (1987).

Clark, J. M., F. C. Hagerman, & R. Gelfand: Breathing patterns during submaximal and maximal exercise in elite oarsmen. *Journal of Applied Physiology.* 55(2):440–446 (1983).

Clausen, J. P.: Effects of physical training on cardiovascular adjustments to exercise in man. *Physiology Reviews.* 57(4): 779–815 (1977).

Comroe, J. H.: *Physiology of Respiration: An Introductory Text.* Chicago: Year Book Medical Publishers (1965).

Cooper Institute for Aerobics Research: *FITNESSGRAM Test Administration Manual* (2nd ed.). Champaign, IL: Human Kinetics (1999).

Cordain, L., & J. Stager: Pulmonary structure and function in swimmers. *Sports Medicine.* 6:271–278 (1988).

Cordain, L., A. Tucker, D. Moon, & J. M. Stager: Lung volumes and maximal respiratory pressures in collegiate swimmers and runners. *Research Quarterly for Exercise and Sport.* 61(1):70–74 (1990).

Coyle, E. F., W. H. Martin III, D. R. Sinacore, M. J. Joyner, J. M. Hagberg, & J. O. Holloszy: Time course of loss of adaptations after stopping prolonged intense endurance training. *Journal of Applied Physiology: Respiratory, Environmental and Exercise Physiology.* 57(6):1857–1864 (1984).

Davies, C. T. M.: The oxygen-transporting system in relation to age. *Clinical Science.* 42:1–13 (1972).

Davies, C. T. M., P. E. DiPrampero, & P. Cerretelli: Kinetics of cardiac output and respiratory gas exchange during exercise and recovery. *Journal of Applied Physiology.* 32(5): 618–625 (1972).

Dempsey, J. A.: Is the lung built for exercise? *Medicine and Science in Sports and Exercise.* 18(2):143–155 (1986).

Dempsey, J. A., & R. F. Fregosi: Adaptability of the pulmonary system of changing metabolic requirements. *American Journal of Cardiology.* 55:59D–67D (1985).

Dempsey, J. A., N. Gledhill, W. G. Reddan, H. V. Foster, P. G. Hanson, & A. D. Claremont: Pulmonary adaptation to exercise: Effects of exercise type and duration, chronic hypoxia and physical training. In P. Milvy (ed.), The Marathon: Physiological, Medical, Epidemiological, and Psychological Studies. *Annals of the New York Academy of Sciences.* 301: 243–261 (1977).

DeVries, H. A., & G. M. Adams: Comparison of exercise responses in old and young men. II. Ventilatory mechanics. *Journal of Gerontology.* 27(3):349–352 (1972).

Dicker, S., G. K. Lofthus, N. W. Thorton, & G. A. Brooks: Respiratory and heart rate responses to tethered controlled frequency breathing swimming. *Medicine and Science in Sports and Exercise.* 12(1):20–23 (1980).

Donevan, R. E., W. H. Palmer, C. J. Varvis, & D. V. Bates: Influence of age on pulmonary diffusing capacity. *Journal of Applied Physiology.* 14(4):483–492 (1959).

Ekelund, L. G.: Circulatory and respiratory adaptation during prolonged exercise. *Acta Physiologica Scandinavica* (Suppl. 292). 70:1–38 (1967).

Ekelund, L. G., & A. Holmgren: Central hemodynamics during exercise. *Circulation Research* (Suppl. 1). 20–21:1–33 (1967).

Ericsson, P., & L. Irnell: Spirometric studies of ventilatory capacity in elderly people. In J. R. Edge, K. K. Pump, J. Arias-Stella, et al., *Aging Lung: Normal Function.* New York: MSS Information Corporation, 209–222 (1974).

Eriksson, B. O.: Effects of physical training on hemodynamic response during submaximal and maximal exercise in 11–13 year old boys. *Acta Physiological Scandinavica.* 87: 27–39 (1973).

Eriksson, B. O.: Physical training, oxygen supply and muscle metabolism in 11–13 year old boys. *Acta Physiologica Scandinavica* (Suppl.). 384:1–48 (1972).

Fahey, T. D., A. D. Valle-Zuris, G. Oehlsen, M. Trieb, & J. Seymour: Pubertal stage differences in hormonal and hematological responses to maximal exercise in males. *Journal of Applied Physiology: Respiratory, Environmental and Exercise Physiology.* 46(4):823–827 (1979).

Ferris, B. G., D. O. Anderson, & R. Zickmantel: Prediction values for screening tests of pulmonary function. *American Review of Respiratory Diseases.* 91:252–261 (1965).

Fleck, S. J., & W. J. Kraemer: *Designing Resistance Training Programs.* Champaign, IL: Human Kinetics (1987).

Fringer, M. N., & G. A. Stull: Changes in cardiorespiratory parameters during periods of training and detraining in young adult females. *Medicine and Science in Sports.* 6(1): 20–25 (1974).

Green, J. S., & S. F. Crouse: Endurance training, cardiovascular function and the aged. *Sports Medicine.* 16(5):331–341 (1993).

Grimby, G.: Respiration in exercise. *Medicine and Science in Sports.* 1(1):9–14 (1969).

Grover, R. F.: Adaptation to high altitude. In L. J. Folinsbee, J. A. Wagner, J. F. Borgia, B. L. Drinkwater, J. A. Gliner, & J. F. Bedi (eds.), *Environmental Stress: Individual Human Adaptations.* New York: Academic Press (1978).

Gurtner, H. P., P. Walser, & B. Fässler: Normal values for pulmonary hemodynamics at rest and during exercise in man. *Progress in Respiration Research.* 9:295–315 (1975).

Guyton, A. C.: *Textbook of Medical Physiology* (7th edition). Philadelphia: Saunders (1986).

Haffor, A. A., A. C. Harrison, & P. A. Catledge Kirk: Anaerobic threshold alterations caused by interval training in 11-year-olds. *Journal of Sports Medicine and Physical Fitness.* 30(1):53–56 (1990).

Hannon, J. P.: Comparative altitude adaptability of young men and women. In L. J. Folinsbee, J. A. Wagner, J. F. Borgia, B. L. Drinkwater, J. A. Gliner, & J. F. Bedi (eds.), *Environmental Stress: Individual Human Adaptations.* New York: Academic Press (1978).

Hanson, P., A. Claremont, J. Dempsey, & W. Reddan: Determinants and consequences of ventilatory responses to competitive endurance running. *Journal of Applied Physiology: Respiratory, Environmental and Exercise Physiology.* 52(3): 615–623 (1982).

Haymes, E. M., & C. L. Wells: *Environment and Human Performance.* Champaign, IL: Human Kinetics (1986).

Hill, A. R., J. M. Adams, B. E. Parker, & D. F. Rochester: Short-term entrainment of ventilation to the walking cycle in humans. *Journal of Applied Physiology.* 65(2):570–578 (1988).

Holmer, I., & L. Gullstrand: Physiological responses to swimming with a controlled frequency of breathing. *Scandinavian Journal of Sports Science.* 2(1):1–6 (1980).

Jain, S. K., & C. K. Gupta: Age, height, and body weight as determinants of ventilatory "norms" in healthy men above forty years of age. In J. R. Edge, K. K. Pump, J. Arias-Stella, et al., *Aging Lung: Normal Function.* New York: MSS Information Corporation, 190–202 (1974a).

Jain, S. K., & C. K. Gupta: Lung function studies in healthy men and women over forty. In J. R. Edge, K. K. Pump, J. Arias-Stella, et al., *Aging Lung: Normal Function.* New York: MSS Information Corporation, 182–189 (1974b).

Jasinskas, C. L., B. A. Wilson, & J. Hoare: Entrainment of breathing rate to movement frequency during work at two intensities. *Respiration Physiology.* 42:199–209 (1980).

Johnson, B. D., & J. A. Dempsey: Demand vs. capacity in the aging pulmonary system. In J. O. Holloszy (ed.), *Exercise and Sport Sciences Reviews.* 19:171–210 (1991).

Jones, N. L.: Exercise testing in pulmonary evaluation: Rationale, methods and the normal respiratory response to exercise. *New England Journal of Medicine.* 293(11):541–544 (1975).

Kao, F. F.: *An Introduction to Respiratory Physiology.* New York: American Elsevier (1974).

Kaufmann, D. A., E. W. Swenson, J. Fencl, & A. Lucas: Pulmonary function of marathon runners. *Medicine and Science in Sports.* 6(2):114–117 (1974).

Kay, J. D. S., E. Strange Petersen, & H. Vejby-Christensen: Breathing in man during steady-state exercise on the bicycle at two pedalling frequencies, and during treadmill walking. *Journal of Physiology.* 251:645–656 (1975).

Kenney, R. A.: *Physiology of Aging: A Synopsis.* Chicago: Year Book Medical Publishers (1982).

Koistinen, P. O., H. Rusko, K. Irjala, A. Rajamki, K. Penttinen, V-P. Sarparanta, J. Karpakka, & J. Leppaluoto: EPO, red cells, and serum transferrin receptor in continuous and intermittent hypoxia. *Medicine and Science in Sports and Exercise.* 32(4):800–804 (2000).

Koyal, S. N., B. J. Whipp, D. Huntsman, G. A. Bray, & K. Wasserman: Ventilatory responses to the metabolic acidosis of treadmill and cycle ergometry. *Journal of Applied Physiology.* 40(6):864–867 (1976).

Krahenbuhl, G. S., J. S. Skinner, & W. M. Kohrt: Developmental aspects of maximal aerobic power in children. In R. L. Terjung (ed.), *Exercise and Sport Sciences Reviews.* 13: 503–538 (1985).

Lavoie, J.-M., & R. R. Montpetit: Applied physiology of swimming. *Sports Medicine.* 3:165–189 (1986).

Leff, A. R., & P. T. Schumacker: *Respiratory Physiology: Basics and Applications.* Philadelphia: Saunders (1993).

Leith, D. G., & M. Bradley: Ventilatory muscle strength and endurance training. *Journal of Applied Physiology.* 41(4): 508–516 (1976).

Levine, B. D., & J. Stray-Gundersen: "Living high—training low": Effect of moderate-altitude acclimatization with low-altitude training on performance. *Journal of Applied Physiology.* 83(1):102–112 (1997).

Loat, C. E. R., & E. C. Rhodes: Relationship between the lactate and ventilatory thresholds during prolonged exercise. *Sports Medicine.* 15(2):104–115 (1993).

Maclennan, S. E., G. A. Silvestri, J. Ward, & D. A. Mahler: Does entrained breathing improve the economy of rowing? *Medicine and Science in Sports and Exercise.* 26(5):610–614 (1994).

Magel, J. R., & K. Lange Andersen: Pulmonary diffusing capacity and cardiac output in young trained Norwegian swimmers and untrained subjects. *Medicine and Science in Sports.* 1(3):131–139 (1969).

Mahler, D. A., C. R. Shuhart, E. Brew, & T. A. Stukel: Ventilatory responses and entrainment of breathing during rowing. *Medicine and Science in Sports and Exercise.* 23(2):186–192 (1991).

Malina, R. M., & C. Bouchard: *Growth, Maturation and Physical Activity.* Champaign, IL: Human Kinetics (1991).

McCafferty, W. B.: *Air Pollution and Athletic Performance.* Springfield, IL: Thomas (1981).

McDonough, P., & R. J. Moffatt: Smoking-induced elevations in blood carboxyhaemoglobin level. *SportsMedicine.* 27(5): 275–283 (1999).

Mostyn, E. M., S. Helle, J. B. L. Gee, L. G. Bentiveglio, & D. V. Bates: Pulmonary diffusing capacity of athletes. *Journal of Applied Physiology.* 18(4):687–695 (1963).

Niinimaa, V., & R. J. Shepard: Training and oxygen conductance in the elderly. I. The respiratory system. *Journal of Gerontology.* 33(3):354–361 (1978).

Pardy, R. L., S. N. A. Hussain, & P. T. Macklein: The ventilatory pump in exercise. *Clinics in Chest Medicine.* 5(1):35–49 (1984).

Paterson, D. H., T. M. McLellan, R. S. Stella, & D. A. Cunningham: Longitudinal study of ventilation threshold and maximal O_2 uptake in athletic boys. *Journal of Applied Physiology.* 62(5):2051–2057 (1987).

Pearce, D. H., & H. T. Milhorn: Dynamic and steady-state respiratory responses to bicycle exercise. *Journal of Applied Physiology: Respiratory, Environmental and Exercise Physiology.* 42(6):959–967 (1977).

Plunkett, B. T., & W. G. Hopkins: Investigation of the side pain "stitch" induced by running after fluid ingestion. *Medicine and Science in Sports and Exercise.* 31(8):1169–1175 (1999).

Pollock, M. L., T. K. Cureton, & L. Greninger: Effects of frequency of training on working capacity, cardiovascular function, and body composition of adult men. *Medicine and Science in Sport.* 1(2):70–74 (1969).

Powers, S. K., & R. E. Beadle: Onset of hyperventilation during incremental exercise: A brief review. *Research Quarterly for Exercise and Sport.* 56(4):352–360 (1985).

Powers, S. K., D. Martin, & S. Dodd: Exercise-induced hypoxemia in elite endurance athletes: Incidence, causes and impact on $\dot{V}O_{2max}$. *SportsMedicine.* 16(1):14–22 (1993).

Prefaut, C., F. Durand, P. Mucci, & C. Caillaud: Exercise-induced arterial hypoxemia in athletes: A review. *Sports Medicine.* 30(1):47–61 (2000).

Rasmussen, B., K. Klausen, J. P. Clausen, & J. Trap-Jensen: Pulmonary ventilation, blood gases, and blood pH after training of the arms or the legs. *Journal of Applied Physiology.* 38(2):250–256 (1975).

Ratzin Jackson, C. G., & B. J. Sharkey: Altitude, training, and human performance. *SportsMedicine.* 6:279–284 (1988).

Reid, J. G., & J. M. Thomson: *Exercise Prescription for Fitness.* Englewood Cliffs, NJ: Prentice Hall (1985).

Reuschlein, P. S., W. G. Reddan, J. Burpee, J. B. L. Gee, & J. Rankin: Effect of physical training on the pulmonary diffusing capacity during submaximal work. *Journal of Applied Physiology.* 24(2):152–158 (1968).

Robinson, E. P., & J. M. Kjeldgaard: Improvement in ventilatory muscle function with running. *Journal of Applied Physiology: Respiratory, Environmental and Exercise Physiology.* 52(6):1400–1406 (1992).

Robinson, S.: Experimental studies of physical fitness in relation to age. *Arbeitsphysiologie.* 10:251–323 (1938).

Rowell, L. B.: Circulation. *Medicine and Science in Sports.* 1(1):15–22 (1969).

Rowell, L. B., H. L. Taylor, Y. Wang, & W. S. Carlson: Saturation of arterial blood with oxygen during maximal exercise. *Journal of Applied Physiology.* 19(2):284–286 (1964).

Rowland, T. W.: Developmental aspects of physiological function relating to aerobic exercise in children. *SportsMedicine.* 10(4):255–266 (1990).

Rowland, T. W., J. A. Auchmachie, T. J. Keenan, & G. M. Green: Physiologic responses to treadmill running in adult and prepubertal males. *International Journal of Sports Medicine.* 8(4):292–297 (1987).

Rowland, T. W., & G. M. Green: Physiological responses to treadmill exercise in females: Adult-child differences. *Medicine and Science in Sports and Exercise.* 20(5):474–478 (1988).

Saltin, B.: Physiological effects of physical conditioning. *Medicine and Science in Sports.* 1(1):50–56 (1969).

Saltin, B., G. Bloomqvist, J. H. Mitchell, R. L. Johnson, K. Wildenthal, & C. B. Chapman: Response to exercise after bed rest and after training. *Circulation* (Suppl. VII). 38(5): VII-1–VII-78 (1968).

Saris, W. H. M., A. M. Noordeloos, B. E. M. Ringnalda, M. A. Van't Hof, & R. A. Binkhorst: Reference values for aerobic power of healthy 4- to 18-year-old Dutch children: Preliminary results. In R. A. Binkhorst, H. C. G. Kemper, & W. H. M. Saris (eds.), *Children and Exercise XI.* Champaign, IL: Human Kinetics, 15:151–160 (1985).

Sawka, M. N., R. G. Knowlton, & R. M. Glaser: Body temperature, respiration, and acid-base equilibrium during prolonged running. *Medicine and Science in Sports and Exercise.* 12(5):370–374 (1980).

Seals, D. R., B. F. Hurley, J. Schultz, & J. M. Hagberg: Endurance training in older men and women. II. Blood lactate response to submaximal exercise. *Journal of Applied Physiology: Respiratory, Environmental and Exercise Physiology.* 57(4):1030–1033 (1984).

Segal, S. S.: Convection, diffusion, and mitochondrial utilization of oxygen during exercise. In D. R. Lamb & C. V. Gisolfi (eds.), *Energy Metabolism in Exercise and Sport.* Dubuque, IA: Brown & Benchmark, 269–338 (1992).

Shapiro, W., C. E. Johnston, R. A. Dameron, & J. L. Patterson: Maximum ventilatory performance and its limiting factors. *Journal of Applied Physiology.* 19(2):197–203 (1964).

Shepard, R. J.: *Physical Activity and Aging.* Chicago: Year Book Medical Publishers, 40–44; 85–95 (1978).

Skinner, J. S., & T. H. McLellan: The transition from aerobic to anaerobic metabolism. *Research Quarterly for Exercise and Sport.* 51(1):234–298 (1980).

Slonim, N. B., & L. H. Hamilton: *Respiratory Physiology* (3rd edition). St. Louis: Mosby (1976).

Stanescu, S., Q. St. Dutu, Z. Jienescu, L. Hartia, N. Nicolescu, & F. Sacerdoteanu: Investigations into changes of pulmonary function in the aged. In J. R. Edge, K. K. Pump, & J. Aris-Stella et al., *Aging Lung: Normal Function.* New York: MSS Information Corporation, 171–181 (1974).

Storstein, O., & A. Voll: New prediction formulas for ventilation measurements: A study of normal individuals in the age group 20–59 years. In J. R. Edge, K. K. Pump, & J. Aris-Stella et al., *Aging Lung: Normal Function.* New York: MSS Information Corporation, 156–170 (1974).

Turner, J. M., J. Mead, & M. E. Wohl: Elasticity of human lungs in relation to age. *Journal of Applied Physiology.* 25(6):664–671 (1968).

Vaccaro, P., & D. H. Clarke: Cardiorespiratory alterations in 9 to 11 year old children following a season of competitive swimming. *Medicine and Science in Sports.* 10(3):204–207 (1978).

Vaccaro, P., C. W. Zauner, & W. F. Updyke: Resting and exercise respiratory function in well trained child swimmers. *Journal of Sports Medicine and Physical Fitness.* 17: 297–306 (1977).

Wagner, P. D.: Central and peripheral aspects of oxygen transport and adaptation with exercise. *SportsMedicine.* 11(3):133–142 (1991).

Walsh, M. L., & E. W. Banister: Possible mechanisms of the anaerobic threshold: A review. *SportsMedicine.* 5:269–302 (1988).

Wasserman, K.: Breathing during exercise. *New England Journal of Medicine.* 298(14):780–785 (1978).

Wasserman, K., A. L. VanKessel, & G. G. Burton: Interaction of physiological mechanisms during exercise. *Journal of Applied Physiology.* 22(1):71–85 (1967).

Wasserman, K., & B. J. Whipp: Exercise physiology in health and disease. *American Review of Respiratory Disease.* 112:219–249 (1975).

Weston, A. R., G. MacKenzie, A. Tufts, & M. Mars: Optimal time of arrival for performance at moderate altitude (1700 m). *Medicine and Science in Sports and Exercise.* 33(2): 298–302 (2001).

Whipp, B. J.: The hyperpnea of dynamic muscular exercise. In R. S. Hutton (ed.), *Exercise and Sport Science Reviews* (Vol. 5). Santa Barbara, CA: Journal Publishing Affiliates (1977).

Whipp, B. J., & S. A. Ward: Ventilatory control dynamics during muscular exercise in men. *International Journal of Sports Medicine.* 1:146–159 (1980).

Whipp, B. J., S. A. Ward, N. Lamarra, J. A. Davis, & K. Wasserman: Parameters of ventilatory and gas exchange dynamics during exercise. *Journal of Applied Physiology: Respiratory, Environmental and Exercise Physiology.* 52(6): 1506–1513 (1982).

Wilmore, J. H., J. Royce, R. N. Girandola, F. I. Katch, & V. L. Katch: Physiological alterations resulting from a 10-week program of jogging. *Medicine and Science in Sports.* 2(1): 7–14 (1970).

Younes, M., & G. Kivinen: Respiratory mechanics and breathing pattern during and following maximal exercise. *Journal of Applied Physiology: Respiratory, Environmental and Exercise Physiology.* 57(6):1773–1782 (1984).

Zauner, C. W., & N. Y. Benson: Physiological alterations in young swimmers during three years of intensive training. *Journal of Sports Medicine and Physical Fitness.* 21: 179–185 (1981).

Zauner, C. W., M. G. Maksud, & J. Milichna: Physiological considerations in training young athletes. *SportsMedicine.* 8(1):15–31 (1989).

Zempel, C.: Hypoxic isn't: Exploding the myth. *Triathlete.* Nov/Dec 20–21 (1989).

Zwiren, L. D., K. J. Cureton, & P. Hutchinson: Comparison of circulatory responses to submaximal exercise in equally trained men and women. *International Journal of Sports Medicine.* 4:255–259 (1983).

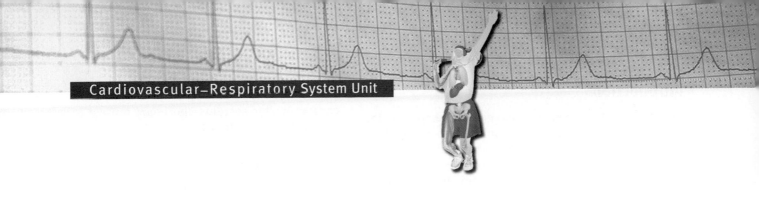

Chapter 12

The Cardiovascular System

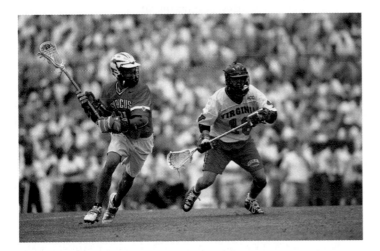

After studying the chapter, you should be able to

- Explain the functions of the cardiovascular system.
- Identify the various components of the cardiovascular system.
- Distinguish among the vessels that comprise the vascular system, and compare the pressure, velocity, and resistance in each type of vessel.
- Explain how electrical excitation is spread through the conduction system of the heart.
- Explain the relationships among the electrical, pressure, contractile, and volume changes throughout the cardiac cycle.
- Calculate mean arterial pressure, total peripheral resistance, and cardiac output.
- Describe the hormonal mechanisms by which blood volume is maintained.
- Explain how the cardiovascular system is regulated.
- Describe the measurement of maximal oxygen consumption, cardiac output, stroke volume, heart rate, and blood pressure.

Introduction

Chapter 10 described how oxygen is taken into the body and made available for delivery to the cells of the body. The ability of the body to circulate oxygen (and other substances) depends on the proper functioning of the cardiovascular system. In many ways the cardiovascular system and the respiratory system operate in a parallel fashion, because they have a common mission—to deliver oxygen to working muscles—and are driven by similar mechanisms. This chapter provides an overview of the cardiovascular system, discusses basic principles of cardiovascular dynamics, and outlines techniques currently used to assess cardiovascular function.

Overview of the Cardiovascular System

The *cardiovascular system* includes the heart, blood vessels, and blood. Its primary functions are

1. transporting oxygen and nutrients to the cells of the body and transporting carbon dioxide and waste products from the cells;

2. regulating body temperature, pH levels, and fluid balance; and

3. protecting the body from blood loss and infection.

The heart is the pump that provides the force to circulate the blood throughout the vessels of the circulatory system. The blood vessels serve as conduits for the blood as it travels through the body. The blood is responsible for the transport of gases and nutrients within the cardiovascular system.

Figure 12.1 provides a schematic overview of the cardiovascular system. *Arteries* carry blood away from the heart, and *veins* return blood to the heart. The *capillary beds* serve as the site of exchange for gases and nutrients between the blood and the tissues of the body.

The Heart

The heart is a hollow muscular organ located in the thoracic cavity. It weighs approximately 250–350 g and is 12–14 cm long, about the size of a clenched fist

---

Intercalated Discs The junction between cardiac muscle cells that forms the mechanical and electrical connection between the two cells.

Syncytium The individual cells of the myocardium that function collectively as a unit during depolarization.

(Marieb, 2001). It serves as the double pump for the cardiovascular system. The heart muscle is referred to as the *myocardium.*

Macroanatomy of the Heart

The heart contains four chambers and is functionally separated into the right and left heart. The right side pumps blood to the lungs (pulmonary circulation), and the left side pumps blood to the entire body (systemic circulation). The two sides of the heart are separated by the interventricular septum. The upper chambers, called *atria* (*atrium* is the singular), receive the blood; the lower chambers, called *ventricles,* eject blood from the heart (Figure 12.2a on page 322). Blood is ejected from the right ventricle to the pulmonary artery and from the left ventricle to the aorta.

One-way valves control blood flow through the heart. The *atrioventricular (AV) valves* separate the atrium and ventricle on each side of the heart; specifically, the tricuspid valve separates the atrium and ventricle on the right side of the heart, and the bicuspid (or mitral) valve separates the atrium and ventricle on the left side of the heart. The *semilunar valves* control blood flow from the ventricles; specifically, the aortic semilunar valve allows blood to flow from the left ventricle into the aorta, and the pulmonary semilunar valve allows blood to flow from the right ventricle into the pulmonary artery.

Figure 12.2a depicts the chambers and valves of the heart and diagrams the flow of blood through the heart. Figure 12.2b summarizes the blood flow through the heart.

Microanatomy of the Heart

Cardiac muscle cells are both similar to and different from skeletal muscle cells. Both types of muscle cells are striated in appearance because they contain the contractile proteins, actin and myosin. The primary difference between cardiac and skeletal muscle cells is that cardiac muscle cells are highly interconnected; that is, the cell membranes of adjacent cardiac cells are functionally linked by **intercalated discs.** These junctions between cells form the electrical connection between two cells. This connection allows the electrical activity in one cell to pass to the adjacent cell. Thus, the individual cells of the myocardium function collectively; when one cell is stimulated electrically, the stimulation will spread cell to cell over the entire area. The result is that the cells of the myocardium function as a unit during depolarization, which is called a **syncytium.** There are two functional syncytia, atrial and ventricular, and each contracts as a unit.

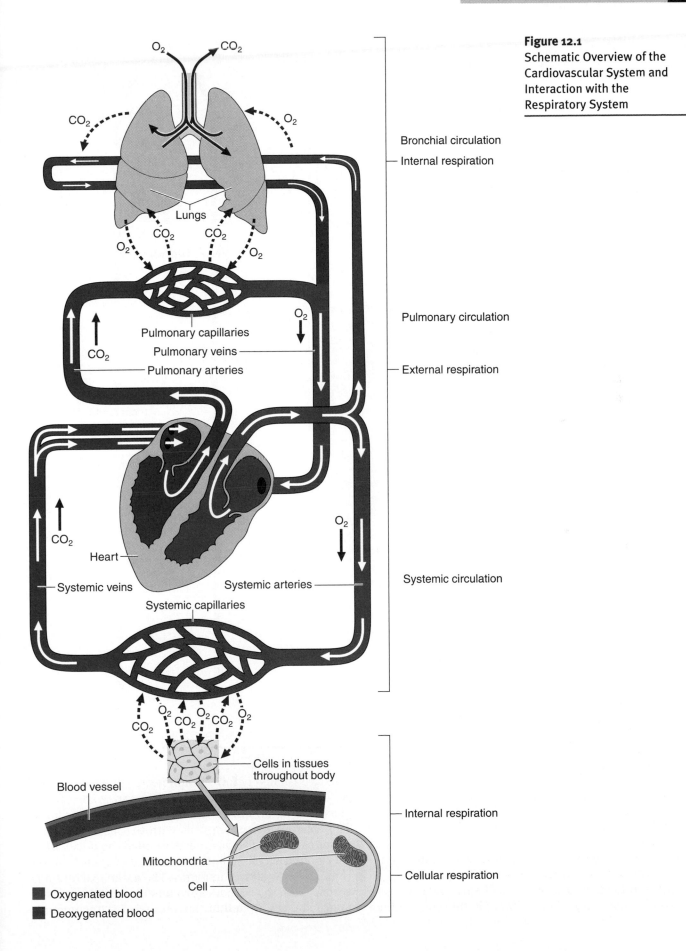

Figure 12.1
Schematic Overview of the Cardiovascular System and Interaction with the Respiratory System

Bronchial circulation

Internal respiration

O_2 CO_2

CO_2 O_2

Lungs

CO_2 CO_2

O_2 O_2

Pulmonary capillaries

Pulmonary veins

Pulmonary arteries

CO_2

O_2

Pulmonary circulation

External respiration

Heart

CO_2

O_2

Systemic veins

Systemic arteries

Systemic capillaries

Systemic circulation

O_2 O_2 O_2

CO_2 CO_2 CO_2

Cells in tissues throughout body

Blood vessel

Internal respiration

Mitochondria

Cellular respiration

Cell

■ Oxygenated blood
■ Deoxygenated blood

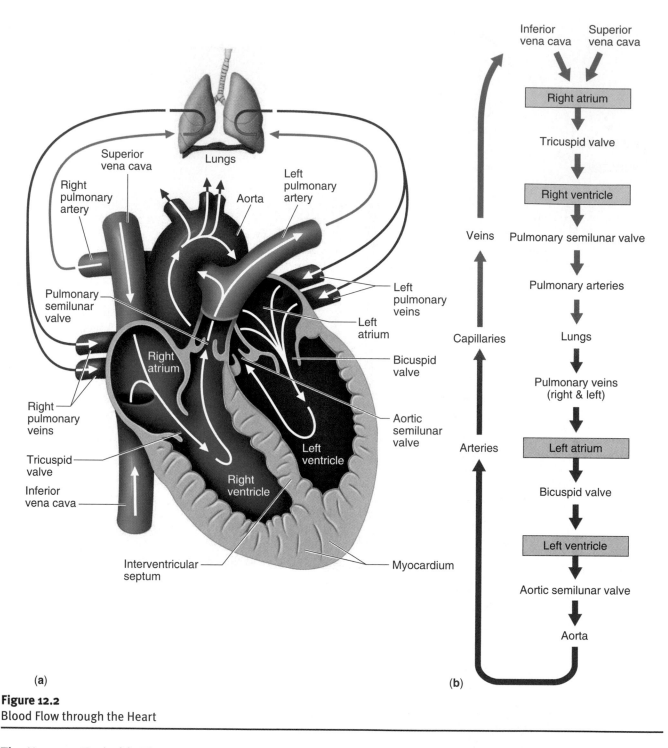

(a)   (b)

Figure 12.2
Blood Flow through the Heart

The Heart as Excitable Tissue

Cardiac muscle cells are excitable cells that are polarized in the resting state and contract when they become depolarized. As a result of contraction, blood is ejected from the chambers. Individual myocardial cells function together to produce a coordinated contraction of the entire organ.

In addition to muscle cells, the heart contains specialized conducting cells. Although the conducting cells are relatively few in number (compared to muscle cells), they are essential because they spread the electrical signal quickly throughout the myocardium. The conduction system cells with the fastest spontaneous rate of depolarization are called the *pacemaker* cells and are located in the *sinoatrial* (*SA*) *node* in the right atria. As shown in Figure 12.3a, the excitation is spread from the SA node throughout the right atria by internodal tracts and to the left atria by Bachmann's

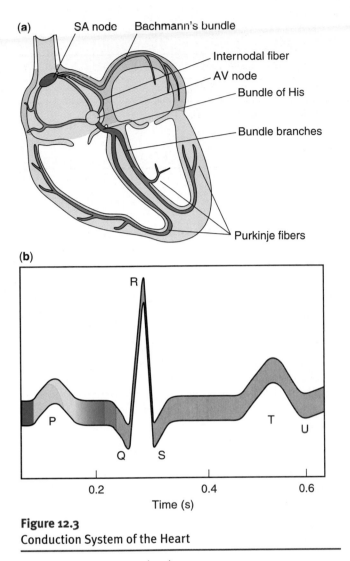

(a)

SA node   Bachmann's bundle

Internodal fiber

AV node

Bundle of His

Bundle branches

Purkinje fibers

(b)

R

P

Q   S

T

U

0.2   0.4   0.6

Time (s)

Figure 12.3
Conduction System of the Heart

Source: Modified from Netter (1987).

Table 12.1
Electrical Events Associated with ECG

Wave (Complex)	Atrial	Ventricular
P	depolarization	
Ta/QRS	repolarization	depolarization
T		repolarization

mal conditions. Cells in each area of the conduction system have their own inherent rate of depolarization. For the SA node the intrinsic rate of depolarization is 60–100 times·min^{-1}. The AV node discharges at an intrinsic rate of 40–60 times·min^{-1} and the Purkinje fibers at a rate of 15–40 times·min^{-1} (Guyton, 1991). In an individual with a diseased SA node, the AV node takes over the pacemaking. Thus, if the only thing you knew about an individual was that he or she had a heart rate of 40 b·min^{-1}, you could not tell whether the person was a highly trained endurance athlete, because endurance training results in a lowering of heart rate, or someone in need of an artificial pacemaker implant.

Electrocardiogram

An *electrocardiogram* (ECG) provides a graphic illustration of the electrical current generated by excitation of the heart muscle. Figure 12.3b presents an ECG tracing that is color-coded to match the conduction system in Figure 12.3a (Netter, 1987). Table 12.1 summarizes the electrical activity in the heart.

The P wave in Figure 12.3b represents atrial depolarization, which causes atrial contraction. The spread of the electrical signal through the conduction system of the atria is indicated by green in Figures 12.3a and 12.3b. Repolarization of the atria, called a Ta wave, is normally not detectable on a resting ECG, but occurs during the time period concurrent with the QRS complex and may be evident during exercise. The electrical signal reaches the AV node at the end of the P wave (yellow). Excitation of the bundle of His and bundle branches (red) occurs in the middle of the PR interval, followed by excitation of the Purkinje fibers (purple). Notice that excitation of the various portions of the conduction system requires very little time and that activation of the entire conduction system precedes the QRS complex. The QRS complex reflects depolarization of the muscle fibers in the ventricles, which occurs after the electrical signal has traveled through the specialized conduction system.

bundle. Because the atrial and ventricular syncytia contract separately, an action potential in the atria does not lead directly to the contraction of cardiac cells in the ventricles. The signal is spread from the atria to the ventricles via the *atrioventricular (AV) node*. Once the AV node is depolarized, the electrical signal continues down the specialized conduction system consisting of the bundle of His, the left and right bundle branches, and the Purkinje fibers. The electrical excitation then spreads out from the conducting system to excite all of the myocardial (muscle) cells. Remember that the excitation is spread first by the conduction system and then by cell-to-cell contact: The excitation is passed from muscle cell to muscle cell within the ventricles since the conduction system does not reach each individual cell.

As mentioned earlier, the cells of the SA node are considered the pacemaker cells of the heart because they have the fastest rate of depolarization under nor-

Table 12.2

Typical Resting Cardiovascular Values for Males and Females of Various Ages

Cardiovascular Value	Age of Males (yr)			Age of Females (yr)		
	10–15	20–30	50–60	10–15	20–30	50–60
Heart rate HR (b·min^{-1})	82	72	80	85	76	82
Stroke volume SV (mL·b^{-1})	50	90	70	40	75	62
Cardiac output (L·min^{-1})	4.0	6.5	5.5	3.4	5.5	5.0

Sources: Åstrand (1952); Fleg, et al. (1995); Ogawa, et al. (1992); Spina, et al. (1992, 1993a, b).

The T wave reflects repolarization of the muscle fibers in the ventricles and is followed by relaxation in preparation to start the cycle all over again.

Although the SA node can depolarize spontaneously, the firing of the SA node is influenced by neural and hormonal factors. Additionally, heart rate varies with age. Table 12.2 presents typical resting heart rate (HR) values in healthy individuals of various ages. Factors that affect heart rate are discussed in greater detail later in this chapter.

Cardiac Cycle

In order to successfully function as a pump, the heart must have alternating times of relaxation and contraction. The relaxation phase, called *diastole,* is the period when the heart fills with blood. The contraction phase, called *systole,* is the period when blood is ejected from the heart. The **cardiac cycle**—one complete sequence of contraction and relaxation of the heart—includes all events associated with the flow of blood through the heart and is marked by dramatic changes in pressure and blood volume. Figure 12.4 summarizes the position of the heart valves throughout the phases of the cardiac cycle and provides information regarding ventricular pressure (indicated by arrows) and volume (indicated by cavity size) at each phase. Although only the right side of the heart is shown in this figure, the events are the same for both sides of the heart.

The ventricular-filling period (VFP) (Figure 12.4a) occurs when the ventricles are at rest (ventricular diastole) and the AV valves are open. The ventricles fill as blood is returned to the atria and flows down into the ventricles because of the force of gravity. Atrial contraction also pushes a small volume of additional blood into the ventricles at the end of diastole. Blood

---

Cardiac Cycle One complete sequence of contraction and relaxation of the heart.

---

volume in the ventricles is greatest at the end of ventricular filling, but pressure remains relatively low because the ventricles are relaxed.

Systole (the contraction phase) is divided into two periods, the isovolumetric contraction period (ICP) and the ventricular ejection period (VEP). During the ICP (Figure 12.4b) both the AV valves and the semilunar valves are closed. Thus, blood volume in the ventricles remains constant despite the high pressure generated by the contraction of the ventricular myocardium. Once pressure in the ventricles exceeds pressure in the aorta, the semilunar valves are forced open. Blood is then ejected from the ventricles, initiating the VEP and causing ventricular volume to decrease (Figure 12.4c).

During the isovolumetric relaxation period (IRP) both the AV and the semilunar valves are closed (Figure 12.4d). Thus, ventricular volume is unchanged, and pressure is low because the ventricles are relaxed.

Figure 12.5, on page 326, summarizes the cardiac cycle. This diagram integrates information about the electrocardiogram; the pressure in the left atrium, the left ventricle, and aorta; the left ventricular volume; the heart phase; the period of the cardiac cycle; and the position of the heart valves. Notice that Figure 12.5 is directly related to Figure 12.4. In both figures, diastole is shown in blue and systole is shown in green. The position of the AV and semilunar valves is shown in Figure 12.4 and in Figure 12.5.

Figure 12.5 begins arbitrarily during the VFP of ventricular diastole. The AV valves are open, allowing blood to flow from the atria into the ventricle; therefore, ventricular volume is increasing. As the atrium contracts, more blood is forced into the ventricle, causing a small increase in ventricular volume and ventricular pressure.

Following the QRS complex, there is an immediate and dramatic increase in ventricular pressure as the myocardium contracts. Notice, however, that the ventricular volume does not change. This is the isovolumetric contraction period. Locate Point A on the

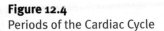

Figure 12.4
Periods of the Cardiac Cycle

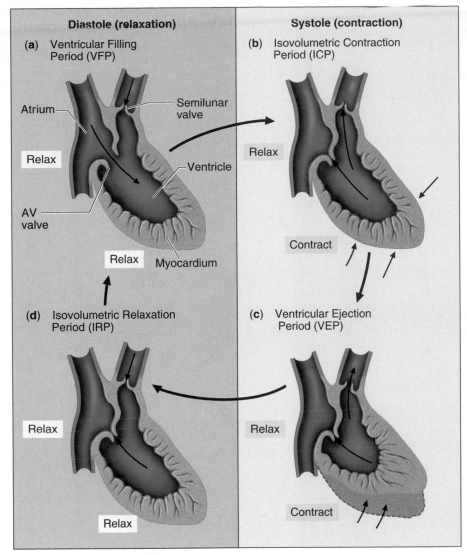

graph of ventricular pressure in Figure 12.5. This is the point where pressure in the ventricle exceeds pressure in the aorta, and the aortic semilunar valve is forced open. Follow the dashed lines downward to the row for the semilunar valves in the chart at the bottom of the figure, and note that these valves are now opened. Also note that this dashed line coincides with the start of a rapid decrease in ventricular volume. Once the valves are open, blood is forced out of the ventricles; thus, blood volume in the ventricle decreases. This is the VEP.

When pressure in the ventricles falls below pressure in the aorta, the semilunar valves close. Refer to Point B on the pressure curve of Figure 12.5 and again follow the dashed line downward, noting ventricular volume and valve position. As pressure continues to decrease, ventricular volume remains constant, because all the valves are closed and no blood

can enter or leave the ventricles. This is known as the IRP.

Following the T wave (ventricular repolarization), the ventricles relax and begin to fill with blood: The AV valves are open, and ventricular volume is increasing. This is the VFP. This cycle of diastole followed by systole followed by diastole continues with each beat of the heart.

Diastole provides time for the cardiac cells to relax and the ventricles to fill, thereby directly affecting the amount of blood that is pumped during the subsequent systole. Furthermore, it is during diastole that the myocardium is supplied with its blood supply, known as the *coronary circulation*.

Systole is the contraction period of the heart, first isometrically (ICP) and then dynamically (VEP). The volume of blood ejected from the ventricles determines the cardiovascular system's ability to meet the

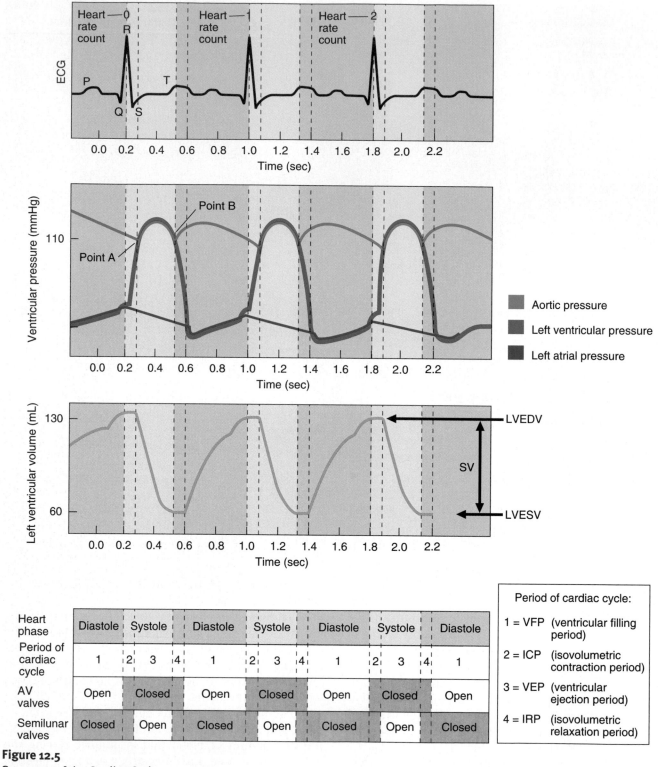

Figure 12.5

Summary of the Cardiac Cycle

The periods of the cardiac cycle are labeled as 1, VFP; 2, ICP; 3, VEP; and 4, IRP.

demands of the body. The volume of blood in the left ventricle at the end of diastole is termed **left ventricular end–diastolic volume (LVEDV)** and is labeled in Figure 12.5. Similarly, the volume of blood in the left ventricle at the end of systole is termed **left ventricular end–systolic volume (LVESV)**. The amount of blood ejected from the heart with each beat is called **stroke volume (SV)**.

Before going to the next section, study Figures 12.4 and 12.5. Be sure you understand what is happening with the ECG, with ventricular, atrial, and aortic pressure, with ventricular volume, and with the heart valves at each period of the cardiac cycle. Now, find your radial pulse and begin counting: 0, 1, 2, 3, ... All the events described in this section occur every time you feel a pulse, which is once every 0.8 sec, assuming you have a resting heart rate of 75 b·min^{-1}. **Heart rate (HR)** is thus defined as the number of cardiac cycles per minute, expressed as beats per minute (b · min^{-1}).

Stroke Volume

As mentioned previously, stroke volume (SV) is the volume of blood ejected from the ventricles with each beat, expressed as milliliters per beat (mL·b^{-1}) or milliliters (mL). The amount of blood ejected from the heart is determined
by three factors:

1. The volume of blood returned to the heart (preload).

2. The force of contraction (contractility).

3. The resistance presented to the contracting ventricle (afterload).

The volume of blood returned to the heart is called **preload** and is critical to determining the amount of blood ejected from the heart (the heart cannot eject blood that is not there). Under resting conditions the heart ejects approximately 50–60% of the blood that is returned; this is known as the **ejection fraction (EF)**. Figure 12.6 depicts changes in the volume of blood in the ventricles throughout the cardiac cycle and defines specific volumes and capacities associated with the ventricles. The LVEDV is approximately 130 mL of blood under resting conditions. Following systole the LVESV is approximately 60 mL of blood. Stroke volume can then be calculated as

12.1 stroke volume (mL) = left ventricular end–diastolic volume (mL) − left ventricular end–systolic volume (mL)

or

$$SV = LVEDV - LVESV$$
$$130 \text{ mL} - 60 \text{ mL} = 70 \text{ mL}$$

Thus, 70 mL of blood was ejected from the heart at rest.

The ejection fraction (EF) can now be calculated from the information as follows:

12.2 ejection fraction (%) = stroke volume (mL) ÷ left ventricular end–diastolic volume (mL) × 100

or

$$EF = \frac{SV}{LVEDV} \times 100$$

Example
- - - - - - - - - - - - - - - -

Calculate the ejection fraction for the previous example.

$$EF = [(70 \text{ mL}) \div (130 \text{ mL})] \times 100 = 54\% \quad \text{✚}$$

Notice in Figure 12.6 that the SV can increase by either an increased LVEDV (which encroaches into diastolic reserve volume) or decreased LVESV (which encroaches into systolic reserve volume) or a combination of the two. However, the entire blood volume cannot be ejected; thus, there is always a residual volume of blood in the heart (Brechar and Galletti, 1963; Clark, 1975). Because the subdivisions of ventricular volume parallel those of the lungs, it may be helpful to refer back to Figure 10.4.

Functional residual capacity is equal to the residual volume and the systolic reserve volume. Total ventricular capacity is the sum of residual volume, systolic reserve volume, stroke volume, and diastolic reserve volume and represents the maximal amount of blood the ventricles can hold.

As the volume of blood returned to the heart (LVEDV) increases, the SV increases. This phenomenon

---

Left Ventricular End–Diastolic Volume (LVEDV) The volume of blood in the left ventricle at the end of diastole.

Left Ventricular End–Systolic Volume (LVESV) The volume of blood in the left ventricle at the end of systole.

Stroke Volume (SV) Amount of blood ejected from the ventricles with each beat of the heart.

Heart Rate (HR) The number of cardiac cycles per minute.

Preload Volume of blood returned to the heart.

Ejection Fraction (EF) The percentage of LVEDV that is ejected from the heart.

Figure 12.6
Subdivisions of Ventricular Volume

Source: G. A. Brechar & P. M. Galletti. Functional anatomy of cardiac pumping. In W. F. Hamilton (ed.), *Handbook of Physiology, Section 2: Circulation.* Washington, D.C.: American Physiological Society (1963). Reprinted by permission.

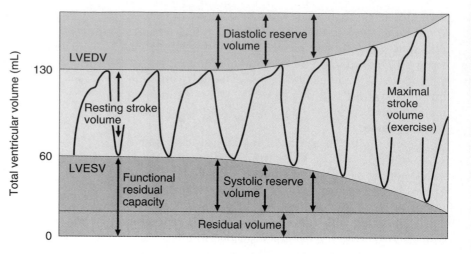

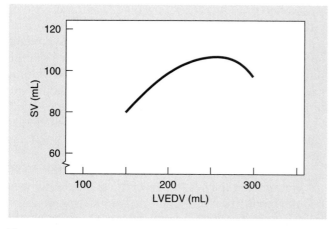

Figure 12.7
Frank-Starling Law of the Heart

is known as the Frank-Starling law of the heart. The relationship is shown in Figure 12.7. Answer the Question of Understanding box below to ensure your understanding of this figure. Check your answer in Appendix D.

Contractility of the myocardium is determined primarily by neural innervation. Sympathetic nerve fibers, as described in Chapter 2, cause an increase in contractility of the myocardium independent of the volume of blood returned to the heart.

Contractility The force of contraction of the heart.

Afterload Resistance presented to the contracting ventricle.

Cardiac Output The amount of blood pumped per unit of time, in liters per minute.

The **afterload,** or the resistance presented to the contracting ventricle, is determined primarily by the blood pressure in the aorta. As blood pressure increases, resistance increases and less blood is ejected from the ventricles for any force of contraction—that is, stroke volume decreases as afterload increases. The stroke volume decreases in this way because the increased pressure in the aorta causes the semilunar valves to remain closed longer and to close sooner. The valve is thus open for less time, thereby causing a decrease in ejection time and a subsequent decrease in stroke volume. Table 12.2 on page 324 presents typical values for stroke volume at rest in healthy individuals of various ages.

Cardiac Output

Cardiac output, $\dot{Q}$, is the amount of blood pumped per unit of time, normally reported in liters per minute. It represents the total blood flow of the entire cardiovascular system and represents the body's ability to meet changing metabolic needs during rest and exercise. Cardiac output is calculated as

12.3 cardiac output (mL·min^{-1}) = stroke volume (mL·b^{-1}) × heart rate (b·min^{-1})

or

$$\dot{Q} = SV \times HR$$

A Question of Understanding

Using Figure 12.7, answer the following questions:

1. What is the SV associated with an LVEDV of 150 mL? Of 200 mL? Of 250 mL? Of 300 mL?
2. What is the EF for each SV?

At rest the total blood volume (~5 L) is approximately equal to the cardiac output. Table 12.2 presents typical values for cardiac output at rest in healthy individuals of various ages.

Example

Calculate $\dot{Q}$ for an individual with a HR of 64 b·min^{-1} and a SV of 100 mL of blood.

$$\dot{Q} = SV \times HR = (100 \text{ mL·b}^{-1}) \times (64 \text{ b·min}^{-1})$$
$$= 6400 \text{ mL·min}^{-1}$$

Because $\dot{Q}$ is usually reported in liters, this value is divided by 1000 and is reported as 6.4 L·min^{-1}. Notice that although SV is usually expressed as milliliters (mL), it is actually measured in milliliters per beat (mL·b^{-1}) since by definition SV must be per beat.   ✛

The Question of Understanding box asks you to do some simple calculations to check your understanding of these formulas. Check your answers in Appendix D.

Coronory Circulation

The energy necessary for cardiac function is supplied through aerobic metabolism, which means that the heart is richly supplied with blood vessels to deliver oxygen. The myocardial blood flow required to provide the necessary amount of oxygen at rest is about 250 mL·min^{-1}, which represents approximately 4% of the normal resting cardiac output (Rowell, 1986). The coronary circulation provides blood to the myocardium. Blood is supplied to the heart by two major coronary arteries, the right and left coronary artery, that originate at the root of the aorta. The left coronary artery divides into the left circumflex and anterior descending arteries. The right coronary artery divides into the marginal artery and the posterior interventricular artery. The myocardium is supplied with a dense distribution of

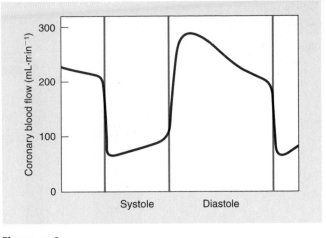

Figure 12.8
Coronary Blood Flow through the Cardiac Cycle

Source: A. C. Guyton. *Textbook of Medical Physiology.* Philadelphia: Saunders (1991), p. 238. Modified and reprinted by permission.

arterioles and capillaries, approximately 3000 to 4000 capillaries per square millimeter of cardiac muscle (Rowell, 1986). The venous blood from the coronary circulation is returned to the right atrium via the coronary sinus.

Blood flow through the coronary circulation is affected greatly by the phase of the cardiac cycle. Figure 12.8 depicts coronary blood flow throughout the cardiac cycle. Because of the high intramyocardial pressure during systole, the coronary arteries are compressed, and blood flow to the myocardium is decreased, demonstrating that the myocardium receives the largest portion of its blood flow during diastole (Guyton, 1991).

The coronary circulation is very effective in the extraction of oxygen as the blood flows through the capillary beds. Under resting conditions 60–70% of the available oxygen is extracted.

Myocardial Oxygen Consumption

Oxygen consumption is determined by oxygen extraction (a-vO$_2$ diff) and blood flow ($\dot{Q}$). Clearly, the metabolic demands of the myocardium are increased during exercise—that is, myocardial oxygen consumption increases during exercise. As mentioned previously (see "Coronary Circulation"), oxygen extraction of the coronary circulation is nearly optimal at rest (60–70%); thus, the increased myocardial oxygen consumption of the myocardium is supported almost entirely by increased blood flow to the myocardium.

The coronary blood flow must be regulated to meet the demands of the myocardium for oxygen. In

A Question of Understanding

Using your knowledge of the components of cardiac output, perform the necessary calculations to determine the missing values.

	HR (b·min^{-1})	SV (mL·b^{-1})	$\dot{Q}$ (L·min^{-1})
Mike	80	90	
Keiko	60	120	
Kirk	122	146.5	
Don	72		6.34
Nora		98	5.68

Figure 12.9
Vascular System

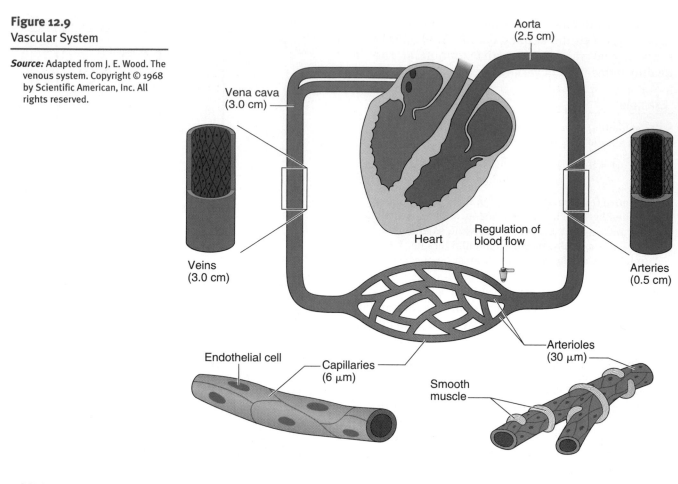

addition to an increased heart rate, an increased blood flow is achieved by two mechanisms:

1. The greater force of myocardial contraction that results from exercise causes more blood to be forced into the coronary circulation, thus increasing blood flow and helping to meet the metabolic demands of the myocardium.

2. By-products of cellular work cause vasodilation of the arterioles that supply the myocardium. Thus, as the heart works harder and produces more by-products, the arterioles dilate, which decreases resistance and effectively increases blood flow to support the work of the myocardium.

Myocardial oxygen consumption increases as heart rate increases. Because heart rate increases in relation to the intensity of exercise, so also does myocardial oxygen consumption (Kitamura, et al., 1972).

Myocardial oxygen consumption can be estimated from the *rate-pressure product (RPP)*, which is the product of heart rate (HR) and systolic blood pressure (SBP):

12.4 rate-pressure product (units) = [systolic blood pressure (mmHg) × heart rate (b·min^{-1})] ÷ 100

or

$$RPP = (SBP \times HR) \div 100$$

RPP provides a good estimate of myocardial oxygen consumption under a wide range of conditions, including dynamic and static exercise.

The Vascular System

The *vascular system* is composed of vessels that transport the blood throughout the body. Each portion of the vascular system has a specific structure and function that is related to the overall function of the cardiovascular system. The components of the vascular system are illustrated in Figure 12.9.

Arteries

The arteries are thick-walled conduits that carry blood from the heart to the various organs (see Figure 12.9). They contain a large amount of elastic tissue that allows them to distend when blood is ejected during systole and to recoil during diastole. Blood flow in the arteries is pulsatile owing to the pumping action of the heart.

Table 12.3
Typical Resting Blood Pressure Values for Males and Females of Various Ages

Blood Pressure Value	Age of Males (yr)			Age of Females (yr)		
	10–15	20–30	50–60	10–15	20–30	50–60
Systolic blood pressure SBP (mmHg)	100	120	134	84	120	130
Diastolic blood pressure DBP (mmHg)	60	80	84	40	74	84
Mean arterial pressure MAP (mmHg)	73	93	97	55	88	92

Sources: Fleg, et al. (1995); Ogawa, et al. (1992); Spina, et al. (1993a, b).

As the left ventricle ejects blood into the aorta, the blood stretches its elastic walls. *Blood pressure (BP)* is the force exerted on the wall of the blood vessel by the blood. The peak pressure is referred to as **systolic blood pressure (SBP)** because it is essentially caused by the contraction of the heart (systole). During relaxation of the heart (diastole), the arterial walls recoil, maintaining pressure on the blood that remains in the vessels. Thus, although the blood pressure drops during diastole, there is always some pressure in the arteries, and this pressure is known as **diastolic blood pressure (DBP)**. *Mean arterial pressure (MAP)* represents the mean driving force of blood throughout the arterial system. Typical blood pressure values for males and females are given in Table 12.3. The measurement of blood pressure is detailed later in this chapter. At this point it is important only to realize that both a first (DBP_1) and second (DBP_2) diastolic pressure can be obtained. Which one is used is important in determing mean arterial pressure.

At rest and during recovery from exercise, mean arterial pressure is determined by first calculating pulse pressure, which is equal to the difference between SBP and DBP_2 ($PP = SBP - DBP_2$). Mean arterial pressure is then calculated as

12.5a mean arterial pressure (mmHg) = pulse pressure (mmHg) ÷ 3 + diastolic blood pressure (mmHg)

or

$$MAP = \frac{PP}{3} + DBP_2$$

MAP is not simply computed as the average of SBP and DBP because diastole lasts longer than systole and is thus weighted more heavily in the computation of MAP. During exercise MAP can be computed according to a modified equation which uses DBP_1, (Robinson, et al., 1988):

12.5b mean arterial pressure (mmHg) = pulse pressure (mmHg) ÷ 2 + diastolic blood pressure (mmHg)

or

$$MAP = \frac{PP}{2} + DBP_1$$

This formula provides a more accurate measurement of MAP during exercise conditions because it gives less weight to DBP. Although both systole and diastole time shorten owing to an increased heart rate, diastole shortens proportionally more.

Arterioles

The *arterioles,* also called **resistance vessels,** are smaller than the arteries and are the major site of resistance in the vascular system (see Figure 12.9). Because of the increased resistance in the arterioles, the pulsatile arterial blood flow becomes continuous before it reaches the capillaries. The arterioles are able to absorb the pulsatile force of the blood flow because of the large amount of elastic tissue they contain. The importance of the elastic tissue in absorbing force can

Systolic Blood Pressure (SBP) The force exerted on the wall of the blood vessels by the blood as a result of contraction of the heart (systole).

Diastolic Blood Pressure (DBP) The force exerted on the wall of the blood vessels by blood during relaxation of the heart (diastole).

Resistance Vessels Another name for arterioles due to their ability to vasodilate and vasoconstrict; changing diameter allows them to control the flow of blood.

Figure 12.10
Anatomy of the Microcirculation

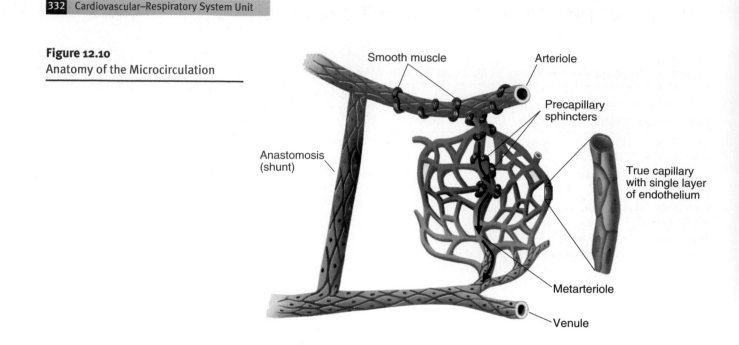

Smooth muscle

Arteriole

Precapillary
sphincters

Anastomosis
(shunt)

True capillary
with single layer
of endothelium

Metarteriole

Venule

be seen by considering an analogy of bouncing a bas-ketball on a gymnasium floor or on a wrestling mat. The ball rebounds from the gym floor at an angle and height that is proportional to the force imparted by your muscle action. However, the same force will not produce much (if any) rebound from the wrestling mat. The elastic tissue in the walls of the arteries ab-sorbs the energy from the pulsatile blood flow in a similar way that the mat absorbs energy from the bas-ketball. In an individual with reduced elasticity, or hardening of the arteries (called arteriosclerosis), the arteries, like the gym floor, are not able to distend as readily and blood pressure is elevated.

The smooth muscle surrounding arterioles is in-nervated by sympathetic neurons. The smooth muscle is able to change the diameter of the vessel by the processes of *vasoconstriction* (contraction of smooth muscle, causing decreased vessel diameter) and *va-sodilation* (relaxation of smooth muscle, causing in-creased vessel diameter). In fact, the vasoconstriction and vasodilation of the smooth muscles surrounding the arterioles is primarily responsible for determining blood flow distribution to various organs. For in-stance, if vasodilation occurs in the arterioles to the skeletal muscle of the legs, blood flow to this area in-creases. Likewise, if vasoconstriction occurs in the ar-terioles that supply the gastrointestinal tract, blood flow to this area decreases.

The degree to which a given arteriole vasodilates or vasoconstricts depends upon the balance of two mechanisms: local control and neural control. When tissue is metabolically active, it produces metabolic by-products that act locally to cause vasodilation, thereby increasing blood flow to the metabolically ac-tive area. In contrast, stimulation of the sympathetic

nervous system generally causes vasoconstriction of arterioles.

Capillaries

The *capillaries* perform the ultimate function of the cardiovascular system: exchanging gases and nutri-ents between the blood and tissues. The walls of the capillaries are composed of a single layer of epithelial tissue called the *endothelium* (see Figure 12.10). The diameter of the capillaries is very small, often neces-sitating that the red blood cells pass through in single file. Within a single capillary, there is increased re-sistance to flow because of its small diameter.

Blood flow through the capillaries depends on the other vessels that make up the microcirculation. As shown in Figure 12.10, the *microcirculation* includes several vessels: arterioles, venules, arteriovenous anastomoses, metarterioles, and true capillaries (Strand, 1983; Vander, et al., 1990). The *anastomoses* are wide, connecting channels that act as shunts be-tween the arterioles and venules. These vessels are particularly abundant in the skin and play an impor-tant role in thermoregulation. When the anastomoses are open, large volumes of blood can be directed to blood vessels close to the surface of the skin, facilitat-ing heat dissipation (Strand, 1983). The *metarteriole* is a short vessel that connects the arteriole with the venule, creating a shortcut through the capillary bed. The metarteriole gives rise to the capillaries. *True capillaries* vary in number depending on the capillary bed and usually contain a precapillary sphincter, which controls the flow of blood into the true capillar-ies. These *sphincters* are smooth muscles that open and close in response to local chemical conditions

(Vander, et al., 1990). Thus, a capillary bed can be perfused with blood or be almost entirely bypassed, depending on the needs of the tissue it supplies.

The exchange of gases and nutrients in the capillaries depends on diffusion. In order for a substance to diffuse from a capillary into a cell, it must cross two membranes: the endothelium of the capillary and the cell membrane. Substances pass from the capillary to the interstitial space by the process of diffusion. Movement from the interstitial space to the cell may occur by diffusion, or it may require carrier-mediated transport. The movement of gases and nutrients into and out of the capillaries depends on the concentration gradient or pressure gradient of the substance or gas that is diffusing.

As first discussed in Chapter 10, oxygen and carbon dioxide diffuse down pressure gradients. Oxygen diffuses down its pressure gradient from systemic capillaries into muscle cells. Hence, there is less oxygen in the veins draining skeletal muscles than in the arteries supplying them. The difference in the oxygen content of the arteries and veins is termed *a-vO₂ difference* and it reflects the oxygen taken up by the skeletal muscles.

Fluids also pass through the capillary membrane. The movement of fluids is determined by two opposing forces: hydrostatic pressure and osmotic pressure. *Hydrostatic pressure* is created by blood pressure and acts to "push" fluid out of the capillaries. *Osmotic pressure,* caused by the larger concentration of proteins in the capillaries, acts to "pull" water into the capillaries. The net result of these opposing forces is the loss of approximately 3 L of fluid a day from the plasma into the interstitial spaces (Marieb, 2001). This fluid is returned to the blood via the lymphatic system. Any change in hydrostatic pressure or the osmolarity of the blood will alter fluid exchange between the blood and the interstitial fluid.

Venules

The venules are small vessels on the venous side of the vascular system. These vessels contain some smooth muscles that can influence capillary pressure. The venules and capillaries constitute the microcirculation where nutrient exchange occurs. Venules empty into the veins.

Veins

Veins, also called **capacitance vessels,** serve as low-resistance conduits that return blood to the heart (Figure 12.9). They contain smooth muscle innervated by the sympathetic nervous system; thus, they can also change their diameter. Contraction of smooth muscle

around the veins is known as *venoconstriction;* relaxation of the veins is known as *venodilation.* Because of the ability of the veins to expand (distensibility), they are capable of pooling large volumes of blood—up to 60% of the total blood volume at rest—and are sometimes referred to as a blood reservoir. The amount of blood in the veins varies with posture and activity. If blood accumulates in the veins and is not returned to the heart, ventricular end–diastolic volume decreases, with the result that stroke volume decreases. Conversely, if venoconstriction occurs, it can significantly increase ventricular end–diastolic volume and thereby lead to an increase in stroke volume, according to the Frank-Starling law of the heart.

The skeletal muscle pump and the respiratory pump help to increase venous return by "massaging" blood back toward the heart. The one-way valves in the veins also help regulate venous pressure and are particularly helpful in counteracting the upright posture, because they prevent the backward flow of blood. Additionally, the increased sympathetic nervous activity during exercise helps to increase venous return via venoconstriction.

Blood

Blood is the fluid that circulates through the heart and the vasculature, and it is responsible for the transport of nutrients and gases. Blood contains living blood cells suspended in a nonliving fluid matrix called plasma. Blood cells can be identified as erythrocytes (red blood cells, RBC) or leukocytes (white blood cells, WBC). Blood cells account for 38–45% of the total blood volume in adult females and 43–48% of the total blood volume in adult males. The ratio of blood cells to total blood volume is known as **hematocrit** and is usually expressed as a percentage.

As discussed in the respiratory section, it is the RBCs that transport oxygen from the lungs to the cells by binding the oxygen to the hemoglobin. Leukocytes are less numerous than erythrocytes, accounting for about 1% of total blood volume. However, these blood cells are essential to the body's defense against disease.

Plasma accounts for approximately 55% of the volume of blood. It is composed primarily of water, which

---

Capacitance Vessels Another name for veins, owing to their distensibility, which enables them to pool large volumes of blood and become reservoirs for blood.

Hematocrit The ratio of blood cells to total blood volume, expressed as a percentage.

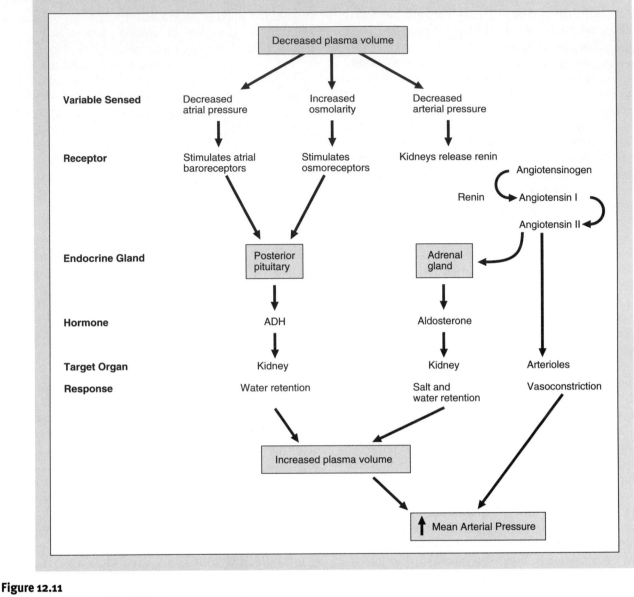

Figure 12.11
Hormonal Control of Blood Volume

accounts for 90% of its volume, and contains over 100 dissolved solutes, including proteins, electrolytes, and respiratory gases. The composition of plasma can vary greatly, depending on the needs of the body. Plasma also plays an important role in thermoregulation, helping to distribute heat throughout the body.

This information can be practically applied to the effects of blood donation on an exerciser. One pint of blood (about 450–500 mL) is typically donated. Because total blood volume is approximately 5000 mL (5 L), the amount of blood donated results in roughly a 10% reduction in blood volume. This amount, however, will represent a greater percentage in small in-

dividuals with less blood (typically women). The blood plasma volume is reestablished in approximately 24 hr, whereas red blood cells are replaced in about 6 weeks. Given the reduction in plasma volume, it seems prudent for endurance athletes to avoid donating blood during the competitive phases of the training cycle. Training intensity may need to be slightly reduced pending complete RBC replacement for fitness participants or athletes who do donate blood. Also, strenuous activities should be avoided for 24 hr after giving blood to allow the body to replace the majority of the lost fluids. Plenty of water should be ingested following blood donation.

Hormonal Control of Blood Volume

As just discussed, blood volume is decreased following blood donation. It can also be decreased due to profuse sweating and/or dehydration. Blood volume varies considerably among individuals and is affected by fitness status and hydration level. Healthy adult men have an average blood volume of approximately 75 mL of blood per kg of body weight, or about 5–6 L of blood. Healthy adult women have approximately 65 mL of blood per kg of body weight, which equals 4–4.5 L of blood for the average size woman. Children typically have about 60 mL of blood per kg of body weight, with total volume varying depending on the size of the child.

Blood volume plays an important role in maintaining stroke volume, cardiac output, and blood pressure. Under normal conditions blood volume is maintained within physiological limits by homeostatic mechanisms involving the endocrine system and urinary system. The major hormones involved in maintaining blood volume are antidiuretic hormone (ADH), released from the posterior pituitary gland, and aldosterone, released from the adrenal cortex. Figure 12.11 outlines the hormonal mechanisms responsible for responding to a reduction in blood volume.

Plasma volume reduction causes a decrease in atrial and arterial pressure. This reduction is sensed by atrial baroreceptors (*atrial* means "in the atrium"; *baro* means "pressure") and arterial receptors within the kidneys. Atrial baroreceptor activation leads to the release of ADH from the posterior pituitary gland, which causes the tubules of the kidneys to reabsorb water, thus increasing plasma volume.

A reduction in blood volume is also associated with an increase in plasma osmolarity. For example, with profuse sweating more water than solutes is lost; thus, the osmolarity of the blood increases. An increase in osmolarity of the blood stimulates osmoreceptors in the hypothalamus, which signals the posterior pituitary gland to release ADH. ADH causes the kidneys to retain water and thus leads to an increase in blood volume.

At the same time the receptors in the kidneys respond to a decrease in arterial pressure by releasing renin. Renin is an enzyme that is necessary for the conversion of angiotensinogen to angiotensin I, which is then converted to angiotensin II. Angiotensin II signals the adrenal cortex to release aldosterone. Aldosterone causes the kidneys to retain salt and water. Angiotensin II also has a vasoconstrictor effect on arterioles, thus helping to increase blood pressure.

Cardiovascular Dynamics

This section deals with the different components of the cardiovascular system and how they function together to meet the changing demands of the body. There is a vast amount of integration and interdependence within the cardiovascular system. Specifically, both the heart and the vasculature respond independently to various conditions but are interrelated because the response of the heart affects the vessels, and vice versa.

In differentiating the response of the heart and the vessels, we commonly refer to central and peripheral circulatory responses. *Central circulatory responses* are those directly related to the heart—heart rate, stroke volume, cardiac output, etc. *Peripheral circulatory responses* are those occurring in vessels—vasodilation, vasoconstriction, venous return, etc.

Cardiac Output ($\dot{Q}$)

The volume of air or blood flow can be described by the basic formula presented in Chapter 10 (Eq. 10.1, $F = \Delta P/R$). Applied to the cardiovascular system, this equation is

12.6 cardiac output ($L \cdot min^{-1}$) = mean arterial blood pressure (mmHg) ÷ total peripheral resistance ($mmHg \cdot mL^{-1} \cdot min^{-1}$)

or

$$\dot{Q} = \frac{MAP}{TPR}$$

In this formula, cardiac output represents the blood flow for the entire cardiovascular system, mean arterial pressure reflects the pressure gradient, and total peripheral resistance refers to the factors that oppose blood flow in the entire system. The equation should really use the difference in pressure (ΔP), that is, the difference between mean arterial pressure and the pressure in the right atrium (where blood is flowing to). However, since pressure in the right atrium is so low (less than 4 mmHg), it is considered negligible and is not usually given in the formula. Thus, the pressure used is simply mean arterial pressure.

Total peripheral resistance (TPR), or simply **resistance (R),** represents the factors that oppose blood flow. It is expressed in millimeters of mercury per milliliter per minute ($mmHg \cdot mL^{-1} \cdot min^{-1}$) or more simply as TPR units. The majority of the resistance in the vascular tree results from the friction against the vessel walls, and it varies depending on the size of the vessel. The three primary factors that affect resistance and

---

Total Peripheral Resistance (TPR) or Resistance (R) The factors that oppose blood flow.

their mathematical relationship are described by Poiseuille's law, which states:

12.7 $\text{resistance} = \dfrac{\text{length} \times \text{viscosity}}{(\text{radius})^4}$

Thus, the more viscous the blood is, the greater resistance to flow it provides. The longer the blood vessel, the greater the friction that will result between the walls of the vessel and the blood. However, under normal conditions vessel length and blood viscosity do not change substantially. The radius of the vessel, however, can change considerably owing to vasodilation or vasoconstriction. Furthermore, because the resistance is inversely related to the fourth power of the radius, a small change in vessel diameter can result in a large change in blood flow. Thus, vessel radius is by far the most important factor determining resistance to blood flow. Recall that vessel diameter is affected by local metabolic conditions (local control) and neural innervation (reflex control).

Total peripheral resistance (TPR) can be calculated by rearranging the formula $\dot{Q} = \text{MAP} \div \text{TPR}$ to solve for TPR, provided that the flow rate ($\dot{Q}$) and blood pressure (MAP) are known. The formula for TPR becomes

12.8 total peripheral resistance (TPR units) = mean arterial blood pressure (mmHg) ÷ cardiac output (L·min^{-1})

or

$$\text{TPR} = \frac{\text{MAP}}{\dot{Q}}$$

Example

Assume that normal resting blood pressure is 110/80 (MAP = 90 mmHg), normal cardiac output is 5.4 L·min, and central venous pressure is zero. Calculate TPR for the entire cardiovascular system.
The calculation is

$$\text{TPR} = \frac{\text{MAP}}{\dot{Q}} = \frac{90 \text{ mmHg}}{5.4 \text{ L·min}} = 16.67 \text{ (TPR units)}$$

This calculation can also be arranged to indicate that MAP is the product of $\dot{Q}$ and TPR. This equation then becomes

$$\text{MAP} = \dot{Q} \times \text{TPR}$$

The Question of Understanding box provides an example to calculate TPR. Check your answer in Appendix D.

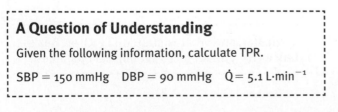

A Question of Understanding

Given the following information, calculate TPR.

SBP = 150 mmHg   DBP = 90 mmHg $\dot{Q}$ = 5.1 L·min^{-1}

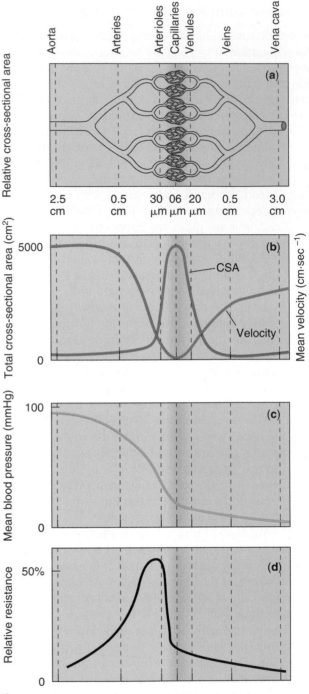

Figure 12.12

Relationships among Cross-Sectional Area of Blood Vessels, Blood Pressure, and Resistance

Source: J. T. Shepherd & P. M. Vanhoutte. *The Human Cardiovascular System.* New York: Raven Press (1980). Reprinted by permission.

Principles of Blood Flow

Figure 12.12 presents the relationships among the cross-sectional area of the blood vessels, blood velocity, blood pressure, and resistance throughout the vascular system. The diameter of the various vessels is shown in Figure 12.12a, and the total cross-sectional area of the various vessels is shown in Figure 12.12b. Thus, although a single capillary is incredibly small, approximately 6 μm (see Figure 12.12a), there are so many capillaries that the total cross-sectional area far exceeds that of the other vessels. The blue curve in Figure 12.12b depicts the velocity of blood in the various vessels—that is, the rate of movement or speed at which blood flows. The velocity of a fluid in a closed system varies inversely with the total cross-sectional area at any given point. Therefore, the velocity of blood flow decreases dramatically in the capillaries. This decreased velocity allows adequate time for the exchange of respiratory gases and nutrients.

Figure 12.12c depicts the change in the mean blood pressure throughout the vascular system. The driving force for the blood is the contraction of the myocardium. Blood flows because of a pressure gradient. Thus, blood flows through the vascular tree because pressure is highest in the aorta and major arteries and lowest in the great veins and right atrium of the heart. Pressure continues to decrease as the blood travels further from the heart, reaching a low of approximately 4 mmHg in the right atrium. In fact, one-way venous valves and muscle and respiratory pump activity are needed to help return blood to the heart.

Resistance to blood flow is shown in Figure 12.12d. Notice that the majority of the resistance is encountered in the arterioles. As the blood enters the capillaries, the resistance decreases.

Regulation of the Cardiovascular System

The regulation of the cardiovascular system is accomplished by interrelated and overlapping mechanisms, including mechanical events, neural control, and neurohormonal control. Mechanical events, such as muscle action, influence venous return and thereby help regulate stroke volume and cardiac output. This regulation is particularly important during exercise. The neural and neurohormonal mechanisms of cardiovascular control are more complex and are discussed in detail in the following sections.

Neural Control

Three cardiovascular centers are located within the medulla oblongata of the brain stem (Figure 12.13). The cardioaccelerator and cardioinhibitor centers innervate the heart. As the names imply, the *cardioaccelerator center* sends signals, via sympathetic accelerator nerves, that cause the heart rate to increase and the force of contraction to strengthen. The *cardioinhibitor center,* also called the vagal nucleus,

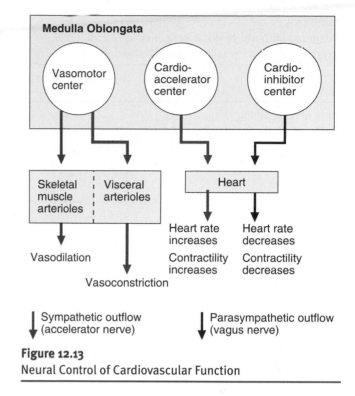

Figure 12.13
Neural Control of Cardiovascular Function

sends signals via the vagus nerve that result in a decreased heart rate.

The *vasomotor center* innervates the smooth muscles of the arterioles via sympathetic nerves. Activation of these sympathetic fibers results in a different response depending on location of the arterioles. The arterioles that supply skeletal muscles vasodilate when stimulated, whereas the arterioles in visceral beds constrict under sympathetic influence. This response ensures that activation of the sympathetic nervous system increases blood flow to skeletal muscles and decreases blood flow in nonessential areas in situations where movement may be required. If all of the arterioles were to dilate during sympathetic stimulation, the blood volume and pressure would be inadequate to meet the circulatory demands of the body.

In summary, activation of sympathetic nervous outflow leads to increased heart rate, increased contractility, vasodilation in the arterioles of skeletal muscle, and vasoconstriction in visceral arterioles. Activation of the parasympathetic nervous system leads to a decrease in each of the above. Table 12.4 summarizes these cardiovascular responses.

Anatomical Sensors and Factors Affecting Control of the Cardiovascular System

The cardiovascular centers—and therefore, the sympathetic and parasympathetic outflow from those centers—are influenced by several factors. These factors

Table 12.4

Summary of Cardiovascular Response to Stimulation of Sympathetic and Parasympathetic Activation

Response	Sympathetic Stimulation	Parasympathetic Stimulation
Rate of contraction	↑	↓
Force of contraction	↑	↓
Excitability	↑	↓
Conductivity	↑	↓
Metabolism	↑	↓

Source: McNaught & Callander (1983).

operate in a variety of circumstances, including exercise. Figure 12.14 schematically presents the most important factors influencing the cardiovascular centers. These factors are described in detail in the following subsections.

Higher Brain Centers

The cardiovascular medullary centers are influenced by several higher brain centers, including the cerebral cortex and the hypothalamus. Emotional influences arising from the cerebral cortex can affect cardiovascular function at rest. Additionally, input from the motor cortex, which is relayed through the hypothalamus, can influence cardiovascular function during exercise, leading to an increase in heart rate and vasodilation in active muscle. The influence of the cortex and hypothalamus on the cardiovascular centers during exercise is often termed "central command," suggesting that the signal to alter cardiovascular variables comes from the central nervous system.

Body temperature also affects the cardiovascular centers through the influence of the hypothalamus. An increase in body temperature results in an increased heart rate, increased cardiac output, and vasodilation in the arterioles of the active muscles and skin.

Systemic Receptors

Systemic receptors are found in the great veins, the heart, and the arterial system. These receptors provide sensory information to the cardiovascular control centers that leads to reflex action.

Baroreceptors Baroreceptors are located in the aorta and carotid bodies. These receptors are sensitive to an increase in mean arterial pressure and cause a reflex decrease in mean arterial pressure owing to a decrease in heart rate and, thus, cardiac out-

put. The decrease in heart rate is mediated through an increased parasympathetic outflow and a simultaneous decrease in sympathetic outflow to the heart. This reflex control of blood pressure is called the *baroreceptor reflex*.

Because this reflex attempts to keep the mean arterial blood pressure down, you may wonder how anyone can become hypertensive or why mean arterial blood pressure goes up during exercise. In the first situation, the action of the baroreceptors is mediated by a set point. If something causes the resting blood pressure to be elevated (and no one knows precisely what causes this elevation), the baroreceptors fire for about 24 hr, trying to bring the mean arterial pressure down. If they are unsuccessful, they simply reset at a level above the current value. In the case of exercise, the relatively weak parasympathetic system is simply overwhelmed by the more powerful sympathetic system. The baroreceptor reflex is, however, very important in achieving recovery to baseline values after exercise.

Stretch Receptors Stretch receptors are located in the right atrium of the heart and are stimulated by an increase in venous return. The signal is transmitted to the cardiovascular centers in the medulla, where they cause an increase in sympathetic outflow and a decrease in parasympathetic outflow. This results in an increased rate and force of contraction of the heart and leads to increased cardiac output. This sequence is called the *Bainbridge reflex*.

Chemoreceptors

Chemoreceptors are located in the aortic and carotid arteries. They are sensitive to arterial blood PO_2, PCO_2, and H^+. An increase in PCO_2 and H^+ or a decrease in PO_2 causes a reflex vasoconstriction of arterioles.

Muscle Joint Receptors

Muscle receptors include mechanical (*mechanoreceptors*) and metabolic (*metaboreceptors*) receptors. They are located in the joints and muscles, and they send impulses to the brain, where the impulses synapse with the cardiovascular centers. These receptors are stimulated by muscle contraction and lead to an increased rate and force of heart contraction and vasodilation in active muscle. Vasoconstriction occurs in inactive skeletal muscles.

Neurohormonal Control

The endocrine system also plays an important role in the regulation of the cardiovascular system.

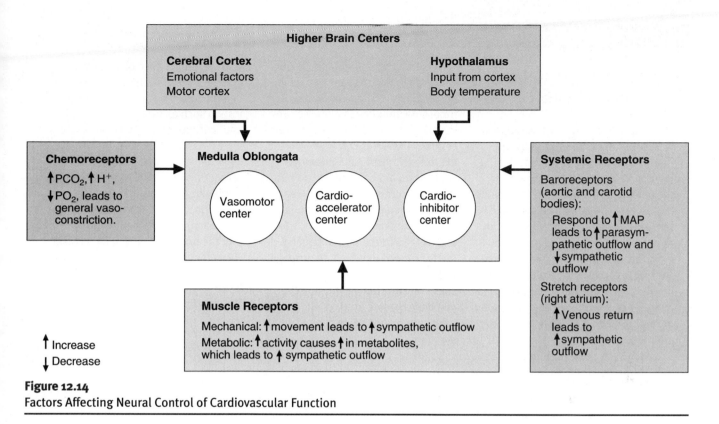

Figure 12.14
Factors Affecting Neural Control of Cardiovascular Function

Considerable control is exerted by components of the autonomic nervous system and the hormones of the adrenal medulla. The previous section discussed the influence of the sympathetic nervous system on the heart and the blood vessels. The sympathetic nervous system also innervates the adrenal medulla, causing the adrenal glands to release the hormones epinephrine and norepinephrine. These hormones circulate in the bloodstream and travel to the target organs, namely, the heart and the blood vessels. Generally, epinephrine and norepinephrine have the same effect on the target organs as the sympathetic nerve fibers innervating them.

In addition to the adrenal hormones, aldosterone and ADH are involved in maintaining blood volume and blood pressure as described in the section on blood volume.

Assessment of Cardiovascular Variables

The assessment and monitoring of cardiovascular variables is routine in sports and fitness settings. The following variables are measured so that one can assess fitness, prescribe exercise, and monitor physiological responses to exercise. Most of these variables can be assessed at rest and during submaximal or maximal exercise.

Cardiac Output

Recall that cardiac output ($\dot{Q}$) is equal to the product of stroke volume and heart rate (Eq. 12.3). However, because stroke volume has historically been very difficult to measure, cardiac output has been calculated from another known relationship described by the **Fick equation**. This equation states that

12.9 cardiac output (L·min^{-1}) = oxygen consumption (mL·min^{-1}) ÷ arteriovenous oxygen difference (mL·L^{-1})

or

$$\dot{Q} = \frac{\dot{V}O_2}{\text{a-v}O_2 \text{ diff}}$$

The direct determination of cardiac output via the Fick equation requires that oxygen consumption and arteriovenous oxygen difference both be measured. Many laboratories can directly measure oxygen consumption and this test is described thoroughly in Chapter 5. The assessment of arteriovenous oxygen difference (a-vO$_2$ diff), however, is more problematic.

Fick Equation An equation used to calculate cardiac output from oxygen consumption and arteriovenous oxygen difference (a-vO$_2$ diff).

Focus on Application

✴ Are All Elevations In Heart Rate Equal?

Heart rate (HR) can be elevated by a variety of factors mediated by the neural and hormonal systems (see Figures 12.13 and 12.14). One of these factors is movement (exercise), but others may be emotion or high temperatures. Does an individual derive the same benefit from HR that is elevated by emotion or heat as from HR that is elevated by exercise? That is, is it possible to improve cardiovascular function while sitting in a sauna or hot tub or when frightened, angry, or anxious?

It is true that a regular, sustained elevation in HR is recognized as important in improving cardiovascular fitness (techniques of exercise prescription based on HR are fully described in Chapter 14). However, the exercise HR responses primarily serve as an indicator of the training stimulus to the body—the increase in energy expenditure or metabolism (oxygen consumption). Heart rate and oxygen consumption rise in a directly proportional fashion during exercise. When emotion or temperature cause an elevation in HR, however, minimal changes occur in energy expenditure, hence there is no training stimulus.

The preeminence of an increase in oxygen consumption has been demonstrated by individuals on medication such as beta blockers, which markedly suppress HR at rest and during exercise, and by those with constant heart-rate pacemakers. Individuals in both of these groups routinely show improvements in exercise capacity and fitness as a result of exercise programs despite the fact that the exercise-induced increase in HR is dampened.   ✴

Source:
Franklin & Munnings (1998).

This test requires a sample of arterial blood from an artery and a sample of mixed venous blood from the vena cava or right atrium.

Because cardiac output is difficult to measure directly without expensive laboratory equipment, it is often estimated from the relationship between cardiac output and oxygen consumption. Estimates of exercise cardiac output can be derived if oxygen consumption is known. This estimate is based on a mathematically established relationship between cardiac output and oxygen consumption. Cardiac output at light to moderate workloads (under 70% $\dot{V}O_2max$) can be calculated according to the following formulas (Åstrand, et al., 1964).

12.10a men: $\quad y = 6.55 + 4.35x$

12.10b women: $\quad y = 3.66 + 6.81x$

where y = predicted cardiac output (in liters per minute) and x = measured oxygen consumption (in liters per minute). The Question of Understanding box provides an opportunity for you to do a sample calculation. Check your answer in Appendix D.

Stroke Volume

Advances in technology have made the assessment of stroke volume (SV) more readily available, particularly during exercise. Stroke volume can now be measured using Doppler echocardiography. **Doppler echocardiography** is a technique that calculates stroke volume from measurements of aortic cross-sectional area (CSA) and time-velocity integral (TVI) of the blood flow in the ascending aorta (Figure 12.15). The formula is

12.11 stroke volume (mL) = cross-sectional area (cm^2) × time-velocity integrals (cm)

or

$$SV = CSA \times TVI$$

Note that, for conversion purposes, $cm^3 = mL$.

Two-dimensional echocardiography is used to measure aortic diameter (Figure 12.15a). Cross-sectional area is then calculated from a geometric model using the following formula:

12.12 cross-sectional area (cm^2) = diameter^2 (cm) × π/4

or

$$CSA = d^2 \times \frac{\pi}{4}$$

Doppler ultrasound is used to assess blood flow velocity in the ascending aorta (Figure 12.15b). From the Doppler waveforms a time-velocity integral is obtained.

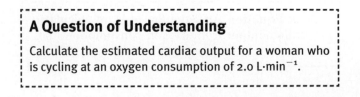

A Question of Understanding

Calculate the estimated cardiac output for a woman who is cycling at an oxygen consumption of 2.0 L·min^{-1}.

Doppler Echocardiography A technique that calculates stroke volume from measurements of aortic cross-sectional area and time-velocity integrals in the ascending aorta.

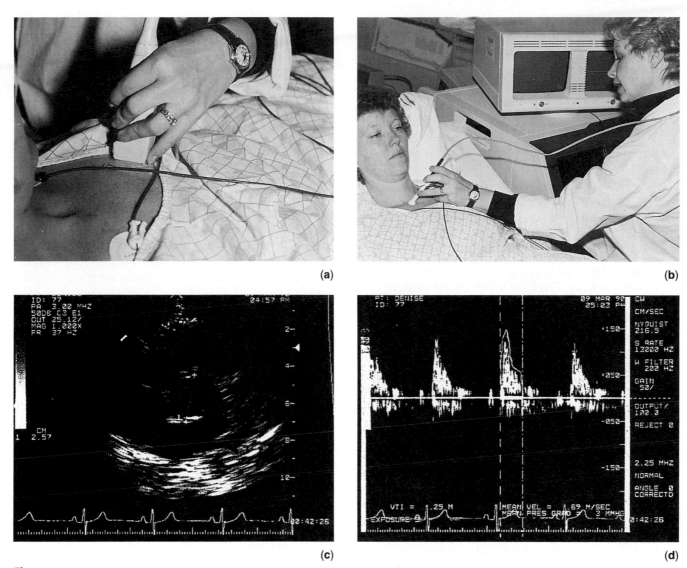

Figure 12.15
Determination of Aortic Diameter and Blood Velocity

Ultrasound technician obtains aortic diameter (a) and Doppler waveforms from the suprasternal
notch (b). Print-out of aortic diameter (c) and Doppler waveforms (d).

Example

Using the information provided in Figures 12.15c and
d, calculate SV.
  The calculations are

$$CSA = 2.57^2 \times \frac{\pi}{4} = 5.18 \ cm^2$$

$$SV = (5.18 \ cm^2) \times (25 \ cm) = 129.5 \ mL \qquad +$$

Heart Rate

In a laboratory setting heart rate is often obtained by
measuring the R-R interval from an ECG recording
(Figure 12.16). The first step is to calculate the distance the ECG paper travels in one minute based on

the speed of the paper. The distance between cycles is
then measured. Because you now know the number of
cycles that occurred within the distance measured,
you can solve for the b·min^{-1} by solving for X in the
following equation:

12.13 HR b·min^{-1} = [number of beats ÷ distance
the cycles occupy (mm)] = [X b·min^{-1} ÷
distance the paper travels in one minute
(mm·min^{-1})]

Example

Using the ECG strip in Figure 12.16, calculate the
heart rate.
  Step 1: Using the paper speed, calculate the
distance the paper travels in one minute. Paper speed

Figure 12.16
ECG Used to Calculate Heart Rate

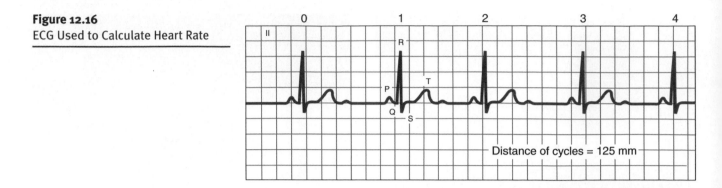

Distance of cycles = 125 mm

equals 25 mm·sec^{-1}. Since there are 60 sec·min^{-1}, 25 mm·sec^{-1} × 60 sec·min^{-1} = 1500 mm·min^{-1}.

Step 2: Measure the distance between 4 cycles, which in this case is 125 mm.

Step 3: Since 4 cycles (1 box = 5 mm) occurred within the time period required for the ECG paper to travel 125 mm, you calculate how many beats will occur in one minute by solving for X in the equation:

$$\frac{4}{125} = \frac{X}{1500}$$

$$125X = 6000, X = 6000/125 = 48 \text{ b·min}^{-1} \quad ✛$$

Heart rate can also be recorded by wireless telemetry, such as a heart rate watch. The transmitter is worn around the chest of the individual, and the heart rate signal is transmitted to a small receiver that looks very similar to a watch.

Heart rate is often measured during exercise to monitor exercise intensity. However, during most exercise sessions, sophisticated and expensive heart rate–measuring devices are not available. Instead, heart rate is assessed by counting the pulse, sometimes called palpation. The pulse can be counted at the carotid or radial artery. Each individual should receive instruction for and have practice in counting his or her pulse if it is to be used to accurately monitor exercise intensity.

To measure an exercise heart rate, the subject usually ceases exercise and finds the pulse as quickly as possible. The pulse count begins with zero and is counted for a set period of time, usually 6, 10, or 15 sec. This pulse count is then multiplied by 10, 6, or 4, respectively, to obtain a per-minute heart rate. Less than 1 min is used for counting because heart rate drops quickly following exercise; thus, the count must be obtained as quickly as possible.

Maximal Oxygen Consumption

Maximal oxygen consumption ($\dot{V}O_2$max) is the greatest amount of oxygen that the body can take in, transport, and utilize during heavy exercise. It is abbreviated as $\dot{V}O_2$max to indicate the maximal volume of

oxygen consumed. The body relies on the respiratory system to bring in the oxygen from the environment, the cardiovascular system to transport the oxygen, and the cells to extract the oxygen and use it in the production of energy (ATP). Thus, the assessment of maximal oxygen consumption provides a means for quantifying the functional capacity of the entire cardiovascular system. $\dot{V}O_2$max is often considered the single most important variable in describing an individual's fitness level and is routinely used to describe an individual's cardiorespiratory capacity.

The limit of circulatory function is reached at the highest attainable oxygen consumption and, rearranging the Fick equation (Eq. 12.9), is expressed in the following equation:

12.14a maximal oxygen uptake (mL·min^{-1})
= [maximal heart rate (b·min^{-1}) × stroke volume (L·b^{-1}) × maximal arteriovenous oxygen difference (mL·L^{-1})]

or

$\dot{V}O_2$max = (HRmax) × (SV max)
× (a-vO$_2$ diff max)

The equation may be simplified to

12.14b $\dot{V}O_2$max = ($\dot{Q}$ max) × (a-vO$_2$ diff max)

Although $\dot{V}O_2$max can be calculated from the variables in Equation 12.14a, it is most often measured with laboratory equipment, namely, open-circuit indirect spirometry, also called metabolic equipment. The assessment of oxygen consumption is described in detail in Chapter 5. Although oxygen is utilized only in aerobic metabolic production of ATP, the delivery of oxygen is primarily limited by the cardiovascular system. Thus, $\dot{V}O_2$max is considered to be a cardiovascular variable.

Factors Limiting $\dot{V}O_2$max

At some point an individual can no longer continue to increase the intensity of the exercise load or to work

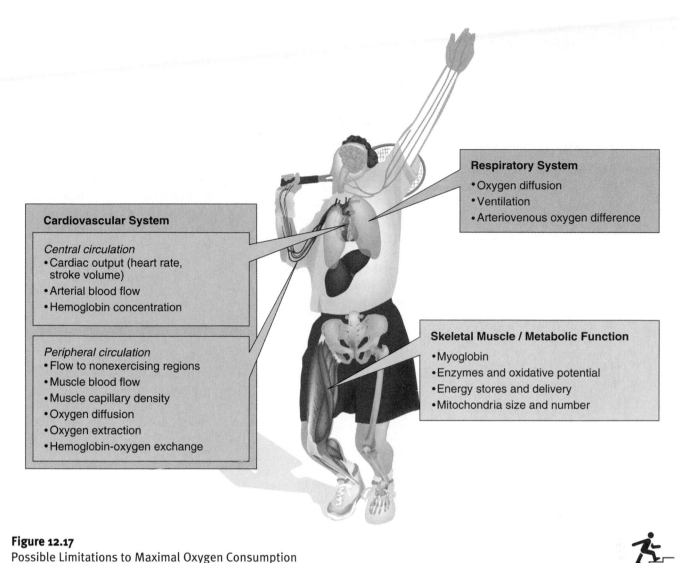

Respiratory System
- Oxygen diffusion
- Ventilation
- Arteriovenous oxygen difference

Cardiovascular System

Central circulation
- Cardiac output (heart rate, stroke volume)
- Arterial blood flow
- Hemoglobin concentration

Peripheral circulation
- Flow to nonexercising regions
- Muscle blood flow
- Muscle capillary density
- Oxygen diffusion
- Oxygen extraction
- Hemoglobin-oxygen exchange

Skeletal Muscle / Metabolic Function
- Myoglobin
- Enzymes and oxidative potential
- Energy stores and delivery
- Mitochondria size and number

Figure 12.17
Possible Limitations to Maximal Oxygen Consumption

Source: Modified from Rowell (1993).

at maximum effort because the body can no longer provide enough oxygen to support an additional workload. But what specifically limits $\dot{V}O_2$max? Figure 12.17 summarizes possible limitations to oxygen consumption within the major systems involved in providing oxygen during exercise.

Theoretically, maximal oxygen uptake could be limited by any system (or step) along the pathway of bringing oxygen into the body and delivering it to the mitochondria for the production of ATP. Thus, any of the following systems may limit $\dot{V}O_2$max:

1. the respiratory system, because of inadequate ventilation, oxygen diffusion limitations, or an inability to maintain the gradient for the diffusion of O_2 (a-vO_2 diff);

2. the cardiovascular system, because of inadequate blood flow ($\dot{Q}$) or oxygen-carrying capacity (Hb);

3. the metabolic functions within skeletal muscle, such as an inability to produce additional ATP because of limited number of mitochondria, limited enzyme levels or activity, or limited substrates.

Indeed, there is evidence to suggest that each of these systems may limit $\dot{V}O_2$max in certain conditions (Bergh, et al., 2000). For example, a reduction in the partial pressure of oxygen (PO_2) at altitude or the disease condition of asthma will cause a reduction in $\dot{V}O_2$max. Pharmacological agents (such as beta-blockers) that limit cardiac output will cause a decrease in $\dot{V}O_2$max, as will a reduction in hemoglobin associated with anemia. Certain diseases in which muscle enzymes involved in metabolism are deficient can also result in reduced $\dot{V}O_2$max.

Although it is important to understand the importance of each of these systems in achieving

Focus on Research

Pulmonary Ventilation

Powers, S. K., J. Lawler, J. A. Dempsey, S. Dodd, and G. Landry. Effects of incomplete pulmonary gas exchange on $\dot{V}O_2$max. *Journal of Applied Physiology.* 66:2491–2495 (1989).

Pulmonary ventilation is not thought to limit $\dot{V}O_2$max in most individuals. Arterial oxygen saturation (SaO_2%) decreases only slightly during maximal exercise in most individuals. Researchers have shown, however, that the SaO_2% does decrease signif-icantly in trained athletes with exercise-induced hypoxemia (EIH; see Chapter 11). Thus, the pulmonary system appears to limit maximal oxygen consumption in these athletes. To investigate the possibility that $\dot{V}O_2$max may be limited by different factors in trained versus untrained subjects, Powers and colleagues had normally trained and highly trained individuals perform a $\dot{V}O_2$max test under two conditions. During one trial the subjects inhaled room air (20.93% O_2), and during the other trial subjects inhaled oxygen-enriched air (26% O_2). The figure below presents the results of this study.

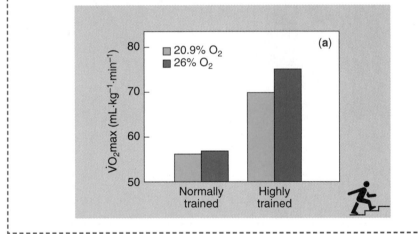

There are two important points to take from these data:

1. Highly trained individuals have a higher $\dot{V}O_2$max than normally trained individuals. This is true regardless of the concentration of oxygen that was inspired.
2. Breathing oxygen-enriched air had little effect on normally trained individuals but resulted in an increased $\dot{V}O_2$max in the highly trained group. This supports the theory that the pulmonary system is not a limiting factor in $\dot{V}O_2$max in normally trained individuals but does limit $\dot{V}O_2$max in some highly trained athletes. The most probable explanation for this difference is that in highly trained athletes there is insufficient time for the hemoglobin to become fully saturated as it passes through the pulmonary capillaries because of the extremely high cardiac output in these individuals.

In addition to the points made above, this research emphasizes the highly integrated function of the systems of the body in supplying oxygen for the production of ATP to support maximal exercise.

---

maximal oxygen uptake and to understand that under some circumstances each of these systems may limit the $\dot{V}O_2$max, the question remains: What limits $\dot{V}O_2$max in healthy humans performing maximal exercise? This question has energized exercise physiologists for decades, beginning with the work of A. V. Hill in the 1920s, and it continues to engender lively debate among physiologists today (Bassett and Howley, 2000; Bergh, et al., 2000; Grassi, 2000; Saltin, 1985).

The current evidence suggests that maximal oxygen uptake is limited by the ability of the cardiorespiratory system to deliver oxygen to the muscle, rather than the ability of the muscle mitochondria to utilize oxygen (Bergh, et al., 2000; Rowell, 1993; Saltin, 1985). More specifically, it appears that cardiac output is the limiting factor in $\dot{V}O_2$max (Bergh, et al., 2000; Saltin, 1985).

Research evidence suggests that oxygen uptake is not limited by pulmonary ventilation in normal, healthy athletes without exercise-induced hypoxemia (Chapter 11). Generally, the functional capacity of the respiratory system is considered to exceed the demands of maximal exercise (Rowell, 1993). The only respiratory variable likely to impose a limitation on oxygen transport is a-vO_2 diff. And, some physiologists consider it to be a cardiovascular variable (in addition to, or instead of, being a respiratory variable).

Many researchers report that skeletal muscles possess a greater ability to use oxygen than can be met by the respiratory and cardiovascular systems (Rowell, 1993; Saltin, 1985). Not all researchers agree with this view, though, and some have proposed that failure of muscle performance may explain exhaustion during maximal exercise (Noakes, 1988).

Possibly, the factors limiting $\dot{V}O_2$max vary with the fitness level of the individual. According to this hypothesis, in the untrained individual the respiratory capacity for gas exchange exceeds the cardiovascular system's capacity to deliver oxygen. A training program results in little change in the respiratory capacity but large changes in the cardiovascular capacity. Thus, in highly trained individuals the increased cardiovascular capacity may exceed the respiratory capacity (Dempsey, 1986). In this case the respiratory system becomes the factor limiting $\dot{V}O_2$max.

Heritability of $\dot{V}O_2$max

Genetics have been suspected as an important component in determining an individual's $\dot{V}O_2$max. Research studies confirm that genotype contributes to individual differences in $\dot{V}O_2$max, but estimates of the genetic influence determining $\dot{V}O_2$max are quite modest. The estimated genetic effect on $\dot{V}O_2$max expressed per kilogram of body weight is less than 40% of individual differences, and it is less than 25% when $\dot{V}O_2$max is expressed relative to fat-free mass (Malina and Bouchard, 1991).

Genetic variation apparently accounts for a substantial fraction of the individual differences in the response to exercise training. Individual differences in sensitivity to exercise training are largely inherited differences, with some individuals being "high responders" and others being "low responders" (Bouchard, et al., 1992; Malina and Bouchard, 1991). Different genetic sensitivity to exercise among individuals helps explain the individualization principle of training, which states that even when individuals engage in similar training programs, different results should be expected.

Field Tests of Cardiorespiratory Capacity ($\dot{V}O_2$max)

Several techniques may be used to assess cardiorespiratory endurance and estimate cardiorespiratory capacity ($\dot{V}O_2$max). They include submaximal cycle ergometer tests, step tests, and distance walks or runs. By far the most practical and inexpensive method, especially when large numbers of individuals must be measured and evaluated in a short period of time (such as in a school setting), is the distance run. Walking tests are recommended for testing the elderly or other very sedentary adults. Three tests will be presented here: the 1-mi walk/run, the progressive aerobic cardiovascular endurance run (PACER) (Cooper Institute for Aerobics Research, 1999), and the Rockport Fitness Walking Test (RFWT) (Kline, et al., 1987).

Both the mile walk/run and the RFWT cover the same distance. The mile test allows the individual to walk, if necessary; but the intent is to cover the distance

as fast as possible, and that goal is best accomplished by running the entire distance. Thus, the individual is asked to perform at a high percentage of his or her maximal capacity for the entire duration of the test. The RFWT, however, is specifically designed for walking, although the fastest sustainable walking speed is the goal. Depending on the age and fitness level of the participant, this speed may or may not represent a high percentage of maximal aerobic capacity.

Unlike the previous tests, the PACER is a multistage fitness test adapted from the 20-m shuttle run—developed in Europe by Léger and his colleagues (1982, 1988). It most closely resembles a graded exercise test that would be done on a treadmill in a laboratory setting. It begins with a light workload and progresses, by small increments, until the individual can no longer complete the required number of laps per minute. This test is run between two lines marked 20 m apart on a smooth unobstructed surface. Running from one line to the other constitutes one lap. The initial speed is set at $8.5 \cdot \text{km} \cdot \text{hr}^{-1}$, and the individual should complete 7 laps in 1 min if that speed is to be achieved. Each minute the speed increases $0.5 \text{ km} \cdot \text{hr}^{-1}$. For the first 15 min the lap count is 7, 8, 8, 9, 9, 10, 10, 11, 11, 11, 12, 12, 13, 13, 13. Thus, this test does not require a sustained high-intensity effort but a gradual progression from submaximal to maximal effort. Pacing is accomplished by prerecorded music or beeps (Cooper Institute for Aerobics Research, 1999).

The equations used to estimate maximal oxygen consumption from the RFWT and the PACER test are given in Appendix B. The estimate from the mile run is as follows:

12.15 $\dot{V}O_2$max $= 0.21(\text{age} \times \text{sex}) - 0.84(\text{BMI})$
$- 8.41(\text{MT}) + 0.34(\text{MT}^2) + 108.94$
SEE $= 4.8 \text{ ml} \cdot \text{kg}^{-1} \cdot \text{min}^{-1}$

where age is the age of the individual in years; sex is 0 if female or 1 if male; BMI is the body mass index, which is weight (in kilograms) divided by height squared (in meters squared); MT is the time it takes the individual to run a mile (in minutes).

Example
- - - - - - - - - - - - - - - - - - -

Estimate $\dot{V}O_2$max given the following data.

age = 15 yr   BMI = 24.3

sex = female   MT = 8.75 min

The calculation is

$\dot{V}O_2$max $= (0.21)(15 \times 0) - (0.84)(24.3) - (8.41)(8.75)$
$+ 0.34(8.75^2) + 108.94 = 40.97 \text{ mL} \cdot \text{kg}^{-1} \cdot \text{min}^{-1}$ ✛

Notice that the equation includes an indication of the standard error of the estimate (SEE). This

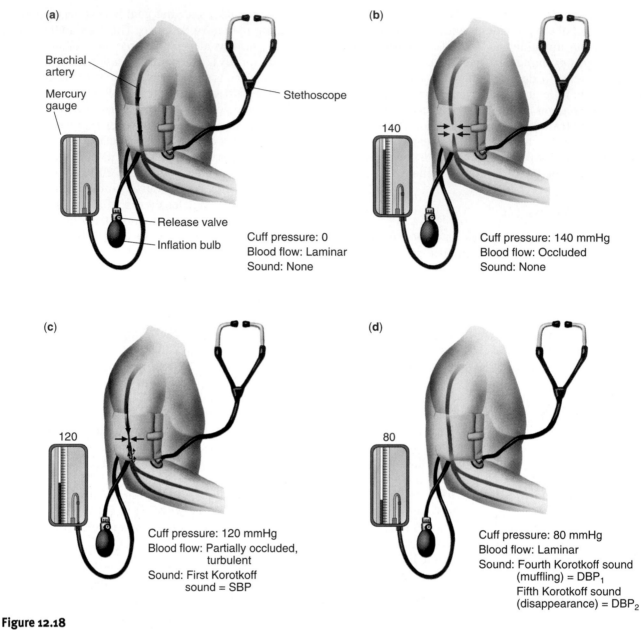

(a)

Brachial artery

Mercury gauge

Stethoscope

Release valve

Inflation bulb

Cuff pressure: 0
Blood flow: Laminar
Sound: None

(b)

140

Cuff pressure: 140 mmHg
Blood flow: Occluded
Sound: None

(c)

120

Cuff pressure: 120 mmHg
Blood flow: Partially occluded,
  turbulent
Sound: First Korotkoff
  sound = SBP

(d)

80

Cuff pressure: 80 mmHg
Blood flow: Laminar
Sound: Fourth Korotkoff sound
  (muffling) = DBP_1
  Fifth Korotkoff sound
  (disappearance) = DBP_2

Figure 12.18
Assessment of Blood Pressure

value means that as estimates, not measured values, the calculated results could be expected to vary from the measured value by that much. These errors are generally acceptable, ranging from 3 to 5 mL·kg·min. Norms are available for evaluation of the results of these field tests (Cooper Institute for Aerobics Research, 1999).

Blood Pressure

In well-equipped laboratories and hospitals, blood pressure can be measured directly by an intra-arterial transducer. A small transducer is inserted

into the artery, and systolic blood pressure and diastolic blood pressure are recorded for every beat of the heart. Although this procedure provides valuable information, it is not practical for routine use owing to the dangers of the invasive procedure.

By far the most common technique of obtaining blood pressure measurements is the *auscultation method.* The indirect method of auscultation uses a sphygmomanometer, as diagramed in Figure 12.18. This instrument consists of a cuff containing an inflatable bag and a mercury or aneroid manometer to measure pressure in the bag (Figure 12.18a). Blood pressure is determined in the following steps.

Table 12.5
Guidelines for Type of Blood Pressure Cuff

Size (Upper Arm Circumference) (cm)	Type of Cuff	Bladder Size (cm)
33–47	Large adult	33 or 42 × 15
25–35	Adult	24 × 12.5
18–26	Child	21 × 10

Source: Adams (1990).

1. The subject is allowed to rest quietly while the arm is measured and a proper cuff size is selected (see Table 12.5). The blood pressure cuff is secured around the upper arm, and the stethoscope is placed just below the antecubital space over the brachial artery (see Figure 12.18a). The movement of the blood through the brachial artery at this point in time is not impeded. Therefore, the blood flow is laminar, and the pulse cannot be heard through the stethoscope.

2. The blood pressure cuff is then inflated to a pressure greater than systolic blood pressure (usually around 140 mmHg at rest), using the inflation bulb (Figure 12.18b). During this time no sound is detected when a person listens to the brachial artery with a stethoscope, because blood flow is occluded.

3. The pressure inside the cuff is slowly released (at the rate of 2 or 3 mmHg·sec^{-1}), using the release valve attached to the inflation bulb. When the pressure within the cuff falls just below the systolic blood pressure, blood flows through the artery and can be heard through the stethoscope with each heartbeat. The sounds heard are referred to as *Korotkoff sounds* and are created by the movement of blood through the partially compressed blood vessel. The pressure at which the first Korotkoff sound is heard represents the systolic blood pressure (SBP) (see Figure 12.18c).

4. The pressure inside the cuff continues to be released; the Korotkoff sounds are heard clearly now (see Figure 12.18d). As the pressure continues to be released, there is a muffling of the Korotkoff sounds, which is taken to be the fourth Korotkoff sound and is called the first measure of diastolic blood pressure (DBP$_1$). The disappearance of the Korotkoff sounds represents the fifth Korotkoff sound and indicates the second measure of diastolic blood pressure (DBP$_2$). The pressure at the fifth Korotkoff sound (DBP$_2$) is considered the best measure of diastolic blood pressure in normal adults at rest. However, DBP$_1$ is recom-

mended for children, for adults during exercise, and for adults if DBP$_2$ is lower than 40 mmHg (American Society of Hypertension, 1992).

Summary

1. The primary functions of the cardiovascular system are transporting oxygen and nutrients to the cells of the body and transporting carbon dioxide and waste products from the cells; regulating body temperature, pH levels, and fluid balance; and protecting the body from blood loss and infection.

2. The heart is the muscular organ that serves as the pump for the cardiovascular system; the heart muscle is referred to as the myocardium.

IP *Cardiovascular–Anatomy Review: The Heart* (pages 1–5)

3. The cells of the heart, called cardiac muscle cells, are functionally linked by intercalated discs. When one cell is depolarized, the stimulation spreads over the entire myocardium.

IP *Cardiovascular–Anatomy Review: The Heart* (pages 6–7); *Cardiovascular–Cardiac Action Potential* (pages 1–10)

4. The heart has its own conduction system, consisting of the sinoatrial (SA) node, internodal fibers and Bachmann's bundle, the atrioventricular (AV) node, the bundle of His, the left and right bundle branches, and Purkinje fibers, all of which rapidly spread the electrical signal throughout the heart.

IP *Cardiovascular–Intrinsic Conduction System* (pages 1–7)

5. The cardiac cycle refers to the alternating periods of relaxation and contraction of the heart. The contraction phase is called systole, and the relaxation phase is called diastole. There are known relationships among the electrical, pressure, volume, and contractile events throughout the cardiac cycle.

IP *Cardiovascular–Cardiac Cycle* (pages 1–9)*

6. The volume of blood ejected from the heart with each beat is known as stroke volume. The amount of blood ejected from the heart each minute is called cardiac output. Under resting conditions the heart ejects approximately 60% of the blood that is returned to it; this percentage represents the ejection fraction.

IP *Cardiovascular–Cardiac Output* (pages 1–10)*

*This topic is available on the InterActive Physiology®
Sampler CD that comes with the purchase of a new copy of
this book.*

7. Blood pressure is the force exerted on the wall of the blood vessel by the blood it contains. Blood flow is the actual volume of blood flowing through a vessel, organ, or the entire circulation system per unit of time. Resistance is the opposition to blood flow created by the friction that the blood encounters.

IP *Cardiovascular–Measuring Blood Pressure* (pages 1–13)*; *Factors Affecting Blood Pressure* (pages 1–15)

8. Primary control of the cardiovascular system resides in the medulla oblongata (cardioaccelerator, cardioinhibitor, and vasomotor centers). Factors affecting these centers include
   a. higher brain centers that exert conscious and unconscious control;
   b. baroreceptors that are sensitive to mean arterial pressure;
   c. stretch receptors that sense blood return to the right atrium; and
   d. chemoreceptors that sense the PO_2, PCO_2, and H^+.

IP *Cardiovascular–Blood Pressure Regulation* (pages 1–31)

9. Maximal oxygen consumption ($\dot{V}O_2$max) is the highest amount of oxygen that the body can take in, transport, and utilize. The assessment of maximal oxygen consumption provides a means for quantifying the functional capacity of the entire cardiovascular system.

This topic is available on the InterActive Physiology® Sampler CD that comes with the purchase of a new copy of this book.

Review Questions

1. Diagram the conduction system of the heart, and describe how activation of the SA node leads to contraction of the heart.

2. Describe the electrical events in the heart in relation to pressure in the left ventricle, the volume of blood in the left ventricle, and the position of the heart valves.

3. Identify the different vessels of the peripheral circulation, and describe the velocity and pressure in each. What accounts for the differences?

4. Describe the hormonal mechanisms by which the body attempts to compensate for a decrease in plasma volume.

5. Discuss the neurohormonal regulation of the cardiovascular system and the factors that affect such regulation.

6. Why is maximal oxygen consumption ($\dot{V}O_2$max) considered to be a cardiovascular variable?

7. What are the possible factors limiting maximal oxygen consumption? What are the most likely factors limiting it?

8. Explain the steps involved in attaining an accurate measurement of blood pressure.

For further review and additional study tools, go to The Physiology Place (www.physiologyplace.com) and the Student Study Guide for Exercise Physiology for Health, Fitness and Performance *by Sharon A. Plowman and Denise L. Smith.*

Passport to the Internet

Visit the following Internet sites to explore further topics and issues related to the cardiovascular system. To visit an organization's web site, go to www.physiologyplace.com and click on "Passport to the Internet."

The American College of Sports Medicine Home page of the professional organization for individuals in sports medicine and exercise science. Spend some time exploring this site and discovering the multitude of resources available.

National Heart, Lung, and Blood Institute (NHLBI) The NHLBI is a part of the federal government's National Institutes of Health. This site contains medical alerts, professional and general health-related information, and research and training information for biomedical investigators and students.

The American Heart Association Visit one of the most complete sites for the latest information on cardiorespiratory health promotion. Investigate the latest findings and ongoing research dedicated to understanding cardiovascular disease. While there, go to www.choosetomove.org and investigate this special program dedicated to helping women establish physical activity as a habit.

References

American College of Sports Medicine: *Resource Manual for Guidelines for Exercise Testing and Prescription.* Malvern, PA: Lea & Febiger (1993).

American Society of Hypertension, Public Policy Position Paper: Recommendations for Routine Blood Pressure Measurement by Indirect Cuff Sphygmomanometry. *American Journal of Hypertension.* 5:207–209 (1992).

Adams, G. M.: *Exercise Physiology Laboratory Manual.* Dubuque, IA: Brown (1990).

Åstrand, P., T. E. Cuddy, B. Saltin, & J. Stenberg: Cardiac output during submaximal and maximal work. *Journal of Applied Physiology.* 19(2):268–274 (1964).

Åstrand, P.: Experimental Studies of Physical Working Capacity in Relation to Sex and Age. *University Microfilms International* (1952).

Bassett, D. R., & E. T. Howley: Limiting factors for maximum oxygen uptake and determinants of endurance performance. *Medicine and Science in Sports and Exercise.* 32: 85–88 (2000).

Bergh, U., B. Ekblom, & P.-O. Åstrand: Maximal oxygen uptake: "Classical" versus "contemporary" viewpoints. *Medicine and Science in Sports and Exercise.* 32:85–88 (2000).

Bouchard, C., F. T. Dionne, J. Simoneau, & M. R. Boulay: Genetics of aerobic and anaerobic performances. In J. O. Holloszy (ed.), *Exercise and Sport Sciences Reviews.* Baltimore: Williams & Wilkins (1992).

Brechar, G. A., & P. M. Galletti: Functional anatomy of cardiac pumping. In W. F. Hamilton (ed.), *Handbook of Physiology, Section 2: Circulation.* Washington, D.C.: American Physiological Society (1963).

Clark, D. H.: *Exercise Physiology.* Englewood Cliffs, NJ: Prentice Hall (1975).

Cooper Institute for Aerobics Research. FITNESSGRAM®: *Test Administration Manual* (2nd edition). Champaign, IL: Human Kinectics (1999).

Dempsey, J. A.: Is the lung built for exercise? *Medicine and Science in Sports and Exercise.* 18(2):143–155 (1986).

Fleg, J. L., F. O'Connor, G. Gerstenblith, L. C. Becker, J. Clulow, S. P. Schulman, & E. G. Lakatta: Impact of age on the cardiovascular response to dynamic upright exercise in healthy men and women. *Journal of Applied Physiology.* 78(3):890–900 (1995).

Franklin, B.A., & F. Munnings: A common misunderstanding about heart rate and exercise. *ACSM's Health and Fitness Journal.* 2(1):18–19 (1998).

Grassi, B.: Skeletal muscle $\dot{V}O_2$ on kinetics: Set by O_2 delivery or by O_2 utilization? New insights into an old issue. *Medicine and Science in Sports and Exercise.* 32:108–116 (2000).

Guyton, A. C.: *Textbook of Medical Physiology* (8th edition). Philadelphia: Saunders (1991).

Kitamura, K., C. R. Jorgensen, F. L. Gobel, H. L. Taylor, & Y. Wang: Hemodynamics correlates of myocardial oxygen consumption during upright exercise. *Journal of Applied Physiology.* 32:516–522 (1972).

Kline, G. M., J. P. Porcari, R. Huntermeister, P. S. Freedson, A. Ward, R. F. McCarron, J. Ross, & J. M. Rippe: Estimation of $\dot{V}O_2$max from a one-mile track walk, gender, age and body weight. *Medicine and Science in Sports and Exercise.* 19:253–259 (1987).

Léger, L. A., & J. Lambert: A maximal multistage 20-m shuttle run test to predict $\dot{V}O_2$max. *European Journal of Applied Physiology.* 49:1–12 (1982).

Léger, L. A., D. Mercier, C. Gadoury, & J. Lambert: The multistage 20 metre shuttle run test for aerobic fitness. *Journal of Sports Sciences.* 6:93–101 (1988).

Malina, R. M., & C. Bouchard: *Growth, Maturation, and Physical Activity.* Champaign, IL: Human Kinetics (1991).

Marieb, E. N.: *Human Anatomy and Physiology* (5th edition). San Francisco, CA: Benjamin Cummings (2001).

McNaught, A. B., & R. Callander: *Illustrated Physiology.* New York: Churchill Livingstone (1983).

Ogawa, T., R. J. Spina, W. H., Martin, W. M. Kohrt, K. B. Schechtman, J. O. Holloszy, & A. A. Ehsani: Effects of aging, sex, and physical training on cardiovascular responses to exercise. *Circulation.* 86:494–503 (1992).

Netter, F. H.: *The CIBA Collection of Medical Illustrations.* New York: CIBA Pharmaceutical Company (1987).

Noakes, T. D.: Implications of exercise testing for prediction of athletic performance: A contemporary perspective. *Medicine and Science in Sports and Exercise.* 20(4):319–330 (1988).

Ramsbottom, R., J. Brewer, & C. Williams: A progressive shuttle run test to estimate maximal oxygen uptake. *British Journal of Sports Medicine.* 22(4):141–144 (1988).

Robinson, T. E., D. Y. Sue, A. Huszczuk, D. Weiler-Ravell, & J. E. Hansen: Intra-arterial and cuff blood pressure responses during incremental cycle ergometry. *Medicine and Science in Sports and Exercise.* 20(2):142–149 (1988).

Rowell, L. B.: *Human Cardiovascular Control.* New York: Oxford University Press (1993).

Rowell, L. B.: *Human Circulation Regulation During Physical Stress.* New York: Oxford University Press (1986).

Saltin, B.: Hemodynamic adaptations to exercise. *American Journal of Cardiology.* 55:42D–47D (1985).

Shepherd, J. T., & P. M. Vanhoutte: *The Human Cardiovascular System.* New York: Raven Press (1980).

Spina, R. J., T. Ogawa, W. H. Martin III, A. R. Coggan, J. O. Holloszy, & A. A. Ehsani: Exercise training prevents decline in stroke volume during exercise in young healthy subjects. *Journal of Applied Physiology.* 72(6):2458–2462 (1992).

Spina, R. J., T. Ogawa, W. M. Kohrt, W. H. Martin III, J. O. Holloszy, & A. A. Ehsani: Differences in cardiovascular adaptations to endurance exercise training between older men and women. *Journal of Applied Physiology.* 75(2): 849–855 (1993a).

Spina, R. J., T. Ogawa, T. R. Miller, W. M. Kohrt, & A. A. Ehsani: Effect of exercise training on left ventricular performance in older women free of cardiopulmonary disease. *American Journal of Cardiology.* 71:99–104 (1993b).

Strand, F. L.: *Physiology: A Regulatory Systems Approach.* Dubuque, IA: Brown (1983).

Wood, J. E.: The venous system. *Scientific American.* 218(1): 86–96 (1968).

Vander, A. J., J. H. Sherman, & D. S. Luciano: *Human Physiology: The Mechanisms of Body Function.* New York: McGraw-Hill (1990).

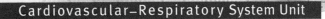

Chapter 13

Cardiovascular Responses to Exercise

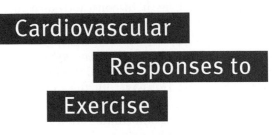

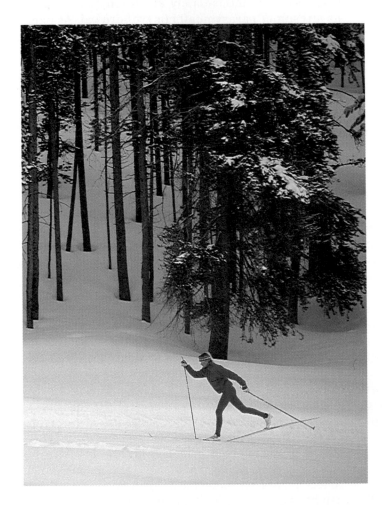

After studying the chapter, you should be able to

- Graph and explain the pattern of response for the major cardiovascular variables during short-term, light to moderate submaximal aerobic exercise.

- Graph and explain the pattern of response for the major cardiovascular variables during long-term, moderate to heavy submaximal aerobic exercise.

- Graph and explain the pattern of response for the major cardiovascular variables during incremental aerobic exercise to maximum.

- Graph and explain the pattern of response for the major cardiovascular variables during dynamic resistance exercise.

- Graph and explain the pattern of response for the major cardiovascular variables during static exercise.

- Compare and contrast the response of the major cardiovascular variables to short-term, light to moderate submaximal aerobic exercise; incremental aerobic exercise to maximum; dynamic resistance exercise; and static exercise.

- Discuss the similarities and differences between the sexes in the cardiovascular response to the various classifications of exercise.

- Discuss the similarities and differences between young and middle-aged adults in the cardiovascular response to the various classifications of exercise.

351

Introduction

All types of human movement, no matter what the mode, duration, intensity, or pattern, require an expenditure of energy above resting values. Much of this energy will be provided through the use of oxygen. In order to supply the working muscles with the needed oxygen, the cardiovascular and respiratory systems must work together. The response of the respiratory system during exercise was detailed in Chapter 11. This chapter describes the parallel cardiovascular responses to dynamic aerobic activity, static exercise, and dynamic resistance exercise.

Cardiovascular Responses to Aerobic Exercise

Aerobic exercise requires more energy—and, hence, more oxygen (and thus the use of the term *aerobic,* with oxygen)—than either static or dynamic resistance exercise. How much oxygen is needed depends primarily on the intensity at which the activity is performed and secondarily on the duration of the activity. Like the discussion on respiration, this discussion will categorize the exercises performed as being short-term (5–10 min), light (30–49% of maximal oxygen consumption, $\dot{V}O_2$max) to moderate (50–74% of $\dot{V}O_2$max) submaximal exercise; long-term (greater than 30 min), moderate to heavy submaximal (60–85% of $\dot{V}O_2$max) exercise; or incremental exercise to maximum (increasing from ~30 to 100% $\dot{V}O_2$max).

Short-Term, Light to Moderate Submaximal Aerobic Exercise

At the onset of short-term, light- to moderate-intensity exercise, there is an initial increase in cardiac output ($\dot{Q}$) to a plateau at steady state (see Figure 13.1a). Cardiac output plateaus within the first 2 min of exercise, reflecting the fact that cardiac output is sufficient to transport the oxygen needed to support the metabolic demands (ATP production) of the activity. Cardiac output increases owing to an initial increase in both stroke volume (SV) (Figure 13.1b) and heart rate (HR) (Figure 13.1c). Both variables level off within 2 min.

During exercise of this intensity the cardiorespiratory system is able to meet the metabolic demands of the body; thus, the term **steady state** or steady rate

---

Steady State A condition in which the energy expenditure provided during exercise is balanced with the energy required to perform that exercise and factors responsible for the provision of this energy reach elevated levels of equilibrium.

---

is often used to describe this type of exercise. During steady state exercise, the exercise is performed at an intensity such that energy expenditure is balanced with the energy required to perform the exercise. The plateau evidenced by the cardiovascular variables (in Figure 13.1) indicates that a steady state has been achieved.

The increase in stroke volume results from an increase in venous return, which, in turn, increases the left ventricular end–diastolic volume (LVEDV) (preload). The increased preload stretches the myocardium and causes it to contract more forcibly in accordance with the Frank-Starling law of the heart described in Chapter 12. Contractility of the myocardium is also enhanced by the sympathetic nervous system, which is activated during physical activity. Thus, an increase in the left ventricular end–diastolic volume and a decrease in the left ventricular end–systolic volume (LVESV) account for the increase in stroke volume during light to moderate dynamic exercise (Poliner, et al., 1980). Heart rate increases immediately at the onset of activity as a result of parasympathetic withdrawal. As exercise continues, further increases in heart rate are due to the action of the sympathetic nervous system (Rowell, 1986).

Systolic blood pressure (SBP) will rise in a pattern very similar to that of cardiac output: There is an initial increase and a plateau once steady state is achieved (Figure 13.1d). The increase in systolic blood pressure is brought about by the increase in cardiac output. Systolic blood pressure would be even higher if not for the fact that resistance decreases, thereby partially offsetting the increase in cardiac output. When blood pressure (BP) is measured intra-arterially, diastolic blood pressure (DBP) does not change. When it is measured by auscultation it either does not change or may go down slightly. Diastolic blood pressure remains relatively constant because of peripheral vasodilation, which facilitates blood flow to the working muscles. The small rise in systolic blood pressure and the lack of a significant change in diastolic blood pressure cause the mean arterial pressure (MAP) to rise only slightly, following the pattern of systolic blood pressure.

Total peripheral resistance (TPR) decreases owing to vasodilation in the active muscles (Figure 13.1e). The vasodilation of vessels in the active muscles is brought about primarily by the influence of local chemical factors (lactate, K^+, and so on), which reflect increased metabolism. The decrease in TPR can be calculated using Equation 12.8:

$$TPR = \frac{MAP}{\dot{Q}}$$

Figure 13.1
Cardiovascular Responses to
Short-Term, Light to Moderate
Aerobic Exercise

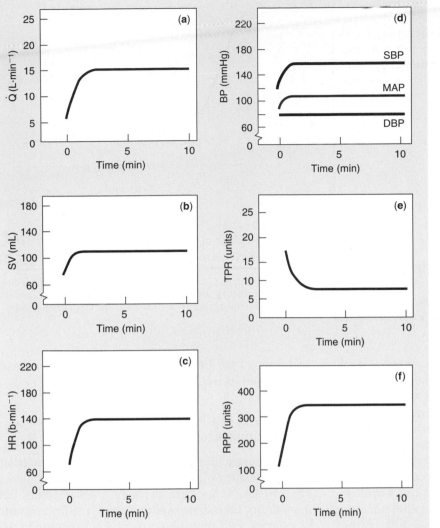

Example

Calculate TPR by using the following information from Figures 13.1a and 13.1d:

$$MAP = 110 \text{ mmHg} \qquad \dot{Q} = 15 \text{ L·min}^{-1}$$

The computation is

$$TPR = \frac{110 \text{ mmHg}}{15 \text{ L·min}^{-1}} = 7.33 \text{ (TPR units)}$$

Thus, TPR is 7.33 for light dynamic exercise.   ✛

The decrease in total peripheral resistance has two important implications. First, the vasodilation in the active muscle that causes the decrease in resistance has the effect of increasing blood flow to the active muscle, thereby increasing the availability of oxygen and nutrients. Second, the decrease in resistance keeps mean arterial pressure from increasing dramatically. The increase in mean arterial pressure is determined by the relative changes in cardiac output and total peripheral resistance. Since cardiac output increases more than resistance decreases, mean arterial pressure increases slightly during dynamic exercise. However, the increase in mean arterial pressure would be much greater if resistance did not decrease.

Myocardial oxygen consumption increases during dynamic aerobic exercise because the heart must do more work to pump an increased cardiac output to the working muscles. The rate-pressure product will increase in relation to increases in heart rate and systolic blood pressure, reflecting the greater myocardial oxygen demand of the heart during exercise (Figure 13.1f). The Question of Understanding box on page 354 provides an example of normal responses to exercise. Refer back to it as each category of exercise is discussed and check your answers in Appendix D.

The actual magnitude of the change for each of the variables shown in Figure 13.1 depends on the

A Question of Understanding

The following measurements were obtained on a 42-year-old man at rest and during light aerobic exercise, during heavy aerobic exercise, during maximal dynamic aerobic exercise, and during sustained static contractions at 50% MVC.

Condition	HR (b·min⁻¹)	SBP (mmHg)	DBP (mmHg)	$\dot{Q}$ (L·min⁻¹)
Rest	80	134	86	6
Light aerobic	130	150	86	10
Heavy aerobic	155	170	88	13
Maximal aerobic	180	200	88	15
Sustained static	135	210	100	8

Calculate MAP, TPR, and RPP for each condition.

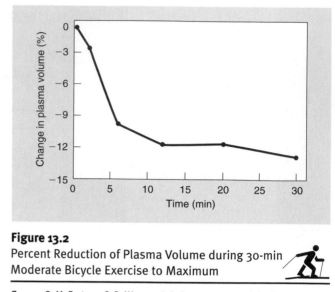

Figure 13.2

Percent Reduction of Plasma Volume during 30-min Moderate Bicycle Exercise to Maximum

Source: S. M. Fortney, C. B. Wenger, J. R. Bove, & E. R. Nadel. Effect of blood volume on sweating rate and body fluids in exercising humans. *Journal of Applied Physiology.* 51(6):1594–1600 (1981). Reprinted by permission.

workload, environmental conditions, and the genetic makeup and fitness level of the individual.

Blood volume decreases during dynamic aerobic exercise. Figure 13.2 shows the percent reduction of plasma volume during 30 min of moderate bicycle exercise (60–70% $\dot{V}O_2max$) in a warm environment (Fortney, et al., 1981). The largest changes occur during the first 5 min of exercise, which is consistent with short-term exercise. Following the initial rapid decrease, plasma volume stabilizes. This rapid decrease in plasma volume suggests that it is fluid shifts, rather than fluid loss, that accounts for the initial decrease in plasma volume (Wade and Freund, 1990). The magnitude of the decrease in plasma volume is dependent upon the intensity of exercise, environmental factors, and the hydration status of the individual.

Figure 13.3 illustrates the distribution of cardiac output at rest and during light exercise. Notice that cardiac output increases from 5.8 L·min⁻¹ to 9.4 L·min⁻¹ in this example (the increase in $\dot{Q}$ is illustrated by the increased size of the pie chart). The most dramatic change in cardiac output distribution with light exercise is the increased percentage (47%) and the actual amount of blood flow (4500 mL) that is directed to the working muscles. Skin blood flow also increases to meet the thermoregulatory demands of exercise. The absolute amount of blood flow to the coronary muscle also increases although the percentage of cardiac output remains relatively constant. The absolute amount of cerebral blood flow remains constant, which means that the percentage of cardiac output distributed to the brain decreases. Both renal

and splanchnic blood flow are modestly decreased during light exercise.

Long-Term, Moderate to Heavy Submaximal Aerobic Exercise

The cardiovascular responses to long-term, moderate to heavy exercise (60–85% of $\dot{V}O_2max$) are shown in Figure 13.4. As for light to moderate workloads, cardiac output increases rapidly during the first minutes of exercise and then plateaus and is maintained at a relatively constant level throughout exercise (Figure 13.4a). Notice, however, that the absolute cardiac output attained is higher during heavy exercise than it was during light to moderate exercise. The initial increase in cardiac output is brought about by an increase in both stroke volume and heart rate.

Stroke volume exhibits a pattern of initial increase, plateaus, and then displays a negative (downward) drift. Stroke volume increases rapidly during the first minutes of exercise and plateaus at a maximal level after a workload of approximately 40–50% of $\dot{V}O_2max$ has been achieved (P. Åstrand, et al., 1964) (Figure 13.4b). Thus, during work that requires more than 50% of $\dot{V}O_2max$, the stroke volume response is not intensity dependent. Stroke volume remains relatively constant during the first 30 min of heavy exercise.

As for light to moderate exercise, the increase in stroke volume results from an increased venous return, leading to the Frank-Starling mechanism, and increased contractility owing to sympathetic nerve

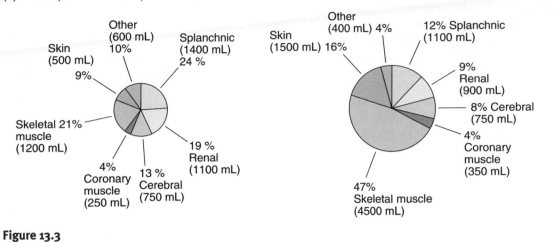

(a) Rest $(\dot{Q} = 5.8\ L{\cdot}min^{-1})$

Other (600 mL) 10%
Skin (500 mL) 9%
Splanchnic (1400 mL) 24 %
Skeletal 21% muscle (1200 mL)
4% Coronary muscle (250 mL)
13 % Cerebral (750 mL)
19 % Renal (1100 mL)

(b) Light Exercise $(\dot{Q} = 9.4\ L{\cdot}min^{-1})$

Other (400 mL) 4%
Skin (1500 mL) 16%
12% Splanchnic (1100 mL)
9% Renal (900 mL)
8% Cerebral (750 mL)
4% Coronary muscle (350 mL)
47% Skeletal muscle (4500 mL)

Figure 13.3
Distribution of Cardiac Output at Rest and during Light Exercise

Source: Data from Anderson (1968).

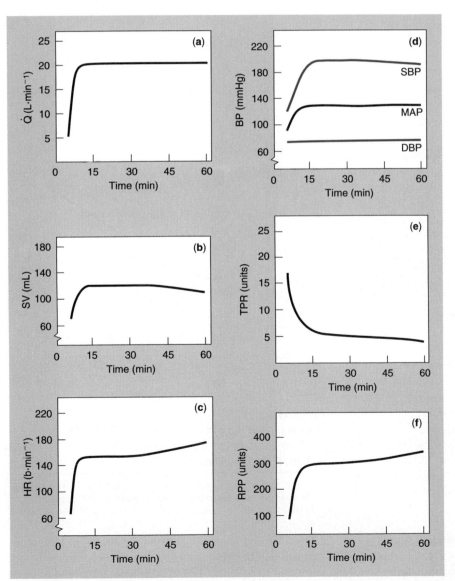

Figure 13.4
Cardiovascular Responses to Long-Term, Moderate to Heavy Submaximal Aerobic Exercise

stimulation. Thus, changes in stroke volume occur because left ventricular end–diastolic volume increases and left ventricular end–systolic volume decreases (Poliner, et al., 1980). Left ventricular end–diastolic volume increases because of the return of blood to the heart by the active muscle pump, increased venoconstriction (which decreases venous pooling, thereby increasing venous return), and increased cardiac output. Left ventricular end–systolic volume decreases owing to augmented contractility of the heart, which effectively ejects more blood from the ventricle, leaving a smaller residual volume.

However, if exercise continues beyond approximately 30 min, stroke volume gradually drifts downward although it remains elevated above resting values. The downward shift in stroke volume after approximately 30 min is most likely due to thermoregulatory stress; plasma loss and a redirection of blood to the cutaneous vessels in an attempt to dissipate heat (Rowell, 1986). This effectively reduces venous return and thus causes the reduction in stroke volume.

Heart rate displays a pattern of initial increase, plateaus at steady state, and then shows a positive drift. Heart rate increases sharply during the first 1–2 min of exercise, with the magnitude of the increase depending on the intensity of exercise (Figure 13.4c). The increase in heart rate is brought about by parasympathetic withdrawal and activation of the sympathetic nervous system. After approximately 30 min of heavy exercise heart rate begins to drift upward. The increase in heart rate is proportional to the decrease in stroke volume, so cardiac output is maintained during exercise.

The changes observed in cardiovascular variables, notably in heart rate and stroke volume, during prolonged, heavy submaximal exercise without a change in workload are known as **cardiovascular drift.** Cardiovascular drift is probably associated with rising body temperature during prolonged exercise. The combination of exercise and heat stress produces competing regulatory demands—specifically, competition between skin and muscle for large fractions of cardiac output. Stroke volume decreases as a result of vasodilation, a progressive increase in the fraction of blood being directed to the skin in an attempt to dissipate heat from the body, and a loss of plasma volume (Rowell, 1974; Sjogaard, et al., 1988).

The magnitude of cardiovascular drift is heavily influenced by fluid ingestion. Figure 13.5 presents data from a study in which subjects cycled for 2 hr with and without fluid replacement (Hamilton, et al.,

> **Cardiovascular Drift** The changes in observed cardiovascular variables that occur during prolonged, heavy submaximal exercise without a change in workload.

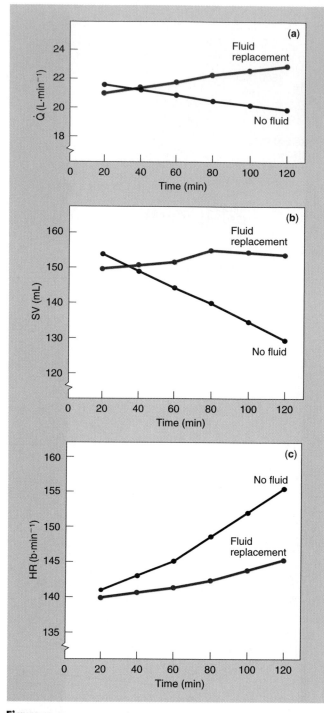

Figure 13.5

Cardiovascular Response to Long-Term, Moderate to Heavy Exercise (70–76% $\dot{V}O_2$max) with and without Fluid Replacement

Source: M. T. Hamilton, J. G. Alonso, S. J. Montain, & E. F. Coyle. Fluid replacement and glucose infusion during exercise prevents cardiovascular drift. *Journal of Applied Physiology.* 71:871–877 (1985). Reprinted by permission.

1991). Values are for minutes 20 through 120; thus, the initial increase in each of the variables is not shown in this figure. When subjects consumed enough water to completely replace the water lost through

Focus on Research

Interval Exercise versus Steady State Exercise

Foster, C., K. Meyer, N. Georgakopoulos, A. J. Ellestad, D. J. Fitzgerald, K. Tilman, H. Weinstein, H. Young, & H. Roskamm: Left ventricular function during interval and steady state exercise. *Medicine and Science in Sports and Exercise.* 31(8):1157–1162 (1999).

Throughout this book, we examine the exercise response to various categories of exercise, with this chapter looking specifically at the cardiovascular responses. Most studies that have examined the cardiovascular response to exercise have used continuous activity. Yet many clinical populations (for example, people undergoing cardiac rehabilitation) and many athletic populations utilize interval training. So how do these activities compare in terms of cardiovascular responses?

Foster and colleagues set out to answer this question by comparing the cardiovascular responses of a group of adults (mean age = 52.9 yr) in two separate 15-minute cycling trials—one involving steady state exercise, the other utilizing interval exercise. Participants cycled at 170 W for the full 15 minutes in one trial and alternated 1-min "hard" (220 W) and "easy" (120 W) periods in the second trial, resulting in an equal power output (170 W) for both trials. Cardiovascular measurements were obtained before exercise (0 minutes) and after minutes 4, 7, 12, and 15.

As can been seen from the results, no significant difference was noted between the steady state exercise and the interval exercise for any of the variables. The authors concluded that heart function during interval exercise is remarkably similar to

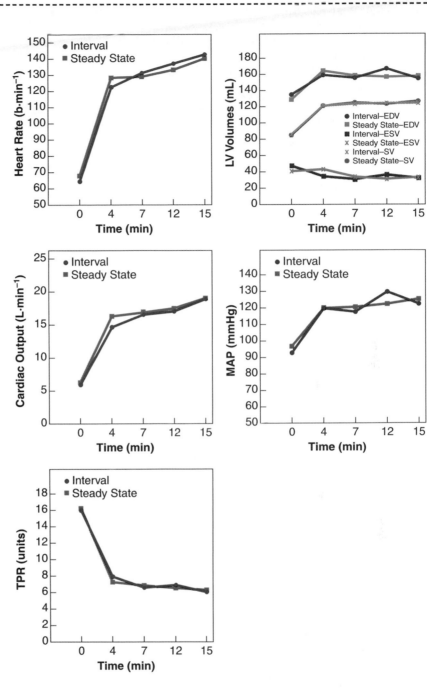

continuous steady state exercise at the same average power output, when moderate duration and evenly timed hard and easy periods are utilized. The results provide good news for individuals with low levels of fitness who may not be able to perform

15 minutes of continuous activity when starting an exercise program. Fitness professionals can assure such clients that alternating periods of "hard" and "easy" work results in cardiovascular responses similar to those resulting from sustained exercise.

sweat, cardiac output remained nearly constant throughout the first hour of exercise and actually increased during the second hour (Figure 13.5a). Cardiac output was maintained in the fluid replacement

trial because stroke volume did not drift downward (Figure 13.5b). Heart rate was significantly lower when fluid replacement occurred (Figure 13.5c). This information can be used by coaches and fitness

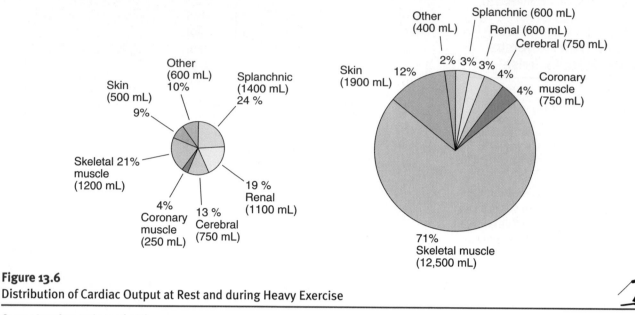

(a) Rest ($\dot{Q}$ = 5.8 L·min⁻¹)

Other (600 mL) 10%
Skin (500 mL) 9%
Splanchnic (1400 mL) 24 %
Skeletal muscle 21% (1200 mL)
Coronary muscle (250 mL) 4%
Cerebral (750 mL) 13 %
Renal (1100 mL) 19 %

(b) Heavy Exercise ($\dot{Q}$ = 17.5 L·min⁻¹)

Other (400 mL) 2%
Splanchnic (600 mL) 3%
Renal (600 mL) 3%
Cerebral (750 mL) 4%
Skin (1900 mL) 12%
Coronary muscle (750 mL) 4%
Skeletal muscle (12,500 mL) 71%

Figure 13.6
Distribution of Cardiac Output at Rest and during Heavy Exercise

Source: Data from Anderson (1968).

leaders. If your clients exercise for prolonged periods, they must replace the fluids that are lost during exercise, or performance will suffer.

Refer back to the cardiovascular responses illustrated in Figure 13.4. Systolic blood pressure responses to long-term, moderate to heavy dynamic exercise are characterized by an initial increase, a plateau at steady state, and a negative drift. Systolic blood pressure increases rapidly during the first 1–2 min of exercise, with the magnitude of the increase dependent upon the intensity of the exercise (Figure 13.4d). Systolic blood pressure then remains relatively stable or drifts slightly downward as a result of continued vasodilation and a resultant decrease in resistance (Ekelund and Holmgren, 1967). Diastolic blood pressure does not change or changes so little that it has no physiological significance during prolonged exercise in a thermoneutral environment. But it may decrease slightly when exercise is performed in a warm environment owing to increased vasodilation as a result of heat production. Because of the increased systolic blood pressure and the relatively stable diastolic blood pressure, mean arterial pressure increases modestly during prolonged activity. Again, as in light to moderate exercise, the magnitude of the increase in mean arterial pressure is mediated by a large decrease in resistance that accompanies exercise.

Total peripheral resistance exhibits a curvilinear decrease during long-term heavy exercise (Figure 13.4e) because of vasodilation in active muscle and because of vasodilation in the cutaneous vessels in order to dissipate the heat produced by mechanical work (Rowell, 1974). Finally, because both heart rate and

systolic blood pressure increase substantially during heavy work, the rate-pressure product increases markedly (Figure 13.4f). The initial increase in rate-pressure product occurs rapidly with the onset of exercise and plateaus at steady state. An upward drift in rate-pressure product may occur after approximately 30 min of exercise as a result of heart rate increasing to a greater extent than systolic blood pressure decreases. The high rate-pressure product reflects the large amount of work the heart must perform to support heavy exercise.

During prolonged exercise, particularly if performed in the heat, there is continued loss of total body fluid owing to profuse sweating. Total body water loss during long-duration exercise varies from 900 to 1300 mL·hr⁻¹, depending on work intensity and environmental conditions (Wade and Freund, 1990). If fluid is not replaced during long-duration exercise, there is a continued reduction in plasma volume throughout exercise.

Figure 13.6 illustrates the distribution of cardiac output at rest and during heavy exercise. Notice that cardiac output increases from 5.8 L·min⁻¹ at rest to 17.5 L·min⁻¹ in this example. The most dramatic change in cardiac output distribution with heavy exercise is the dramatic increase in blood flow to the working muscle, which now receives 71% of cardiac output. Skin blood flow is also increased to meet the thermoregulatory demands of exercise. The absolute amount of blood flow to the coronary muscle again increases although the percentage of cardiac output remains relatively constant. The absolute amount of cerebral blood flow remains constant, which means that the

Figure 13.7
Cardiovascular Response to Incremental Maximal Exercise

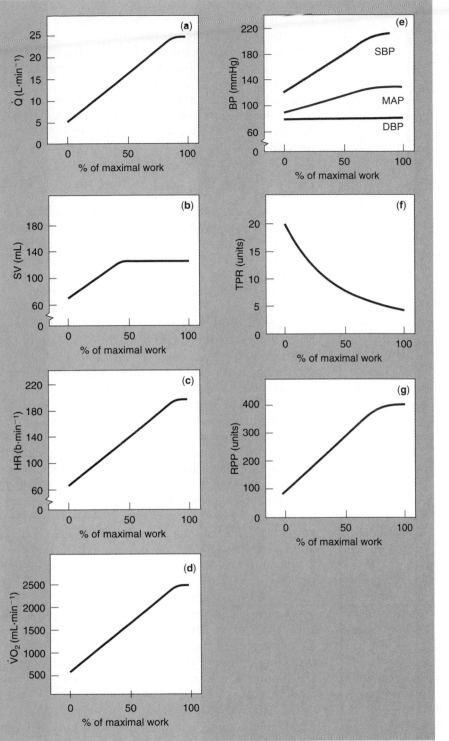

percentage of cardiac output distributed to the neural tissue decreases. Both renal and splanchnic blood flow are further decreased as exercise intensity increases.

Incremental Aerobic Exercise to Maximum

An incremental exercise to maximum bout consists of a series of progressively increasing work intensities that continue until the individual can do no more. The length of each work intensity (stage) varies from 1 to 3 min to allow for the achievement of a steady state, at least at the lower workloads.

Cardiac output displays a rectilinear increase and plateaus at maximal exercise (Figure 13.7a). The initial increase in cardiac output reflects an increase in stroke volume and heart rate; however, at workloads

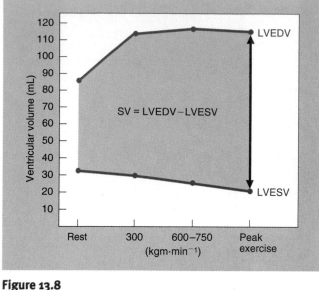

Figure 13.8

Changes in LVEDV and LVESV That Account for Change in SV during Incremental Exercise

Source: Based on data from Poliner, et al. (1980).

greater than 40–50% $\dot{V}O_2$max, the increase in cardiac output is achieved solely by an increase in heart rate. As shown in Figure 13.7b, in normally active individuals stroke volume increases rectilinearly initially and then plateaus at approximately 40–50% of $\dot{V}O_2$max (P. Åstrand, et al., 1964; Higginbotham, et al., 1986). Stroke volume may actually decrease slightly near the end of maximal exercise in untrained and moderately trained individuals (Gledhill, et al., 1994).

Figure 13.8 indicates the changes in left ventricular end–diastolic volume and left ventricular end–systolic volume that account for changes in stroke volume during progressively increasing exercise (Poliner, et al., 1980). Left ventricular end–diastolic volume increases largely because of the return of blood to the heart by the active muscle pump and the increased sympathetic outflow to the veins causing venoconstriction and augmenting venous return. Left ventricular end–systolic volume decreases because of augmented contractility of the heart, which ejects more blood from the ventricle and leaves less in the ventricle.

Heart rate increases in a rectilinear fashion and plateaus at maximal exercise (Figure 13.7c). The myocardial cells are capable of contracting at over 300 b·min^{-1} but rarely exceeds 210 b·min^{-1} because a faster heart rate would not be of any benefit since there would be inadequate time for ventricular filling. Thus, stroke volume and ultimately cardiac output would be decreased. Consider the simple analogy of a bucket brigade. Up to a certain point it is very useful to increase the speed of passing the bucket; however,

there is a limit to this speed because some time must be allowed for the bucket to be filled with water.

The maximal amount of oxygen an individual can take in, transport, and utilize ($\dot{V}O_2$max) is another variable that is usually measured during an incremental maximal exercise test (Figure 13.7d). Although $\dot{V}O_2$max is considered primarily a cardiovascular variable, it also depends on the respiratory and metabolic systems. As noted in Chapter 12, $\dot{V}O_2$max can be defined by rearranging the Fick equation (Eq. 12.9) to the following equation, as described in Equation 12.14b.

13.1 $\dot{V}O_2\text{max} = (\dot{Q}\,\text{max}) \times (\text{a-vO}_2\,\text{diff max})$

The changes in cardiac output during a maximal incremental exercise test have just been described (a rectilinear increase). The changes in the a-vO$_2$ diff were discussed in Chapter 11 (an increase plateauing at approximately 60% of $\dot{V}O_2$max). Reflecting these changes, oxygen consumption ($\dot{V}O_2$) also increases in a rectilinear fashion and plateaus at maximum ($\dot{V}O_2$max) during an incremental exercise test to maximum. The plateauing of $\dot{V}O_2$ is one of the primary indications that a true maximal test has been achieved.

The arterial blood pressure responses to incremental dynamic exercise to maximum are shown in Figure 13.7e. Systolic blood pressure increases rectilinearly and plateaus at maximal exercise, often reaching values in excess of 200 mmHg in very fit individuals. The increase in systolic blood pressure is caused by the increased cardiac output, which outweighs the decrease in resistance. Systolic blood pressure and heart rate are two variables that are routinely monitored during an exercise test to ensure the safety of the participant. If either of these variables fails to rise with an increasing workload, cardiovascular insufficiency and an inability to adequately profuse tissue may result, and the exercise test should be stopped.

Diastolic blood pressure typically remains relatively constant or changes so little it has no physiological significance, although it may decrease at high levels of exercise. Diastolic pressure remains relatively constant because of the balance of vasodilation in the vasculature of the active muscle and vasoconstriction in other vascular beds. Diastolic pressure is most likely to decrease when exercise is performed in a hot environment; under these conditions skin vessels are more dilated, and there is decreased resistance to blood flow.

An excessive rise in either systolic blood pressure (over 260 mmHg) or diastolic blood pressure (over 115 mmHg) indicates an abnormal exercise response and is also reason to consider stopping an exercise test or exercise session (American College of Sports Medicine [ACSM], 2000). Individuals who exhibit an exaggerated blood pressure response to exercise are

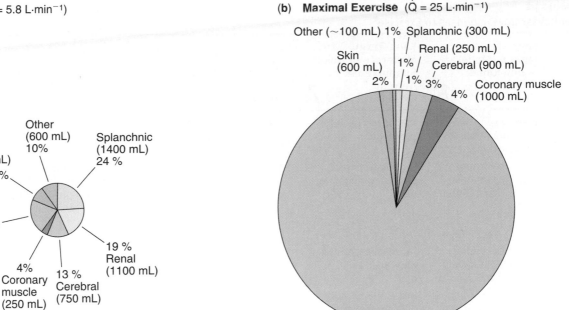

Figure 13.9
Distribution of Cardiac Output at Rest and during Maximal Exercise

Source: Data from Anderson (1968).

two to three times more likely to develop hypertension than those with a normal exercise blood pressure response (ACSM, 1993).

Total peripheral resistance decreases in a negative curvilinear pattern and reaches its lowest level at maximal exercise (Figure 13.7f). Decreased resistance reflects maximal vasodilation in the active tissue in response to the need for increased blood flow that accompanies maximal exercise. Also, the large drop in resistance is important in keeping mean arterial pressure from exhibiting an exaggerated increase. The rate-pressure product increases in a rectilinear fashion plateauing at maximum in an incremental exercise test (Figure 13.7g), paralleling the increases in heart rate and systolic blood pressure.

The reduction in plasma volume seen during submaximal exercise is also seen in incremental exercise to maximum. Because the magnitude of the reduction depends on the intensity of exercise, the reduction is greatest at maximal exercise. A decrease of 10–20% can be seen during incremental exercise to maximum (Wade and Freund, 1990).

Considerable changes in blood flow occur during maximal incremental exercise. Figure 13.9 illustrates the distribution of cardiac output at rest and at maximal exercise. Maximum cardiac output in this example is 25 L·min⁻¹. Again, the most striking characteristic of this figure is the tremendous amount of cardiac output that is directed to the working muscles (88%). At maximal exercise skin blood flow is reduced in order to direct the necessary blood to the muscles. Renal and splanchnic blood flow also decrease considerably. Blood flow to the brain and cardiac muscle is maintained.

Table 13.1 summarizes the cardiovascular responses to exercise that have been discussed in these sections.

Upper-Body versus Lower-Body Aerobic Exercise

Upper-body exercise is routinely performed in a variety of industrial, agricultural, military, and sporting activities. There are some important differences in the cardiovascular responses, depending on whether exercise is performed on an arm ergometer (using muscles of the upper body) or a cycle ergometer (using muscles of the lower body). Figure 13.10 presents data from a study that compared cardiovascular responses to incremental exercise to maximum in able-bodied individuals using the upper body and lower body. Notice that a higher peak $\dot{V}O_2$ was achieved during lower-body

Table 13.1

Cardiovascular Responses to Exercise*

	Short-Term, Light to Moderate Submaximal Aerobic Exercise	Long-Term, Moderate to Heavy Submaximal Aerobic Exercise[†]	Incremental Aerobic Exercise to Maximum	Static[††] Exercise	Resistance[††] Exercise
$\dot{Q}$	Increases rapidly; plateaus at steady state within 2 min	Increases rapidly; plateaus	Rectilinear increase with plateau at max	Modest gradual increase	Modest gradual increase
SV	Increases rapidly; plateaus at steady state within 2 min	Increases rapidly; plateaus; negative drift	Increases initially; plateaus at 40–50% $\dot{V}O_2$max	Relatively constant at low workloads; decreases at high workloads; rebound rise in recovery	Little change, slight decrease
HR	Increases rapidly; plateaus at steady state within 2 min	Increases rapidly; plateaus; positive drift	Rectilinear increase with plateau at max	Modest gradual increase	Increases gradually with numbers of reps
SBP	Increases rapidly; plateaus at steady state within 2 min	Increases rapidly; plateaus; slight negative drift	Rectilinear increase with plateau at max	Marked steady increase	Increases gradually with numbers of reps
DBP	Shows little or no change	Shows little or no change	Shows little or no change	Marked steady increase	No change or increase
MAP	Increases rapidly; plateaus at steady state within 2 min	Increases initially; little if any drift	Small rectilinear increase	Marked steady increase	Increases gradually with numbers of reps
TPR	Decreases rapidly; plateaus	Decreases rapidly; plateaus; slight negative drift	Curvilinear decrease	Decreases	Slight increase
RPP	Increases rapidly; plateaus at steady state within 2 min	Increases rapidly; plateaus; positive drift	Rectilinear increase with plateau at max	Marked steady increase	Increases gradually with numbers of reps

* Resting values are taken as baseline.

[†] The difference between a plateau during the short-term, light to moderate and long-term, moderate to heavy submaximal exercise response is one of magnitude; that is, a plateau occurs at a higher value with higher intensities.

[††] The magnitude of a plateau change depends on the %MVC/load.

exercise. By comparing cardiovascular responses at any given level of oxygen consumption, these data also allow for the comparison of cardiovascular responses to submaximal upper- and lower-body exercise. When the oxygen consumption required to perform a submaximal workload is the same, cardiac output is similar for upper- and lower-body exercise (Figure 13.10a). However, the mechanism to achieve the required increase in cardiac output is not the same. As shown in Figures 13.10b and 13.10c, upper-body exercise results in a lower stroke volume and a higher heart rate at any given submaximal workload (Clausen, 1976; Miles, et al., 1989; Pendergast, 1989). Systolic, diastolic, and mean arterial blood pressures (Figure 13.10d), total peripheral resistance (Figure 13.10e), and rate-pressure product (Figure 13.10f) are significantly higher in upper-body exercise than in lower-body exercise performed at the same oxygen consumption.

There are several likely reasons for the differences in cardiovascular responses to upper-body and lower-body exercise. The elevated heart rate is thought to reflect a greater sympathetic stimulation during upper-body exercise (P. O. Åstrand and Rodahl, 1986; Davies, et al., 1974; Miles, et al., 1989). Stroke volume is less during upper-body exercise than during lower-body exercise because of the absence of the skeletal muscle pump augmenting venous return from the legs. The greater sympathetic stimulation that occurs during upper-body exercise may also be partially responsible for the increased blood pressure and total peripheral resistance seen with this type of activity. Additionally, upper-body exercise is usually performed using an arm-cranking ergometer, which involves a static component because the individual must grasp the hand crank. Static tasks are known to cause exaggerated blood pressure responses.

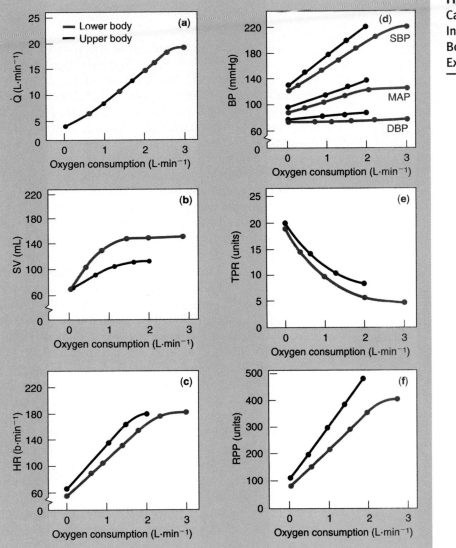

Figure 13.10
Cardiovascular Response to
Incremental Maximal Upper-
Body and Lower-Body
Exercise

When maximal exercise is performed by using upper-body exercise, $\dot{V}O_2$max values are approximately 30% lower than when maximal exercise is performed by using lower-body exercise (Miles, et al., 1989; Pendergast, 1989). Maximal heart rate values for upper-body exercise are 90–95% of those achieved for lower-body exercise, and stroke volume is 30–40% less during maximal upper-body exercise. Maximal systolic blood pressure and the rate-pressure product are usually similar for both forms of exercise, but diastolic blood pressure is typically 10–15% higher during upper-body exercise (Miles, et al., 1989).

The different cardiovascular responses to a given level of exercise for upper-body work and lower-body work suggest that exercise prescriptions for arm work cannot be based on data obtained from testing with leg exercises. Furthermore, the greater cardiovascular strain associated with upper-body work must be kept in mind when one prescribes exercise for individuals with cardiovascular disease.

Sex Differences during Aerobic Exercise

The pattern of cardiovascular responses to aerobic exercise is similar for both sexes, although the magnitude of the response may vary between the sexes for some variables. Differences in body size and structure are related to many of the differences in cardiovascular responses evidenced between the sexes.

Submaximal Exercise

Females have a higher cardiac output than males during submaximal exercise when work is performed at the same *absolute workload* (P. Åstrand, et al., 1964; Becklake, et al., 1965; Freedson, et al., 1979).

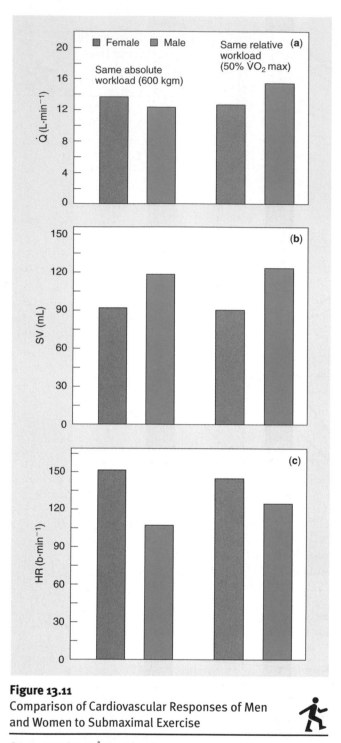

Figure 13.11

Comparison of Cardiovascular Responses of Men and Women to Submaximal Exercise

Source: Data from P. Åstrand (1952).

Females have a lower stroke volume and a higher heart rate than males during submaximal exercise when exercise is performed at the same absolute workload (P. Åstrand, et al., 1964). The higher heart rate more than compensates for the lower stroke volume in females, resulting in the higher cardiac output seen at the same absolute workload. Thus, if a male

and female perform the same workout, the female will typically be stressing the cardiovascular system to a greater extent.

This relative disadvantage to the woman results from several factors. First, females typically are smaller than males; they have a smaller heart and less muscle mass. Second, they have a lower oxygen-carrying capacity than males. Finally, they typically have lower aerobic capacity ($\dot{V}O_2$max). Therefore, researchers commonly discuss exercise response in terms of *relative workload,* that is, how individuals compare when they are both working at the same percentage of their $\dot{V}O_2$max.

The importance of distinguishing between relative and absolute workloads when comparing males and females is shown in Figure 13.11. This figure compares the cardiovascular response of men and women to the same absolute workload (600 kgm) on the left side of the graph and the same relative workload (50% of $\dot{V}O_2$max) on the right side of the graph. Cardiac output is higher in women during the same absolute workload. However, cardiac output (Figure 13.11a) is less for women when the same relative workload is performed. Stroke volume (Figure 13.11b) is lower in women than in men whether the workload is expressed on an absolute or relative basis. Notice that the values are very similar for both conditions, suggesting that stroke volume has plateaued as would be expected at 50% of $\dot{V}O_2$max in both conditions. The difference in heart rate between the sexes (Figure 13.11c) is smaller when exercise is performed at the same relative workload.

Males and females display the same pattern of response for blood pressure; however, males tend to have a higher systolic blood pressure than females at the same relative workloads (Malina and Bouchard, 1991; Ogawa, et al., 1992). Much of the difference in the magnitude of the blood pressure response is attributable to differences in resting systolic blood pressure. Diastolic blood pressure response to submaximal exercise is very similar for both sexes. Thus, mean arterial blood pressure is slightly greater in males during submaximal work at the same relative workload. The pattern of response for resistance is similar for males and females, although males typically have a lower resistance owing to their greater cardiac output. Males and females both exhibit cardiovascular drift during heavy, prolonged submaximal exercise.

Incremental Exercise to Maximum

The cardiovascular response to incremental exercise is similar for both sexes, although, again, there are differences in the maximal values attained. Maximal oxygen consumption ($\dot{V}O_2$max) is higher for males

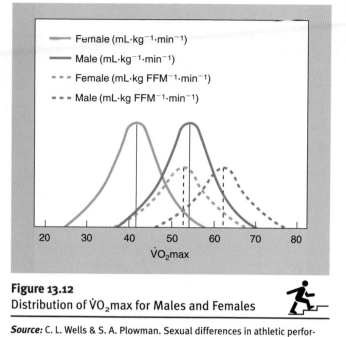

Figure 13.12
Distribution of $\dot{V}O_2$max for Males and Females

Source: C. L. Wells & S. A. Plowman. Sexual differences in athletic performance: Biological or behavioral? *Physician and Sports Medicine.* 11(8): 52–63 (1983). Reprinted by permission.

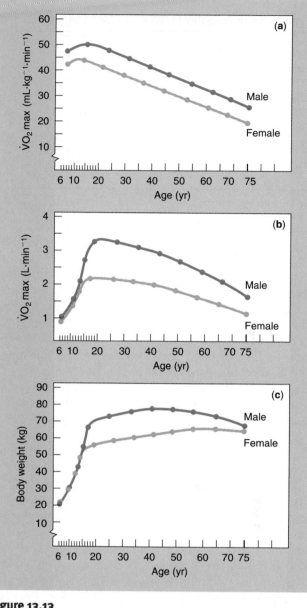

Figure 13.13
Maximal Oxygen Consumption ($\dot{V}O_2$max) and Weight for Males and Females from 6–75 Years

Source: E. Shvartz & R. C. Reibold. Aerobic fitness norms for males and females aged 6 to 75 years: A review. *Aviation, Space, and Environmental Physiology.* 61:3–11 (1990). Reprinted by permission.

than for females. When $\dot{V}O_2$max is expressed in absolute values (liters per minute), males typically have values that are 40–60% higher than in females (P. Åstrand, 1952; Sparling, 1980). When differences in body size are considered and $\dot{V}O_2$max values are reported on the relative basis of body weight (in milliliters per kilogram per minute), the differences between the sexes decreases to 20–30%. If differences in body composition are considered and $\dot{V}O_2$max is expressed relative to fat-free mass (in milliliters per kilogram of fat-free mass per minute), the difference between the sexes is reduced to 0–15% (Sparling, 1980). Reporting $\dot{V}O_2$max relative to fat-free mass is important in terms of understanding the influence of adiposity and fat-free mass in determining $\dot{V}O_2$max. However, it is not a very practical way to express $\dot{V}O_2$max because, in reality, consuming oxygen in relation to only the fat-free mass is not an option. Individuals cannot leave their fat mass behind when exercising.

Figure 13.12 represents the distribution of $\dot{V}O_2$max values for males and females expressed per kilogram of weight and per kilogram of fat-free mass. This figure demonstrates the important point that there is considerable variability in $\dot{V}O_2$max for both sexes. Thus, although males generally have a higher $\dot{V}O_2$max than females, some females will have a higher $\dot{V}O_2$max than the average man.

Figure 13.13 shows the differences in $\dot{V}O_2$max, expressed in relative terms (Figure 13.13a) and absolute terms (Figure 13.13b) and body weight (Figure

13.13c) between the sexes across the age span. Differences in $\dot{V}O_2$max between the sexes is largely explained by differences in the size of the heart (and thus maximal cardiac output) and differences in the oxygen-carrying capacity of the blood. Males have approximately 6% more red blood cells and 10–15% more hemoglobin than females; thus, males have a greater oxygen-carrying capacity than females (P. Åstrand and Rodahl, 1986).

Table 13.2
Cardiovascular Variables for Women When Compared to Men

		Exercise Condition		
Variable	Rest	Absolute, Submaximal	Relative, Submaximal	Incremental, Maximal
$\dot{V}O_2max$	—	—	—	Lower
$\dot{Q}$	Lower	Higher	?	Lower
SV	Lower	Lower	Lower	Lower
HR	Higher	Higher	Higher	Similar

Source: Wells (1991).

Males typically have maximal cardiac output values that are 30% higher than those of females (Wells, 1985). Maximal stroke volume is higher for men, but the increase in stroke volume during maximal exercise is achieved by the same mechanisms in both sexes (Sullivan, et al., 1991). Furthermore, if maximal stroke volume is expressed relative to body weight, there is no difference between the sexes. The maximal heart rate is similar for both sexes.

Males and females display the same pattern of blood pressure response; however, males attain a higher systolic blood pressure than females at maximal exercise (Malina and Bouchard, 1991; Ogawa, et al., 1992; Wanne and Haapoja, 1988). Diastolic blood pressure response to maximal exercise is similar for both sexes. Thus, mean arterial blood pressure is slightly greater in males at the completion of maximal work. The pattern of response for resistance and rate-pressure product is the same for both sexes. Resistance is greatly reduced during maximal exercise in both sexes. Because the heart rate response is similar and because systolic blood pressure is greater in males, males tend to have a higher rate-pressure product at maximal exercise levels than do females.

Table 13.2 summarizes the differences between the sexes in cardiovascular variables at various exercise levels.

Responses of Children to Aerobic Exercise

The responses of children to cardiovascular exercise are similar to the responses of adults. However, there are differences in the magnitude of the responses primarily because of differences in body size and structure.

Submaximal Exercise

The pattern of cardiac output response to submaximal dynamic exercise is similar in children and adults, with cardiac output increasing rapidly at the onset of exercise and plateauing when steady state is achieved. However, children have a lower cardiac output than adults at all levels of exercise, primarily because children have a lower stroke volume than adults at any given level of exercise (Bar-Or, 1983; Rowland, 1990). The lower stroke volume in children is compensated for, to some extent, by a higher heart rate. Stroke volume in girls is less than that in boys at all levels of exercise (Bar-Or, 1983).

The magnitude of the cardiovascular response depends on the intensity of the exercise. Table 13.3 reports the cardiac output, stroke volume, and heart rate values of children 8–12 years old during treadmill exercise at 40%, 53%, and 68% of $\dot{V}O_2max$ (Lussier and Buskirk, 1977). Both cardiac output and heart rate increase in response to increasing intensities of exercise. Stroke volume peaks at 40% of $\dot{V}O_2max$ and changes little with increasing exercise intensity. This is consistent with the finding that stroke volume plateaus at 40–50% of $\dot{V}O_2max$ in adults (P. Åstrand, et al., 1964).

Although the pattern of response in children is similar to that of adults, a careful review of Table 13.3 reveals that the values for cardiac output and stroke volume are much smaller in children. As children grow and mature, cardiac output and stroke volume increase at rest and during exercise. The heart rate response, by contrast, is higher in the younger children (Bar-Or, 1983; Cunningham et al., 1984).

Systolic blood pressure in children increases during exercise, as it does in adults, and depends on the intensity of the exercise. Boys tend to have a higher systolic blood pressure than girls (Malina and Bouchard, 1991). The magnitude of the increase in systolic pressure at submaximal exercise is less in children than in adults (James, et al., 1980; Wanne and Haapoja, 1988). The failure of systolic blood pressure to reach adult levels is probably the result of lower cardiac output in children. As children mature, the increases in systolic blood pressure during

Table 13.3

Cardiovascular Responses in Children to Submaximal Exercise of Various Intensities

Variable	Intensity of Exercise (% $\dot{V}O_2$max)		
	40%	53%	68%
$\dot{Q}$ (L·min^{-1})	6.7	7.6	8.5
SV (mL·b^{-1})	53	51	49
HR (b·min^{-1})	126	149	173

Source: Lussier & Buskirk (1977).

exercise become greater. Diastolic pressure changes little during exercise but is lower in children than adults (James, et al., 1980; Wanne and Haapoja, 1988).

Similar decreases in resistance occur in children as in adults, owing to vasodilation in working muscles. Myocardial oxygen consumption and, thus, rate-pressure product increase in children during exercise. However, the work of the heart reflects the higher heart rate and lower systolic blood pressure for children than for adults. Blood flow through the exercising muscle appears to be greater in children than in adults, resulting in a higher a-vO$_2$ diff and thereby compensating partially for the lower cardiac output (Rowland, 1990; Rowland and Green, 1988). Children appear to exhibit cardiovascular drift during heavy, prolonged exercise, just as adults do (Asano and Hirakoba, 1984).

Incremental Exercise to Maximum

The cardiovascular responses to incremental exercise to maximum are similar for children and adults; however, children achieve a lower maximal cardiac output and a lower maximal stroke volume. Maximal heart rate is higher in children than in adults and is not age dependent until the late teens (Cunningham, et al., 1984; Rowland, 1996).

The maximal oxygen consumption that is typically attained by children between the ages of 6 and 18 is shown in Figure 13.14. As children grow, their ability to take in, transport, and utilize oxygen improves. This improvement represents dimensional and maturational changes—specifically, heart volume, maximal stroke volume, maximal cardiac output, blood volume and hemoglobin concentration, and a-vO$_2$ diff increase.

The rate of improvement in absolute $\dot{V}O_2$max (expressed in liters per minute) is similar for boys and girls until approximately 12 yr of age (Figure 13.14a). Maximal oxygen uptake continues to increase in boys until the age of 18; it remains relatively constant in girls between the ages of 14 and 18.

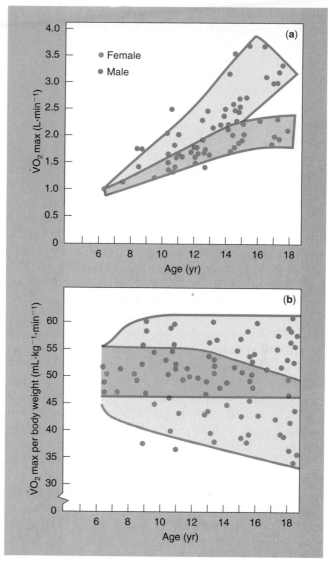

Figure 13.14

Maximal Oxygen Consumption ($\dot{V}O_2$max) of Children

(a) Changes in $\dot{V}O_2$max in children and adolescents during the ages of 6–18 are expressed in absolute terms. The dots represent means from various studies. The outer lines indicate normal variability in values. (b) Changes in $\dot{V}O_2$max in children and adolescents during the ages of 6–18 are expressed relative to body weight. The dots represent means from various studies. The outer lines indicate normal variability in reported values.

Source: O. Bar-Or. Physiologic principles to clinical applications. *Pediatric Sports Medicine for the Practitioner.* New York: Springer-Verlag (1983). Reprinted by permission.

When $\dot{V}O_2$max is expressed relative to body weight (expressed in milliliters per kilogram of body weight per minute), it remains relatively constant throughout the years between 8 and 16 for boys (Figure 13.14b). However, there is a tendency for the $\dot{V}O_2$max expressed per kilogram of body weight per minute to decrease in girls as they enter puberty, and their adiposity increases (Figure 13.14b). As children mature, they also grow; and the developmental changes indicated previously are largely offset if $\dot{V}O_2$max is described per kilogram of body weight. Notice that in both parts of Figure 13.14 there is a large area of overlap for reported values of $\dot{V}O_2$max for boys and girls. This reflects the large variability in $\dot{V}O_2$max among children.

One major difference between children/adolescents and adults is the meaning of $\dot{V}O_2$max. In adults $\dot{V}O_2$max reflects both physiological function (cardiorespiratory power) and cardiovascular endurance (the ability to perform strenuous, large-muscle exercise for a prolonged period of time) (Taylor, et al., 1955). In children, $\dot{V}O_2$max is not as directly related to cardiorespiratory endurance as it is in adults (Bar-Or, 1983; Krahenbuhl, et al., 1985; Rowland, 1990). Figure 13.15b shows performance as determined by the number of stages or minutes completed in the PACER test (Léger, et al., 1988). This progressive, aerobic cardiovascular endurance run (PACER) was fully described in Chapter 12. Recall that a higher number of laps completed is positively associated with a higher $\dot{V}O_2$ max. Figure 13.15a shows that for boys the mean value of $\dot{V}O_2$max, expressed in $mL \cdot kg^{-1} \cdot min^{-1}$, changes very little from age 6 to 18 yr. However, mean performance on the PACER test (Figure 13.15b) shows a definite linear improvement with age. The girls show the same trend as the boys prior to puberty; but thereafter, $\dot{V}O_2$max declines steadily and PACER performance plateaus. Similar results are seen in treadmill endurance times and other distance runs (Cumming, et al., 1978). Thus, in general, endurance performance improves progressively throughout childhood, at least until puberty; but directly determined $\dot{V}O_2$max, expressed relative to body size, does not. Furthermore, at any given age the relationship between $\dot{V}O_2$max and endurance performance is weak.

The reason for the weak association between $\dot{V}O_2$max and endurance performance in young people is unknown. The most frequent suggestion is that children use more aerobic energy (require greater oxygen) at any submaximal pace than adults do. This phenomenon is called *running economy* and is fully discussed in the unit on metabolism. More important than the actual oxygen consumption at a set pace, however, may be the percentage of $\dot{V}O_2$max that value represents, and more so in children than adolescents (McCormack, et al., 1991). Other factors that may impact endurance running performance in children and adolescents include body composition, particularly the percentage body fat component; sprint speed, possibly as a reflection of a high percentage of muscle

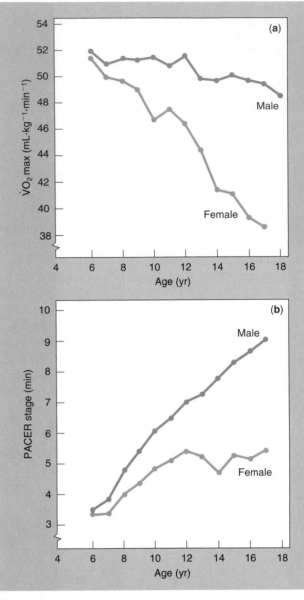

Figure 13.15
Maximal Oxygen Consumption ($\dot{V}O_2$max) and Endurance Performance in Children and Adolescents

Source: L. A. Léger, D. Mercer, C. Gadoury, & J. Lambert. The multistage 20 metre shuttle run test for aerobic fitness. *Journal of Sports Sciences.* 6:93–101 (1988). Modified and reprinted by permission.

fibers differentiated for speed and power; and various aspects of body size (Cureton, Baumgartner, et al., 1991; Cureton, Boileau, et al., 1977; Mayhew and Gifford, 1975; McVeigh, et al., 1995). There is also the possibility that many children and adolescents are not motivated to perform exercise tests and so do not perform well despite high $\dot{V}O_2$max capabilities.

Figure 13.16 presents the arterial blood pressure response of children and adolescents to incremental maximal exercise. The blood pressure response is

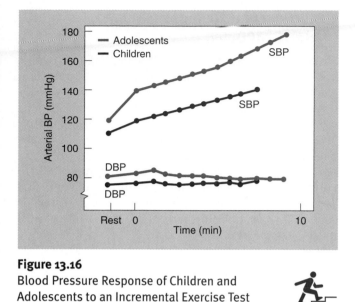

Figure 13.16

Blood Pressure Response of Children and
Adolescents to an Incremental Exercise Test

Source: D. A. Riopel, A. B. Taylor, & A. R. Hohn. Blood pressure, heart rate,
pressure-rate product and electrocardiographic changes in healthy children during treadmill exercise. *American Journal of Cardiology.* 44(4):
697–704 (1979). Reprinted by permission.

Table 13.4

Cardiovascular Responses to Maximal Exercise in Pre- and
Postpubescent Children

	Boys		Girls	
Variable	10 yr	15 yr	10 yr	15 yr
$\dot{Q}$ (L·min^{-1})	12	18	11	14
SV (mL·b^{-1})	60	90	55	70
HR (b·min^{-1})	200	200	200	200
$\dot{V}O_2$ (L·min^{-1})	1.7	3.5	1.5	2.0
SBP (mmHg)	144	174	140	170
DBP (mmHg)	64	64	64	64
MAP (mmHg)	105	110	103	117.5
TPR (units)	7.0	6.1	9.4	8.4
RPP (units)	290	350	280	340

Source: P. Åstrand (1952); Rowland (1990).

similar for children and adults; however, there are
again age- or size-related quantitative differences.
For a given level of exercise, a small child responds
with a lower systolic and diastolic blood pressure than
does an adolescent, and an adolescent responds with
lower blood pressure than an adult. The lower blood
pressure response in young children is consistent with
their lower stroke volume response. Typically, boys
have a higher peak systolic blood pressure than girls
(Riopel, et al., 1979; Wade and Freund, 1990). This
difference too is most likely attributable to differences
in stroke volume.

Table 13.4 reports typical cardiovascular responses to maximal exercise in pre- and postpubescent children.

Responses of the Elderly to Aerobic Exercise

Aging is associated with a loss of function in many systems of the body. Thus, aging is characterized by a decreased ability to respond to physiological stress (Skinner, 1993). There is considerable debate, though,
about what portion of the loss of function that charac-
terizes aging represents an inevitable age-related
loss, what portion is related to disease, and what portion is attributable to the sedentary lifestyle that so
often accompanies aging, because each causes similar decrements in function.

There are many examples of older adults who remain active into their later years and who perform
amazing athletic feats. For example, Mavis Lindgren

began an exercise program of walking when she was
in her early sixties. She slowly increased her training
volume and began jogging. At the age of 70 she completed her first marathon. In the next 12 years she
raced in over fifty marathons (Nieman, 1990). Many
studies of physical activity suggest that by remaining
active in the older years, individuals can markedly reduce loss of cardiovascular function, even if they don't
run a marathon.

Submaximal Exercise

At the same absolute submaximal workload, cardiac
output and stroke volume are lower in older adults,
but heart rate is higher when compared with those
variables for younger adults. The pattern of systolic
and diastolic pressure is the same for younger and
older individuals. The difference in resting blood
pressure is maintained throughout exercise, so that
older individuals have a higher systolic, diastolic, and
mean blood pressure at any given level of exercise
(Ogawa, et al., 1992). The higher blood pressure response is related to a higher total peripheral resistance in older individuals, resulting from a loss of
elasticity in the blood vessels. Because heart rate and
systolic blood pressure are higher for any given level
of exercise in the elderly, myocardial oxygen consumption, and thus rate-pressure product, will also
be higher in older individuals than in younger adults.

Incremental Exercise to Maximum

Maximal cardiac output is lower in older individuals
than in younger adults. This results from a lower
maximal heart rate and a lower maximal stroke

Table 13.5

Cardiovascular Responses to Maximal Exercise in Young and Older Adults

Variable	Men		Women	
	25 yr	65 yr	25 yr	65 yr
$\dot{Q}$ (L·min^{-1})	25	16	18	12
SV (mL·b^{-1})	128	100	92	75
HR (b·min^{-1})	195	155	195	155
$\dot{V}O_2$ (L·min^{-1})	3.5	2.5	2.5	1.5
SBP (mmHg)	190	200	190	200
DBP (mmHg)	70	84	64	84
MAP (mmHg)	130	143	128	143
TPR (units)	5.2	8.9	7.1	11.9
RPP (units)	371	310	371	310

Source: Ogawa, et al. (1992).

volume. Maximal stroke volume decreases with advancing age, and the decline is of similar magnitude for both men and women, although women have a much smaller maximal stroke volume initially. Maximal heart rate decreases with age but does not vary significantly between the sexes. A decrease of approximately 10% per decade, starting at approximately age 30, has been reported for $\dot{V}O_2$max in sedentary adults (I. Åstrand, 1960; Heath, et al., 1981). Figures 13.13a and 13.13b depict the change in $\dot{V}O_2$max from childhood to age 75.

As with resting blood pressure, systolic and aerobic blood pressure responses to maximal exercise are typically higher in older individuals than in younger individuals of similar training (Ogawa, et al., 1992). Maximal systolic blood pressure may be 20–50 mmHg higher in older individuals, whereas maximal diastolic blood pressure may be 15–20 mmHg higher. As a result of an elevated systolic and diastolic blood pressure, mean arterial blood pressure is considerably higher at maximal exercise in the elderly than in younger adults.

Total peripheral resistance decreases during aerobic exercise in the elderly, but not to the same extent that it does in younger individuals. This difference is a consequence of the loss of elasticity of the connective tissue in the vasculature that accompanies aging. Since the decrease in maximal heart rate for older individuals is greater than the increase in maximal systolic blood pressure when compared with those variables for younger adults, older individuals have a lower rate-pressure product at maximal exercise than younger individuals have. Table 13.5 presents typical cardiovascular values at maximal exercise in young and old adults of both sexes.

Cardiovascular Responses to Static Exercise

Static work occurs repeatedly during daily activities, such as lifting and carrying heavy objects, and is a common form of activity encountered in many occupational settings, particularly manufacturing jobs where lifting is common. Additionally, a large number of sports and recreational activities have a static component associated with their performance. For example, weight-lifting, rowing, and racquet sports all involve static exercise. The magnitude of the cardiovascular response to static exercise is affected by several factors, but most noticeably by the intensity of muscle contraction.

Intensity of Muscle Contraction

The cardiovascular response to static exercise depends on the intensity of contraction, provided the contraction is held for a specified time period. The intensity of a static contraction is expressed as a percentage of maximal voluntary contraction (% MVC). Figure 13.17 illustrates the cardiovascular response to static contractions of the forearm (handgrip) muscles at 10, 20, and 50% MVC. Notice that at 10 and 20% MVC the contraction could be held for 5 min, but at 50% MVC the contraction could be held for only 2 min. Thus, as with aerobic exercise, intensity and duration are inversely related. Also note that the data presented in this figure are from handgrip exercises. Although the pattern of response appears to be similar for different muscle groups, the actual values may vary considerably depending on the amount of active muscle involved.

Cardiac output increases during static contractions owing to an increase in heart rate, with the magnitude of the increase dependent upon the intensity of exercise. Stroke volume (Figure 13.17b) remains relatively constant during low-intensity contractions and decreases during high-intensity contractions. There is a marked increase in stroke volume immediately following the cessation of high-intensity contractions (Lind, et al., 1964; Smith, et al., 1993). This is the same rebound rise in recovery as seen in a-$\dot{V}O_2$ diff, $\dot{V}_E$, and $\dot{V}O_2$ (Chapter 11). The reduction in stroke volume during high-intensity contractions is probably the result of both a decreased preload and an increased afterload. Preload is decreased because of high intrathoracic pressure, which compresses the vena cava and thus decreases the return of venous blood to the heart. Because arterial blood pressure is markedly elevated during static contractions (increased afterload), less blood will be ejected at a given force of contraction. Heart

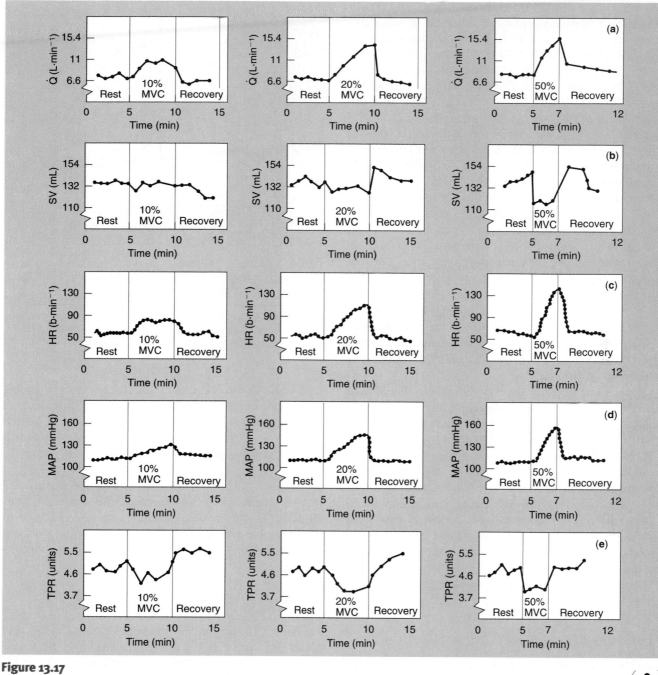

Figure 13.17
Cardiovascular Response to Varying Intensities
of Handgrip Exercise

Source: Modified from A. R. LInd, S. H. Taylor, P. W. Humphreys, B. M. Kennelly, & K. W. Donald. The circulatory effects of sustained voluntary muscle contraction. *Clinical Science.* 27:229–244. Reprinted by permission of the
Biochemical Society and Portland Press (1964).

rate (Figure 13.17c) increases during static exercise. The magnitude and the rate of the increase in heart rate depends on the intensity of contraction. The greater the intensity, the greater the heart rate response.

Static exercise is characterized by a rapid increase in both systolic pressure and diastolic pressure, termed the **pressor response,** which appears to be inappropriate for the amount of work produced by

---

Pressor Response The rapid increase in both systolic pressure and diastolic pressure during static exercise.

the contracting muscle (Lind, et al., 1964). Since both systolic and diastolic pressures increase in static exercise, there is a marked increase in mean arterial pressure (Figure 13.17d) (Donald, et al., 1967; Lind, et al., 1964; Seals, et al., 1985; Tuttle and Horvath, 1957). As in any muscular work, static exercise increases metabolic demands of the active muscle. However, in static work high intramuscular tension results in mechanical constriction of the blood vessels, which impedes blood flow to the muscle. The reduction in muscle blood flow during static exercise results in a buildup of local by-products of metabolism. These chemical by-products [H^+, adenosine diphosphate (ADP), and others] stimulate sensory nerve endings, which leads to a pressor reflex, causing a rise in mean arterial pressure (pressor response). This rise is substantially larger than the increase during aerobic exercise requiring similar energy expenditure (Asmussen, 1981; Hanson and Nagle, 1985). Notice in Figure 13.17d that holding a handgrip dynamometer at 20% MVC for 5 min results in an increase of 20–30 mmHg in mean arterial pressure and holding 50% MVC for 2 min caused a 50-mmHg increase in mean arterial pressure!

Total peripheral resistance, indicated by TPR in Figure 13.17e, decreases during static exercise, although not to the extent seen in dynamic aerobic exercise. The failure of resistance to decrease markedly helps to explain the higher blood pressure response to static contractions. The high blood pressure generated during static contractions helps overcome the resistance to blood flow owing to mechanical occlusion. Because systolic blood pressure and heart rate both increase during static exercise, there is a large increase in myocardial oxygen consumption and thus rate-pressure product.

Table 13.1 on page 362 summarizes cardiovascular responses to static exercise.

Blood Flow during Static Contractions

Blood flow to the working muscle is impeded during static contractions because of mechanical constriction of the blood vessel supplying the contracting muscle (Freund, et al., 1979; Sjogaard, et al., 1988). Figure 13.18 depicts blood flow in the quadriceps muscle when a 5% and 25% MVC contraction were held to fatigue. The 5% MVC load could be held for 30 min; the 25% load could be held for only 4 min. Quadriceps blood flow is greater during the 5% MVC, suggesting that at 25% MVC there is considerable impedance to blood flow. In fact, blood flow during the 25% MVC load was very close to resting levels despite the metabolic work done by the muscle. The response seen during recovery suggests that when contraction ceases, a mechanical occlusion to the muscle is

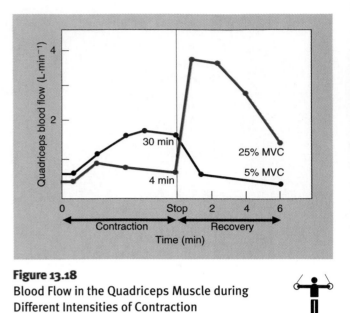

Figure 13.18
Blood Flow in the Quadriceps Muscle during Different Intensities of Contraction

Source: G. Sjogaard, G. Savard, & C. Juel. Muscle blood flow during isometric activity and its relation to muscle fatigue. *European Journal of Physiology.* 57:327–335 (1988). Reprinted by permission.

released. The marked increase in blood flow during recovery compensates for the reduced flow during sustained contraction. The relative force at which blood flow is impeded varies greatly among different muscle groups (Lind and McNichol, 1967; Rowell, 1993).

There is also mechanical constriction during dynamic aerobic exercise. However, the alternating periods of muscular contraction and relaxation that occur during rhythmical activity allow—and, indeed, encourage—blood flow, especially through the venous system.

Comparison of Aerobic and Static Exercise

Figure 13.19 compares the heart rate (13.19a) and blood pressure (13.19b) responses to fatiguing handgrip (static) exercise (30% MVC held to fatigue) and a maximal treadmill (dynamic aerobic) test to fatigue. Aerobic exercise (treadmill) is characterized by a large increase in heart rate, which contributes to an increased cardiac output. Aerobic exercise also shows a modest increase in systolic blood pressure and a relatively stable or decreasing diastolic blood pressure. Aerobic exercise is said to impose a "volume load" on the heart. Increased venous return leads to increased stroke volume, which contributes to an increased cardiac output. In contrast, fatiguing static exercise (handgrip) is characterized by a modest increase in heart rate but a dramatic increase in blood pressure (pressor response). Mean blood pressure increases as a result of increased systolic and diastolic blood

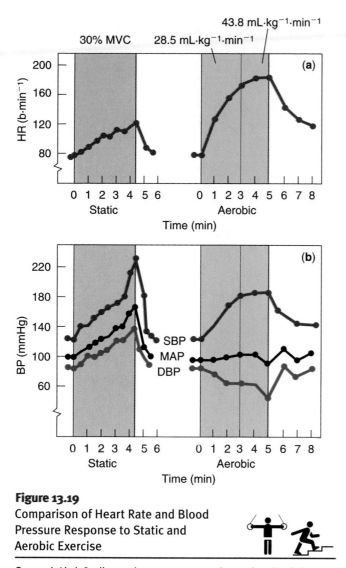

Figure 13.19
Comparison of Heart Rate and Blood
Pressure Response to Static and
Aerobic Exercise

Source: A. Lind. Cardiovascular responses to static exercise. *Circulation.*
XLI(2) (1970). Reproduced with permission. Copyright 1970 American
Heart Association.

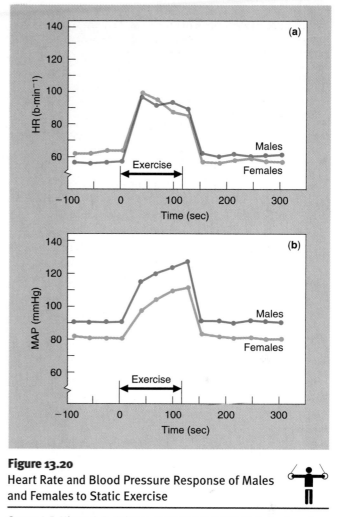

Figure 13.20
Heart Rate and Blood Pressure Response of Males
and Females to Static Exercise

Source: J. E. Misner, S. B. Going, B. H. Massey, T. E. Ball, M. G. Bemben, &
L. K. Essandoh. Cardiovascular response in males and females to sustained maximal voluntary static muscle contraction. *Medicine and
Science in Sports and Exercise.* 22(2):194–199 (1990). Reprinted by permission of Williams & Wilkins.

pressure. Static exercise is said to impose a "pressure
load" on the heart. Increased mean arterial pressure
means that the heart must pump harder to overcome
the pressure in the aorta.

Sex Differences in Responses to Static Exercise

The heart rate response to static exercise (Figure
13.20a) is similar in males and females (Misner, et al.,
1990). However, as shown in Figure 13.20b, when a
group of young adult, healthy subjects held maximal
contractions of the handgrip muscles for 2 min, the
blood pressures reported for women were significantly lower than those reported for men (Misner, et
al., 1990). Stroke volume and cardiac output responses in women during maximal static contraction
of the finger flexors were similar to the responses

observed in the men, but no direct comparisons between men and women were made for these variables
(Smith, et al., 1993). There are no comparable data
available for boys and girls.

Cardiovascular Responses to Static Exercise in Older Adults

Many studies have described the cardiovascular responses to static exercise in the elderly (Goldstraw
and Warren, 1980; Petrofsky and Lind, 1975; Sagiv,
et al., 1988; VanLoan, et al., 1989). As an example,
Figure 13.21 depicts the cardiovascular responses of
young and old men to sustained handgrip and leg
extension exercise over a range of submaximal static
workloads (VanLoan, et al., 1989). Note that cardiac output (Figure 13.21a) and stroke volume

Figure 13.21
Cardiovascular Response of
Males by Age to Static Exercise

Source: M. D. VanLoan, et al. Age as a factor in the
hemodynamic responses to isometric exercise.
*Journal of Sports Medicine and Physical
Fitness.* 29(3):262–268 (1989). Reprinted by
permission.

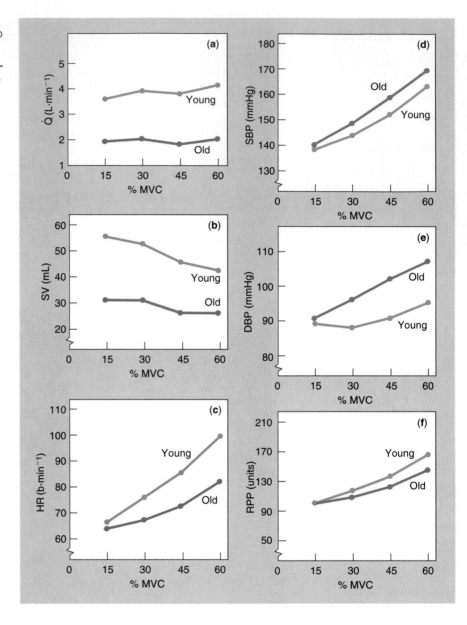

(Figure 13.21b) values are lower than normally reported owing to the measurement technique. However, concentrating on the relative differences between the responses of the young and older subjects reveals that cardiac output, stroke volume, and heart rate (Figure 13.21c) were lower for the older men than the younger men at each intensity. In contrast, blood pressure responses (Figures 13.21d and 13.21e) were higher for the older men at each intensity. As with dynamic aerobic exercise the differences in the cardiovascular responses between the two age groups are probably due to an age-related increase in resistance due to a loss of elasticity in the vasculature and a decreased ability of the myocardium to stretch and contract forcibly (VanLoan, et al., 1989). The rate-pressure product (Figure 13.21f) was higher for

the younger subjects than for the older subjects at 30, 45, and 60% MVC. The small difference in rate-pressure product reflected a higher heart rate in younger subjects at each intensity of contraction, which was not completely offset by a lower systolic blood pressure in the younger subjects.

Cardiovascular Responses to Dynamic Resistance Exercise

Weight-lifting or resistance exercise includes a combination of dynamic and static contractions (Hill and Butler, 1991; MacDougall, et al., 1985). At the beginning of the lift, a static contraction exists until muscle force exceeds the load to be lifted and movement occurs, which leads to a dynamic concentric (shortening) contraction as the lift continues. This is then followed by a dynamic eccentric (lengthening) contraction during the lowering phase (McCartney, 1999). Furthermore, there is always a static component associated with gripping the barbell. During dynamic resistance exercise there is a dissociation between the energy demand and the cardiorespiratory system. In contrast, during dynamic endurance activity the cardiorespiratory system is directly tied to the use of oxygen for energy production. In part, the reason for this dissociation between oxygen use and cardiovascular response to resistance exercise is that much of the energy required for resistance exercise comes from anaerobic (without oxygen) sources. Another important difference between resistance exercise and aerobic exercise that affects cardiovascular responses is the mechanical constriction of blood flow during resistance exercise because of the static nature of the contraction.

The magnitude of the cardiovascular response to resistance exercise depends on the intensity of the load (the weight lifted) and the number of repetitions performed.

Constant Repetitions/Varying Load

The cardiovascular responses also depend on the way in which the load and repetitions are combined. As expected, cardiovascular responses are greater when heavier loads are lifted, assuming the number of repetitions are held constant (Fleck, 1988; Fleck and Dean, 1987). For example, when subjects performed ten repetitions of three different weights (identified as light, moderate, and heavy), blood pressure was highest *at the completion* of the heaviest set (Wescott and Howes, 1983). Systolic blood pressure increased 16%, 22%, and 34% during the light, moderate, and heavy sets, respectively. Diastolic blood pressure, measured by auscultation, did not change significantly with any of the sets. There is disagreement about the diastolic blood pressure response to resistance exercise; some authors report an increase and others report no change (Fleck, 1988; Fleck and Dean, 1987; Wescott and Howes, 1983). These discrepancies may reflect differences in measurement techniques (namely, auscultation and intra-arterial assessment) and timing of the measurement.

Resistance Exercise to Fatigue

A different pattern of response is seen when a given load is performed to fatigue. In this case the individual is performing maximal work regardless of the load. Figure 13.22 shows the cardiovascular

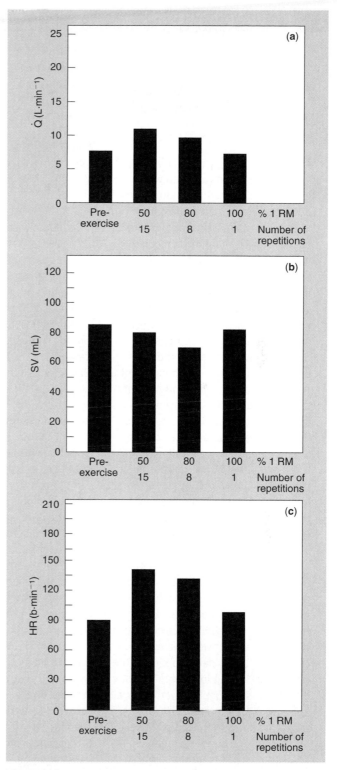

Figure 13.22
Cardiovascular Response at the Completion of Fatiguing Resistance Exercise (concentric knee extension exercise)

Source: Based on data from Falkel, et al. (1992).

Focus on Application

✳ Cardiovascular Demands of Shoveling Wet, Heavy Snow

Variable	Snow Shoveling	Snow Blower	Treadmill (max)
Heart rate (b·min^{-1})	175 ± 15	124 ± 18	179 ± 17
Systolic blood pressure (mmHg)	198 ± 17	161 ± 14	181 ± 25
Rate-pressure product	347	199.6	324
$\dot{V}O_2$ (mL·kg^{-1}min^{-1})	19.95 ± 2.8	8.4 ± 2.5	32.55 ± 6.3
Rating of perceived exertion	16.7 ± 1.7	9.9 ± 1.0	17.9 ± 1.5

As the text has described, upper-body exercise is associated with greater cardiovascular strain (exemplified by higher heart rates and higher blood pressures at any given submaximal level of oxygen consumption) than lower-body exercise. Similarly, it was emphasized that both static and dynamic resistance exercise are characterized by modest increases in heart rate but exaggerated increases in blood pressure. Snow shoveling presents the shoveler with the unique combination of a predominantly upper-body activity that has both static and dynamic components. In addition, snow shoveling is always done in the cold (and sometimes in frigid conditions), and often when the individual is under the added stress of digging out to get somewhere on time. It is not unusual to hear about individuals collapsing and dying of heart attacks while clearing snow.

Franklin and his colleagues performed an experiment to determine the specific demands of snow shoveling on the heart. Ten sedentary, healthy, young adult males cleared two 15-m paths of wet, heavy snow that was 5–13 cm deep outside in the cold (2 degrees C) for 10 min. For one trial they used a 1.4 kg plastic shovel. They were told to repeatedly lift-throw the snow to the side at a self-selected rate. The group mean was 12 ± 2 loads per minute at approximately 7.3 kg per load for a total of 872.7 kg (1920 lb) over the 10-min time span. For the second trial they used a motorized snow blower. Ten to 15 min of rest was permitted between the randomly assigned trials. On another day, each participant underwent a treadmill maximal oxygen consumption test in the laboratory. The results are presented in the accompanying table.

After only 2 min of snow shoveling, the subjects' average heart rate was 85% of the treadmill HRmax. The HR continued to increase until it reached 98% HRmax. Systolic blood pressure during the snow shoveling exceeded the treadmill maximum by 9.3%. The total body oxygen consumption was only 61.3% $\dot{V}O_2$max, but the myocardial oxygen consumption, as indicated by the rate-pressure product, was 107% of that required during maximal treadmill work. The disproportionate increase in myocardial oxygen demand relative to total body oxygen demand during shoveling was attributed to several factors: a reduced myocardial efficiency of arm exercise, a large static exercise component, the Valsalva maneuver, and the inhalation of cold air that could cause a spasm or constriction in the coronary arteries. These results clearly indicate that shoveling wet, heavy snow even for a short time period (10 min) places a tremendous physiological demand on the heart.

By comparison, using the snow blower resulted in elevations to only 69% HRmax, 89% maximal systolic blood pressure, 25% $\dot{V}O_2$max, and 61% maximal myocardial oxygen consumption, as reflected by the rate-pressure product. Whereas the manual shoveling was perceived as "very heavy" work, using the snow blower resulted in a "fairly light" rating.

The healthy, but untrained subjects in this study completed the shoveling without any adverse cardiac or musculoskeletal complications. Such work, especially if continued for 20–60 min would provide a heavy but acceptable workout. However, these results suggest that individuals with a history of heart disease, symptoms suggestive of cardiac disorder (dizziness, chest pain, abnormal electrocardiograms) or one or more major coronary risk factor (see Chapter 16) should avoid the work, or take precautions when faced with the task of clearing wet, heavy snow. These precautions include:

1. Take frequent breaks or use a work–rest approach.
2. Use both arms and legs in the lift-throw action.
3. Regulate body temperature with a hat, scarf over the mouth, and layers that can easily be added or removed.
4. Avoid large meals, alcohol consumption, and smoking immediately before and after shoveling.
5. Consider using a motorized snow blower. ✳

Sources:

Franklin (1997); Franklin, et al. (1995).

response at the completion of leg extension exercise performed to fatigue. Subjects performed 50%, 80%, and 100% of their one repetition maximum (1 RM) as many times as they could, and cardiovascular variables were recorded at the end of each set (Falkel, et al., 1992). Subjects could perform the 100% load only one time, of course; but they could perform the 80% and 50% loads an average of 8 and 15 times, respectively. Thus, the greatest volume of work was performed when the lightest load was lifted the greatest number of times. Cardiac output *at the completion* of the set was highest when the lightest load was lifted for the greatest number of repetitions (Figure 13.22a).

The stroke volume achieved at the end of a set was similar for each condition (Figure 13.22b) and was slightly below resting levels. This is in contrast to significant increases in stroke volume measures typically obtained during aerobic exercise. Thus, dynamic resistance exercise does not produce the stroke volume overload that dynamic endurance exercise does (Hill and Butler, 1991; McCartney, 1999).

Heart rate was highest after completion of the set using the lightest load and lifting it the greatest number of times (Figure 13.22c). Heart rate was lowest when the single repetition using the heaviest weight was performed. Heart rates between 130 and 160 b·min^{-1} have been reported during resistance exercise (Hill and Butler, 1991). There is some evidence that the heart rate and blood pressure attained at fatigue are the same when loads between 60% and 100% of 1 RM are used, regardless of the number of times the load can be performed (Nau, et al., 1990).

When the load is heavy, MAP and HR increase gradually with succeeding repetitions in a set to failure (Fleck and Dean, 1987; MacDougall, et al., 1985). Figure 13.23a shows the mean arterial blood pressure, measured intra-arterially, *during a set* of leg press exercises that represented 95% of one repetition maximum, and Figure 13.23b shows the heart rate during these exercises. In this study peak systolic blood pressure averaged 320 mmHg, and peak diastolic blood pressure averaged 250 mmHg! The dramatic increase in blood pressure during dynamic resistance exercise results from the mechanical compression on the blood vessels and performance of the Valsalva maneuver (as explained in Chapter 11). Total peripheral resistance is higher during dynamic resistance exercise than during dynamic aerobic exercise because of the vasoconstriction caused by the pressor reflex. In fact, some studies have reported a slight increase in total peripheral resistance during resistance exercise, rather than the decrease that is observed with aerobic exercise (Lentini, et al., 1993;

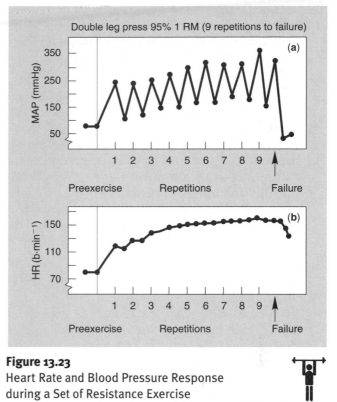

Figure 13.23
Heart Rate and Blood Pressure Response during a Set of Resistance Exercise

Source: J. D. MacDougall, D. Tuxen, D. G. Sale, J. R. Moroz, & J. R. Sutton. Arterial blood pressure response to heavy resistance exercise. *Journal of Applied Physiology.* 58(3):785–790 (1985). Reprinted by permission.

McCartney, 1999; Miles, et al., 1987). Myocardial oxygen consumption and, thus, the rate-pressure product can reach extremely high levels because of the tachycardia and exaggerated systolic blood pressure response. Dynamic resistance exercise causes large (about 15%) but transient decreases in plasma volume (Hill and Butler, 1991). The cardiovascular response of children to resistance exercise is similar to that of adults, with heart rate and blood pressure increasing progressively throughout a set (Nau, et al., 1990).

A summary of cardiovascular responses to resistance exercise is included in Table 13.1 on page 362.

Summary

1. During short-term, light to moderate aerobic exercise, cardiac output, stroke volume, heart rate, systolic blood pressure, and rate-pressure product increase rapidly at the onset of exercise and reach steady state within approximately 2 min. Diastolic blood pressure remains relatively unchanged, and resistance decreases rapidly and then plateaus.

IP *Cardiovascular–Blood Pressure Regulation* (page 9); *Cardiovascular–Cardiac Output* (pages 1–10); *Cardiovascular–Factors that Affect Blood Pressure* (pages 1–4; 13–14); *Cardiovascular–utoregulation and Capillary Dynamics* (pages 1–12)**

2. During long-term, moderate to heavy aerobic exercise, cardiac output, stroke volume, heart rate, systolic blood pressure, and rate-pressure product increase rapidly. Once steady state is achieved, cardiac output remains relatively constant owing to the downward drift of stroke volume and the upward drift of heart rate. Systolic blood pressure and resistance may also drift downward during prolonged, heavy work. This cardiovascular drift is associated with rising body temperature.

3. During incremental exercise to maximum, cardiac output, heart rate, systolic blood pressure, and rate-pressure product increase in a rectilinear fashion with increasing workload. Stroke volume increases initially and then plateaus at a workload corresponding to approximately 40–50% of $\dot{V}O_2$ max in normally active adults and children. Diastolic blood pressure remains relatively constant throughout an incremental exercise test. Resistance decreases rapidly with the onset of exercise and reaches its lowest value at maximal exercise.

4. The decrease in resistance that accompanies aerobic exercise has two important implications. First, the decrease in resistance allows greater blood flow to the working muscles. Second, the decrease in resistance keeps blood pressure from rising excessively. The increase in cardiac output would produce a much greater rise in blood pressure if it were not for the fact that there is a simultaneous decrease in resistance.

5. Blood volume decreases during aerobic exercise. The majority of the decrease occurs within the first 10 min of activity and depends on exercise intensity. A decrease of 10% of blood volume is not uncommon.

6. Stroke volume initially increases during dynamic aerobic exercise and then plateaus at a level that corresponds to 40–50% of $\dot{V}O_2$max. The increase in stroke volume results from changes in left ventricular end–diastolic volume and left ventricular end–systolic volume. Left ventricular end–diastolic volume increases primarily because the active muscle pump returns blood to the heart. Left ventricular end–systolic volume decreases owing to augmented contractility of the heart, thus ejecting more blood and leaving less in the ventricle.

7. The pattern of cardiovascular response is the same for both sexes. However, males have a higher cardiac output, stroke volume, and systolic blood pressure at maximal exercise. Additionally, males have a higher $\dot{V}O_2$max. Most of these differences are attributable to differences in body size and heart size between the sexes and to the greater hemoglobin concentration of males.

8. The pattern of cardiovascular response in children is similar to the adult response. However, children have a lower cardiac output, stroke volume, and systolic blood pressure at an absolute workload and at maximal exercise. Most of these differences are attributable to differences in body size and heart size.

9. As adults age, their cardiovascular responses change. Maximal cardiac output, stroke volume, heart rate, and $\dot{V}O_2$max decrease. Maximal systolic blood pressure, diastolic blood pressure, and mean arterial pressure increase.

10. Static exercise is characterized by modest increases in heart rate and cardiac output and exaggerated increases in systolic blood pressure, diastolic blood pressure and mean arterial pressure, known as the pressor response.

11. Dynamic resistance exercise results in a modest increase in cardiac output, an increase in heart rate, little change or a decrease in stroke volume, and a large increase in blood pressure.

*This topic is available on the InterActive Physiology® Sampler CD that comes with the purchase of a new copy of this book.

Review Questions

1. Graph and explain the pattern of response for each of the major cardiovascular variables during short-term, light to moderate aerobic exercise. Explain the mechanisms responsible for each response.

2. Graph and explain the pattern of response for each of the major cardiovascular variables during long-term, moderate to heavy aerobic exercise. Explain the mechanisms responsible for each response.

3. Graph and explain the pattern of response for each of the major cardiovascular variables during incremental aerobic exercise to maximum. Explain the mechanisms responsible for each response.

4. Graph and explain the pattern of response for each of the major cardiovascular variables during

static exercise. Explain the mechanisms responsible for each response.

5. Graph and explain the pattern of response for each of the major cardiovascular variables during dynamic resistance exercise. Explain the mechanisms responsible for each response.

6. Discuss the change that occurs in total peripheral resistance during exercise, and explain its importance for blood flow and blood pressure. Why is resistance altered in older adults?

7. Describe the pressor response to static exercise, and explain the mechanisms by which blood pressure is elevated.

For further review and additional study tools, go to The Physiology Place (www.physiologyplace.com) and the Student Study Guide for Exercise Physiology for Health, Fitness, and Performance by Sharon A. Plowman and Denise L. Smith.

Passport to the Internet

Visit the following Internet sites to explore further topics and issues related to understanding cardiovascular response to exercise. To visit an organization's web site, go to www.physiologyplace.com and click on "Passport to the Internet."

The American College of Sports Medicine Home page of the professional organization for individuals in sports medicine and exercise science. Spend some time exploring this site and discovering the multitude of resources available.

Masters Athlete Physiology & Performance This site is the springboard to an ever-growing body of literature on the physiological basis for endurance performance and training. Many exercise physiologists started out as athletes whose desire for better performance drove them to explore how the human machine worked. This site begins with the basics and allows the reader to explore topics in greater depth.

The American Heart Association Visit one of the most complete sites for the latest information on cardiorespiratory health promotion. Investigate the latest findings and ongoing research dedicated to understanding cardiovascular disease. While there, go to www.choosetomove.org and investigate this special program dedicated to helping women establish physical activity as a habit.

The Nicholas Institute of Sports Medicine and Athletic Trauma (NISMAT) The Nicholas Institute of Sports Medicine and Athletic Trauma (NISMAT) is the first hospital-based facility dedicated to the study of sports medicine in the United States. This site has various resources related to cardiovascular and muscular issues.

Inner Learning Online This interactive web site contains an inner exploration of the human anatomy. Each topic has animations, graphics, and numerous descriptive links.

References

American College of Sports Medicine: *Guidelines for Exercise Testing and Prescription* (6th edition). Philadelphia: Lea & Febiger (2000).

American College of Sports Medicine: Position stand: Physical activity, physical fitness, and hypertension. *Medicine and Science in Sports and Exercise.* 25(10):1-X (1993).

Anderson, K. L.: The cardiovascular system in exercise. In H. B. Falls (ed.), *Exercise Physiology.* New York: Academic Press (1968).

Asano, K., & K. Hirakoba: Respiratory and circulatory adaptation during prolonged exercise in 10–12 year-old children and adults. In J. Ilmarinen, & I. Valimaki (eds.), *Children and Sports.* Berlin: Springer-Verlag (1984).

Asmussen, E.: Similarities and dissimilarities between static and dynamic exercise. *Circulation Research* (Suppl. I). 48(6):3–10 (1981).

Åstrand, I.: Aerobic work capacity in men and women with special reference to age. *Acta Physiologica Scandinavica* (Suppl. 169). 49:1–92 (1960).

Åstrand, P.: Experimental Studies of Physical Working Capacity in Relation to Sex and Age. *University Microfilms International* (1952).

Åstrand, P., T. E. Cuddy, B. Saltin, & J. Stenberg: Cardiac output during submaximal and maximal work. *Journal of Applied Physiology.* 19(2):268–274 (1964).

Åstrand, P. O., & K. Rodahl: *Textbook of Work Physiology.* New York: McGraw-Hill (1986).

Bar-Or, O.: Physiologic principles to clinical applications. *Pediatric Sports Medicine, for the Practitioner.* New York: Springer-Verlag (1983).

Becklake, M. R., H. Frank, G. R. Dagenais, G. L. Ostiguy, & C. A. Guzman: Influence of age and sex on exercise cardiac output. *Journal of Applied Physiology.* 20(5):938–947 (1965).

Clausen, J. P.: Circulatory adjustments to dynamic exercise and effect of physical training in normal subjects and in patients with coronary artery disease. *Progressive Cardiovascular Disease.* 18:459–495 (1976).

Cumming, G. R., D. Everatt, & L. Hastman: Bruce treadmill test in children: Normal values in a clinic population. *American Journal of Cardiology.* 41:69–75 (1978).

Cunningham, D. A., D. H. Paterson, C. J. R. Blimkie, & A. P. Donner: Development of cardiorespiratory function in circumpubertal boys: A longitudinal study. *Journal of Applied Physiology: Respiratory Environment Exercise Physiology.* 56(2):302–307 (1984).

Cureton, K. J., T. A. Baumgartner, & B. McManis: Adjustment of 1-mile run/walk test scores for skinfold thickness in youth. *Pediatric Exercise Science.* 3:152–167 (1991).

Cureton, K. J., R. A. Boileau, T. G. Lohman, & J. E. Misner: Determinants of distance running performance in children: Analysis of a path model. *Research Quarterly.* 48(2): 270–279 (1977).

Davies, C. T. M., J. Few, K. G. Foster, & A. J. Sargeant: Plasma catecholamine concentration during dynamic exercise involving different muscle groups. *European Journal of Applied Physiology.* 32:195–206 (1974).

Donald, K. W., S. R. Lind, G. W. McNichol, P. W. Humphreys, S. H. Taylor, & H. P. Stauton: Cardiovascular responses to sustained (static) contractions. *Circulation Research* (Suppl. I). 15–32 (1967).

Ekelund, L. G., & A. Holmgren: Central hemodynamics during exercise. *Circulation Research* (Suppl. I). 33–43 (1967).

Falkel, J. E., S. J. Fleck, & T. F. Murray: Comparison of central hemodynamics between powerlifters and bodybuilders during resistance exercise. *Journal of Applied Sport Science Research.* 6(1):24–35 (1992).

Fleck, S. J.: Cardiovascular adaptations to resistance training. *Medicine and Science in Sports and Exercise.* 20: S146–S151 (1988).

Fleck, S. J., & L. S. Dean: Resistance-training experience and the pressor response during resistance exercise. *Journal of Applied Physiology.* 63:116–120 (1987).

Fortney, S. M., C. B. Wenger, J. R. Bove, & E. R. Nadel: Effect of blood volume on sweating rate and body fluids in exercising humans. *Journal of Applied Physiology.* 51(6): 1594–1600 (1981).

Franklin, B. A.: Prevention of heart attacks during snow shoveling. *ACSM's Health & Fitness Journal.* 1(6):20–23 (1997).

Franklin, B. A., P. Hogan, K. Bonzheim, D. Bakalyar, E. Terrien, S. Gordon, & G. C. Timmis: Cardiac demands of heavy snow shoveling. *Journal of the American Medical Association.* 273:880–882 (1995).

Freedson, P., V. L. Katch, S. Sady, & A. Weltman: Cardiac output differences in males and females during mild cycle ergometer exercise. *Medicine and Science in Sports.* 11(1): 16–19 (1979).

Freund, P. R., S. F. Gobbs, & L. B. Rowell: Cardiovascular responses to muscle ischemia in man, dependency on muscle mass. *Journal of Applied Physiology.* 45:762–767 (1979).

Gledhill, N., D. Cox, & R. Jamnik: Endurance athletes' stroke volume does not plateau: Major advantage is diastolic function. *Medicine and Science in Sports and Exercise.* 26: 1116–1121 (1994).

Goldstraw, P. W., & D. J. Warren: The effect of age on the cardiovascular responses to isometric exercise: A test of autonomic function. *Gerontology.* 31:54–58 (1989).

Hamilton, M. T., J. G. Alonso, S. J. Montain, & E. F. Coyle: Fluid replacement and glucose infusion during exercise prevents cardiovascular drift. *Journal of Applied Physiology.* 71:871–877 (1991).

Hanson, P., & F. Nagle: Isometric exercise: Cardiovascular responses in normal and cardiac populations. *Cardiology Clinics.* 5(2):157–170 (1985).

Heath, G. W., J. M. Hagberg, A. A. Ehsani, & J. O. Holloszy: A physiological comparison of young and older endurance athletes. *Journal of Applied Physiology.* 51:634–640 (1981).

Higginbotham, M. B., K. G. Morris, R. S. Williams, P. A. McHale, R. E. Coleman, & F. R. Cobb: Regulation of stroke volume during submaximal and maximal upright exercise in normal man. *Circulation Research.* 58:281–291 (1986).

Hill, D. W., & S. D. Butler: Haemodynamic responses to weightlifting exercise. *Sports Medicine.* 12(1):1–7 (1991).

James, F. W., S. Kaplan, C. J. Glueck, J. Y. Tsay, M. J. S. Knight, & C. J. Sarwar: Responses of normal children and young adults to controlled bicycle exercise. *Circulation.* 61:902–912 (1980).

Krahenbuhl, G. S., J. S. Skinner, & W. M. Kohrt: Developmental aspects of maximal aerobic power in children. In R. L. Terjung (ed.), *Exercise and Sport Science Reviews.* 13: 503–538 (1985).

Léger, L. A., D. Mercer, C. Gadoury, & J. Lambert: The multistage 20 metre shuttle run test for aerobic fitness. *Journal of Sports Sciences.* 6:93–101 (1988).

Lentini, A. C., R. S. McKelvie, N. McCartney, C. W. Tomlinson, & J. D. MacDougall. Left ventricular responses in healthy young men during heavy-intensity weight-lifting exercise. *Journal of Applied Physiology.* 75:2703–2710 (1993).

Lind, A.: Cardiovascular responses to static exercise. *Circulation.* XLI(2): (1970).

Lind, A. R., & G. W. McNichol: Circulatory responses to sustained handgrip contractions performed during other exercise. *Journal of Physiology.* 192:595–607 (1967).

Lind, A. R., S. H. Taylor, P. W. Humphreys, B. M. Kennelly, & K. W. Donald. The circulatory effects of sustained voluntary muscle contraction. *Clinical Science.* 27:229–244 (1964).

Lussier, L., & E. R. Buskirk: Effects of an endurance training regimen on assessment of work capacity in prepubertal children. *Annals of the New York Academy of Sciences.* 734–777 (1977).

MacDougall, J. D., D. Tuxen, D. G. Sale, J. R. Moroz, & J. R. Sutton: Arterial blood pressure response to heavy resistance exercise. *Journal of Applied Physiology.* 58(3):785–790 (1985).

Malina, R. M., & C. Bouchard: *Growth, Maturation and Physical Activity.* Champaign, IL: Human Kinetics (1991).

Mayhew, J. L., & P. B. Gifford: Prediction of maximal oxygen intake in preadolescent boys from anthropometric parameters. *Research Quarterly.* 46(3):302–311 (1975).

McCartney, N. Acute responses to resistance training and safety. *Medicine and Science in Sports and Exercise.* 31(1):31–37 (1999).

McCormack, W. P., K. J. Cureton, T. A. Bullock, & P. G. Weyand: Metabolic determinants of 1-mile run/walk performance in children. *Medicine and Science in Sport and Exercise.* 23(5):611–617 (1991).

McVeigh, S. K., A. C. Payne, & S. Scott: The reliability and validity of the 20-meter shuttle test as a predictor of peak oxygen uptake in Edinburgh school children, ages 13 to 14 years. *Pediatric Exercise Science.* 7:69–79 (1995).

Miles, D. S., M. H. Cox, & J. P. Bomze: Cardiovascular responses to upper body exercise in normal and cardiac patients. *Medicine and Science in Sport and Exercise.* 21(5):s126–s131 (1989).

Miles, D. S., J. J. Owens, J. C. Golden, & R. W. Gotshall. Central and peripheral hemodynamics during maximal leg extension exercise. *European Journal of Applied Physiology.* 56:12–17 (1987).

Misner, J. E., S. B. Going, B. H. Massey, T. E. Ball, M. G. Bemben, & L. K. Essandoh: Cardiovascular response in males and females to sustained maximal voluntary static muscle contraction. *Medicine and Science in Sports and Exercise.* 22(2):194–199 (1990).

Nau, K. L., V. L. Katch, R. H. Beekman, & M. Dick II: Acute intra-arterial blood pressure response to bench press weight lifting in children. *Pediatric Exercise Science.* 2:37–45 (1990).

Ogawa, T., R. J. Spina, W. H. Martin, W. M. Kohrt, K. B. Schechtman, J. O. Holloszy, & A. A. Ehsani: Effects of aging, sex, and physical training on cardiovascular responses to exercise. *Circulation.* 86:494–503 (1992).

Nieman, D.: *Fitness and Sports Medicine.* Palo Alto, CA: Bull Publishing (1990).

Pendergast, D. R.: Cardiovascular, respiratory, and metabolic responses to upper body exercise. *Medicine and Science in Sport and Exercise.* 21(5):s122–s125 (1989).

Petrofsky, J. S., & A. R. Lind: Aging, isometric strength and endurance, and cardiovascular responses to static effort. *Journal of Applied Physiology.* 38(1):91–95 (1975).

Poliner, L. R., G. J. Dehmer, S. E. Lewis, R. W. Parkey, C. G. Blomqvist, & J. T. Willerson: Left ventricular performance in normal subjects: A comparison of the responses to exercise in the upright supine positions. *Circulation.* 62:528–534 (1980).

Riopel, D. A., A. B. Taylor, & A. R. Hohn: Blood pressure, heart rate, pressure-rate product and electrocardiographic changes in healthy children during treadmill exercise. *American Journal of Cardiology.* 44:697–704 (1979).

Rowell, L.: Human cardiovascular adjustments to exercise and thermal stress. *Physiological Reviews.* 54:75–159 (1974).

Rowell, L. B.: *Human Cardiovascular Control.* New York: Oxford University Press: (1993).

Rowell, L. B.: *Human Circulation: Regulation During Physical Stress.* New York: Oxford University Press (1986).

Rowell, L. B., H. J. Marx, R. A. Bruce, R. D. Conn, & F. Kusumi: Reductions in cardiac output, central blood volume, and stroke volume with thermal stress in normal men during exercise. *Journal of Clinical Investigation.* 45(11):1801–1816 (1966).

Rowland, T. W.: *Developmental Exercise Physiology.* Champaign, IL: Human Kinetics (1996).

Rowland, T. W.: *Exercise and Children's Health.* Champaign, IL: Human Kinetics (1990).

Rowland, T. W., & G. M. Green: Physiological responses to treadmill exercise in females: Adult-child differences. *Medicine and Science in Sports and Exercise.* 20(5):474–478 (1988).

Sagiv, M., E. Goldhammer, E. G. Abinader, & J. Rudoy: Aging and the effect of increased after-load on left ventricular contractile state. *Medicine and Science in Sport and Exercise.* 20(3):281–284 (1988).

Sawka, M. N.: Upper body exercise: Physiology and practical considerations. *Medicine and Science in Sport and Exercise.* 21(5):s119–s120 (1989).

Seals, D. R., R. A. Washburn, & P. G. Hanson: Increased cardiovascular response to static contraction of larger muscle groups. *Journal of Applied Physiology.* 54(2):434–437 (1985).

Shvartz, E., & R. C. Reibold: Aerobic fitness norms for males and females aged 6 to 75 years: A review. *Aviation, Space, and Environmental Physiology.* 61:3–11 (1990).

Sjogaard, G., G. Savard, & C. Juel: Muscle blood flow during isometric activity and its relation to muscle fatigue. *European Journal of Physiology.* 57:327–335 (1988).

Skinner, J. S: *Exercise Testing and Exercise Prescription for Special Cases* (2nd edition). Philadelphia: Lea & Febiger (1993).

Smith, D. L., J. E. Misner, D. K. Bloomfield, & L. K. Essandoh: Cardiovascular responses to sustained maximal isometric contractions of the finger flexors. *European Journal of Applied Physiology.* 67:48–52 (1993).

Sparling, P. B.: A meta-analysis of studies comparing maximal oxygen uptake in men and women. *Research Quarterly for Exercise and Sport.* 51(3):542–552 (1980).

Sullivan, M. J., F. R. Cobb, & M. B. Higginbotham: Stroke volume increases by similar mechanisms during upright exercise in normal men and women. *American Journal of Cardiology.* 67:1405–1412(1991).

Taylor, H. L., E. Buskirk, & A. Henshel: Maximal oxygen intake as an objective measure of cardio-respiratory performance. *Journal of Applied Physiology.* 8:73–80 (1955).

Tuttle, W. W., & S. M. Horvath: Comparison of effects of static and dynamic work on blood pressure and heart rate. *Journal of Applied Physiology.* 10(2):294–296 (1957).

VanLoan, M. D., B. H. Massey, R. A. Boileau, T. G. Lohman, J. E. Misner, & P. L. Best: Age as a factor in the hemodynamic responses to isometric exercise. *Journal of Sports Medicine and Physical Fitness.* 29(3):262–268 (1989).

Wade, C. E., & B. J. Freund: Hormonal control of blood volume during and following exercise. In C. V. Gisolfi, & D. R. Lamb (eds.), *Perspectives in Exercise Science and Sports Medicine.* 3:1405–1412 (1990).

Wanne, O. P. S., & E. Haapoja: Blood pressure during exercise in healthy children. *European Journal of Applied Physiology.* 58:62–67 (1988).

Wells, C. L.: *Women, Sport and Performance* (2nd edition). Champaign, IL: Human Kinetics (1991).

Wells, C. L., & S. A. Plowman: Sexual differences in athletic performance: Biological or behavioral? *Physician and Sports Medicine.* 11(8):52–63 (1983).

Wescott, W., & B. Howes: Blood pressure response during weight training exercise. *National Strength and Conditioning Association Journal.* January–February: 67–71 (1983).

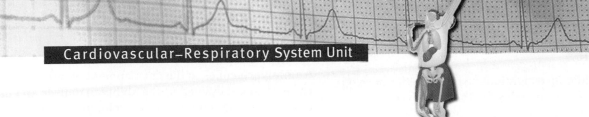

Chapter 14

Cardiorespiratory Training Principles and Adaptations

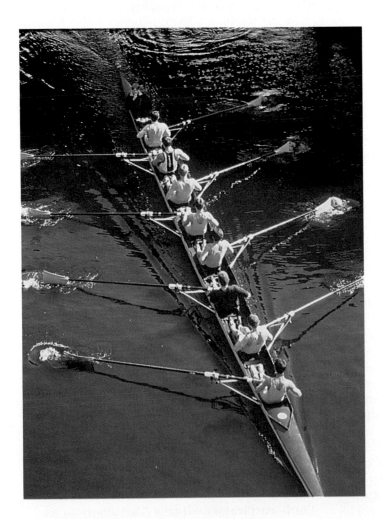

After studying the chapter, you should be able to

- Discuss the application of each of the training principles to the development of a cardiorespiratory training program.

- Explain how the FIT principle is related to the overload principle.

- Differentiate among the methods used to classify exercise intensity.

- Calculate training intensity ranges by using the percentage of maximal heart rate, the percentage of heart rate reserve, and the percentage of oxygen consumption reserve methods.

- Discuss the merits of specificity of modality and cross training in bringing about cardiovascular adaptations.

- Identify central and peripheral cardiovascular adaptations that occur at rest, during submaximal exercise, and at maximal exercise following a dynamic endurance or dynamic resistance training program.

Introduction

Early scientific investigations leading to the development of training principles for the cardiovascular system almost always had as the desired end point the improvement of physical fitness, operationally defined as an improvement of maximal oxygen consumption ($\dot{V}O_2$max). Such studies formed the basis for the guidelines developed by the American College of Sports Medicine (ACSM), originally published in 1978 as "the recommended quantity and quality of exercise for developing and maintaining fitness in healthy adults" and revised in 1998 to "the recommended quantity and quality of exercise for developing and maintaining cardiorespiratory and muscular fitness, and flexibility in healthy adults." In the years following 1978 these guidelines were increasingly applied not only to healthy adults intent on becoming more fit but also to individuals wishing solely to receive health benefits from exercise training. Although there is sufficient evidence to support the view that health benefits will accrue when fitness is improved, health and fitness are not the same thing. The quantity and quality of exercise required to develop or maintain cardiorespiratory fitness may not be (and probably is not) the same as that required to improve and maintain cardiorespiratory health (ACSM, 1998; Haskell, 1994). Furthermore, most exercise science or physical education college majors and competitive athletes who want or need high levels of fitness can handle physically rigorous and time-consuming training programs. However, these programs carry the risk of injury and are often psychologically intimidating to those who are sedentary, elderly, or obese. Thus, what constitutes an optimal cardiovascular training program—which maximizes the benefit while minimizing the time, effort, and risk—will vary with both the population and the intended goal. These factors, plus the realization that meaningful health benefits can be achieved with moderate levels of physical activity, led to the recommendation published in the Surgeon General's Report on Physical Activity and Health (U.S. Department of Health and Human Services, 1996) (Appendix C, summarized in Table 14.1) that individuals of all ages should accumulate a minimum of 30 min of physical activity of moderate intensity on most, if not all, days of the week. This recommendation should be viewed as a baseline and is intended primarily for previously sedentary individuals. The report goes on to acknowledge and encourage individuals who already include moderate activity in their daily lives to increase the duration of their moderate activity and/or include vigorous activity 3 to 5 days per week in order to obtain additional health and fitness benefits. These levels coincide with the American College of Sports Medicine guidelines also presented in Table 14.1.

This chapter addresses the application of the training principles to the development of **cardiorespiratory fitness,** defined as the ability to deliver and use oxygen during intense and prolonged exercise or work. The discussion relies heavily on the cardiorespiratory portion of the 1998 ACSM guidelines.

Where possible, we will cite variations for the upper and lower extremes in order to acknowledge that these guidelines do not represent a threshold below which no benefits are achieved. There is a point of diminishing return, where more exercise is not necessarily better; nevertheless, some activity is always better than no activity.

Application of the Training Principles

Specificity

Any activity that involves large muscle groups and is sustained for prolonged periods of time has the potential to increase cardiorespiratory fitness. Such modes of exercise include aerobics, bicycling, cross-country skiing, dancing (various forms), jogging, roller blading, rowing, speed skating, stair climbing or stepping, swimming, and walking. Sports in which the action is basically high energy and nonstop, such as field hockey, lacrosse, and soccer, can also positively benefit the cardiovascular system (ACSM, 1998; Pollock, 1973).

For the fitness participant the choice of exercise modalities should be based on interest, availability, and risk of injury. If the activity is enjoyable to the individual, it is more likely that he or she will adhere to the program. Although jogging or running may be the most time-efficient way to achieve cardiorespiratory fitness, these activities are not enjoyable for many individuals, and they have a relatively high incidence of overuse injuries. Therefore, other options should be available in fitness programs.

Although many different modalities can improve cardiovascular function, the greatest improvements in performance occur in the modality that was used for training—that is, there is *modality specificity.* For example, individuals who train by swimming improve more in swimming than in running (Magel, et al., 1975), and individuals who train by bicycling improve more in cycling than running (Pechar, et al., 1974; Roberts and Alspaugh, 1972). This modality specificity has two important practical applications. First, to determine whether an individual is improving, he or she should be tested in the modality that is used

---

Cardiorespiratory Fitness The ability to deliver and use oxygen under the demands of intensive, prolonged exercise or work.

Table 14.1
Physical Activity and Exercise Prescription for Health and Physical Fitness

Source	Frequency	Intensity	Duration	Modality	
				Cardiorespiratory	Neuromuscular
Surgeon General's Report (1995)	Most, if not all days of the week	Moderate[†]	Accumulate 30 min·d^{-1}	Any physical activity burning $\approx$ 150 kcal·d^{-1} or 2 kcal·kg·d^{-1}	
American College of Sports Medicine (1998)	3–5 d·wk^{-1}	55*/65–90% HRmax 40*/50–85% HRR 40*/50–85% $\dot{V}O_2R$	Continuous 20–60 min or Intermittent ($\geq$10 min bouts)	Rhythmical, aerobic, large muscles	Dynamic resistance: 1 set of 8–12 (or 10–15*) reps; 8–10 lifts; 2–3 d·wk^{-1} Flexibility: Major muscle groups ROM; 2–3 d·wk^{-1}

* Intended for least fit individuals.

† Examples include touch football, gardening, wheeling self in wheelchair, walking at pace of 20 min·mi^{-1}, shooting baskets, bicycling at 6 mi·hr^{-1}, social dancing, pushing a stroller 1.5 mi·30 min^{-1}, raking leaves, water aerobics, swimming laps.

for training. Second, the more the individual is concerned with sports competition rather than fitness or rehabilitation, the more important the mode of exercise becomes; that is, the competitive rower, whether competing on open water or on an indoor ergometer, should do most of his or her training in that modality. Running, however, does seem to be less specific than most other modalities; running forms the basis of many sports other than track or road races (Pechar, et al., 1974; Roberts and Alspaugh, 1972; Wilmore, et al., 1980).

Having just emphasized the importance of modality specificity for competitive athletes, we must now make a case for cross training. Originally, the term *cross training* referred to the development or maintenance of muscle function in one limb by exercising the contralateral limb or upper limbs as opposed to lower limbs (Housh and Housh, 1993; Kilmer, et al., 1994; Pate, et al., 1978). Such training remains important, especially in situations where one limb has been injured or placed in a cast. As used here, however, the term **cross training** means the development or maintenance of cardiovascular fitness by alternating between or concurrently training in two or more modalities. The interest in cross training comes from two primary sources. The first is the prevention of detraining in injured athletes, particularly those injuries associated with high-mileage running. The second is in the growth of multisport competitions such as biathlons and triathlons.

Theoretically, there is merit to the application of specificity *and* cross training to a training program. Any form of aerobic endurance exercise will affect both central and peripheral cardiorespiratory functioning. The central cardiovascular system is comprised of the heart and oxygen delivery components. **Central cardiovascular adaptations** are adaptations that occur in the heart and contribute to an increased ability to deliver oxygen. Central cardiovascular adaptations are the same regardless of modality provided the heart is stressed to the same extent; that is, central cardiovascular adaptations are the same regardless of whether the activity is running, skiing, or roller blading. Thus, many modalities can have the same overall training benefit by leading to central cardiovascular adaptations.

The peripheral cardiovascular system is involved in oxygen extraction in the musculature; and, which muscles are exercised does vary from modality to modality. **Peripheral cardiovascular adaptations** are adaptations that occur in the vasculature or the muscles that contribute to an increased ability to

> **Cross Training** The development or maintenance of cardiovascular fitness by alternating between or concurrently training in two or more modalities.
>
> **Central Cardiovascular Adaptations** Adaptations that occur in the heart and contribute to an increased ability to deliver oxygen.
>
> **Peripheral Cardiovascular Adaptations** Adaptations that occur in the vasculature or the muscles that contribute to an increased ability to extract oxygen.

Table 14.2
Situations in Which Cross Training Is Beneficial

Reason	Fitness Participant	Competitive Athlete
Multisport participation		General preparation phase, specific preparation phase, competitive phase
Injury or rehabilitation; fitness maintenance	As needed	As needed
Inclement weather	As needed	As needed
Baseline or general conditioning	Always	General preparation phase
Recovery	After intense workout	After intense workout or competition
Prevention of boredom and burnout	Always	Transition phase

Source: Kibler & Chandler (1994).

extract oxygen. Peripheral cardiovascular adaptations are specific to the modality and the specific muscles used in an exercise. For example, additional capillaries will be formed to carry oxygen to habitually active muscles but not to habitually inactive ones. Other factors within the exercising muscles such as mitochondrial density and enzyme activity will also impact upon the body's ability to reach a high $\dot{V}O_2$max. Specificity of modality operates because peripheral adaptations occur in the muscles that were trained. Thus, the specific activity—or closely related activities that mimic the muscle action of the primary sport—are needed to maximize peripheral adaptations. Examples of mimicking muscle action are side sliding or cycling for speed skating and water running in a flotation vest for jogging or running.

In one study endurance-trained runners were divided into three groups. One-third continued to train by running, one-third trained on a cycle ergometer, and one-third trained by deep water running. The intensity, frequency, and duration of workouts in each modality were equal. After 6 weeks, the $\dot{V}O_2$max of all three groups had decreased slightly (approximately 4%), and performance in a 2-mi run had improved slightly (approximately 1%) (Eyestone, et al., 1993). Thus, running performance was maintained by each of the modalities. On the other hand, arm ergometer training has not been shown to maintain training benefits derived from leg ergometer activity (Pate, et al., 1978). Apparently, then, the closer the activities are in terms of muscle action, the greater the potential benefit of cross training is.

Table 14.2 lists several situations, in addition to the maintenance of fitness when injured, where cross training may be beneficial (Kibler and Chandler, 1994; O'Toole, 1992). Note that the multisport athlete may or may not be limited to the sports in which he or she is competing. For example, although a duathlete needs to train for both running and cycling, this training will have the benefits of both specificity and cross training. In addition, this athlete may also cross train by doing other activities such as roller blading or speed skating. Note also that cross training can be recommended at any time for a fitness participant, but its value to a healthy competitive athlete is sporadic during the season. Cross training is most valuable to a single-sport competitive athlete during the transition (active rest) phase but may also be beneficial during the general conditioning phase.

Overload

Overload of the cardiovascular system is achieved by manipulating the intensity, duration, and frequency of the training bouts. These variables are easily remembered by the *FIT acronym* (F = frequency, I = intensity, and T = time or duration). However, as the most critical component, intensity will be discussed first.

Intensity

Intensity, both alone and in conjunction with duration, is very important in improving $\dot{V}O_2$max. The intensity of an exercise may be described in relation to heart rate, oxygen consumption, or rating of perceived exertion (RPE). Laboratory studies typically use $\dot{V}O_2$, but heart rate and RPE are more practical for individuals anywhere.

Figure 14.1a shows the relationship between change (Δ) in $\dot{V}O_2$max and exercise intensity. At exercise levels greater than 100% (supramaximal exercise), where the amount of training decreases, improvement falls somewhat. Interval training, in which the individual alternates work and rest intervals, permits greater amounts of exercise to be completed at 90–100% $\dot{V}O_2$max and, therefore, results in the greatest improvement in $\dot{V}O_2$max. However, the rate of improvement may be higher with continuous, nonstop

Figure 14.1

Changes in $\dot{V}O_2$max Based on Frequency, Intensity, and Duration of Training and on Initial Fitness Level

Source: H. A. Wenger & G. J. Bell. The interactions of intensity, frequency and duration of exercise training in altering cardiorespiratory fitness. *Sports Medicine.* 3:346–356 (1986). Reprinted by permission of Adis International, Inc.

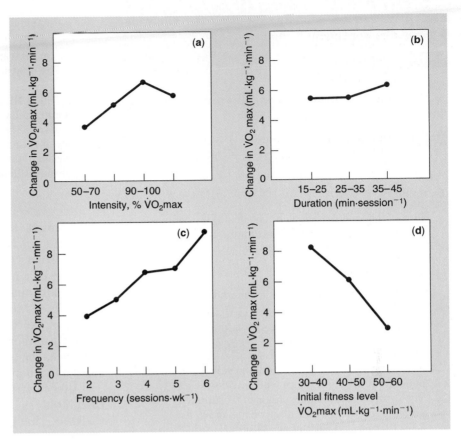

Table 14.3

Classification of Intensity of Exercise Based on 20–60 Min of Endurance Training

	Relative Intensity		
Classification of Intensity	**% HRmax**	**% HRR / % $\dot{V}O_2$R**	**Rating of Perceived Exertion**
Very light	< 35	< 20	< 10
Light	35–54	20–39	10–11
Moderate	55–69	40–59	12–13
Hard	70–89	60–84	14–16
Very Hard	≥ 90	≥ 85	17–19
Maximal	100	100	20

Source: American College of Sports Medicine (1998).

effort. Adaptation at submaximal workloads is not as intensity-dependent.

Table 14.3 includes techniques used to classify intensity and suggested percentages for activity that varies from very light to very heavy (American College of Sports Medicine, 1998). Note that these percentages and classifications are intended to be used when the exercise duration is 20–60 min, and the exercisers are healthy adults.

Heart Rate Methods   Exercise intensity can be expressed either as a percentage of maximal heart rate (% HRmax) or as a percentage of heart rate reserve (% HRR). Both techniques, which are explained in succeeding paragraphs, require that maximal heart rate be known or estimated. The methods are most accurate if the maximal heart rate is actually measured during a maximal graded exercise test. However, if such a test cannot be performed, maximal heart rate can be estimated by using the following general age-dependent formula:

14.1a maximal heart rate (b·min^{-1})
$$= 220 - \text{age (yr)}$$

For obese individuals the following equation is more accurate (Miller, et al., 1993):

14.1b maximal heart rate (b·min^{-1})
$$= 200 - [0.5 \times \text{age (yr)}]$$

Example

For a 28-yr-old female with a normal body composition, find her predicted or estimated HRmax.
The calculation is

$$\text{HRmax} = 220 - \text{age} = 220 - (28 \text{ yr}) = 192 \text{ b·min}^{-1}$$

If the female is obese, her estimated maximal heart rate is

$$\text{HRmax} = 200 - (0.5 \times \text{age}) = 200 - (0.5 \times 28 \text{ yr})$$
$$= 186 \text{ b·min}^{-1}$$

Because these values are estimated values, based on population averages, there will be wide variability. The estimated value may either overestimate or underestimate the true HRmax by as much as 10–12 b·min^{-1} (Miller, et al., 1993). ✢

Once a maximal heart rate is available, calculate the % HRmax as follows:

14.1c Target exercise heart rate = maximal heart rate (b·min^{-1}) × percentage of heart rate max (expressed as a decimal)

or

$$\text{TExHR} = \text{HRmax} \times \% \text{ HRmax}$$

1. Determine the desired intensity of the workout.
2. Use Table 14.3 to find the % HRmax associated with the desired exercise intensity.
3. Multiply the percentages (as decimals) times the HRmax.

Example

Determine the target HR training range for the nonobese 28-yr-old woman in the previous example who wants to perform a moderate workout.

1. Because the desired intensity for this example is a moderate workout, you would consult Table 14.3 and determine that a moderate workout ranges from 55–69% HRmax.
2. Multiply the percentages (as decimals) times the HRmax.

maximal heart rate (b·min^{-1})	192	192
desired intensity (decimal)	× .55	× .69
target training range (to closest b·min^{-1})	106	133

Thus a HR of 106 b·min^{-1} represents 55% of HRmax and a HR of 133 b·min^{-1} represents 69% of HRmax. So, in order to be exercising between 55% and 69% of HRmax, which represents a moderate workload, this individual should keep her heart rate between 106 and 133 b·min^{-1}. ✢

It is always best to provide the potential exerciser with a target range rather than just a lower threshold heart rate. In fact, the term *threshold* may be a misnomer since no particular percentage has been shown to be a minimally necessary threshold stimulus for all individuals in all situations (Haskell, 1994). Additionally, a range allows for the heart rate drift that occurs in exercise after about 30 min and for variations in weather, terrain, fluid replacement, and other influences on the individual. The upper limit can serve as a boundary against overexertion.

Alternatively, a target heart rate range can be calculated as a percentage of heart rate reserve (% HRR). This technique of calculating training heart rate is also called the *Karvonen method*. It involves a little more mathematics but has the added advantage of taking resting heart rate into consideration. The steps are as follows:

1. Determine the heart rate reserve (HRR) by subtracting the resting heart rate from the maximal heart rate.

14.2a Heart rate reserve (b·min^{-1}) = maximal heart rate (b·min^{-1}) − resting heart rate (b·min^{-1})

or

$$\text{HRR} = \text{HRmax} - \text{RHR}$$

The resting heart rate is best determined when the individual is truly resting, such as immediately on awakening in the morning. However, for purposes of exercise prescription this should be a standing resting heart rate. Heart rates taken prior to an exercise test are anticipatory, not resting, and will be abnormally high.

2. Determine the desired intensity of the workout.
3. Use Table 14.3 to find the % HRR associated with the desired exercise intensity.
4. Multiply the percentages (as decimals) for the upper and lower exercise limits by the HRR using Equation 14.2b and add RHR.

14.2b Target exercise heart rate (b·min^{-1}) = [heart rate reserve (b·min^{-1}) × percentage of heart rate reserve (expressed as a decimal)] + resting heart rate (b·min^{-1})

or

$$\text{TExHR} = (\text{HRR} \times \% \text{ HRR}) + \text{RHR}$$

Example

Determine the appropriate HR range for a moderate workout for a 28-yr-old using the HRR method, assuming a RHR of 80 b·min^{-1}.

1. Determine the HRR:

   192 b·min^{-1} − 80 b·min^{-1} = 112 b·min^{-1}

2. Determine the desired intensity of the workout. Again, using Table 14.3, 40–59% of HRR corresponds to a moderate workout. This reinforces the point that the % HRmax does not equal % HRR.

3. Multiply the percentages (as decimals) for the upper and lower exercise limits by the HRR. Thus:

HRR	112	112
desired intensity (decimal)	× .4	× .59
	45	66

4. Add RHR as follows:

target HR training range (b·min^{-1})	45	66
	+ 80	+ 80
	125	146

Thus, a HR of 125 b·min^{-1} represents 40% of HRR and a HR of 146 b·min^{-1} represents 59% of HRR. So, in order to be exercising between 40 and 59% of HRR, which represents a moderate workload, this individual should keep her heart rate between 125 and 146 b·min^{-1}. ✛

This heart rate range (125–146 b·min^{-1}), although still moderate, is different from the one calculated by using % HRmax because of the influence of the resting heart rate.

A Question of Understanding

Calculate the target HR range for a light workout for two individuals, using the % HRmax and % HRR methods and the following information.

	Age	RHR
Lisa	50	62
Susie	50	82

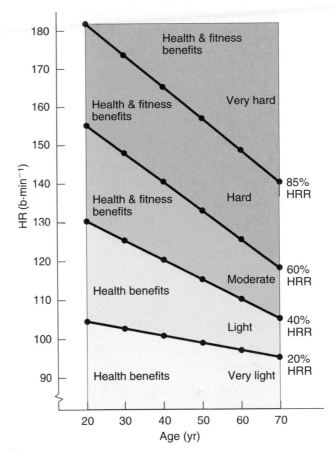

Figure 14.2

Age-Related Changes in Training Heart Rate Ranges Based on the Heart Rate Reserve (Karvonen) Method

Note: Calculations are based on RHR = 80 b·min^{-1}, HRmax = 220 − age.

Work through the problem presented in the Question of Understanding box, paying careful attention to the influence of resting heart rate in determining the training heart rate range when using the heart rate reserve (Karvonen) method. Check your answer in Appendix D.

Because maximal heart rate is age dependent, declining in a rectilinear fashion with advancing age, the heart rate, calculated by either the maximal heart rate or heart rate reserve method, needed to achieve a given intensity level will decrease with age. Figure 14.2 exemplifies these decreases for light, moderate, and heavy exercise using the percent of heart rate reserve method and the expected benefits within each range.

Oxygen Consumption/% $\dot{V}O_2R$ Methods   In a laboratory setting where an individual has been tested for $\dot{V}O_2$max and equipment is available for monitoring $\dot{V}O_2$ during training bouts, % $\dot{V}O_2R$ may be used. Oxygen reserve is parallel to heart rate reserve; that is, it is the difference between a resting and maximal value, in this case calculated according to the formula:

14.3a Oxygen consumption reserve $(mL \cdot kg^{-1} \cdot min^{-1})$ = maximal oxygen consumption $(mL \cdot kg^{-1} \cdot min^{-1})$ – resting oxygen consumption $(mL \cdot kg^{-1} \cdot min^{-1})$

or

$$\dot{V}O_2R = \dot{V}O_2max - \dot{V}O_2rest$$

Target exercise oxygen consumption is then determined by the equation:

14.3b Target exercise oxygen consumption $(mL \cdot kg^{-1} \cdot min^{-1})$ = [oxygen consumption reserve $(mL \cdot kg^{-1} \cdot min^{-1})$ × percentage of oxygen consumption reserve (expressed as a decimal)] + resting oxygen consumption $(mL \cdot kg^{-1} \cdot min^{-1})$

or

$$TEx\dot{V}O_2 = (\dot{V}O_2R \times \% \dot{V}O_2R) + \dot{V}O_2rest$$

The following steps are used to calculate training intensity using this method.

1. Determine the desired intensity of the workout.
2. Use Table 14.3 to find the $\% \dot{V}O_2R$ associated with the desired exercise intensity.
3. Multiply the percentage (as a decimal) of the desired intensity times the $\dot{V}O_2max$.
4. Add the resting oxygen consumption to the obtained values. Note that this may be an individually measured value or the estimated $3.5\ mL \cdot kg^{-1} \cdot min^{-1}$ that represents 1 MET.
5. Because oxygen drifts, as does heart rate, it is best to use a target range.

Example

Determine the $\dot{V}O_2R$ that corresponds to a moderate workout intensity for an individual with a $\dot{V}O_2max$ of $43\ ml \cdot kg^{-1} \cdot min^{-1}$.

1. Based on Table 14.3 it is determined that a moderate workout corresponds to 40–59% of $\dot{V}O_2R$.
2. Determine the $\dot{V}O_2R$:

   $43\ mL \cdot kg^{-1} \cdot min^{-1} - 3.5\ mL \cdot kg^{-1} \cdot min^{-1} =$
   $39.5\ mL \cdot kg^{-1} \cdot min^{-1}$

3. Multiply the percentages (as decimals) times the $\dot{V}O_2R$.

$\dot{V}O_2R$ $(mL \cdot kg^{-1} \cdot min^{-1})$	39.5	39.5
desired intensity	× .4	× .59
	15.8	23.31
resting $\dot{V}O_2$ $(mL \cdot kg^{-1} \cdot min^{-1})$	+ 3.5	+ 3.5
target training range $(mL \cdot kg \cdot min^{-1})$	19.3	26.81

Table 14.4
Time a Selected $\% \dot{V}O_2max$ Can Be Sustained during Running

% $\dot{V}O_2max$	Time (min)
100	8–10
97.5	15
90	30
87.5	45
85	60
82.5	90
80	120–210

Source: Daniels & Gilbert (1979).

Thus, this individual would work at a workload that elicited an oxygen consumption of approximately 19.3–26.8 $mL \cdot kg^{-1} \cdot min^{-1}$ in order to achieve a moderate workout.

Basing the intensity of a workout on $\% \dot{V}O_2R$ is not a very practical option because most people do not have access to the needed equipment. However, the technique is modifiable for individuals who wish to use it. The first way in which it may be made practical is to use the formula in Appendix B (The Calculation of Oxygen Consumed Using Mechanical Work or Speed of Movement) to solve for the workload (velocity of level or inclined walking or running; resistance for arm or leg cycling; height or cadence for bench stepping). Then the exerciser can be given a prescription in terms of minutes per mile, cadence of stepping at a particular height, or load setting at a specific revolutions per minute pace.

The second way to make this approach feasible in practice is to utilize the direct relationship between heart rate and oxygen consumption.

Look closely again at Table 14.3. Note that the column for $\% \dot{V}O_2R$ is also the column for % HRR; that is, any given % HRR represents an equivalent $\% \dot{V}O_2R$. Thus, an individual who is working at 50% HRR is also working at 50% $\dot{V}O_2R$. Therefore, heart rate can be used to indicate oxygen consumption when an individual is training or competing.

Historically, $\% \dot{V}O_2max$ had been used as the equivalent of % HRR (Londeree, et al., 1995; Parker, et al., 1989). However, that was recently shown to be inaccurate, especially in low fit individuals and at low exercise intensities. The equivalency between $\% \dot{V}O_2R$ and % HRR has been demonstrated experimentally in both young and elderly males and females and for the modalities of cycle ergometry and treadmill walking and running (Swain, 2000).

Table 14.4 provides information on how long running can be continued at a specific percentage of maximal oxygen consumption. The Question of Understanding box below provides an example of how this information (Table 14.3) can be used in training and in a running competition. Take the time now to work through the situation described in the box.

Rating of Perceived Exertion Methods The third way exercise intensity can be prescribed is by a subjective impression of the overall effort, strain, and fatigue during the activity. This impression is known as a **rating of perceived exertion.** Perceived exertion is typically measured by using either Borg's 6–20 RPE scale or the revised 0–10+ Category Ratio Scale (Borg, 1998). Both scales are presented in Table 14.5 in a format that indicates how they relate to each other. The RPE scale is designed so that these perceptual ratings rise in a rectilinear fashion with heart rate,

Table 14.5
Scales for Ratings of Perceived Exertion

RPE Scale		CR-10 Scale	
6		0.0	
7	Very, very light	0.0	
8		0.5	Just noticeable
9	Very light	1.0	Very weak
10		1.5	
11	Fairly light	2.0	Light/weak
12		3.0	Moderate
13	Somewhat hard	3.5	
		4.0	Somewhat strong
14		4.5	
		5.0	
15	Hard	5.5	
		6.0	
16		6.5	Very strong
		7.0	
17	Very hard	7.5	
		8.0	
18		9.0	
19	Very, very hard	10.0	Extremely strong
20		10^+ (~12)	Highest possible

oxygen consumption, and mechanical workload during incremental exercise. It is thus the primary scale used for cardiovascular exercise prescription (Table 14.3). The CR-10 scale increases in a positively accelerating curvilinear fashion and closely parallels the physiological responses of pulmonary ventilation and blood lactate. The use of the scales for metabolic exercise prescription is described in Chapter 6.

The classification of exercise intensity and the corresponding relationships between % HRmax, % $\dot{V}O_2R$, % HRR, and RPE presented in Table 14.3 have been derived from and are intended for use with land-based activities in moderate environments.

Whether a water activity is performed horizontally, as in swimming, or vertically, as in running or water aerobics, postural and pressure changes shift the blood volume centrally and necessitate adjustments in blood pressure, cardiac output, resistance, and respiration. Although there is a large variation among individuals in the magnitude of change in the cardiovascular system, the most consistent changes are lower submaximal HR (8–12 b·min^{-1}) at any given $\dot{V}O_2$, a lower HRmax (~15 b·min^{-1}), and a lower

---

A Question of Understanding

Four friends from work meet at the track for a noontime workout. The physiological characteristics are as follows. (The estimated $\dot{V}O_2$max values have been calculated from a 1-mi running test.)

Individual	Age (yr)	Estimated $\dot{V}O_2$max (mL·kg^{-1}·min^{-1})	Resting HR (b·min^{-1})
Janet	23	52	60
Juan	35	64	48
Mark	22	49	64
Gail	28	56	58

The following oxygen requirements have been calculated for a given speed based on the equations that are presented in Appendix B.

Speed (mph)	Oxygen Requirement (mL·kg^{-1}·min^{-1})
4	27.6
5	30.3
6	35.7
7	41.0
8	46.4
9	51.7

The friends wish to do a moderate workout and run together. Assume temperate weather conditions.

1. At what speed should they be running?
2. What heart rate should be achieved by each runner at that pace?

Check your answers with the ones provided in Appendix D.

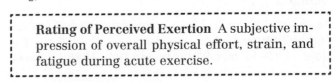

Rating of Perceived Exertion A subjective impression of overall physical effort, strain, and fatigue during acute exercise.

$\dot{V}O_2$max when exercise is performed in the water. A greater reliance on anaerobic metabolism is evident, and the RPE is higher in water than at the same workload used on land (Svedenhag and Seger, 1992). The lower HR is probably a compensation for the increased stroke volume that occurs when blood is shifted centrally. As a result, the HR prescription should be about 10% lower for water workouts than for land-based workouts. Thus, if an individual would normally work out at 75% HRmax on land, the prescription for an equivalent workout in the water should be 65% HRmax. Another way to achieve the adjustment, if an estimated HRmax is being used, is to start with 205 b·min^{-1} minus age rather than 220 b·min^{-1} minus age. Either of these changes should effectively reduce the RPE as well.

Regardless of the method chosen to prescribe exercise intensity, it is important to consider three factors.

1. Exercise intensity should generally be prescribed within a range. Many activities will require different levels of exertion throughout the activity. This is particularly true of games and athletic activities, but it also applies to activities like jogging and bicycling where changes in terrain can greatly affect exertion. In addition, a range allows for the cardiovascular and oxygen consumption drifts that occur during prolonged exercise.

2. Exercise intensity must be considered in conjunction with duration and frequency.

   a. Intensity cannot be prescribed without regard to duration. These two variables are inversely related: In general, the more intense an activity is, the shorter its duration should be.

   b. The appropriate intensity of exercise also depends on the fitness level of the individual and, to some extent, on the point the individual has reached in his or her fitness program. Individuals should begin an exercise program at a low exercise intensity and gradually increase intensity in a steploading progression until the desired level is achieved.

3. Using heart rate or perceived exertion to monitor training sessions, rather than merely time over distance, allows the influence of weather, terrain, and surfaces and the way the individual is responding to be taken into account in the assessment of adaptation to a training program.

Duration

As shown in Figure 14.1b, improvements in $\dot{V}O_2$max can be achieved when exercise is sustained for durations of 15–45 min (Wenger and Bell, 1986). Slightly

greater improvements are achieved from the longer sessions (35–45 min) than from shorter sessions (either 15–25 or 25–35 min). Indeed, greater improvements in $\dot{V}O_2$max can be achieved if the sessions are long (35–45 min) and the intensity moderate to heavy (50–90%) than if the sessions are short (25–35 min) and the intensity very hard to maximal (90–100%). Apparently, the total volume of work done is more important in determining cardiorespiratory adaptations than either intensity or duration of the exercise considered individually. This is good news, because the risk of injury is lower in moderate-intensity, long-duration activity than in high, near maximal, short-duration activity; and the compliance rate is higher. Thus, most adult fitness programs should emphasize moderate- to heavy-intensity workouts (55–89% HRmax; 40–84% HRR or $\dot{V}O_2$max) for a duration of 20–60 min (ACSM, 1998).

This does not mean that exercise sessions of less than 20 min are not valuable either in terms of $\dot{V}O_2$max or health benefits, or that the 20 min must be accumulated during one exercise session. An accumulation of 30 min of activity spread throughout the day may be sufficient to achieve health benefits. For example, two groups of adult males participated in a walk-jog program at 65–75% HRmax, for 5 days per week for 8 weeks (De Busk, et al., 1990). The only variation between the groups was that one did the 30-min workout continuously and the other participated in 10-min sessions at three different times throughout the day. Both groups increased their $\dot{V}O_2$max significantly (although the 30-min consecutive group did so to a greater extent) and lost equal amounts of weight—an important health benefit.

Thus, for the individual who claims he or she does not have time to exercise, the suggestion of a 10-min walk in the morning (perhaps to work or taking the kids to school), at noon (to a favorite restaurant and back), and in the evening (perhaps walking home from work or taking the kids for a walk) might make it easier for the person to achieve a total of 30 min of activity. Once again, some activity is better than no activity, especially if the goal is health benefits rather than improved performance.

A recognition of the benefit of split sessions is particularly important for those in a rehabilitation program and for children. The injured person may simply not be able to exercise for a long period of time, but short bouts may be possible if they are spread throughout the day. Children tend to be sporadic exercisers by nature, and getting them to exercise continuously for 20 min is often difficult (Corbin and Pangrazi, 1994). Because many elementary schools only have physical education classes scheduled for 20 min, a program of running for 20 min would mean the children would do nothing else, which is not pedagogically sound. Thus, some portion of each class should be devoted to fitness development, and the children should be encouraged to be active outside school.

Frequency

If the total work done or the number of exercise sessions is held constant, there is basically no difference in the improvement of $\dot{V}O_2$max over 2, 3, 4, or 5 days (Pollock, 1973). However, when these conditions are not adhered to, there does seem to be an advantage to more frequent training. As seen in Figure 14.1c, the improvement in $\dot{V}O_2$max is proportional to the number of training sessions per week (Wenger and Bell, 1986). In general, training less than 2 days per week does not result in improvements in $\dot{V}O_2$max. Likewise, further improvement in $\dot{V}O_2$max is not meaningful if exercise participation is increased from 4 to 5 days a week. Although there is the potential for further improvement in $\dot{V}O_2$max if a 6th day of training is added, a 6th day is not generally recommended for those pursuing fitness goals because of a higher incidence of injury and fatigue. The optimal frequency for all intensities appears to be 4 days per week.

The ACSM recommendation for healthy individuals is a frequency of 3–5 days per week. However, individuals with very low fitness levels may wish to start a program of only 2 days per week if they are attempting to meet the ACSM intensity and duration guidelines or to be active daily in less-intense and shorter-duration bouts of exercise following the Surgeon General's recommendation. Athletes in training may feel compelled to train 6 days per week as a way of increasing the total training volume. In this case "easy" and "hard" days should be interspersed within most microcycles. Cross training may also be employed.

Individualization

Fitness programs should be individualized to the participant. Not only will individual goals vary, but also individuals will respond to and adapt to exercise differently. One of the major determinants of the individual's response is genetics, which was discussed in Chapter 12. Another major determinant is initial fitness level. Figure 14.1d clearly shows that independent of frequency, intensity, or duration, the greatest improvements in $\dot{V}O_2$max occur in those individuals with the lowest initial-fitness level. Thus, both absolute and relative increases in $\dot{V}O_2$max are inversely related to initial fitness level. Although improvements in $\dot{V}O_2$max are smallest in highly fit individuals, at this level small changes may have a significant influence

on performance (that is, many athletic events are won by fractions of a second).

The initial fitness level generalization also applies to health benefits. Health benefits are greatest when a person moves from a low-fitness to a moderately fit category. This progress can be accomplished by most sedentary individuals if they participate in a regular, low-to-moderate–endurance exercise program (Haskell, 1994).

Rest/Recovery/Adaptation

Adaptation can be categorized into several stages. The initial stage usually lasts 4 to 6 weeks, although this duration varies considerably among individuals. This stage should include low-level aerobic activities that cause a minimum of muscle soreness or discomfort. In fact, it is often prudent to begin an exercise program at an intensity lower than the desired exercise range. The duration of the aerobic exercise session should be at least 10 min and should gradually be increased. For individuals with very low levels of fitness a discontinuous training program may be warranted, wherein the individual completes several repetitions of exercise, each lasting 2–5 min (ACSM, 2000). Frequency may vary from short, light daily activity to longer exercise sessions two or three times per week.

Adaptation has occurred when the same amount of work can be accomplished in less time, when the same amount of work can be accomplished with less physiological (homeostatic) disruption, when the same amount of work can be accomplished with a lower perception of fatigue or exertion, or when more work can be accomplished. During the improvement stage of a training program, significant improvements in physiological function indicate that the body is adapting to the stress of the training program.

Progression

Once adaptation occurs, the workload must be increased if further improvement is desired. The workload can be increased by manipulating the frequency, intensity, and duration of the exercise. Increasing any of these variables will effectively increase the volume of exercise and will thus provide the overload necessary for further adaptation. The rate of progression depends on the individual's needs or goals, fitness level, health status, and age but should always be done in a steploading fashion of 2 or 3 weeks of increase followed by a decrease for recovery and regeneration before increasing training volume again.

The improvement stage of a training program typically lasts for 4 to 5 months and is characterized

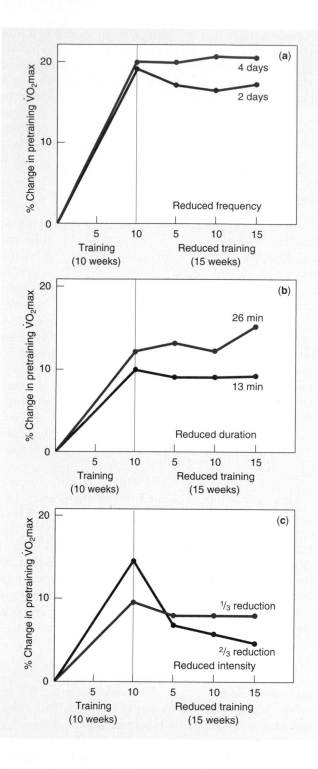

Figure 14.3
Effects of Reducing Exercise Frequency, Intensity, and Duration on Maintenance of $\dot{V}O_2$max

(a) Improvements in $\dot{V}O_2$max during 10 weeks of training (bicycling and running) for 40 min a day, 6 days a week were maintained when training intensity and duration were maintained, but the frequency was reduced from 6 days a week to 4 or even 2 days per week. (b) $\dot{V}O_2$max was maintained when frequency of training and intensity were maintained, but training duration was reduced to 13 min. $\dot{V}O_2$max continued to improve when training duration was reduced to 26 min. (c) $\dot{V}O_2$max was maintained when frequency and duration were maintained and intensity was reduced by one-third. $\dot{V}O_2$max was not maintained when training was reduced by two-thirds.

Sources: Hickson & Rosenkoetter (1981); Hickson, Foster, et al. (1985); Hickson, Kanakis, et al. (1982).

themselves several times until the desired level of fitness or performance is achieved. Each time an exercise program is modified, there will be a period of adaptation that may be followed by further progression if desired.

Maintenance

Athletes tend to vary their training levels according to a general conditioning phase (off-season), specific conditioning phase (preseason), competitive phase (in-season), and transition phase (active rest), with the active rest and in-season phases being the times when they can shift to a maintenance schedule. For the rehabilitation or fitness participant, maintenance typically begins after the first 6 months of training. Achieving the maintenance stage indicates that the individual has reached a personally acceptable level of cardiorespiratory fitness and is no longer interested in increasing the conditioning load (ACSM, 2000).

Once a desired level of aerobic fitness has been attained, this level can be maintained by either continuing the same volume of exercise or by decreasing the volume of training, as long as intensity is maintained. Figure 14.3 shows the results of research that investigated changes in $\dot{V}O_2$max with 10 weeks of relatively intense interval training and a subsequent 15-week reduction in training frequency (14.3a), duration (14.3b), or intensity (14.3c) (Hickson and Rosenkoetter, 1981; Hickson, Foster, et al., 1985; Hickson, Kanakis, et al., 1982). When training frequency was reduced from 6 days per week to 4 or 2 days per week and intensity and duration were held constant, training-induced improvements in $\dot{V}O_2$max were maintained. Similarly, when training duration was reduced from 40 to 26 or 13 min, improvements in

by relatively rapid progression. For an individual with a low fitness level, the progression from a discontinuous activity to a continuous activity should occur first. Then the duration of the activity should be increased to 20–30 min. Frequency can then be increased. Intensity should be the last variable to be increased.

The principles of adaptation and progression are intertwined. Adaptation and progression may repeat

Focus on Application

✳ Manipulation of Training Overload in a Taper

Peaking for performance often involves manipulating the training principles of specificity, overload, and maintenance within a periodization plan. This can be exemplified by a study in which 18 male and 6 female distance runners were pretested, matched, and then divided into three groups. The run taper group systematically reduced its weekly training volume to 15% of their previous training volume over a 7-day period, performing 30% of the calculated reduced training distance on day 1, and then 20%, 15%, 12%, 10%, 8%, and 5% on each succeeding day. Training consisted of 400-m intervals at close to 5-km pace (~100% $\dot{V}O_2$ peak) resulting in a HR of 170–190 $b \cdot min^{-1}$ with recovery to 100–110 $b \cdot min^{-1}$ before the next interval. The cycle taper group performed approximately the same number of intervals for the same duration as paired athletes in the run taper group, at the same work

and recovery heart rates. The control group continued normal training, of which 6–10% of the weekly training distance was interval/fartlek work. All subjects participated in a 10-min submaximal treadmill run, an incremental treadmill test to volitional fatigue in which the grade remained constant at 0% and the speed increased, and a 5-km time trial on the treadmill.

At the same absolute speed during the submaximal run, the run taper group (and 7 of the 8 individual runners) exhibited a 5% reduction (2.4 $mL \cdot kg^{-1} \cdot min^{-1}$) in oxygen consumption and a decrease of 7% (0.9 $kcal \cdot min^{-1}$) in calculated energy expenditure. No changes were evident in either the cycle taper or control group. Both maximal treadmill speed (2%) and total exercise time (4%) increased for the run taper group without concomitant increase in $\dot{V}O_2$max or HRmax. No changes occurred in any maximal value for the cycle run or control groups. The run taper group (all 8 individuals) significantly improved 5-km performance by a mean of 2.8 ± 0.4%, or an average of almost 30 sec. No improvement in

performance was seen in either the cycle run or control groups.

These results clearly demonstrate the benefits of a 7-day taper in which intensity is maintained, training volume drastically reduced, and specificity of training utilized. Of the variables measured, the most likely explanation for the improved 5-km performance was the increase in submaximal running economy (decreased submaximal oxygen and energy cost). It should also be noted, however, that all three groups maintained their $\dot{V}O_2$max values. This cross-training benefit exhibited by the cycle taper group is particularly important. Distance runners often have nagging injuries. These results imply that a non–weight-bearing taper may be used in such cases and allow the runner to possibly heal (or at least not aggravate an injury) while maintaining cardiovascular fitness. Performance enhancement, however, appears to necessitate mode specificity during the taper. ✳

Source:

Houmard, et al. (1994).

$\dot{V}O_2$max were maintained. However, when intensity was reduced by two-thirds, improvements in $\dot{V}O_2$max were not maintained. These results indicate that intensity plays a primary role in maintaining cardiovascular fitness. Thus, although total volume of exercise is important in the attainment of a given fitness level, intensity is important in the maintenance of the achieved fitness level. During the maintenance phase of a training program, cross training becomes particularly beneficial, especially on days when a high-intensity workout is not called for.

Retrogression/Plateau/Reversibility

At one or more points in the training process, an individual will fail to improve (plateau) or will exhibit a performance or physiological decrement (retrogression), despite progression of the training program. When a pattern of nonimprovement occurs, it is

important to check for other signs of overtraining (see Chapter 2). A shift of training emphasis or the inclusion of more easy days is then warranted. Remember that a reduction in the frequency of training does not necessarily lead to detraining and may actually enhance performance.

If training is discontinued for any reason, detraining will occur. This principle, often referred to as the *reversibility concept,* holds that when a training program is stopped or reduced, the body systems readjust in accordance with the decreased physiological stimuli. Increases in $\dot{V}O_2$max with low to moderate exercise programs are completely reversed when training is stopped. Values of $\dot{V}O_2$max decrease rapidly during a month of detraining, followed by a slower rate of decline during the second and third month (Bloomfield and Coyle, 1993).

Figures 14.4a–14.4d depict the time course for detraining for several cardiovascular variables in

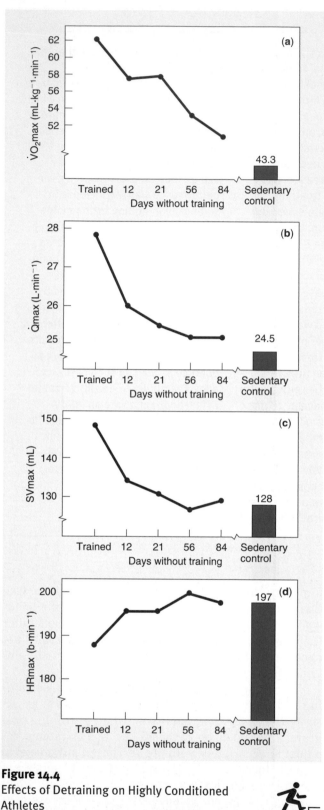

Figure 14.4
Effects of Detraining on Highly Conditioned Athletes

Source: E. F. Coyle, W. H. Martin, D. R. Sinacore, M. J. Joymer, J. M. Hagberg, & J. O. Holloszy. Time course of loss of adaptations after stopping prolonged intense endurance training. *Journal of Applied Physiology.* 57:1857–1864 (1984). Reprinted by permission.

highly trained individuals who became sedentary. Notice that there is a decline in $\dot{V}O_2$max by almost 15% during the 84 days of detraining. However, this study did not measure $\dot{V}O_2$max before training; thus, we cannot conclude that $\dot{V}O_2$max returned to baseline values (as happens with low to moderate levels of training). In fact, the $\dot{V}O_2$max of these previously highly trained individuals was significantly higher following 84 days of detraining (50.8 mL·kg^{-1}·min^{-1}) than the $\dot{V}O_2$max of age-matched untrained individuals (43.3 mL·kg^{-1}·min^{-1}) (Coyle, Martin, et al., 1984). The stroke volume and cardiac output of the trained subjects decreased during the 84 days of detraining (Figures 14.4c and 14.4d), reaching values that were similar to those for untrained individuals.

The higher $\dot{V}O_2$max in detrained athletes than in untrained subjects is due to an augmented ability of the muscles to extract oxygen, as evidenced by a greater capillary density in the trained athletes than in the sedentary controls. The reduction of stroke volume observed with detraining is largely a result of reduced blood volume, which occurs with detraining, and not a deterioration of heart function (Coyle, Hemmert, et al., 1986). The cardiovascular changes with detraining appear to be the same for males and females (Drinkwater and Horvath, 1972).

Warm-Up and Cool-Down

A warm-up period allows the body to adjust to the cardiovascular demands of exercise. At rest the skeletal muscles receive about 15–20% of the blood pumped from the heart; during moderate exercise they receive approximately 70% of cardiac output. This increased blood flow is important in warming the body since the blood carries heat from the metabolically active muscle to the rest of the body.

A warm-up period of 5–10 min should precede the conditioning portion of an exercise session (ACSM, 2000). The warm-up should gradually increase in intensity until the desired intensity of training is achieved. For many activities the warm-up period simply continues into the aerobic portion of the exercise session. For example, if an individual is going for a noontime run and wants to run at an 8-min-mi pace, he may begin with a slow jog for the first few minutes (say a 10-min-mi pace), increase to a faster pace (say a 9-min-mi pace), and then proceed into the desired pace (the 8-min-mi pace).

A warm-up period has the following beneficial effects on cardiovascular function.

- It increases blood flow to the active skeletal muscles.

- It increases blood flow to the myocardium.

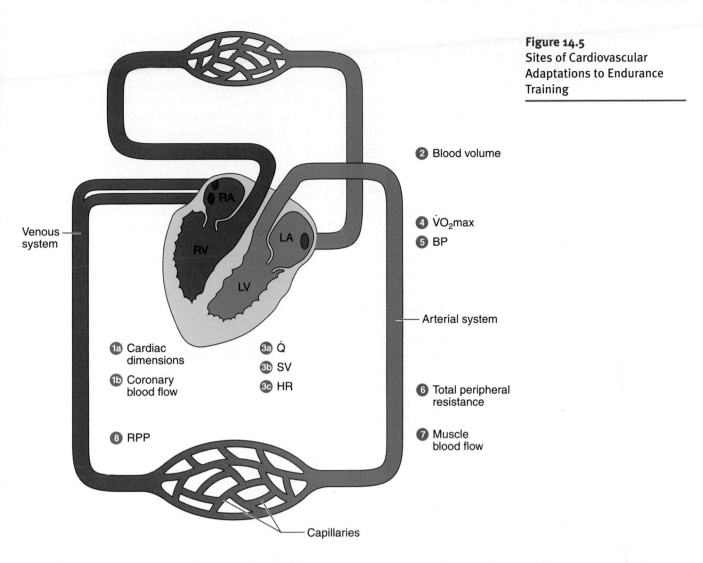

Figure 14.5
Sites of Cardiovascular Adaptations to Endurance Training

2 Blood volume

4 $\dot{V}O_2$max

5 BP

Venous system

RA

LA

RV

LV

Arterial system

1a Cardiac dimensions

1b Coronary blood flow

3a $\dot{Q}$

3b SV

3c HR

6 Total peripheral resistance

7 Muscle blood flow

8 RPP

Capillaries

- It increases the dissociation of oxyhemoglobin.
- It leads to earlier sweating, which plays a role in temperature regulation.
- It may reduce the incidence of abnormal rhythms in the conduction system of the heart (dysrhythmias), which can lead to abnormal heart function (Barnard, et al., 1973).

The cool-down period should follow the conditioning period of the exercise session. The primary cardiovascular advantage to a cool-down period is that it prevents venous pooling and thus reduces the risk of fainting by keeping the muscle pump active when the venous system is dilated immediately after strenuous exercise.

Cardiovascular Adaptations to Aerobic Endurance Training

Regular physical activities result in improvements in cardiovascular function, which is most readily demonstrated by an increase in the functional capacity of the cardiovascular system (that is, an increase in $\dot{V}O_2$max). The magnitude of the improvement is determined by the training program—specifically by the frequency, intensity, and duration of the exercise and the initial-fitness status of the individual. Changes in cardiovascular function are evident at rest, during submaximal exercise, and during maximal exercise.

Figure 14.5 provides an overview of the cardiovascular system with numbers added to indicate sites where cardiovascular adaptations occur as a result of endurance training. The following subsections refer to that numerical sequence.

Cardiac Dimensions (1a)

Cardiac dimensions and mass increase with endurance training (Huston, et al., 1985; Keul, et al., 1981; Longhurst, et al., 1981). These changes are associated with high cardiac outputs during sustained dynamic aerobic exercise. Endurance training exposes the heart to conditions of increased ventricular filling, with subsequent high stroke volume and cardiac output. This chronic exposure to high levels of ventricular filling (large left ventricular end–diastolic volume) is known as *volume overload* (Morganroth, et al., 1975). Chronic volume overload results in an increased left ventricular end–diastolic diameter (Huston, et al., 1985; Keul, et al., 1981) and left ventricular mass (Cohen and Segal, 1985; Longhurst, et al., 1981).

Coronary Blood Flow (1b)

Endurance training results in an increase in the size of the coronary vascular bed (Blomqvist and Saltin, 1983). This increase in capillarization may be related to an increase in heart weight as a result of training (Schaible and Schever, 1981). Although there is some evidence that exercise training can lead to the development of *coronary collateral circulation,* defined as the ability to supply areas of the myocardium with blood through small new growth anastomoses, this finding is suspect in humans (Connor, et al., 1976; Eckstein, 1957; Ferguson, et al., 1974). There is better evidence that coronary collateral circulation is caused by myocardial hypoxia that occurs with coronary artery disease (Zoll, et al., 1951). One of the difficulties in determining the extent to which exercise training affects coronary collateral circulation is the inability to distinguish the effects of disease states and a sedentary lifestyle.

The internal diameter of the coronary arteries also may be increased by endurance training. Several studies (including the classic autopsy report of Clarence DeMar, winner of seven Boston marathons) have shown that habitual exercise is related to a larger cross-sectional arterial size. DeMar's arteries were reportedly two to three times normal size (Currens and White, 1961). Conversely, a study that compared ultramarathoners with sedentary individuals did not show any difference in the internal diameter of the coronary arteries in the two groups at rest (Haskell, et al., 1993). However, the capacity of the coronary arteries to dilate was two times greater in the marathoners than in the sedentary individuals (13.2 mm^2 versus 6 mm^2). The ability to dilate arteries while exercising may be even more important than the resting diameter, because the myocardial demand for oxygen is low during rest and high during exercise, as evidenced by the low rate-pressure product (RPP) seen at rest and the high RPP during exercise.

Blood Volume (2)

Blood volume increases as a result of endurance training. Highly trained endurance athletes have a 20–25% larger blood volume than untrained subjects.

The increase in blood volume is primarily due to an expansion of plasma volume. This training-induced increase in blood volume has been reported for both males and females and appears to be independent of age (Convertino, 1991). Changes in plasma volume occur soon after the initiation of an endurance training program, with changes between 8% and 10% occurring within the first week (Convertino, Brock, et al., 1980) followed by a plateauing of plasma volume. For up to 10 days of training an expansion of plasma volume accounts for changes in blood volume, with little or no change in red blood cell mass (Convertino, 1991; Convertino, Brock, et al., 1980).

Tests of hematocrit and hemoglobin concentration during this time period are often low, because the red blood cells and hemoglobin are diluted by the larger plasma volume. At times this condition has been labeled as *sports anemia,* but this term is a misnomer, since the number of red blood cells is almost the same or may actually be increased above pretraining levels. Thus, this condition represents no reason for alarm and may be beneficial. The lower hematocrit as a result of elevated plasma volume and normal or slightly elevated number of red blood cells means that the blood is less viscous, which decreases resistance to flow and facilitates the transportation of oxygen.

After 1 month of training, the increase in blood volume is distributed more equally between increases in plasma volume and red blood cell mass (Convertino, 1991; Convertino, Mack, et al., 1991). Blood volume and plasma volume return to pretraining levels when exercise is discontinued. Figure 14.6 depicts these changes in blood volume, plasma volume, and red blood cell volume during 8 days of exercise training and after 7 days of cessation of exercise.

Cardiac Output (3a)

Resting cardiac output is not changed following a training program; however, it is achieved by a larger stroke volume and a lower heart rate (Saltin, 1969). Cardiac output at an absolute submaximal workload is decreased or unchanged with training (Åstrand and Rodahl, 1986; Mitchell and Raven, 1994). Maximal cardiac output is increased at maximal levels of exercise following an endurance exercise training program (Figure 14.7a on page 400). The increase in cardiac output seen at maximal exercise is the result of an increase in stroke volume, since maximal heart rate does not change with training to a degree that has any physiological meaning. The magnitude of the increase in cardiac output depends on the level of training. Elite endurance athletes may have cardiac output values in excess of 35 L·min^{-1}.

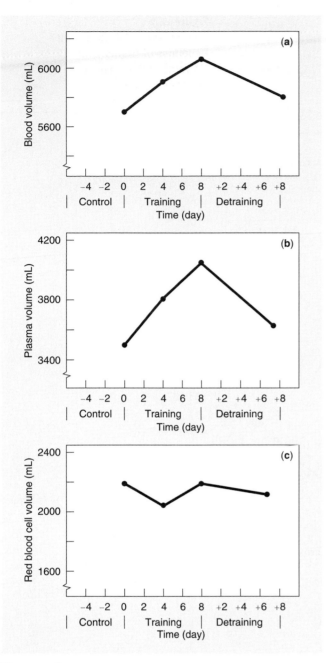

Figure 14.6
Changes in Blood Volume as a Result of Training and Detraining

Source: V. A. Convertino, P. J. Brock, L. C. Keil, E. M. Bernauer, & J. E. Greenleaf. Exercise training-induced hypervolemia: Role of plasma albumin, renin, and vasopressin. *Journal of Applied Physiology.* 48:665–669 (1980). Reprinted by permission.

Stroke Volume (3b)

As shown in Figure 14.7b, endurance training results in an increased stroke volume at rest, during submaximal exercise, and during maximal exercise. The increase in stroke volume results from increased plasma volume, increased cardiac dimensions, increased venous return, and an enhanced ability of the ventricle to stretch and accommodate increased venous return (Mitchell and Raven, 1994; Smith and Mitchell, 1993). Since several of these are structural changes, they will exert their influence whether the individual is resting or working.

It has traditionally been assumed that the pattern of stroke volume response during incremental work to maximum, described as an initial rectilinear rise that plateaus at about 40–50% of $\dot{V}O_2$max, was similar regardless of training status. However, as shown in Figure 14.8 on page 401, evidence now suggests that stroke volume does not plateau in *highly trained* endurance athletes (68.6 mL·kg^{-1}·min^{-1}). Research studies report that stroke volume continues to increase throughout an incremental test to maximum in young through elderly endurance-trained adults (Gledhill, et al., 1994; Wiebe, et al., 1999). Enhanced ventricular filling (increased LVEDV) and emptying (decreased LVESV) both contribute to the augmented stroke volume in these highly trained athletes, although ventricular filling appears to have the greater influence (Gledhill, et al., 1994).

Heart Rate (3c)

Resting heart rate is lower following endurance training (Figure 14.7c). Although *bradycardia* is technically defined as a resting heart rate of less than 60 b·min^{-1}, the term is sometimes used to mean the reduction in resting heart rate that occurs as a result of exercise training. Bradycardia is one of the classic and most easily assessed indicators of training adaptation. The heart rate response to an absolute submaximal amount of work is significantly reduced following endurance training. Maximal heart rate is unchanged or slightly decreased (2–3 b·min^{-1}) with endurance training (Ekblom, et al., 1968; Saltin, 1969).

Maximal Oxygen Consumption (4)

Maximal oxygen consumption ($\dot{V}O_2$max) increases as a result of endurance training (Figure 14.7d). The magnitude of the increase depends on the type of program followed. Improvements of 5–30% are commonly reported, with improvements of 15% routinely found for training programs that meet the recommendations of the ACSM (1998). There are rapid improvements in $\dot{V}O_2$max during the first 2 months of an endurance training program. Following this period, improvements continue to occur, but at a slower rate. This pattern appears to be independent of gender and

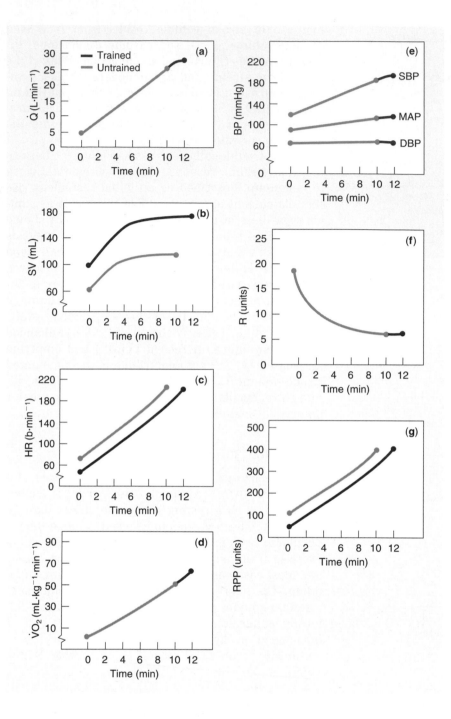

Figure 14.7
Comparison of Cardiovascular
Response of Trained and
Untrained Individuals to
Incremental Exercise to
Maximum

is consistent over a wide age range, although elderly individuals may take longer to adapt to endurance training (ACSM, 1998; Cunningham and Hill, 1975; Seals, et al., 1984).

The improvement in $\dot{V}O_2$max is the result of central and peripheral cardiovascular adaptations. Recall that $\dot{V}O_2$max can be calculated as the product of cardiac output and arteriovenous oxygen difference (a-vO_2 diff) (Equation 12.14b). Increased maximal cardiac output as a result of endurance training was discussed in a previous subsection, and it represents a central adaptation that supports the training-induced improvement in $\dot{V}O_2$max. The a-vO_2 diff reflects oxygen extraction by the working tissue and thus represents a peripheral adaptation that supports the improvement in $\dot{V}O_2$max (see Chapter 11). The changes in cardiac output are a more consistent training adaptation than the changes in a-vO_2 diff, and stroke volume appears to be the principal factor in the increase in cardiac output.

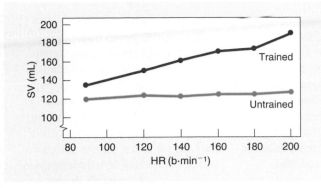

Figure 14.8
Stroke Volume Response in Trained and
Untrained Subjects

Source: N. Gledill, D. Cox, & R. Jamnik. Endurance athletes' stroke volume
does not plateau: Major advantage is diastolic function. *Medicine and
Science in Sports and Exercise.* 26:1116–1121 (1994). Modified and
reprinted by permission of Williams & Wilkins.

Figure 14.9 presents a compilation of data regarding $\dot{V}O_2$max of various athletic groups (Wilmore
and Costill, 1988). Several conclusions can be drawn
from this graph. First, even in the athletic population
the male-female difference is maintained, with males
generally having a greater $\dot{V}O_2$max than females. Second, there is considerable variability in $\dot{V}O_2$max
among athletes. Third, $\dot{V}O_2$max is related to the demands of the sport. Athletes whose performance depends on the ability of the cardiovascular system to
sustain dynamic exercise consistently have higher
$\dot{V}O_2$max values than athletes whose sport performance is based primarily on motor skills, such as
baseball. What is unclear from Figure 14.9 is the relative influence of genetics and training in determining
an individual's $\dot{V}O_2$max. Genetics set the upper limit
on the $\dot{V}O_2$max that can ultimately be achieved by any
individual. Thus, although all individuals are able to
increase $\dot{V}O_2$max with training, an individual with a
greater genetic potential is more likely to excel at
sports that require a high $\dot{V}O_2$max. Furthermore, individuals differ in their sensitivity to training, in part
because of different genetic makeup (Bouchard and
Persusse, 1994).

Blood Pressure (5)

As indicated in Figure 14.7e and as most studies report, there is little or no change in arterial blood pressure (SBP, DBP, MAP) at rest, during submaximal exercise, or during maximal exercise in normotensive
individuals following an endurance training program
(Seals, et al., 1984). However, because the maximal
amount of work that can be done increases with

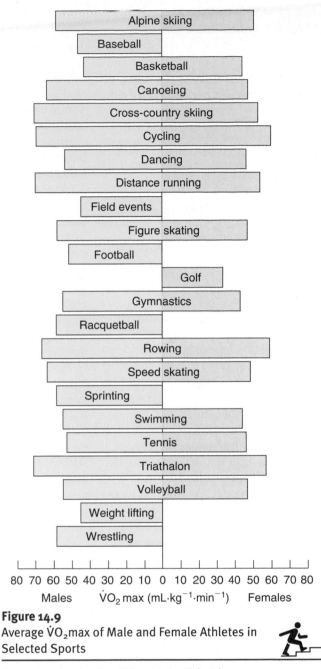

Figure 14.9
Average $\dot{V}O_2$max of Male and Female Athletes in
Selected Sports

Source: Based on data from Wilmore & Costill (1988).

exercise training, a trained individual is capable of
doing more work. Thus, maximal systolic blood pressure may be higher for this individual at maximal exercise. This difference is usually small between
sedentary and normally fit individuals.

Total Peripheral Resistance (6)

Resistance is unchanged at rest or during an absolute
submaximal workload following a training program

Benefits of Lifestyle versus Structured Exercise Training

Dunn, A. L., M. E. Garcia, B. H. Marcus, J. B. Kampert, H. D. Kohl, III, & S. N. Blair: Six-month physical activity and fitness changes in Project Active, a randomized trial. *Medicine and Science in Sports and Exercise.* 30(7): 1076–1083 (1998).

Dunn, A. L., B. H. Marcus, J. B. Kampert, M. E. Garcia, H. W. Kohl, III, & S. N. Blair: Comparison of lifestyle and structured interventions to increase physical activity and cardiorespiratory fitness: A randomized trial. *Journal of the American Medical Association.* 281(4):327–334 (1999).

Preprofessional students involved in athletics or high-intensity personal exercise training programs often find it difficult to accept that the level of activity recommended in the Surgeon General's Report (Table 14.1) can have any meaningful impact on measures of cardiorespiratory fitness or physiological variables. A study conducted at the Cooper Institute for Aerobics Research (and reported in these two articles) provides evidence for the effectiveness of this approach. Subjects were randomized into either a structured intervention program or lifestyle activity intervention program. Individuals in the structured group were given free memberships to the Cooper Fitness Center and trained with a designated exercise leader. Their program began with 30 min of walking 3 days per week, but after 3 weeks they were allowed to select any available aerobic program and eventually progressed to 5 days per week. The lifestyle group received curricular material at weekly meetings centered around individual motivational readiness and behavioral motivation techniques. They were asked to accumulate no fewer than 30 min of at least moderate-intensity activity most days in any way that could be adapted to their individual lifestyle and to progress at their own rate. After 6 months both groups were put on maintenance programs, during which they were requested simply to continue their respective activities. Direct leadership and the number of group meetings were reduced. Selected cardiovascular results are presented in the accompanying table.

As anticipated, the greatest changes were made in the initial 6 months in both groups. Both interventions were effective in increasing physical activity, as indicated by the increases in energy expenditure and walking and the decreases in sitting. However, the structured group increased hard activity more than the lifestyle group and hence improved more than the lifestyle group in physical fitness. The improvement was measured by a greater decrease in HR during submaximal treadmill walking and a greater increase in $\dot{V}O_2$peak. In the ensuing 18 months, both groups decreased physical activity (energy expenditure) and physical fitness ($\dot{V}O_2$peak) from the 6-month level but maintained significant improvements over their initial values. Although the absolute magnitude of the changes is not great, it is important to realize that during the first 6 months only 32% and 27% of the lifestyle and structure groups attained the level of activity suggested by the Surgeon General's Report. During the maintenance phase, these numbers were reduced to 20% in each group. Those in both groups who reported that they were active 70% or more of the weeks had at least twice as much improvement as those who did not.

The "take home" messages from this study are that even under the conditions of well-designed and well-delivered external intervention, getting all individuals to include minimal but meaningful levels of activity into their lives is difficult. However, in previously sedentary healthy adult males and females, lifestyle intervention can be as effective as a structured exercise program in improving physical activity and cardiorespiratory fitness.

	Lifestyle 6 months	Lifestyle 24 months	Structured 6 months	Structured 24 months
Activity energy expenditure (kcal·kg^{-1}·d^{-1})	+1.53[a]	+0.84[a]	+1.34[a]	+0.69[a]
Achieve SG goal (2 kcal·kg^{-1}·d^{-1})	32%	20%	27%	20%
Walking (min·d^{-1})	+19.80[a]	+13.07	+16.52[a]	+26.75[a]
Sitting (hr·wk^{-1})	−5.27[a]	−1.18	−6.88[a]	−6.85[a,b]
Treadmill time (min)	+0.46[a]	+0.23[a]	+0.92[a]	+0.37[a]
Submaximal HR (b·min^{-1})	−4.75[a]	−2.62[a]	−10.22[a,b]	−4.88[a]
$\dot{V}O_2$peak (mL·kg^{-1}·min^{-1})	+1.58[a]	+0.77[a]	+3.64[a,b]	+1.34[a]
SBP (mmHg)		−3.63[a]		−3.26[a]
DBP (mmHg)		−5.38[a]		−5.14[a]
Body fat (%)		−2.39[a]		−1.85[a]

[a] Significant difference each group compared to its own baseline

[b] Significant difference between groups at 6 or 24 months

Table 14.6
Cardiovascular Adaptations to Dynamic Aerobic Exercise

	Rest	Absolute Submaximal Exercise	Maximal Exercise
$\dot{Q}$	Unchanged	Decreased or unchanged	Increased
SV	Increased	Increased	Increased
HR	Decreased	Decreased	Unchanged or slight decrease
SBP	Little or no change	Little or no change	Little increase or no change
DBP	Little or no change	Little or no change	Little decrease or no change
MAP	Little or no change	Little or no change	Little increase or no change
$\dot{V}O_2$	—	—	Increased
TPR	Unchanged	Unchanged	Decreased
RPP	Decreased	Decreased	Unchanged or slight increase

(Figure 14.7f). However, a further reduction in total peripheral resistance occurs in athletes at maximal exercise. For this reason, athletes can generate significantly higher cardiac outputs at similar arterial pressures during maximal exercise. Much of the additional decrease in the total peripheral resistance at maximal exercise is due to the increased capillarization of the skeletal muscle (Blomqvist and Saltin, 1983).

Muscle Blood Flow (7)

Muscle blood flow is unchanged at rest following exercise training. Active muscle blood flow increases during maximal exercise as a result of endurance training. The effect of endurance training on muscle blood flow at submaximal levels is unclear (Åstrand and Rodahl, 1986).

Rate-Pressure Product (8)

Myocardial oxygen consumption, indicated by the rate-pressure product, is lower at rest and during submaximal exercise following endurance training (Figure 14.7g). This result reflects the greater efficiency of the heart, since fewer contractions are necessary to eject the same amount of blood during submaximal exercise following an endurance training program (Mitchell and Raven, 1994). Because maximal heart rate is unchanged and systolic blood pressure is either unchanged or increases slightly with exercise training, it follows that the maximal rate-pressure product is unchanged or increases slightly following a training program. Table 14.6 summarizes the training adaptations that occur within the cardiovascular system as a result of a dynamic aerobic exercise program.

Cardiovascular Adaptations to Dynamic Resistance Training

Low-volume dynamic resistance training (few repetitions and low weight) has not been shown to make any consistent or significant changes in cardiovascular variables. Thus, the changes described in the following sections depend on high-volume (high–total workload) dynamic resistance training programs (Stone, et al., 1991).

Cardiac Dimensions

Dynamic resistance-trained athletes often have increased left ventricular wall and septal thicknesses, although this is not a consistent finding in short-term training studies (Keul, et al., 1981; Longhurst, et al., 1981; Morganroth, et al., 1975). When the increase in wall thickness is reported relative to body surface area or lean body mass, the increase is greatly reduced or even nonexistent (Fleck, 1988a). The increase in wall thickness results from the work the heart must do to overcome the high arterial pressures (increased pressure afterload) encountered during resistance training, and it depends on the training intensity and volume.

Stroke Volume and Heart Rate

Resting stroke volume in highly trained dynamic resistance athletes has been reported to be greater than normal and not different from normal (Effron, 1989; Fleck, 1988b). Because stroke volume is so seldom measured during resistance activities, the changes that occur in the stroke volume response to resistance activities as a result of training are not known (Sjogaard, et al., 1988).

Highly trained dynamic resistance athletes have average or below average resting heart rates (Stone, et al., 1991). Heart rate at a specified submaximal dynamic resistance workload is lower following resistance training (Fleck and Dean, 1987).

Blood Pressure

Dynamic resistance-trained athletes do not have elevated resting blood pressures, provided that they are not chronically overtrained, do not have greatly increased muscle mass, or are not using anabolic steroids. This information contradicts the popular misconception that resistance-trained individuals have a higher resting blood pressure than endurance-trained or untrained individuals. Indeed, most scientific investigations report that highly trained resistance athletes have average or lower-than-average systolic and diastolic blood pressures (Fleck, 1988b). Resistance-trained individuals also exhibit a lower blood pressure response to the same relative workload of resistance exercise than untrained individuals, even though the trained individuals are lifting a greater absolute load.

Dynamic resistance training has not been shown to consistently lower blood pressure in hypertensive individuals. Therefore, resistance training is not recommended as the only exercise modality for hypertensives unless it is in the form of circuit training. *Circuit training* relies on high repetitions, low loads, and short rest periods set up in a series of stations. A *supercircuit* integrates aerobic endurance activities between the stations.

The rate-pressure product, which reflects myocardial oxygen consumption, is decreased at rest following strength training, during weight lifting or circuit training, and during aerobic exercise to which a resistance component has been added (such as holding hand weights while walking) (Fleck, 1988b; Stone, et al., 1991). Researchers have suggested that these results occur because of a reduction in peripheral resistance.

Maximal Oxygen Consumption

Small increases (4–9%) in $\dot{V}O_2$max have been reported following circuit training and Olympic-style weight-lifting programs (Gettman, 1981; Stone, et al., 1991). However, other studies have failed to identify any increase in $\dot{V}O_2$max with resistance training (Hurley, et al., 1984). $\dot{V}O_2$max probably doesn't change much because of the low percentage of $\dot{V}O_2$max that is achieved during a resistance training program. Weight training may impact the central cardiovascular variables as described earlier (that is,

resulting in a reduced resting heart rate), but it does not enhance peripheral cardiovascular adaptations (that is, a-vO_2 diff). Thus, individuals should not rely on resistance training programs to improve cardiorespiratory fitness; instead, a dynamic resistance training program should be used in conjunction with an aerobic endurance training program.

The Influence of Age and Sex on Cardiovascular Training Adaptations

There are few data available regarding the influence of age and sex on cardiovascular adaptations to dynamic resistance exercise. Therefore, this section will address only cardiovascular adaptations to aerobic endurance exercise.

Sex Differences in Adaptations

Research evidence suggests that there are no differences between the sexes in central or peripheral adaptations to aerobic endurance training. Both sexes exhibit similar cardiovascular adaptations at rest, during submaximal exercise, and at maximal exercise (Drinkwater, 1984; Mitchell, et al., 1992). Maximal cardiac output is higher in both sexes owing to an increased stroke volume following training; however, the absolute value achieved by a woman is less than that attained by a similarly trained man.

When males and females of similar fitness level train at the same frequency, intensity, and duration, there are no differences in the relative increase in $\dot{V}O_2$max (Lewis, et al., 1986; Mitchell, et al., 1992). As shown earlier in Figure 13.12, there is considerable overlap in $\dot{V}O_2$max between the sexes. Thus, a well-trained female may have a higher $\dot{V}O_2$max than a sedentary or even normally active male; however, a female will always have a lower $\dot{V}O_2$max than a similarly trained male.

The blood pressure (SBP, DBP, MAP) response to exercise is unchanged following an endurance training program for both sexes. Males and females show the same adaptations in total peripheral resistance and rate-pressure product. The effects of endurance training on cardiovascular variables at maximal exercise are reported in Table 14.7 for the two sexes. In summary, the trainability of females does not differ from that of their male counterparts, and similar benefits can and should be gained by regular activity by both sexes (Hanson and Nedde, 1974). However, the absolute values achieved for maximal oxygen consumption, cardiac output, and stroke volume will generally be lower in females owing to their smaller body size and heart size.

Table 14.7
Comparison of Cardiovascular Responses to Maximal Exercise in Sedentary and Trained
Young Adults (20–30 yr)

Variable	Men		Women	
	Sedentary	Trained	Sedentary	Trained
$\dot{Q}max$ (L·min^{-1})	22	30	16	20
SVmax (mL·b^{-1})	115	155	80	105
HRmax (b·min^{-1})	195	195	195	195
$\dot{V}O_2max$ (mL·kg^{-1}·min^{-1})	50	65	37	52
SBP (mmHg)	200	200	190	190
DBP (mmHg)	70	70	66	66
MAP (mmHg)	135	135	128	128
TPR (units)	6.1	4.5	8.0	6.4
RPP (units)	390	390	370	370

Adaptations in Children

There is relatively little information available regarding cardiovascular adaptations in children and adolescents as a result of endurance training, especially in children of a very young age. However, it has been documented that endurance training results in an increase in left ventricular mass and heart volume in children, as it does in adults (Bar-Or, 1983; Greenen, et al., 1982). The increase in heart size is associated with an increase in resting stroke volume (Gutin, et al., 1988), a decrease in resting heart rate, but no change in cardiac output (Eriksson and Koch, 1973). Research also suggests an increased blood volume and hemoglobin level in young endurance athletes compared with sedentary children (Koch and Rocher, 1980; Zauner, et al., 1989). There has been some speculation that children are more likely to respond to endurance training at a certain age or maturity level, but no level or age has yet been clearly identified (Cunningham, et al., 1984; Pate and Ward, 1990; Rowland, 1990).

At submaximal levels of exercise, cardiac output is unchanged or slightly decreased in youngsters after endurance training (Bar-Or, 1983; Soto, et al., 1983). This result is due to an increase in submaximal stroke volume and a decrease in heart rate (Bar-Or, 1983; Lussier and Buskirk, 1977). Neither systolic nor diastolic blood pressure changes significantly as a result of endurance training during submaximal work (Lussier and Buskirk, 1977).

At maximal work, cardiac output increases in children and adolescents as a result of endurance training. This result is due to an increased maximal stroke volume and stable maximal heart rate (Eriksson and Koch, 1973; Lussier and Buskirk, 1977).

Children and adolescents in a wide variety of training programs, in either school or community-based settings, have consistently shown improvements in endurance performance. Such improvements have occurred whether endurance performance was measured as an increase in the workload performed (longer treadmill times or distances run, more distance covered in a set amount of time, higher work output on a cycle ergometer, or longer rides at the same load setting) or as a faster time for a given distance (Cooper, et al., 1975; Daniels and Oldridge, 1971; Daniels, et al., 1978; Duncan, et al., 1983; Dwyer, et al., 1983; Goode, et al., 1976; Graunke, et al., 1990; Mosellin and Wasmund, 1973; Siegel and Manfredi, 1984). Given the lack of association between endurance performance and $\dot{V}O_2max$ in children, it should come as no surprise that endurance performance improvements are not always accompanied by a comparable improvement in $\dot{V}O_2max$ (Daniels and Oldridge, 1971; Daniels, et al., 1978). Furthermore, although children and adolescents who participate in organized athletic activities have higher $\dot{V}O_2max$ values than those who do not engage in such activities, the relationship between measures of physical activity (such as self-report questionnaires, heart rate monitoring, and motion detection devices) and measures of $\dot{V}O_2max$ is generally only low to moderate (Morrow and Freedson, 1994; Vaccaro and Mahon, 1987).

Because of these findings, researchers have hotly debated whether children and adolescents could improve $\dot{V}O_2max$ as a result of training. At this time the consensus is that children can improve $\dot{V}O_2max$ values; the key to this adaptation lies in the training program being of sufficient intensity, duration, and frequency. Precisely what constitutes an adequate intensity for the exercise prescription of children and

Table 14.8

Comparison of Cardiovascular Responses to Maximal Exercise in Sedentary and Trained Elderly Individuals (60–70 yr)

Variable	Men		Women	
	Sedentary	Trained	Sedentary	Trained
$\dot{Q}max$ ($L \cdot min^{-1}$)	16	19.4	12	15
SVmax ($mL \cdot b^{-1}$)	100	125	75	90
HRmax ($b \cdot min^{-1}$)	155	155	155	155
$\dot{V}O_2max$ ($mL \cdot kg^{-1} \cdot min^{-1}$)	28	48	22	35
SBP (mmHg)	190	190	190	190
DBP (mmHg)	84	84	84	84
MAP (mmHg)	138	138	138	138
TPR (units)	8.6	7.3	11.5	9.2
RPP (units)	290	290	290	290

adolescents is unknown, but intensities recommended for adults appear to be effective. For these intensities, improvements of 10–15% in $\dot{V}O_2max$ are typical.

Adaptations in the Elderly

Elderly males and females respond to endurance exercise training with adaptations similar to those seen in younger adults (Hagberg, et al., 1989; Heath, et al., 1981; Ogawa, et al., 1992). Left ventricular wall thickness and myocardial mass are greater in elderly athletes than in elderly sedentary individuals, although these training adaptations may not be as pronounced or as quickly achieved as in younger adults (Green and Crouse, 1993; Heath, et al., 1981; Ogawa, et al., 1992).

Left ventricular–end diastolic volume and ejection fraction increase as a result of endurance training in older individuals. These changes lead to an enhancement of myocardial contractile function, especially the Frank-Starling mechanism, and assist in maintaining cardiac outputs in the active elderly (Green and Crouse, 1993).

Resting cardiac output is unchanged as a result of endurance training in the elderly. Elderly athletes with an extensive history of endurance training consistently show lower resting heart rates than their sedentary counterparts. However, short-term training programs sometimes show the expected decrease in resting heart rates and sometimes do not. Resting stroke volume typically increases, but the increase is generally small (Green and Crouse, 1993).

As for normotensive individuals of other ages, endurance training does not affect systolic blood pressure, diastolic blood pressure, or mean arterial blood pressure at rest in elderly people. Both hemoglobin levels and blood volume increase in the elderly as a result of endurance training, as does the density of capillaries supplying blood to the active musculature (Green and Crouse, 1993).

Most training studies indicate that no change occurs in cardiac output during any given submaximal workload. The components of cardiac output, however, often change reciprocally with the expected decrease in heart rate and increase in stroke volume. Again, the stroke volume changes tend to be small and do not always reach statistical significance. Submaximal values for systolic blood pressure, mean arterial blood pressure, and total peripheral resistance are lower in elderly athletes than in nonathletes and decrease as a result of endurance training (Green and Crouse, 1993).

Maximal cardiac output may be increased by exercise training in elderly individuals. This increase is completely accounted for by an increase in maximal stroke volume, since maximal heart rate is unchanged. The reported effects of endurance training on blood pressures and systematic vascular resistance are inconsistent, although the majority of the evidence suggests no change in these variables (Green and Crouse, 1993).

The results of training status on cardiovascular responses to maximal exercise in the elderly, including $\dot{V}O_2max$, are shown in Table 14.8 for both men and women. $\dot{V}O_2max$ is higher in trained than in untrained elderly. Thus, training programs can result in increases in $\dot{V}O_2max$ in the elderly. The magnitude of the increase in $\dot{V}O_2max$ depends on the initial fitness level of the individual and the training program followed. Research suggests, though, that healthy, elderly untrained males and females can improve their $\dot{V}O_2max$ by 15–30% with training (Hagberg, et al., 1989; Ogawa, et al., 1992; Seals, et al., 1984).

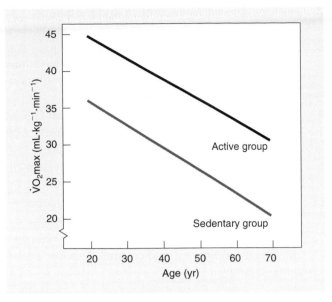

Figure 14.10

Age-Related Decline in $\dot{V}O_2$max in Highly Active and Sedentary Women

Source: S. A. Plowman, B. L. Drinkwater, & S. M. Horvath. Age and aerobic power in women: A longitudinal study. *Journal of Gerontology.* 34(4): 512–520 (1979). Copyright © The Gerontological Society of America. Reprinted by permission.

One study using a short-duration exercise program (9 weeks) of endurance training reported that a low-intensity exercise prescription (30–45% HRR) was as effective as a high-intensity exercise prescription (60–75% HRR) in eliciting improvements in $\dot{V}O_2$max (Badenhop, 1983). However, a 1-yr training program found that 6 months of training at low intensities (40% HRR) resulted in a 10.5% improvement in $\dot{V}O_2$max. When the training program was progressively changed to a high-intensity program (85% HRR) and the duration was extended, the elderly subjects increased their $\dot{V}O_2$max by another 16.5%. This research suggests that elderly individuals respond to exercise training in much the same way that younger individuals do.

When initiating a training program with elderly people, it is important to begin at low intensities to avoid injury. However, significant improvements in function can be gained by low-intensity programs. After individuals become accustomed to the program, the training program can be upgraded to an intense training program if desired. Note that the rate of adaptation, though, may be slower in older individuals (ACSM, 1998).

Although elderly athletes are more similar to younger individuals than to their sedentary counterparts, and training programs tend to show that the same beneficial changes occur in the elderly that

occur in younger subjects, exercise training does not stop the effects of aging on the cardiovascular system. At best, exercise training can only lessen the age-related losses in cardiovascular function. This conclusion is exemplified in Figure 14.10, where the average rate of decline in $\dot{V}O_2$max is shown for both an active, highly fit (HF) group of females and a relatively sedentary, low-fitness (LF) comparison group (Plowman, et al., 1979). The first thing to notice is that the HF group had higher $\dot{V}O_2$max values than the LF group in every decade. Indeed, the active 45-yr-old group had $\dot{V}O_2$max values that equaled those of the inactive 20-yr-olds. Second, $\dot{V}O_2$max expressed per kilogram of body weight declined with age, and the rate of decline was similar in the two groups.

Summary

1. What constitutes an optional cardiovascular training program depends on the age and health status of the individual and the goal of the program.

2. Any activity that involves large muscle groups and is sustained for prolonged periods of time has the potential to increase cardiovascular fitness. The choice of exercise modalities should be based upon interest, availability, and low risk of injury.

3. Training using different exercise modalities causes the same overall benefits by leading to central cardiovascular adaptations. However, peripheral cardiovascular adaptations are specific to the muscles being exercised.

4. Intensity is very important in improving maximal oxygen consumption ($\dot{V}O_2$max) primarily in conjunction with duration, which determines training volume. Intensity can be prescribed in relation to heart rate, oxygen consumption, or rating of perceived exertion (RPE). Training intensity is the most important factor in maintaining cardiovascular fitness.

5. The Surgeon General's Report recommends an accumulation of 30 min of physical activity on most, if not all, days of the week for all previously sedentary individuals to obtain meaningful health benefits.

6. The American College of Sports Medicine (ACSM) recommends the following training goals to develop and maintain cardiorespiratory fitness in healthy adults: frequency of 3–5 days per week; intensity of 55/65–90% HRmax; 40/50–85% $\dot{V}O_2$R or HRR; duration of 20–60 min of continuous aerobic activity.

7. The absolute and relative increases in $\dot{V}O_2$max and the health benefits are inversely related to initial fitness level. That is, the greatest improvements in fitness and health benefits occur when very sedentary individuals begin a regular, low- to moderate-endurance exercise program. Thus, meaningful health benefits can be achieved with minimal increases in activity or fitness by those who need it most.

8. Endurance training results in an increase in cardiac dimensions, mass, and the size of the coronary vascular bed. The internal diameter of the coronary arteries may also increase as result of training. More importantly, the arteries are more distensible during exercise as a result of training.

9. Endurance training results in an increase in blood volume, with highly trained endurance athletes having 20–25% greater blood volume than untrained subjects. Changes in plasma volume occur early in a training program, with changes between 8 and 10% occurring within the first week. Early changes (1 month) are due almost entirely to increases in plasma volume, whereas increases in red blood cells and hemoglobin occur later.

10. Cardiac output at rest and at an absolute submaximal workload is unchanged following an endurance training program. However, cardiac output at the same relative workload and at maximal exercise is greater following an endurance training program.

11. Stroke volume is greater at rest, at submaximal exercise (absolute and relative workloads), and at maximal exercise following an endurance training program.

12. Heart rate is lower at rest and during an absolute submaximal workload following endurance training. It is unchanged at the same relative submaximal workload and at maximal exercise.

13. There is little or no change in blood pressure at rest, during submaximal exercise, or during maximal exercise in normotensive individuals following an endurance training program.

14. $\dot{V}O_2$max increases as a result of endurance training; improvements of 15% are routinely reported with training programs that meet the recommendations of ACSM.

Review Questions

1. How is overload manipulated to bring about cardiorespiratory adaptation?

2. Differentiate between central and peripheral cardiovascular adaptations.

3. Compare and contrast cardiac output, stroke volume, heart rate, and blood pressure adaptations to endurance training at rest and during submaximal and maximal exercise.

4. Discuss the impact of an individual's initial-fitness level on expected improvements in fitness and health-related benefits.

5. Describe the physiological benefits of a warm-up and a cool-down period.

6. Explain the changes in blood volume that occur as a result of an endurance training program.

7. Compare and contrast cardiovascular adaptations to aerobic endurance and dynamic resistance training.

For further review and additional study tools, visit The Physiology Place. (www.physiologyplace.com) and the Student Study Guide for Exercise Physiology for Health, Fitness, and Performance *by Sharon A. Plowman and Denise L. Smith.*

Passport to the Internet

Visit the following Internet sites to explore further topics and issues related to cardiorespiratory training. To visit an organization's web site, go to www.physiologyplace.com and click on "Passport to the Internet."

Runner's World **Magazine** Includes training pace calculator based on individual race times for different types of workouts such as long slow distance, tempo runs, repeat 800s, and so on.

Fitness for Children Training programs, stories and advice for children, written at a child's level.

President's Council on Physical Fitness & Sports Exercise, physical activity and health information for individuals of all ages.

The National Center on Physical Activity and Disability Includes resources on how to adapt exercise and physical activity equipment.

Physical Education and Fitness Information and links to items of interest to physical educators including health and fitness programming ideas.

References

American College of Sports Medicine: *Guidelines for Exercise Testing and Prescription* (6th edition). Philadelphia: Lea & Febiger (2000).

American College of Sports Medicine: Position stand on the recommended quantity and quality of exercise for developing and maintaining fitness in healthy adults. *Medicine and Science in Sports and Exercise.* 10(3):vii–x (1978).

American College of Sports Medicine: Position stand on the recommended quantity and quality of exercise for developing and maintaining cardiorespiratory and muscular fitness and flexibility in healthy adults. *Medicine and Science in Sports and Exercise.* 30(6):975–985 (1998).

Åstrand, P. O., & K. Rodahl: *Textbook of Work Physiology.* New York: McGraw-Hill (1986).

Badenhop, D. T., P. A. Cleary, S. F. Schaal, E. L. Fox, & R. L. Bartels: Physiological adjustments to higher- or lower-intensity exercise in elders. *Medicine and Science in Sports and Exercise.* 15(6):496–502 (1983).

Barnard, R. J., G. W. Gardner, N. V. Diasco, R. N. MacAlpin, & A. A. Kattus: Cardiovascular responses to sudden strenuous exercise—Heart rate, blood pressure and ECG. *Journal of Applied Physiology.* 34:833–837 (1973).

Bar-Or, O.: *Pediatric Sports Medicine for the Practitioner.* New York: Springer-Verlag (1983).

Blomqvist, C. G., & B. Saltin: Cardiovascular adaptations to physical training. *Annual Review of Physiology.* 45:169 (1983).

Bloomfield, S., & E. F. Coyle: Bedrest, detraining, and retention of training-induced adaptations. In American College of Sports Medicine (ed.), *Resource Manual for Guidelines for Exercise Testing and Prescription.* Philadelphia: Lea & Febiger (1993).

Borg, G.: *Borg's Perceived Exertion and Pain Scales.* Champaign, IL: Human Kinetics (1998).

Bouchard, C., & L. Persusse: Heredity, activity level, fitness, and health. In C. Bouchard, R. J. Shephard, & T. Stephens (eds.), *Physical Activity, Fitness, and Health, International Proceedings and Consensus statement.* Champaign, IL: Human Kinetics (1994).

Cohen, J. L., & K. R. Segal: Left ventricular hypertrophy in athletes: An exercise-echocardiographic study. *Medicine and Science in Sports and Exercise.* 17:695–700 (1985).

Connor, J. F., F. LaCamera, E. J. Swanick, M. J. Oldham, D. W. Holzaepfel, & O. Lyczkowskyj: Effects of exercise on coronary collateralization—Angiographic studies of six patients in a supervised exercise program. *Medicine and Science in Sports.* 8(3):145–151 (1976).

Convertino, V. A.: Blood volume: Its adaptation to endurance training. *Medicine and Science in Sports and Exercise.* 23:1338–1348 (1991).

Convertino, V. A., P. J. Brock, L. C. Keil, E. M. Bernauer, & J. E. Greenleaf: Exercise training–induced hypervolemia: Role of plasma albumin, renin, and vasopressin. *Journal of Applied Physiology.* 48:665–669 (1980).

Convertino, V. A., G. W. Mack, & E. R. Nadel: Elevated central venous pressure: A consequence of exercise training–induced hypervolemia? *American Journal of Physiology.* 29:R273–R277 (1991).

Cooper, K. H., J. G. Purdy, A. Friedman, R. L. Bohannon, R. A. Harris, & J. A. Arends: An aerobics conditioning program for the Fort Worth, Texas, School District. *Research Quarterly.* 46:345–380 (1975).

Corbin, C. B., & R. P. Pangrazi: Toward an understanding of appropriate physical activity levels for youth. *Physical Activity and Fitness Research Digest.* 1(8):1–8 (1994).

Coyle, E. F., M. K. Hemmert, & A. R. Coggan: Effects of detraining on cardiovascular responses to exercise: Role of blood volume. *Journal of Applied Physiology.* 60:95–99 (1986).

Coyle, E. F., W. H. Martin, D. R. Sinacore, M. J. Joymer, J. M. Hagberg, & J. O. Holloszy: Time course of loss of adaptations after stopping prolonged intense endurance training. *Journal of Applied Physiology.* 57:1857–1864 (1984).

Cunningham, D. A., & J. S. Hill: Effect of training on cardiovascular response to exercise in women. *Journal of Applied Physiology.* 39:891–895 (1975).

Cunningham, D. A., D. H. Paterson, & C. J. R. Blinkie: The development of the cardiorespiratory system in growth and development. In R. A. Boileau (ed.), *Advances in Pediatric Sport Sciences* (Vol. 1). Champaign, IL: Human Kinetics, 85–116 (1984).

Currens, J. G., & P. D. White: Half century of running: Clinical, physiologic and autopsy findings in the case of Clarence De Mar, "Mr. Marathoner." *New England Journal of Medicine.* 265:988–993 (1961).

Daniels, J., & J. Gilbert: *Oxygen Power: Performance Tables for Distance Runners.* Tempe, AZ: Author (1979).

Daniels, J., & N. Oldridge: Changes in oxygen consumption of young boys during growth and running training. *Medicine and Science in Sports.* 3:161–165 (1971).

Daniels, J., N. Oldridge, F. Nagle, & B. White: Differences and changes in $\dot{V}O_2$ among young runners 10 to 18 years of age. *Medicine and Science in Sports.* 10:200–203 (1978).

De Busk, R. F., U. Hakanssan, M. Sheehan, & W. L. Haskell: Training effects of long versus short bouts of exercise. *American Journal of Cardiology.* 65:1010–1013 (1990).

Drinkwater, B. L.: Women and exercise: Physiological aspects. *Exercise and Sport Sciences Reviews.* 12:21–52 (1984).

Drinkwater, B. L., & S. M. Horvath: Detraining effects on young women. *Medicine and Science in Sports and Exercise.* 4:91–95 (1972).

Ducan, B., W. T. Boyce, R. Itami, & N. Puffengarger: A controlled trial of a physical fitness program for fifth grade students. *Journal of School Health.* 53:467–471 (1983).

Dwyer, T., W. E. Coonan, D. R. Leitch, B. S. Hetzel, & R. A. Boghurst: An investigation of the effects of daily physical activity on the health of primary school students in South Australia. *International Journal of Epidemiology.* 12:308–313 (1983).

Eckstein, R. W.: Effects of exercise and coronary heart narrowing on coronary collateral circulation. *Circulation Research.* 5:230–235 (1957).

Effron, M. B.: Effects of resistance training on left ventricular function. *Medicine and Science in Sports and Exercise.* 21:694–697 (1989).

Ekblom, B., P. O. Astrand, B. Saltin, J. Stenberg, & B. Wallstrom: Effect of training on circulatory response to exercise. *European Journal of Applied Physiology.* 24:518–528 (1968).

Eriksson, B. O., & G. Koch: Effects of physical training on hemodynamic response during submaximal and maximal exercise in 11 to 13 year old boys. *Acta Physiologica Scandinavia.* 87:27–39 (1973).

Eyestone, E. D., G. Fellingham, J. George, & A. G. Fisher: Effect of water running and cycling on maximum oxygen consumption and 2-mile run performance. *American Journal of Sports Medicine.* 21(1):41–44 (1993).

Ferguson, F. J., R. Petitclerc, G. Choquette, L. Chaniotis, P. Gauthier, R. Hout, C. Allard, L. Jankowski, & L. Campeau: Effect of physical training on treadmill exercise capacity, collateral circulation and progression of coronary disease. *American Journal of Cardiology.* 34:764–769 (1974).

Fleck, S. J.: Cardiovascular adaptations to resistance training. *Medicine and Science in Sports and Exercise.* 20:S146–S151 (1988a).

Fleck, S. J.: Cardiovascular responses to strength training. In P. V. Komi (ed.), *Strength and Power in Sport.* Champaign, IL: Human Kinetics, 305–319 (1988b).

Fleck, S. J., & L. S. Dean: Resistance-training experience and the pressor response during resistance exercise. *Journal of Applied Physiology.* 63:116–120 (1987).

Gettman, L. R: Circuit weight-training: A critical review of its physiological benefits. *The Physician and Sports Medicine.* 9(1):44–59 (1981).

Gledhill, N., D. Cox, & R. Jamnik: Endurance athletes' stroke volume does not plateau: Major advantage is diastolic function. *Medicine and Science in Sports and Exercise.* 26:1116–1121 (1994).

Goode, R. C., A. Virgin, T. T. Romet, P. Crawford, J. Duffin, T. Palland, & Z. Woch: Effects of a short period of physical activity in adolescent boys and girls. *Canadian Journal of Applied Sport Sciences.* 1:241–250 (1976).

Graunke, J. M., S. A. Plowman, & J. R. Marett: Evaluation of a fitness based physical education curriculum for the high school freshman. *Illinois Journal of Health, Physical Education, Recreation and Dance.* 27:24–27 (1990).

Green, J. S., & S. F. Crouse: Endurance training, cardiovascular function and the aged. *Sports Medicine.* 16(5):331–341 (1993).

Greenen, D. L., T. B. Gilliam, D. Crowley, C. Moorehead-Steffens, & A. Rosenthal: Echocardiographic measures in 6 to 7 year old children after an 8 month exercise program. *American Journal of Cardiology.* 49:1990–1995 (1982).

Gutin, B., N. Mayers, J. A. Levy, & M. V. Herman: Physiologic and echocardiographic studies of age-group runners. In E. W. Brown & C. F. Branta (eds.), *Competitive Sports for Children and Youth.* Champaign, IL: Human Kinetics, 115–128 (1988).

Hagberg, J. M., J. E. Graves, M. Limacher, D. R. Woods, S. H. Leggett, C. Cononie, J. J. Gruber, & M. L. Pollock: Cardiovascular responses of 70- to 79-yr-old men and women to exercise training. *Journal of Applied Physiology.* 66:2589–2594 (1989).

Hanson, J. S., & W. H. Nedde: Long-term physical training effect in sedentary females. *Journal of Applied Physiology.* 37:112–116 (1974).

Haskell, W. L.: Health consequences of physical activity: Understanding and challenges regarding dose response. *Medicine and Science in Sports and Exercise.* 26(6):649–660 (1994).

Haskell, W. L., C. Sims, J. Myll, W. M. Bortz, F. G. St. Goar, & E. L. Alderman: Coronary artery size and dilating capacity in ultra distance runners. *Circulation.* 87(4):1076–1082 (1993).

Heath, G. W., J. M. Hagberg, A. A. Ehsani, & J. O. Holloszy: A physiological comparison of young and older endurance athletes. *American Physiological Society.* 51(3):634–640 (1981).

Hickson, R. C., C. Foster, M. L. Pollock, T. M. Galassi, & S. Rich: Reduced training intensities and loss of aerobic power, endurance, and cardiac growth. *Journal of Applied Physiology.* 58:492–499 (1985).

Hickson, R. C., C. Kanakis, J. R. Davis, A. M. Moore, & S. Rich: Reduced training duration effects on aerobic power, endurance, and cardiac growth. *Journal of Applied Physiology.* 53(1):225–229 (1982).

Hickson, R. C., & M. A. Rosenkoetter: Reduced training frequencies and maintenance of increased aerobic power. *Medicine and Science in Sports and Exercise.* 13:13–16 (1981).

Houmard, J. A., B. K. Scott, C. L. Justice, & T. C. Chenier: The effects of taper on performance in distance runners. *Medicine and Science in Sports and Exercise.* 26(5): 624–631 (1994).

Housh, D. J., & T. J. Housh: The effects of unilateral velocity—Specific concentric strength training. *Journal of Orthopaedic and Sports Physical Therapy.* 17(5):252–260 (1993).

Hurley, B. F., D. R. Seals, A. A. Ehsani, L. J. Cartier, G. P. Dalsky, J. M. Hagberg, & J. O. Holloszy: Effects of high-intensity strength training on cardiovascular function. *Medicine and Science in Sports and Exercise.* 16(5):483–488 (1984).

Huston, T. P., J. C. Puffer, & W. MacMillan: The athletic heart syndrome. *New England Journal of Medicine.* 313:24–32 (1985).

Keul, J., H. H. Dickhuth, G. Simon, & M. Lehmann: Effect of static and dynamic exercise on heart volume, contractility, and left ventricular dimensions. *Circulation Research.* 48:I162–I170 (1981).

Kibler, W. B., & T. J. Chandler: Sport-specific conditioning. *American Journal of Sports Medicine.* 22(3):424–432 (1994).

Kilmer, D. D., M. A. McCrory, N. C. Wright, S. G. Aitkens, & E. M. Bernaver: The effect of a high resistance exercise program in slowly progressive neuro-muscular disease. *Archives of Physical Medicine and Rehabilitation.* 75(5):560–563 (1994).

Koch, G., & L. Rocher: Total amount of hemoglobin, plasma and blood volumes, and intravascular protein masses in trained boys. In K. Berg & B. O. Erickson (eds.), *Children and Exercise IX.* Baltimore: University Park Press, 109–115 (1980).

Lewis, D. A., E. Kamon, & J. L. Hodgson: Physiological differences between genders. Implications for sports conditioning. *Sports Medicine.* 3:357–369 (1986).

Londeree, B. R., T. R. Thomas, G. Ziogas, T. D. Smith, & Q. Zhang: % VO$_2$max versus % HRmax regressions for six modes of exercise. *Medicine and Science in Sports and Exercise.* 27:458–461 (1995).

Longhurst, J. C., A. R. Kelly, W. J. Gonyea, & J. H. Mitchell: Chronic training with static and dynamic exercise: Cardiovascular adaptation and response to exercise. *Circulation Research.* 48:I171 (1981).

Lussier, L., & E. R. Buskirk: Effects of an endurance training regimen on assessment of work capacity in prepubertal children. *Annals of the New York Academy of Sciences,* 734–747 (1977).

Magel, J. R., G. F. Foglia, W. D. McArdle, B. Gutin, G. S. Pechar, & F. I. Katch: Specificity of swim training on maximum oxygen uptake. *Journal of Applied Physiology.* 38(1):151–155 (1975).

Miller, W. C., J. P. Wallace, & K. E. Eggert: Predicting max HR and the HR-V̇O$_2$ relationship for exercise prescription in obesity. *Medicine and Science in Sports and Exercise.* 25:1077–1081 (1993).

Mitchell, J. H., & P. Raven: Cardiovascular adaptation to physical activity. In C. R. Bouchard, R. J. Shepard, & T. Stephens (eds.), *Physical Activity, Fitness, and Health: International Proceedings and Consensus Statement.* Champaign, IL: Human Kinetics, 286–301 (1994).

Mitchell, J. H., C. Tate, P. Raven, F. Cobb, R. Kraus, R. Moreadith, M. O'Toole, B. Saltin, & N. Wenger: Acute response and chronic adaptation to exercise in women. *Medicine and Science in Sports and Exercise* (Suppl.). 24(6):258–265 (1992).

Morganroth, J., B. J. Maron, W. L. Henry, & S. E. Epstein: Comparative left ventricular dimensions in trained athletes. *Annals of Internal Medicine.* 82:521 (1975).

Morrow, J. R., & P. S. Freedson: Relationship between habitual physical activity and aerobic fitness in adolescents. *Pediatric Exercise Science.* 6:315–329 (1994).

Mosellin, R., & U. Wasmund: Investigations on the influence of a running-training program on the cardiovascular and motor performance capacity in 53 boys and girls of a second and third primary school class. In O. Bar-Or (ed.), *Pediatric Work Physiology: Proceedings of the Fourth International Symposium.* Natanya, Israel: Wingate Institute (1973).

Ogawa, T., R. J. Spina, W. H. Martin, W. M. Kohrt, K. B. Schechtman, J. O. Holloszy, & A. A. Ehsani: Effects of aging, sex, and physical training on cardiovascular responses to exercise. *Circulation.* 86:494–503 (1992).

O'Toole, M.: Prevention and treatment of injuries to runners. *Medicine and Science in Sports and Exercise* (Suppl.). 24(9):5360–5363 (1992).

Parker, S. B., B. F. Hurley, D. P. Hanlon, & P. Vaccaro: Failure of target heart rate to accurately monitor intensity during aerobic dance. *Medicine and Science in Sports and Exercise.* 21(2):230–234 (1989).

Pate, R. R., R. D. Hughes, J. V. Chandler, & J. L. Ratliffe: Effects of arm training on retention of training effects derived from leg training. *Medicine and Science in Sports.* 10(2):71–74 (1978).

Pate, R. R., & D. S. Ward: Endurance exercise trainability in children and youth. In W. A. Grana, K. A. Lombardo, B. J. Sharkey, & J. A. Stone (eds.), *Advances in Sports Medicine and Fitness.* 3:37–55 (1990).

Pechar, G. S., W. D. McArdle, F. I. Katch, J. R. Magel, & J. Deluca: Specificity of cardiorespiratory adaptation to bicycle and treadmill training. *Journal of Applied Physiology.* 36(6):753–756 (1974).

Plowman, S. A., B. L. Drinkwater, & S. M. Horvath: Age and aerobic power in women: A longitudinal study. *Journal of Gerontology.* 34(4):512–520 (1979).

Pollock, M. L.: The quantification of endurance training programs. In J. H. Wilmore (ed.), *Exercise and Sport Sciences Reviews.* 1:155–188 (1973).

Roberts, J. A., & J. W. Alspaugh: Specificity of training effects resulting from programs of treadmill running and bicycle ergometer riding. *Medicine and Science in Sports.* 4(1):6–10 (1972).

Rowland, T. W.: *Exercise and Children's Health.* Champaign, IL: Human Kinetics (1990).

Saltin, B.: Physiological effects of physical conditioning. *Medicine and Science in Sports.* 1:50–56 (1969).

Schaible, T. F., & J. Schever: Cardiac function in hypertrophied hearts from chronically exercised female rats. *Journal of Applied Physiology.* 50:1140–1145 (1981).

Seals, D. R., J. M. Hagberg, B. F. Hurley, A. A. Ehsani, & J. O. Holloszy: Endurance training in older men and women. *Journal of Applied Physiology.* 57(4):1024–1029 (1984).

Siegel, J. A., & T. G. Manfredi: Effects of a ten month fitness program on children. *The Physician and Sports Medicine.* 12:91–97 (1984).

Sjogaard, G., G. Savard, & C. Juel: Muscle blood flow during isometric activity and its relation to muscle fatigue. *European Journal of Applied Physiology.* 57:327–335 (1988).

Smith, M. L., & J. H. Mitchell: Cardiorespiratory adaptations to exercise training. In American College of Sports Medicine (ed.), *Resource Manual for Guidelines for Exercise Testing and Prescription.* Philadelphia: Lea & Febiger (1993).

Soto, K. I., C. W. Zauner, & A. B. Otis: Cardiac output in preadolescent competitive swimmers and in untrained normal children. *Journal of Sports Medicine.* 23:291–299 (1983).

Stone, M. H., S. J. Fleck, N. T. Triplett, & W. J. Kraemer: Health- and performance-related potential of resistance training. *Sports Medicine.* 11(4):210–231 (1991).

Svedenhag, J., & J. Seger: Running on land and in water: Comparative exercise physiology. *Medicine and Science in Sports and Exercise.* 24(10):1155–1160 (1992).

Swain, D. P.: Energy cost calculations for exercise prescription: An update. *Sports Medicine.* 30(1):17–22 (2000).

U.S. Department of Health and Human Services: *Physical Activity and Health: A Report of the Surgeon General.* Atlanta, GA: U.S. Department of Health and Human Services, Centers for Disease Control and Prevention, National Center for Chronic Disease Prevention and Health Promotion (1996).

Vaccaro, P., & A. Mahon: Cardiorespiratory responses to endurance training in children. *Sports Medicine.* 4:352–363 (1987).

Wells, C. L., & S. A. Plowman: Sexual differences in athletic performance: Biological or behavioral? *The Physician and Sports Medicine.* 11(8):52–63 (1983).

Wenger, H. A., & G. J. Bell: The interactions of intensity, frequency and duration of exercise training in altering cardiorespiratory fitness. *Sports Medicine.* 3:346–356 (1986).

Wiebe, C. G., N. Gledhill, V. K. Jamnik, & S. Ferguson: Exercise cardiac function in young through elderly endurance trained women. *Medicine and Science in Sports and Exercise.* 31(5):684–691 (1999).

Wilmore, J. H., & D. L. Costill: *Training for Sport and Activity: The Physiological Basis of the Conditioning Process* (3rd edition). Dubuque, IA: Brown (1988).

Wilmore, J. H., J. A. Davis, R. S. O'Brien, P. A. Vodak, G. R. Walder, & E. A. Amsterdam: Physiological alterations consequent to 20-week conditioning programs of bicycling, tennis, and jogging. *Medicine and Science in Sports and Exercise.* 12(1):1–8 (1980).

Zauner, C. W., M. G. Maksud, & J. Melichna: Physiological considerations in training young athletes. *Sports Medicine.* 8:15–31 (1989).

Zoll, P. M., S. Wessler, & M. J. Schlesinger: Interarterial coronary anastomoses in the human heart with particular reference to anemia and relative anoxia. *Circulation.* 4:797–815 (1951).

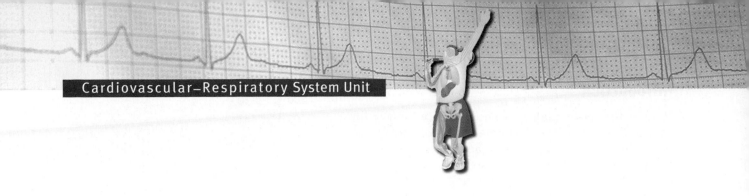

Chapter 15

Thermoregulation

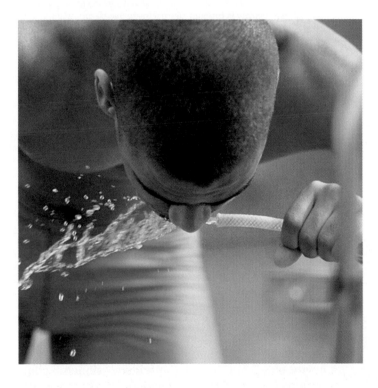

After studying the chapter, you should be able to

- Identify environmental factors that affect human thermoregulation and be able to use indices of heat stress and windchill to assess the risk associated with exercise under various conditions.

- Describe thermal balance and discuss factors that contribute to heat gain and heat loss.

- List and define the mechanisms by which heat is lost from the body.

- Identify the factors that influence heat exchange between an individual and the environment.

- Describe the challenges facing the cardiovascular system when exercise is performed in a hot environment and in a cold environment.

- Differentiate between the different types of heat illness in terms of symptoms, causes, and first aid.

- Identify ways in which an exercise leader can prevent heat and cold injuries and illness.

Introduction

Human thermoregulatory responses rely heavily on the cardiovascular system to maintain body temperature. This chapter will address the issue of exercise in environmental extremes, emphasizing the role of the cardiovascular system in mediating the body's response to exercise under such conditions.

Exercise in Environmental Extremes

Exercise in conditions of environmental extremes can present a serious challenge to the thermoregulatory and cardiovascular systems of the body. If the cardiovascular system is unable to meet the concurrent demands of supplying adequate blood to the muscles and maintaining thermal balance, heat illness may ensue. Heat illness covers a spectrum of disorders from heat cramps to life-threatening heat exhaustion. Cold conditions can also pose problems. If an exerciser is unprepared or inadequately clothed for exercise in cold environments, heat loss can exceed heat production, leading to cold-induced injury.

Exercise professionals have a responsibility to understand the problems associated with exercise in extreme environmental conditions because they may affect an individual's performance or place an exerciser at risk for injury or illness. An understanding of the body's response to extreme environmental conditions provides a basis for minimizing performance decrements and avoiding injury or illness in those who train and compete in adverse conditions (Vogel, Rock, et al., 1993).

Basic Concepts

If you are to understand the body's response to exercise in different environments, you must first understand basic environmental measures and the way that body temperature is assessed.

Measurement of Environmental Conditions

Environmental conditions that affect human thermoregulation are ambient temperature (T_{amb}), relative

---

Relative Humidity The moisture in the air relative to how much moisture, or water vapor, can be held by the air at any given ambient temperature.

Heat Stress Index A scale used to determine the risk of heat stress from measures of ambient temperature and relative humidity.

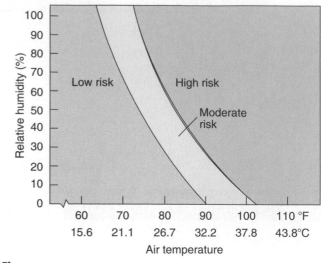
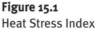

Figure 15.1
Heat Stress Index

Low risk: Use discretion, especially if unconditioned or unacclimatized; little danger of heat stress for acclimatized individuals who hydrate adequately.

Moderate risk: Heat-sensitive and nonacclimatized individuals may suffer; avoid strenuous activity in the sun; take adequate rest periods and replace fluids.

High risk: Extreme heat stress conditions exist; consider canceling all exercise.

Source: Modified from Armstrong & Hubbard (1985).

---

humidity, and wind speed. Ambient temperatures are most often measured with a mercury thermometer. **Relative humidity** indicates the moisture in the air relative to how much moisture, or water vapor, can be held by the air at any given ambient temperature. Thus, 70% humidity means that the air contains 70% of the moisture that it is capable of holding. The **heat stress index** is a scale used to determine the risk of heat stress from measures of ambient temperature and relative humidity (Figure 15.1).

Wind speed affects the amount of heat lost from the body and is used in the calculation of the windchill factor. Table 15.1 presents the revised windchill chart, adopted by the U. S. National Weather Service in the fall of 2001. The revised windchill chart measures the wind velocity at a height of 1.3 m (5 ft), as opposed to a height of 8.7 m (33 ft) in the original windchill chart (developed in the 1940s). The windchill chart was developed as a public health tool to reduce frostbite and hypothermia by providing information that can be used to inform people how to dress appropriately based on readily available environmental data.

Measurement of Body Temperature

Exercise physiologists differentiate temperatures at different portions of the body, most commonly using

Table 15.1

Windchill Index

Wind Speed (mi·hr⁻¹)	Thermometer Reading*																
	40	35	30	25	20	15	10	5	0	−5	−10	−15	−20	−25	−30	−35	−40
5	36	31	25	19	13	7	1	−5	−11	−16	−22	−28	−34	−40	−46	−52	−57
10	34	27	21	15	9	3	−4	−10	−16	−22	−28	−35	−41	−47	−53	−59	−66
15	32	25	19	13	6	0	−7	−13	−19	−26	−32	−39	−45	−51	−58	−64	−71
20	30	24	17	11	4	−2	−9	−15	−22	−29	−35	−42	−48	−55	−61	−68	−74
25	29	23	16	9	3	−4	−11	−17	−24	−31	−37	−44	−51	−58	−64	−71	−78
30	28	22	15	8	1	−5	−12	−19	−26	−33	−39	−46	−53	−60	−67	−73	−80
35	28	21	14	7	0	−7	−14	−21	−27	−34	−41	−48	−55	−62	−69	−76	−82
40	27	20	13	6	−1	−8	−15	−22	−29	−36	−43	−50	−57	−64	−71	−78	−84
45	26	29	12	5	−2	−9	−16	−23	−30	−37	−44	−51	−58	−65	−72	−79	−86
	Low risk					Moderate risk					High risk						

Low Risk: Use discretion; little danger if properly clothed.

Moderate Risk: Postpone exercise if possible. Proper clothing is essential. Individuals at risk should take added precautions against overexposure.

High Risk: There is great danger from cold exposure; consider canceling all exercise.

*Note that this table uses °F; see Appendix A for conversion.

Source: U. S. National Weather Service (2001).

core (T_{co}) and *skin temperature* (T_{sk}). Even this distinction is simplistic because core temperature and skin temperature will each vary depending on the specific site that is measured. Core temperature is normally maintained within fairly narrow limits of approximately 36.1–37.8°C (97–100°F) (Marieb, 2001). Skin temperatures, however, are considerably cooler, averaging approximately 33.3°C (91.4°F). They are also more variable because they are greatly influenced by environmental conditions.

Measurements of body temperature are most commonly obtained from a thermometer placed in the oral cavity. However, this method is affected by many factors, including breathing rate and fluid ingestion, and it is not the method of choice among physiologists. Core temperature is most accurately assessed by measuring the temperature of the blood as it enters the right atrium or measuring esophageal temperatures. These are invasive procedures, however, and are not practical for routinely measuring core temperature. Therefore, rectal temperatures (T_{re}) are often used in laboratory settings to assess core body temperature.

Although rectal temperature is a reliable way to measure body temperature, it is not applicable for mass testing, nor is it routinely used to assess temperatures in exercise participants or athletes. Despite the importance of assessing body temperature in preventing and treating heat illness, there is no readily available, accurate, and convenient way of assessing core temperature in many situations, including athletic events. Often practitioners must rely on oral temperatures despite problems associated with this method. Other times medical personnel will obtain rectal temperatures. And in some instances tympanic membrane temperatures (T_{tym}) may be assessed, although it is not clear that tympanic thermometry can actually detect exercise-induced heat stress.

Skin temperatures are not routinely measured in field settings, but they are important because they determine the amount of heat that will be exchanged with the environment. Heat moves down a thermal gradient. Therefore, more heat will be lost from the body when the body is considerably hotter than the environment (larger gradient) than when the two temperatures are similar (smaller gradient). In the same way, more heat will be gained by the body when the environment is considerably hotter than the body. Skin temperatures are assessed via thermocouples attached to the skin.

Figure 15.2
Thermal Balance

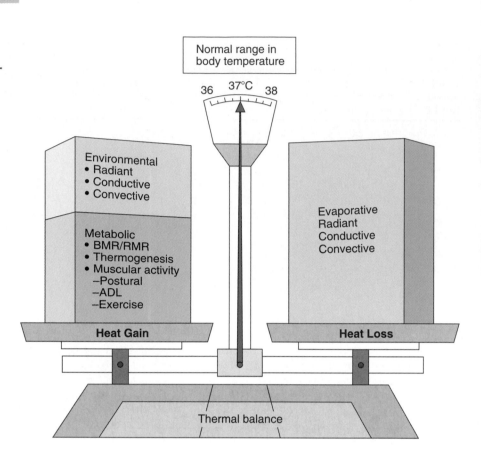

Thermal Balance

The temperature of the body is the result of a balance between heat gain and heat loss (Figure 15.2). Although heat can be gained from the environment, the majority of heat is typically produced by the body as a result of metabolic activity. Heat is a by-product of cellular respiration; at rest the body liberates approximately 60–75% of the energy from aerobic metabolism as heat (see Chapter 5). The minimum energy required to meet the metabolic demands of the body at rest is called *basal metabolic rate* (BMR) or *resting metabolic rate* (RMR) and accounts for a large proportion of heat production.

The ingestion of food increases the body's production of heat and is known as *thermogenesis* (see Chapter 9). Also, any muscular activity will increase heat production, including activity related to muscle tone and posture; activities of daily living (ADL), such as bathing, dressing, and meal preparation; and planned exercise. Because metabolism is greatly increased during physical activity, heat production is also increased dramatically.

Heat can be exchanged (gained or lost) from the body by four processes: radiation, conduction, convection, and evaporation. The effectiveness of these processes depends on environmental conditions—namely, ambient temperature, relative humidity, and wind speed.

Radiant heat loss occurs through the emission of electromagnetic heat waves to the environment and depends on the thermal gradient between the body and the environment. When the environmental temperature equals skin temperature, no heat is lost through radiation. If the environmental temperature exceeds skin temperature, radiation will add to the heat load of the body.

Conduction involves the direct transfer of heat from one molecule to another. In terms of human temperature regulation, conduction involves warming molecules of air and other surfaces in contact with the skin. The effectiveness of conductive heat loss is determined by the thermal gradient between the skin and the molecules in contact with the skin and by the thermal properties of the molecules in contact with the skin. Because water can absorb and conduct heat much better than air, submersion in water is an effective way to lower the body temperature.

Convective heat loss depends on the movement of the molecules in contact with the skin. When there is a breeze, heat loss is enhanced, because the warmer molecules are moved away from the skin. Thus the

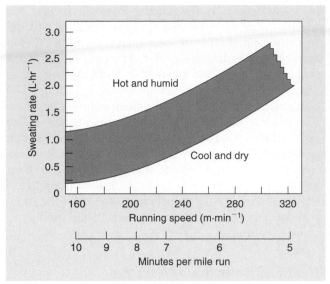

Figure 15.3
Estimated Sweating Rate at Various Running Speeds

Source: M. N. Sawka & K. B. Pandolf. Effects of body water loss on physiological function and exercise performance. In C. V. Gisolfi & D. R. Lamb (eds.), *Perspectives in Exercise Science and Sports Medicine. Vol 3: Fluid Homeostasis During Exercise.* Carmel, IN: Cooper Publishing Group; 97–151 (1993). Reprinted by permission.

thermal gradient is maintained so that more heat can be lost by conduction.

Evaporation is the conversion of liquid into vapor. The evaporation of unnoticed water from the skin, called *insensible perspiration,* contributes to heat dissipation under resting conditions. The evaporation of sweat is a major mechanism for cooling the body under exercise conditions. Sweat is a hypotonic solution (99% water) derived from plasma and released from eccrine glands located throughout the body but concentrated on the forehead, hands, and feet (Marieb, 2001).

During heavy exercise, the sweat rate of an individual can increase dramatically. Sweat rates vary considerably among individuals, depending on genetics and fitness level. For any one individual, sweat rate depends on environmental conditions, exercise intensity, fitness level, degree of acclimatization, and hydration status. Figure 15.3 provides an estimate of hourly sweating rates for running at various speeds under different environmental conditions (Sawka and Pandolf, 1990; Shapiro, et al., 1982). Notice how common it is for sweating rates to exceed $1 \; \text{L·hr}^{-1}$ of sweat. Clearly, this water loss will lead to a decrease in total body water and plasma volume and will result in deleterious effects on cardiovascular function if fluid is not replaced.

The evaporation of sweat represents the primary defense against heat stress. Sweating itself does not cool the body; the sweat must be evaporated. The evaporation of sweat produces a cooling of the body because energy is needed to convert the liquid sweat into a vapor, and this energy is extracted from the immediate surroundings. The amount of energy needed for the evaporation of sweat can be quantified: 580 kcal of heat energy is released for each liter of water that is vaporized (Åstrand and Rodahl, 1986).

When the body is in thermal balance, the amount of heat produced and the amount of heat lost are equal. So if they are added, the sum is equal to zero, and body temperature is constant. This can be explained by the following formula (Winslow, et al., 1939):

15.1 $M \pm R \pm C \pm K - E = 0$

where M is metabolic heat production, R is radiant heat exchange, C is convective heat exchange, K is conductive heat exchange, and E is evaporative heat loss.

The plus or minus sign for radiant, convective, and conductive processes indicates that heat can be lost or gained by the body through these mechanisms. When the environment is hotter than the skin temperature, heat is gained by the body (a plus sign in the equation). When skin temperature is higher than the environment temperature, heat is lost from the body (a negative sign in the equation). Evaporation cannot add to the heat load of the body. This mechanism can only dissipate heat; thus, there is only a negative sign in the equation for evaporation.

Heat Exchange

The exchange (transfer) of heat between the body and the environment occurs by the mechanisms just described: conduction, convection, radiation, and evaporation. Heat exchange is represented schematically in Figure 15.4. These four mechanisms are important in dissipating heat to the environment under most conditions. However, under certain conditions—namely, high ambient temperatures—conduction, convection, and radiation may actually add heat to the body.

The effectiveness of heat exchange between an individual and the environment is affected by five factors:

1. the thermal gradient;
2. the relative humidity;
3. air movement;
4. the degree of direct sunlight; and
5. the clothing worn by the individual.

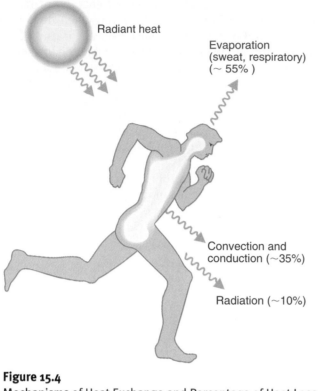

Radiant heat

Evaporation
(sweat, respiratory)
(~ 55%)

Convection and
conduction (~35%)

Radiation (~10%)

Figure 15.4
Mechanisms of Heat Exchange and Percentage of Heat Loss

Source: Modified from Gisolfi & Wenger (1984).

The greater the difference between two temperatures—called the *thermal gradient*—the greater the heat loss is from the warmer of the two. Typically, the body is warmer than the environment, so heat moves down its thermal gradient to the environment. More heat is lost on cooler days because the thermal gradient is greater.

High humidity decreases evaporative heat loss from the body because the air is already largely saturated with water vapor. Relative humidity is the primary factor that determines the effectiveness of evaporative cooling (Vogel, Rock, et al., 1993). As a result, on humid days evaporative cooling is limited. Although the exerciser may sweat profusely, the sweat cannot evaporate as effectively.

Air movement increases convective heat loss from the skin to the environment. Thus, on windy days more heat is lost from the body.

Direct sunlight can add considerably to the radiant heat load of an individual. Conversely, shade or cloud cover can often provide significant relief from heat.

Clothing can also influence the effectiveness of heat transfer with the environment. In cold weather, clothing protects against excessive heat loss. However, clothing can also interfere with heat dissipation in hot weather by decreasing convective heat loss. Clothing that is lightweight, nonrestrictive, and light in color promotes heat loss; heavy, dark clothing interferes with the dissipation of heat. Football uniforms, especially the protective padding, are an example of heavy, restrictive clothing. Helmets, in particular, limit heat loss by encapsulating the head. The color of the clothing is also a consideration. Dark colors absorb light and thereby add to the radiant heat load; light colors reflect light. Thus, dark-colored uniforms can contribute to the heat stress of athletes as they play on a synthetic field that radiates heat in the hot fall sun. Short shirts and the use of mesh materials are attempts to aid in heat dissipation under these conditions.

Heat Exchange during Exercise

Heat production and heat transfer occur by the same mechanisms during exercise as they do at rest. However, during exercise the total body metabolism may increase to 15–20 times the resting rate (Sawka and Pandolf, 1990). Under these conditions, metabolic heat production may increase to an extent that heat production is greater than heat dissipation; thus, the body will store heat and body temperature will increase, a condition known as *hyperthermia*.

Metabolic heat from the muscles is transported to the core of the body and skin by the blood. Heat is also transferred to the skin and exchanged with the environment by conduction, convection, radiation, and evaporation. There are two physiological mechanisms that allow the body to dissipate heat in an attempt to maintain thermal balance during exercise: an increase in sweating rate and vasodilation of the cutaneous vessels. The evaporation of sweat increases evaporative cooling and is the primary mechanism by which the body cools itself during exercise in warm temperatures. Vasodilation in the cutaneous vessels brings the warmer blood close to the body's surface so that heat can be dissipated to the environment via conduction, radiation, and convection, assuming that ambient temperature is cooler than the body.

Figure 15.5 on page 420 depicts the relative importance of the heat exchange mechanisms during 60 min of cycling exercise (900 kpm·min^{-1}) at various ambient temperatures. Total heat loss (THL) remains relatively constant across a wide range of ambient temperatures. The fact that metabolic heat production (M) exceeds the total heat loss accounts for the increase in temperature that is observed with exercise. An important point to realize from Figure 15.5 is that the increase in body temperature (depicted as heat storage) is relatively constant over a wide range in ambient temperatures as long as the work rate is held

Focus on Research

Heat Dissipation and Age

Tankersley, C. G., et al. Sweating and skin blood flow during exercise: The effects of age and maximal oxygen uptake. *Journal of Applied Physiology.* 71(1):236–242 (1991).

The two primary physiological mechanisms to dissipate heat are an increase in sweat rate and an increase in skin blood flow. It has long been known that the ability to dissipate heat during exercise in hot environments declines with increasing age. However, for many years it was unclear what physiological mechanisms caused the alterations in sweat rate and skin blood flow that occur as a person ages. The obvious way to explore an answer to this question is to design a study that compares younger adults with their older counterparts. However, one inherent difficulty in such studies is that older adults typically have a lower $\dot{V}O_2$max. It is known that an increase in $\dot{V}O_2$max is associated with an earlier onset of sweating, presumably because in a trained individual the body has adapted to maintain thermal balance more effectively. Thus, it has been unclear whether aging itself or the age-related decline in $\dot{V}O_2$max is responsible for the decrease in sweating, and thus heat loss in older exercisers.

To overcome these difficulties, Tankersley and colleagues designed a study that compared young normally fit individuals to a group of older normally fit individuals and to a group of older highly fit individuals during 20 min of submaximal exercise (67.5% of $\dot{V}O_2$max). Thus, the younger group could be compared to an older group with a lower $\dot{V}O_2$max (the normally fit older group) and an older group with a similar $\dot{V}O_2$max (the highly fit older group). The graphs below present the esophageal temperature, chest sweating rate, and forearm blood flow in the three groups.

The graphs indicate the following:

1. Esophageal temperature during the exercise was not different among the three groups working at the same relative workload. However, because the normally fit older group had the lowest $\dot{V}O_2$max, they were working at a lower absolute workload and thus should be producing less metabolic heat. Therefore, the fact that the increase in temperature among the three groups was similar may indicate an impaired ability to dissipate heat in the normally fit older group compared to the two groups with a higher $\dot{V}O_2$max.
2. In general, the average forearm blood flow and chest sweating rates for the highly fit older individuals was intermediate to those in the normally fit older group and the normally fit younger group.
3. The normally fit older individuals had a lower forearm blood flow and lower sweating response during most of the exercise protocol compared to the normally fit younger individuals.

These results suggest that younger and older subjects matched for similar $\dot{V}O_2$max have similar heat loss responses to submaximal exercise. Therefore, it appears that the decrease in $\dot{V}O_2$max that typically accompanies aging is primarily responsible for the changes in sweating and blood flow that are reported in older adults. A person who maintains a high fitness level as he or she ages is not likely to experience these detrimental changes in the thermoregulatory response to aging.

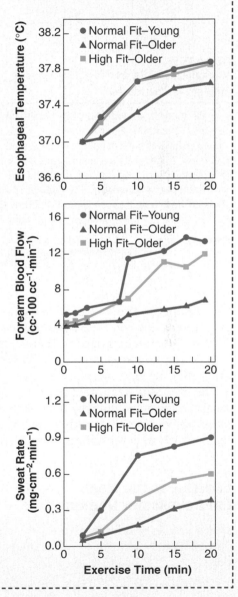

constant. This is true because metabolic heat production depends on the amount of work being done regardless of temperature. The total heat loss also remains the same. Thus, the difference between metabolic heat production and total heat loss—that is, heat storage—is constant. Although total heat loss remains relatively constant, it is achieved by different mechanisms at different ambient temperatures. At

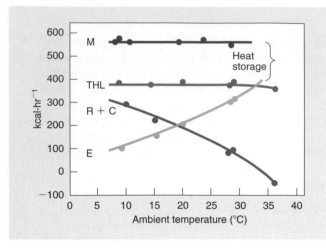

Figure 15.5

Mechanisms of Heat Loss during Exercise at Different Ambient Temperatures

M = metabolic heat production, THL = total heat loss, R + C = heat loss by radiation and conduction, E = heat loss by evaporation. Exercise was performed for 60 min at work rate of 900 kpm·min⁻¹ at each ambient temperature. Notice that the metabolic heat produced and the total heat loss (and thus the heat storage) is constant over a wide range of temperatures although it is achieved via different mechanisms. Evaporative heat loss becomes increasingly important as ambient temperature increases.

Source: C. V. Gisolfi & C. B. Wenger. Temperature regulation during exercise: Old concepts, new ideas. *Exercise and Sport Sciences Reviews.* 12:339–372 (1984). Reprinted by permission of Williams & Wilkins.

high temperatures evaporative heat loss dominates, and radiant and convective heat losses become less effective. This combination is effective, however, only as long as the humidity is low enough to allow sweat to evaporate. In high humidity, evaporative heat loss is ineffective, and heat storage (body temperature) increases. This explains why temperature and humidity must be considered together (using the heat index; Figure 15.1) in determining when activity is safe.

Exercise in the Heat: Cardiovascular Demands

There are several interrelated problems that the cardiovascular system faces under hyperthermic conditions.

1. There is a competition for blood flow between the skin and the muscles. The muscles need increased blood flow to meet the demands of metabolic activity, and the skin needs increased blood flow to dissipate heat from the core of the body. The combined needs of the skin and muscle for blood flow may exceed the cardiac output.

2. Vasodilation in the cutaneous vessels effectively decreases venous return, thus decreasing stroke volume. Therefore, cardiac output may be reduced at a time when the demands for flow are greatest (Rowell, 1986).

3. There is a reduction in plasma volume, which contributes to the reduction in stroke volume, and, hence, cardiac output.

4. The body must maintain an adequate blood pressure to perfuse the vital organs, including the brain, kidneys, and liver. The ability to maintain blood pressure is challenged by widespread vasodilation in the skeletal muscle beds and cutaneous vessels, thus decreasing total peripheral resistance.

As seen in Figure 15.6a, during short-term, light submaximal exercise cardiac output increases to a similar degree whether exercise is performed in a hot or a thermoneutral environment (Rowell, 1974). However, cardiac output in a hot environment is achieved by a higher heart rate and a lower stroke volume than in a thermoneutral environment. The reduction in stroke volume during hot conditions occurs because of vasodilation in the cutaneous vessels, which decreases central venous volume. Mean arterial pressure is similar to or slightly lower in hot environments than in thermoneutral environments because of vasoconstriction in the kidneys and digestive tract. During light exercise in a hot environment, rectal temperature is similar to values achieved in a thermoneutral environment (Seals, 1983).

During prolonged, heavy submaximal exercise in the heat, cardiac output increases less than when exercise is performed in a thermoneutral environment (see Figure 15.6). Cardiac output in hot environments fails to reach levels attained under thermoneutral conditions during heavy exercise because stroke volume declines progressively as the severity of exercise increases. Although heart rate is higher under hot conditions, the increase is not able to compensate for the reduction in stroke volume during heavy exercise. Thus, cardiac output is lower in hot conditions.

During long-term, heavy submaximal exercise in the heat, vasoconstriction occurs in the digestive and renal areas in an attempt to maintain mean arterial blood pressure. In fact, vasoconstriction may result in ischemia and even tissue damage under severe conditions (Rowell, 1986). The regulatory mechanisms that maintain blood pressure are stressed by the excessive water loss that occurs through profuse sweating (see Figure 15.3). If this fluid is not replaced, stroke volume, cardiac output, and blood pressure will decrease. Additionally, performance will suffer, and heat illness becomes increasingly likely.

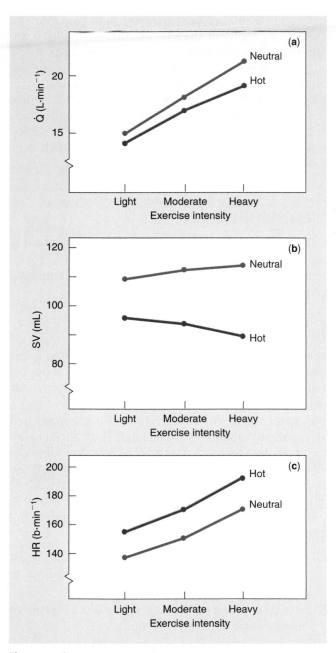

Figure 15.6
Cardiovascular Responses to Hot or Thermoneutral
Conditions

Source: L. B. Rowell. Human cardiovascular adjustments to exercise and
thermal stress. *Physiological Reviews.* 54:75–159 (1974). Reprinted by
permission.

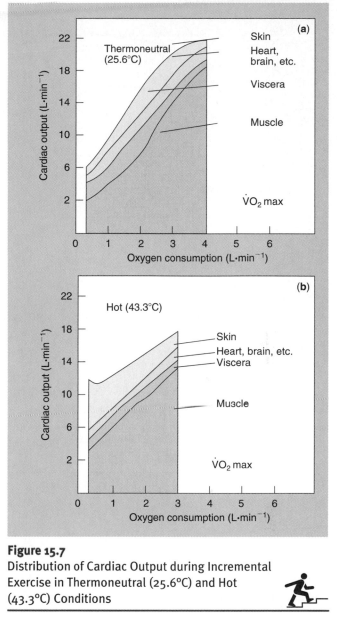

Figure 15.7
Distribution of Cardiac Output during Incremental
Exercise in Thermoneutral (25.6°C) and Hot
(43.3°C) Conditions

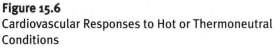

Source: Modified from Rowell (1986).

Maximal cardiac output is lower during incremental exercise to maximum when performed under hot conditions than under thermoneutral conditions. This decrease results from a lower stroke volume, because maximal heart rate is unchanged, although maximal heart rate may occur earlier when exercise is performed in the heat. The estimated distribution of cardiac output during an incremental exercise test performed under neutral and hot conditions is presented in Figure 15.7.

When exercise is performed in the hot environment, it cannot be performed for as long as in cooler conditions. Consequently, $\dot{V}O_2$max is lower in the hot environment (Figure 15.7b). Cardiac output increases during exercise in both conditions. However, cardiac output at $\dot{V}O_2$max is less when exercise is performed in the hot environment, presumably because blood is displaced in cutaneous veins, thus decreasing venous return and stroke volume. Blood flow to the active skeletal muscles increases throughout exercise in both conditions. However, blood flow to skeletal muscle

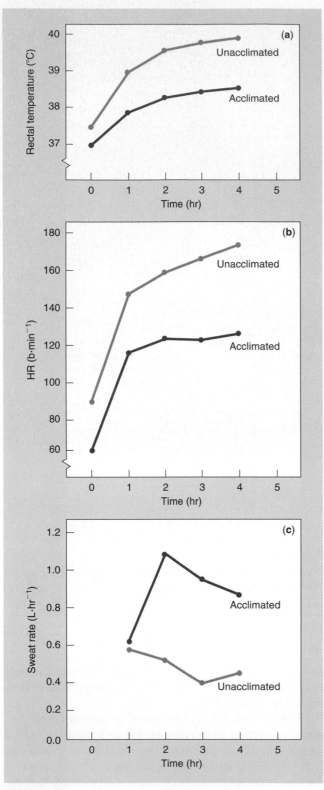

Figure 15.8
Comparison of Rectal Temperature, Heart Rate, and Sweat Loss in Acclimated and Unacclimated Individuals during Long-Term, Moderate to Heavy Submaximal Exercise

Source: Based on data in Wyndham (1964).

represents a smaller proportion of total blood flow in the hot environment than in the thermoneutral environment, because skin blood flow accounts for a larger portion of the blood flow. At $\dot{V}O_2$max in the hot condition, visceral blood flow is severely reduced in an effort to support the muscles with adequate blood flow and maintain blood pressure. The lower cardiac output and the decrease in blood flow when maximal exercise is performed in a hot environment both contribute to a lower $\dot{V}O_2$max.

Factors Affecting Cardiovascular Response to Exercise in the Heat

Several factors affect an individual's response to exercise in the heat. This section will discuss four of them: acclimatization, cardiovascular fitness, body composition, and hydration level.

Acclimatization

Acclimatization refers to adaptive changes that occur when an individual undergoes prolonged or repeated exposure to a stressful environment; these changes reduce the physiological strain produced by such an environment. Acclimatization to heat is accomplished by repeated exposure to heat sufficient to increase core body temperature and elicit moderate to profuse sweating (Werner, 1993). Light to moderate exercise in the heat for 1–2 hr a day can lead to positive adaptations within a few days.

Acclimatization to heat involves three underlying mechanisms:

1. Cardiovascular changes occur that decrease heart rate and cardiovascular strain at a given level of exercise in the heat.

2. Sweating patterns are altered such that sweating begins earlier.

3. There is a higher sweating rate for a given core temperature that can be maintained for longer periods of time (Wenger, 1988).

Figure 15.8 presents changes in rectal temperature, heart rate, and sweating rate during 4 hr of aerobic exercise before and after acclimatization (Wenger, 1988). These data reinforce the point that the benefits of heat acclimatization are lowered thermal and cardiovascular strain. Proper acclimatization

> **Acclimatization** The adaptive changes that occur when an individual undergoes prolonged or repeated exposure to a stressful environment; these changes reduce the physiological strain produced by such an environment.

ensures that individuals can perform longer and more safely in the heat.

Fitness Level

Aerobic fitness improves an individual's thermoregulatory function and heat tolerance (Wenger, 1988). Endurance training results in a lower resting core temperature, a larger plasma volume, an earlier onset of sweating, and a smaller decrease in plasma volume during exercise (Drinkwater, 1984; Werner, 1993). Therefore, individuals who are aerobically fit are better able to handle the cardiovascular demands associated with exercise in hot conditions than sedentary individuals. High-intensity interval training in thermoneutral conditions also decreases the time required for acclimatization to exercise in a hot environment (Cohen and Gisolfi, 1982).

Body Composition

Excessive body fat is a liability in terms of thermoregulation during exercise in the heat. Greater adiposity contributes to heat stress by two primary mechanisms. First, it interferes with the dissipation of heat; body fat acts to insulate the core. Second, body fat adds to the metabolic cost of activity by adding weight to the body that must be moved. Heat illness is more common in overweight individuals and more likely to be fatal to these individuals (Henshell, 1967).

Hydration Level

An individual's level of hydration has a large impact on exercise tolerance and on the cardiovascular responses to long-term exercise in the heat. Body water accounts for 65–70% of the total body mass of an average adult. During long-term exercise in the heat, profuse sweating leads to large losses of total body water and a reduction in plasma volume if fluid is not replaced (Wade and Freund, 1990). The loss of plasma volume has negative effects on the thermoregulatory and cardiovascular systems and contributes to performance decrements and heat illness. Figure 13.5 presented the differences in cardiovascular responses to long-term exercise with and without fluid replacement. When fluid was replaced, cardiac output and stroke volume could be maintained throughout exercise. However, when water was not replaced, there was a considerable negative drift in stroke volume and a positive drift in heart rate.

Thirst is an inadequate mechanism to fully replace the fluid lost during exercise. Even when unlimited access to water is provided, individuals will not voluntarily consume enough water to replace water loss, and a relative state of dehydration occurs. **Voluntary dehydration** refers to the exercise-induced dehydration that develops despite an individual's access to unlimited water. Thus, the coach or exercise leader needs to encourage participants to consume water beyond what thirst dictates. Experts recommend that 400–500 mL of water be ingested prior to activity and that another 200–400 mL be consumed every 15–30 min of activity (Nieman, 1990; Vogel, Rock, et al., 1993). The goal is to replace all water lost through sweating or to consume the maximal amount that can be tolerated (American College of Sports Medicine [ACSM], 1996). Regardless of acclimatization or fitness level, an individual must be well hydrated prior to and during exercise in a warm environment (Coyle and Montain, 1993; Sawka and Wenger, 1993).

Influence of Age and Sex on the Exercise Response in Heat

Sex Differences in Exercise Response in Heat

The majority of scientific evidence suggests that the response of individuals to exercise in a hot environment depends more on the state of their cardiovascular system than upon their sex (Drinkwater, 1984; Stephenson and Kolka, 1993, 1988). Early studies suggested that women experienced more heat strain than men when both performed the same absolute work. However, these studies failed to control for differences in aerobic fitness levels. The women were working at a higher percentage of maximal effort, and core temperature response to exercise is related more to relative exercise intensity than absolute intensity (Drinkwater, 1984). More recent studies that have matched subjects for fitness level, body size, body fat, and degree of heat acclimatization have found few thermoregulatory differences between the sexes, particularly if the phase of the menstrual cycle was controlled for (Stephenson and Kolka, 1988).

There does appear to be a difference between the sexes in sweating response. Males begin sweating at a lower core temperature and have a greater sweat rate in humid conditions than similarly trained females (Avellini, Kamon, et al., 1980; Drinkwater, 1984). Whether this difference is an asset or a liability to males is unknown. Some researchers have argued that males are inefficient and wasteful in terms of sweat production and that females have the

---

Voluntary Dehydration Exercise-induced dehydration that develops despite an individual's access to unlimited water.

advantage of sweating less and, thus, decreasing blood volume to a lesser extent (Avellini, Shapiro, et al., 1980; Wyndham, Morrison, et al., 1965). Others counter that higher sweat rates might be advantageous in situations where evaporative heat loss is important (Frye and Kamon, 1981). Although the sweating response is slightly different in males and females, heart rate and core temperature responses to exercise in the heat are similar (Frye and Kamon, 1983). Heat acclimatization produces similar results in both sexes (Frye and Kamon, 1983).

One of the confounding factors that needs to be considered regarding the thermoregulatory response of females is the phase of the menstrual cycle. Core temperature is greater, at rest and during exercise, during the luteal than the follicular phase of the menstrual cycle (days 14–28) (Pivarnik, et al., 1992; Stephenson and Kolka, 1993).

Exercise Response of Older Adults in the Heat

Cardiac output increases above resting levels during exercise in the heat for both young and older individuals. However, at higher workloads the increase in cardiac output is not as great when exercise is performed in the heat as when it is performed under thermoneutral conditions (see Figure 15.6). The increase in cardiac output during exercise in a hot environment is less in older persons than in younger individuals of similar fitness levels (Kenney and Anderson, 1988). Furthermore, it appears that young adults increase cardiac output by augmenting heart rate, but older individuals increase cardiac output by increasing stroke volume (Kenney and Anderson, 1988). This result helps explain why differences exist in cardiac output at higher workloads; apparently, there is a limit to the extent to which older individuals can increase stroke volume.

Exercise-induced reductions in plasma volume are greater in older individuals than in young individuals when they exercise in hot and humid conditions. When exercising at the same relative workload, young and older individuals demonstrate similar changes in systolic, diastolic, and mean arterial blood pressure. There is no difference in core temperature between young and older individuals when they exercise in the heat. Acclimatization to heat results in similar changes in older individuals and in young people (Pandolf, et al., 1988).

Exercise Response of Children in the Heat

Several age-related differences in thermoregulatory responses place children at a disadvantage compared with adults when they exercise in the heat (Bar-Or,

Table 15.2

Responses of Children Relative to Adults to Exercise in the Heat

Characteristic	Response of Children Compared with Response of Adults
Cardiac output/O_2 uptake	Lower
Metabolic heat of locomotion	Higher
Sweating rate	Lower
Sweating threshold	Higher
Exercise tolerance time	Lower
Rise in core temperature	Faster
Acclimatization to heat	Slower

Source: Modified from Bar-Or (1984).

1984; Bar-Or and Baranowski, 1994). Table 15.2 summarizes the cardiovascular responses of children, relative to adults, during exercise in the heat. As discussed in Chapter 13, children have a lower cardiac output than adults at any given level of oxygen consumption. This lower cardiac output proves to be a detriment for children exercising in the heat because of the demands for increased blood flow during exercise-induced heat stress. Children also have a smaller plasma volume than adults from which to draw fluids. Thus, they have a reduced sweating capacity compared with that of adults. This is true when sweat rate is reported in absolute values, per surface area, and per sweat gland. Additionally, the sweating threshold is higher in children than in adults (Bar-Or, 1984).

As a result of these differences in responses, children have a shorter tolerance time for exercise performed in the heat and experience a faster increase in core temperature when dehydration is a factor than adults. Thus, special concerns exist when children and adults exercise together in hot environments. Activity should be restricted for children to 30 min or less if the thermal conditions represent moderate or high risk (see Figure 15.1).

Children need a long and gradual acclimatization program to ensure that they are physiologically prepared for exercise in the heat (Rowland, 1990). Children subjectively feel acclimatized before physiological acclimatization has occurred, and thus, they are likely to try to do too much too soon.

Heat Illness

The magnitude of cardiovascular stress placed on the body by exercise in the heat was addressed by Rowell (1986):

Focus on Application

✳ Working under Extremes

Many occupational workers, such as construction workers, miners, and hazardous material crews, are routinely required to perform muscular work under extreme conditions. Probably no workers are exposed to higher thermal environments than are firefighters. Firefighters produce large amounts of metabolic heat and are often exposed to very high temperatures. Firefighters wear vapor-impermeable gear weighing approximately 20 kg and perform heavy muscular work, often in temperatures ranging from 100°C to 400°C. Thus, it is not surprising that firefighters experience severe cardiac strain. In fact, the leading cause of death in the line of duty among firefighters is myocardial infarction. It accounts for approximately 50% of the line-of-duty deaths each year—far more than deaths due to burn injuries (fewer than 10% in most years).

To better understand the magnitude of the cardiovascular stress, Smith et al. (2001) had firefighters perform three trials of a standardized set of firefighting tasks in a training building that contained live fires. Each set of drills took approximately 7 min to complete. A 10-min rest period was provided between the second and third trials, during which firefighters removed their helmet, face mask, and coats in an attempt to cool the body and were strongly encouraged to consume cold water. As seen in the accompanying graphs, HR increased quickly during the first trial and reached age-predicted maximal values by the end of the third trial. Stroke volume increased following the first trial but was significantly below resting values by the end of the third trial. Stroke volume was lower following several minutes of firefighting due to profuse sweating and vasodilation of cutaneous vessels. This occurred despite the attempt to cool the body and replace fluid during the 10-min rest period.

Because of the severe cardiovascular strain associated with firefighting and the risk of myocardial infarction, many fire departments are initiating fitness programs for their personnel. Aerobic fitness programs help lessen the cardiovascular strain associated with firefighting by increasing plasma volume and improving heart function.   ✳

Source:

Smith, et al. (2001).

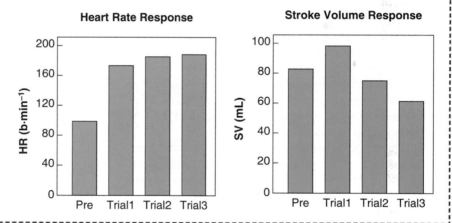

Heart Rate Response — HR (b·min⁻¹): Pre, Trial1, Trial2, Trial3

Stroke Volume Response — SV (mL): Pre, Trial1, Trial2, Trial3

Probably the greatest stress ever imposed on the human cardiovascular system is the combination of exercise and hyperthermia. Together these stresses can present life-threatening challenges, especially in highly motivated athletes who drive themselves to extremes in hot environments.

When the cardiovascular system is unable to meet the thermoregulatory and metabolic demands of the body, heat illness ensues. **Heat illness** represents a spectrum of disorders that range in intensity and severity from mild cardiovascular and central nervous system disruptions (for instance, hypotension and fainting) to severe cell damage, including the brain, kidney, and liver (heatstroke) (Hubbard and Armstrong, 1988). Heat illness may manifest itself in a number of ways; from least to most serious, heat illness can be categorized as heat cramps, heat syncope, heat exhaustion, and heatstroke.

Types of Heat Illness

Heat Cramps

Heat cramps are an acute disorder consisting of brief, recurrent, and excruciating pain in the voluntary muscles of the legs, arms, or abdomen. Typically, the

> **Heat Illness** A spectrum of disorders that range in intensity and severity from mild cardiovascular and central nervous system disruptions to severe cell damage, including the brain, kidney, and liver.

muscles have recently been engaged in intense physical activity. Heat cramps may result from a fluid-electrolyte imbalance.

Heat Syncope

Heat syncope is a temporary disorder characterized by circulatory failure due to pooling of blood in the peripheral veins and the subsequent decrease in ventricular filling, which leads to a decrease in cardiac output (Wenger, 1988). Thus, the individual feels light-headed and may faint. Heat syncope occurs most often when individuals perform strenuous and unaccustomed exercise or when they perform exercise during a sudden rise in temperature and/or humidity (Hubbard and Armstrong, 1988). Moving the individuals to a cooler location and having them rest in a recumbent position is the appropriate first aid treatment for heat syncope.

Heat Exhaustion

Heat exhaustion is characterized by a rapid and weak pulse, fatigue, weakness, profuse sweating, psychological disorientation, and fainting. The skin is often pale and clammy, and body temperature is near normal or moderately elevated (usually below 39.5°C). Heat exhaustion is caused by an acute fluid loss and the inability of the cardiovascular system to adequately compensate for the concurrent demands of muscle and skin blood flow.

Children may be more susceptible to heat exhaustion because they have a smaller plasma pool from which to decrease fluids. Thus, they have a potential for greater deficiency of peripheral blood supply during strenuous activity in the heat than adults (Zwiren, 1992).

Individuals suffering from heat exhaustion should be moved to a cool place, given fluids, and encouraged to lie down. In severe cases of heat exhaustion, a person may require intravenous administration of fluids and electrolytes.

Heatstroke

Heatstroke is a serious medical emergency; it is characterized by elevated skin and core temperatures (core temperature may exceed 40°C), tachycardia (rapid heart rate), vomiting, diarrhea, hallucinations, and coma. Because sweating has stopped, the skin is usually dry, hot, and red. Heatstroke represents a failure of the thermoregulatory mechanisms; thus, core temperature increases rapidly to dangerous levels. If heatstroke is suspected, the individual should be cooled as quickly as possible (using water, ice, or a fan) and medical personnel notified immediately. Heat stroke is a life-threatening medical emergency.

Prevention of Heat Illness

Although exercise professionals should be able to recognize and respond to heat illness, they should preferably prevent heat injuries by using sound judgment and observing some basic recommendations. The American College of Sports Medicine (ACSM) has published a position stand, "The Prevention of Thermal Injuries During Distance Running" (1987), that outlines strategies to decrease thermal injuries during road races. The following list provides basic recommendations for people who exercise in hot environments (Vogel, Rock, et al., 1993).

1. Allow adequate time for acclimatization (10–14 days).
2. Exercise during cooler parts of the day (early morning or evening).
3. Limit or defer exercise if the heat stress index is in the high-risk zone (see Figure 15.1).
4. Adequately hydrate prior to exercise and replace fluid loss during exercise. Monitor daily body weight changes closely, because they reflect acute water loss.
5. Wear clothing that is light in color and loose fitting, with large areas of skin exposed to the air to enhance evaporation.

Exercise in the Cold

Cold weather can cause significant injuries to individuals who are unprepared or inadequately equipped for exercise training or competition. Although cold-related injuries are less common than heat-related injuries, they can be serious. The most common instances of individuals' exercising in the cold are in sporting events and wilderness experiences. Sporting events include winter sports, such as skiing and ice skating, and athletic contests, such as football. During most of these activities, hypothermia is not a major threat, because individuals typically have proper clothing, are producing a great deal of metabolic heat, and have access to shelter if it is necessary. Wilderness activities, such as hiking and backpacking, present more risk because exposure can often be prolonged.

Exposure to cold results in several physiological responses that alter thermal balance: Heat production increases, and heat loss is minimized by vasoconstriction. Heat production increases owing to nonshivering thermogenesis, shivering thermogenesis, and exercise metabolism. *Nonshivering thermogenesis* refers to increased metabolic heat production from sources other than muscular contraction. Circulating hormones—namely, catecholamines, glucocorticoids, and thyroxine—increase metabolic rate during cold exposure (Toner and McArdle, 1988). Muscular tensing without noticeable shivering accounts for over 30% of the increase in heat liberation in response to cold exposure (Toner and McArdle, 1988). This response is sometimes called *preshivering*. Shivering can also contribute significantly to heat production. Exercise significantly increases metabolic heat.

To a large extent, cool temperatures are useful as a means of dissipating the large amount of heat produced by exercise. Very often, individuals who are exposed to the cold will voluntarily increase muscular activity as a means to increase heat production and thus feel more comfortable. Heat loss is minimized by widespread vasoconstriction, which decreases blood flow to the periphery in an attempt to maintain core temperature.

Despite the compensatory mechanisms, there are situations in which exercise in the cold leads to heat loss that exceeds heat production and body temperature drops. When an individual is exposed to cold environments and heat loss is greater than heat production, serious injuries can result. The two most common cold-induced injuries of concern to exercise professionals are hypothermia and frostbite (Vogel, Rock, et al., 1993).

Cold-Induced Injuries

Hypothermia, defined as a core temperature less than 35°C, is a lowering of the body temperature to the point that it affects normal function (Bar-Or and Baranowski, 1994). This condition is potentially fatal. The lowering of body temperature occurs when heat loss exceeds heat production. The magnitude of heat loss is affected by temperature, wind speed, and how wet the individual becomes. The windchill chart (Table 15.1) takes into account the combined effects of temperature and windspeed and should be consulted before activity is performed in the cold.

Heat production increases greatly during exercise. Thus, hypothermia is seldom a concern provided that the exerciser is properly clothed and is not exposed to the environment for prolonged periods of time. However, during long-term events, such as a marathon, hypothermia may occur owing to a reduction in heat production and an increase in heat loss. For instance, many runners will run the second half of a race at a slower pace; thus, heat production will decrease. At this time the runner may also have removed some clothing, because of greater heat production earlier in the run, and may be wet due to accumulated sweat, thus increasing the rate of conductive and evaporative heat loss.

As body temperature decreases, physical signs of hypothermia can be observed. Early signs of hypothermia include a depression of heart rate, respiration, and reflexes. Mild hypothermia is marked by a loss of judgment and an inability to reason. The person often complains of being cold and focuses attention on getting warm. As hypothermia progresses, fine motor skills are affected, and speech may become slurred. Severe hypothermia is characterized by agitation and inappropriate behavior (Vogel, Rock, et al., 1993). Mild hypothermia can be managed by warming the individual with blankets and warm beverages. However, moderate and severe cases of hypothermia should be treated by medical personnel. Because a person suffering from hypothermia often has an impaired ability to reason, the person should not be left alone.

Frostbite is the consequence of water crystallization within tissues that causes cellular dehydration and leads to tissue destruction (Vogel, Rock, et al., 1993). Insufficiently insulated skin can be frostbitten, leading to permanent circulatory damage and possible amputation. Activities that involve speed (such as running, skiing, and cycling) can create windchill conditions that increase the likelihood of frostbite.

Prevention of Cold-Induced Injuries

Preventing injury is preferable to treating injury. To avoid injury, individuals should exercise in appropriate clothing. Windproof and water-repellent outer garments are necessary. Layering loose-fitting clothing is more advantageous than wearing a single layer of heavy, bulky clothes. The layer next to the skin should be a material that wicks moisture away from the skin. Cotton should not be worn next to the skin because it holds moisture, which will draw heat away from the body.

Exercisers should consider warming up inside, but just to the point where they begin to sweat so that they aren't wet when they go outside. If possible, they should run into the wind first and return with the wind at their back. Exercisers should also avoid periods in which there is a decrease in metabolic heat production that is not compensated for by additional clothing or by leaving the cold environment. For instance, the cool-down period at the end of exercise is potentially dangerous because heat production in the exerciser has now decreased, although heat loss remains high. Additionally, the exerciser may be fatigued, which further exacerbates the condition. Thus, the exerciser should consider cooling down inside as well as warming up inside.

Influence of Age and Sex on Cold Tolerance

Body size and composition are important factors influencing an individual's response to cold exposure. Body fat provides protection against heat loss and can thus be advantageous when an individual is exposed to cold (Toner and McArdle, 1988). Because women on average have a greater percentage of body fat than men, they may tolerate cold better. Because children have a larger surface area per kilogram of body weight, they have a greater rate of heat loss in the cold than adults. To compensate for this loss, children have a greater degree of vasoconstriction in the periphery to protect core temperature. This compensatory factor, however, increases the risk of frostbite in the extremities (Bar-Or and Baranowski, 1994). Children also cool faster in water because of their higher surface area and smaller amount of subcutaneous fat than adults. Thus, special attention should be paid when children are swimming on cool days or when water temperatures are cool.

– – – – – –
Summary

1. Environmental conditions that affect human thermoregulation are ambient temperature (T_{amb}), relative humidity, and wind speed. The heat stress index assesses the risk of thermal injury from measures of ambient temperature and relative humidity. The windchill index assesses the risk of cold-induced injury from wind speed and ambient temperature.

   IP *Cardiovascular–Cardiac Output* (pages 1–10)*; *Cardiovascular–Factors that Affect Blood Pressure* (pages 13–14).

2. The temperature of the body is the result of a balance between heat gain and heat loss. The major contributor of heat gain is heat produced by the body as a result of metabolic heat production. Heat can be lost from the body by four processes: radiation, conduction, convection, and evaporation.

3. The evaporation of sweat is the primary defense against heat stress. For each liter of water that is vaporized, 580 kcal of heat energy is released.

4. The effectiveness of heat exchange depends on the thermal gradient, relative humidity, air movement, degree of direct sunlight, and clothing worn.

5. There are several interrelated problems that challenge the cardiovascular system under hyperthermic conditions.

   a. There is a competition for blood flow between the skin and the muscles.

   b. Vasodilation in the cutaneous vessels effectively decreases venous return and, thus, stroke volume.

   c. Adequate blood pressure must be maintained to perfuse the vital organs.

   d. There is a reduction in plasma volume, which contributes to the reduction in cardiac output.

6. An individual's response to exercise is influenced by the degree of acclimatization, cardiovascular fitness, body composition, and hydration level.

7. Scientific evidence suggests that the response of males and females to exercise in a hot environment is similar, although males appear to have a greater sweat rate.

8. Children are at greater risk of heat stress than adults when exercising in hot environments.

9. When the cardiovascular system is unable to meet the thermoregulatory and metabolic demands of the body, heat illness ensues. Heat illness represents a spectrum of disorders that range in intensity and severity; it includes heat cramps, heat syncope, heat exhaustion, and heatstroke.

10. During exercise in the cold, heat loss may exceed heat production. When heat loss is greater than heat production, serious injuries can result. The two most common cold-induced injuries of concern to exercise professionals are hypothermia and frostbite.

This topic is available on the InterActive Physiology® Sampler CD that comes with the purchase of a new copy of this book.

Review Questions

1. Diagram the thermal balance that is typically maintained at rest. Indicate how this balance is altered during exercise in hot and cold environments.

2. Identify the factors that influence heat exchange, and discuss how each factor facilitates or impedes the transfer of heat to and from the body.

3. Describe the cardiovascular response to incremental exercise in a hot environment. Explain why these responses occur.

4. What is the importance of acclimatization? How much time is needed for acclimatization to occur?

5. Explain the influence of hydration level on an individual's response to exercise in the heat. What is necessary to maintain adequate hydration during exercise?

6. Discuss the effects of fitness level and body composition on an individual's response to exercise in the heat.

7. Provide a definition, cause, and treatment for each of the following: heat cramps, heat syncope, heat exhaustion, and heatstroke.

8. Identify ways in which the likelihood of heat illness can be minimized.

9. Explain the underlying cause of hypothermia and frostbite. Suggest ways in which these conditions can be prevented.

For further review and additional study tools, go to The Physiology Place (www.physiologyplace.com) and the Student Study Guide for Exercise Physiology for Health, Fitness, and Performance by Sharon A. Plowman and Denise L. Smith.

Passport to the Internet

Visit the following Internet sites to explore further topics and issues related to thermoregulation. To visit an organization's web site, go to www.physiologyplace.com and click on "Passport to the Internet."

The American College of Sports Medicine As the leading professional organization for individuals in sports medicine and exercise science, the ACSM issues position statements on a number of topic critical to the study of exercise physiology. Search out the ACSM's position stands titled "The Prevention of Thermal Injuries during Distance Running" and "Exercise and Fluid Replacement."

Gatorade Sport Science Institute Members can access extensive information on sports nutrition and research. Read about the importance of hydration, and explore current research in the area.

References

American College of Sports Medicine: Position stand: The prevention of thermal injuries during distance running. *Medicine and Science in Sports and Exercise.* 19(5):529–533 (1987).

American College of Sports Medicine: Position stand: Exercise and fluid replacement. *Medicine and Science in Sports and Exercise.* 28(1):i–vii (1996).

Armstrong, L. E., & R. W. Hubbard: High and dry. *Runners World.* June:38–45 (1985).

Åstrand, P. O., & K. Rodahl: *Textbook of Work Physiology.* New York: McGraw-Hill (1986).

Avellini, B. A., E. Kamon, & J. T. Krajewski: Physiological responses of physicaOlly fit men and women to acclimation to humid heat. *Journal of Applied Physiology.* 49:254–261 (1980).

Avellini, B. A., Y. Shapiro, K. B. Pandolf, N. A. Pimental, & R. F. Goldman: Physiological responses of men and women to prolonged dry heat exposure. *Aviation Space Environmental Medicine.* 51:1081–1085 (1980).

Bar-Or, O.: Children and physical performance in warm and cold environments. In R. A. Boileau (ed.), *Advances in Pediatric Sport Sciences. Vol. 1: Biological Issues.* Champaign, IL: Human Kinetics, 117–130 (1984).

Bar-Or, O.: Children's responses to exercise in hot climates: Implications for performance and health. *Sports Science Exchange.* 7(2):1–4 (1994).

Bar-Or, O., & T. Baranowski: Physical activity, adiposity, and obesity among adolescents. *Pediatric Exercise Science.* 6(4): 348–360 (1994).

Cohen, J. S., & C. V. Gisolfi: Effects of interval training on work-heat tolerance of young women. *Medicine and Science in Sports and Exercise.* 14:46–52 (1982).

Coyle, E. F., & S. J. Montain: Thermal and cardiovascular responses to fluid replacement during exercise. In C. V. Gisolfi, D. R. Lamb, & E. R. Nadel (eds.), *Perspectives in Exercise Science and Sports Medicine. Vol. 6: Exercise, Heat, and Thermoregulation.* Indianapolis: Benchmark Press, 179–213 (1993).

Drinkwater, B. L.: Women and exercise: Physiological aspects. *Exercise and Sport Sciences Reviews.* 12:21–52 (1984).

Frye, A. J., & E. Kamon: Responses to dry heat of men and women with similar aerobic capacities. *Journal of Applied Physiology.* 50:65–70 (1981).

Frye, A. J., & E. Kamon: Sweating efficiency in acclimated men and women exercising in humid and dry heat. *Journal of Applied Physiology.* 54:972–977 (1983).

Gisolfi, C. V., & C. B. Wenger: Temperature regulation during exercise: Old concepts, new ideas. *Exercise and Sport Sciences Reviews.* 12: 339–372 (1984).

Henshell, A.: Obesity as an occupational hazard. *Canadian Journal of Public Health.* 58:491–497 (1967).

Hubbard, R. W., & L. E. Armstrong: The heat illnesses: Biochemical ultrastructural and fluid-electrolyte considerations. In K. B. Pandolf, M. N. Sawka, & R. R. Gonzalez (eds.), *Human Performance Physiology and Environmental Medicine at Terrestrial Extremes.* Dubuque, IA: Brown & Benchmark, 305–360 (1988).

Kenney, W. L., & R. K. Anderson: Responses of older and younger women to exercise in dry and humid heat without fluid replacement. *Medicine and Science in Sports and Exercise.* 20:155–160 (1988).

Marieb, E. N.: *Human Anatomy and Physiology* (5th edition). Redwood City, CA: Benjamin/Cummings (2001).

Nieman, D.C.: *Fitness and Sports Medicine: An Introduction.* Palo Alto, CA: Bull Publishing (1990).

Pandolf, K. B., B. S. Cadarette, M. N. Wawka, A. J. Young, R. P. Francesconi, & R. R. Gonzalez: Thermoregulatory responses of matched middle-aged and young men during dry-heat acclimation. *Journal of Applied Physiology.* 65(1): 65–71 (1988).

Pivarnik, J. M., C. J. Marichal, T. Spillman, & J. R. Marrow, Jr.: Menstrual cycle phase affects temperature regulation during endurance exercise. *Journal of Applied Physiology.* 72:543–548 (1992).

Rowell, L. B.: Human cardiovascular adjustments to exercise and thermal stress. *Physiological Reviews.* 54:75–159 (1974).

Rowell, L. B.: *Human Circulation Regulation During Physical Stress.* New York: Oxford University Press (1986).

Rowland, T. W.: *Exercise and Children's Health.* Champaign, IL: Human Kinetics (1990).

Sawka, M. N., & K. B. Pandolf: Effects of body water loss on physiological function and exercise performance. In C. V. Gisolfi & D. R. Lamb (eds.), *Perspectives in Exercise Science and Sports Medicine. Vol. 3: Fluid Homeostasis During Exercise.* Indianapolis: Benchmark Press, 1–38 (1990).

Sawka, M. N., & C. B. Wenger: Physiological responses to acute exercise-heat stress. In C. V. Gisolfi, D. R. Lamb, & E. R. Nadel (eds.), *Perspectives in Exercise Science and Sports Medicine. Vol. 6: Exercise, Heat, and Thermoregulation.* Indianapolis: Benchmark Press, 97–151 (1993).

Seals, D. R.: Influence of aging on autonomic-circulatory control at rest and during exercise in humans. In C. V. Gisolfi, D. R. Lamb, & E. R. Nadel (eds.), *Perspectives in Exercise Science and Sports Medicine. Vol. 6: Exercise, Heat, and Thermoregulation.* Indianapolis: Benchmark Press, 257–297 (1993).

Shapiro, Y., K. B. Pandolf, & R. F. Goldman: Predicting sweat loss response to exercise, environment and clothing. *European Journal of Applied Physiology.* 48:83–96 (1982).

Smith, D. L., T. S. Manning, & S. J. Petruzzello: The effect of strenuous live-fire drills on cardiovascular and psychological responses of recruit firefighters. *Ergonomics.* 44(3): 244–254 (2001).

Stephenson, L. A., & M. A. Kolka: Effect of gender, circadian period and sleep loss on thermal responses during exercise. In K. B. Pandolf, M. N. Sawka, & R. R. Gonzalez (eds.), *Human Performance Physiology and Environmental Medicine at Terrestrial Extremes.* Dubuque, IA: Brown & Benchmark, 267–304 (1988).

Stephenson, L. A., & M. A. Kolka: Thermoregulation in women. *Exercise and Sport Sciences Reviews.* 21:231–262 (1993).

Toner, M. M., & W. D. McArdle: Physiological adjustments of man to the cold. In K. B. Pandolf, M. N. Sawka, & R. R. Gonzalez (eds.), *Human Performance Physiology and Environmental Medicine at Terrestrial Extremes.* Dubuque, IA: Brown & Benchmark, 361–400 (1988).

Wade, C. E., & B. J. Freund: Hormonal control of blood volume during and following exercise. In C. V. Gisolfi & D. R. Lamb (eds.), *Perspectives in Exercise Science and Sports Medicine. Vol. 3: Fluid Homeostasis During Exercise.* Indianapolis: Benchmark Press, 201–246 (1990).

Wenger, C. B.: Human heat acclimatization. In K. B. Pandolf, M. N. Sawka, & R. R. Gonzalez (eds.), *Human Performance Physiology and Environmental Medicine at Terrestrial Extremes.* Dubuque, IA: Brown & Benchmark, 153–198 (1988).

Werner, J.: Temperature regulation during exercise: An overview. In C. V. Gisolfi, D. R. Lamb, & E. R. Nadel (eds.), *Perspectives in Exercise Science and Sports Medicine. Vol. 6: Exercise, Heat, and Thermoregulation.* Indianapolis: Benchmark Press, 49–79 (1993).

Winslow, C. E. A., A. P. Gagge, & L. P. Herrington: Influence of air movement upon heat losses from clothed human body. *American Journal of Physiology.* 127:505 (1939).

Wyndham, C. H., J. F. Morrison, & C. G. Williams: Heat reaction of male and female Caucasians. *Journal of Applied Physiology.* 20:357–364 (1965).

Wyndham, C. H., N. B. Strydom, J. F. Morrison, C. G. Williams, G. A. G. Bredell, M. J. E. Von Rahden, L. D. Holdsworth, C. H. Van Graan, A. J. Van Rensburg, and A. Munro: Heat reactions of Caucasians and Bantu in South Africa. *Journal of Applied Physiology.* 19:598–606 (1964).

Zwiren, L. D.: Children and exercise. In R. J. Shephard & H. S. Miller (eds.), *Exercise and the Heart in Health and Disease.* New York: Dekker, 105–163 (1992).

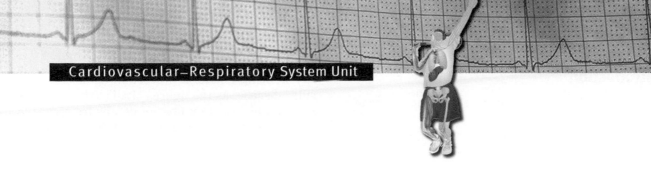

Chapter 16

Cardiovascular Disease Risk Factors and Physical Activity

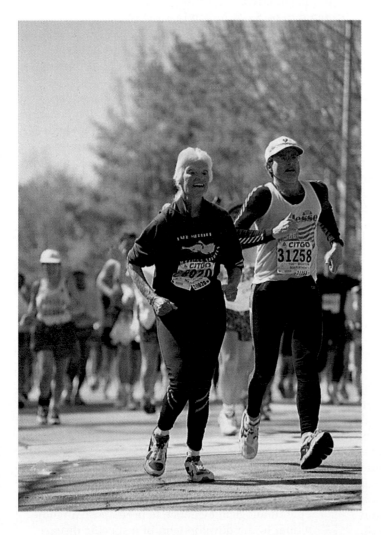

After studying the chapter, you should be able to

- Identify the cardiovascular risk factors and classify them as major risk factors that can or cannot be modified, contributing risk factors, or nontraditional risk factors.

- Describe the relationship between each risk factor and cardiovascular disease. Identify how exercise training impacts each of the risk factors.

- Track the cardiovascular risk factors from childhood to adulthood.

Introduction

Earlier in this unit a distinction was made between the application of the training principles for the achievement of health and for the achievement of fitness. The health factor of primary concern is cardiovascular disease. Cardiovascular disease (CVD) includes, but is not limited to, coronary heart disease (which can lead to myocardial infarctions or heart attacks), cerebrovascular disease (which can lead to strokes), hypertension, congestive heart failure, atherosclerosis and aneurysms, peripheral vascular diseases (which can lead to claudication, or severe calf pain during walking), and rheumatic heart diseases. Coronary heart disease (CHD) is the most prevalent of the subdivisions of cardiovascular disease (American Heart Association, 1993). This chapter will explore the relationships between physical activity and cardiovascular disease.

Physical Activity and Cardiovascular Risk Factors

Between 1980 and 1990 the total number of deaths from cardiovascular disease declined steadily in males from 510,000 per year to 450,000 per year in the United States. For females the death rate increased from 490,000 per year in 1980 to about 502,000 in 1988 and then decreased to approximately 478,000 per year in 1990. However, the age-adjusted death rate from cardiovascular disease again increased slightly from 1992–1993 (the last year for which date were available). Cardiovascular disease remains the leading cause of death in the United States, accounting for approximately 40% of all deaths (Hahn, et al., 1998; Hanson, 1993). This is true for both males and females and for all races (white, African American, Hispanic, Asian, and Native American). Someone dies from cardiovascular disease every 34 sec in the United States alone (American Heart Association, 1993). Worldwide, cardiovascular disease is also increasing as a cause of illness and death. It is projected that the proportion of worldwide deaths from cardiovascular disease will increase from 28.9% in 1990 to 36.3% in 2020 (Hanson, 1993).

Although in the United States the vast majority of deaths due to CVD (83%) occur in individuals over the age of 65, many individuals under the age of 65 have cardiovascular disease or acute heart attacks that do not immediately result in death. For example, 5% of all heart attacks occur in individuals under the age of 40, and 45% occur in people under the age of 65. Thus, old age increases the possibility of death from cardiovascular disease, but being young is not an automatic protection from impairment or death.

Nor is being female a protection against cardiovascular disease, as the figures cited earlier emphasize. In fact, the actual number of deaths from cardiovascular disease was higher in females than in males from 1984 to 1990. This result, however, is at least partially a reflection of a higher population of females than males. When prorated per 100,000 population, the age-adjusted death rates show that men do have a higher rate of death from cardiovascular disease, by approximately 50%, than women. At the same time, though, women who have had heart attacks are more likely to die from them within a few weeks to a year, or to suffer a second heart attack, than men who have had heart attacks (American Heart Association, 1993).

If the data are further subdivided by sex and race, the order from highest to lowest death rate is black males, white males, black females, and white females. Figures are unavailable for the other races (American Heart Association, 1993). The economic cost of cardiovascular disease, including all medical care and lost productivity resulting from disability, was estimated to be $128 billion in 1994 (American Heart Association, 1994), but had escalated to $286.5 billion in 1999 (U.S. Department of Health and Human Services, Centers for Disease Control and Prevention [CDC], 1999).

Because of the statistics just listed, age, race, and sex are considered to be risk factors for coronary heart disease. A **risk factor** is defined as an aspect of personal behavior or lifestyle, an environmental exposure, or an inherited characteristic that has been shown by epidemiological evidence to predispose an individual to the development of a specific disease (Caspersen and Heath, 1993). Table 16.1 lists various classifications of risk factors for coronary heart disease (American Heart Association, 1993). Note that the three factors already identified, along with heredity, constitute risk factors that cannot be changed. The point at which age becomes a risk factor for males is 45 yr; it is 55 yr for females, or the time of menopause without estrogen replacement. Heredity is interpreted as a family history (parent or sibling) with premature (less than 55 yr of age if male; less than 65 yr of age if female) cardiovascular disease or death from cardiovascular disease, especially heart attack or stroke. A family history of coronary revascularization (bypass surgery), diabetes mellitus, hypertension, and/or high

---

Risk Factor An aspect of personal behavior or lifestyle, an environmental exposure, or an inherited characteristic that has been shown by epidemiological evidence to predispose an individual to the development of a specific disease.

Table 16.1

Coronary Heart Disease Risk Factors

Factors That Cannot Be Changed	Major Factors That Can Be Modified	Contributing and Selected Nontraditional Factors
Age	Cholesterol-lipid fractions	Apolipoproteins
Heredity	Cigarette smoking	Fibrinogen levels
Race	Diabetes mellitus	Fibrinolytic activity
Sex	Hypertension	Stress
	Obesity	
	Physical inactivity	

cholesterol levels (hyperlipidemia) also increases the risk of coronary heart disease.

The major risk factors are, to some degree, modifiable through diet, exercise, medication, or other lifestyle changes. This section will discuss each of these risk factors and the role of physical activity or exercise training in modifying each. Each major risk factor acts independently and will be discussed separately, but many are also interrelated and act jointly. Furthermore, the list of contributing and nontraditional factors could be much longer, because the traditional factors predict only slightly more than 50% of the incidence of coronary heart disease. Particularly interesting potential additions to the list of nontraditional risk factors include homocysteine, a procoagulant (proclotting) factor that may also induce direct injury to blood vessel endothelium (Gordon, 1998; Hanson, 1993) and C-reactive protein. Infection, smoking, diabetes, and dental disease all increase proinflammatory cytokines. Proinflammatory cytokines increase the amount of C-reactive protein, which is thought to be a marker indicating systemic inflammation. Proinflammatory cytokines also increase coagulation and unfavorably impact blood lipids. Serum homocysteine levels appear to be reduced by B vitamins (B_6, B_{12}, and folate, in particular), while proinflammatory cytokines may be reduced by aspirin, other nonsteroidal antiinflammatory drugs, and antioxidants (Gordon, 1998, Hanson, 1993).

Major Modifiable Risk Factors

Cholesterol-Lipid Fractions

Lipids, or fats, are by definition water-insoluble substances. They may be classified as simple (or neutral) fats, compound fats, or derived fats. The primary simple fat is triglyceride. Compound fats are combinations of a neutral fat and another substance such as phosphate (phospholipid), glucose (glucolipid), or protein (lipoprotein). Derived fats originate from simple and compound fats. Chief among them is **cholesterol,** a derived fat that is essential for the body but may be detrimental in excessive amounts.

Combining fats with another substance makes the compound water-soluble, and it is through such compounds—specifically **lipoproteins**—that fat is transported in the bloodstream. The protein portions of lipoproteins are called **apolipoproteins.** Five types of lipoproteins circulate in blood, namely chylomicrons, very low density lipoproteins, intermediate-density lipoproteins, low-density lipoproteins, and high-density lipoproteins. *Chylomicrons* are microscopic fat particles formed after digestion that enter the bloodstream via the lymphatic system. Triglycerides and some cholesterol are transported in the blood, from the small intestines or liver to adipose tissue or muscle for storage or use as fuel, by chylomicrons and *very low density lipoproteins* (VLDL). The VLDL from which the triglyceride has been removed is degraded into an *intermediate-density lipoprotein* (IDL), which in turn is converted in the liver to a **low-density lipoprotein (LDL).** LDL is composed of protein, a small portion of triglyceride, and a large portion of cholesterol. LDL transports 60–70% of the total cholesterol in the body to all cells except liver cells. The major apolipoprotein of LDL is called *Apo-B.*

The process of atherosclerosis begins when the following conditions are present: more cholesterol is made available to the cells than is needed; an area of injury is present in the wall of the artery; and LDL is oxidized (modified) by free radicals (see the Focus on Application box in Chapter 6) and interacts with macrophage immune cells responding to the arterial wall injury and to chronically elevated levels of LDL. Initial injury to the endothelium of the arterial wall may result from chemical irritants in tobacco smoke,

Cholesterol A derived fat that is essential for the body but may be detrimental in excessive amounts.

Lipoprotein Water-soluble compound composed of apolipoprotein and lipid components that transport fat in the bloodstream.

Apolipoprotein The protein portion of lipoproteins.

Low-Density Lipoprotein (LDL) A lipoprotein in blood plasma composed of protein, a small portion of triglyceride, and a large portion of cholesterol whose purpose is to transport cholesterol to the cells.

hypertension and resultant turbulent blood flow, high cholesterol levels, immune complexes, vasoconstrictor substances, homocysteine, and viral or bacterial infection. An inflammatory response on the part of the immune system is a normal reaction to such an injury. The process may begin in childhood and progress for years before any symptoms of disease occur (Squires, 1998). It is important to distinguish *atherosclerosis* from *arteriosclerosis*. **Arteriosclerosis** encompasses the natural aging changes that occur in blood vessels—namely, thickening of the wall, loss of elastic connective tissue, and hardening of the vessel wall. **Atherosclerosis** is a pathological process that results in the buildup of *plaque* (composed of connective tissue, smooth muscle cells, cellular debris, and cholesterol) inside the blood vessels.

Ultimately, the buildup of plaque, often in conjunction with a blood clot (thrombus), will obstruct blood flow. The primary sites of plaque growth are the aorta and the carotid, coronary, femoral, and iliac arteries. Depending on the amount of obstruction, the result can be pain (angina pectoris in the heart or claudication in the legs) or a heart attack or stroke.

High-density lipoprotein (HDL) is a lipoprotein in blood plasma composed primarily of protein and a minimum of cholesterol or triglyceride. The purpose of HDL is to transport cholesterol from the tissues to the liver. HDL carries cholesterol away from the tissue to the liver, where the cholesterol can be broken down and eliminated in the bile. There is also some speculation that HDL may block or in some way interfere with the deposition of cholesterol in the arterial wall lining. The subfraction of HDL that protects from CVD is HDL_2. The major apolipoprotein of HDL is called *Apo-A1* (Squires and Williams, 1993).

Triglycerides (but not the associated VLDLs) represent a risk factor by themselves—that is, they act as an independent risk factor (Summary of the Third Report of the National Cholesterol Education Program [NCEP], 2001). Chylomicrons are not thought to be

---

Arteriosclerosis The natural aging changes that occur in blood vessels—namely thickening of the walls, loss of elastic connective tissue, and hardening of the vessel wall.

Atherosclerosis A pathological process that results in the buildup of plaque inside the blood vessels.

High-Density Lipoprotein (HDL) A lipoprotein in blood plasma composed primarily of protein and a minimum of cholesterol or triglyceride whose purpose is to transport cholesterol from the tissues to the liver.

Table 16.2

Classification of Total, LDL, HDL Blood Cholesterol Levels, and Triglycerides

Lipid and Category	Level for Adults ($mg \cdot dL^{-1}$)	Level for Children and Adolescents ($mg \cdot dL^{-1}$)
Total cholesterol		
Desirable	< 200	< 170
Borderline	200–239	170–199
High	≥ 240	≥ 200
LDL cholesterol		
Optimal	< 100	< 110
Near optimal	100–129	
Borderline high	130–159	110–129
High	160–189	130
Very high	≥ 190	
HDL cholesterol		
Low	< 40	
High	≥ 60	
Triglyceride level		
Normal	< 150	
Borderline high	150–199	
High	200–499	

Sources: Summary of the Third Report of the National Cholesterol Education Program (2001); U. S. Department of Health and Human Services (1991).

atherosclerotic. There is abundant evidence, however, that an elevated total cholesterol (TC) level is independently and directly related to the incidence of CHD. A classification system for TC is presented in Table 16.2 (Summary of the Third Report of the National Cholesterol Education Program, 2001; U.S. Department of Health and Human Services, 1991). In the United States, an adult level of 240 $mg \cdot dL^{-1}$ represents twice the risk as a value of 200 $mg \cdot dL^{-1}$. Therefore, these values have been taken as representing high-risk and desirable levels, respectively. They apply to all adults regardless of age or sex. (The information on children will be considered later.) The term *hyperlipidemia* (excessive fat in the blood) is commonly used to describe this risk factor.

Not only is the total amount of cholesterol important, but also the fractions of LDL and/or HDL in that total are important. High levels of LDL and/or Apo-B are positively related to CHD. High levels of HDL and/or Apo-A1 are inversely related to CHD. Optimal levels of LDL are 100 $mg \cdot dL^{-1}$ or less. Low levels of HDL are 40 $mg \cdot dL^{-1}$ or less. An HDL level greater than or equal to 60 mg·dL^{-1} is actually so good that it is said to be a negative risk factor (see Table 16.2). Some consider a decrease in Apo-A1 and/or an increase in Apo-B to be independent risk factors (U.S. Department of Health and Human Services, 1991; Wood and Stefanik, 1990). However, specific levels have not been agreed on and so the apolipoproteins are considered here to be nontraditional risk factors.

The impact of exercise on lipid levels may be both transient (a last-bout effect from a single bout of exercise) and chronic (a consistent adaptation resulting from exercise training). Triglycerides, total cholesterol, and LDL all decease the 24–48 hours following vigorous aerobic exercise, and HDL may increase. Many of these changes appear to require 9–12 months of training to become more or less permanent (Thomas and LaFontaine, 1998).

Cross-sectional studies in adults have generally shown that active individuals have lipid profiles indicating a reduced risk for CHD. This result is true at least as far as TC (lower in more active) and HDL (higher in more active) are concerned. However, there is little, if any, difference in LDL levels between active and inactive individuals. Cross-sectional studies, however, are by their very design difficult to interpret, because the element of self-selection is always a danger. Perhaps individuals who have a good cholesterol profile are simply more likely to be active. This problem can be overcome by the use of training studies. In general, exercise training studies have supported a reduction in TC levels, but often not to statistically significant levels. Likewise, LDL levels have not shown significant reductions as a result of exercise training. On the other hand, all studies with a duration of greater than 12 weeks and a training volume of the equivalent of at least 15 km·wk^{-1} of running or 1000–1200 kcal·wk^{-1} of aerobic activity have shown a significant increase in HDL levels. There is probably a dose-response relationship such that more vigorous activity and a higher total calorie expenditure will exhibit greater HDL increases. Triglycerides are also consistently reduced (Wood and Stefanik, 1990).

The direct impact of exercise training on the process of atherosclerosis has been difficult to document in humans. However, in a 1992 study (Schuler, et al., 1992) one group of patients was placed on a low-fat diet (less than 20% of total calories, less than 200 mg of cholesterol), and a high-intensity daily aerobic exercise program (75% HRmax). This study showed that 32% of the subjects experienced a regression in their coronary atherosclerotic lesion, 45% stayed the same, and only 23% exhibited a progression in their lesions. These figures were significantly better than the changes in the control group, who were advised to eat less fat and to exercise but were left to their own initiatives. Other studies have supported this tendency (Froelicher, 1990; LaFontaine, 1994; Squires and Williams, 1993; Wood and Stefanik, 1990). Individuals who participate exclusively in anaerobic training programs, including dynamic resistance training, appear to have lipid profiles similar to those of untrained individuals (Thomas and LaFontaine, 1998).

Although the results from exercise training studies are not as conclusive as might be desired, they are sufficient for the National Institutes of Health to support the statement that "the appropriate use of physical activity is considered an essential element in the nonpharmacologic therapy of elevated serum cholesterol" (U.S. Department of Health and Human Services, 1991). Physical activity, of course, is to be used in conjunction with a low-fat diet and weight loss.

Cigarette Smoking

Nearly 20% of the deaths from cardiovascular disease can be directly attributed to cigarette smoking (American Heart Association, 1993). Smoking one pack a day doubles the risk compared to not smoking, while smoking more than one pack a day triples the risk. Breathing second-hand smoke also increases the risk of heart disease (American Heart Association, 1994). Cigar and pipe smokers have a higher risk of CVD than nonsmokers but less than that of cigarette smokers.

The chemicals in cigarettes, particularly nicotine, stimulate the sympathetic nervous system, causing an acute increase in heart rate and blood pressure, thus making the heart work harder. The carbon monoxide produced binds with hemoglobin, thus reducing oxygen transport. The atherosclerotic process is accelerated because smoking injures the arterial wall lining, increases the levels of circulating TC, and decreases the amount of HDL.

Smoking also causes blood platelets to adhere to each other, speeds up the rate of internal blood clotting, and makes the clots that do form tougher to dissolve. Prostacyclin, which is partially responsible for blood vessel dilation, is decreased. Capillaries and small arteries constrict and may spasm shut. Thus, the possibility of a thrombis (clot) or an embolism (moving clot) blocking an artery already narrowed by atherosclerosis is enhanced.

Narrowing of blood vessels to the arms and legs also makes smokers vulnerable to peripheral vascular disease, which may lead to gangrene and amputation. Certain life-threatening dysrhythmias of the heartbeat can also occur. Thus, smoking both operates independently and contributes to other CHD risk factors (American Heart Association, 1994; Caspersen and Heath, 1993; Squires and Williams, 1993; Wood and Stefanik, 1990).

The relationship between exercise training and smoking is only indirect. One study of over 3000 individuals showed a consistent and statistically significant inverse relationship between the number of cigarettes smoked and the level of physical activity in both males and females (Dannenberg, et al., 1989). Another study (a random sampling of Peachtree Road Race runners) indicated that 85% of both men and women had never smoked. In addition, 81% of the men and 75% of the women who had smoked when they began running had since stopped. Only 1% of the men and 2% of the women who were nonsmokers began to smoke after beginning to run (Koplan, et al., 1982). Although these results are encouraging, there is no direct cause-and-effect relationship. You probably know someone who is active or a good athlete who also smokes. Individuals must make a conscious decision to not smoke. It takes 15 years of abstinence for the risk of former smokers to approach that of lifelong nonsmokers (Hahn, et al., 1998).

Diabetes Mellitus

Diabetes mellitus is a complex metabolic disorder characterized by the inability to use carbohydrates effectively (glucose intolerance). The 1997 classification divides diabetes into four categories according to etiology (cause): Type 1, Type 2, gestational (onset during pregnancy), and other. Only Type 1 and Type 2 will be considered here. Type 2 accounts for 90–95% of all cases of diabetes in the United States.

Type 1 diabetes is most common in childhood and adolescence but is occurring more frequently in older individuals. In Type 1 diabetes, an environmentally triggered autoimmune process destroys the insulin-producing beta cells in the pancreas. Thus, an external source of insulin must be supplied.

Type 2 diabetes is a progressive disease whose diagnosis is often delayed for years. The underlying causes of Type 2 diabetes are insulin resistance (an inability to achieve normal rates of glucose uptake in response to insulin) and defective secretion of insulin by pancreatic beta cells. Insulin resistance typically precedes the onset of Type 2 diabetes and is characterized by slight elevations in blood sugar level (impaired glucose tolerance) that get progressively higher until a level denoting actual diabetes is attained.

The upper limit for normal fasting glucose is <110 mg·dL^{-1}. Values between 110 and 125 mg·dL^{-1} are designated as impaired fasting glucose (IFG). The threshold for the diagnosis of diabetes is 126 mg·dL^{-1} (American College of Sports Medicine [ACSM], 2000; Colberg, 2001; Grundy, et al., 1999). Insulin resistance develops from obesity (predominantly abdomi-

nal visceral obesity) and a lack of physical activity superimposed on a genetic predisposition (ACSM, 2000; Grundy, et al., 1999). Type 2 diabetes used to occur predominantly in adults over the age of 40 but in recent years has become more and more prevalent in younger individuals, including children and adolescents. Early in the progression of Type 2 diabetes, insulin may be produced in sufficient or even excessive amounts. Thus, individuals with Type 2 diabetes are initially not insulin dependent, but eventually approximately 40% of these individuals will require insulin injections. Among the multitude of pathological complications resulting from diabetes is an acceleration of atherosclerosis, impaired myocardial contraction, poor peripheral perfusion, and alterations in blood coagulation mechanisms, including increased fibrinogen levels (Hanson, 1993). Impaired fasting glucose, Type 1 diabetes, and Type 2 diabetes are all independent risk factors for cardiovascular disease (ACSM, 2000; Grundy, et al., 1999).

One of the acute effects of submaximal dynamic endurance exercise is an increase in non–insulin-dependent uptake of glucose into the active skeletal muscle. This effect continues postexercise while the depleted stores of glucose (as glycogen) are restored. Additionally, studies have shown an increased insulin sensitivity as a result of exercise training. These changes are transient last-bout or augmented last-bout effects persisting from 12 to 72 hours, so they rely on a constant pattern of exercise. However, they are often sufficient to permit a reduction in the amount of daily insulin that needs to be injected in Type 1 diabetics. Regular exercise training, along with body weight or fat loss, has been shown to restore near-normal glucose tolerance and to increase insulin sensitivity in individuals with Type 2 diabetes (Hanson, 1993). The favorable change in glucose tolerance is also a last-bout effect with a window of approximately 72 hours (ACSM, 2000).

The use of exercise training for individuals with diabetes requires close monitoring and should be done in conjunction with medical personnel. Individuals with diabetes, especially Type 1 individuals, often exhibit abnormal blood pressure and other cardiovascular responses to exercise. Insulin injection (amount and site that avoids working muscles) and carbohydrate ingestions must be carefully adjusted to prevent the exercising diabetic from developing hypoglycemia (ACSM 2000; Colberg, 2001; Hanson, 1993).

Hypertension

One in every four American adults has *hypertension* (American Heart Association, 1993). However, there is wide variation based on race and sex. The

Focus on Research

Understanding Short-Term Inactivity

Arciero, P. J., D. L. Smith, & J. Calles-Escandon. Effects of short-term inactivity on glucose tolerance, energy expenditure, and blood flow in trained subjects. *Journal of Applied Physiology.* 74(4):1365–1373 (1998).

Endurance training improves glucose tolerance and enhances insulin sensitivity. This means that if a trained individual ingests a given amount of glucose, that glucose is transported into the cells more readily, leaving less glucose in the blood than in the blood of an untrained individual. Insulin plays an important role in moving glucose from the blood to the cells by enhancing glucose transporters on the cell membrane (GLUT-4 transporters) and possibly by increasing blood flow. The reversibility principle states that when training is discontinued, adaptations are lost. The reversibility of metabolic adaptations can occur quickly; in fact, it is known that 7–10 days of detraining reduces glucose tolerance. However, it was not known whether this decrease is attributable to changes in GLUT-4 transporters only or whether blood flow is also altered in 7–10 days of detraining. Arciero and colleagues (1998) designed a study to determine whether 7–10 days of detraining (from a highly trained state) resulted in changes in blood flow that were associated with a decline in glucose tolerance and insulin sensitivity.

Arciero and coworkers tested highly trained male endurance athletes on two occasions: one when the participants were in a highly trained state, and one after they refrained from exercise training for a period of 7–10 days (detrained). During the testing period, the athletes ingested a known amount of glucose (75 g) and had blood samples taken for the next 3 hr—this is known as an oral glucose tolerance test (OGTT). Blood flow was measured in the forearm and calf before and during the OGTT. The graphs below present blood glucose and blood insulin data that were obtained in the trained and detrained state.

These data reveal the following:

1. There was a greater blood glucose response following the ingesting of 75 g of glucose in the detrained state compared to the trained state, despite higher insulin levels. This is consistent with earlier studies that showed that endurance training increases glucose tolerance.

2. Calf blood flow was lower in the detrained state than in the trained state after ingestion of the OGTT. Resting calf blood flow was not different between the two conditions.

These data suggest that blood flow may be an important element in enhancing the ability of muscles to extract glucose from the blood in the trained state. As with most research, this study invites future inquiry, specifically to explore the relationship between blood flow and glucose tolerance in different populations and at different points in a training or detraining program.

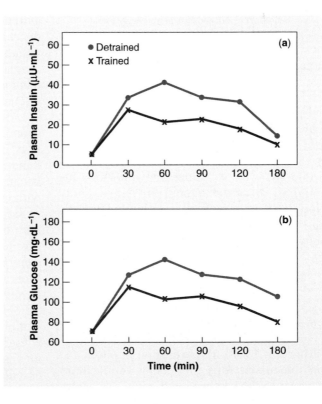

Table 16.3

Classification of Blood Pressure for Adults, Children, and Adolescents

Category	Systolic (mmHg)	Diastolic (mmHg)
Adults (≥ 19 yr)		
Normal	< 130	< 85
High Normal	130–139	85–89
Hypertension		
Stage I (mild)	140–159	90–99
Stage II (moderate)	160–179	100–109
Stage III (severe)	190–209	110–119
Stage IV (very severe)	≥ 210	≥ 120
Children (3–12)*		
Mild-moderate	≥ 130	≥ 86
Severe	≥ 144	≥ 96
Adolescents†		
Mild-moderate	≥ 144	≥ 90
Severe	≥ 160	≥ 104

* Values less than the 90th percentile for age and sex can be considered normal, and values between the 90th and 95th percentile abnormal.

† Values at or above the 95th percentile for age and sex indicate hypertension.

Source: National High Blood Pressure Education Program (1993).

age-adjusted prevalence from hypertension is 33.5% for black males, 29.5% for black females, 24.85% for white males, and 21.0% for white females (Hall, 1999). The various stages of hypertension are presented in Table 16.3. These values are applicable to both sexes and all races throughout the entire adult life span. Note that the cutoff for defining **hypertension,** or high blood pressure, is 140/90 mmHg but readings between 130/85 and 140/90 mmHg represent values where lifestyle modifications should begin. All stages of hypertension are associated with an increased risk of cardiovascular disease. The higher the stage of hypertension, the higher the risk of CHD is and the more aggressive the monitoring and treatment need to be (National High Blood Pressure Education Program, 1993). Hypertension imposes an afterload on the heart, thus increasing ventricular muscle hypertrophy (thickness) and reducing early diastolic filling. Hypertension is a leading factor in arterial wall injury and calcium deposition in the coronary arteries, as well as thickening and stiffening of

smaller blood vessels. The process of atherosclerosis occurs in hypertensive individuals at a rate that is 2–3 times that of normotensive individuals (Kannel and Wilson, 1999; Stewart, 1998).

Ninety to 95% of the cases of hypertension have no known cause. Such hypertension is called *primary* or *essential hypertension.* However, for hypertension to occur, either cardiac output ($\dot{Q}$) or total peripheral resistance (TPR), or both, must be elevated. The most likely scenario is a transient increase in $\dot{Q}$ followed by an elevation in TPR, both brought about by overactivity of cardiac sympathetic nerves (Izzo, 1999), that attempts to decrease $\dot{Q}$ and is itself sustained. The resultant high blood pressure may injure the artery linings and begin the process of atherosclerosis (Hagberg, 1990).

The role of exercise training in the treatment of moderate hypertension is well substantiated by research. Individuals who are at high risk for developing hypertension—because of either genetics, body composition, primary disease status, or exaggerated blood pressure response to acute exercise—can reduce the risk by participating in an endurance training program. Most, albeit not all, hypertensive individuals in well-designed and controlled studies have decreased both systolic and diastolic pressures by about 10 mmHg with aerobic endurance exercise programs. Light to moderate exercise (40–60% $\dot{V}O_2$max) has been shown to be equal to or better than higher-intensity programs.

Most studies have found that blood pressure responds quickly to exercise training; that is, the reduction in blood pressure occurs within 3 weeks to 3 months after the start of the training, often does not become fully normalized, and does not reduce further with continued training. If the training is stopped, the resting blood pressure returns to the elevated level. It may be that at least part of the reduction in blood pressure is a function of each individual exercise session rather than a permanent training adaptation, for even single sessions of submaximal exercise result in a reduced blood pressure for 1–9 hr postexercise (ACSM, 1993; Hagberg, 1990). That is, blood pressure exhibits a last-bout or augmented last-bout effect rather than a chronic adaptation to training. This means that maintenance of the training program is essential for keeping blood pressure lowered. These training changes seem to occur across the age spectrum of 15–79 yr and apply equally to males and females (American Heart Association, 1994), although females generally demonstrate a greater reduction in blood pressure than males who follow a similar training program (ACSM, 1993; Hagberg, 1990).

Dynamic aerobic endurance exercise training can also benefit individuals with severe or very

---

Hypertension High blood pressure, defined as values equal to or greater than 140/90 mmHg.

severe hypertension. In this case, however, pharmacological therapy should be initiated first and then an exercise program added. Such a sequencing leads to a further reduction in blood pressure and ultimately a decreased reliance on antihypertensive medication (ACSM, 1993; Hagberg, 1990; Simons-Morton, 1999).

The pressor response accompanying dynamic resistance training has always been of great concern, and individuals with hypertension have historically been discouraged from doing weight lifting. Studies on resistance exercise, however, have failed to substantiate an adverse effect on blood pressure. At the same time, dynamic resistance training (with the exception of circuit weight training) has not consistently been shown to lower blood pressure in individuals with hypertension, although a recent meta-analysis found an average reduction of approximately 5 mmHg in systolic blood pressure and 4 mmHg in diastolic blood pressure with no difference between normotensive individuals and hypertensive individuals (Kelley, 1997). Therefore, although the cardiovascular changes elicited by endurance training are more desirable than the changes brought about by resistance training, dynamic resistance training can be done by hypertensive individuals as part of a comprehensive training program. Strength training should not be the only exercise program, though, and it is best if added after 2 or 3 months of typical aerobic endurance training (Caspersen and Heath, 1993).

Obesity

The relationship between obesity and CHD is both independent of and interrelated with the other cardiovascular risk factors in a progressive disease process known as *Metabolic Syndrome* (Gordon, 1998; Kannel and Wilson, 1999; Welk and Blair, 2000). Syndrome X occurs in the presence of high amounts of visceral abdominal fat. Under the stimulation of the enzyme lipoprotein lipase, visceral abdominal adipocytes readily release free fatty acids (FFA) into the circulation. Two fates are possible for the FFA: (1) the FFA may be transported to the liver (where they are converted to VLDL and ultimately LDL cholesterol); or (2) they may be taken up by other cells, including skeletal muscle cells, and oxidized to provide ATP energy by cellular respiration. This enhancement of lipid oxidation may lead to a reduction in the use of glucose as a fuel. At the same time, the increased FFA levels act directly in the liver to inhibit insulin clearance, resulting in hyperinsulinemia. Hyperinsulinemia combined with high levels of blood glucose lead to a reduction in insulin sensitivity. This combination (high glucose and

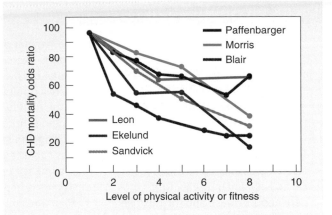

Figure 16.1

Relationship between Activity Level and Mortality from Coronary Heart Disease

Source: W. S. L. Haskell. Health consequence of physical activity: Understanding and challenges regarding dose response. *Medicine and Science in Sports and Exercise.* 26(6):649–660 (1994). Reprinted by permission of Williams & Wilkins.

decreased insulin sensitivity) can hasten the development of Type 2 diabetes. Hyperinsulinemia also increases sodium retention and in susceptible salt-sensitive individuals may precipitate hypertension. Thus, high visceral abdominal obesity is directly related to *dyslipidemia* (low HDL and high triglycerides), reduced glucose tolerance, insulin resistance, and hypertension, which together form a cluster of risk factors for cardiovascular disease (Buemann and Tremblay, 1996; Gordon, 1998; Kannel and Wilson, 1999; Welk and Blair, 2000).

The impact of exercise training on visceral and total body obesity is detailed in the metabolic unit of this text. The impact of exercise training on each of the other risk factors in the cluster of Metabolic Syndrome is described in the appropriate sections of this chapter. Suffice it to say that in general, physical activity and exercise training bring about beneficial changes that limit the progression of Metabolic Syndrome, with or without changes in total body weight and composition (Buemann and Tremblay, 1996; Welk and Blair, 2000).

Physical Inactivity

Figure 16.1 shows the relationship between level of physical activity or fitness ($\dot{V}O_2max$) on the horizontal axis and the CHD mortality odds ratio on the vertical axis (Haskell, et al., 1993). The odds ratio was computed by dividing the rate of deaths from CHD for more active or more fit individuals by the rate of

Focus on Application

✳ The Impact of a Change in Physical Fitness on Cardiovascular Disease Mortality

The text of this chapter describes the inverse relationship between physical activity and mortality from coronary heart disease and the positive impacts of exercise training on each cardiovascular disease risk factor. The studies cited in the chapter relating physical activity or physical fitness to mortality, however, generally utilized only a single baseline evaluation of activity or fitness with subsequent follow-up to determine the incidence of death from cardiovascular causes. Although extremely important, these results could have been influenced both by genetics and by changes in risk factor status between the baseline testing and time of death. Conversely, the studies of exercise training had both pretraining and posttraining evaluations but did not examine the overall impact on

cardiovascular mortality. From a public health, exercise professional, and personal perspective, the overall goal of exercise training is to enhance both the quality and quantity of life. It is important to determine whether improving and maintaining physical fitness can attain these goals. Therefore, a linkage between the two types of studies is important.

Blair and colleagues (1995) studied the mortality rates and relative risk of death ratios from cardiovascular disease of 9777 men who had at least two complete examinations at the Cooper Institute for Aerobics Research between 1970 and 1989. The average interval between the two testing sessions was 4.0 ± 4.1 yr, and the average follow-up for mortality was 5.1 ± 4.2 yr, but the range was 1–18 yr for both. Treadmill time to volitional fatigue, converted to maximal oxygen uptake, was the measure of cardiovascular physical fitness. Individuals whose results fell into the bottom quintile (lowest 20%) based on age-adjusted results (< 35 mL·kg^{-1}·min^{-1}, 20–39 yr;

< 32.2 mL·kg^{-1}·min^{-1}, 40–49 yr; < 29.4 mL·kg^{-1}·min^{-1}, 50–59 yr; < 24.5 mL·kg^{-1}·min^{-1}, 60+ yr) were labeled unfit. Everyone else, that is, individuals in quintiles (Q) 2, 3, 4, and 5, was labeled fit. Men who were unfit at both testing times had the highest death rate from CVD; men who were fit at both testing times had the lowest death rate; and men who changed fitness status between testing sessions had intermediate death rates, as shown in panel (a) of the accompanying graph. Although the values for the men who changed fitness status appear to be similar, these must be interpreted relative to the direction of the change. The unfit men who moved out of the lowest quintile died at a rate less than half that of those who remained unfit, whereas those who moved from fit to unfit increased their death rate by approximately 25%. When changes in status occurred among the four upper quartiles, a dose-response relationship was seen. A low mortality rate was evident in men who remained in quintiles 2 and 3; a lower

death for the least active or least fit individuals. A definite inverse relationship is shown in the graph. That is, the more active or fit individuals have lower odds of death from CHD than the least active or least fit individuals. Of course, the relationship is not a perfect one and offers no guarantee for any given individual, but physical activity does tip the odds in a favorable direction for the population as a whole. Additional evidence suggests that even individuals with documented CHD can benefit from physical activity and reduce their likelihood of additional heart attacks or sudden death (Schuler, et al., 1992).

The degree of risk for those who are inactive, about twice that of those without the risk factor, is approximately the same for physical inactivity as for systolic hypertension, cigarette smoking, and hyperlipidemia. However, the number of individuals who are sedentary is substantially more than the number possessing the other risk factors. Only about 10% of Americans report exercising daily for at least 30 min. Therefore, potentially more benefit overall could be

achieved by increasing the activity level of U.S. citizens than by changing any other single risk factor (American Heart Association, 1993; Caspersen and Heath, 1993; Froelicher, 1990).

The mechanisms by which physical activity achieves its protective effect are many and varied. Some are independent and a direct result of the adaptive changes that occur in the cardiovascular system and its neural control that were documented earlier in this unit. For example, the increases in parasympathetic tone and decreases in sympathetic response will lower the resting and exercise heart rates in physically active individuals and possibly impact hypertension. These changes also will enhance the electrical stability of the myocardial cells, reducing the risk of potentially fatal conduction system defects and coronary vessel spasms. Other mechanisms are indirect and linked to the different risk factors (Caspersen and Heath, 1993). The impact of physical activity or exercise training is briefly summarized in Table 16.4 on page 442.

mortality rate was seen in men who moved from quintiles 2 and 3 to 4 and 5; and the lowest mortality rate was seen in men in the upper two quintiles (4 and 5) who remained there.

The comparable results in terms of relative risk are shown in panel (b) of the graph. The unfit men who moved into the fit category reduced their risk of death from cardiovascular disease by 52% (relative risk = .48). After adjustment for potential confounders, each minute of increase in treadmill time (equivalent to a $\dot{V}O_2$max increase of only 1.75 mL·kg^{-1}·min^{-1} in the protocol used) was associated with a reduced risk of 8.6% for CVD mortality. Those who changed from fit to unfit exhibited a risk less than half that of the consistently unfit, but almost twice that of those who remained fit.

The message is clear. Individuals who are unfit must be encouraged and helped to attain at least a minimal level of fitness. This minimal level can be achieved by following the recommendations in the Surgeon General's Report: engaging in at least 30 min of moderate physical activity on most, if not all, days of the week. Individuals who are already fit must be equally encouraged and helped to maintain or improve their level of fitness. Although Blair and his colleagues' results were compiled only on men (because of an insufficient number of women subjects), Manson and colleagues (1999) have reported similar findings from the Nurses' Health Study, which followed 72,488 women 40–65 yr of age.

It is never too late to try to become fit; it is never too soon to make a lifetime commitment to activity and fitness.

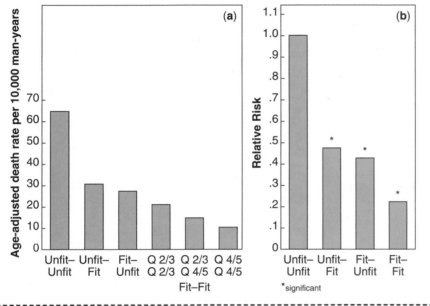

*significant

Sources:

Blair, et al. (1995); Manson, et al. (1999).

One of the most important facts about activity or exercise training is that the greatest health benefits occur when very sedentary individuals increase their endurance activity levels even minimally (Blair and Minocha, 1989).

Contributing and Selected Nontraditional Risk Factors

Fibrinogen

As previously mentioned, one of the major dangers of the buildup of atherosclerotic plaque is that a clot might form and block the already narrowed blood vessel. *Fibrinogen* is a protein present in blood plasma that, under the proper physiological circumstances, is converted into *fibrin* threads that form the basis of a blood clot. In addition, fibrinogen increases blood platelet aggregation and blood viscosity. Thus, fibrinogen is a thrombotic marker. High levels of fibrinogen increase the likelihood of internal clot formation. Environmental factors that increase plasma fibrinogen levels include aging, cigarette smoking, a high body mass index, high LDL levels, and chronic inflammation (Wu, 1997). Thus, much of the relationship between smoking and CHD and some of the association between psychological stress and CHD may be mediated through plasma fibrinogen levels. Prospective studies suggest that individuals with the highest fibrinogen levels (highest tertile) have an increased risk of coronary heart disease similar to the increased risk for those in the highest tertile of plasma cholesterol (Meade, 1995). An elevation of plasma fibrinogen levels of approximately 50 mg·dL^{-1} increases the risk of cardiovascular disease by factors of about 2.5 and 3.0 in adult females and males, respectively (Wu, 1997). Despite these strong associations, it is still uncertain whether elevated fibrinogen levels are a cause or a consequence of atherosclerosis (Hennekens, 1998).

A single bout of exercise has no documented effect on fibrinogen levels. There is only weak evidence from

Table 16.4

Summary of Impact of Physical Activity or Exercise Training on Modifiable CHD Risk Factors

Risk Factor	Impact of Exercise Training
Cholesterol-lipid fractions	↑ HDL fraction ↓ TC (maybe)
Cigarette smoking	Indirect
Hypertension	↓ SBP; ↓ DBP (incomplete normalization)
Physical inactivity	Directly eliminates
Diabetes mellitus	↑ glucose tolerance ↑ insulin sensitivity
Obesity	↓ body fat ↓ visceral abdominal fat
Stress	Unknown on hostility component of type A behavior; TABP may ↓
Fibrinogen levels and fibrinolytic activity	↓ fibrinogen levels ↑ fibrinolytic activity

Note: The impact is the same for children, adolescents, and adults except for stress and fibrinogen level and fibrinolytic activity, where insufficient information is available.

Increased = ↑, Decreased = ↓.

one study that dynamic endurance exercise training decreases fibrinogen level in older (over 60 yr) but not younger (24–36 yr) males (Stratton, et al., 1991).

Fibrinolytic Activity

Fibrinolytic activity refers to the breakdown of fibrin clots. Enhanced fibrinolytic activity could potentially reduce the risk of clots and, hence, CHD. Conversely, an inhibition of fibrinolysis increases the risk of arterial thrombosis. High visceral abdominal obesity is directly related to reduced fibrinolytic activity. Prospective studies have reported that elevated levels of plasminogen activator inhibitor (PAI-1), a protein that inhibits fibrinolytic activity, is associated with increased risk of initial and recurrent myocardial infarction (Meade, 1995).

A single dynamic aerobic endurance exercise bout (but not static exertion) has consistently been shown to increase fibrinolytic activity (Drygas, 1988). The change is greater in active than in sedentary individuals, and high-intensity exercise produces more change than moderate-intensity exercise. The effect of exercise training is less certain; but there is some minimal evidence that training enhances fibrinolytic activity (Beumann and Tremblay, 1996; Carroll, et al.,

2000; Davis, et al., 1976; El-Sayed, et al., 2000; Ferguson, et al, 1987; Szymanski and Pate, 1994; Szymanski, et al., 1994; Wood and Stefanik, 1990).

Stress

Stress is probably the most controversial of the CHD risk factors. Many factors affect how stress impacts an individual, and these factors are difficult to identify and measure. How any given stressor is perceived will depend not just on the stressor but also on characteristics of the individual being stressed. For example, what vulnerabilities does the individual have, or what coping strategies are available to the individual?

The response to the stressor will vary according to the individual's psychological and physiological level of reactivity. For example, among the acute physiological responses to fear or anger, mediated through the neural and hormonal systems, are an increase in heart rate, blood pressure, respiratory rate, and blood viscosity, and a decrease in clotting time and the breakdown of fats for use as a fuel. In the short-term, these responses, if appropriate to the level of need, are good. After all, the individual might have to fight (and, if wounded, would need to clot blood quickly to prevent too great a loss of blood) or flee (and have sufficient energy and oxygen-carrying capacity to do so). However, if they are excessive, or if they become chronic, these responses form a possible mechanism for the development of hypertension, atherosclerosis, thrombogenesis, and clinical heart disease.

The consequences of both the stressor and the response to the stressor can also vary, from extremely positive and health enhancing to illness or injury or, ultimately, death. Such things as adaptation to exercise training for an improved fitness level can enhance health. Conversely, as has been documented in several cases, bad news can precipitate sudden death from a heart attack in susceptible individuals (Caspersen and Heath, 1994; Landers, 1994; Plowman, 1994).

The type of stress primarily implicated in cardiovascular disease is psychosocial or emotional stress and not physical stress. Although life events, daily hassles, and occupational stresses, among other factors, have been considered in studies of stress, most emphasis has been placed on behavioral patterns known as Type A and Type B. The **Type A behavior pattern (TABP)** is characterized by hard-driving

---

Type A Behavior Pattern (TABP) Behavior that is characterized by hard-driving competitiveness; time urgency, haste, and impatience; a workaholic lifestyle; and hostility.

competitiveness; time urgency, haste, and impatience; a workaholic lifestyle; and hostility. The **Type B behavior pattern (TBBP)** is characterized by relaxation without guilt and no sense of time urgency.

Research in the 1970s showed a positive relationship between Type A behavior and CHD. Research in the 1980s and 1990s, however, seemed to pinpoint only the hostility component. As a psychological concept, hostility includes cynicism, anger, mistrust, and aggression and is frequently associated with situations of "high demand and low control" or social isolation. Without hostility, the other Type A personality traits are now thought to be relatively benign (Landers, 1994; Plowman, 1994). The impact of stress may be direct through neurohormonal changes (especially in catecholamine and serotonin levels) or indirect by the use of unhealthy coping strategies, such as overeating, smoking, or excessive alcohol intake (Gordon, 1998).

Three studies have investigated the impact exercise training has on TABP, and none of them isolated the component of hostility. Two of the three did show, however, a decrease in TABP with dynamic endurance exercise training. These studies involved both higher-intensity and longer-duration exercise than the study that showed no significant response (Landers, 1994).

On the other hand, an acute bout of exercise is well established as an effective stress management technique. Thus, as with the influence of exercise on several of the other risk factors, it may be the short-term last-bout effect rather than the long-term chronic adaptation that is most important (Berger, 1994).

Children and the Cardiovascular Risk Factors

The concern about cardiovascular disease risk factors for children is not that children exhibit clinical cardiovascular disease but that cardiovascular disease is a lifelong process that begins in childhood. Therefore, if risk factors can be prevented, modified, or counteracted in childhood, it may be possible to prevent or at least delay or reduce the severity of cardiovascular problems in adulthood.

In relation to physical activity the intent is to establish patterns of participation in children that will continue into and throughout adulthood. To a large extent, the success of this strategy depends on a phenomenon called *tracking*. In this context **tracking** means that a characteristic is maintained, in terms of relative rank, over a long time span or even a lifetime. The easiest nonrisk factor to relate tracking to is

height. Children in the upper percentiles of height at a very young age tend to maintain that position and be taller than average adults. Thus, in relation to children, it is important to be able to determine the presence or absence of the modifiable risk factors, the tracking strength of the risk factors, and the impact of physical activity and exercise training on both the short-term risk factor reductions and long-term lifestyle modifications (Rowland, 1991; Rowland and Freedson, 1994).

Cholesterol-Lipid Fractions

At birth, total cholesterol levels are approximately 70 mg·dL^{-1}, with 35 mg·dL^{-1} of that total being HDL. During the first few weeks of life the level of TC rises rapidly to between 100 and 150 mg·dL^{-1}. By 2 yr and until adulthood the average value for males is about 160 mg·dL^{-1} and for females about 165 mg·dL^{-1} with HDL levels of between 50 and 55 mg·dL^{-1}. At puberty males show a decline of HDL and females a decline in LDL values. In general, cholesterol levels do track from childhood to adulthood, but not all children with high juvenile levels of cholesterol will have elevated adult levels. In one study 43% of the children who had cholesterol values above the 90th percentile also had adult values above the 90th percentile and 81% had values above the 50th percentile (Armstrong and Simons-Morton, 1994; Mahoney, et al., 1991).

Values that represent acceptable, borderline, and high-risk levels for children are included in Table 16.2. As for adults, high TC, high-LDL, and low-HDL levels have been found to be related to the magnitude of early atherosclerotic lesions. Autopsy reports have confirmed that early signs of atherosclerosis are present in children as young as 3 yr and frequently evident by age 10. Poor lipid profiles often run in families owing to both shared genetics and common lifestyle factors (U.S. Department of Health and Human Services, 1991). Insufficient evidence is available regarding the role of the apolipoproteins in children.

As with adults, cross-sectional studies have consistently reported that trained adolescents have higher

---

Type B Behavior Pattern (TBBP) Behavior associated with characteristics of relaxation without guilt and no sense of time urgency.

Tracking A phenomenon in which a characteristic is maintained, in terms of relative rank, over a long time span or even a lifetime.

HDL values than untrained adolescents but that TC levels do not differ with training status. Other studies have found similar, but less consistent, evidence between active and inactive children. The few short-term (8–12 weeks) aerobic exercise training studies that have investigated lipid changes in children and adolescents have found no significant changes in blood lipid profiles following training. The impact of dynamic resistance training on lipid levels in children and adolescents has not been adequately addressed (Armstrong and Simons-Morton, 1994).

Cigarette Smoking

An estimated 2.2 million U.S. adolescents, 12–17 yr old, smoke. Every day another 3000 young people begin to smoke. Seventy-five percent of adult smokers started smoking before age 18, and 90% started smoking prior to age 21 (American Heart Association, 1993). Each year from 1991 to 1996, cigarette smoking rates increased in the United States among 8th, 10th, and 12th grade students (Hennekens, 1998). Thus, smoking definitely tracks from adolescence to adulthood. The physiological effects and the indirect relationship between activity and smoking are the same no matter what the age of the smoker.

One study of Finnish youth showed that over a 6-yr span, with individuals who were 12, 15, and 18 yr old at the beginning of the study, higher activity levels were related to less smoking in both boys and girls. Almost half of those who were sedentary smoked, but only about 10% of those who were active smoked (Raitakari, et al., 1994). A primary goal of physical education and exercise science professionals must be to encourage an active lifestyle and discourage the onset of smoking in children and adolescents (U.S. Department of Health and Human Services, 1991).

Diabetes Mellitus

Children with Type 1 and Type 2 diabetes are at risk of prematurely developing atherosclerosis. Furthermore, diabetes tracks into adulthood. The importance and cautions of physical activity and exercise training for individuals with diabetes was discussed in the section on adults but are also applicable here.

Hypertension

Hypertension is evident in children as young as 6 yr of age. Between 6 and 17 yr of age, as many as 2.8 million children are estimated to be hypertensive (American Heart Association, 1993). Table 16.3 gives systolic and diastolic values taken to represent normal,

high-normal, and hypertensive blood pressures (Scott, 1993). Note that in children these values are lower than in adults. The change in blood pressure with growth (age 2–18) is presented in Figure 16.2 (National Heart, Lung and Blood Institute's Task Force on Blood Pressure Control in Children [NHLBI], 1977). Because blood pressure changes so much with age, it may be better to use those values higher than the 90th percentile, especially at younger ages, as the criterion for hypertension rather than the absolute values presented in Table 16.3.

Although childhood blood pressures do not predict adult blood pressures, there is a definite tendency for both systolic and diastolic blood pressures to track from childhood to adulthood. In one study, children with blood pressures at the 90th percentile had three times the risk of having high adult systolic blood pressure and twice the risk of having high adult diastolic blood pressure as those whose childhood values were at the 50th percentile (Mahoney, et al., 1991).

Results from dynamic aerobic endurance training studies show consistent reductions in both systolic and diastolic blood pressure in hypertensive children, although, as with adults, these reductions rarely achieve normal blood pressure levels. Dynamic resistance training used by itself, in one reported study, did not bring about a reduction in either systolic or diastolic pressure. However, when weight training was instituted after a period of aerobic endurance training that resulted in reduced blood pressures, the reduction in blood pressure was maintained with just the weight training. Therefore, as with adults, the best procedure is to begin young hypertensives on a dynamic endurance activity regimen and add resistance training several months later, if desired (Alpert and Wilmore, 1994).

Obesity

Close to 25% of all American children are obese. The number increased from the 1960s to the 1980s and has shown no signs of reversing (U.S. Department of Health and Human Services, 1991). Unfortunately, obesity does show evidence of tracking. Obese children are at an increased risk of becoming obese adults. Also, obese children are at greater risk for health problems, including those that relate to CHD. Research shows that 60% of overweight children between the ages of 5 and 10 have at least one other major risk factor (CDC, 1999). As for adults, the relationship between exercise training and body weight or body fat reduction is detailed in the metabolic unit of this text (Chapter 9). In general, obese adolescents appear to be less active than nonobese adolescents. In children, as well as in adults, aerobic exercise

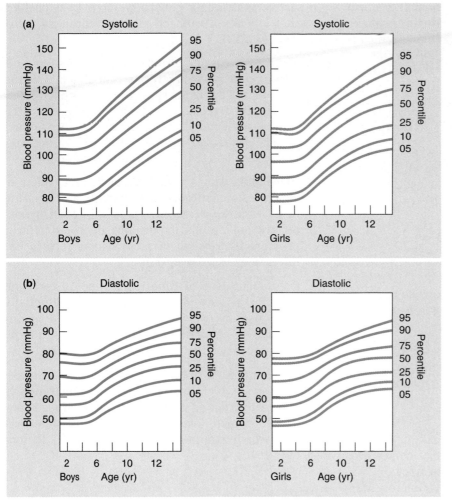

Figure 16.2

Age-Related Changes in Blood Pressure in Boys and Girls

Source: NHLBI (1993).

training has been shown to reduce body fat and/or increase fat-free mass (Bar-Or and Baranowski, 1994).

Physical Inactivity

At least as important as the level of physical fitness achieved and the amount of physical activity engaged in is the establishment of a physically active lifestyle in young people. The health outcomes depend more on the constancy of physical activity throughout life than on any changes that may occur as a result of exercise training. One cannot deposit the benefits of physical activity into a fitness bank to withdraw at a later date. Furthermore, genetics has a definite impact on fitness scores. It is a hard but sad truth that some individuals will score high on fitness tests without doing any activity, but others who are very active may never achieve high fitness scores. It is the pattern of consistent activity that is most important for both types of individuals and everyone in between.

Significant tracking of physical activity was observed in a Finnish study of both boys and girls, with 44% remaining active from age 12 to 18 years, from 15 to 21 years, and from 18 to 24 years. Physical inactivity tracked even better, with 57% remaining inactive over the 6 years of the study. Those who remained active had better risk factor profiles than their inactive counterparts. They smoked less (as mentioned earlier), were less fat, had higher HDL cholesterol and lower TC values, and exhibited favorable differences in insulin levels. They also consumed a healthier diet, which would, of course, have affected these results. Further tracking evidence to older ages is needed (Raitakari, et al., 1994).

In general, whether the investigations of tracking of physical activity has occurred from early to middle childhood, childhood to adolescence, within adolescence, from adolescence to adulthood, or within adulthood, the results have indicated low to moderate stability for both males and females as indicated by statistical correlations (r values) of < .30 to .60. Physical fitness has shown a similar pattern but with a wider range that included some high (r > .70) stability results. Interestingly, attributes of neuromuscular fitness such as strength, power, and flexibility, have tended to show a higher stability than the primary cardiovascular measurement of maximal oxygen consumption (Janz, et al., 2000; Malina, 1996; Pate, et al., 1999; Raudsepp and Pall, 1998; Twisk, et al., 2000).

Stress, Fibrinogen, and Fibrinolytic Activity

Insufficient information is available on stress, fibrinogen, and fibrinolytic activity in children and adolescents to link them directly to CHD risk or establish the influence of physical activity or exercise training on these factors.

Summary

1. Cardiovascular disease is a major cause of death in the United States, accounting for approximately 40% of all deaths.

2. Cardiovascular risk factors are classified as nonmodifiable (age, heredity, race, and sex); major (hyperlipidemia, cigarette smoking, diabetes mellitus, hypertension, obesity, physical inactivity); contributing and nontraditional (apolipoproteins, fibrin level, fibrinolytic activity, stress).

3. Triglycerides and a small amount of cholesterol are transported from the small intestines or liver to adipose tissue or muscles by chylomicrons and very low density lipoproteins (VLDL).

4. VLDLs are degraded into intermediate-density lipoproteins (IDL), which, in turn, are converted to low-density lipoproteins (LDL) in the liver. LDL transports 60–70% of the total cholesterol (TC) in the body to all cells except liver cells.

5. High-density lipoproteins (HDL) may block cholesterol uptake at the cellular or tissue level. HDL definitely carry cholesterol away from the sites of deposit to the liver, where the cholesterol can be broken down and eliminated in the bile.

6. Arteriosclerosis is characterized by a thickening of the arterial wall, loss of elastic connective tissue, and hardening of the vessel wall.

7. Atherosclerosis is a pathological process that results in the buildup of plaque (composed of connective tissue, smooth muscle cells, cellular debris, and cholesterol) inside the vessel. The buildup of plaque obstructs blood flow and increases the risk of thrombosis. Depending on the amount of obstruction, the result can be pain, a heart attack, or a stroke.

8. Active individuals generally have lipid profiles that indicate a reduced risk for coronary heart disease (CHD).

9. The atherosclerotic process is accelerated in individuals who smoke cigarettes. Smoking injures the arterial wall lining, increases the levels of circulating TC, and decreases the amount of HDL. Smoking also causes blood platelets to adhere to each other, speeds up the rate of internal blood clotting, and makes the clots that do form tougher to dissolve.

10. Individuals who are at high risk for developing hypertension can reduce the risk by participating in an endurance training program. Most hypertensive individuals experience decreased blood pressure as a result of a consistent aerobic endurance exercise program.

11. Only about 10% of Americans report exercising daily for at least 30 min. Therefore, potentially more benefit overall could be achieved by increasing the activity level of U.S. citizens than by changing any other single CHD risk factor.

12. Metabolic Syndrome is a progressive disease process in which high visceral abdominal obesity is directly related to dyslipidemia, reduced glucose tolerance, insulin resistance, and hypertension, which together form a cluster of risk factors for CVD.

Review Questions

1. Identify risk factors that cannot be changed, and discuss their relationship with cardiovascular disease.

2. Identify the major risk factors, and discuss their relationship with cardiovascular disease.

3. Identify contributing and nontraditional risk factors, and discuss their relationship with cardiovascular disease.

4. Discuss Metabolic Syndrome.

5. What is the impact of exercise training on each CHD risk factor?

6. What is the importance of identifying cardiovascular disease risk factors in children?

For further review and additional study tools, go to The Physiology Place (www.physiologyplace.com) and the Student Study Guide for Exercise Physiology for Health, Fitness, and Performance *by Sharon A. Plowman and Denise L. Smith.*

Passport to the Internet

Visit the following Internet sites to explore further topics and issues related to cardiorespiratory health and disease. To visit an organization's web site, go to www.physiologyplace.com and click on "Passport to the Internet."

Source for President's Council on Physical Fitness and Sports *Physical Activity and Fitness Research Digests* 1996–present.

Centers for Disease Control and Prevention National Center for Chronic Disease Prevention and Health Promotion

Centers for Disease Control and Prevention National Center for Health Statistics

American Heart Association Heart and Stroke Guide, Risk Awareness

American Heart Association Journal *Circulation* **online** Scientific statements archived (1965) to current issues.

Online version of the Merck Manual Comprehensive reference for anatomy, physiology, and diseases by system

References

Alpert, B. S., & J. H. Wilmore: Physical activity and blood pressure in adolescents. *Pediatric Exercise Science.* 6(4): 361–380 (1994).

American College of Sports Medicine: Position stand: Exercise and Type 2 diabetes. *Medicine and Science in Sports and Exercise.* 32(7):1345–1360 (2000).

American College of Sports Medicine: Position stand: Physical activity, physical fitness, and hypertension. *Medicine and Science in Sports and Exercise.* 25(10):I–IX (1993).

American Heart Association: *Heart and Stroke Facts.* Dallas: Author (1994).

American Heart Association: *Heart and Stroke Facts: 1994 Statistical Supplement.* Dallas: Author (1993).

Armstrong, N., & B. Simons-Morton: Physical activity and blood lipids in adolescents. *Pediatric Exercise Science.* 6(4):381–405 (1994).

Bar-Or, O., & T. Baranowski: Physical activity, adiposity, and obesity among adolescents. *Pediatric Exercise Science.* 6(4):348–360 (1994).

Berger, B. G.: Coping with stress: The effectiveness of exercise and other techniques. *Quest.* 46:100–119 (1994).

Blair, S. N., H. W. Kohl, C. E. Barlow, R. S. Paffenbarger, L. W. Gibbons, & C. A. Macera: Changes in physical fitness and all-cause mortality: A prospective study of healthy and unhealthy men. *Journal of the American Medical Association.* 273(14):1093–1098 (1995).

Blair, S. N., & H. C. Minocha: Physical fitness and all-cause mortality: A prospective study of healthy men and women. *Journal of the American Medical Association.* 262: 2395–2401 (1989).

Buemann, B., & A. Tremblay: Effects of exercise training on abdominal obesity and related metabolic complications. *SportsMedicine.* 21(3):191–212 (1996).

Carroll, S., C. B. Cooke, & R. J. Butterly: Leisure time physical activity, cardiorespiratory fitness, and plasma fibrinogen concentrations in nonsmoking middle-aged men. *Medicine and Science in Sports and Exercise.* 32(3):620–626 (2000).

Caspersen, C. J., & G. W. Heath. The risk factor concept of coronary heart disease. In J. L. Durstine, A. C. King, P. L. Painter, J. L. Roitman, L. D. Zwireu, & W. L. Kenney (eds.), *American College of Sports Medicine: Resource Manual for Guidelines for Exercise Testing and Prescription* (2nd edition). Philadelphia: Lea & Febiger (1993).

Centers for Disease Control and Prevention: Obesity epidemic increases dramatically in the United States. www.cdc.gov/nccdphp/dnpa/obesity-epidemic.htm (1999).

Colberg, S. R.: Exercise: A diabetes "cure" for many? *ACSM's Health and Fitness Journal.* 5(2):20–26 (2001).

Dannenberg, A. L., J. B. Keller, P. W. F. Wilson, & W. P. Castelli: Leisure time physical activity in the Framingham offspring study. *American Journal of Epidemiology.* 129: 76–88 (1989).

Davis, G. L., C. F. Abildgaard, E. M. Bernauer, & M. Brittan: Fibrinolytic and hemostatic changes during and after maximal exercise in males. *Journal of Applied Physiology.* 40(3):287–292 (1976).

Drygas, W. K.: Changes in blood platelet function, coagulation, and fibrinolytic activity in response to moderate, exhaustive, and prolonged exercise. *International Journal of Sports Medicine.* 9:67–72 (1988).

El-Sayed, M. S., C. Sale, P. G. W. Jones, & M. Chester: Blood hemostasis in exercise and training. *Medicine and Science in Sports and Exercise.* 32(5):918–925 (2000).

Ferguson, E. W., L. L. Bernier, G. R. Bauta, J. Yu-Yahiro, & E. B. Schoomaker: Effects of exercise and conditioning on clotting and fibrinolytic activity in men. *Journal of Applied Physiology.* 62(4):1416–1421 (1987).

Froelicher, V. F.: Exercise, fitness, and coronary heart disease. In C. Bouchard, R. J. Shephard, T. Stephens, J. R. Sutton, & B. D. McPherson (eds.), *Exercise, Fitness, and Health: A Consensus of Current Knowledge.* Champaign, IL: Human Kinetics, 429–451 (1990).

Gordon, N. F.: Conceptual basis for coronary artery disease risk factor assessment. In J. L. Roitman (ed.) *ACSM's Resource Manual for Guidelines for Exercise Testing and Prescription* (3rd edition). Philadelphia: Lippincott, Williams & Wilkins, 3–12 (1998).

Grundy, S. M., I. J. Benjamin, G. L. Burke, A. Chait, R. H. Eckel, B. V. Howard, W. Mitch, S. C. Smith, & J. R. Sowers: Diabetes and cardiovascular disease: A statement for healthcare professionals from the American Heart Association. *Circulation.* 100:1134–1146 (1999).

Hagberg, J. M.: Exercise, fitness and hypertension. In C. Bouchard, R. J. Shephard, T. Stephens, J. R. Sutton, & B. D. McPherson (eds.), *Exercise, Fitness, and Health: A Consensus of Current Knowledge.* Champaign, IL: Human Kinetics (1990).

Hahn, R. A., G. W. Heath, & M.-H. Chang: Cardiovascular disease risk factors and preventive practices among adults—United States, 1994: A behavioral risk factor atlas. *Morbidity and Mortality Weekly Report (MMWR).* 47 (SS-5): 35–69 (1998).

Hall, W. D.: Geographic patterns of hypertension in the United States. In J. L. Izzo & H. R. Black (eds.), Council on High Blood Pressure Research, American Heart Association, *Hypertension Primer* (2nd edition). Baltimore: Lippincott, Williams & Wilkins, 226–228 (1999).

Hanson, P.: Pathophysiology of chronic diseases and exercise. In J. L. Durstine, A. C. King, P. L. Painter, J. L. Rostman, L. K. Zwireu, & W. L. Kenney (eds.), *American College of Sports Medicine Resource Manual for Guidelines for Exercise Testing and Prescription* (2nd edition). Philadelphia: Lea & Febiger, 187–196 (1993).

Haskell, W. L., C. Sims, J. Myll, W. M. Bortz, F. G. St. Goar, & E. L. Alderman: Coronary artery size and dilating capacity in ultra distance runners. *Circulation.* 87(4):1076–1082 (1993).

Haskell, W. S. L.: Health consequence of physical activity: Understanding and challenges regarding dose response. *Medicine and Science in Sports and Exercise.* 26(6):649–660 (1994).

Hennekens, C. H.: Increasing burden of cardiovascular disease: Current knowledge and future directions for research on risk factors. *Circulation.* 97:1095–1101 (1998).

Izzo, J. L.: The sympathetic nervous system in human hypertension. In J. L. Izzo & H. R. Black (eds.), Council on High Blood Pressure Research, American Heart Association, *Hypertension Primer* (2nd edition). Baltimore: Lippincott, Williams & Wilkins, 109–112 (1999).

Janz, K. F., J. D. Dawson, & L. T. Mahoney: Tracking physical fitness and physical activity from childhood to adolescence: The Muscatine study. *Medicine and Science in Sports and Exercise.* 32(7):1250–1257 (2000).

Kannel, W. B., & P. W. F. Wilson: Cardiovascular risk factors and hypertension. In J. L. Izzo & H. R. Black (eds.), Council on High Blood Pressure Research, American Heart Association, *Hypertension Primer* (2nd edition). Baltimore: Lippincott, Williams & Wilkins, 199–202 (1999).

Kelley, G.: Dynamic resistance exercises and resting blood pressure in adults: A meta-analysis. *Journal of Applied Physiology.* 82(5):1559–1565 (1997).

Koplan, J. P., K. E. Powell, R. K. Sikes, R. W. Shirley, & C. C. Campbell: An epidemiological study of the benefits and risks of running. *Journal of the American Medical Association.* 248:3118–3121 (1982).

LaFontaine, T.: Preventing the progression of or reversing coronary atherosclerosis. *American College of Sports Medicine Certified News.* 4(3):1–6 (1994).

Landers, D. M.: Performance, stress, and health: Overall reaction. *Quest.* 46:123–135 (1994).

Mahoney, L. T., R. M. Lauer, J. Lee, & W. R. Clarke: Factors affecting tracking of coronary heart disease risk factors in children: The Muscatine study. In Hyperlipidemia in Childhood and the Development of Atherosclerosis. *Annals of the New York Academy of Sciences.* 623:120–132 (1991).

Malina, R. M.: Tracking of physical activity and physical fitness across the lifespan. *Research Quarterly for Exercise and Sport.* 67 (supplement to No. 3):48–57 (1996).

Manson, J. E., F. B. Hu, J. W. Rich-Edwards, G. A. Colditz, M. J. Stamfer, W. C. Willett, F. E. Speizer, & C. H. Hennekens: A prospective study of walking as compared with vigorous exercise in the prevention of coronary heart disease in women. *New England Journal of Medicine.* 341:650–658 (1999).

Meade, T. W.: Fibrinogen in ischaemic heart disease. *European Heart Journal.* 16 (supplement A):31–35 (1995).

National High Blood Pressure Education Program: National Institutes of Health; National Heart, Lung, and Blood Institute: *The Fifth Report of the Joint Committee on Detection, Evaluation, and Treatment of High Blood Pressure.* Washington, D.C. (1993).

National Heart, Lung, and Blood Institute's Task Force on Blood Pressure Control in Children: Report of the task force on blood pressure control in children. *Pediatrics Supplement.* 59(5):797–820 (1977).

Pate, R. R., S. G. Trost, M. Dowda, A. E. Ott, D. S. Ward, R. Saunders, & G. Felton: Tracking of physical activity, physical inactivity, and health-related physical fitness in rural youth. *Pediatric Exercise Science.* 11:364–376 (1999).

Plowman, S. A.: Stress, hyperactivity, and health. *Quest.* 46:78–99 (1994).

Raitakari, O. T., K. V. K. Porkka, S. Taimela, R. Telama, L. Rasaneu, & J. S. A. Viikari: Effects of persistent physical activity and inactivity on coronary risk factors in children and young adults: The cardiovascular risk in young Finns study. *American Journal of Epidemiology.* 140(3):195–208 (1994).

Raudsepp, L., & P. Pall: Reproducibility and stability of physical activity in children. *Pediatric Exercise Science.* 10: 320–326 (1998).

Rowland, T. W.: *Exercise and Children's Health.* Champaign, IL: Human Kinetics (1990).

Rowland, T. W.: Influence of physical activity and fitness on coronary risk factors in children: How strong an argument? *Pediatric Exercise Science.* 3(3):189–191 (1991).

Rowland, T. W., & P. S. Freedson: Physical activity, fitness, and health in children: A close look. *Pediatrics.* 93(4):669–672 (1994).

Schuler, G., R. Hainbrecht, G. Schlierf, J. Niebauer, K. Haver, J. Neumann, E. Hoberg, A. Drinkmann, F. Bacher, M. Grunze, & W. Kubler: Regular physical exercise and low-fat diet: Effects on progression of coronary artery disease. *Circulation.* 86:1–11 (1992).

Scott, C. B.: Blood pressure and exercise. *American College of Sports Medicine Certified News.* 3(2):1–5 (1993).

Simons-Morton, D. G.: Physical activity, fitness and blood pressure. In J. L. Izzo & H. R. Black (eds.), Council on High

Blood Pressure Research, American Heart Association, *Hypertension Primer* (2nd edition). Baltimore: Lippincott, Williams & Wilkins, 259–262 (1999).

Squires, R. W.: Coronary atherosclerosis. In J. L. Roitman (ed.) *ACSM's Resource Manual for Guidelines for Exercise Testing and Prescription* (3rd edition). Philadelphia: Lippincott, Williams & Wilkins, 225–230 (1998).

Squires, R. W., & W. L. Williams: Coronary atherosclerosis and acute myocardial infarction. In J. L. Durstine, A. C. King, P. L. Painter, J. L. Roctman, L. D. Zwiren, & W. L. Kenney (eds.), *American College of Sport Medicine Resource Manual for Guidelines for Exercise Testing and Prescription* (2nd edition). Philadelphia: Lea & Febiger, 129–150 (1993).

Stewart, K. J.: Exercise and hypertension. In J. L. Roitman (ed.) *ACSM's Resource Manual for Guidelines for Exercise Testing and Prescription* (3rd edition). Philadelphia: Lippincott, Williams & Wilkins, 275–280 (1998).

Stewart, K. J.: Weight training in coronary artery disease and hypertension. *Progress in Cardiovascular Disease.* 35(2):159–168 (1992).

Strand, F.: *Physiology: A Regulatory Systems Approach.* New York: Macmillan (1978).

Stratton, J. R., W. L. Chandler, R. S. Schwartz, M. D. Cerqueira, W. C. Levy, S. E. Kahn, V. G. Larson, K. C. Cain, J. C. Beard, & I. B. Abrass: Effects of physical conditioning on fibrinolytic variables and fibrinogen in young and old healthy adults. *Circulation.* 83:1692–1697 (1991).

Summary of the Third Report of the National Cholesterol Education Program (NCEP): Expert panel on detection, evaluation and treatment of high blood cholesterol in adults (adult treatment panel II). *Journal of the American Medical Association.* 285:2486–2497 (2001).

Szymanski, L. M., & R. R. Pate: Effects of exercise intensity, duration, and time of day on fibrinolytic activity in physically active men. *Medicine and Science in Sports and Exercise.* 26(9):1102–1108 (1994).

Szymanski, L. M., R. R. Pate, & J. L. Durstine: Effect of maximal exercise and venous occlusion on fibrinolytic activity in physically active and inactive men. *Journal of Applied Physiology.* 77(5):2305–2310 (1994).

Tanaka, H., D. R. Bassett, E. T. Howley, D. L. Thompson, M. Ashraf, & F. L. Rawson: Swimming training lowers the resting blood pressure in individuals with hypertension. *Journal of Hypertension.* 15:651–657 (1997).

Thomas, T. R., & T. LaFontaine: Exercise and lipoproteins. In J. L. Roitman (ed.) *ACSM's Resource Manual for Guidelines for Exercise Testing and Prescription* (3rd edition). Philadelphia: Lippincott, Williams & Wilkins, 294–301 (1998).

Twisk, J. W. R., H. C. G. Kemper, & W. vanMechelen: Tracking of activity and fitness and the relationship with cardiovascular risk factors. *Medicine and Science in Sports and Exercise.* 32(8):1455–1561 (2000).

U.S. Department of Health and Human Services, Centers for Disease Control and Prevention: *Chronic diseases and their risk factors: The nation's leading cause of death.* Author. (1999).

U.S. Department of Health and Human Services, Public Health Service, National Institutes of Health: Report of the expert panel on blood cholesterol levels in children and adolescents. *National Institutes of Health Publication.* No. 91-2732 (1991).

Welk, G. J., & S. N. Blair: Physical activity protects against the health risks of obesity. *President's Council on Physical Fitness and Sports Research Digest.* Series 3 (12):1–8 (2000).

Wood, P. D., & M. L. Stefanick: Exercise, fitness, and atherosclerosis. In C. Bouchard, R. J. Shephard, T. Stephens, J. R. Sutton, & B. D. McPherson (eds.), *Exercise, Fitness, and Health: A Consensus of Current Knowledge.* Champaign, IL: Human Kinetics, 409–423 (1990).

Wu, K. K.: Hemostatic tests in the prediction of atherothrombotic disease. *International Journal of Clinical and Laboratory Research.* 27:145–152 (1997).

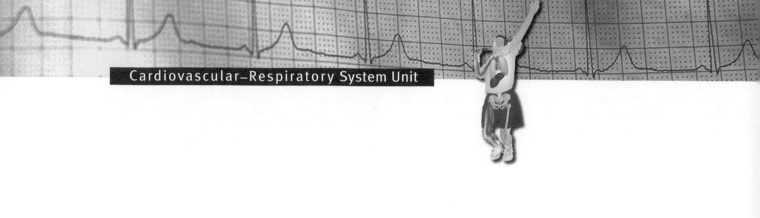

Chapter 17

The Immune System,
Exercise,
Training, and Illness

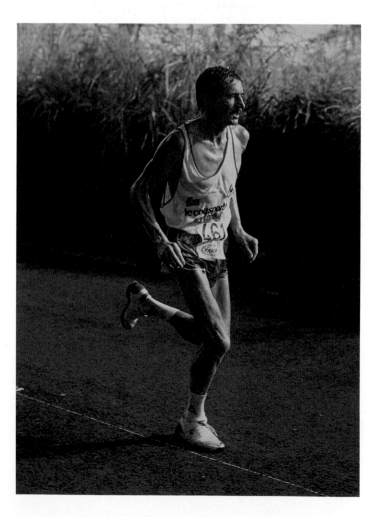

After studying the chapter, you should be able to

- Identify the primary cells of the innate and adaptive branches of the immune system and indicate the mechanisms by which they lead to antigen destruction.

- Describe the sequence of events in inflammation.

- Differentiate between the immune response to moderate aerobic exercise and exhaustive exercise.

- Describe the cytokine theory of overtraining.

- Respond to the question: Does exercise increase or decrease the likelihood of illness?

- Describe the role of physical activity in the life of an individual infected with HIV.

450

Introduction

Exercise training has many health benefits; often active individuals, perhaps yourself included, claim they feel better and are healthier than their sedentary friends. They claim these benefits not just because they have altered their risk factors for major diseases, but also because they have experienced fewer colds, flu, sore throats, and other common illnesses. On the other hand, it is not unusual to hear that an Olympic or professional athlete has gotten out of a sick bed to compete or isn't competing because of illness, not injury. So which is it? Does exercise training make an individual more resistant to infections or illness, or does exercise training make the most fit individuals the most susceptible to infection? To answer these questions, we must explore the relationship between exercise training and the immune system. In addition, the role of exercise and exercise training in individuals with known infections is of concern (whether it be a simple cold or HIV/AIDS). Should they or should they not be active?

A definitive response to each of these questions is not yet possible. This chapter, however, provides what is known about the functioning of the immune system, explores the acute immune response to exercise, considers adaptations in the immune system that occur as a result of exercise training, and, finally, addresses beneficial and detrimental influences of exercise on immune function and disease susceptibility.

The Immune System

Humans are constantly exposed to bacteria, viruses, and parasites that are capable of causing serious disease. The fact that we are not normally overcome by these foreign invaders is a testimony to the importance and efficiency of the body's defense mechanisms, comprised primarily of the immune system. The **immune system** is a complex yet precisely ordered system of cells, hormones, and chemicals that regulate susceptibility to, severity of, and recovery from infection and illness (Marieb, 2001; Nash, 1994). *Immunology* is the study of the physiological responses by which the body destroys or neutralizes foreign matter (Smith, 1995).

In its organization and operation, the immune system can be considered parallel to the nervous and endocrine systems. For example, all three systems consist of identifiable cells and chemical substances. All three systems react to stimuli; each possesses a network that allows for communication within itself and with the other systems; and all three control and interact with other cells and organs. One major difference, however, is a gradient of mobility. The nervous system functions through fixed nerves and locally released neurotransmitters; the major endocrine glands are also fixed in place, but their hormones travel throughout the body primarily via the bloodstream; the immune system consists predominantly of free mobile cells that move within and outside the bloodstream, although some may be anatomically specific (Roitt, et al., 1998).

As with the nervous and hormonal systems, it is important to understand first the parts and processes of the immune system before studying how it functions. Figure 17.1 presents a general structural outline of the basics of the immune system. All immune responses are intended to recognize a threat to the body and react to eradicate that threat while minimizing damage. In general, the threat or stimulus to the immune system is an infectious microbe or pathogen; such microorganisms include bacteria, fungi, parasites, protozoa, and viruses. Some pathogens (all viruses, some bacteria and small protozoan parasites) invade the body's cells and replicate there, while others (most bacteria and larger parasites) reside primarily in body fluids and extracellular spaces. The site of the infection and the specific pathogen determine how the immune system responds.

Structure and Function of the Immune System

Cells

The primary immune cells are *leukocytes,* more commonly known as white blood cells. Leukocytes are subdivided into *lymphocytes* and *phagocytes.* In turn, there are three major subdivisions of each of these.

B lymphocytes and *T lymphocytes* (*B cells* and *T cells*) specifically recognize individual pathogens. Any molecular pathogen that can be specifically recognized by B cells and/or T cells is called an *antigen.* Both B cells and T cells are derived from bone marrow cells, but B cells mature in the bone marrow, whereas T cells mature in the thymus. Each B and T cell is genetically programmed to recognize only one particular antigen. Once an antigen is recognized, B cells proliferate into plasma cells that produce an antibody to act immediately and memory cells that will ultimately provide lasting immunity. Vaccinations confer immunity against diseases such as polio or measles by altering an antigen in such a way that it becomes harmless but still brings about an antibody reaction.

> **Immune System** A precisely ordered system of cells, hormones, and chemicals that regulate susceptibility to, severity of, and recovery from infection and illness.

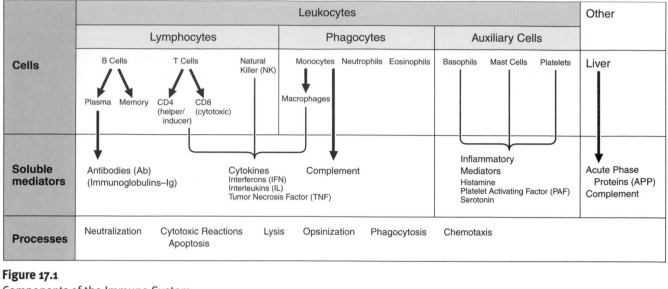

Figure 17.1
Components of the Immune System

Source: Based on Roitt et al. (1998).

Antigens recognized by T cells have been processed first in some way. Sensitized T cells enlarge and divide into two functionally separate classifications: (1) CD8, cytotoxic or killer cells, which destroy infected cells directly; and (2) CD4, helper or inducer cells, which stimulate the action of cytotoxic cells and increase antibody production by B plasma cells. Through a variety of feedback mechanisms, both CD4 and CD8 cells can also act as suppressor T cells that inhibit cytotoxic T cells and antibody production, thus preventing excessive destruction (Roitt, et al., 1998). Although they are classified as large granular lymphocytes, *natural killer (NK) cells* are different from other lymphocytes in that they act spontaneously against any target, apparently by recognizing surface changes on a variety of tumor cells and virally infected cells. As their name would imply, these cells directly destroy infected host cells.

Phagocytes are leukocytes that bind to pathogenic microorganisms and antigens, internalize them, and then kill them. When they are in the bloodstream, mononuclear phagocytes are called *monocytes;* when they migrate into tissue, they evolve into *macrophages.* It is macrophages that often "process" an antigen and then present it to T lymphocytes. *Neutrophils* are the most abundant blood leukocytes. Large numbers are necessary because when neutrophils engulf and destroy foreign material, they also die. *Eosinophils* are specialized to act against large extracellular parasites.

The role of the *auxiliary cells* is to release mediators to produce inflammation. *Mast cells* lie close to blood vessels; *basophils* and *platelets* circulate in the blood. The main purpose of inflammation is to attract leukocytes and their resultant soluble mediators to a site of infection.

Soluble Mediators

Soluble mediators are intervening agents that are dissolved in a solution. They are substances produced primarily, but not exclusively, by immune cells that act either directly on the target pathogen or indirectly by signaling other immune cells to act or release additional mediators. Each immune cell produces and secretes only one particular set of mediators, although more than one cell type may produce the same classification of mediator. The list of soluble mediators presented in Figure 17.1 is representative, not exhaustive.

Antibodies produced by B plasma cells are also known as *immunoglobulins (Ig).* Antibodies do not directly destroy antigens; rather, they identify the invader by forming an antigen-antibody (An·Ab) complex, and they then activate other soluble mediators and immune cells that perform the actual destruction. *Cytokines* are proteins or peptides that are involved in communication between immune cells (especially lymphocytes and phagocytes) and other cells of the body. Table 17.1 presents the major cytokines involved in the exercise immune response. Cytokines stimulate the proliferation of various immune cells and are important regulators of inflammation and the immune response. Among the principle types of cytokines are *interferons (IFNs),* which are important in limiting the spread of certain viral infections;

interleukins (ILs), each of which acts on a specific group of immune cells to divide and differentiate; and *tumor necrosis factors (TNFs)*, which are particularly important in dealing with inflammation and cytotoxic reactions. Cytokines are thought to be important in the exercise immune response because certain ones (IL-1, IL-6, IFNγ, and TNFα) are proinflammatory factors that probably play a role in coordinating the responses to muscle damage that may result from strenuous exercise. Other cytokines (IL-4, IL-10, and possibly IL-6 in a dual role) are anti-inflammatory and as such suppress activity of inflammatory cells allowing normal structure and function to be restored. The release of these anti-inflammatory cytokines follows the proinflammatory response to vigorous physical activity (Moldoveanu, et al., 2001).

Complement is a group of serum proteins whose overall function is to control inflammation. Complement activation results in a series of reactions, including increased blood flow to the site and increased permeability of capillaries to plasma molecules, which ultimately leads to destruction of the stimulating antigen (Mackinnon, 1999; Marieb, 2001; Vander, et al., 2001).

Acute phase proteins (APP) are produced and secreted from the liver, as are some complement proteins (Mackinnon, 1992; Marieb, 2001). APP are stimulated by proinflammatory cytokines and are so named because they increase rapidly during an infection. One example of an APP is C-reactive protein (CRP). Elevated levels of C-reactive protein represent a possible risk factor for cardiovascular disease. APP stimulate an increase in the number of leukocytes and play an important role in tissue repair following muscle cell damage.

Inflammatory mediators are molecules that, as the name implies, control the development of inflammation. The three selected factors identified in Figure 17.1, *histamine, platelet activating factor (PAF)*, and *serotonin*, all bring about increased vascular permeability and smooth muscle contraction. Other inflammatory mediators, not released from basophils, mast cells, or platelets, include *fibrinopeptides* (the substance removed from fibrinogen during blood coagulation) and *fibrin breakdown products* plus *prostaglandins (PGE₂)*. These substances make the actions of the other inflammatory mediators more effective.

Processes

There are numerous ways in which the immune system can deal with pathogens. These defense mechanisms vary according to the type of pathogen and its particular life cycle stage. *Cytotoxic reactions* are those in which whole cells are killed, primarily by punching holes in their outer membranes. A target cell may be signaled to self-destruct, a process that is termed *apoptosis*. *Lysis* is a form of cytotoxic reaction in which a cell is killed by destruction of the cell membrane. *Neutralization* is a process that occurs when antibodies block the binding site on antigens so that they cannot bind to tissues and cause damage. *Opsinization* is the process of coating the membrane of an antigen, making it easier for phagocytes to adhere to and engulf the antigen. *Phagocytosis* is the process of engulfing and digesting a pathogen. Additionally, intracellular granules (small grainlike bodies) may be released. This is called a *respiratory oxidative burst* and is a potent killer.

Functional Organization of the Immune System

Functionally, the immune system can be divided into two separate but interrelated and overlapping

Table 17.1

Major Cytokines Involved in the Exercise Immune Response

Cytokine	Released From	Primary Function
Interleukin IL-1α, IL-1β	Macrophages	T cell activation Macrophage function Proinflammatory Fever
IL-2	T cells	T cell activation T cell proliferation
IL-4	T cells	Anti-inflammatory
IL-6	Activated T cells Macrophages	T and B cell growth Stimulates acute phase proteins Anti-inflammatory Proinflammatory
IL-10	T cells B cells Macrophages Mast cells	Anti-inflammatory, immunosuppressive
Interferon IFNα	Leukocytes	Antiviral activity Stimulates cytotoxicity
IFNγ	T cells, NK cells	Stimulates cytotoxicity Macrophage activation Proinflammatory
Tumor necrosis factor TNFα	Macrophages, NK cells	Stimulates cytotoxicity against tumor cells Proinflammatory

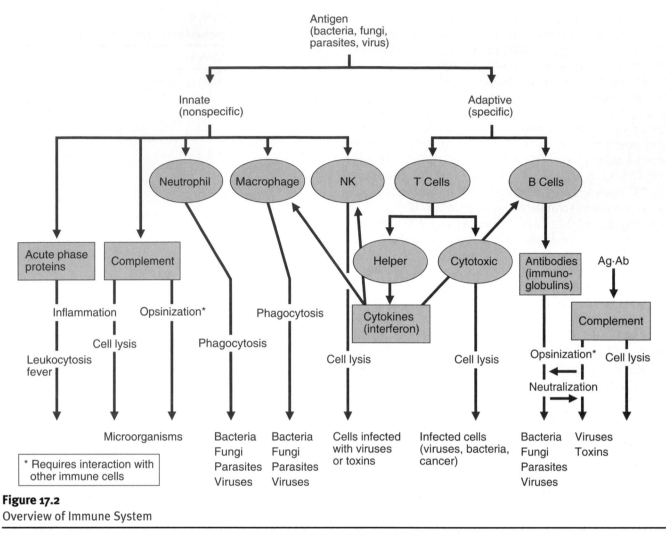

Figure 17.2
Overview of Immune System

Sources: Modified from Marieb (2001) and Smith (1995).

branches: the innate (nonspecific) and the adaptive (specific) branches (Marieb, 2001; Smith, 1995). This organization is presented in Figure 17.2. The cells of the immune system are represented by circles, and the soluble mediators (chemicals) by boxes. The processes or mechanisms of destruction are given within the arrows that point to the pathogen destroyed by a given mechanism.

The Innate Branch

The *innate branch* protects against foreign substances or cells without having to recognize them. It is nonselective; thus it provides an initial line of defense against microbial invasion. The innate system consists of both a cellular component and physical barriers. Intact skin and mucous membranes are the major physical barriers. The primary cells of the innate

system are the NK lymphocytes, neutrophils, and macrophages. Complement and acute phase proteins are the major soluble mediators, and the processes by which the innate system works are lysis, opsinization, and phagocytosis.

Inflammation

Central to the functioning of the innate branch of the immune system is the *inflammatory response* (Figure 17.3). The cells of the immune system are widely dispersed in the body. When an injury (thermal or physical) or infection occurs, it is necessary to concentrate immune cells at the site of the emergency, much as fire trucks, ambulances, and police cars with their respective personnel converge on a disaster area. As shown in Figure 17.3, four processes combine to accomplish this convergence:

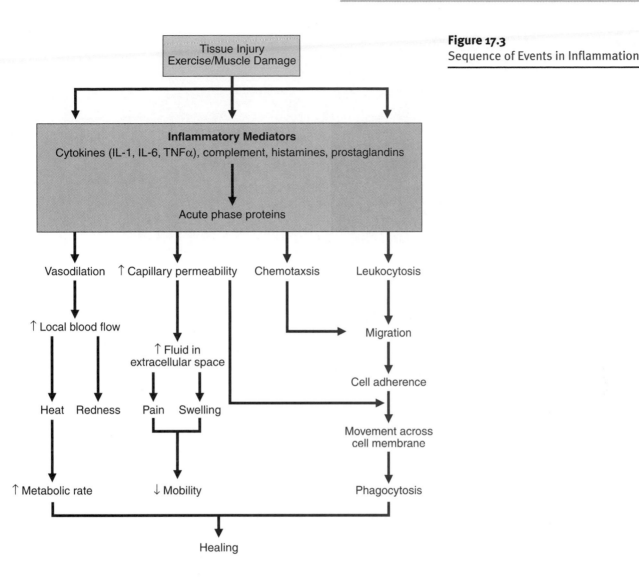

Figure 17.3
Sequence of Events in Inflammation

1. vasodilation and an increased blood supply to the area;

2. increased capillary permeability;

3. chemotaxis; and

4. leukocytosis (an increased number of leukocytes).

The first two are self-explanatory. *Chemotaxis* is the increased directional migration of immune cells. Figure 17.4 depicts the sequence of events by which muscular damage can initiate chemotaxis and set the stage for repair of the damaged tissue (Marieb, 2001). Chemotaxis occurs in response to the release of chemotactic factors, inflammatory mediators, and acute phase proteins. Neutrophils are the first cells to arrive at the injury site and do so within an hour. Neutrophils are followed by monocytes, which become macrophages once they enter the tissue. Macrophages dominate at the site of the injury 5–6 hr after the initi-

ation of the inflammatory response. Upon arrival, these phagocytes adhere to the walls of the capillaries. Eventually the phagocytes push between the endothelial cells in the capillary and cross the membrane. They then squeeze through the cell membrane and move to the actual site of the inflammation. Once at the site, both neutrophils and macrophages phagocytize the foreign antigens and/or cellular debris.

Inflammation is characterized by redness, heat, swelling, and pain. The increased blood flow to the tissues resulting from vasodilation leads to the redness and heat. The increased capillary permeability allows fluid to seep into extracellular spaces, creating swelling that activates pain receptors. The pain and swelling can result in lack of mobility. Although immobility is generally viewed as inconvenient, it forces the injured part to rest, which aids in healing. Thus, inflammation can destroy foreign pathogens, prevent the spread of damaging agents, dispose of cellular debris, and set the stage

Figure 17.4
Events by Which Tissue
Damage Leads to Increased
Leukocytes in Tissues

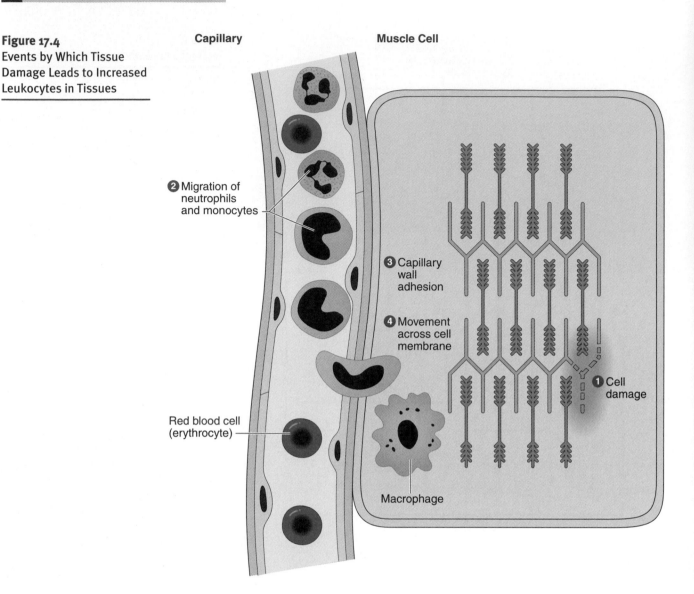

Capillary

Muscle Cell

2 Migration of
neutrophils
and monocytes

3 Capillary
wall
adhesion

4 Movement
across cell
membrane

1 Cell
damage

Red blood cell
(erythrocyte)

Macrophage

The Adaptive Branch

for tissue repair. Although classified as part of the innate system, inflammation is also an important component of the adaptive immune response.

In contrast to the innate branch, the *adaptive branch* of the immune system requires that the immune cells recognize a foreign material and react specifically and selectively to destroy it. The adaptive branch is antigen specific, is systemic, and has memory. The adaptive branch includes humoral (from the Latin word *humor,* meaning "fluids") and cell-mediated immunity. *Humoral immunity* is provided by the antibodies produced from B cells. The antibodies circulate in the blood and lymph, where they bind to bacteria, toxins, and free viruses; inactivate them temporarily; and mark them for destruction by phagocytes or complements. *Cell-mediated immunity* is provided by T

lymphocytes that directly attack and lyse cells infected by viruses, parasites, cancer cells, or grafts; release chemical mediators to enhance inflammation; and activate lymphocytes and macrophages.

The body's ability to mount a specialized immune response is based on specific proteins called *major compatibility proteins (MHC)* that exist on the membranes of the body's own cells and pathogens. MHCs are different in each individual, except identical twins. Thus, in the case of an organ transplant, the immune system must be suppressed; otherwise, the recipient's immune system would not recognize the donor MHC (unless the donor were a twin). An "attack" resulting in the "rejection" of the organ would occur. As can be seen in Figure 17.2, the major cells of the adaptive branch are the B and T cells. The major soluble mediators are antibodies, cytokines, and complement. The processes of action include lysis, neutralization, opsinization, and, indirectly,

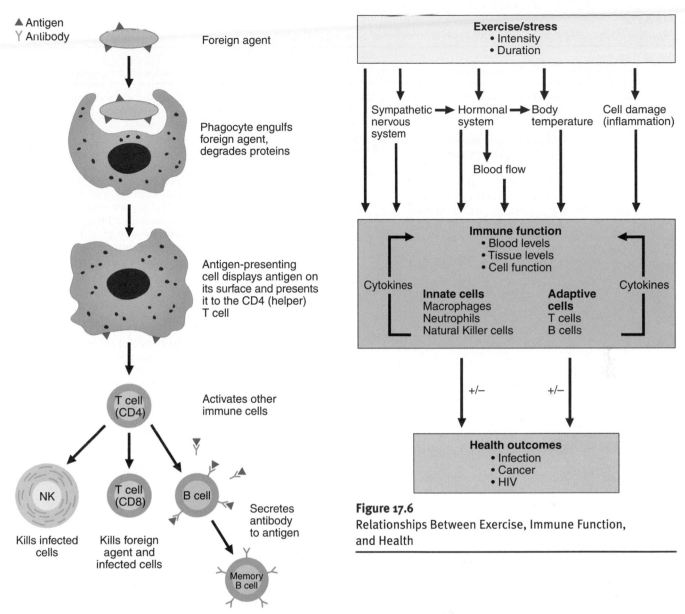

▲ Antigen
Y Antibody

Foreign agent

Phagocyte engulfs
foreign agent,
degrades proteins

Antigen-presenting
cell displays antigen on
its surface and presents
it to the CD4 (helper)
T cell

T cell
(CD4)

Activates other
immune cells

NK

T cell
(CD8)

B cell

Secretes
antibody
to antigen

Kills infected
cells

Kills foreign
agent and
infected cells

Memory
B cell

Figure 17.5
Central Role of Macrophages in the Innate and Adaptive
Immune Response

Exercise/stress
• Intensity
• Duration

Sympathetic
nervous
system → Hormonal
system → Body
temperature

Cell damage
(inflammation)

Blood flow

Immune function
• Blood levels
• Tissue levels
• Cell function

Cytokines

Innate cells
Macrophages
Neutrophils
Natural Killer cells

**Adaptive
cells**
T cells
B cells

Cytokines

+/−   +/−

Health outcomes
• Infection
• Cancer
• HIV

Figure 17.6
Relationships Between Exercise, Immune Function,
and Health

structures and substances in the immune system
overlap and are in some ways redundant. This ensures an effective immune response to most pathogens the body encounters and is essential to the
health of the individual.

The Immune Response to Exercise

An acute bout of exercise causes an immune response. Exercise physiologists, other exercise professionals, clinicians, and the general public are all interested in understanding the relationship between
exercise and immune function. Indeed, a great deal of
research has been directed at this issue. Yet, much remains unanswered about the relationship between
exercise and immune function. Figure 17.6 depicts
the complexities encountered in trying to address this

phagocytosis. Figure 17.5 provides an overview of
how the innate and adaptive branches work together
for a generalized immune response, emphasizing the
role of macrophages in phagocytosizing the foreign
invader and activating the adaptive immune response
by serving as antigen-presenting cells.

The body's myriad of defenses against tissue
injury and infection is amazing and, admittedly, can
be overwhelming. Table 17.2 provides a glossary of
the cells, soluble mediators, and processes that play
an important role in the immune response.
It is helpful to remember that the functions of the

Table 17.2

Glossary of Cells, Molecules, and Processes Involved in the Immune Response

Branch of Immune System	Processes	Cells	Molecules/Chemical Factors
Innate and adaptive	*Lysis* is the killing of a cell via destruction of the cell membrane. *Phagocytosis* is the process of engulfing and digesting an antigen. *Inflammation* is the process that prevents the spread of damaging agents, disposes of pathogens and cellular debris, and sets the stage for tissue repair.	*Macrophages* are immune cells that (1) phagocytize pathogens, (2) present parts of the engulfed antigen on its plasma membrane to activate the T cell response, and (3) secrete cytokines. They are important in both the innate and adaptive immune responses.	*Antigens* are substances capable of provoking an immune response. *Complement* is a group of approximately 20 plasma proteins. When activated, complement lyses microorganisms, enhances phagocytosis, and enhances the inflammatory response. Complement may be activated and function in either the innate or adaptive immune response. *Cytokines* are chemicals released from sensitized T cells, NK cells, and activated macrophages to help regulate the immune response.
Innate		*Natural killer (NK)* cells are innate immune cells that destroy virus-infected and cancerous body cells by cell lysis. *Neutrophils* are innate immune cells that phagocytize pathogens.	*Acute phase proteins (APPs)* are blood proteins produced in the liver that function in the innate immune response. APPs are important in the response to infection and inflammation.
Adaptive	*Neutralization* is a process that occurs when antibodies block the binding site on antigens so that they cannot bind to tissues and cause damage. *Opsinization* is the process of coating the membrane of an antigen, making it easier for phagocytes to adhere to and engulf the antigen.	*B cells* are lymphocytes that are part of the adaptive immune response and are responsible for the production of antibodies to a specific antigen. *T cells* are lymphocytes that are responsible for cell-mediated responses of the adaptive immune system. Functionally, there are two classes of T cells: cytotoxic T cells (CD8 cells), which destroy virus-infected and cancer cells directly via cell lysis; and helper T cells (CD4 cells), regulatory cells that influence the activity of cytotoxic T cells, B cells, NK, and macrophages. Both cytotoxic and helper T cells can act as suppressor cells once the infection is controlled.	*Antibodies* are proteins produced by B cells to attack antigens.

important question (Woods, Davis, Smith, et al., 1999). As with the effect of exercise on the other systems of the body, the immune response to exercise depends on the intensity and duration of the exercise and the immune system variable being measured. Furthermore, the physiological stress of exercise may well be additive with other stresses in one's life. Further complicating the relationship between exercise and immune function is the vast array of immune functions. Exercise appears to affect all of the cells of the immune system, but it appears that they are affected in different ways. Furthermore, each cell of the immune system may perform several functions, and exercise may affect these functions differently. When researchers investigate the effect of exercise on immune function, they may report changes in blood levels of an immune cell, tissue levels of an immune cell, or functioning of an immune cell. Although it is

Focus on Research

What Causes the Immune Exercise Response?

Rhind, S. G., G. A. Gannon, P. N. Shek, I. K. M. Brenner, Y. Severs, J. Zamecnik, A. Buguet, V. M. Natale, R. J. Shephard, & M. W. Radomski: Contribution of exertional hyperthermia to sympathoadrenal-mediated lymphocyte subset redistribution. *Journal of Applied Physiology*. 87(3):1178–1185 (1999).

It is known that aerobic exercise causes leukocytosis (an increase in circulating leukocytes). It is also known that leukocytes respond differently to exercise; some leukocytes increase in number and remain elevated during recovery, whereas other leukocytes increase during exercise but decrease during recovery. Furthermore, studies have clearly demonstrated that the changes that occur in immune cells depend on exercise intensity and duration. In addition to describing the exercise response, researchers have long been interested in determining the mechanisms responsible for the changes in leukocyte number and distribution in response to exercise. The most frequently proposed mechanism is the action of the sympathoadrenal-mediated stress hormones. However, increase in body temperature (exertional hyperthermia) has also been proposed as a possible mechanism. To understand the relative influence of these mechanisms more completely, Rhind and colleagues (1999) designed a study to examine changes

in stress hormone levels and lymphocyte redistribution during exercise with and without a rise of rectal temperature. In order to achieve this goal, Rhind and colleagues had the participants perform exercise while immersed in water. One trial was performed in cold water (18°C), and the other trial was performed in hot water (39°C). This allowed the participants to perform the same amount of exercise during the two trials. However, rectal temperature increased only during the trial that was performed in hot water. The accompanying graphs present changes in the stress hormones (epinephrine, norepinephrine, and cortisol) and changes in immune cells (total leukocyte number and lymphocyte number).

These results demonstrate convincingly that hyperthermia has an effect on hormone concentrations (increases in epinephrine, norepinephrine, and cortisol were all significantly higher in the hot trial) and, thus, on leukocyte number and distribution (both total leukocyte number and lymphocyte number were higher in the hot trial). Furthermore, these data suggest that the influence of hyperthermia on leukocyte number and distribution is indirect, meaning that it is not the increase in temperature itself that influences leukocytes, but rather that the increase in temperature affects the hormonal system, which in turn affects the immune system. This research reinforces the interdependence of several systems of the body.

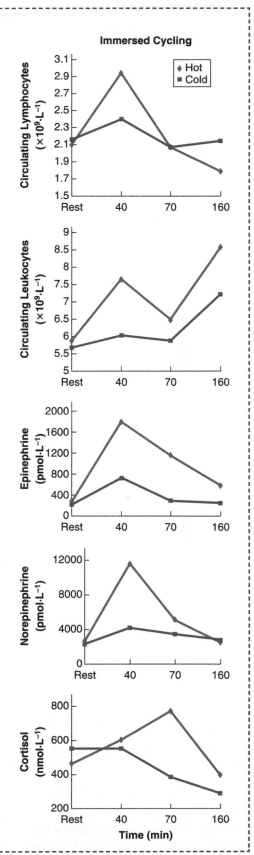

Table 17.3

Exercise Response of Immune Cells to Medium-Duration (< 45 min), Moderate- and High-Intensity Aerobic Exercise

Variable Exercise Intensity	During Exercise or Immediate Postexercise	Recovery
Total Leukocytes		
Moderate-intensity	↑ 0–40%	Unknown
High-intensity	↑ 50%	↑ 50–100% 2 hr postexercise
Innate Immune System		
Neutrophils		
Moderate-intensity	↑ 30–50%	Unknown
High-intensity	↑ 30–150%	Unknown up to 2 hr postexercise 25–100% 2–4 hr postexercise
Monocytes		
Moderate-intensity	No Change	Unknown
High-intensity	↑ 0–20%	↑ 0–50% 2 hr postexercise
Natural Killer cells		
Moderate-intensity	↑ 0–50%	Normal by 1 hr postexercise
High-intensity	↑ 100–200%	↓ 40% 2–4 hr postexercise
Adaptive Immune System		
T cells		
Moderate-intensity	No change	Unknown
High-intensity	↑ 100%	↓ 30% 1–2 hr postexercise
B cells		
Moderate-intensity	No change	Unknown
High-intensity	No change	↓ 0–25% 1–2 hr postexercise
Serum Ig		
Moderate-intensity	No change	No change
High-intensity	No change	No change
Salivary IgA		
Moderate-intensity	No change	No change
High-intensity	No change	No change

Source: Based on data from Mackinnon (1999).

interesting to know how exercise affects individual cells of the immune system, most people are more interested in how exercise relates to health outcomes, such as the rate and severity of an infection or the incidence and progression of a tumor. Such studies are very difficult to conduct in humans. Therefore, the majority of data relating exercise to disease or infection in humans is based on epidemiological evidence, whereas experiments relating exercise to health outcomes are often performed in laboratory animals. A final challenge to understanding the relationship between exercise and immune function, one that is also depicted in Figure 17.6, is the number of possible mechanisms that may mediate the effect of exercise on the immune system. Exercise may alter immune function by any combination of the mechanisms listed below (Pedersen and Ullum, 1994; Woods, Davis, Smith, et al., 1999):

1. by directly stimulating immune function;

2. by stimulating the sympathetic nervous system;

3. by altering hormones (especially epinephrine, norepinephrine, cortisol, growth hormone, prolactin, and thyroxine);

4. by increasing body temperature; and

5. by exercise-induced cell damage (and the release of acute phase proteins).

Another important factor that must be considered is the recovery period from exercise. Exercise may alter immune function for several hours or days. In fact, it is the suppression of several immune cells in the postexercise period that is most often proposed as the link to the incidence of upper respiratory tract infection among high-volume, endurance-trained athletes (Mackinnon, et al., 1987; Nieman, 1997; Tomasi, et al., 1982).

Clearly the type of exercise that is performed affects the exercise response of the immune system. Prolonged aerobic exercise has received the greatest research attention relative to the immune system. Prolonged aerobic exercise has been the focus of research because there are epidemiological data linking high-volume endurance training with a greater incidence of upper respiratory tract infection. Thus, in this section we will deviate from the categories typically used in this textbook and describe the immune response relative to "medium-duration" (< 45 min) moderate- and high-intensity, aerobic exercise; "prolonged" (1–3 hr) moderate- and high-intensity exercise; and intense interval exercise. Mackinnon (1999) has recently provided a summary of the research findings in exercise immunology based on these categories.

Medium-Duration (<45 min), Moderate- to High-Intensity Aerobic Exercise

Table 17.3 reports the changes in immune cell numbers (reported as a percentage) during or immediately postexercise and during recovery from medium-duration, moderate-, and high-intensity exercise (Mackinnon, 1999). Exercise results in *leukocytosis,* an increased number of white blood cells. Leukocytosis is evident during most forms of physical activity and depends on the intensity and duration of the exercise. In most cases, the leukocytosis persists for at least 1–4 hr postexercise.

Neutrophils increase in number as a result of endurance exercise. The increases are greater following high-intensity exercise than following moderate exercise. The increase in neutrophils is evident for 2–4 hr postexercise and is likely evident during moderate exercise, although research data are lacking. In addition to increasing cell numbers, it appears that medium-duration aerobic exercise enhances neutrophil function. Both the phagocytic activity and the oxidative burst activity of the neutrophils are reported to be enhanced (Marieb, 2001; Woods, Davis, Smith, et al., 1999).

The circulating levels of monocytes are not altered by medium-duration, moderate exercise but increase modestly during high-intensity exercise (Mackinnon, 1999). This elevation persists for at least 2 hr

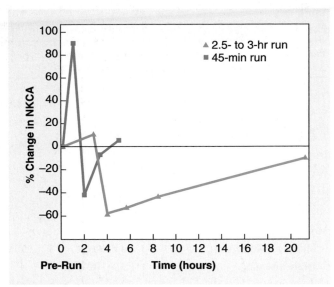

Figure 17.7
Natural Killer Cell Activity (NKCA) during and following Exercise of Different Durations

NKCA is greater following 45 min of running (~80% $\dot{V}O_2$max) than following 2.5–3 hr of running (~76% $\dot{V}O_2$max). However, NKCA is suppressed longer following prolonged running (2.5–3 hr) than 45 min of running.

Source: Modified from Woods, et al. 1999. Based on data from Nieman et al., 1995; Nieman et al., 1990.

postexercise. You will recall that when monocytes leave the bloodstream they are transformed to macrophages, which perform several roles in the immune response. Research suggests that macrophage functions are enhanced following medium-duration exercise. These functions include phagocytic activity, oxidative burst activity, and antitumor activity (Nieman, 1997; Woods, Ceddia, et al., 1997; Woods and Davis, 1994; Woods, Davis, Mayer, et al., 1993; Woods, Davis, Smith, et al., 1999).

The circulating levels of natural killer (NK) cells increase during medium-duration bouts of both moderate- and high-intensity exercise, with the more intense exercise causing a larger increase in NK cell numbers. Of greater importance, however, is the differential response seen during recovery. Following moderate-intensity exercise, blood levels of NK cells return to normal within 1 hr. Following high-intensity exercise, in contrast, NK cell levels drop approximately 40% below normal levels and remain depressed for 2–4 hr. Natural killer cell activity (NKCA) mimics the changes in NK cell numbers (Mackinnon, 1999; Woods, Davis, Smith, et al., 1999). Figure 17.7 depicts the change in NKCA following both 45 min of intense (80% $\dot{V}O_2$max) and 2.5–3 hr of running (~76% $\dot{V}O_2$max) and during recovery. For now, concentrate on the 45-min bout of ex-

Table 17.4

Exercise Response of Immune Cells to Prolonged (1–3 hr) Moderate- and High-Intensity Aerobic Exercise

Variable Exercise Intensity	During Exercise or Immediate Postexercise	Recovery
Total Leukocytes		
Moderate-intensity	↑ 25–50%	↑ 25–65% 2 hr postexercise
High-intensity	↑ 200–300%	↑ 200–300% 2–6 hr postexercise
Innate Immune System		
Neutrophils		
Moderate-intensity	↑ 20–50%	↑ 50–150% 2 hr postexercise
High-intensity	↑ 300%	↑ 300–400% 2–6 hr postexercise
Monocytes		
Moderate-intensity	No change	No change
High-intensity	↑ 50–100%	↑ 50–100% 2–3 hr postexercise
Natural Killer cells		
Moderate-intensity	↑ 70–100%	↓ 0–50% 1–2 hr postexercise
High-intensity	↑ 100–200%	↓ 30–60% 1–2 hr postexercise
Adaptive Immune System		
T cells		
Moderate-intensity	↑ 20–30%	↓ 20% 2 hr postexercise
High-intensity	↑ 30–60%	↓ 30–40% 1–6 hr postexercise
B cells		
Moderate-intensity	No change	No change
High-intensity	No change	No change
Serum Ig		
Moderate-intensity	No change	No change
High-intensity	No change	No change
Salivary IgA		
Moderate-intensity	No change	No change
High-intensity	↓ 20–60%	↓ 20–60% 1 hr postexercise

Source: Based on data from Mackinnon (1999).

ercise. Notice that there is a large increase in NKCA immediately postexercise, followed by a reduction in NKCA below preexercise levels and a subsequent return to preexercise values by the fourth hour (Nieman, Ahle, et al., 1995; Nieman, Buckley, et al., 1995; Nieman, Johanssen, et al., 1990; Woods, Davis, Smith, et al., 1999).

T cell numbers do not change during moderate-intensity, medium-duration exercise but increase markedly as a result of high-intensity exercise. During recovery from intense exercise there is a suppression in T cell numbers that is evident for 1–2 hr of recovery (Mackinnon, 1999). As with NK cells, this suppression in T cells postexercise may have implications for susceptibility to infection.

B cell numbers do not appear to change immediately after medium-duration bouts of moderate- or high-intensity dynamic exercise. However, B cell numbers decrease 1–2 hr following intense exercise. Daughter cells of the B cells, plasma cells, produce antibodies (immunoglobulins) that lead to destruction of antigens. It appears that there is no change in serum or salivary levels of immunoglobulins following aerobic exercise lasting less than 45 min (Mackinnon, 1999).

Prolonged (1–3 hr), Moderate- to High-Intensity Aerobic Exercise

Table 17.4 reports the changes in immune cell numbers during or immediately postexercise and during recovery from prolonged, moderate- and high-intensity aerobic exercise (Mackinnon, 1999). As stated earlier, exercise results in leukocytosis, which depends on the intensity and duration of the exercise. Prolonged, high-intensity exercise results in the greatest leukocytosis immediately postexercise and in recovery.

Neutrophils increase in number as a result of aerobic exercise. The increases are greater following high-intensity exercise, and prolonged, high-intensity exercise causes a significantly greater increase in neutrophils than shorter exercise bouts of the same intensity. Large increases in neutrophil numbers are evident for 2–6 hr following high-intensity exercise. Despite the increase in neutrophil number following prolonged, moderate- and high-intensity exercise, there is evidence that neutrophil function may not respond uniformly (Mackinnon, 1999). Prolonged moderate-exercise is associated with enhanced neutrophil function (phagocytic activity, oxidative burst activity, and antimicrobial activity). In contrast, prolonged, high-intensity exercise is associated with a suppression of neutrophil function (Nieman, 1997; Woods, Davis, Smith, et al., 1999).

The circulating levels of monocytes are not altered by moderate-intensity, aerobic exercise but increase substantially during intense aerobic exercise. The elevation persists for at least 2 hr postexercise. Furthermore, the increase in monocytes following prolonged, high-intensity exercise is considerably greater than the increase in monocytes following medium-duration, high-intensity exercise, as is the postexercise elevation (Mackinnon, 1999). Research suggests that macrophage function is enhanced following prolonged, moderate-intensity, aerobic exercise. However, the effect of high-intensity exercise on macrophage function is unclear. It appears that some functions are enhanced (phagocytosis, lysing, and antiviral activity), whereas other activities (oxidative burst) may be suppressed (Kohut, et al., 1998; Nieman, 1997; Woods, Ceddia, et al., 1997; Woods, Davis, Smith, et al., 1999).

The circulating levels of NK cells increase considerably following prolonged bouts of both moderate and high-intensity, aerobic exercise, with the intense exercise causing a larger increase in NK cell numbers. Notice, however, that following prolonged exercise there is a reduction in NK cell numbers. This reduction is evident following moderate- as well as high-intensity exercise, although high-intensity exercise is associated with a greater reduction in NK cell numbers. As with medium-duration exercise, NKCA mimics the changes in NK cell numbers. Look again at Figure 17.7, this time paying attention to the change in NKCA following 2.5–3 hr of intense (76% $\dot{V}O_2$max) running and during recovery (Nieman, Ahle, et al., 1995;

Table 17.5
Exercise Response of Immune Cell Counts to Intense Interval Exercise

Variable	During Exercise or Immediate Postexercise	Recovery
Total Leukocyte Number	↑ 65–80%	↑ 75% 2–6 hr postexercise
Innate Immune System		
Neutrophils	↑ 25%	↑ 60–100% 2–6 hr postexercise
Monocytes	↑ 40–50%	↑ 15–60% 2–6 hr postexercise
Natural Killer cells	↑ 100–200%	Normal by 1–2 hr postexercise
Adaptive Immune System		
T cells	↑ 60–100%	↓ 30–40% 1–2 hr postexercise
B cells	↑ 0–7%	Normal by 1–6 hr postexercise

Source: Based on data from Mackinnon (1999).

Nieman, Buckley, et al., 1995; Nieman, Johanssen, et al., 1990; Woods, Davis, Smith, et al., 1999). Notice that there is a smaller increase in NKCA immediately postexercise for the prolonged run (2.5–3 hr) compared to the shorter run (45 min). However, during recovery from the prolonged run there is a severe and persistent reduction in NKCA below preexercise levels. NKCA remained suppressed in excess of 20 hr following the prolonged, high-intensity run.

T cell numbers increase following prolonged, moderate-intensity and high-intensity exercise. During recovery from prolonged exercise (both moderate- and high-intensity) T cell numbers are suppressed. B cell numbers do not appear to change immediately after prolonged bouts of moderate- or high-intensity exercise. There is also no change noted during recovery from exercise. Salivary levels of immunoglobulin A (IgA), however, appear to be depressed following prolonged, high-intensity exercise (Mackinnon, 1999; Tomasi, et al., 1982).

Intense, Interval Exercise

Table 17.5 reports the changes in immune cell numbers during or immediately postexercise and during recovery from intense, interval exercise (Mackinnon, 1999). As stated previously, exercise

Table 17.6
Selected Cytokine Responses to Exercise

Cytokine	Exercise Response
IL-1	May ↑ in blood after moderate-intensity exercise ↑ 100% in urinary excretion after endurance exercise ↑ 100% in skeletal muscle up to 5 days after eccentric exercise
IL-2	No change after exercise
IL-6	No change after moderate exercise ↑ 150% after endurance exercise
IFNα	↑ after endurance exercise
INFγ	No change after endurance exercise
TNFα	No change in blood after moderate exercise; may be decreased after high-intensity exercise ↑ 100% in urinary excretion after endurance exercise

Source: Based on data from Mackinnon (1999).

results in leukocytosis, which persists for at least 2–6 hr postexercise.

Neutrophils increase in number as a result of intense, interval exercise and remain elevated for 2–6 hr postexercise. Likewise, the circulating levels of monocytes increase following intense, interval exercise and remain elevated for 2–6 hr postexercise. NK cell numbers increase markedly following intense interval exercise but return to preexercise levels within 2 hr postexercise.

T cell numbers increase following intense interval exercise. During recovery from intense interval exercise, there is a suppression of T cell numbers that is evident for 1–2 hr of recovery. B cell numbers increase immediately after intense interval exercise but return to normal levels within 1–6 hr postexercise.

Cytokine Response to Exercise

The response of various cytokines to exercise is of interest because the cytokines regulate much of the function of the immune system. Although this is an important area of research, relatively few studies have been conducted in this area, largely because of technical difficulties in obtaining these measures. Table 17.6 presents what is currently known about the cytokine response to exercise (Mackinnon, 1999). Notice that currently there is not enough information to categorize the cytokine response to various durations and intensities of exercise.

In summary, an acute bout of exercise has profound effects on many immune variables, including cell number and function and circulating levels of cytokines. In general, it appears that moderate exercise causes transient increases in immune function, with immune cell number and function returning to baseline within a couple of hours. Strenuous exercise, however, is associated with greater disruption of the immune system and results in a decrease in some cells and cellular function (especially NK cells and T cells) and this suppression may last for many hours into recovery. In fact, it is this reduction in cell number and function that provides the theoretical link to the greater incidence of upper respiratory tract infection that is reported in high-volume, endurance-trained individuals.

Hormonal Control of Immune Response to Exercise

As stated previously, moderate, aerobic exercise enhances immune function, and the cells of the immune system return to resting levels soon after exercise. Severe exhaustive, aerobic exercise, by contrast, is associated with an enhanced immune function that is followed by a suppression of cell activity.

The differential response of enhanced immune function following moderate exercise and suppression of some components of immune function following severe exercise depends largely on the hormones epinephrine and cortisol. During exercise at greater than 60% of $\dot{V}O_2max$, epinephrine and cortisol levels in the blood begin to increase rapidly, reaching their highest level following maximal exercise. Epinephrine is associated with a substantial increase in the number of lymphocytes in the blood. Cortisol causes an increase in the number of neutrophils but a decrease in the number of lymphocytes. Immediately following exercise, the blood concentrations of epinephrine fall rapidly to preexercise levels, whereas cortisol levels remain elevated for 2 hr or more (see Chapter 2). Thus, researchers hypothesize that following intense exercise, epinephrine is responsible for the increase in circulating lymphocytes, and the longer-acting cortisol is responsible for the prolonged increase in neutrophils and the decrease in lymphocytes (Nieman, 1994).

Training Adaptations in Immune Function

Table 17.7 presents a summary of training adaptations in the immune system of moderately trained and highly trained or overtrained individuals. The resting

Table 17.7
Effect of Moderate and Intense Training/Overtraining on Immune Function and Resistance to Illness

	Moderate Training	Intense Training/Overtraining
Cells		
Leukocytes	No change in resting number	↓ Resting number in circulation of athletes after intense exercise
Neutrophils	No change in resting number	No change in resting number (or decrease) ↓ Activation at rest and after exercise
NK cells	No change in resting number ↑ NKCA at rest	↓ Resting number in circulation ↓ NKCA at rest
T cells	No change	No change, or decrease
B cells	No change in resting number	No change in resting number
Chemical Mediators		
Cytokines	No change in resting concentration ↑ Resting IL-1 in plasma of athletes compared with nonathletes	No change in resting concentrations ↑ Resting 1L-1 in plasma of athletes compared with nonathletes
APP	↓ Acute phase protein release after exercise	↓ Acute phase protein release after exercise
Antibodies (Ig)	No change in serum and secretory Ig levels ↑ Specific antibody response	↓ Serum Ig levels in athletes after intensified training ↓ Salivary IgA levels in athletes after intensified training
Resistance to Illness	↑ Survival rate following viral infection ↑ Survival rate following bacterial infection ↓ Incidence of cancer ↓ Incidence of URTI	↑ Incidence of URTI ↑ Rate of paralysis following polio infection

Sources: Based on data from Mackinnon (2000, 1999) and Nieman (1997).

immune system of moderately trained aerobic athletes is usually within normal parameters, although neutrophil function and serum immunoglobulins may be relatively low (Mackinnon, 2000; Nieman, 1994; Shephard, et al., 1995). In general, moderate training appears to enhance some functions of the immune system, especially natural killer cell count and activity (Mackinnon, 2000; Shephard, et al., 1995; Woods, Davis, Smith, et al., 1999). In contrast, strenuous training or overtraining is associated with a suppression of several immune variables. Most notable among the changes in the immune function following severe training is a suppression of leukocyte numbers, a decrease in neutrophil function, a decrease in natural killer cell activity, and a reduction in lymphocytes (B cells, T cells, and NK cells) (Mackinnon, 2000, 1999; Nieman, 1997; Woods, Davis, Smith, et al., 1999). As seen in Table 17.7, there are also training-induced adaptations in several cytokines, acute phase proteins, and antibodies (immunoglobulins). Intense training or

Table 17.8
Cytokine Training Adaptations

Cytokine	Training Adaptation
IL-1	May be higher at rest in endurance-trained athletes
IL-2	Unknown
IL-6	Higher at rest in endurance-trained athletes
IFN	No change
TNFα	Higher at rest in endurance-trained athletes

Source: Based on data from Mackinnon (1999).

overtraining is associated with a reduction in acute phase proteins, serum Ig, salivary IgA, and complement (Mackinnon, 1999; Nieman, 1997; Woods, Davis, Smith, et al., 1999). Table 17.8 presents some additional information about training adaptations in selected cytokines, although there is insufficient

Focus on Application

✳ Dietary Supplementation and the Exercise Immune Response

In the pursuit of optimal fitness or performance, individuals often push the limits of the various systems of the body, including the immune system. The possibility that nutritional supplements stabilize or enhance the immune system's response to exercise in active individuals is intriguing and attractive. Three dietary interventions or manipulations have begun to receive attention: (1) carbohydrate (CHO) supplementation, (2) branched chain amino acid (BCAA)/glutamine supplementation, and (3) vitamin C and E supplementation (Mackinnon, 1999).

1. *Carbohydrate supplementation.* There are three situations in which carbohydrate supplementation has been reasonably well established as beneficial: an increase from 55 to 70% of total calories during training to replenish and maintain glycogen levels;

carbohydrate loading before endurance competition to increase glycogen stores to maintain a high-intensity during the event; and ingestion of carbohydrate to provide blood-borne glucose as a readily available energy supply during a competitive endurance event. From the standpoint of the immune system, the latter two appear to be particularly relevant. Several studies have shown that a 5–6% CHO drink taken during prolonged strenuous exercise (cycling, rowing, and running) maintains blood glucose levels (Bishop, et al., 2000; Henson, et al., 2000; Nieman, et al., 1997). In turn, the maintenance of blood glucose levels blunts the large increase in stress hormones (which probably control the immune response) thus blunting the changes in circulating leukocytes (neutrophils, NK cells, and monocytes), soluble mediators (pro- and anti-inflammatory cytokines and IgA) as well as some processes (phagocytosis and respiratory oxidative bursts) but not others (NK cell activity). This

blunting means less of a suppression of immune function and possibly a minimization of inflammation. However, the precise clinical benefits of CHO supplementation (in terms of infection or illness) have not been established. Thus, while the current evidence is insufficient to recommend CHO ingestion during and immediately postexercise specifically to benefit the immune system, the possibility that it might strengthens the importance of adequate CHO intake (especially if taken in fluid form) for the endurance exercise participant (Nieman, 2000).

2. *BCAA/glutamine supplementation.* Glutamine is the most abundant amino acid in human muscle and plasma. Hence, skeletal muscle, not food intake, is the primary source of glutamine in the body. It is comprised of glutamate (a product of the transamination of 12 different amino acids) and NH_4 (ammonium). Glutamine is both an energy source and a precursor of substances essential for immune cell (especially lymphocyte and monocyte) replication (Field, et

research to categorize these as responses to moderate or severe training (Mackinnon, 1999).

One of the greatest challenges in this area of research is to define more clearly what constitutes "moderate" training, and what constitutes "strenuous" training. Furthermore, there is a need to understand more fully whether strenuous training in itself results in immune suppression or whether immune suppression occurs only if the training is so severe as to qualify as overtraining.

Cytokine Hypothesis of Overtraining

Chapter 2 discussed the overtraining syndrome (OTS) in the context of Selye's theory of stress and presented the signs and symptoms of the OTS. This section will present a hypothesis of overtraining which proposes that Selye's third stage (the Stage of Exhaustion) is

largely adaptive, in the sense that the individual is forced to attempt to survive or recover as opposed to improve. If the cause of the excessive stress is not removed, the attempts at survival invoke an immune system response, mediated primarily by cytokines, which in turn triggers actions by the neural and hormonal systems.

There is often a fine line between high-intensity/high-volume training, such as shock microcycles, which is followed by sufficient rest during restoration cycles that brings about positive training adaptations and high-intensity/high-volume training followed by insufficient rest and recovery, which can precipitate overreaching or overtraining. The cytokine hypothesis of overtraining argues that the latter (high-intensity/high-volume training with insufficient recovery) produces tissue trauma in muscles and joints (Smith, 2000). This trauma results in activation of al., 2000). Macrophages cannot synthesize cytokines or function effectively if glutamine is in short supply. The liver also uses glutamine during exercise in the production and release of the antioxidant glutathione as well as acute phase proteins. Limited data have shown that glutamine levels decrease following high intensity or prolonged exercise and that some athletes suffering from the OTS demonstrate low glutamine levels (Walsh, et al., 1998). More recently (Smith and Norris, 2000), the ratio of glutamine (Gm) to glutamate (Ga) or (Gm/Ga) has been proposed as a means of tracking training tolerance. That is, a high Gm/Ga is hypothesized to indicate adaptive tolerance to the training load whereas a low ratio may indicate intolerance and possibly overtraining. While theoretically attractive, only minimal evidence exists to show that direct supplementation by glutamine or indirect supplementation with BCAA positively impacts glutamine levels, the incidence of upper respiratory tract infections (URTI), and lymphocyte responses (Bassit, et al., 2000; Mackinnon 1999, Walsh, 1998). At present these results are deemed insufficient to conclude that such supplementation is warranted. However, they do provide additional support for the necessity of an adequate intake of high quality protein during hard endurance exercise training.

3. *Vitamin C and E supplementation.* Vitamin C supplementation (600 mg·d^{-1} for 3 wk) has been shown to reduce the incidence of URTI in ultraendurance runners compared with nonsupplemented nonathletes, but not in marathoners or sedentary controls randomly assigned to either a 2-month regimen of 1000 mg·d^{-1} or a placebo. In addition, no alteration was seen in immune response after 2.5 hr of intensive running following 8 days of 1000 mg·d^{-1} supplementation. Conversely, after 48 days of 800 IU·d^{-1} of vitamin E supplementation or placebo, the response to 45 min of downhill running indicated that IL-1 and IL-6, but not TNFα, was lower in the supplemented individuals. In a related study, the exercise neutrophil increase was blunted in elderly but not young adults (Mackinnon 1999). These data were interpreted to mean that vitamin E might reduce inflammation after eccentric exercise. Thus, although the benefit of vitamin C for the immune system remains controversial, that of vitamin E looks promising.

Much work remains before it is established that dietary supplements are effective in moderating or eliminating some of the possibly negative effects of high-intensity exercise on immune function. In the meantime, following the nutrition guideline established for the metabolic system in training and competition that are detailed in Chapter 7 seems to be prudent in terms of the immune system as well.

Sources:

Bassit, et al. (2000); Bishop, et al. (2000); Field, et al. (2000); Henson, et al. (2000); MacKinnon (1999); Nieman (2000); Nieman, et al. (1997); Smith & Norris (2000); Walsh, et al. (1998).

immune cells (especially monocytes) and the release of several proinflammatory cytokines, namely IL-1, IL-6, and TNFα. The elevated levels of cytokines then play a central role in coordinating the body's response to the stress of training by affecting the central nervous system (CNS), the endrocrine system, and the production of acute phase proteins by the liver.

Activation of the CNS by proinflammatory cytokines provides a mechanism for explaining many of the psychological and behavioral, as well as physiological, signs and symptoms of the OTS. The binding of cytokines in the hypothalamus inhibits the hypothalamus-pituitary-gonadal axis, possibly leading to amenorrhea. Conversely, such binding activates the hypothalamus-pituitary-adrenal axis and the sympathetic nervous system, resulting in the release of epinephrine, norepinephrine, and cortisol. These stress hormones not only bring about physical changes but also are associated with mood changes, depression, and anxiety. The activation of other discrete portions of the hypothalamus may account for changes in appetite, sleep, and body core temperature. The hippocampal area of the brain is important in learning and memory. Cytokine stimulation of the hippocampus may therefore explain loss of attention and the return of previously corrected errors.

Figure 17.8 proposes a model by which tissue trauma resulting from training causes either local inflammation (which ultimately leads to adaptation and improvement) or systemic inflammation (which may lead to the OTS). In both cases, the cytokines are central in bringing about the inflammatory response, but the magnitude of the response varies. With high-intensity/high-volume training and insufficient rest, there is greater tissue trauma, causing greater activation of cytokines for a longer period of time, which

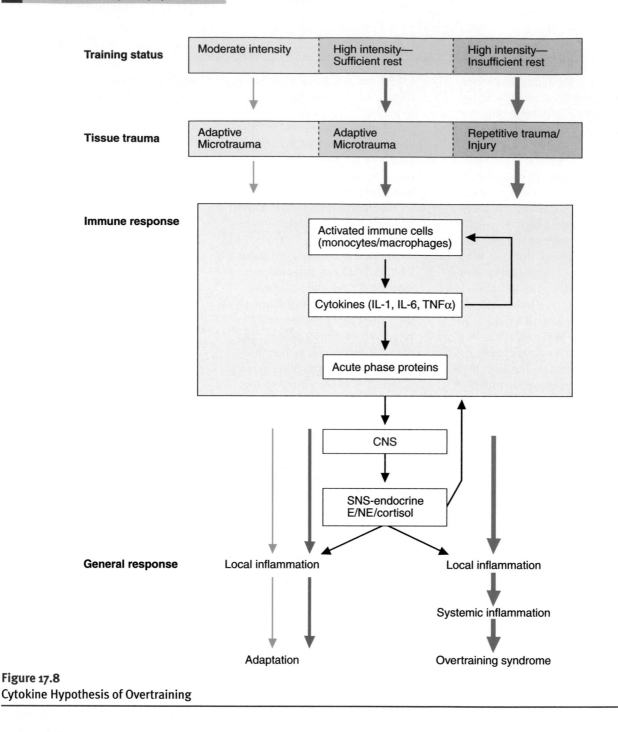

Figure 17.8
Cytokine Hypothesis of Overtraining

mediates greater neurohormonal response and ultimately leads from local to systemic inflammation. Systemic inflammation, regardless of the cause, is associated with many of the same symptoms that define the OTS. Notice in Figure 17.8 that the training status and resulting tissue trauma sections are divided by dashed lines, indicating that these categories may represent more of a continuum than discrete categories. Note also that this is a hypothesis that requires more experimental evidence to be completely accepted.

Selected Interactions of Exercise and Immune Function

Exercise, the Immune System, and Upper Respiratory Tract Infection

Many people believe that individuals who exercise regularly are less likely to acquire a cold or the flu, whereas others believe that highly trained, competitive athletes are more susceptible to upper respiratory tract infections (URTI). This section provides

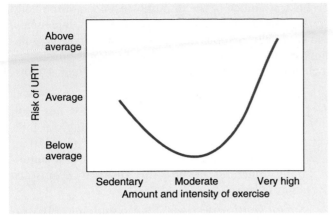

Figure 17.9

J-Shaped Model of Relationship between Exercise Intensity and URTI

Source: D. C. Nieman. The effects of moderate exercise training on natural killer cells and acute upper respiratory tract infections. *International Journal of Sports Medicine.* 111:467–473 (1990). Reprinted by permission of Williams & Wilkins.

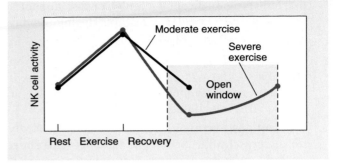

Figure 17.10

The "Open Window" Hypothesis

The open window is a period after severe exercise when NK cell activity decreases. During this period, microbial agents can establish an infection.

Source: Adapted from B. K. Pedersen & H. Ullum. NK cell response to physical activity: Possible mechanisms of action. *Medicine and Science in Sports and Exercise.* 26(2):140–146 (1994). Reprinted by permission of Willimas & Wilkins.

scientific evidence to suggest that both positions may be correct. It appears that the relationship between exercise and URTI is mediated by exercise intensity (Mackinnon, 1999; Nieman, Johanssen, et al., 1990; Nieman, Miller, et al., 1993).

A J-shaped model of relationship between exercise intensity and risk of URTI (see Figure 17.9) has been proposed to explain the risk of URTI infections among exercisers (Nieman, Johanssen, et al., 1990; Woods, Davis, Smith, et al., 1999). This model suggests that a moderate exercise session is beneficial, but exhaustive exercise may be detrimental. Figure 17.10 presents the "open window" hypothesis, which suggests that the suppression of immune function is greater and more prolonged following severe exercise than following moderate exercise (Pedersen and Ullum, 1994). Notice the similarities between the theoretical curve depicted in Figure 17.10 and Figure 17.7, which depicts NK cell activity. The suppression of the T cells and NK cells during recovery may provide a period of increased susceptibility (the "open window") for infection. This hypothesis, however, is not universally accepted. It may be that changes in immune cell number and function that are measured in recovery have little or no effect on health outcomes, such as infections (Rowbottom and Green, 2000).

Moderate exercise, then, appears to enhance immune function and may play an important role in determining an individual's susceptibility to infection. There is insufficient evidence, however, to recommend any given laboratory test of immune function to

ascertain whether an individual is at high risk for an infectious episode from overtraining or psychological stress.

Because endurance athletes often do not have the option of training moderately, the precautions listed below can help lessen the risk of URTI in competitive endurance athletes (Brenner, et al., 1994; Heath, et al., 1992; Nieman, 1994). The guidelines that follow the precautions also suggest when exercise training is and is not appropriate. The precautions are as follows:

1. Eat a well-balanced diet. Improper nutrition can compound the negative influence of heavy exertion on the immune system.

2. Minimize other life stresses. Psychological stress may be additive.

3. Avoid overtraining and chronic fatigue. Get plenty of rest, and space vigorous workout and race events as far apart as possible.

4. Get a flu shot. Flu shots are especially important for athletes competing in the winter.

5. Avoid excessive muscular soreness. Soreness may require immune system involvement, which could decrease its ability to ward off viruses.

6. Try to avoid being around sick people.

The guidelines for postponing training are as follows:

1. Maintain training if the URTI is only minor, without a systemic infection (fever, aching muscles,

extreme fatigue, swollen glands), or just stop for a couple of days. Use decongestants during the day and antihistamines at night.

2. If the URTI has the positive systemic infection signs listed above, stop training for 2–4 weeks. If training is not stopped, viral cardiomyopathy or severe viral infection may result.

3. If symptoms are above the neck (runny or stuffy nose, scratchy throat), begin sessions with short or light activity. If symptoms worsen, stop; if symptoms lessen, continue. If symptoms are below the neck (muscle ache, vomiting, diarrhea, fever), stop training until the symptoms go away.

Exercise, the Immune System, and Cancer

The NK cells and macrophages are important cells in the innate immune system involved in the defense against the development and spread of malignancies (Woods and Davis, 1994). Acute dynamic aerobic physical exercise causes an increase in these cells. Therefore, there is a theoretical, but largely undocumented, link between physical activity and cancer. Furthermore, epidemiological studies have found a relationship between physical activity and cancer (Blair and Minocha, 1989; Sternfeld, 1992). Physical activity is associated with lower prevalence and mortality rates for cancers involving the colon, breast, prostate, and lung. The mechanisms responsible for the effects of exercise on cancer are unknown but may include a better overall lifestyle for the exercisers, lower body fat, decreased stool transit time, and enhancement of antioxidant enzyme systems (Woods and Davis, 1994).

NK cells are known to be important in the control of tumor metastases (Hoffman-Goetz, 1994; Marieb, 2001). Exercise training enhances NK activity and thus may play a role in the control of tumor metastasis.

Macrophages represent an important group of cells because of the central role they play in resistance to infection, surveillance against cancer, and the regulation of adaptive immunity. However, the impact of exercise-induced changes in macrophage function on defense against cancer is just beginning to be studied (Woods and Davis, 1994).

Exercise, the Immune System, and AIDS

Acquired immune deficiency syndrome (AIDS) is a disease caused by the human immunodeficiency virus (HIV) and characterized by severe CD4 cell depletion. Estimates suggest that 42 million people are infected with HIV worldwide (Brenner, et al., 1994). This virus infects the CD4-bearing T cells (helper T cells), which orchestrate much of the immune response of the body. As the infection progresses, there is greater depletion of the CD4 cells, leading ultimately to immunodysregulation (Brenner, et al., 1994). HIV infection is considered a chronic disease involving three stages (Phair, 1990):

1. *Healthy carrier:* During this stage the virus infects relatively few CD4-bearing cells and is not clinically detectable except by blood testing. An individual may remain in this stage for up to 10 yr. These individuals are viral carriers and potentially infectious despite the absence of outward signs of infection.

2. *Symptomatic infections:* Mild symptoms of HIV infection, such as fatigue, intermittent fever, and weight loss, become evident during this phase. The CD4 count is further diminished.

3. *AIDS:* Severe CD4 cell depletion and the presence of major complications resulting from opportunistic infection or malignancy. At this stage of the disease, the entire health of the individual is compromised.

During the early stages of the disease, when individuals are asymptomatic, moderate aerobic exercise training appears to be a useful strategy; some evidence suggests that exercise training may delay the progression of the disease (Brenner, et al., 1994). These data may reflect the immune benefits of exercise training (increased number of CD4 cells) and/or psychological benefits of exercise training (Brenner, et al., 1994; Mackinnon, 1992). Furthermore, evidence suggests that exercise may be a safe activity throughout the course of the disease.

On the basis of research to date, some broad recommendations for exercise training can be made (Brenner, et al., 1994). In general, before initiating an exercise program, all HIV-infected individuals should follow these guidelines:

1. Have a complete physical examination.

2. Discuss exercise plans with a physician and/or exercise specialist.

3. Comply with ACSM testing and prescription guidelines.

Healthy, asymptomatic HIV-positive individuals should follow these guidelines:

1. Continue unrestricted exercise activity.

2. Continue with competition.

3. Avoid overtraining.

Individuals in the stage defined as symptomatic infection should follow these steps:

1. Continue exercise training.

2. Terminate competition.

3. Avoid exhaustive exercise.

Individuals diagnosed as having AIDS should follow these guidelines:

1. Remain physically active.
2. Continue exercise training on a symptom-limited basis.
3. Avoid strenuous exercise.
4. Reduce or curtail exercise during acute illness.

Summary

1. The immune system can be functionally divided into the innate and the adaptive branches. The innate branch protects against foreign substances or cells without having to recognize them. The adaptive branch of the immune system requires that the immune cells recognize a foreign material and react specifically and selectively to destroy it.

2. Moderate aerobic exercise leads to an increase in the number and activity of neutrophils; an increase in the number, percentage, and activity of NK cells; an increase in phagocytic activity and secretion of cytokines from macrophages; an increase in the number of acute phase proteins; and an increase in the number of B and T cells.

3. Exhaustive aerobic exercise is associated with a reduction in NK cell number and activity and a decrease in lymphocytes and neutrophils.

4. The depressed levels of NK cells following strenuous exercise is a likely explanation of the vulnerability to acute infection that is associated with high-level competition and chronic overtraining.

5. Hormonal control of the immune response is mediated primarily by the action of epinephrine and cortisol.

6. Severe exercise training is associated with immunosuppression and an increased risk of URTI.

7. Physical activity is associated with lower prevalence and mortality rates for cancers involving the colon, breast, prostate, and lung.

8. Exercise training appears to be beneficial to individuals infected with HIV.

Review Questions

1. Graphically present the two branches of the immune system, emphasizing how the two branches work together.

2. Identify the primary cells of the innate and adaptive branches of the immune system, and indicate the mechanisms by which each leads to antigen destruction.

3. Describe the sequence of events in inflammation.

4. Describe the immune response to moderate aerobic exercise and to a severe exercise bout.

5. Differentiate between the training adaptations of the immune system to a moderate training program and the immune system's adaptations to overtraining.

6. Describe the cytokine hypothesis of overtraining.

7. Describe the relationship between exercise and the incidence of URTI.

8. Describe the relationship between physical activity levels and the risk of various cancers.

9. Describe the role of physical activity in the life of an individual infected with the HIV.

For further review and additional study tools, go to The Physiology Place (www.physiologyplace.com) and the Student Study Guide for Exercise Physiology for Health, Fitness, and Performance *by Sharon A. Plowman and Denise L. Smith.*

Passport to the Internet

Visit the following Internet sites to explore further topics and issues related to the immune response. To visit an organization's web site, go to www.physiologyplace.com and click on "Passport to the Internet."

WebMD Visit WebMD and conduct a search of the site for information related to HIV disease and the immune response. Seek out information on the effect of exercise and nutrition in the fight against HIV infection. Go to http://my.webmd.com/content/article/ 1680. 50211 for a glossary of terms that might be used in connection with a discussion of an HIV vaccine.

Centers for Disease Control and Prevention The CDC maintains the most comprehensive database on numerous diseases that threaten to compromise the immune system. For more information on various threats, check out Divisions of HIV/AIDS Prevention and the National Center for HIV, STD, and TB Prevention.

CancerLinksUSA CancerLinksUSA.com is a noncommercial site founded to provide support and information to cancer patients and their caregivers.

References

Bassit, R. A., L. A. Sawada, R. F. P. Bacura, F. Navarro, & L. F. B. P. Costa Rosa: The effect of BCAA supplementation upon the immune response of triathletes. *Medicine and Science in Sports and Exercise.* 32(7):1214–1219 (2000).

Bishop, N. C., A. K. Blannin, E. Armstrong, M. Rickman, & M. Gleeson: Carbohydrate and fluid intake affect the saliva flow rate and IgA response to cycling. *Medicine and Science in Sports and Exercise.* 32(12): 2046–2051 (2000).

Blair, S. N., & H. C. Minocha: Physical fitness and all-cause mortality: A prospective study of healthy men and women. *Journal of the American Medical Association.* 262: 2395–2401 (1989).

Brenner, I. K. M., P. N. Shek, & R. J. Shephard: Infection in athletes. *Sports Medicine.* 17(2):86–107 (1994).

Calabrese, L. H., & A. LaPerriere: Human immunodeficiency virus infection, exercise and athletics. *Sports Medicine.* 15(1):6–13 (1993).

Centers for Disease Control and Prevention. http://www.cdc.gov/hiv/ pubs/facts.htm

Dale, D. A., & M. M. McCarthy: The leukocytosis of exercise: A review and model. *Sports Medicine.* 6:333–363 (1988).

Davis, J. M., M. L. Kohut, D. A. Jackson, L. M. Hertler-Colbert, E. P. Mayer, & A. Ghaffar: Exercise effects on lung tumor metastases and *in vitro* alveolar macrophage anti-tumor cytotoxicity. *American Journal of Physiology.* 274: R1454–R1459 (1998).

Dziedziak, W.: The effect of incremental cycling on the physiological functions of peripheral blood granulocytes. *Biology of Sport.* 7:239–247 (1990).

Fehr, H. G., H. Lotzerich, & H. Michna: Influence of physical exercise on peritoneal macrophage functions: Histochemical and phagocytic studies. *International Journal of Sports Medicine.* 9:77–81 (1988).

Fehr, H. G., H. Lotzerich, & H. Michna: Human macrophage function and physical exercise: Phagocytic and histochemical studies. *European Journal of Applied Physiology.* 58: 613–617 (1989).

Field, C. J., I. Johnson, & V. C. Pratt: Glutamine and arginine: Immunonutrients for improved health. *Medicine and Science in Sports and Exercise.* 32(7) Suppl. S377–S388 (2000).

Gabriel, H., H. J. Muller, A. Urhausen, & W. Kinderman: Suppressed PMA-induced oxidative burst and unimpaired phagocytosis of circulating granulocytes one week after a long endurance exercise. *International Journal of Sports Medicine.* 15:441–445 (1994).

Gray, A. B., R. D. Telford, M. Collins, M. S. Baker, & M. J. Weidemann: Granulocyte activation induced by intense interval running. *Journal of Leukocyte Biology.* 53:591–597 (1993).

Gumprez, J. E., & P. Parham: The enigma of the natural killer cell. *Nature.* 378:245–248 (1995).

Heath, G. W., C. A. Macera, & D. C. Nieman: Exercise and upper respiratory tract infections: Is there a relationship? *Sports Medicine.* 14(6):353–365 (1992).

Henson, D. A., D. C. Nieman, S. L. Nehlsen-Cannarella, O. R. Fagoaga, M. Shannon, M. R. Bolton, J. M. Davis, C. T. Gaffney, W. J. Kelln, M. D. Austin, J. M. E. Hjertman, & B. K. Schilling: Influence of carbohydrate responses to 2h of rowing. *Medicine and Science in Sport and Exercise.* 32(8): 1384–1389 (2000).

Hoffman-Goetz, L.: Exercise, natural immunity, and tumor metastasis. *Medicine and Science in Sports and Exercise.* 26(2):157–163 (1994).

Kohut, M. L., J. M. Davis, D. A. Jackson, et al.: Exercise effects on IFN-β expression and viral replication in lung macrophages following HSV-1 infection. *American Journal of Physiology.* (*Lung Cell. Mol. Physiol.* 19). 275: L1089–L1094 (1998).

Kokot, K., R. M. Schaefer, M. Teschner, U. Gilge, R. Plass, & A. Heiland: Activation of leukocytes during prolonged physical exercise. *Advances in Experimental Biology.* 240: 57–63 (1988).

Mackinnon, L. T.: *Advances in Exercise Immunology.* Champaign, IL: Human Kinetics (1999).

Mackinnon, L. T.: Chronic exercise training effects on immune function. *Medicine and Science in Sports and Exercise.* 32(7):S369–S376 (2000).

Mackinnon, L. T.: Current challenges and future expectations in exercise immunology: Back to the future. *Medicine and Science in Sports and Exercise.* 26(2):191–194 (1994).

Mackinnon, L. T.: *Exercise and Immunology.* Champaign, IL: Human Kinetics (1992).

Mackinnon, L. T., T. W. Chick, A. Van As, & T. B. Tomasi: The effect of exercise on secretory and natural immunity. *Advances in Experimental Medicine and Biology.* 216:869–876 (1987).

Marieb, E. N.: *Human Anatomy and Physiology* (5th edition). Redwood City, CA: Benjamin/Cummings (2001).

Moldoveanu, A. I., R. J. Shephard, & P. N. Shek: The cytokine response to physical activity and training. *Sports Medicine.* 31(2):115–144 (2001).

Muns, G., I. Rubinstein, & P. Singer: Neutrophil chemotactic activity is increased in nasal secretions of long-distance runners. *International Journal of Sports Medicine.* 17:56–59 (1996).

Nash, M. S.: Exercise and immunology. *Medicine and Science in Sports and Exercise.* 26(2):125–127 (1994).

Nieman, D. C.: Exercise, upper respiratory tract and the immune system. *Medicine and Science in Sports and Exercise.* 26(2):128–139 (1994).

Nieman, D. C.: Immune response to heavy exertion. *Journal of Applied Physiology.* 82(5):1385–1394 (1997).

Nieman, D. C.: Is infection risk linked to exercise workload? *Medicine and Science in Sports and Exercise.* 32(7). Suppl.: S406–S411 (2000).

Nieman, D. C., J. C. Ahle, D. A. Henson, et al.: Indomethacin does not alter natural killer cell response to 2.5 h of running. *Journal of Applied Physiology.* 79:748–755 (1995).

Nieman, D. C., D. A. Henson, E. B. Garner, D. E. Butterworth, B. J. Warren, A. Utter, J. M. Davis, O. R. Fagoaga, & S. L. Nehlsen-Cannarella: Carbohydrate affects natural killer cell redistribution but not activity after running. *Medicine and Science in Sports and Exercise.* 29(10):1318–1324 (1997).

Nieman, D. C., K. S. Buckley, D. A. Henson, et al.: Immune function in marathon runners versus sedentary controls.

Medicine and Science in Sport and Exercise. 27:5986–5992 (1995).

Nieman, D. C., L. M. Johanssen, J. W. Lee, & K. Arabatzis: Infectious episodes in runners before and after the Los Angeles Marathon. *Journal of Sports Medicine and Physical Fitness.* 30:316–328 (1990).

Nieman, D. C., A. R. Miller, D. A. Henson, B. J. Warren, G. Gusewitch, B. J. Johnson, J. M. Davis, D. E. Butterworth, & S. L. Nehlsen-Cannarella: Effects of high- vs moderate-intensity exercise on natural killer activity. *Medicine and Science in Sports and Exercise.* 25(10):1126–1134 (1993).

Nieman, D. C., S. L. Nehlsen-Cannarella, P. A. Markoff, et al.: The effects of moderate exercise training on natural killer cells and acute upper respiratory tract infections. *International Journal of Sports Medicine.* 11:467–473 (1990).

Ortega, E., M. E. Collazos, C. B. Barriga, & M. De La Fuenta: Stimulation of the phagocytic function in guinea pig peritoneal macrophages by physical activity stress. *European Journal of Applied Physiology.* 54:323–327 (1992).

Ortega, E., M. A. Forner, & C. B. Barriga: Exercise-induced stimulation of murine macrophage chemotaxis: Role of corticosterone and prolactin as mediators. *Journal of Physiology (London).* 498:729–734 (1997).

Pavlidis, N., & M. Chirigos: Stress-induced impairment of macrophage tumoricidal function. *Psychosomatic Medicine.* 42:47–53 (1980).

Pedersen, B. K., & H. Ullum: NK cell response to physical activity: Possible mechanisms of action. *Medicine and Science in Sports and Exercise.* 26(2):140–146 (1994).

Phair, J. D.: The natural history of HIV infection. In M. A. Sande & P. A. Volberding (eds.), *The Medical Management of AIDS.* Philadelphia: Saunders (1990).

Roitt, I., J. Brostoff, & D. Male: *Immunology* (4th edition). Baltimore: Mosby (1998).

Rowbottom, D. G., & K. J. Green: Acute exercise effects on the immune system. *Medicine and Science in Sports and Exercise.* 32(7):S396–S405 (2000).

Shephard, R. J.: *Physical Activity, Training and the Immune Response.* Carmel, IN: Cooper Publishing Group, 56–64 (1997).

Shephard, R. J., S. Rhind, & P. N. Shek: The impact of exercise on the immune system: NK cells, interleukins 1 and 2, and related responses. In J. O. Holloszy (ed.), *Exercise and Sport Sciences Reviews.* Baltimore: Williams & Wilkins (1995).

Smith, D. J., & S. R. Norris: Changes in glutamine and glutamate concentrations for tracking tolerance. *Medicine and Science in Sports and Exercise.* 32(3):684–689 (2000).

Smith, J. A.: Guidelines, standards, and perspectives in exercise immunology. *Medicine and Science in Sports and Exercise.* 27(4):497–506 (1995).

Smith, J. A., R. D. Telford, I. B. Mason, & M. J. Weidemann: Exercise, training and neutrophil microbicidal activity. *International Journal of Sports Medicine.* 11:179–187 (1990).

Smith, L. L.: Cytokine hypothesis of overtraining: A physiological adaptation to excessive stress. *Medicine and Science in Sports and Exercise.* 32(2):317–331 (2000).

Sternfeld, B.: Cancer and the protective effect of physical activity: The epidemiological evidence. *Medicine and Science in Sports and Exercise.* 24:1195–1209 (1992).

Tomasi, T. B., F. B. Trudeau, D. Czerwinski, & S. Erredge: Immune parameters in athletes before and after strenuous exercise. *Journal of Clinical Immunology.* 2:173–178 (1982).

Vander, A. J., J. H. Sherman, & D. S. Luciano: *Human Physiology* (8th edition). New York: McGraw-Hill (2001).

Walsh, N. P., A. K. Blannin, P. J. Robson, & M. Gleeson: Glutamine, exercise, and immune function. *Sports Medicine.* 26(3):177–191 (1998).

Wood, P. D., & M. L. Stefanick: Exercise, fitness, and atherosclerosis. In C. Bouchard, R. J. Shephard, T. Stephens, J. R. Sutton, & B. D. McPherson (eds.), *Exercise, Fitness, and Health: A Consensus of Current Knowledge.* Champaign, IL: Human Kinetics, 409–423 (1990).

Woods, J. A., M. A. Ceddia, C. Kozak, & B. Wolters: Effect of exercise on the macrophage MHC II response to inflammation. *International Journal of Sports Medicine.* 18:483–488 (1997).

Woods, J. A., & J. M. Davis: Exercise, monocyte/macrophage function, and cancer. *Medicine and Science in Sports and Exercise.* 26(2):147–157 (1994).

Woods, J. A., J. M. Davis, E. P. Mayer, A. Ghaffar, & R. R. Pate: Effects of exercise on macrophage activation for antitumor cytotoxicity. *Journal of Applied Physiology.* 76: 2177–2185 (1994).

Woods, J. A., J. M. Davis, E. P. Mayer, A. Ghaffar, & R. R. Pate: Exercise increases inflammatory macrophage antitumor cytotoxicity. *Journal of Applied Physiology.* 75: 879–886 (1993).

Woods, J. A., J. M. Davis, J. A. Smith, & D. C. Nieman: Exercise and cellular innate immune function. *Medicine and Science in Sport and Exercise.* 31(1):57–66 (1999).

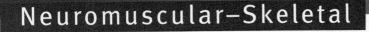

Neuromuscular–Skeletal
System Unit

Neuromuscular–Skeletal System

- Locomotion (exercise)
- Movement brought about by muscular contraction (under neural stimulation acting on bony levers of skeletal system)

Cardiovascular–Respiratory System

Metabolic System

The contraction of skeletal muscles, pulling on the bony levers of the body, causes movement. The nervous system provides the electrical signal that causes the contraction of skeletal muscle. Hence, exercise is, by definition, the direct result of neuromuscular activity. This unit will address how the skeletal, muscular, and neural systems function together to bring about movement of any type, including exercise. These systems are not the only body systems that play a role in exercise and other movement, however. In order for muscles to contract, they must continually produce energy (ATP), which means that the metabolic system is also responsible for muscle contraction and, therefore, exercise. Furthermore, the cardiorespiratory system is responsible for supplying the muscle cells with oxygen, which supports the production of ATP necessary for continued contractions.

Chapter 18

Skeletal System

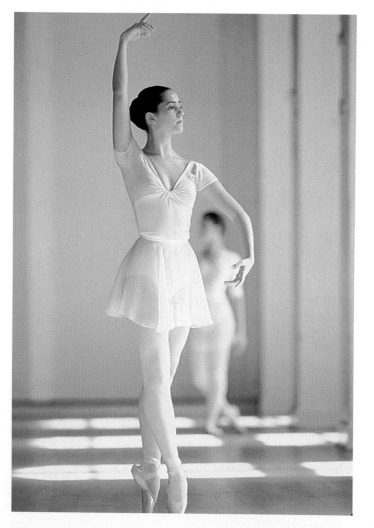

After studying the chapter, you should be able to

- Differentiate between cortical and trabecular bone.
- Define bone remodeling, and explain how bone mineral density is affected by the balance of bone resorption and deposition.
- Describe the hormonal control of bone remodeling and growth.
- Explain the criterion method of assessing bone mineral density.
- Identify age-related changes in bone mineral density.
- Identify sex-related differences in bone mineral density.
- Discuss the factors involved in the attainment of peak bone mineral density.
- Discuss the factors involved in the rate of bone loss in adults.
- Apply the training principles to the development of an exercise program to enhance bone health.
- Describe the skeletal adaptations that occur as a result of an exercise training program.
- Identify the risk to bone health associated with athletic amenorrhea.
- Describe micro- and macrotrauma skeletal injuries, and suggest ways of minimizing their prevalence.

Introduction

The skeletal system includes the bones and cartilage that provide the framework for the muscles and organs of the body. The skeletal system is not only taken for granted but also generally neglected in exercise physiology textbooks. This neglect is no longer acceptable: Research indicates that the skeletal system adapts to exercise training in much the same way as other body systems and that a healthy skeleton is important in preventing major health problems, including osteoporosis.

Exercise physiologists are concerned with such issues as the prevention and treatment of osteoporosis (in amenorrheic athletes and the elderly) and the impact of heavy training on the skeleton of growing prepubescent athletes. This chapter will address these important issues. But first we must review the basic concepts of skeletal physiology in order to understand the influence of activity on bone.

Skeletal Tissue

Bone tissue, also called *osseous tissue,* is a dynamic, living tissue that is constantly undergoing change. In fact, adults recycle 5–7% of their bone mass every week (Marieb, 2001). **Bone remodeling** refers to the continual process of bone breakdown (resorption) and formation (deposition of new bone). Bone remodeling plays an important role in regulating blood calcium levels and in replacing old bone with new bone to ensure the integrity of the skeletal system. The mass and shape of the bones depend largely on the stress placed on them. The more the bones are stressed (by mechanical loading in the form of activity), the more they increase in volume and mass, specifically at the site of mechanical loading. The concept that bone adapts to changes in mechanical loading is referred to as *Wolff's Law* (Beck and Marcus, 1999).

Functions

The skeletal system provides a number of important functions that can be classified as either structural or physiological. Structurally, the skeletal system provides rigid support and protection for the vital organs and allows for locomotion. Physiologically, skeletal tissue provides a site for blood formation (hema-

---

Bone Remodeling The continual process of bone breakdown (resorption) and formation (deposition of new bone).

---

topoiesis), plays a role in the immune function (by providing the site for white blood cell formation), and serves as a dynamic storehouse for calcium and phosphate, which are essential for nerve conduction, heart and muscle contraction, blood clotting, and energy formation (Bailey and McColloch, 1990; Marieb, 2001).

The ability of the bone to perform its structural functions is directly related to its role as a storehouse for calcium. Because calcium is essential for many processes within the body, bone will be broken down (resorbed) to maintain blood calcium levels; that is, the body will sacrifice bone mineral (calcium) if it is needed to maintain blood calcium levels.

Levels of Organization

An understanding of the functions of the skeletal system and the way that the skeletal system responds to training is best pursued by examining the skeletal system at the organ and tissue levels.

Bones as Organs

The human body contains over 200 different bones joined together at articulations known as joints. *Joints* enable movement by providing junctions for bones whereby they move when muscles exert force on them. The skeleton is typically divided into two categories: the central or axial skeleton includes the bones of the skull, vertebral column, ribs, and sternum; and the peripheral or appendicular skeleton includes the bones of the hips, shoulders, and extremities. There are several different shapes of bone— long, short, flat, and irregular—and each shape is specific to its function. Furthermore, as described by Wolff's Law, each bone's shape reflects its response to the stress placed on it.

Bone Tissue

There are two types of bone tissue: cortical and trabecular bone. *Cortical bone,* also called compact, dense, or lamellar bone, is densely packed and makes up the majority of the skeleton (around 80%). *Trabecular bone,* also called spongy or cancellous bone, is more porous and surrounded by cortical bone. Individual bones are composed of both types of bone tissue; however, the relative proportion of trabecular and cortical bone varies. Table 18.1 presents relative percentages of trabecular and cortical bone tissue in various bones of the body. In general, bones of the axial skeleton have a much greater percentage of trabecular bone, whereas bones of the appendicular skeleton have a greater percentage of cortical bone.

Table 18.1
Composition of Various Bones

Measurement Site	Cortical Percentage	Trabecular Percentage
Calcaneus	5	95
Lumbar spine		
Anterior-posterior view	50	50
Lateral view	10	90
Proximal femur	60	40
Total body	80	20

Source: Highet (1989).

Figure 18.1 is a diagram of the humerus, a typical long bone. Note that it is composed of both cortical and trabecular bone. The shaft is composed primarily of cortical bone, and the epiphyses have a greater percentage of trabecular bone.

Cortical bone is composed of *osteons,* which are the functional units of bone (Haversian system). Osteons are organized into concentric layers of matrix called lamellae, which are surrounded by widely dispersed cells. The matrix is the intercellular space, and it is made up of organic and inorganic substances.

Trabecular bone is composed of branching projections or struts, called *trabeculae,* which form a latticelike network of interconnecting spaces. Its appearance is responsible for another one of its names, spongy bone. Trabecular bone has the same cells and matrix elements as cortical bone, but it has a greater degree of porosity. About 80–90% of the volume of cortical bone is calcified; only 15–25% of trabecular bone is calcified (the remaining volume is occupied by bone marrow, blood vessels, and connective tissue) (Baron 1993). Therefore, cortical bone is best suited for structural support and protection, and trabecular bone is best suited for bone's physiological functions.

Owing to its large surface area, trabecular bone is able to remodel more rapidly than cortical bone. It is also in the trabecular bone that the greatest age-related loss in bone mineral density occurs. Therefore, most osteoporotic fractures occur in areas composed predominantly of trabecular bone (wrist, hip, and spine).

Bone Development

Bone development can be divided into three processes: bone growth, bone modeling, and bone remodeling. Each process occurs at different times throughout an individual's life.

Growth

Bone growth refers to the increase in size of bone owing to an increasing number of bone cells (Frost, 1991a). There are two types of bone growth. The first is called *appositional growth,* which indicates that a bone increases in thickness or mass. The second type of bone growth, *longitudinal growth,* occurs at the epiphyseal plate until a person reaches adult height. This is an area of interest owing to the concern of stunting a child's growth as a result of excessive exercise.

The longitudinal growth of bones results from the longitudinal growth of cartilage, which is later replaced by bone. During the process of growth, bone is also remodeling itself—that is, it is changing its shape and thickness. Bone growth and remodeling are two processes that are distinct but closely related. In general, *growth* refers to the longitudinal growth of bone, and *remodeling* describes the balance between bone resorption and bone formation. If bone formation exceeds resorption, this process would also represent *growth.*

Modeling

Bone modeling is the process of altering the shape of bone by bone resorption and bone formation (Frost, 1991a). *Micromodeling* is the microscopic level of cell organization that occurs during formation; it determines what kind of tissue will be formed (Frost, 1991a). *Macromodeling* controls if, when, and where new tissue will form or old tissue will be removed (Frost, 1991a). This process ensures that the shape of the bone is matched to the role that bone will serve (Frost, 1988, 1991a, 1991b; Lanyon, 1989; Marcus, 1987).

Remodeling

As noted earlier, bone remodeling refers to the continual process of bone turnover, maintenance, replacement, and repair (Frost, 1991a). It reflects the balance between the coupled processes of bone resorption and bone formation. This ongoing process occurs because of the coupled action of bone cells.

Bone Cells   There are three types of bone cells: osteoclasts, osteoblasts, and osteocytes. The cells are the living part of bone. Although the cells represent a small fraction—less than 2% (Teitelbaum, 1993)—of

> **Bone Modeling**   The process of altering the shape of bone by bone resorption and bone deposition.

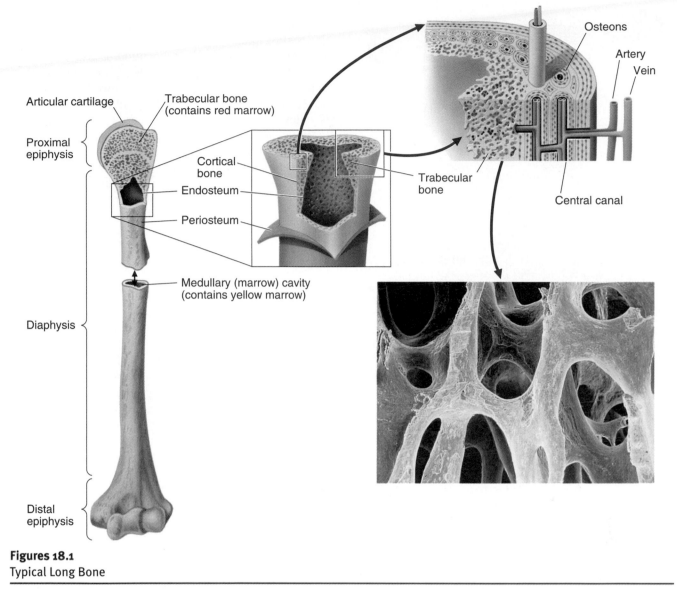

Articular cartilage

Proximal epiphysis

Trabecular bone (contains red marrow)

Cortical bone

Endosteum

Periosteum

Trabecular bone

Osteons

Artery

Vein

Central canal

Medullary (marrow) cavity (contains yellow marrow)

Diaphysis

Distal epiphysis

Figures 18.1
Typical Long Bone

Structure and cross-sectional view of bone.

the total composition of bone, they are responsible for its remodeling.

Osteoclasts are large, multinucleated bone cells that cause the resorption of bone tissue. Also called bone-destroying cells, osteoclasts secrete digestive enzymes that destroy and disintegrate (phagocytize) bone matrix. As the bone is degraded, the mineral salts (primarily calcium and phosphate) are dissolved and move into the bloodstream. **Osteoblasts** are bone cells that cause the deposition of bone tissue. Also called bone-forming cells, osteoblasts produce an organic bone matrix that will become calcified and harden when minerals are deposited in it. The hardening of the bone matrix is known as ossification. **Osteocytes** are mature osteoblasts surrounded by calcified bone that help regulate the process of bone

remodeling. Osteocytes appear to initiate the process of calcification.

The actions of the osteoclasts and the osteoblasts are coupled; they work together to remodel bone. In fact, osteoclasts must first cause bone resorption before the osteoblasts can form new bone. Figure 18.2

Osteoclasts   Bone cells that cause the resorption of bone tissue (bone-destroying cells).

Osteoblasts   Bone cells that cause the deposition of bone tissue (bone-forming cells).

Osteocytes   Mature osteoblasts surrounded by calcified bone that help regulate the process of bone remodeling.

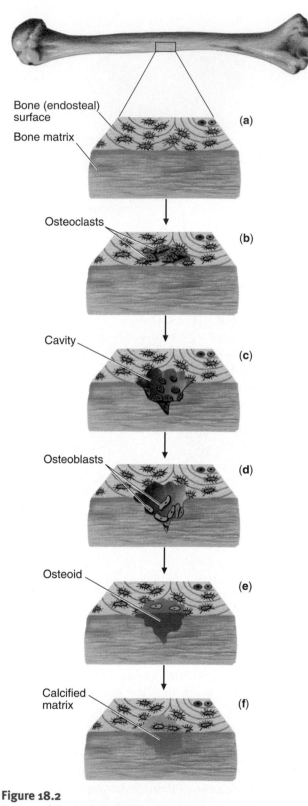

Bone (endosteal) surface

Bone matrix

Osteoclasts

Cavity

Osteoblasts

Osteoid

Calcified matrix

Figure 18.2
Stages of Bone Remodeling

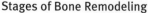

(a) Resting cell surface. (b) Osteoclasts (multinucleated) are activated and begin dissolving bone (minerals released to the blood). (c) Osteoclasts produce a cavity in the blood matrix. (d) Osteoblasts appear. (e) Osteoblasts secrete the osteoid (uncalcified matrix). (f) The matrix is calcified.

outlines the major events of a bone-remodeling cycle (Marcus, 1987; Parfitt, 1987; Teitelbaum, 1993). From the resting phase (Figure 18.2a), the osteoclasts are stimulated and cause the resorption of bone, resulting in a cavity (Figures 18.2b and 18.2c). Osteoblasts then appear and deposit bone matrix where the cavity exists (Figure 18.2d). The matrix is called *osteoid* until it is calcified (Figure 18.2e). Calcification of the new bone occurs as calcium and phosphate minerals are deposited in the osteoid (Figure 18.2f). The bone then returns to the resting or quiescent phase.

Bone remodeling may result in greater bone mass, the same bone mass, or a reduction in bone mass. Through young adulthood, typically, more bone is formed than is resorbed; thus, there is an increase in bone mass. This increased mass strengthens the bone and accounts for the increase in bone mineral density that occurs during this period of life. When bone remodeling is in equilibrium, the amount of bone resorbed is equal to the amount of bone formed; thus, bone mineral density remains relatively constant. In the elderly and as a result of some disease conditions the amount of bone resorbed is greater than the amount of bone formed, and a decrease in bone mineral density occurs.

The remodeling of bone provides the means for skeletal growth, particularly during developmental years, and for the constant turnover of bone that occurs throughout life. Bone remodeling is a complex process that is regulated by hormonal and local factors, which in turn affect bone cells and the process of bone resorption and formation (Canalis, 1990).

Hormonal Control Bone remodeling reflects the interrelationship between the structural and physiological functions of bone. Calcium not only is necessary to provide structural integrity of bone, but also is essential to the proper functioning of the heart, skeletal muscles, and nervous tissue. Only about 1 g of calcium (less than 1%) is present in the extracellular fluid of the body, compared to approximately 1150 g of calcium present in bone tissue. Blood calcium levels are normally maintained within the range of 9–11 mg·dL^{-1} of blood (Bailey and McColloch, 1990; Marieb, 2001).

The skeletal system, the digestive system, and the urinary system operate together, under hormonal control, to maintain blood calcium levels. Because of the importance of calcium in so many vital processes of the body, bone mass is broken down to maintain blood calcium within normal limits. Thus, blood calcium is the variable that is closely regulated. As introduced in Chapter 2, the primary hormones involved in regulating blood calcium levels and bone remodeling are parathyroid hormone (PTH), calcitonin, and vitamin D (calcitrol).

Excess calcium in the blood leads to the release of calcitonin (from the thyroid gland), which causes deposition of calcium in the bone (Marieb, 2001). This deposition has the effect of decreasing blood calcium levels and simultaneously increasing bone mineral density. Conversely, when blood calcium levels drop below normal values, parathyroid hormone stimulates osteoclast activity, causing calcium to be released from its storage site, the skeletal system. This release of calcium from the bone causes blood calcium levels to increase and bone mineral density to decrease. Table 18.2 provides a summary of the effect of calcitonin and PTH on bone and blood calcium levels. Vitamin D (calcitrol) is important for the absorption of calcium from the intestines. Thus, it leads to an increased blood level of calcium.

Other hormones that play an important role in skeletal health are the sex steroids (estrogen and testosterone) and growth hormone. These hormones stimulate the protein formation necessary for bone growth and are responsible for the closure of the epiphyseal plate, which will ultimately determine bone length and thus a person's height (Bailey and McColloch, 1990). Estrogen is important in promoting calcium retention and acts as an inhibiting agent of parathyroid hormone. The loss of the protective role of estrogen on the skeletal system has important consequences for women after menopause or during secondary amenorrhea. A decrease in estrogen has the net result of increasing bone resorption. Hormones are themselves stimulated by other factors, including physical activity.

Assessment of Bone Health

The strength and health of bone are determined by bone mass, external geometry, and internal microstructure (Beck and Marcus, 1999; Frost, 1997). However, it is difficult to quantify measures of external geometry and microstructure. Therefore, measures of bone mass and bone mineral density are most often used to describe bone health. *Bone mineral content (BMC)* refers to the absolute amount of **hydroxyapatite**—calcium and phosphate salts that are responsible for the hardness of the bone matrix—measured in grams. *Bone mineral density (BMD)* is defined as the relative value of bone mineral per measured bone area, expressed as grams per centimeter squared ($g \cdot cm^{-2}$) or milligrams per centimeter cubed ($mg \cdot cm^{-3}$), depending on the technology used to assess area. Bone mineral density is used clinically to provide an operational definition of osteopenia and osteoporosis (Jones, Harris, et al., 1989). **Osteopenia** is a condition of decreased bone mineral density and is diagnosed when BMD is greater than

Table 18.2

Effect of Calcitonin and PTH on Bone and Blood Calcium Levels

Hormone	Stimulus for Release	Effect on Bone	Effect on Blood Calcium Levels
Calcitonin	Increased blood calcium levels	Bone deposition (increased calcium)	Decreased blood calcium levels
Parathyroid hormone (PTH)	Decreased blood calcium levels	Bone resorption (decreased calcium)	Increased blood calcium levels

one standard deviation (SD) below (but not more than 2.5 SD below) values for young, normal adults. **Osteoporosis** is a condition of porosity and decreased BMD that is defined as BMD greater than 2.5 SD below values for young, normal adults. Established osteoporosis refers to the condition of osteoporosis as defined above, and one or more fractures (Kanis, et al., 1993).

Laboratory Measures

Bone mineral content and bone mineral density are measured only in laboratory or clinical settings, primarily because of the cost of equipment and safety considerations. The results, however, are worth the effort because they have dramatically increased the amount of information that is available to researchers, clinicians, and those involved in fitness professions. Two laboratory measures are absorptiometry and biochemical markers.

Hydroxyapatite Calcium and phosphate salts that are responsible for the hardness of the bone matrix.

Osteopenia A condition of decreased bone mineral density (BMD), diagnosed when BMD is greater than one standard deviation (SD) below (but not more than 2.5 SD below) values for young, normal adults.

Osteoporosis A condition of porosity and decreased bone mineral density that is defined as a BMD greater than 2.5 SD below values for young, normal adults.

Figure 18.3

Dual Energy X-ray Absorptiometer

Subject is positioned for the acquisition of total body scan.

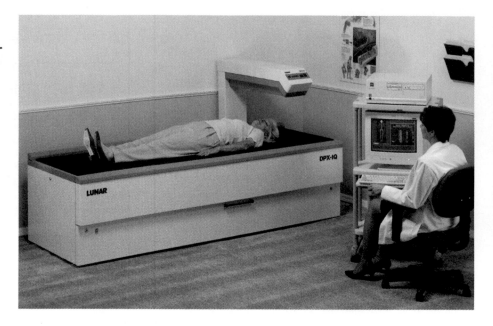

Absorptiometry

During the past 30 yr a large number of studies have investigated bone mineral density using the accurate, noninvasive techniques of single- and dual-photon absorptiometry (SPA and DPA, respectively). However, dual-energy, X-ray absorptiometry (DXA) has become the standard or criterion measure to assess bone mineral density, and most investigations now rely on this technique (Genant, et al., 1993). Dual-energy X-ray absorptiometry (DXA) uses an X-ray beam to measure regional and whole-body mineral content (Figure 18.3). This technology decreases the time necessary for a scan and also decreases the subject's exposure to radiation. Figure 18.4 provides a computer-generated printout of whole-body BMD and various regions of the body for a 37-yr-old active female. Figure 18.4a represents regions of the body that are individually analyzed for BMD. The total body BMD is compared with standard references in Figure 18.4b. The dark area represents an average range across the age span of 20–100 yr. Notice that the individual in the example is above average for total body BMD as represented by the asterisk (located at the intersection of age 37 yr and BMD 1.197 $g \cdot cm^{-2}$).

Regional BMDs are provided in Figure 18.4c along with comparisons with young adult normative data. Notice that each region of the body has a unique BMD value because of the composition of the bone and the stress (load) placed on it. For example, the legs have a BMD of 1.229 $g \cdot cm^{-2}$, whereas the pelvis has a BMD of 1.217 $g \cdot cm^{-2}$. These values correspond to 106 and 110% of young adult values, respectively.

Figure 18.5 provides a total body scan of an individual with low BMDs. Work through the problem in the Question of Understanding box to be sure that you understand the differences in total body and regional BMDs in these examples. Check your answer in Appendix D.

In addition to the total body scans just discussed, clinicians often measure BMD at specific sites, such as the hip or spine, where osteoporotic fractures are more likely to occur. By scanning just a small area of the body (e.g., a hip or spine) a better quality scan can be obtained. Figures 18.6a and 18.6b on page 484 present a hip and spine scan, respectively, for an active, older woman. These techniques enable researchers to investigate differences in bone mineral density at various sites, among various individuals, and as a result of adaptation to long-term exercise training.

Biochemical Markers

Some researchers are using sophisticated blood analysis techniques in an attempt to quantify changes in

---

A Question of Understanding

Figure 18.4 gives bone mineral data for a 37-yr-old active female. Figure 18.5 gives bone mineral data for a 69-yr-old osteoporotic woman. Study these printouts carefully and answer the following questions.

1. What is the BMD and percentage of young healthy values for the (a) arms, (b) pelvis, (c) spine, and (d) total body for each of these individuals?
2. What implications do these results have for the likelihood of each individual having an osteoporotic fracture?

(a)

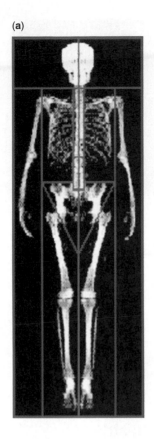

(b) Total comparison to reference

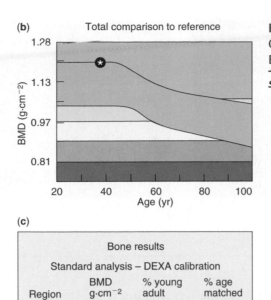

(c)

Bone results			
Standard analysis – DEXA calibration			
Region	BMD g·cm⁻²	% young adult	% age matched
Head	2.323	—	—
Arms	0.977	116	117
Legs	1.229	106	108
Trunk	0.971	106	108
Ribs	0.711	—	—
Pelvis	1.217	110	112
Spine	1.289	113	116
Thoracic	1.185	—	—
Lumbar	1.507	—	—
Total	1.197	106	108

Figure 18.4
Computer-Generated Printout of Whole Body BMD for Young, Healthy Female

Source: Data from the University of Connecticut Health Center, Osteoporosis Research Center.

(a)

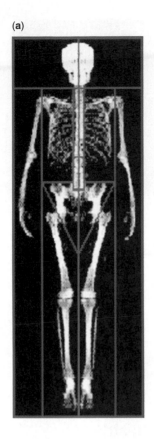

(b) Total comparison to reference

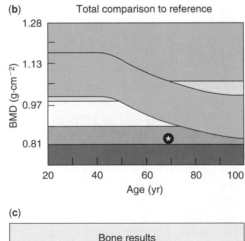

(c)

Bone results			
Standard analysis – DEXA calibration			
Region	BMD g·cm⁻²	% young adult	% age matched
Head	1.897	—	—
Arms	0.631	75	88
Legs	0.733	63	76
Trunk	0.677	74	88
Ribs	0.575	—	—
Pelvis	0.717	65	80
Spine	0.718	63	78
Thoracic	0.710	—	—
Lumbar	0.732	—	—
Total	0.847	75	88

Figure 18.5
Computer-Generated Printout of Whole Body BMD for an Older, Osteopenic Female

Source: Data from the University of Connecticut Health Center, Osteoporosis Research Center.

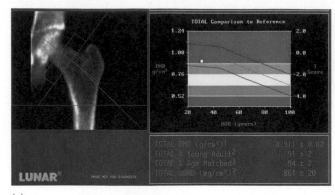
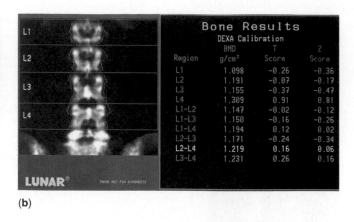

(a)

(b)

Figure 18.6
DXA Scan. (a) Hip (head of femur). (b) Spine.

blood levels of hormones, ions, and proteins (for example, osteocalcin) unique to bone following an acute bout of exercise (Nishiyama, et al., 1988). For example, osteocalcin may be an indicator of bone formation, and as such, it could be used as a marker of bone turnover. The use of biochemical markers represents an exciting area of bone research, but it is in the very early stages of development.

Field Tests

There are currently no field tests to measure bone mineral density. However, because the actions and adaptations of muscles and bones are so interdependent, some scientists speculate that measures of muscular strength might also give an indication of bone mineral density.

Significant positive correlations have been found between lumbar spine BMD and back extensor strength, grip strength and forearm BMD, back strength and hip BMD, and hip adductor strength and hip BMD (Snow-Harter and Marcus, 1991). These relationships make intuitive sense because the action of the muscle on bone would be expected to be site-specific. However, significant positive relationships have also been found between biceps brachii strength and spine BMD, biceps strength and hip BMD, and dominant grip strength and spine BMD (Snow-Harter, et al., 1990). These relationships imply that site specificity is not absolute.

Arm activity may require sufficient simultaneous trunk stabilization so that enough force is exerted on the spine and hips to cause bone density to increase. Unfortunately, these relationships are not very strong, with correlations falling in the range of 0.35–0.50.

Because strength measures are relatively easy to do as part of a physical fitness assessment, it would be convenient to be able to get an estimate of BMD from strength tests. However, the relationships are simply not strong enough as currently assessed to be able to do so. The relationships between muscle strength and BMD do hold some promise for yielding estimates of BMD; but for now, we cannot assume that muscle strength indicates BMD.

Factors Influencing Bone Health

Bone health is determined largely by the attainment of peak bone mass and the rate of bone loss. Both of these processes are influenced by age and sex.

Age-Related Changes in Bone

Bone is a dynamic tissue that changes in density throughout its life. As shown in Figure 18.7, a characteristic pattern exists between bone mass and age for males and females (Ott, 1990). Approximately the first 20 yr of life are characterized by active growth in bone mass. The skeletal consolidation phase occurs during early adulthood, and this is the time when peak bone mass occurs. Shortly after the attainment of peak bone mass, a loss of bone mass begins. Following the rapid-loss phase, the rate of bone loss decreases (Teitelbaum, 1993).

Sex Differences in Bone Mineral Density

There are systematic differences in BMD between males and females. As shown in Figure 18.7, total BMD changes throughout the life span for both sexes. Bone mineral density increases throughout childhood and early adult life for males and females; however, the peak bone mineral density achieved by females is less than that achieved by males (Ott, 1990). In addition to differences in total BMD between males and

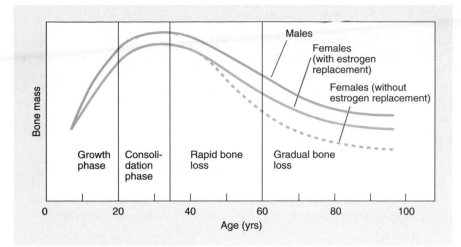

Figure 18.7
Comparison of BMD for Females and Males

Table 18.3
Comparison of Adult Male and Female BMD at Various Sites

	Males	**Females**
Hip (gm·cm^{-2})	1.033	.942
Spine (L2–L4) (gm·cm^{-2})	1.115	1.079
Radius (gm·cm^{-2})	.687	.579

Source: Beck and Marcus (1999).

Table 18.4
NIH Consensus Statement: Optimal Daily Calcium Intake

Age Group	Optimal Calcium Intake (mg)
Infant	
Birth–6 months	400
6 months–1 yr	600
Children	
1–5 yr	800
6–10 yr	800–1200
Adolescents and Young Adults	
11–24 yr	1200–1500
Men	
25–65 yr	1000
Over 65 yr	1500
Women	
25–60 yr	1000
Postmenopausal (under 65 yr), on estrogen	1000
Postmenopausal, not on estrogen	1500
Over 65 years	1500
Pregnant or nursing	1200–1500

Source: NIH Consensus Conference (1994).

females, BMD also varies according to the site where it is measured. Table 18.3 provides a comparison of adult BMD at various sites for men and women (Beck and Marcus, 1999).

Additionally, at the time of menopause women lose the protective influence of estrogen, and the rate of bone loss is accelerated if estrogen is not pharmacologically replaced. The loss of the protective influence of estrogen explains the prevalence of osteoporotic fractures in women.

Development of Peak Bone Mass

Peak bone mass is attained during the mid-30s for both sexes. However, 95% of peak bone mass is achieved by age 20 (Beck and Marcus, 1999). Peak bone mass developed during young adulthood is influenced by mechanical factors, nutrition, hormonal levels, and genetics (Ott, 1990). The mechanical factors affecting bone are physical activity and gravity. These forces are generally accepted as necessary stimuli for bone formation and growth (Malina and Bouchard, 1991). Although there is still much research to be done before specific exercise prescriptions can be developed for the skeletal system, children and adolescents should be encouraged to engage in physical activity to promote bone health as well as to promote

other positive changes and development within the body. Specifically, children and adolescents should be encouraged to participate in high-impact activities for bone development (Grimston, et al., 1993).

Adequate nutrition is necessary in order to develop a strong skeletal system. A nutrient that is essential to bone health, and often deficient in young athletes, is calcium. Table 18.4 shows the recommended optimal dietary intake of calcium. Unfortunately, many

Mechanical Stress and Bone Mass Density

Snow, C. M., C. J. Rosen, & T. L. Robinson: Serum IGF-1 is higher in gymnasts than runners and predicts bone and lean mass. *Medicine and Science in Sports and Exercise.* 32(11): 1902–1907 (2000).

Although it is well established that bone responds to mechanical stress, notably to physical activity, the mechanisms by which bone responds to exercise are not fully understood. The hormone insulin-like growth factor (IGF) is known to be anabolic to muscle, and there is a positive relationship between muscle and bone. To investigate this relationship further, Snow and colleagues (2000) examined the relationship between plasma IGF-1 and BMD in collegiate runners and gymnasts. As shown in the graphs, the gymnasts had higher BMD values than the runners at several sites. The gymnasts also had higher IGF-1 values than the runners.

Analysis of the data revealed that the correlations between BMD and IGF-1 were significant at the spine (r = .43), femoral neck (r = .55), and trochanter (.41). Although a significant correlation does not prove cause and effect, the authors speculated that the lower BMD in the runners may be due, in part, to the lower IGF-1 levels. Furthermore, the IGF-1 levels may partially explain the relationship between bone and muscle mass. This research is important because it shows that the type of mechanical stress affects BMD, and it provides a possible explanation for how the different exercise stresses lead to differences in BMD. Specifically, this study suggests that the hormonal system, through IGF-1, mediates bone's adaptation to exercise.

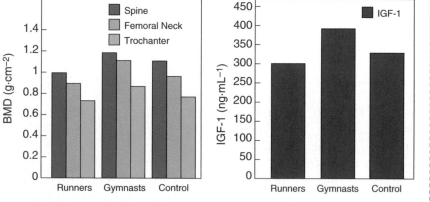

individuals fall well below recommendations, particularly young women who are concerned about weight control. For instance, they may eliminate dairy products from their diet because they are high in fat. But dairy products also are an excellent source of calcium. Thus, while trying to maintain weight, these athletes may be negatively affecting the attainment of peak bone mass. Exercise professionals should be careful to consider the need for dietary calcium when counseling young athletes (particularly females) about weight management (Loucks, 1988). The availability of the many low-fat dairy products makes including calcium in the diet easier.

As mentioned previously, adequate levels of the hormone estrogen are also needed to attain peak bone mass. Thus, athletes who are amenorrheic are likely to develop a lower peak bone mass than athletes with normal menstrual function (American College of Sports Medicine [ACSM], 1997).

Finally, genetic makeup is an important determinant of BMD. In other words, there are genetically determined limits to the amount of BMD that an individual can attain. But the only way to achieve genetic potential is to pay careful attention to the factors that an individual can modify, namely, nutritional status, hormonal status, and activity level.

Exercise Response

There is skeletal adaptation to exercise training; therefore, logic implies that there must also be an exercise response occurring within the skeletal system to bring about training adaptations. Unfortunately, researchers have not yet found a way to quantify the acute effects of exercise on the skeletal system. Some research has been conducted on the effects of exercise on biochemical markers of bone activity and the response of hormones known to be involved with bone remodeling (Lindsay, 1993; Nishiyama, et al., 1988). However, human research in this area is limited.

Application of the Training Principles

Given that exercise physiologists generally agree that physical activity has a positive effect on bone health, the logical question is: What is an appropriate exercise prescription for increasing or maintaining bone

Table 18.5
Recommended Activities for Skeletal Health

	Children and Young Adults	Adults, Premenopausal	Adults, Below-Normal BMD	Adults, Very Low BMD
Goal	To attain peak bone mass	To slow the rate of bone loss and prevent musculoskeletal injury	To decrease risk of injury and/or slow rate of bone loss	To avoid injury
Type of activity	High-impact-loading movements Dynamic resistance exercise	Moderate-impact-loading movements Dynamic resistance exercise	Low- to moderate-impact-loading movements	Low-impact-loading movements
Example	Sprinting, jumping, track and field, volleyball, basketball, gymnastics, soccer, weight training, rope skipping	Walking, jogging, running, hiking, stair climbing, stepping (machines), dancing, weight training, rope skipping, skiing	Stair climbing (machine), hiking, cross-country skiing, weight training	Walking, water aerobics, swimming, stationary cycling

health? Unfortunately, the answer to that question is not fully known. However, several recommendations can be made on the basis of available research.

Specificity

The specificity principle applies to the specific bones being stressed, the composition of the bone being stressed (cortical versus trabecular), and the type of activity being performed. Research data suggest that the type of exercise or activity performed greatly influences skeletal adaptations. **Weight-bearing exercise** refers to movement in which the body weight is supported by muscles and bones, thereby working against the pull of gravity. **Non–weight-bearing exercise,** by contrast, refers to movement in which the body is supported or suspended and thereby not working against the pull of gravity. Weight-bearing or impact-loading activities, such as running, gymnastics, stair climbing, volleyball, or resistance training, are more likely to stimulate an increase in bone mass than non–weight-bearing activities, such as swimming or cycling (Dalsky, 1993; Grimston, et al., 1993; Jacobson, et al., 1984). The type of activity that should be chosen depends on the health and preference of the

individual. A major concern when one is considering exercise for individuals with low bone mineral content is the risk of falling and causing a fracture. Activities that carry a high risk of falls or collisions should not be recommended for certain segments of the population, such as the elderly. Table 18.5 provides some general guidelines for the type of activity that should be considered for various groups (Dalsky, 1993).

Because dynamic resistance training has been associated with positive adaptations in skeletal tissue, as well as muscular fitness, exercise physiologists recommend that individuals engage in dynamic resistance training exercise as a way of maintaining both muscular and skeletal health (Layne and Nelson, 1999). Loading seems to have a localized effect (Wolff's Law); thus, specific sites can be isolated for impact. Conversely, a general dynamic resistance program that works all the major muscles of the body should benefit the total skeleton.

The Question of Understanding box provides you the opportunity to apply the information presented in this section. Check your answer in Appendix D.

Weight-Bearing Exercise   A movement performed in which the body weight is supported by muscles and bones.

Non–Weight-Bearing Exercise   A movement performed in which the body weight is supported or suspended and thereby not working against the pull of gravity.

A Question of Understanding

Use Table 18.5 to answer the following questions.

1. What type of activities would you recommend for your 45-yr-old aunt who has just found out that she has low BMD? How is this program consistent with the goals for this population?
2. Because of your aunt's diagnosis of low BMD, what physical activities and dietary recommendations would you give to your 15-yr-old cousin (your aunt's daughter)? Why?

Focus on Application

✳ Plyometrics

As stated in the text of this chapter, high-impact activities are thought to be the key for bone development. Plyometrics is an exercise training method originally designed to develop explosive power. It consists of exercises involving powerful contractions following dynamic loading or prestretching of the contracting muscles. Plyometrics depth jumps have been shown to produce ground reaction forces of up to seven times body weight. In terms of skeletal loading, ground reaction forces of less than two times body weight are considered to be low intensity; ground reaction forces two to four times body weight fall into the moderate-intensity range; and ground reaction forces greater than four times body weight comprise a high-intensity load (Witzke and Snow, 2000). Thus, plyometrics provides a potentially excellent training modality for building bone mineral density.

Basic plyometric exercises include the following:

- *bounds* for horizontal distance;
- *jumps* for vertical height;
- *hops* for vertical height as rapidly as possible;
- *leaps* for maximal vertical plus horizontal distance;
- *skips* for vertical height plus horizontal distance;
- *ricochets* for rapid leg and foot movement while minimizing vertical and horizontal distance;
- *swings* for trunk movements with involvement of shoulders and arms; and
- *twists* for lateral movement without shoulder or arm involvement.

A program of plyometrics can be used with individuals as young as 12 yr of age if designed carefully and applied progressively (Radcliffe and Farentinos, 1985).

Witzke and Snow (2000) implemented a plyometrics training program in a freshman physical education class (3 d·wk^{-1}, 30–45 min·d^{-1}, for 9 months). All participants volunteered for this class. Despite the fact that the control subjects in a "traditional" physical education class were active for more hours per week outside class than the plyometrics exercisers (5.6 versus 2.6 hr·wk^{-1}), the plyometrics exercisers exhibited greater increases in bone mass measured at all sites. However, the difference between groups was statistically significant at only one site, the greater trochanter. The researchers reported that although some students worked harder in class than others, most enjoyed the plyometrics class and participated in it safely. Only one injury occurred during the entire program. Thus, plyometrics training may be a viable alternative activity for junior-senior high school physical education classes or after-school programs in fitness facilities. The implementation of such programs requires a knowledgeable instructor and a conscientiously constructed training program. ✳

Sources:

Radcliffe & Farentinos (1985); Witze & Snow (2000).

Overload

As mentioned earlier, weight-bearing exercises result in positive adaptations to the skeleton. However, the load that is necessary for positive bone adaptation is not known. The threshold for a stimulus that initiates new bone formation is termed the *minimal effective strain (MES)* (Frost, 1997). It is thought that a load or force that exceeds this threshold, and is repeated a sufficient number of times, will cause osteoblasts to secrete osteoid and lead to the formation of new bone. The MES, and thus the impact load, necessary to induce positive skeletal adaptations in humans is not precisely known, but the stimulus must include forces considerably greater than normally attained by habitual activity. There is strong evidence that weight-bearing, impact-loading exercises can lead to an increase in bone mineral density or a decrease in age-related loss of bone mineral density (Ernst, 1998).

Impact loads, and hence the strain applied to bones, can be manipulated by increasing repetitions or by increasing the intensity as measured by ground reaction force or joint force. For example, running would load the bones by high repetition whereas rope jumping would overload primarily by intensity. For adaptations to skeletal tissue, intensity is apparently more important than repetition (Beck and Marcus, 1999).

Until the amount of exercise needed to impose an overload is known, we cannot determine the rate of adaptation or the progression necessary to induce additional gains in bone density. However, any type of exercise overload (intensity, duration, or frequency) must begin at a level the individual can handle and progress gradually.

Individualization

The individual response principle applies to bone as well as to other systems of the body; that is, different people will respond to the same exercise stress differently, depending on their genetic makeup, hormonal and nutritional status, and so on. Individuals with low

Table 18.6

Effects of Physical Activity and Exercise Training on Bone Health

No or Too Little Activity	Acceptable Amounts of Activity	Too Much, High-Intensity, Long-Duration, Rapid Increment Activity
	Amount of Activity	
←————————————————————————————————→		
Low mineralization and density	Adequate mineralization or enhanced mineralization and density	Osteopenia or osteoporosis in amenorrheic athletes
Aging-associated osteoporosis	Normal rate of growth, stature, and proportion	Fragile bones; increased risk of fracture
Fragile bones; increased fracture potential	Delayed aging-associated osteoporosis	Overuse injuries include those to the elbow (bony spurs or bone disruption at joint surface), the vertebrae (microfractures leading to slippage), the knees (Osgood-Schlatter diseases: inflammation of the bones or cartilage), and the legs and feet (stress reactions and/or fractures)

BMD have the greatest potential for benefit. Therefore, the guidelines for applying this principle as described for aerobic and dynamic resistance activities should be employed.

Retrogression/Plateau/Reversibility

The reversibility principle suggests that if you cease exercising for a period of time, you will lose the benefits of exercising. Studies of immobilized patients (Donaldson, et al., 1970; Vogel and Whittle, 1976) and discontinued training (Dalsky, et al., 1988) indicate that this principle also applies to bone. However, neither the level of activity needed to maintain bone mineral density, the threshold at which bone loss occurs, nor the rate of bone loss is known. Additional research is necessary to determine the level of activity necessary to maintain improvements in bone mineral density that have resulted from exercise training.

Warm-Up and Cool-Down

The effect of warming up and cooling down on bone density is not known. However, warming up and stretching are important to the ligaments and tendons, which are part of the skeletal system.

In summary, the exact exercise prescription for skeletal health is not currently known. However, this should not be used as an excuse not to exercise. Some weight-bearing or impact-loading exercise is better than none. Furthermore, because aerobic and dynamic resistance activities are recommended, it is prudent to use the guidelines given for these modalities until guidelines more specific to skeletal health are developed (ACSM, 2000).

Skeletal Adaptations to Exercise Training

The adaptation of the skeletal system to exercise training is depicted by the continuum in Table 18.6. As the table indicates, the adaptation of bone depends on the amount of activity. In addition, skeletal adaptation depends on the type of bone being measured (trabecular or cortical) and the type of activity employed.

Research clearly indicates that a lack of weight-bearing exercise is detrimental to the skeleton (that is, results in a loss of bone mineral density). This effect has been shown in astronauts and in patients confined to bed rest or immobilized in a cast. Studies have consistently indicated that weight-bearing bones are affected to a greater degree and that trabecular bone (measured in the spine) is lost at a greater rate than cortical bone (Donaldson, et al., 1970; Frost, 1988; Vogel and Whittle, 1976).

Despite the fact that the exact amount and type of exercise needed to develop and maintain a healthy or enhanced skeletal system are unknown, there is evidence that suggests that physical activity, within a reasonable range, does have a positive effect on bone density. There is no consistent evidence that suggests that exercise training affects either skeletal maturation (measured by ossification) in growing children or bone length. Although isolated studies have shown both retarded and accelerated growth in stature in young athletes, the consensus is that youngsters involved in exercise training grow at the same rate and to the same extent as do their sedentary counterparts (Caine, 1990; Malina, 1988; Plowman, et al., 1991; Sprynarova, 1987).

One approach to studying the effect of increased physical activity on bone density is to compare the dominant limb to the nondominant limb in sports such as tennis and baseball. These studies report that the dominant arm has greater bone mineral density or mass than the nondominant arm (Huddleston, et al., 1980; Jones, Priest, et al., 1977). This result appears to be true for both females and males and across a wide age span.

Another approach has been to compare different athletic groups with one another and with control groups. These studies collectively suggest that individuals who are involved in athletics or participate in vigorous fitness training have greater bone mineral density than sedentary controls. Furthermore, individuals who are involved in weight-bearing or impact-loading sports tend to have higher BMD than those involved in non–weight-bearing activities (Jacobson, et al., 1984; Riser, et al., 1990).

Training studies have also been conducted in which sedentary individuals initiated an exercise program. BMD measurements were compared prior to and following the exercise training. In a study that investigated changes in bone mineral content with training and subsequent detraining, Dalsky and colleagues (1988) reported that 22 months of weight-bearing exercise caused a significant increase (6.2%) in lumbar bone mineral content. When subjects discontinued exercise training (or trained less than 3 days per week), however, bone mineral content returned to baseline values. After 1 yr of detraining, bone mineral content was only 1.1% above baseline values. These data suggest that the increase in bone mineral that results from exercise is lost if exercise is not continued; bone responds to activity and inactivity.

A study by Welsh and Rutherford (1996) suggests that elderly men and women respond to exercise in a similar manner. High-impact aerobics, performed 2–3 days per week, resulted in an increase in total body BMD and in hip and spine BMD. The increase in BMD was similar for the males and females who participated in the 12-month study.

A review of 21 longitudinal studies in which participants were randomly assigned to exercise treatment or control groups found that the studies taken collectively strongly suggest that regular physical exercise can delay the physiological decrease in bone mineral density and reduce the risk of osteoporosis. Weight-bearing exercises, including weightlifting, jumping, and running, were associated with the greatest improvements in bone mass (Ernst, 1998).

Skeletal adaptation to exercise depends on the age of the participant. Vigorous exercise helps

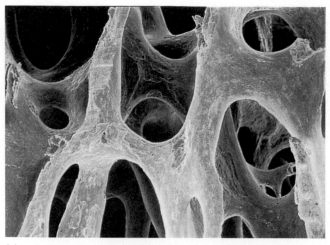

(a)

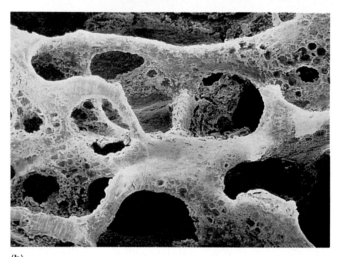

(b)

Figure 18.8
Trabecular Bone

(a) Normal. (b) Osteoporotic.

increase bone mass and strength in children and is thus important in the attainment of peak bone mass. Weight-bearing activities minimize age-related bone loss in aging adults (Frost, 1997). Although the precise mechanisms by which weight-bearing exercise helps improve or maintain BMD are not known, it is clear that increases in mechanical stress on bone lead to multiple physiological changes that increase or maintain bone density (Ernst, 1998; Frost, 1997; Layne and Nelson, 1999).

If some is good, more is not necessarily better when it comes to exercise training and bone health. As indicated in Table 18.6, excessive amounts of physical activity can potentially exceed the adaptive ability of bone, resulting in decreased bone density and/or overuse injuries.

Table 18.7
Risk Factors Associated With Osteoporosis

Risk Factors	Relationship to Disease	Possible Explanations
Genetic		
Race	Whites are more likely to develop disease than African Americans.	Unknown
Sex	Women are four times more likely to develop osteoporosis than men.	Lighter bones of females; rapid bone loss following menopause; longer life span
Heredity	There appears to be a genetic predisposition to the disease.	Unknown
Body build	Petite individuals are at greater risk.	Less peak bone mass to lose
Lifestyle		
Lack of physical activity	Lack of weight-bearing activity increases risk of disease.	No weight-bearing activities to stimulate bone formation
Smoking	Smoking increases risk of disease.	May lower serum estrogen or cause early menopause
Sex hormones (late menarche, amenorrhea, or menopause)	Decrease in sex hormones is associated with increased risk.	Loss of protective effect of estrogen on bone
Nutritional		
Calcium intake	Low calcium level interferes with bone formation.	Insufficient calcium to adequately ossify bone
Alcohol use	Alcohol use may be damaging to bone.	Resulting poor diet from excessive alcohol consumption

Special Applications to Health and Fitness

This section will discuss several topics related to the practical implications of skeletal health of special interest to those involved in health and fitness. These topics include osteoporosis, amenorrhea, and skeletal injuries.

Osteoporosis

Osteoporosis is a serious health problem that affects over 20 million Americans; it is estimated that 10 million individuals already have the disease and that 18 million more have low bone mass, placing them at increased risk for osteoporosis (National Osteoporosis Foundation). *Osteoporosis* means "porous bones," and the condition is characterized by a loss of BMD, resulting in bones that are weak and susceptible to fracture. This disease represents an imbalance between bone resorption and bone formation: Resorption occurs faster than formation, leading to a decrease in BMD. Osteoporosis, as defined earlier, is a condition in which the BMD is greater than 2.5 SD below the young normal adult average (Kanis, et al., 1993). Figure 18.8 presents photographs of normal and osteoporotic trabecular bone. Note the more porous trabeculae in the osteoporotic bone, which weakens the bone.

The most common sites of fracture related to osteoporosis are the hip, spine, and wrist. Approximately 300,000 hip, 700,000 vertebral, and 250,000 wrist fractures each year in the United States are related to osteoporosis. Most hip fractures require surgery, and there is a 15–20% mortality rate following such surgeries. The estimated national direct cost for osteoporotic fractures was $13.8 billion in 1995 (National Osteoporosis Foundation). Spinal vertebral fractures occur when a osteoporotic bone is literally crushed by the weight of the body, resulting in a loss of height, curvature of the spine, and considerable pain.

The cause of osteoporosis is not known. However, several risk factors have been identified, and they are outlined in Table 18.7 (Kleerekoper and Avioli, 1993; Lindsay, 1993; Loucks, 1988). Genetic factors related to the development of osteoporosis include race, sex, family history, and body size. Nutritional factors associated with increased risk of osteoporosis include low calcium intake, excessive alcohol consumption, and consistently high protein intake.

Lifestyle factors associated with osteoporosis include lack of physical activity, smoking, and inadequate levels of estrogen (related to a delayed menarche, amenorrhea, or an early menopause). Several research studies have indicated that the rapid loss of BMD following menopause is related to the decrease in estrogen levels at this time. These findings have led to an increase in the use of estrogen replacement therapy (ERT) for women who are at a higher risk of developing osteoporosis. The low activity levels of females in the United States, particularly older women, also contribute to the risk of developing osteoporosis. Bone mineral content is positively related to long-term physical activity.

In addition to having a positive effect on BMD, exercise may also be helpful in preventing fractures by increasing muscular strength and coordination and thereby decreasing the risk of falling. Individual factors that affect the risk of falling include coordination, sight, and muscular strength. Environmental factors that influence the risk of falling include lighting, floor surface, and footwear. Exercise leaders have a specific responsibility to provide an exercise area that reduces the risk of falling for the elderly.

Physical Activity, Altered Menstrual Function, and Bone Density

The elderly and postmenopausal females are not the only people at risk for developing osteoporosis and subsequent bone fractures; so too are young amenorrheic athletes (ACSM, 1997). **Amenorrhea** is the absence of menses and may be classified as either primary or secondary. *Primary amenorrhea* refers to a late or delayed menarche. Mean menarcheal age in the United States is between 12.3 and 12.8 yr. Menarche is attained later in athletes than in the general population, although the degree of delay varies among sports. In general, swimmers show the least delay (a matter of a couple of months); dancers and gymnasts show delays of approximately 2 yr. Athletes who have been the most successful exhibit the greatest delays in menarche. Furthermore, the higher the level of competition, the higher the percentage of delayed menarche in the athletic population. The cause of the delay in menarche in young athletes has not yet been clearly established (Frisch and McArthur, 1974; Plowman, 1989; Wells and Plowman, 1988).

Delayed menarche has not been associated with either increased or decreased bone mineral density, but it has been weakly (although inconclusively) linked with both secondary amenorrhea and high levels of stress fractures (Wells and Plowman, 1988). *Secondary amenorrhea* refers to the cessation of menstruation or menstrual periods that occur at in-

tervals greater than 90 days after an established periodicity has been achieved. The exact incidence of secondary amenorrhea in athletes is unknown; however, it is generally acknowledged that young, competitive, lean female athletes engaged in high-intensity training are at a greater risk for developing amenorrhea than their sedentary counterparts. Like delayed menarche, this phenomenon is somewhat sport specific, with those at the highest level of international competition showing the greatest vulnerability. In addition, as with delayed menarche, the cause of secondary amenorrhea has not yet been determined (Highet, 1989; Keizer and Rogol, 1990; Sanborn and Wagner, 1986; Sanborn, 1986; Wells and Plowman, 1988).

Although the cause of secondary amenorrhea is not known, its effect on bone is quite clear. Amenorrheic athletes often have *osteopenia,* or decreased levels of bone mineral density (Cann, et al., 1984; Drinkwater, Nilson, Chesnut, et al., 1984; Lindberg, et al., 1984; Marcus, et al., 1985; Rigotti, et al., 1984). The first study to show this effect did so quite accidently when one subgroup of amenorrheic women being studied for spinal mineral content just happened to be athletes (Cann, et al., 1984). Prior to this study, on the basis of the positive protective influence of exercise training on the bone density of postmenopausal women and the findings of enhanced bone mineralization in male athletes, exercise physiologists had simply assumed that female athletes, regardless of their menstrual status, would show the same benefits. When the research study just cited showed that the amenorrheic athletes had 29% less spinal mineralization than normal controls, research in the area was stimulated.

The average results from subsequent studies of amenorrheic athletes are presented in Figure 18.9. The decrease in bone mineralization appears to be greatest in vertebral bone, which is composed primarily of trabecular bone. Indeed, as shown in Figure 18.9, bone density measured at the cortical radius site is not distinguishable among amenorrheic athletes, normally cycling athletes, and sedentary controls, all of which exhibit values in the normal range. But no matter which unit is used to express bone density ($g \cdot cm^{-2}$ or $mg \cdot cm^{-3}$), the bone density at the spinal site is different among the three groups. Other trabecular sites have not shown this deficit in bone mineral density. Therefore, vulnerability is not determined just by whether a bone is cortical or trabecular but is also specific to certain bones; the spine appears to be most vulnerable (Drinkwater, Bruemner, et al., 1990). Although the differences may not appear to be great, a 25-year-old amenorrheic athlete's values in one study were equivalent to those of 51-yr-old women (Drinkwater, Nilson, Chesnut, et al., 1986)!

Amenorrhea   The absence of menses.

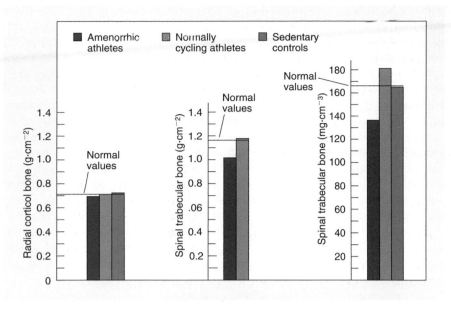

Figure 18.9
Bone Density Comparison in
Amenorrheic and Normally Cycling
Athletes

Horizontal line indicates normal value.

Sources: Cann, et al. (1984); Drinkwater, Nilson,
Chesnut, et al. (1984); Drinkwater, Bruemner,
et al. (1990); Lindberg, Fears, Hunt, et al.
(1984); Marcus, Cann, Madrig, et al. (1985);
Myburg, et al. (1990); and Ragotti, et al.
(1984).

Note that the spinal trabecular values for the normally cycling athletes are not only higher than those for the amenorrheic athletes but are also at or above the normal expected values. Thus, if an athlete who trains hard maintains a normal menstrual cycle, the expected effect of enhanced bone density is maintained.

The factor that is most suspected as the causal link or mechanism in amenorrhea is a deficiency in estrogen (that is, a hypoestrogenic state) (Cann, et al., 1984; Highet, 1989; Marcus, et al., 1985; Rigotti, et al., 1984). Numerous studies have shown that a deficiency in estrogen is associated with both cessation of menstruation and low bone mineral density. Until the late 1980s, when estrogen receptors were discovered on bone, researchers had speculated that estrogen exerted its influence on bone by its effect on calcium balance (Drinkwater, Nilson, et al., 1984). Increased amounts of calcium intake are needed in individuals who are hypoestrogenic. Highly trained hypoestrogenic female athletes often do not take in sufficient calcium. With the discovery of estrogen receptors on bone, however, a direct link was established. A lack of estrogen appears to affect the balance between bone formation and bone resorption, favoring resorption over formation and thus resulting in net loss in bone density. Bone loss continues over time but is most rapid (4–5% per year) immediately after cessation of menstruation (Highet, 1989).

It is important that such bone loss be prevented if at all possible. If an athlete becomes amenorrheic, medical attention should quickly be sought to determine the cause and to determine whether bone density is being lost. If bone density is low, a physician may decide to place the individual on estrogen therapy or encourage training and/or dietary changes that might bring about a resumption of the menses. Generally, these changes include a reduction in training and an increase in caloric intake, with special attention paid to calcium. With a resumption of menstruation, bone density is regained; however, reversal may not be complete (Drinkwater, Bruemner, et al., 1990; Drinkwater, Nilson, Ott, et al., 1986). Therefore, the sooner the amenorrhea can be reversed, the less bone will be lost and the greater the chances will be for better mineralization. Also, if bone loss is reversed as quickly as possible, injuries, especially stress fractures, may be prevented.

Skeletal Injuries

Skeletal injuries can be categorized as resulting from macrotrauma or from microtrauma (Micheli, 1989). *Macrotrauma injuries* are sudden acute incidents, such as a broken leg or clavicle from impact or fractures at the epiphyseal growth plate. Of these macrotrauma injuries, growth plate fractures have the greatest potential for harm. The probability of suffering a growth plate injury is greatest in automobile accidents, falls, contact sports, and dynamic resistance training. Fractures of the growth plate can result in progressive bone shortening, deformity, or joint incongruity. However, the occurrence of acute traumatic growth plate injury is less frequent than other injury types, and most such injuries appear not to result in growth disturbances (Caine, 1990).

Microtrauma injuries are overuse injuries that result from chronic repetitive overtraining (Micheli,

1989). Where the microtrauma is manifested anatomically depends on the sport. Microtrauma injuries to bone generally involve an uncoupling or imbalance between bone resorption and bone deposition called a stress reaction. **Stress reactions** refer to maladaptive areas of bone hyperactivity where the balance between resorption and deposition is progressively lost such that resorption exceeds deposition.

Early minor stress reactions may have no clinical manifestations; that is, the individual feels no pain and exhibits no swelling or tenderness. As the overuse continues and the imbalance becomes more extreme, several clinical symptoms may occur, including degeneration and loosening of portions of bone from the joint capsules, the formation of bone spurs, inflammation of bone and cartilage, and/or stress fractures. A **stress fracture** is a hairline break in bone that occurs in the absence of acute trauma, is clinically symptomatic, and is detectable by X rays or bone scans. Exactly when the bone's stress reaction becomes a stress fracture is often difficult to determine. The typical fine hairline fracture may be undetectable by X rays or bone scans for three or four weeks after pain is evident.

Thus, although exercise training can and does have a beneficial impact on bone growth and health, too much exercise training, usually in the form of repetitive overuse or rapid increments of intensity or duration, can be detrimental. Harm is more likely to be done if the bone already has a low bone mineral density. Concern therefore revolves around two groups, amenorrheic female athletes and young growing athletes of both sexes (Sterling, et al., 1992).

The concern for amenorrheic athletes is well founded: A higher prevalence of stress fractures has been documented in this population than in normally cycling athletes in a variety of sports (Lloyd, et al., 1986; Maffulli, 1990; Micheli, 1989; Myburgh, et al., 1990). The same factors that predispose amenorrheic athletes to osteopenia appear to make them more susceptible to stress fractures.

The exact incidence of microtrauma, including stress fractures, in youth sport participants has been difficult to document, although reports from orthopedists indicate that the number is growing as more

children and adolescents participate in competitive sports (Faulkner, et al., 1993). The time of peak incidence for stress fractures is between the ages of 10 and 15, at the time of peak growth (Lloyd, et al., 1986; Sterling, et al., 1992). Some researchers have suggested that during the growth spurt there is a normal imbalance between bone matrix formation and mineralization. Furthermore, during this growth spurt muscle imbalances can occur around joints as the muscles, tendons, and ligaments are stretched and become progressively tighter when the bones elongate. A muscle that is fatigued from overuse, is weak or out of balance with its antagonist, and/or is inflexible loses its ability to absorb shock; so abnormally high stress is transmitted to the bone. This situation increases the chances not only of stress fractures or other repetitive stress reactions but also of an impact injury (Jones, et al., 1989; Kibler, et al., 1992; Mafulli, 1990).

The primary risk factor for overuse injuries is training error, particularly abrupt increases in intensity, duration, and frequency (Micheli, 1989). Increases greater than 10% per week in workload should be avoided in training the young athlete. Other risk factors include the aforementioned musculoskeletal imbalances of strength, flexibility, or size; errors in technique or skills; anatomical malalignments; footwear that fits improperly; and hard surfaces such as concrete and asphalt for running. Careful attention needs to be given to these factors by parents and individuals involved in youth sports. For example, during periods of rapid growth, intensity of training should be reduced and static stretching programs emphasized.

Although the skeletal system is often taken for granted, it should not be. When it is injured or malfunctioning, we quickly become aware of its importance. Adequate nutrition, reasonable training regimens, and maintenance of normal hormonal levels are keys to good bone health.

Summary

1. The skeletal system serves a number of important functions, including support, protection, movement, mineral storage, and hematopoiesis (blood cell formation).

2. Bone tissue is dynamic, living tissue that is constantly undergoing change. Bone remodeling refers to the continual process of bone resorption and the formation of new bone.

3. Osteoclasts are bone cells that cause the resorption (breakdown) of bone tissue. Osteoblasts are bone-forming cells. Osteocytes are mature osteoblasts that are surrounded by calcified bone.

Stress Reactions Maladaptive areas of bone hyperactivity where the balance between resorption and deposition is progressively lost such that resorption exceeds deposition.

Stress Fracture A fine hairline break in bone that occurs in the absence of acute trauma, is clinically symptomatic, and is detectable by X rays or bone scans.

4. There are two major types of bone tissue, cortical and trabecular bone; they differ in their microscopic appearance.

5. In general, studies suggest that physical activity has a positive effect on bone health. That is, exercise training can enhance the attainment of peak bone mass during late adolescence and early adulthood, can slow the rate of age-related bone loss in later adulthood, and may offset menopausal-related bone loss.

6. Weight-bearing or impact-loading activities produce greater changes in bone mineral density than do non–weight-bearing or weight-supported activities.

7. Appropriate exercise prescription for skeletal health should take into account the current skeletal health of the individual. On the basis of current status and individual desires, activities should be chosen from a continuum of impact-loading activities.

8. *Osteoporosis* means "porous bones," and it is characterized by a loss of bone mineral density, resulting in bones that are weak and susceptible to fracture. It is clinically defined as a bone mineral density greater than 2.5 standard deviations below young, normal adult averages.

9. Amenorrheic athletes are at risk for developing osteopenia, osteoporosis, and subsequent bone fractures. If amenorrhea does occur in an athlete, medical attention should be sought.

Review Questions

1. Compare and contrast cortical and trabecular bone.

2. Diagram the stages of bone remodeling, citing the specific role of the bone cells.

3. What is the relationship between the hormonal control of blood calcium levels and the hormonal control of bone remodeling?

4. Why are osteoporotic fractures more likely to occur in bones with a higher percentage of trabecular bone than cortical bone?

5. Why are women more likely than men to suffer osteoporotic fractures?

6. What can be done during the growth years to optimize the attainment of peak bone mass? Why is the attainment of peak bone mass important?

7. What factors influence skeletal adaptations to exercise?

8. Why should an amenorrheic athlete seek medical advice?

9. Describe the role of physical activity in preventing osteoporosis.

10. Defend or refute the following statements:
    a. Disturbances in bone growth frequently result from overtraining in young athletes.
    b. Young athletes are more susceptible to stress fractures during the time of peak growth than at other times.

For further review and additional study tools, go to The Physiology Place (www.physiologyplace.com) and the Student Study Guide for Exercise Physiology for Health, Fitness, and Performance *by Sharon A. Plowman and Denise L. Smith.*

Passport to the Internet

Visit the following Internet sites to explore further topics and issues related to the skeletal system. To visit an organization's web site, go to www.physiologyplace.com and click on "Passport to the Internet."

The American College of Sports Medicine   As the leading professional organization for individuals in sports medicine and exercise science, the ACSM issues position statements on a number of topics critical to the study of exercise physiology. Search the ACSM's position stand on the "Female Athlete Triad."

The American Orthopaedic Society for Sports Medicine   The American Orthopaedic Society for Sports Medicine (AOSSM) is a national organization of orthopedic surgeons specializing in sports medicine. The AOSSM works closely with many other sports medicine specialists and clinicians, including family physicians, emergency physicians, pediatricians, athletic trainers, and physical therapists, to improve the identification, prevention, treatment, and rehabilitation of sports injuries.

Shape Up America!   A nationwide network of over 40 organizations in the fields of medicine, public health, nutrition, and physical activity united to encourage healthy weight and increased physical activity. Explore the Fitness Center and critique the information provided at this site.

National Osteoporosis Foundation   The National Osteoporosis Foundation (NOF) is the leading nonprofit, voluntary health organization dedicated to promoting lifelong bone health while working to find a cure for the disease through programs of research, education, and advocacy. Explore this site and examine its recommendations for preventing osteoporosis.

References

American College of Sports Medicine: *Guidelines for Exercise Testing and Prescription* (6th edition). Philadelphia: Lea & Febiger (2000).

American College of Sports Medicine: Position stand: Female athlete triad. *Medicine and Science in Sports and Exercise.* 25(5):i–ix (1997).

Bailey, D. A., & R. G. McColloch: Bone tissue and physical activity. *Canadian Journal of Sports Studies.* 15(4):229–239 (1990).

Baron, R.: Anatomy and ultrastructure of bone. In M. J. Favus (ed.), *Primer on the Metabolic Bone Diseases and Disorders of Mineral Metabolism* (2nd edition). New York: Raven Press, 3–10 (1993).

Beck, B., & R. Marcus: Skeletal effects of exercise in men. In E. S. Orwoll (ed.), *Osteoporosis in Men: The Effect of Gender on Skeletal Health.* San Diego: Academic Press, 129–155 (1999).

Broekhoff, J.: The effect of physical activity on physical growth and development. In *Effects of Physical Activity on Children.* American Academy of Physical Education Papers, No. 19. Champaign, IL: Human Kinetics (1986).

Caine, D. J.: Growth plate injury and bone growth: An update. *Pediatric Exercise Science.* 2(3):209–229 (1990).

Canalis, E.: Regulation of bone remodeling. In M. J. Favus (ed.), *Primer of Metabolic Bone Disorders.* Kelseyville, CA: American Society of Bone and Mineral Research Society Office, 23–26 (1990).

Cann, C. E., M. C. Martin, H. K. Genant, & R. B. Jaffe: Decreased spinal mineral content in amenorrheic women. *Journal of the American Medical Association.* 251(5):626–629 (1984).

Dalsky, G. P.: The role of exercise in the prevention and treatment of osteoporosis. *Osteoporosis Report.* 8(4):2–3 (1993).

Dalsky, G. P., K. Stocke, A. Ehsani, E. Slatopolsky, W. Lee, & S. Birge: Weight-bearing exercise training and lumbar bone mineral content in post-menopausal women. *Annals of Internal Medicine.* 108:824–828 (1988).

Donaldson, G. L., S. B. Hulley, J. M. Vogel, R. S. Huttner, J. H. Boyers, & D. E. MacMillan: Effect of prolonged bed rest on bone mineral. *Metabolism.* 19:1071–1084 (1970).

Drinkwater, B. L., B. Bruemner, & C. H. Chestnut III: Menstrual history as a determinant of current bone density in young athletes. *Journal of the American Medical Association.* 263(4):545–548 (1990).

Drinkwater, B. L., K. Nilson, C. H. Chesnut III, W. J. Bremner, S. Shainholtz, & M. B. Southworth: Bone mineral content of amenorrheic and eumenorrheic athletes. *New England Journal of Medicine.* 311(5):277–281 (1984).

Drinkwater, B. L., K. Nilson, S. Ott, & C. H. Chestnut III: Bone mineral density after resumption of menses in amenorrheic athletes. *Journal of the American Medical Association.* 256(3):380–382 (1986).

Ernst, E.: Exercise for female osteoporosis: A systematic review of randomised clinical trials. *Sports Medicine.* 25(6):359–368 (1998).

Faulkner, R. A., D. A. Bailey, D. T. Drinkwater, A. A. Wilkinson, C. S. Houston, & H. A. McKay: Regional and total body bone mineral content and bone mineral density, and total body tissue composition in children 8–16 years of age. *Calcified Tissue International.* 53(2):7–12 (1993).

Frisch, R. E., & J. W. McArthur: Menstrual cycles: Fatness as a determinant of minimum weight for height necessary for their maintenance or onset. *Science.* 185:949–951 (1974).

Frost, H. M.: Vital biomechanics: Proposed general concepts for skeletal adaptations to mechanical usage. *Calcified Tissue International.* 42:145–156 (1988).

Frost, H. M.: Some ABC's of skeletal pathophysiology. The growth/modeling/remodeling distinction. *Calcified Tissue International.* 49:301–302 (1991a).

Frost, H. M.: Some ABC's of skeletal pathophysiology. 7. Tissue mechanisms controlling bone mass. *Calcified Tissue International.* 49:303–304 (1991b).

Frost, H. M.: Why do marathon runners have less bone than weight lifters? A vital-biomechanical view and explanation. *Bone.* 20(3):183–189 (1997).

Genant, H. K., K. G. Faulkner, C. C. Glüer, & K. Engelke: Bone densitometry: Current assessment. *Osteoporosis International.* 3 (Suppl. 1). s91–s97 (1993).

Grimston, S. K., N. D. Willows, & D. A. Hanley: Mechanical loading regime and its relationship to bone mineral density in children. *Medicine and Science in Sports and Exercise.* 25(11):1203–1210 (1993).

Highet, R.: Athletic amenorrhea: An update on etiology, complications and management. *Sports Medicine.* 7:82–108 (1989).

Huddleston, A. L., D. Rockwell, D. N. Kulund, & R. B. Harrison: Bone mass in lifetime tennis athletes. *Journal of the American Medical Association.* 244:1107–1109 (1980).

Jacobson, P. C., W. Beaver, S. A. Grubb, T. N. Taft, & R. V. Talmage: Bone density in women: College athletes and older athletic women. *Journal of Orthopaedic Research.* 2:328–332 (1984).

Jones, B. H., J. M. Harris, T. N. Vinh, & C. Rubin: Exercise-induced stress fractures and stress reactions of bone: Epidemiology, etiology and classification. In K. B. Pandolf (ed.), *Exercise and Sport Sciences Reviews.* Baltimore: Williams & Wilkins. 17:379–422 (1989).

Jones, H. H., J. D. Priest, W. C. Hayes, C. C. Tichenor, & D. A. Nagel: Humeral hypertrophy in response to exercise. *Journal of Bone and Joint Surgery.* 58-A:204–208 (1977).

Kanis, J. A., P. Meunier, L. Alexeera, P. Burkhardt, C. Christiansen, C. Cooper, P. Delmas, O. Johnell, C. Johnston, P. Lips, L. J. Melton, E. Seeman, J. Stephan, & A. Tosteson: *1993 Assessment of Osteoporotic Risk Fracture and Its Role in Screening for Postmenopausal Osteoporosis.* Geneva: World Health Organization (1993).

Keizer, H. A., & A. D. Rogol: Physical exercise and menstrual cycle alterations: What are the mechanisms? *Sports Medicine.* 10(4):218–235 (1990).

Kibler, W. B., T. J. Chandler, & E. S. Stracener: Musculoskeletal adaptations and injuries due to overtraining. In J. O. Holloszy (ed.), *Exercise and Sport Science Reviews.* Baltimore: Williams & Wilkins. 20:99–126 (1992).

Kleerekoper, M., & L. V. Avioli: Evaluation and treatment of postmenopausal osteoporosis. In *Primer on the Metabolic Bone Diseases and Disorders of Mineral Metabolism* (2nd edition). New York: Raven Press, 223–228 (1993).

Layne J. E., & M. E. Nelson: The effects of progressive resistance training on bone mineral density: A review. *Medicine and Science in Sports and Exercise.* 31(1):25–30 (1999).

Lanyon, L. E.: Strain-related bone modeling and remodeling. *Topics in Geriatric Rehabilitation.* 4(2):13–24 (1989).

Lindberg, J. S., W. B. Fears, M. M. Hunt, M. R. Powell, D. Boll, & C. E. Wade: Exercise-induced amenorrhea and bone density. *Annals of Internal Medicine.* 101(5):647–648 (1984).

Lindsay, R.: Prevention of osteoporosis. In *Primer on the Metabolic Bone Diseases and Disorders of Mineral Metabolism* (2nd edition). New York: Raven Press, 240–245 (1993).

Lloyd, T., S. J. Triantafyllou, E. R. Baker, P. S. Houts, J. A. Whiteside, A. Kalenak, & P. G. Stumpf: Women athletes with menstrual irregularities have increased musculo-skeletal injuries. *Medicine and Science in Sports and Exercise.* 18(4):373–379 (1986).

Loucks, A.: Osteoporosis prevention begins in childhood. In E. Brown & C. Branta (eds.), *Competitive Sports for Children and Youth.* Champaign, IL: Human Kinetics (1988).

Maffulli, N.: Intensive training in young athletes: The orthopedic surgeon's viewpoint. *Sports Medicine.* 9(4):229–243 (1990).

Malina, R. M.: Biological maturity status of young athletes. In R. M. Malina (ed.), *Young Athletes: Biological, Psychological and Educational Perspectives.* Champaign, IL: Human Kinetics (1988).

Malina, R. M., & C. Bouchard: *Growth Maturation and Physical Activity.* Champaign, IL: Human Kinetics, 371–390 (1991).

Marcus, R.: Normal and abnormal bone remodeling in man. *Annual Review of Medicine.* 38:129–141 (1987).

Marcus, R. C., C. Cann, P. Madrig, J. Minkoff, M. Goddard, M. Bayer, M. Martin, L. Gaudiani, W. Haskell, & H. Genant: Menstrual function and bone mass in elite women distance runners: Endocrine and metabolic features. *Annals of Internal Medicine.* 102(2):158–163 (1985).

Marieb, E.: *Human Anatomy and Physiology* (5th edition). Redwood City, CA: Benjamin/Cummings (2001).

Micheli, L. T.: Sports injuries in children and adolescence. In D. Nudel (ed), *Pediatric Sports Medicine.* New York: PMA Publishing, 177–192 (1989).

Myburgh, K. H., J. Hutchins, A. B. Fataar, S. F. Hough, & T. D. Noakes: Low bone density is an etiologic factor for stress fractures in athletes. *Annals of Internal Medicine.* 113:754–759 (1990).

National Institutes of Health (NIH) Consensus Conference: Optimal calcium intake. *Journal of the American Medical Association.* 272:1942–1948 (1994).

National Osteoporosis Foundation. http://www.nof.org/osteoporosis/stats.htm.

Nishiyama, S., S. Tomoeda, T. Ohta, A. Higuchi, & I. Matsuda: Differences in basal and postexercise osteocalcin levels in athletic and nonathletic humans. *Calcified Tissue International.* 43:150–154 (1988).

Ott, S.: Editorial: Attainment of peak bone mass. *Journal of Clinical Endocrinology and Metabolism.* 71(5):1082A–1082C (1990).

Parfitt, A. M.: Bone remodeling and bone loss: Understanding the pathophysiology of osteoporosis. *Clinical Obstetrics and Gynecology.* 30(4):789–811 (1987).

Plowman, S. A.: Exercise and puberty: Is there a relationship in the young female athlete? In D. Nudel (ed.), *Pediatric and Adolescent Sports Medicine and Rehabilitation.* New York: PMA Publishing, 215–232 (1989).

Plowman, S. A., N. Y.-S. Lui, & C. L. Wells: Body composition and sexual maturation in premenarcheal athletes and nonathletes. *Medicine and Science in Sports and Exercise.* 23(1):23–29 (1991).

Radcliffe, J. C., & R. C. Farentinos. *Plyometrics: Explosive Power Training.* Champaign, IL: Human Kinetics (1985).

Rigotti, N. A., S. R. Nussbaum, D. B. Herzog, & R. M. Neer: Osteoporosis in women with anorexia nervosa. *New England Journal of Medicine.* 311(25):1601–1606 (1984).

Riser, W. L., E. J. Lee, A. Leblanc, H. B. Poindexter, J. M. Risser, & V. Schneider: Bone density in eumenorrheic female college athletes. *Medicine and Science in Sports and Exercise.* 22:570–574 (1990).

Sanborn, C. F.: Etiology of athletic amenorrhea. In J. L. Pohl & C. H. Brown (eds.), *The Menstrual Cycle and Physical Activity.* Champaign, IL: Human Kinetics, 45–58 (1986).

Sanborn, C. F., & W. W. Wagner: Athletic amenorrhea. In B. L. Drinkwater (ed.), *Female Endurance Athletes.* Champaign, IL: Human Kinetics, 125–148 (1986).

Snow-Harter, C., M. Bouxsen, B. Lewis, S. Charette, P. Weinstein, & R. Marcus: Muscle strength as a predictor of bone mineral density in young women. *Journal of Bone and Mineral Research.* 5:589–595 (1990).

Snow-Harter, C., & R. Marcus: Exercise, bone mineral density, and osteoporosis. In J. O. Holloszy (ed.), *Exercise and Sport Science Reviews.* Baltimore: Williams & Wilkins. 19:351–388 (1991).

Sprynarova, S.: The influence of training on physical and functional growth before, during and after puberty. *European Journal of Applied Physiology.* 56:719–724 (1987).

Sterling, J. C., D. W. Edelstein, R. D. Calvo, & R. Webb II: Stress fractures in the athlete: Diagnosis and management. *Sports Medicine.* 14(5):336–346 (1992).

Teitelbaum, S. L.: Skeletal growth and development. In M. J. Favus (ed.), *Primer on Metabolic Bone Diseases and Disorders of Mineral Metabolism.* Kelseyville, CA: American Society of Bone and Mineral Research Society (1993).

Vogel, J. M., & M. W. Whittle: Bone mineral changes: The second manned skylab mission. *Aviation, Space, and Environmental Medicine.* 13:282–289 (1976).

Wells, C. L., & S. A. Plowman: Relationship between training, menarche, and amenorrhea. In W. W. Brown & C. F. Branta (eds.), *Competitive Sports for Children and Youth: An Overview of Research and Issues.* Champaign, IL: Human Kinetics (1988).

Welsh, L., & O. M. Rutherford: Hip bone mineral density is improved by high-impact aerobic exercise in post-menopausal women and men over 50 years. *European Journal of Applied Physiology and Occupational Physiology.* 74:511–517 (1996).

Witzke, K. A., & C. M. Snow: Effects of plyometric jump training on bone mass in adolescent girls. *Medicine and Science in Sports and Exercise.* 32(6):1051–1057 (2000).

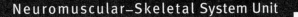
Chapter 19

Skeletal Muscle
System

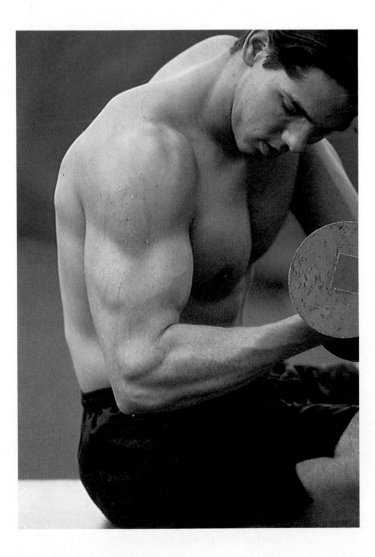

After studying the chapter, you should be able to

- Describe the functions of skeletal muscle tissue.
- Identify the characteristics of muscle tissue that make movement possible.
- Describe the macroscopic and microscopic organization of skeletal muscle tissue.
- Relate the molecular structure of the myofilaments to the sliding-filament theory of muscle contraction.
- Identify the regions of a sarcomere, and explain the changes that occur in these regions during contraction.
- Discuss the importance of specialized organelles, specifically, the sarcoplasmic reticulum, the T tubules, and the myofibrils.
- Explain the events involved in excitation-contraction coupling.
- Describe the sequence of events involved in the generation of force within the contractile elements.
- Differentiate muscle fiber types on the basis of contractile and metabolic properties.
- Discuss the ramifications of fiber type distribution on the likelihood of success in a given athletic event.

Introduction

Muscle contractions provide the basis for all human movement. To understand how movement occurs, you must first appreciate the interactions among the various systems of the body. For instance, the muscle cells (fibers) must be able to produce and utilize ATP to provide the energy for contraction and force production. This process requires that the digestive, respiratory, endocrine, and cardiovascular systems operate effectively to provide the muscle cells with the oxygen and nutrients they require to produce the energy. For the purposes of this chapter, we will assume that these other systems of the body are functioning properly.

Overview of Muscle Tissue

Muscle tissue produces force because of the interaction of its basic contractile elements (myofilaments), which are composed primarily of protein. The function of the muscle tissue ultimately depends on the type of muscle tissue involved: skeletal, smooth, or cardiac muscle. The force of contraction may be used for locomotion (skeletal muscle), the movement of materials through hollow tubes such as the digestive tract or blood vessels (smooth muscle), or the pumping action of the heart (cardiac muscle). However, all muscle tissue has the ability to produce force because of certain basic characteristics common to all types. This chapter will focus on skeletal muscle, as shown in Figure 19.1.

Because skeletal muscles have various characteristics, physiologists refer to them by different names. On the one hand, skeletal muscles are under conscious control, so they are often referred to as voluntary muscles. On the other hand, skeletal muscles are

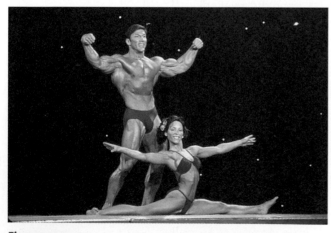

Figure 19.1
Bodybuilders

Bodybuilding poses demonstrate muscle hypertrophy and definition.

sometimes referred to as striated muscle because of the repeating pattern of light and dark bands seen in the microscopic structure of the muscle. Additionally, in order to differentiate skeletal muscle fibers from intrafusal fibers found in sensory organs of the muscle (proprioceptors; see Chapter 22), physiologists sometimes refer to skeletal muscle fibers as extrafusal muscle fibers.

Functions of Skeletal Muscle

Although locomotion is the primary function of muscle tissue, the muscular system also performs other important roles. In addition to locomotion and manipulation, skeletal muscles maintain body posture, assist in venous return of blood to the heart, and play an important role in thermogenesis (heat generation). Heat is a by-product of cellular respiration; and because muscles utilize a great deal of energy for movement, they also generate a great deal of heat. Additionally, muscles act as energy transducers by converting biochemical energy, from ingested food, into mechanical and thermal energy. Skeletal muscles also protect internal organs and make up most of the protein in the body. Because muscles represent such a large amount of protein, they constitute a potential but rarely used form of stored energy. The use of protein as an energy substrate is discussed in the metabolism unit.

Characteristics of Muscle Tissue

Muscle tissue has unique characteristics that are specifically suited to its primary function, namely, converting an electrical signal into a mechanical event (contraction of muscle fibers). The characteristics that allow a muscle to produce movement include irritability, contractility, extensibility, and elasticity.

Irritability refers to the ability of a muscle to receive and respond to stimuli. The stimulus is generally in the form of a chemical message (from a neurotransmitter), and the response is the generation of an electrical current (action potential) along the cell membrane. **Contractility** refers to the ability of a muscle to respond to a stimulus by shortening. It is this shortening that produces force. Muscle tissue is the only tissue with the ability to generate force. **Extensibility** refers

> **Irritability** The ability of a muscle to receive and respond to stimuli.
>
> **Contractility** The ability of a muscle to respond to a stimulus by shortening.
>
> **Extensibility** The ability of a muscle to be stretched or lengthened.

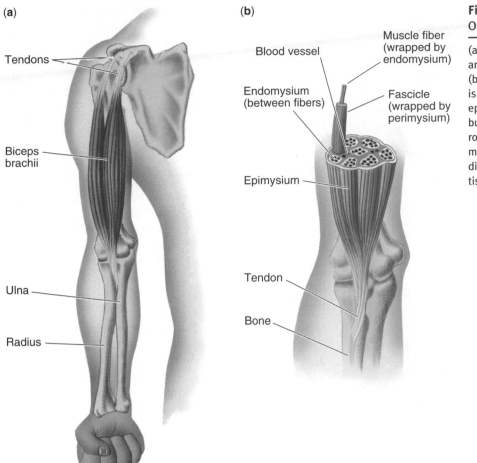

(a)

Tendons

Biceps
brachii

Ulna

Radius

(b)

Blood vessel

Endomysium
(between fibers)

Epimysium

Tendon

Bone

Muscle fiber
(wrapped by
endomysium)

Fascicle
(wrapped by
perimysium)

Figure 19.2
Organization of Skeletal Tissue

(a) Intact skeletal muscle. Biceps brachii
are attached to bones through tendons.
(b) Connective tissue. The entire muscle
is surrounded by connective tissue called
epimysium. The muscle is organized into
bundles called fasciculi, which are surrounded by connective tissue called perimysium. Each fasciculus contains many individual fibers surrounded by connective
tissue called endomysium.

to the ability of a muscle to be stretched or lengthened.
Stretching occurs when a muscle is manipulated by
external force. **Elasticity** refers to the ability of a muscle to return to its resting length after being stretched.
These characteristics of muscles function together to
allow for human movement.

Macroscopic Structure of Skeletal Muscles

There are over 400 skeletal muscles in the human
body, and they account for 40–45% of the adult male
body weight and 23–25% of the adult female body
weight (Fox, 1987; Hunter, 2000). These muscles
function together in a remarkable way to provide
smooth, integrated movement for a wide variety of activities, many of which require little conscious
thought. Muscle action also provides the basis for
sport and fitness activities, and muscle definition itself, as seen in Figure 19.1, has become the goal of the

---

Elasticity The ability of a muscle to return to
resting length after being stretched.

---

sport of bodybuilding. To understand how muscles
function in bodybuilding poses, or in any other activity, it is necessary to look beneath the skin.

Organization and Connective Tissue

Skeletal muscles are organized in a systematic fashion,
as depicted in Figure 19.2. Some of this organization is
apparent to the naked eye, but other aspects of this
organization are apparent only when muscle fibers are
viewed through a simple or an electron microscope.

Skeletal muscles are attached to bones by tendons, an arrangement that allows the contraction of a
muscle to move a bone. Each muscle is bound together by a thick layer (sheath) of connective tissue
called *fascia*. Just beneath the fascia is a more
delicate layer of connective tissue called *epimysium*
that directly covers the muscle.

The interior of the muscle is subdivided into bundles of muscle fibers called *fasciculi* (the singular is
fasciculus or *fascicle*), which are also surrounded by
connective tissue. The sheath of connective tissue that
separates the fasciculi within a skeletal muscle is

Classification	Example	Diagram
Longitudinal	Sartorius	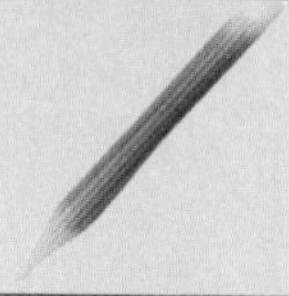
Fusiform	Biceps brachii	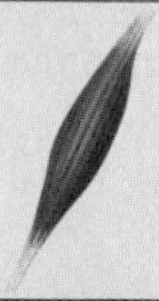
Radiate	Gluteus medius	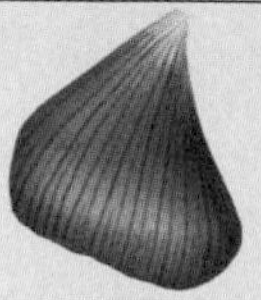
Unipennate	Tibialis posterior	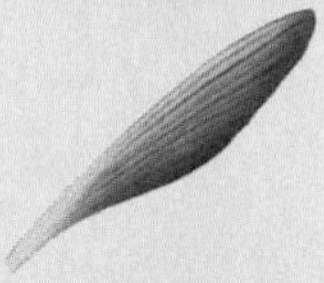
Bipennate	Gastrocnemius	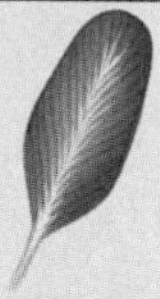
Circular	Orbicular oculi (and sphincters)	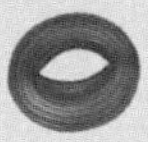

Figure 19.3
Arrangement of Fasciculi

called *perimysium*. The fasciculi are comprised of many individual muscle fibers (cells), each of which is surrounded by its own sheath of connective tissue called *endomysium*.

The three layers of connective tissue (the epimysium, the perimysium, and the endomysium) provide the framework that holds the muscle together. These three layers of connective tissue come together at each end of the muscle to form the tendons that attach the muscle to bone. As a muscle contracts, it pulls on the connective tissue in which it is wrapped, causing the tendon to move the bone to which it is attached.

Architectural Organization

Different arrangements of fasciculi within a muscle account for the different shapes that a muscle may take. Muscles can be described as longitudinal, fusiform, radiate, unipennate, bipennate, or circular, as shown in Figure 19.3. The shape of the muscle

determines its range of motion and influences its power production. The longer and more parallel muscle fibers, as found in longitudinal muscles, allow for greater muscle shortening. Bipennate and multipennate muscles, by contrast, shorten very little, but are more powerful. The relationship between architectural organization and force production is further discussed in Chapter 20.

Microscopic Structure of a Muscle Fiber

Individual muscle fibers are composed primarily of smaller units called myofibrils, which are in turn made up of myofilaments. This organization of skeletal muscle is shown in Figure 19.4, which should be referred to as you read the following sections.

Muscle Fibers

Muscle fibers, also called muscle cells, are long, cylinder-shaped cells ranging from 10–100 μm in diameter and 1–400 mm in length (Hunter, 2000; Marieb, 2001; Vander, et al., 2001; Williams, 1994). The major structures of a muscle fiber and their functions are summarized in Table 19.1 on page 504.

A skeletal muscle fiber contains many nuclei, which are located just below the cell membrane. The *polarized plasma membrane* of a muscle cell is referred to as the *sarcolemma*, and it is the properties of this membrane that account for the irritability of muscle. The *sarcoplasm* of a muscle cell is similar to the cytoplasm of other cells, but it has specific adaptations to serve the functional needs of muscle cells, namely, increased amounts of glycogen and the oxygen-binding protein myoglobin.

The muscle fiber contains the organelles found in other cells (including a large number of mitochondria) along with some specialized organelles. The organelles that are of specific interest are the transverse tubules, the sarcoplasmic reticulum, and the myofibrils. The myofibrils are composed of the protein myofilaments and are responsible for the contractile properties of muscles.

Sarcoplasmic Reticulum and Transverse Tubules

Figure 19.4 illustrates the relationship among the myofibrils, the sarcoplasmic reticulum, and the transverse tubules. The **sarcoplasmic reticulum (SR)** is a

> **Sarcoplasmic Reticulum (SR)** The specialized muscle cell organelle that stores and releases calcium.

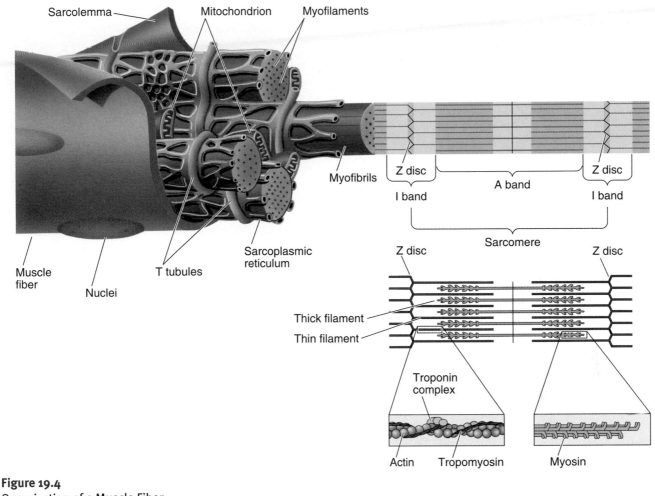

Figure 19.4
Organization of a Muscle Fiber

There is a close anatomical relationship among the organelles, specifically the myofibrils, T tubules, and sarcoplasmic reticulum (SR). The repeating pattern of the myofibrils is due to the arrangement of the myofilaments.

specialized organelle that stores and releases calcium. It is an interconnecting network of tubules running parallel with and wrapped around the myofibrils. (Notice in Figure 19.4 that the sarcolemma has been partially removed in order to illustrate the SR and myofibrils.) The major significance of the sarcoplasmic reticulum is its ability to store, release, and take up calcium and thereby control muscle contraction. Calcium is stored in the portion of the sarcoplasmic reticulum called the *lateral sacs* or *cisterns.*

The **transverse tubules (T tubules)** are organelles that carry the electrical signal from the sarcolemma to the interior of the cell. T tubules are continuous with the sarcolemma and protrude into the sarcoplasm of the cell. Although the T tubules run in close proximity to the sarcoplasmic reticulum and interact with it, they are anatomically separate organelles. As the name implies, the T tubules run perpendicular (transverse) to the myofibril. The spread of an electri-

cal signal (action potential) through the T tubules causes the release of calcium from the lateral sacs of the sarcoplasmic reticulum.

Myofibrils and Myofilaments

Each muscle fiber contains hundreds to thousands of smaller cylindrical units, or rodlike strands, called myofibrils (Figure 19.4). **Myofibrils** are contractile structures composed of myofilaments. These myofibrils, or

Transverse Tubules (T Tubules) Organelles that carry the electrical signal from the sarcolemma into the interior of the cell.

Myofibril Contractile structures composed of myofilaments.

Table 19.1
Summary of Major Components of a Skeletal Muscle Cell

Cell Part	Description	Function
Nucleus	Multinucleated	Is the control center for the cell
Sarcolemma	Polarized cell membrane	Is capable of receiving stimuli from the nervous system
Sarcoplasm	Intracellular material	Holds organelles and nutrients; provides the medium for glycolytic enzymatic reactions
Organelles		
Myofibrils	Rodlike structures composed of smaller units called myofilaments; account for 80% of muscle volume	Contain contractile proteins (myofilaments), which are responsible for muscle contraction
T tubules	Series of tubules that run perpendicular (transverse) to the cell and are open to the external part of cell	Spread polarization from the cell membrane into the interior of cell, which triggers the sarcoplasmic reticulum to release calcium
Sarcoplasmic reticulum	Interconnecting network of tubules running parallel with and wrapped around the myofibrils	Stores and releases calcium
Mitochondria	Sausage or spherical-shaped organelles; numerous in a muscle cell	Are the major site of energy production

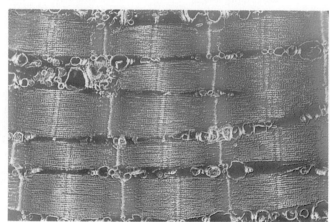

(a)

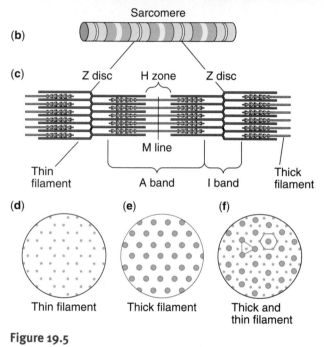

(b) Sarcomere

(c) Z disc · H zone · Z disc

Thin filament · M line · A band · I band · Thick filament

(d) Thin filament (e) Thick filament (f) Thick and thin filament

Figure 19.5
Arrangement of Myofilaments in a Sarcomere

(a) Micrograph of sarcomeres. (b) Model of sarcomeres. (c) Relationship between thick and thin filaments. (d) Cross-sectional view of thin filaments. (e) Cross-sectional view of thick filaments. (f) Cross-sectional view of thick and thin filaments.

simply fibrils, typically lie parallel to the long axis of the muscle cell and extend the entire length of the cell. Myofibrils account for approximately 80% of the volume of a muscle fiber.

As shown in Figure 19.4, each myofibril is composed of still smaller myofilaments (or filaments) that are arranged in a repeating pattern along the length of the myofibril. **Myofilaments** are contractile proteins (thick and thin) that are responsible for muscle contraction. It is the myofilaments that account for the majority of muscle protein. The repeating pattern of these myofilaments along the length of the myofi-

bril gives skeletal muscle its striated appearance. Each repeating unit is referred to as a *sarcomere.*

Sarcomeres

A **sarcomere** is the functional unit (contractile unit) of a muscle fiber. As illustrated in Figure 19.5, each sarcomere contains two types of myofilaments: *thick* filaments, composed primarily of the contractile protein myosin, and *thin* filaments, composed primarily of the contractile protein actin. Thin filaments also contain the regulatory proteins, troponin and tropomyosin.

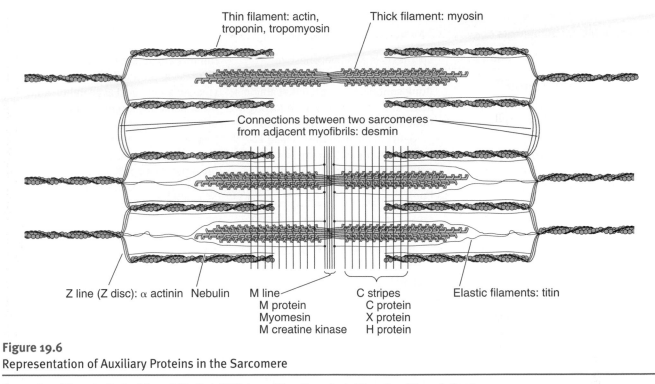

Figure 19.6
Representation of Auxiliary Proteins in the Sarcomere

Source: From "Muscular Basis of Strength" by Rudolf Billeter and Hans Hoppeler. In *Strength and Power in Sport* (p. 45) by P. V. Komi (ed.). Champaign, IL: Human Kinetics. Copyright 1992 by International Olympic Committee. Reprinted by permission.

When myofilaments are viewed under an electron microscope, their arrangement gives the appearance of alternating bands of light and dark striations. The light bands are called *I bands* and contain only thin filaments. The dark bands are called *A bands* and contain thick and thin filaments, with the thick filaments running the entire length of the A band. Thus, it is the length of the thick filament that determines the length of the A band.

The names for the various regions of the sarcomere are not arbitrary; they are derived from the first letter of the German word that describes their appearance. The names for the bands describe the refraction of light through the respective bands. The I band is abbreviated from the word *isotropic,* which means that this area appears lighter because more light is able to pass through it. The A band is so named because of its *anisotropic* properties, meaning that it appears darker because it does not allow as much light to pass through. These properties are directly related to the type of filament present.

Each A band is interrupted in the midsection by an *H zone* (from the German *Hellerscheibe,* for "clear disc"), where there is no overlap of thick and thin filaments. Running through the center of the H zone is a dense line called the *M line* (from the German *Mittelscheibe,* for "middle disc"). The I bands are also interrupted at the midline by a darker area called the *Z disc* (from the German *Zwischenscheibe,* for "between disc"). A sarcomere extends from one Z disc to the successive Z disc. The Z disc serves to anchor the thin filaments to adjacent sarcomeres.

Myofilaments occupy three-dimensional space. The arrangement of the myofilaments at different points in the sarcomere is shown in Figure 19.5d–19.5f. Notice that in regions where the thick and thin filaments overlap, each thick filament is surrounded by six thin filaments, and each thin filament is surrounded by three thick filaments.

A sarcomere consists of more than just contractile and regulatory proteins. Proteins of the cytoskeleton provide much of the internal structure of the muscle cell. Figure 19.6 diagrams the cytoskeleton of the sarcomere and its relationship to the contractile proteins (Billeter and Hoppler, 1992). The M line and the Z disc hold the thick and the thin filaments in place, respectively. The elastic filament helps keep the thick filament in the middle between the two Z discs during contraction.

Myofilaments Contractile (thick and thin) proteins that are responsible for muscle contraction.

Sarcomere The functional unit (contractile unit) of muscle fibers.

Focus on Application

✳ Increasing Protein Synthesis—Interaction of Training and Nutrition

Many athletes, especially those engaged in resistance training, are interested in increasing protein synthesis. Increased protein synthesis increases the amount of contractile proteins and, hence, make the muscles larger and stronger. Protein synthesis is enhanced in several circumstances: (a) following resistance exercise, (b) when amino acid availability is increased, and (c) when blood insulin levels are high. Recent research by Rasmussen et al. (2000) suggests that when these three conditions occur together, the effect on protein synthesis is additive. These researchers had participants ingest a drink containing six essential amino acids and 35 g of sucrose following a bout of resistance training. The participants consumed the drink at either 1 or 3 hr posttraining, and the results were compared to a control group that consumed a flavored placebo drink. The ingestion of sucrose caused an elevation in blood insulin levels.

The combination of essential amino acids, elevated insulin levels, and resistance training stimulated protein synthesis approximately 400% above pre-drink levels when the drink was consumed 1 or 3 hr after resistance exercise. This increase in protein synthesis is greater than that reported following resistance training alone (approximately a 100% increase in protein synthesis), increased amino acid availability alone (approximately a 150% increase in protein synthesis), and the combination of resistance training and increased amino acid availability (approximately a 200% increase in protein synthesis). Based on these results, fitness professionals may recommend that exercise participants who are interested in increasing muscle size consider consuming a drink containing essential amino acids and carbohydrate following resistance-training workouts. The supplement is equally effective if it is consumed 1 or 3 hr after a workout.   ✳

Source:

Rasmussen, et al. (2000).

Molecular Structure of the Myofilaments

The contractile proteins of the myofilaments slide over one another during muscular contraction. Hence, the **sliding-filament theory of muscle contraction** explains how muscles contract. Therefore, it is essential to pay careful attention to the structure of the myofilaments.

Thick Filaments

Thick filaments are composed primarily of myosin molecules (Figure 19.7). Each molecule of myosin has a rodlike tail and two globular heads (Figure 19.7a). A typical thick filament contains approximately 200 myosin molecules (Vander, et al., 2001). These molecules are oriented so that the tails form the central rodlike structure of the filament (Figure 19.7b). The globular myosin heads extend outward and will form *cross-bridges* when they interact with the thin filaments. The myosin heads have two reactive sites: One allows it to bind with the actin filament, and one binds to ATP (Marieb, 2001). It is only when the myosin heads bind to the active sites on actin, forming a cross-bridge, that contraction can occur.

The myosin subunits are oriented in opposite directions along the filament, forming a central section that lacks projecting heads (Figure 19.7c). The result is a bare zone in the middle of the filament, which accounts for the H zone seen in the middle of the A band (Figure 19.7d).

Thin Filaments

Thin filaments are composed primarily of the contractile protein actin. As illustrated in Figures 19.8a and 19.8b, actin is composed of small globular subunits (G actin) that form long strands called fibrous actin (F actin). A filament of actin is formed by two strands of F actin coiled about one another to form a double-helical structure; it resembles two strands of pearls wound around each other and may be referred to as a *coiled coil* (Figure 19.8c). The actin molecules contain active sites to which myosin heads will bind during contraction.

The thin filaments also contain the regulatory proteins called tropomyosin and troponin, which regulate the interaction of actin and myosin. *Tropomyosin* is a long, double-stranded, helical protein that

---

Sliding-Filament Theory of Muscle Contraction The theory that explains muscle contraction as the result of the myofilaments sliding over one another.

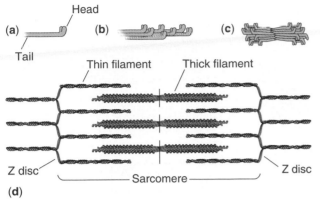

Figure 19.7
Molecular Organization of Thick Filaments

(a) Individual myosin molecules have a rodlike tail and two globular heads. (b) Individual molecules are arranged so that the tails form a rodlike structure and the globular heads project outward to form cross-bridges. (c) Myosin subunits are oriented in opposite directions along the filament forming a central bare zone in the middle of the filament (H zone). (d) Thick filament (myosin) within a single sarcomere showing the myosin heads extending toward the thin filament.

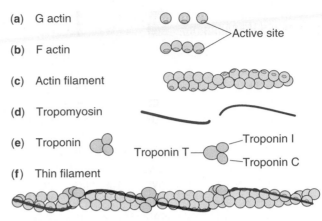

Figure 19.8
Molecular Organization of Thin Filaments

(a) Individual actin subunits (globular, G actin) shown with active site for binding to myosin heads. (b) Fibrous actin (F actin). (c) Actin filament with two strands of fibrous actin wound around itself to form a coiled coil. Active sites are exposed. (d) Tropomyosin is a regulatory protein that covers the binding sites on actin. (e) Troponin is a regulatory protein that when bound to Ca^{2+} removes tropomyosin from its blocking position on actin. (f) The thin filament is composed of actin, tropomyosin, and troponin.

is wrapped about the long axis of the actin backbone (Figure 19.8d). Tropomyosin serves to block the active site on actin, thereby inhibiting actin and myosin from binding under resting conditions.

Troponin is a small, globular protein complex composed of three subunits that control the position of the tropomyosin (Figure 19.9). The three units of troponin are troponin C (Tn-C), troponin I (Tn-I), and troponin T (Tn-T). Tn-C contains the calcium-binding sites, Tn-T binds troponin to tropomyosin, and Tn-I inhibits the binding of actin and myosin in the resting state (Figure 19.9b). When calcium binds to the Tn-C subunit, the troponin complex undergoes a configurational change. Because troponin is attached to tropomyosin, the change in the shape of troponin causes tropomyosin to be removed from its blocking position, thus exposing the active sites on actin (Marieb, 2001; Vander, et al., 2001). Once the active sites are exposed, the myosin heads are able to bind to the actin forming the cross-bridges (Figure 19.9c). Thus, calcium is the key to controlling the interaction of the filaments and, therefore, muscle contraction.

Contraction of a Muscle Fiber

In order for a muscle to contract, an *action potential* must be generated in the motor neuron that innervates the muscle fibers that will contract (Chapter 2). The message from the motor neuron must then be passed to the muscle fiber through the neuromuscular junction. Finally, the action potential must be conducted along the sarcolemma and into the interior of the muscle fiber to stimulate movement of the myofilaments. The process whereby electrical events in the sarcolemma of the muscle fiber are linked to the movement of the myofilaments is called *excitation-contraction coupling.*

As we describe the specific changes that occur during contraction, pay careful attention to three factors: the position of the myofilaments, the location of calcium ions, and the role of ATP.

The Sliding-Filament Theory of Muscle Contraction

A great deal of data has been amassed since the 1950s on the basis of X-ray, light microscopic, and electron microscopic studies to support the sliding-filament theory of muscle contraction. The basic principles of this theory are summarized in three statements:

1. The force of contraction is generated by the process that slides the actin filament over the myosin filament.

2. The lengths of the thick and the thin filaments do not change during muscle contraction.

3. The length of the sarcomere decreases as the actin filaments slide over the myosin filaments and pull the Z discs toward the center of the sarcomere.

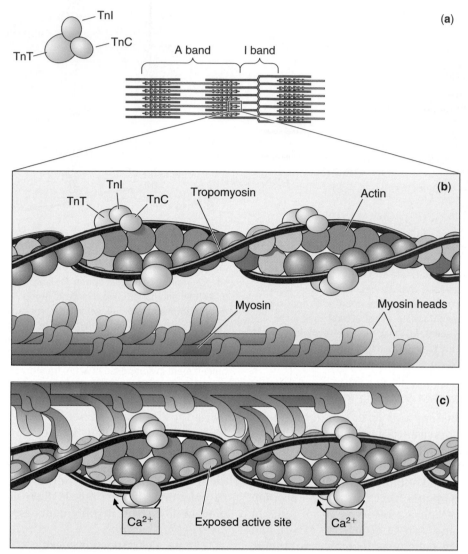

Figure 19.9
Regulatory Function of Troponin and Tropomyosin

(a) Troponin is a small globular protein with three subunits. (b) Resting condition: Tropomyosin blocks the active sites on actin, preventing actin and myosin from binding. (c) Contraction: When troponin binds with Ca^{2+}, it undergoes a configurational change and *pulls* tropomyosin from the blocking position on the actin filament, allowing myosin heads to form cross-bridges with actin.

Excitation-Contraction Coupling

Excitation-contraction coupling refers to the sequence of events by which an action potential (an electrical event) in the sarcolemma of the muscle cell initiates the sliding of the myofilaments, resulting in contraction (a mechanical event). Excitation-contraction coupling can be categorized into three phases:

1. The spread of depolarization
2. The binding of calcium to troponin
3. The generation of force

Figure 19.10 summarizes the events that occur during each phase of excitation-contraction coupling. Excitation-contraction coupling begins with depolarization and spread of an action potential (AP) along the sarcolemma (labeled 2 in Figure 19.10) and continues with the propagation of the action potential into the T tubules (labeled 2). An action potential in the T tubules causes the release of calcium from the lateral sacs of the sarcoplasmic reticulum (labeled 3).

When calcium is released from the sarcoplasmic reticulum (the second phase), it binds to the troponin molecules on the thin filament. The binding

Figure 19.10
Phases of Excitation-Contraction
Coupling

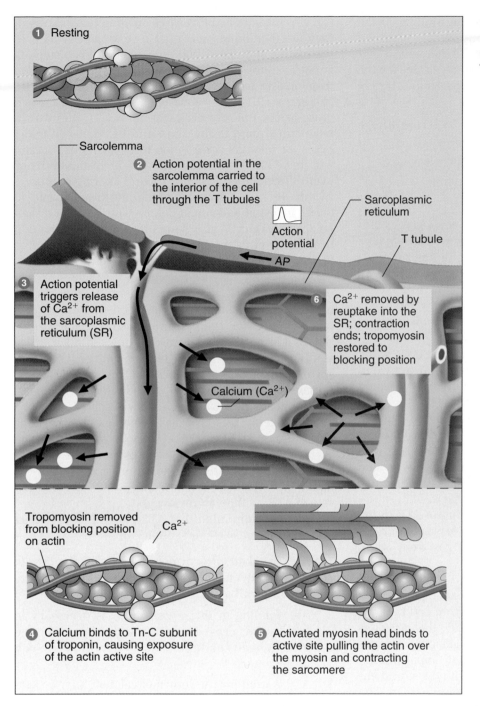

① Resting

Sarcolemma

② Action potential in the sarcolemma carried to the interior of the cell through the T tubules

Action potential

AP

Sarcoplasmic reticulum

T tubule

③ Action potential triggers release of Ca^{2+} from the sarcoplasmic reticulum (SR)

⑥ Ca^{2+} removed by reuptake into the SR; contraction ends; tropomyosin restored to blocking position

Calcium (Ca^{2+})

Tropomyosin removed from blocking position on actin

Ca^{2+}

④ Calcium binds to Tn-C subunit of troponin, causing exposure of the actin active site

⑤ Activated myosin head binds to active site pulling the actin over the myosin and contracting the sarcomere

of calcium to troponin causes troponin to undergo a configurational change, thereby removing tropomyosin from its blocking position on the actin filament (labeled 4 in the figure).

The third phase of excitation-contraction coupling is the cross-bridging cycle (labeled 5 in Figure 19.10). The **cross-bridging cycle** describes the cyclic events that are necessary for the generation of force or tension within the myosin heads during muscle contraction. The generation of tension within the

Excitation-Contraction Coupling The sequence of events by which an action potential in the sarcolemma initiates the sliding of the myofilaments, resulting in contraction.

Cross-Bridging Cycle The cyclic events that are necessary for the generation of force or tension within the myosin heads during muscle contraction.

contractile elements results from the binding of the myosin heads to actin and the subsequent release of stored energy in the myosin heads. As shown in Figure 19.11, four individual steps are necessary for the cross-bridging cycle (Berne and Levy, 1988; Marieb, 2001; Vander, et al., 2001):

1. binding of myosin heads to actin (cross-bridge formation);

2. power stroke;

3. dissociation of myosin and actin; and

4. activation of myosin heads.

The first step in the *cross-bridge cycle* is the binding of activated myosin heads (*M) with the active sites on actin, forming cross-bridges. In Figure 19.11, a centered dot ($\cdot$) is used to indicate binding, and an asterisk (*) is used to indicate activated myosin heads. Thus, A·*M indicates that the activated myosin heads are bound to actin (A), whereas A + M indicates that actin and myosin are unbound.

The second step in the cross-bridging cycle is the power stroke. It is during this step that activated myosin heads swivel from their high-energy, activated position to a low-energy configuration (M with no *). This movement of the myosin cross-bridges results in a slight displacement (sliding) of the thin filament over the thick filament toward the center of the sarcomere. As shown in Figure 19.11, during the second step ADP and P_i are released from the myosin heads, resulting in myosin bound only to actin (A·M).

The third step involves the binding of ATP to the myosin heads and the subsequent dissociation (detachment) of the myosin cross-bridges from actin, thus producing A + M·ATP.

Note the role of ATP in steps 3 and 4. It is the *binding of ATP* molecules to the myosin head, in step 3, that allows the myosin heads to detach from actin. In the fourth step *it is the breakdown of ATP* that provides the energy to activate the myosin heads (*M). The activation of the myosin head is extremely important because it provides the cross-bridges with the stored energy to move the actin during the power stroke. The breakdown of ATP at this step depends on the presence of myosin ATPase (also known as myofibrillar ATPase), as depicted in the following reaction:

$$\text{M}\cdot\text{ATP} \xrightarrow{\substack{\text{myosin} \\ \text{ATPase}}} \text{*M}\cdot\text{ADP} + P_i$$

Notice that the products of ATP hydrolysis, ADP + P_i, remain bound to the myosin heads and that the myosin is now in its high-energy or activated state.

The cross-bridging cycle will continue as long as ATP is available and calcium is bound to troponin (Tn-C), causing the active sites on actin to be exposed. On the other hand, activated myosin will remain in the resting state awaiting the next stimulus if calcium is not available in sufficient concentration to remove tropomyosin from its blocking position on actin [(4b) in Figure 19.11]. Because each cycle of the myosin cross-bridges barely displaces the actin, the myosin heads must bind to the actin and be displaced many times for a single contraction to occur. Thus, myosin will make and break its bond with actin hundreds or even thousands of times during a single muscle twitch. In order for this make-and-break cycle to occur, myosin heads must detach from actin and then be reactivated. This detaching and reactivating process requires the cycle to be repeated and requires the presence of ATP (step 3) (Vander, et al., 2001).

An analogy may be helpful for an understanding of the role of ATP in providing energy to activate the myosin head. Visualize a spring-loaded mousetrap. It takes energy to set the trap, just as it takes the splitting of ATP to set or activate the myosin head. Once set, however, the trap will release energy when it is sprung. In a similar manner, the myosin head possesses stored energy, which will be released when the myosin heads bind to actin and swivel.

Admittedly, this process is complex (and perhaps intimidating at first). Take time to go through the cycle of events presented in Figure 19.11 several times. Try paying attention to different aspects of the figure (the symbols, the wording, the diagrams, the role of ATP) with each review of it.

Also, keep in mind that ATP plays several important roles in muscle contraction.

1. ATP breakdown provides the energy to activate and reactivate the myosin cross-bridge prior to binding with actin.

2. ATP binding to the myosin head is necessary to break the cross-bridge linkage between the myosin heads and the actin so that the cycle can be repeated.

3. ATP is used for the return of calcium into the sarcoplasmic reticulum and restoration of the resting membrane potential once contraction has ended.

The final phase of muscular contraction is muscular relaxation. Relaxation occurs when the nerve impulse ceases and calcium is pumped back into the sarcoplasmic reticulum by active transport. In the absence of calcium, tropomyosin returns to its blocking position on actin, and myosin heads are not able to bind to actin. Note that although we often place considerable emphasis on muscle contraction, the ability to relax a muscle following contraction is just as important.

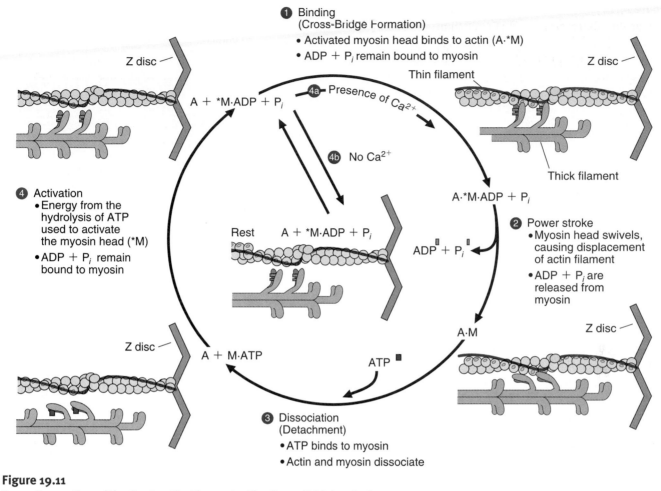

Figure 19.11
Force Generation of the Contractile Elements: The Cross-Bridging Cycle

Changes in the Sarcomere during Contraction

Much of the evidence supporting the sliding-filament theory comes from observation of changes in the length of a sarcomere during muscular contraction. Figure 19.12 provides diagrams of the sarcomere during rest (Figure 19.12a) and during contraction (Figure 19.12b). Notice the following changes in a sarcomere that result from contraction:

1. The A band does not change length, but the Z discs do move closer together. The length of the A band is preserved because the thick filament length does not change.

2. The I band shortens and may disappear. The I band shortens because the thin filaments are pulled over the thick filaments toward the center of the sarcomere. Thus, there is little or no area where the thin filaments do not overlap the thick filaments.

3. The H zone shortens and may disappear because the thin filaments are pulled over the thick filaments toward the center of the sarcomere. If the thin filament overlaps the thick filament for the entire length of the thick filament, there is no H zone.

The shortening of the sarcomere is the result of the attachment of the myosin heads with the active site on actin and the subsequent release of stored energy that swivels the myosin cross-bridges. This step causes the actin to pull the Z disc toward the center of the sarcomere, which, in turn, causes the sarcomere, and hence the muscle fiber, length to decrease.

All-or-None Principle

According to the **all-or-none principle,** when a motor neuron is stimulated, all of the muscle fibers in that

---

All-or-None Principle When a motor neuron is stimulated, all of the muscle fibers in that motor unit contract to their fullest extent or they do not contract at all.

Figure 19.12

Changes in a Sarcomere during Contraction

(a) Sarcomere at rest. (b) During contraction of the sarcomere, the lengths of actin and myosin filaments are unchanged. Sarcomere shortens because actin slides over myosin, pulling Z discs toward the center of the sarcomere. The H zone disappears, the I band shortens, and the A band remains unchanged.

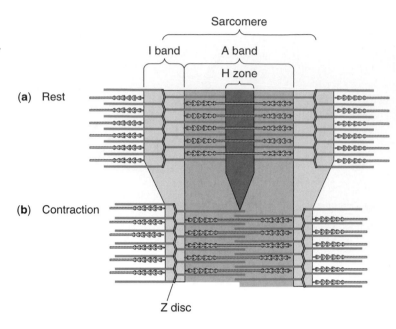

(a) Rest

(b) Contraction

motor unit contract to their fullest extent or they do not contract at all. The minimal amount of stimuli necessary to initiate that contraction is referred to as the *threshold stimulus;* that is, if the threshold of contraction is reached, a muscle fiber will contract to its fullest extent. This phenomenon is related to the electrical properties of the cell membrane and refers to the contractile properties of a motor unit or a single muscle fiber only, not to the entire muscle.

To better understand this principle, consider the analogy of turning on a light switch. If sufficient pressure is applied to the switch (to reach a threshold for flipping it on), the lights will be turned on to their fullest extent. Expanding the analogy to a motor unit, when you turn on a light switch that controls a group of lights (such as the overhead lights in a classroom), all of the lights connected to it will turn on to their fullest extent. You cannot cause the lights to be brighter by pulling (or pushing) the light switch harder. It is an all-or-none response. Either you produce enough force to turn the lights on, or you do not. The same is true for an individual muscle fiber or a motor unit: Either a threshold stimulus is reached and contraction occurs, or a threshold stimulus is not reached and contraction does not occur.

Muscle Fiber Types

Muscle fibers are typically described by two characteristics: their contractile, or twitch, properties and their metabolic properties (Figure 19.13).

Contractile (Twitch) Properties

On the basis of differences in *contractile (twitch) properties,* human muscle fibers can be divided into two types, *slow-twitch (ST)* and *fast-twitch (FT) fibers.* Slow-twitch fibers are sometimes called Type I fibers; fast-twitch fibers are correspondingly called Type II fibers. The difference between ST and FT fibers appears to be almost absolute—like the difference between black and white. Some FT fibers contract and relax slightly faster than other fast-twitch fibers, but both of them are clearly much faster than ST fibers. To understand the difference between twitch speeds, we must consider the integration of muscles and nerves.

Skeletal muscle fibers are innervated by alpha (α) motor neurons, which are subdivided into two categories, α_1 and α_2. The α_1 motor neurons innervate FT fibers, and the α_2 motor neurons innervate ST fibers. Figure 19.14 shows an experiment in which the innervation of muscle fibers was manipulated: The α_1 motor neuron was severed from the FT fibers and connected to the ST fibers, and the α_2 motor neuron was cut from the ST fibers and connected to the FT fibers. What conclusion can we draw from this diagram regarding why a muscle fiber is either ST or FT? Because the ST fiber became an FT fiber when the α_1 motor neuron replaced the α_2 motor neuron and vice versa, it is logical to conclude that the contractile property of muscle depends on the type of motor neuron that innervates the muscle fiber (Noth, 1992).

What cannot be seen from the experiment is that other elements in the muscle, especially the contractile enzyme myosin ATPase, also contribute to the variation in twitch speed (Van deGraaff and Fox,

Muscle Fibers			
Twitch properties	Slow	Fast	
Metabolic properties	Oxidative	Oxidative/ glycolytic	Glycolytic
Name based on twitch and metabolic properties	SO	FOG	FG
Other nomenclature	ST, Type I	FTa, FTA, Type IIA	FTb, FTB, Type IIB
Motor Neurons			
Neuron type	α_2	α_1	α_1
Neuron size	Small	Large	Large
Conduction velocity	Slow	Fast	Fast
Recruitment threshold	Low	High	High

Figure 19.13
Properties of Motor Units

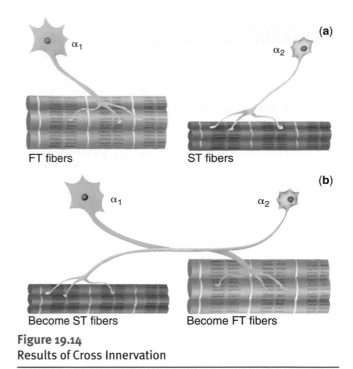

Figure 19.14
Results of Cross Innervation

(a) Under normal conditions α_1 motor neurons innervate FT fibers and α_2 motor neurons innervate ST fibers. (b) If the neurons supplying the muscles are switched (cross-innervated), the muscle fibers acquire the properties of the new motor neuron.

1989). Indeed, when muscle fibers are typed, it is often the amount of stain for myosin ATPase that is used to distinguish twitch speed, since the motor neurons are not typically biopsied. Note that α_2 motor neurons are the smaller of the two nerves and innervate the ST muscle fibers; the α_1 motor neurons are the larger nerves and innervate the FT muscle fibers. The size difference is important because small motor neurons have low excitation thresholds and slow conduction velocities and are thus recruited at low workloads. In contrast, larger motor neurons have a higher excitation threshold and are not recruited until very high force output is needed. Thus, motor neurons are recruited according to the *size principle*. Smaller motor units (α_2 motor neurons innervating ST fibers) are recruited during activities that require low force output (i.e., maintaining posture). As the need for force production increases (e.g., lifting heavy weights), larger motor units (α_1 motor neurons innervating FT fibers) are recruited.

Metabolic Properties

On the basis of differences in *metabolic properties,* human muscle fibers can be described as *glycolytic, oxidative,* or a combination of both, *oxidative/ glycolytic.* All muscle fibers can produce energy both anaerobically (that is, without oxygen, labeled as glycolytic) and aerobically (that is, with oxygen, labeled as oxidative). These processes and terms are fully explained in the unit on metabolism.

Despite the ability of all muscle fibers to produce energy by both glycolytic and oxidative processes, one or the other may predominate or the production may be balanced. Thus, the metabolic properties of muscle fibers do not represent discrete entities as much as a continuum (oxidative to glycolytic), or shades of gray, as opposed to the black-and-white type of dichotomy seen for twitch speed (slow or fast twitch). The metabolic properties are determined by staining for key enzymes in the muscle specimen [often phosphofructokinase (PFK) for glycolytic processes and succinate dehydrogenase (SDH) for oxidative processes] (Saltin, et al., 1977).

Integrated Nomenclature

Slow-twitch fibers rely primarily on oxidative metabolism to produce energy and are therefore referred to as **slow oxidative (SO) fibers.** Fast-twitch fibers that have the ability to work under both oxidative and

> **Slow Oxidative (SO) Fibers** Slow-twitch muscle fibers that rely primarily on oxidative metabolism to produce energy.

Focus on Research

Does Fiber-Type Distribution Affect Maximal Oxygen Uptake?

Bergh, U., A. Thorstensson, B. Sjodin, B. Hulten, K. Piehl, & J. Karlsson: Maximal oxygen uptake and muscle fiber types in trained and untrained humans. *Medicine and Science in Sports and Exercise.* 10(3):151–154 (1978).

Researchers have long been interested in the fiber type distribution of athletes. At the time that Bergh and colleagues undertook this study, researchers knew that aerobically trained individuals were characterized by a high percentage of ST fibers (and hence a lower percentage of FT fibers), and that anaerobically trained individuals (e.g., sprinters) were more likely to have a high percentage of FT fibers. Researchers also knew that aerobic training was associated with a high $\dot{V}O_2$max. $\dot{V}O_2$max is the greatest amount of oxygen an individual can take in and transport and use during strenuous work; it is considered the best measure of an individual's aerobic (or cardiovascular) fitness. Thus, Bergh and colleagues proposed that there would be a relationship between the percentage of slow-twitch fibers and a person's $\dot{V}O_2$max. The results, in the graph, support their hypothesis.

There are two important points that you should take from these data:

1. There is a strong linear relationship between $\dot{V}O_2$max and %ST fibers. This makes sense because the ST fibers have the greatest oxidative ability, that is, the ability to use oxygen to produce large amounts of ATP to support long-duration activities.
2. At any given %ST (above approximately 40%), an athlete has a greater $\dot{V}O_2$max than does a nonathlete. This is consistent with what we know about the trainability of muscle fibers. Endurance training increases the oxidative capacity of muscle, thereby allowing the muscle to use more oxygen and thus achieve a higher $\dot{V}O_2$max.

In addition to the specific points above, this research also reinforces the tremendous amount of interaction among the various systems of the body.

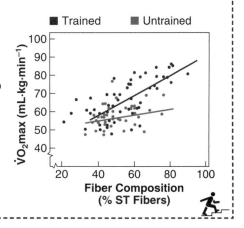

---

glycolytic conditions are called **fast oxidative glycolytic (FOG) fibers.** These fibers are also referred to as fast-twitch A (FTa, FTA, or Type IIA) fibers. Other fast-twitch fibers that perform predominantly under glycolytic conditions are called **fast glycolytic (FG) fibers.** These fibers are also called fast-twitch B (FTb, FTB, or Type IIB) fibers. A third type of fast-twitch fiber (between FTa and FTb, called unclassified, undifferentiated, Type IIC, or FTc) appears to represent a small percentage of total muscle fibers primarily in infants. By the end of the first year of life these Type IIC fibers have largely become differentiated, and by age 6 a normal adult pattern has been established (Baldwin, 1984). Figure 19.13 and Table 19.2 summarize the properties of motor units and muscle fibers (Harris and Dudley, 2000).

A **motor unit** is defined as a motor neuron (α_1 or α_2) and the muscle fibers it innervates. As we have just seen, the twitch speed of a muscle fiber depends largely on the motor neuron that innervates it. Thus, all muscle fibers within a motor unit will be either FT or ST. In addition, because all muscle fibers in a motor unit are recruited to contract together, they will require the same metabolic capabilities as well. Therefore, a motor unit is composed exclusively of SO, FOG, or FG muscle fibers. Thus, when reference is made to muscle fiber types, it also means motor unit types.

Table 19.2 further compares the different muscle fiber types in reference to important structural, neural, functional, and metabolic characteristics (Harris and Dudley, 2000). As the table indicates, the diameters of the individual muscle fibers differ between ST and FT fibers. The size of the muscle fiber is related to the size of the nerve fiber innervating it but primarily reflects the amount of contractile proteins within the muscle cell. ST fibers are smaller than FT fibers and have smaller motor neurons. The larger size of the FT fibers

---

> **Fast Oxidative Glycolytic (FOG) Fibers** Fast-twitch muscle fibers that have the ability to work under oxidative and glycolytic conditions.
>
> **Fast Glycolytic (FG) Fibers** Fast-twitch muscle fibers that perform primarily under glycolytic conditions.
>
> **Motor Unit** A motor neuron and the muscle fibers it innervates.

Table 19.2
Characteristics of Muscle Fibers

	Type I	Type II	
	ST	FTa	FTb
Contractile (Twitch):	ST	FTa	FTb
Metabolic:	SO	FOG	FG
Structural Aspects			
Muscle fiber diameter	Small	Intermediate	Large
Mitochondrial density	High	Intermediate	Low
Capillary density	High	Intermediate	Low
Myoglobin content	High	Intermediate	Low
Functional Aspects			
Twitch (contraction) time	Slow	Fast	Fast
Relaxation time	Slow	Fast	Fast
Force production	Low	Intermediate	High
Fatigability	Low	Intermediate	High
Metabolic Aspects			
Phosphocreatine stores	Low	High	High
Glycogen stores	Low	High	High
Triglyceride stores	High	Intermediate	Low
Myosin-ATPase activity	Low	High	High
Glycolytic enzyme activity	Low	High	High
Oxidative enzyme activity	High	Intermediate	Low

is the result of their having more contractile proteins, which, in turn, enables them to produce greater force. Figure 19.15 indicates differences in force production, twitch speed, and fatigue curves for the three types of muscle fibers (Edington and Edgerton, 1986).

Other structural differences exist between fiber types that can be related directly to their predominant metabolic pathway for energy production. The SO fibers, which rely mainly on oxidative pathways for energy production, have a high number of mitochondria, high capillary density, high myoglobin content, and high oxidative enzyme activity. The FG fibers, which rely primarily on glycolytic pathways for energy production, have few mitochondria, low capillary density, low myoglobin content, and high glycolytic enzyme activity. The FOG fibers possess not only characteristics common to both SO and FG but also characteristics unique to themselves. Specifically, the FOG fibers have intermediate mitochondrial density, capillary density, myoglobin content and oxidative enzyme activity, and high PC stores, glycogen stores, and glycolytic enzyme activity.

The metabolic differences among muscle fibers both require and reflect differences in energy substrate availability. All muscles store and utilize glycogen; but since glycogen is the only substrate (along with its constituent parts—glucose) that can be used

to fuel glycolysis, it makes sense that the FOG and FG fibers would have higher glycogen stores than SO fibers have. Conversely, since triglycerides can only be broken down and used oxidatively, it would be anticipated that SO fibers would have more triglyceride storage than either FG or FOG fibers. Furthermore, FOG fibers would have an intermediate amount of triglycerides—more than FG but less than SO fibers.

Because SO fibers are so well supplied by the cardiovascular system and have ample fuel supplies (that is, energy substrate), particularly from triglycerides, they are very resistant to fatigue. Because the FOG fibers have a substantial oxidative capability and the FG fibers do not, the FG fibers are the quickest to fatigue. The FOG fibers are somewhat less resistant to fatigue than the SO fibers and somewhat more resistant to fatigue than the FG fibers.

Table 19.2 is a convenient way to make logical sense of all of this information and to check your understanding of the characteristics of each fiber type. Take a few minutes now to study this table and interrelate all of the information. Remember that although the fiber types have been labeled at the top of the columns separately for their contractile and metabolic properties, in practice the designations ST and SO, FTa and FOG, FTb and FG are used interchangeably.

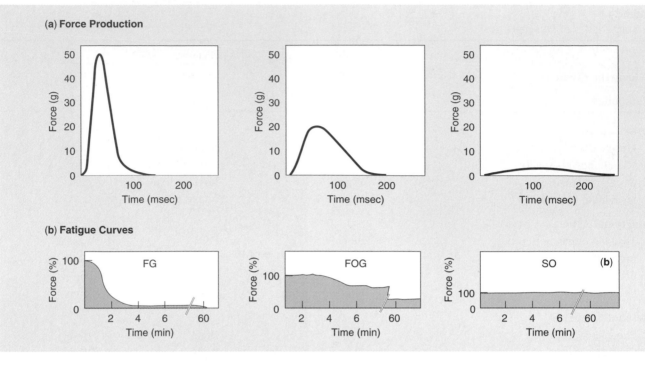

Figure 19.15
Force Production and Fatigue Curves of Fiber Types

Source: Adapted from Edington & Edgerton (1986).

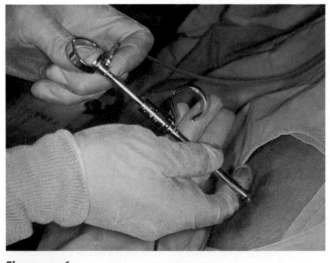

Figure 19.16
Muscle Biopsy

Assessment of Muscle Fiber Type

Muscle fiber type is typically determined by an invasive procedure that involves collecting a small sample of skeletal muscle by a needle biopsy (Figure 19.16). Muscle biopsies are most commonly obtained from the gastrocnemius, vastus lateralis, or deltoid muscles. Prior to the collection of the muscle sample, the skin is thoroughly cleaned and a topical anesthetic is applied to numb the area. A small incision is made through the skin, subcutaneous tissue, and fascia. The biopsy needle is then inserted into the belly of the muscle to extract a small amount of skeletal muscle tissue (approximately 20–40 mg). The small sample of muscle is then frozen in liquid nitrogen and sliced into very thin cross-sections. The cross-sections are then chemically stained so that the muscle fibers can be differentiated into categories. Muscle samples may be stained for the enzyme myosin ATPase and for glycolytic and oxidative enzymes. When the stained muscle fibers are viewed in cross-section under a microscope, the muscle fiber types appear a different color. Figure 19.17 is an example of skeletal muscle that has been histochemically stained, revealing ST and FT fibers. Notice that the different fiber types are intermingled, revealing a mosaic pattern. Counting the number of fibers of each category and dividing by the total number of fibers seen will indicate a percentage of each fiber type (see Question of Understanding box). In addition to counting the number of fibers and expressing them as a percentage, researchers often measure the diameter of the muscle fibers.

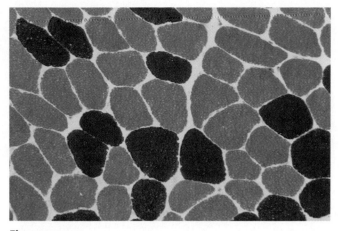

Figure 19.17
Mosaic Pattern of FT and ST Muscle Fibers

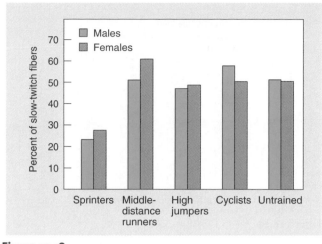

Figure 19.18
Fiber Type Distribution among Athletes

Source: Data from Fox et al. (1993).

Muscle fibers also can be typed noninvasively by nuclear magnetic resonance spectroscopy (NMR), but this is still an expensive, little-used laboratory technique (Boicelli, et al., 1989). Attempts to use the vertical jump as a field measure of fiber type have proven unsuccessful (Costill, 1978).

Knowledge about fiber types is important for at least three reasons.

1. Fiber type differences help explain individual differences in performance and response to training.

2. Fiber type differences help explain what training can and cannot do.

3. The relationship between fiber types, training, and performance in elite athletes helps in the design of training programs for others who wish to be successful in specific events even if they do not know their exact fiber type percentages or distribution.

Distribution of Fiber Types

All of the muscles of the human body are composed of a combination of slow-twitch and fast-twitch muscle fibers arranged in a mosaic pattern. This arrangement is thought to reflect the variety of tasks that human muscles must perform. The relative distribution, or percentage, of these fibers, however, may vary greatly from one muscle to another. For example, the soleus muscle may have as much as 85% ST fibers, and the triceps and ocular muscles may have as few as 30% ST fibers. The distribution may also vary considerably from one individual to another for the same muscle group (Saltin, et al., 1977). In general, the following statements describe the distribution of fiber types.

1. Although distribution of fiber type varies within and between individuals, most individuals possess between 45% and 55% ST fibers.

2. The distribution of fiber types is not different for males and females, although males tend to show greater extremes or variation than females.

3. After early childhood the fiber distribution does not change significantly as a function of age.

4. Fiber type distribution is primarily genetically determined.

5. Muscles that are involved in sustained postural activity have the highest number of slow-twitch muscle fibers.

Fiber Type in Athletes

Few topics have caused as much interest and debate as the topic of fiber type in athletes. Figure 19.18 shows the distribution of fiber types for male and female athletes. Athletes involved in endurance activi-

---

A Question of Understanding

Fiber typing involves determining the percentage of fibers within a sample that are fast twitch or slow twitch. Count how many total fibers are visible in Figure 19.17. Now count how many of those fibers are darkly stained (indicating, in this example, that they are ST fibers). Based on these two numbers, what is the percentage of ST fibers in this muscle sample? What is the percentage of FT fibers in this sample? Check your answer in Appendix D.

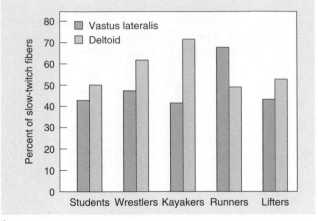

Figure 19.19
Fiber Type Distribution of Different Muscle Groups Among Athletes

Source: Tesch & Karlsson (1985).

ties typically have a higher percentage of slow-twitch fibers; athletes involved in power activities have a higher percentage of fast-twitch muscle fibers. There is, however, a large range of fiber type in each group, indicating that athletic success is not determined solely by fiber type.

Not only do endurance athletes differ in general fiber type from power or resistance athletes, but often these differences are site-specific within athletic groups. The results of one study of fiber type distribution are reported in Figure 19.19 (Tesch and Karlsson, 1985). According to the study, the vastus lateralis muscles of the legs possess a greater percentage of ST fibers in endurance athletes who rely heavily upon the legs for their activity (such as runners). In contrast, athletes whose sport requires endurance of the upper body possess a greater percentage of ST fibers in the deltoid muscle.

An interesting question arises when looking at the fiber type distribution of various athletes: Did training for and participating in a given sport influence the fiber type, or did fiber type influence the type of athletic participation? Available evidence indicates that the distribution of fiber types based on contractile properties (ST or FT) is genetically determined and is not altered in humans by exercise training (Kraemer, 2000; Saltin, et al., 1977; Williams, 1994). There is evidence, however, that training can alter the metabolic properties of the cell (enzyme concentration, substrate storage, and so on). These changes may lead to a conversion of FT fiber subdivisions. Indeed, with

endurance training the oxidative potential of FOG and FG fibers can exceed that of SO fibers of sedentary individuals (Saltin, et al., 1977).

In summary, the distribution of fiber types varies considerably within the muscle groups of an individual and between individuals. The basic distribution of fiber type appears to be genetically determined. Training may alter the metabolic capabilities of muscle fibers (but not the contractile properties), and there remains the possibility that this alteration could be significant enough to change the classification of the FT fibers.

Summary

1. Skeletal muscles provide for locomotion and manipulation, maintain body posture, and play an important role in heat generation.

2. The characteristics that allow a muscle to produce movement include irritability, contractility, extensibility, and elasticity.

IP *Muscular–Contraction of Motor Units* (pages 1–11)*

3. A motor neuron and the muscle fibers it innervates is called a motor unit. Because each muscle fiber in a motor unit is connected to the same neuron, the electrical activity in the motor neuron controls the contractile activity of all the muscle fibers in a given motor unit.

4. Skeletal muscle fibers are bundled together into groups of fibers called fasciculi. A muscle fiber is itself comprised of smaller units called myofibrils, which are, in turn, made up of myofilaments.

IP *Muscular–Anatomy Review: Skeletal Muscle Tissue* (pages 1–13); *Muscular–Sliding Filament Theory* (pages 1–12)

5. There are two types of myofilaments: thick and thin filaments. It is the repeating pattern of these myofilaments along the length of the myofibril that gives skeletal muscle its striated appearance.

6. Each repeating unit is referred to as a sarcomere and represents the functional unit of the muscle.

7. Tropomyosin is a regulatory protein that serves to block the active site on actin, thereby inhibiting actin and myosin from binding under resting conditions. The position of tropomyosin is controlled by troponin.

IP *Muscular–Sliding Filament Theory* (pages 13–16)*

8. Excitation-contraction coupling refers to the sequence of events by which an action potential in the sarcolemma initiates the contractile process of the myofilaments.

9. Excitation-contraction coupling has three phases: the spread of depolarization, the binding of calcium to troponin, the generation of force. The cross-bridging cycle describes the generation of force. This cycle consists of the binding of myosin to actin, the powerstroke, the dissociation of myosin and actin, and the activation of myosin heads.

10. The spread of depolarization (action potential) is carried into the interior of the muscle fiber by the T tubules. As the electrical signal is carried into the cell, it causes the release of calcium, which is stored in the lateral sacs of the sarcoplasmic reticulum.

11. When calcium is released from the sarcoplasmic reticulum, it binds to the troponin molecules, which undergo a configuration change, thereby removing tropomyosin from its blocking position on the actin filament. This removal of tropomyosin allows the myosin cross-bridges (heads) to bind with the actin filaments.

IP *Muscular–Sliding Filament Theory* (pages 13– 16)*

12. The generation of tension within the contractile elements results from the binding of actin and myosin, which causes the release of stored energy in the myosin heads.

IP *Muscular–Sliding Filament Theory* (pages 18– 27)*

13. ATP plays several important roles in muscle contraction. The hydrolysis of ATP provides the energy to activate or reactivate the myosin head prior to binding with actin. ATP binding is also necessary to break the linkage between the myosin cross-bridge and actin so that the cycle can be repeated. ATP is also used to return calcium to the sarcoplasmic reticulum and to restore the resting membrane potential.

IP *Muscular–Sliding Filament Theory* (pages 21–25; 29)*; *Muscular–Muscle Metabolism* (pages 1–8)

14. During relaxation, calcium is pumped back into the sarcoplasmic reticulum (by active transport), and troponin no longer keeps tropomyosin from its blocking position.

15. When a muscle fiber or motor unit is stimulated to contract, it contracts to its fullest extent, or it does not contract at all. This response is referred to as the all-or-none principle.

IP *Muscular–Muscle Metabolism* (pages 24–28)

16. Human muscle fibers can be divided into two different types, ST and FT, on the basis of contractile properties. The FT fibers can be further subdivided into FOG and FG fibers on the basis of metabolic properties.

17. Athletes involved in endurance activities typically have a higher percentage of slow-twitch fibers. Athletes involved in power activities typically have a higher percentage of fast-twitch muscle fibers.

IP *Muscular–Muscle Metabolism* (page 29)

18. Training may alter the metabolic capabilities of muscle fibers (but not the contractile properties), and there remains the possibility that this alteration could be significant enough to change the classification of the FT fibers.

This topic is available on the InterActive Physiology® Sampler CD that comes with the purchase of a new copy of this book.

Review Questions

1. List, in order of largest to smallest, the major components of the whole muscle.

2. What causes the striated appearance of skeletal muscle fibers?

3. What are the T tubules and the sarcoplasmic reticulum? What is the function of each?

4. Relate each region of the sarcomere to the presence of thick and thin myofilaments.

5. Diagram a sarcomere at rest and at the end of a contraction, and identify each of the areas.

6. Describe the role of the regulatory proteins in controlling muscle contraction.

7. Describe the sequence of events in excitation-contraction coupling.

8. Identify the role of ATP in the production of force within the contractile unit of muscle.

9. What is the role of calcium in muscle contraction?

10. Describe the all-or-none principle as it relates to the contraction of a single muscle fiber.

11. Diagram the force production, twitch speed, and fatigue curve for the different fiber types.

12. Discuss the possibility of influencing fiber type distribution by exercise training.

For further review and additional study tools, go to The Physiology Place (www.physiologyplace.com) and the Student Study Guide for Exercise Physiology for Health, Fitness, and Performance *by Sharon A. Plowman and Denise L. Smith.*

Passport to the Internet

Visit the following Internet sites to explore further topics and issues related to the skeletal muscle system. To visit an organization's web site, go to www.physiologyplace.com and click on "Passport to the Internet."

The Nicholas Institute of Sports Medicine and Athletic Trauma (NISMAT) The Nicholas Institute of Sports Medicine and Athletic Trauma (NISMAT) is the first hospital-based facility dedicated to the study of sports medicine in the United States. This site has various resources related to cardiovascular and muscular issues.

Physical Therapy Central This web site offers a resource for physical therapists that can serve as a wonderful study tool for related fields as well. Look under the "Online University" for a connection to the Hosford Muscle Tables. Here you'll find detailed information about the skeletal muscles of the human body, including the identification of each muscle's origin, insertion, action, blood supply, and innervation.

HomeExerciseProgram.com This site is dedicated to helping individuals strengthen and condition back muscles.

Inner Learning Online This interactive web site contains an inner exploration of the human anatomy. Each topic has animations, graphics, and numerous descriptive links.

The Visible Human Project® The Visible Human Project® is the creation of complete, anatomically detailed three-dimensional representations of the normal male and female human bodies. Explore this site and identify the long-term goal of the project and how to access some of the findings.

References

Baldwin, K. M.: Muscle development: Neonatal to adult. In R. L. Terjung (ed.), *Exercise and Sport Sciences Reviews.* Baltimore: Williams & Wilkins. 12:1–19 (1984).

Berne, R. B., & M. N. Levy: *Physiology.* St. Louis: Mosby, 315–342 (1988).

Billeter, R., & H. Hoppler: Muscular basis of strength. In P. V. Komi (ed.), *Strength and Power in Sport.* Oxford: Blackwell Scientific, 39–63 (1992).

Boicelli, C. A., A. M. Baldassarri, C. Borsetto, & F. Conconi: An approach to noninvasive fiber type distribution by nuclear magnetic resonance. *International Journal of Sports Medicine.* 10:53–54 (1989).

Costill, D. L.: *Inside Running: Basics of Sports Physiology.* Indianapolis: Benchmark Press, 1–29 (1986).

Costill, D. L.: Muscle biopsy research: Application of fiber composition to swimming. *Proceedings from Annual Clinic of American Swimming Coaches Association, Chicago.* Ft. Lauderdale: American Swimming Coaches Association (1978).

Edington, D. W., & V. R. Edgerton: *The Biology of Physical Activity.* Boston: Houghton Mifflin (1986).

Fox, E. L., R. W. Bowers, & M. L. Foss: *The Physiological Basis for Exercise and Sport.* Dubuque, IA: Brown & Benchmark, 94–135 (1993).

Fox, S.: *Human Physiology.* Dubuque, IA: Brown (1987).

Harris, R. T., & G. Dudley: Neuromuscular anatomy and physiology. In T. R. Baechle & R. W. Earle (eds.), *Essentials of Strength and Conditioning.* Champaign, IL: Human Kinetics, 15–23 (2000).

Hunter, G. R.: Muscle physiology. In T. R. Baechle & R. W. Earle (eds.), *Essentials of Strength Training and Conditioning.* Champaign, IL: Human Kinetics, 3–13 (2000).

Kraemer, W. J.: Physiological adaptations to anaerobic and aerobic training programs. In T. R. Baechle & R. W. Earle (eds.), *Essentials of Strength Training and Conditioning.* Champaign, IL: Human Kinetics, 137–168 (2000).

Marieb, E.: *Human Anatomy and Physiology* (5th edition). Redwood City, CA: Benjamin Cummings (2001).

Noth, J.: Motor units. In P. V. Komi (ed.), *Strength and Power in Sport.* Oxford: Blackwell Scientific, 21–28 (1992).

Rasmussen, B. B., K. D. Tipton, S. L. Miller, S. E. Wolf, & R. R. Wolfe: An oral essential amino acid-carbohydrate supplement enhances muscle protein anabolism after resistance exercise. *Journal of Applied Physiology.* 88:386–392 (2000).

Saltin, B., J. Henriksson, E. Nygaard, P. Anderson, & E. Jansson: Fiber types and metabolic potentials of skeletal muscles in sedentary man and endurance runners. *Annals of the New York Academy of Sciences.* 301:3–29 (1977).

Tesch, P. A., & J. Karlsson: Muscle fiber types and size in trained and untrained muscles of elite athletes. *Journal of Applied Physiology.* 59:1716–1720 (1985).

Van deGraaff, K. M., & S. I. Fox: *Concepts of Human Anatomy and Physiology* (2nd edition). Dubuque, IA: Brown, 291–355 (1989).

Vander, A. J., J. H. Sherman, & D. S. Luciano: *Human Physiology: The Mechanisms of Body Function* (8th edition). New York: McGraw-Hill (2001).

Williams, J.: Normal musculoskeletal and neuromuscular anatomy, physiology, and responses to training. In S. M. Hasson, *Clinical Exercise Physiology.* St. Louis: Mosby-Year Book Publishers (1994).

Chapter 20

Muscular Contraction
and Movement

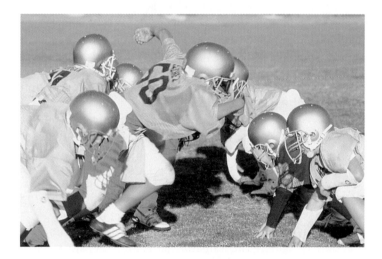

After studying the chapter, you should be able to

- Differentiate between force and load.

- Identify the different types of muscle contraction, and indicate the proper use of the terms to describe muscle fiber contraction or whole-muscle contraction.

- Compare and contrast concentric and eccentric dynamic contractions.

- Describe neural and mechanical factors that affect force development.

- Differentiate between the length-tension relationship as it applies to a muscle fiber and as it applies to a whole muscle.

- Identify possible causes of muscle fatigue, and indicate the most probable cause of muscle fatigue for various types of activity.

- Outline the two primary models that explain delayed-onset muscle soreness, and discuss a possible integration of these two models.

- Refute the popular belief that delayed-onset muscle soreness is caused by an accumulation of lactic acid in the muscle.

- Identify the different laboratory and field methods for assessing muscular function.

- Describe the basic pattern of strength development.

- Compare and contrast the expression of strength in males and in females.

- Describe the factors that affect age-related loss of muscular strength.

- Discuss the heritability of muscle function.

Exercise—The Result of Muscle Contraction

Taber's Cyclopedia Medical Dictionary defines *exercise* as "performed activity of the muscles" (Thomas, 1989). In other words, the contraction of muscles is exercise. Therefore, it is impossible to discuss the exercise response of the neuromuscular system in the same way that it is discussed for the cardiovascular-respiratory or metabolic systems.

Nonetheless, there are enough differences in the contraction of muscles that an endless number of exercises result. For example, imagine a basketball player taking off from the foul line for a slam dunk, a bodybuilder flexing in a pose, a swimmer slicing through the water doing a front crawl stroke, the movement of your eyes across the pages of this book. All of these activities require different muscle actions—explosive dynamic power; controlled static activity; force against a resistance through a large range of motion; highly coordinated, rapid, but minimal force movement. In fact, the list of individual actions involving muscle contractions is practically endless; yet some generalities are apparent, and hence, some classifications can be made. But first, some terms must be clarified.

Tension versus Load

The force developed when a contracting muscle acts on an object is called **muscle tension.** The force exerted on the muscle by the object is called the **load.** The load and muscle tension are opposing forces.

Muscle Tension Force developed when a contracting muscle acts on an object.

Load Force exerted on the muscle.

Contraction Initiation of tension-producing process of the contractile elements within muscle.

Torque The capability of a force to produce rotation of a limb around a joint.

Isotonic Contraction A muscle fiber contraction in which the tension generated by the muscle fiber is constant through the range of motion.

Dynamic Contraction A muscle contraction in which the force exerted varies as the muscle shortens to accommodate change in muscle length and/or joint angle throughout the range of motion while moving a constant external load.

The term **contraction** refers to the initiation of the tension-producing process of the contractile elements within muscle. However, not all contractions produce movement; movement depends on the magnitude of the load exerted and the tension produced by the muscle. In order for a muscle to move a load, the force of muscle tension must exceed the force of the load. Furthermore, muscle tension developed experimentally in an isolated muscle fiber, a motor unit, or even a whole muscle is not necessarily the same as the force developed by an intact muscle in the human body.

All human motion involves rotation of body segments about their joint axes. The capability of a force to produce rotation is referred to as **torque** (Enoka, 1988). Thus, torque is force applied at some distance away from the center of the joint, causing the limb to rotate around the joint. Torque changes as a muscle moves bone through the range of motion.

Classification of Muscle Contractions

A classification of muscle contractions is presented in Table 20.1. This classification is based on three component characteristics: time (as duration and/or velocity), displacement (length change), and force production. As you read this section, consult Table 20.1, and pay careful attention to whether a contraction is being described in an isolated muscle fiber/motor unit or in intact, whole muscles.

As shown in Table 20.1, at the muscle fiber or motor unit level three basic types of contraction are possible: isotonic, isokinetic, and isometric. At the whole muscle level, contractions may be defined as dynamic, isokinematic, or static. The following section describes contractions in a muscle fiber and the corresponding contraction in an intact muscle.

An **isotonic contraction** is a muscle fiber contraction in which the tension generated by the muscle fiber is constant throughout the range of motion. The name *isotonic contraction* indicates that the force production (or tonus) is unchanged (*iso* means "same") when the muscle fiber contracts, causing movement of an external load. In the intact human system such a contraction is practically impossible. What happens in intact whole muscle is that the muscle force varies as the muscle contracts. This variation is necessary to accommodate changes in muscle length and/or joint angles as limbs move through their ranges of motion. Thus, the load is constant, but the force produced to move it through the range of motion is not. Therefore, the term *dynamic,* or *isotorque,* is more accurate to describe contraction within the intact human.

A **dynamic contraction** is a whole muscle contraction that produces movement of the skeleton. If

Table 20.1
Classification of Contractions

Type of Contraction		External Work in Intact Muscle in Humans	Function of Contraction
Muscle Fiber or Motor Unit	**Intact Muscle in Humans**		
Isotonic: constant-force production: shortening, or lengthening	**Dynamic concentric (isotorque):** muscle force varies as muscle shortens to accommodate change in muscle length and/or joint angles as limb moves through ROM while moving a constant external load	Positive: (work = force × distance); external load can be overcome	Acceleration
	Dynamic eccentric: see above, except muscle lengthens	(work = force × negative distance); external load assists lengthening	Deceleration
Isokinetic: constant velocity of lengthening or shortening	**Isokinematic (dynamic):** rate of limb displacement or joint rotation is constant. Velocity varies with joint angle.	Positive or negative: see above	Acceleration or deceleration
Isometric: constant muscle length	**Static:** limb displacement or joint rotation does not occur; little muscle fiber shortening occurs	Zero: (work = force × distance, where distance = 0); external load cannot be overcome	Fixation

Note: ROM = range of motion.
Source: Komi (1984); Williams (1994).

the movement results from a dynamic muscle contraction that produces tension during shortening, it is a **concentric contraction.** Concentric contractions result in positive external work and are primarily responsible for acceleration in movement. The lifting action of the biceps in curling a barbell is an example of a concentric dynamic contraction. The discussion in Chapter 19 of the sliding-filament theory describes this type of contraction.

If movement occurs as a result of a dynamic muscle contraction that produces tension while lengthening, the contraction is referred to as an **eccentric contraction.** Eccentric contractions result in negative work and are primarily responsible for deceleration in movement. The lowering action of the biceps in curling a barbell is an example of an eccentric dynamic contraction. During an eccentric contraction, the cross-bridges are cycling as the filaments are being pulled apart. Because of this action of being pulled apart, strenuous eccentric activities can cause damage to myofibrils. Strenuous eccentric contractions also allow for a greater force of contraction at a lower energy cost than do concentric contractions (Stauber, 1989).

Why can an eccentric contraction produce more force than a concentric one? During a concentric contraction, only about half of the available cross-bridges cycle. During an eccentric contraction, some of the cross-bridges do not cycle but are continually pulled backward. Because the cross-bridges are pulled backward, the myosin heads do not rotate forward, and the actin and myosin remain bound (Stauber, 1989). As the contraction continues, additional cross-bridges are formed in an amount that may exceed the number of cross-bridges in a concentric contraction. Hence, more tension can be produced.

Why does eccentric (negative) work have a lower energy cost than concentric (positive) work? The answer to this question is not completely known, but two possibilities have been suggested (Stauber, 1989). First, fewer muscle fibers are recruited during eccentric than during concentric contractions; fewer fibers use less oxygen, which translates to a smaller energy cost. Second, because some of the cross-bridges do not cycle, less ATP is broken down and used as energy. Researchers estimate that positive work uses three to nine times more energy than negative work. All you have to do is think about climbing up the stairs in a high-rise building and then think about walking down them to believe this estimate.

Concentric Contraction A dynamic muscle contraction that produces tension during shortening.

Eccentric Contraction A dynamic muscle contraction that produces tension (force) while lengthening.

An **isokinetic contraction** is a muscle fiber contraction in which the velocity of contraction is kept constant. Isokinetic contractions are also dynamic contractions in that movement occurs; the force generated is sufficient to overcome the external load. In the intact human, the velocity of the movement actually varies with the joint angle; however, the rate of limb displacement or joint rotation can be held constant with the help of special exercise equipment. Thus, the term **isokinematic** is technically more accurate; the term *isokinetic* is more frequently used, though. What differentiates isokinetic contractions from other forms of dynamic contractions is that the rate of shortening or lengthening (*kinesis* means "motion") is constant (*iso* means "same").

An **isometric contraction** is a muscle fiber contraction that does not result in a length change in muscle fiber. In an isometric contraction, the cross-bridges are cycling—hence producing tension—but sliding of the filaments does not occur. The actual length (*metric*) is constant. This kind of action is possible in an isolated fiber because the fiber can be stabilized at both ends in an experimental apparatus before being stimulated. However, an intact fiber has an elastic element (in connective tissue and joints) to contend with, and so some fiber shortening actually does occur even though no limb displacement or joint rotation occurs. A **static contraction** is a muscle contraction that produces an increase in muscle tension but does not cause meaningful limb displacement or joint rotation and therefore does not result in movement of the skeleton. Thus, the term *static,* meaning "not in motion," is a better descriptor when describing a contraction that occurs in a human. No external work is done by static contractions, but they often perform the important task of fixation or stabilization. For example, gripping a tennis racket or barbell is an example of a static contraction.

Force Development

All types of contractions exert tension; however, the amount of tension that can be generated is not the same for all contractions. In whole muscles, eccentric dynamic contractions produce the greatest force, followed by static contractions, and finally, by dynamic concentric contractions.

The amount of force produced by each type of contraction depends on both neural and mechanical factors (Komi, 1984). This is true for muscle contractions considered on the level of the muscle fiber or of intact, whole muscle. The following section discusses how neural and mechanical factors influence force development in muscle fibers and in whole

muscles. In each section, we first discuss the muscle fiber, and then we describe the relationship in the more complex environment of whole muscles.

Neural Activation

If a single muscle fiber or motor unit is stimulated to contract, it will contract maximally or not contract at all (according to the all-or-none principle of muscle contraction). If a muscle fiber is stimulated to contract, it will produce a twitch and then relax (Figure 20.1a). If a second stimulus is applied before the fiber has completely relaxed, temporal summation results, producing slightly greater tension. If the frequency of stimulation is increased to a sufficient level (so that relaxation is prohibited), the individual contractions blend together to form first an irregular (or unfused) tetanus and then a smooth (fused) tetanus (Figure 20.1b). Unfused tetanic contractions produce greater tension than both single twitches and summations, and fused tetanic contractions produce the highest tension.

In the intact human, muscle contractions are based on tetanic contractions of motor units (Powers and Howley, 1990). Whole muscle contractions do not occur in an all-or-none fashion, as do muscle fiber contractions. Instead, whole muscle contractions can be graded, meaning a muscle contraction can produce little force (for instance, to move your hand while turning a page) or a lot of force (for instance, to lift a heavy barbell). There are two neural factors that determine force production in whole muscle. The first factor is the frequency of stimulation, or *rate-coding* (Enoka, 1988). As shown in Figure 20.1c, as the frequency of stimulation increases so does the force that the muscle produces. Notice that at frequencies less than 50 Hz, a small increase in frequency of firing can produce a large increase in muscle tension (Sale, 1992).

Isokinetic Contraction A muscle fiber contraction in which the velocity of the contraction is kept constant.

Isokinematic Contraction A muscle contraction in which the rate of limb displacement or joint rotation is held constant with the use of specialized equipment.

Isometric Contraction A muscle fiber contraction that does not result in a length change in muscle fiber.

Static Contraction A muscle contraction that produces an increase in muscle tension but does not cause meaningful limb displacement or joint displacement and therefore does not result in movement of the skeleton.

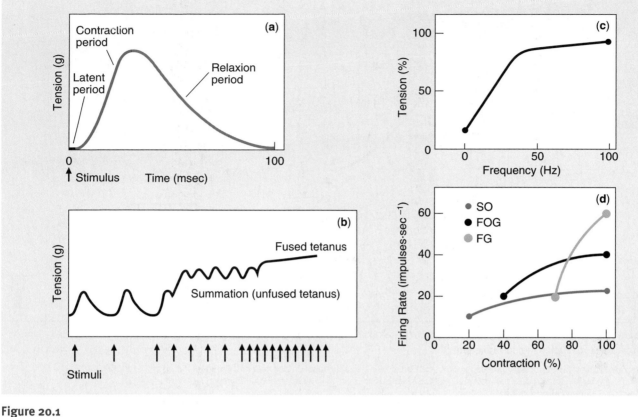

Figure 20.1
Muscle Response to Stimulation

(a) Myogram of a single muscle fiber twitch. (b) Myogram of a series of muscle fiber twitches.
(c) Effect of frequency of stimulation on muscle tension in whole muscle. (d) Effect of firing rate on
muscle tension and fiber type recruitment in whole muscle.

The second neural way of controlling force output is by varying the number of motor units activated, which is called *recruitment,* or *number coding.* In the intact human, some motor units, on an alternating basis, are always contracting. These contractions maintain what is called *muscle tone,* or tonus. When greater tension is needed, more motor units are recruited by the central nervous system. Such activation or recruitment, and the subsequent deactivation or derecruitment, occurs according to the size principle. Remember that smaller motor neurons are easier to stimulate than larger ones. Therefore, in accordance with the size principle, the small α_2 motor neurons innervating SO motor units are recruited first (Sale, 1992) (Figure 20.1d). As the stimulus increases, the larger α_1 motor neurons that innervate the FOG muscle fibers will be activated, followed by the recruitment of FG fibers as the stimulus continues to increase. Thus, the speed continuum of walk, jog, and run is paralleled by a muscle fiber recruitment continuum of SO, FOG, and FG recruitment. Deactivation, once the neural stimulation has been removed,

proceeds in reverse sequence. The larger, faster fibers (FG, then FOG) are inactivated first; finally, the slower, smaller fibers are deactivated until only muscle tonus remains.

Mechanical Factors Influencing Muscle Contractions

There are several mechanical factors that influence the force produced during muscle contractions. This section discusses four of them: length-tension-angle relationships, force-velocity relationships, the elasticity-force relationship, and cross-sectional area/architectural design. Once again, we first discuss how these relationships influence force production in a muscle fiber and then proceed to discuss the more complex situation in whole muscles.

Length-Tension-Angle Relationships First, within a muscle fiber, the amount of tension that can be exerted is related to the initial length of the

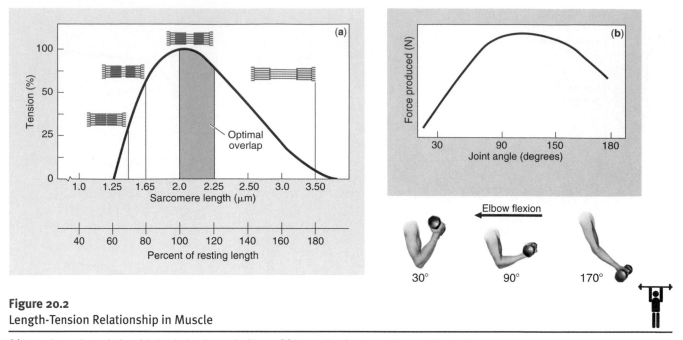

Figure 20.2
Length-Tension Relationship in Muscle

(a) Length-tension relationship in skeletal muscle fibers. (b) Example of a strength curve illustrating the length-tension relationship in whole muscle.

Source: From "Contractile Performance of Skeletal Muscle Fibres" by K. A. Paul Edman. In *Strength and Power in Sport* (p. 103) by P. V. Komi (ed.). Champaign, IL: Human Kinetics. Copyright 1992 by International Olympic Committee. Reprinted by permission.

sarcomeres. As shown in Figure 20.2a, this relationship can basically be described as an inverted U (Edman, 1992). The amount of tension produced is directly related to the degree of overlap of the thick and thin filaments. In elongated fibers there is little overlap of the actin and myosin filaments, making it hard for cross-bridges to form. In shortened fibers, where the thick and thin filaments already overlap almost completely, there is little room for further shortening. Thus, less force is produced in both the elongated and shortened position. In contrast, the maximum number of cross-bridges coincides with the highest force production, which occurs at approximately 100–120% of the resting sarcomere length (Edman, 1992).

In whole muscle, this length-tension relationship holds, but its expression is complicated by many factors. These factors include the cross-sectional area of the muscle, the arrangement of the sarcomere to the line of pull, the level of neural muscle activation, the degree of fatigue, the involvement of the elastic components of muscle, and the biomechanical aspects of how a muscle exerts force at a joint. The biomechanical aspects are most notable and will be considered here.

When whole muscle tension (measured as muscle force or torque) is plotted against the joint angle at which it occurs, *strength curves* are generated (Figure 20.2b). Imagine the muscle action involved in performing a bicep curl. As the barbell is lifted

through the range of motion, different amounts of force are generated in order to compensate for biomechanical differences in joint angle. Of course, the force produced is related to the length of the sarcomere, but force production is also greatly influenced by biomechanical aspects of the joint. Figure 20.2b provides a schematic of a strength curve for this bicep curl (elbow flexion) example. The joint angle is plotted along the horizontal axis, and the force produced by the contracting muscle is plotted along the vertical axis. Notice that the action of raising the barbell proceeds from right to left; that is, the joint angle is greatest in the lowered position (~170°) and least when the barbell is in the raised position (~30°). In this example peak force occurs at approximately 100–120°.

As indicated in Figure 20.3, strength curves can take one of three forms: ascending, descending, or ascending and descending. An ascending strength curve is characterized by an increase in torque as the joint angle increases. A descending strength curve is characterized by a decrease in torque as the joint angle increases. An ascending and descending curve is one where force initially increases and then decreases as a function of joint angle.

Figure 20.4a presents a generalized strength curve for knee flexion. Most studies describe this as an ascending curve, although there is some disparity in the findings (Kulig, et al., 1984). As shown in

Focus on Research

The Benefits of Tapering

Trappe, S., D. Costill, & R. Thomas: Effect of swim taper on whole muscle and single muscle fiber contractile properties. *Medicine and Science in Sports and Exercise.* 33(1):48–56 (2001).

Athletes commonly participate in a taper—that is, a period of reduced training volume—in order to optimize performance for an important athletic event. Although improvements in performance have been documented with a taper, there has been relatively little scientific research to document the underlying mechanisms that result from a taper. Trappe and colleagues investigated the effect of a swim taper on changes in whole muscle function and single muscle cell contractile properties of SO and FOG muscle fibers from the deltoid muscle of highly trained swimmers before and after a 21-day taper. Swim time improved by 4%. The graphs represent whole muscle power and muscle fiber peak force before and after training.

Analysis of the data revealed the following:

1. Whole muscle power increased significantly after the taper.
2. Peak force increased significantly in FOG fibers following the taper, but peak force was not significantly different in SO fibers.
3. Muscle fiber diameter and cross-sectional area increased significantly in FOG fibers following the taper but did not change significantly SO fibers (data not shown).

These data suggest that tapering induces alterations in the contractile properties of single muscle fibers, with the FOG fibers being more affected than SO. The increased size, strength, and power of the FOG fibers may be responsible for the improvement in whole muscle strength and in performance.

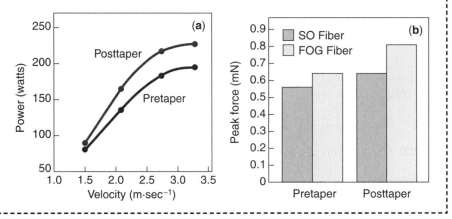

---

the figure, when the joint angle is greatest, the greatest force is exerted. This point also corresponds to the time when the muscles of the hamstrings are longest.

Figure 20.4b presents a generalized strength curve for hip abduction (Kulig, et al., 1984). These curves are generally described as descending. In this case, larger joint angles correspond to lower forces. In this example, the tensor fasciae latae (the muscle responsible for hip abduction) is longest at the lowest joint angle.

Both of these situations—Figures 20.4a and 20.4b—are really consistent: The longer the muscle length, the greater the force that is exerted. However, remember that it is not just, or even primarily, the length of the muscle itself that causes this variation.

There is general agreement that both elbow flexion (Figure 20.4c) and knee extension (Figure 20.4d) exhibit ascending and descending strength curves (Kulig, et al., 1984). The strongest angles for elbow flexion seem to be between 90° and 130°; for knee extension the strongest angles are between 100° and

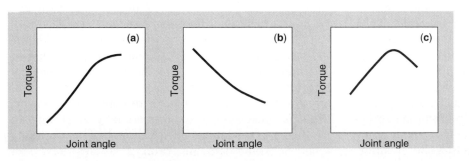

Figure 20.3
Classification of Strength Curves

(a) Ascending. (b) Descending.
(c) Ascending and descending.

Source: K. Kulig, J. G. Andrews, & J. G. Hay. Human strength curves. In R. Terjung (ed.), *Exercise and Sport Sciences Reviews* (Vol. 12). Lexington, MA: Collamore Press, 417–466 (1984). Reprinted by permission of Williams & Wilkins.

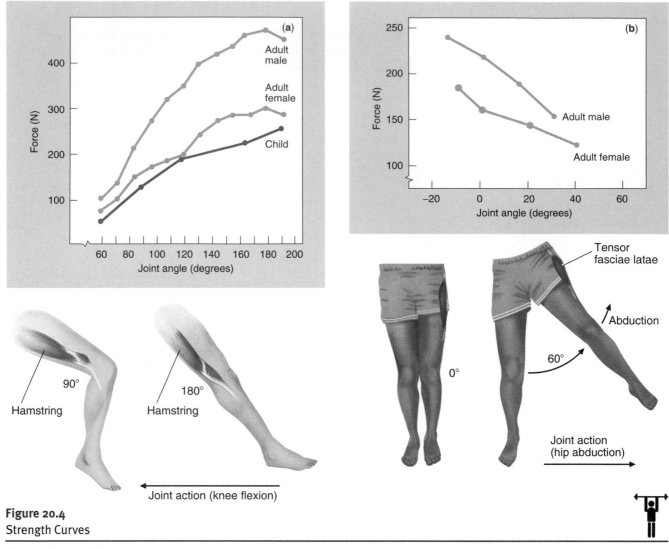

Figure 20.4
Strength Curves

(a) Knee flexion. (b) Hip abduction.

Source: K. Kulig, J. G. Andrews, & J. G. Hay. Human strength curves. In R. Terjung (ed.), *Exercise and Sport Sciences Reviews* (Vol. 12). Lexington, MA: Collamore Press, 417–466 (1984). Reprinted by permission of Williams & Wilkins.

130°. As with the other configurations, the joint angle that coincides with the greatest force production is partially, but not entirely, a result of the muscle length and degree of overlap of the thick and thin filaments.

Although there are some differences, by and large the shapes of the strength curves are consistent for males and females, the young and the old. Injuries typically result in low strength curve values; thus, preinjury strength curves or strength curves from a comparable healthy individual are sometimes used as goals in rehabilitation. Agreed-upon norms for strength curves are not generally available.

Knowledge of strength curves has another practical application. If an individual is going to lift an external load—for example, a barbell through the range of elbow flexion (biceps curl exercise)—he or she is limited by the weight that can be handled at the weakest point. Thus, the stronger angles are not overloaded to the same extent as the weaker angles, and the muscle is taxed maximally only at its "sticking point."

Finally, strength curves have been used in the design of strength training equipment—specifically, variable-resistance equipment (Kulig, et al., 1984). Nautilus developed the variable-radius cam to mimic the strength curve of selected single-joint exercises. The aim is to compensate for changes in mechanical leverage throughout the range of motion of a joint, thereby matching the load to the strength curve so that the muscles are taxed maximally at all angles, not just the sticking point. Although this reasoning appears to be logical, training studies have not

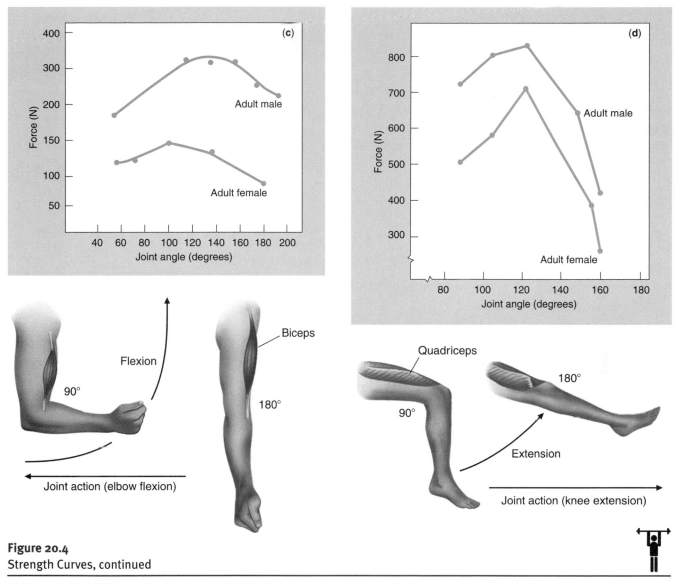

Figure 20.4
Strength Curves, continued

(c) Elbow flexion. (d) Knee extension.

demonstrated that greater benefits are derived from variable-resistance training programs than from traditional free weight programs.

Force-Velocity and Power-Velocity Relationships The second major mechanical factor that influences the expression of muscle force or torque is the velocity at which the shortening occurs.

The relationship between force and velocity is similar for a single muscle fiber (Figure 20.5a) and for an intact whole muscle (Figure 20.5b). The single muscle fiber does not exhibit the smooth hyperbolic curve that an intact muscle does, but both show the basic relationship: The shortening velocity of a muscle increases as the force developed by the muscle decreases, which means that a muscle can shorten

fastest when the load is the lightest. Maximal velocity occurs in an unloaded (zero force) situation, and a maximal load results in no movement (zero velocity). In between these two extremes the velocity gradually decreases in a curvilinear fashion as the load increases. To apply this information, consider a simple example of swinging a bat. As the weight of the bat is increased, the speed with which it can be swung decreases.

If the external force overcomes the ability of the muscle to resist it, the muscle lengthens (eccentric contraction), but only after producing additional tension (Stauber, 1989). The eccentric contraction is seen in Figure 20.5a where the force curve dips below the horizontal axis. Notice that the force produced continues to increase during this eccentric phase. This

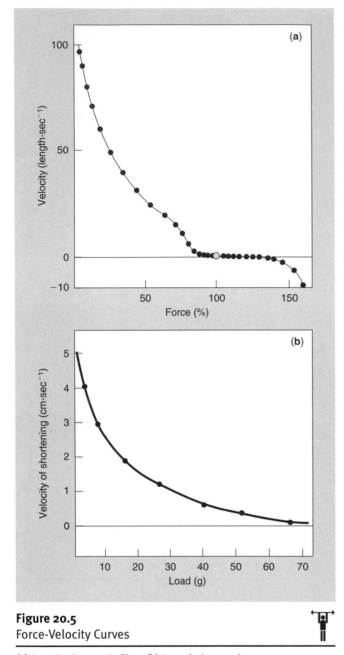

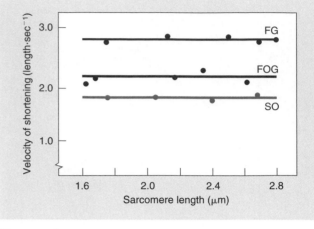

Figure 20.6
Velocity-Length Curves

Source: Reprinted with permission from Edman (1992).

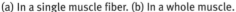

Figure 20.5
Force-Velocity Curves

(a) In a single muscle fiber. (b) In a whole muscle.

Source: From "Contractile Performance of Skeletal Muscle Fibers" by
K. A. Paul Edman. In *Strength and Power in Sport* (p. 105) by P. V. Komi
(ed.). Champaign, Il: Human Kinetics. Copyright 1992 by International
Olympic Committee. Reprinted by permission.

result is consistent with the information presented earlier in this chapter concerning eccentric dynamic contractions.

It is interesting to note that on the cellular level, the maximal velocity of shortening varies among individual muscle fibers, but within the same fibers, maximal velocity of shortening is constant regardless of the sarcomere length (Figure 20.6) (Edman, 1992).

Compare Figure 20.6 with Figure 20.2 (the length-tension curve). From the comparison, it is apparent that the length of the sarcomere influences force production, but it does not affect the velocity of force production. The maximum velocity of shortening does not depend on the number of cross-bridges between the thick and thin filaments but on the maximal cycling rate of the cross-bridges (Edman, 1992).

Figure 20.7 shows the relationship between power and velocity in whole muscles. These data were derived from a study of two different groups of subjects: one group of subjects with more than 50% FT muscle fibers (average = 58.5%) and one group with less than 50% FT fibers (average = 38.3%) (Coyle, et al., 1976). Several conclusions can be drawn from these graphs.

1. Power is positively related to velocity.

2. The shape of the relationship is curvilinear. Consider what this power-velocity relationship means if a heavier (as opposed to lighter) bat can be swung quickly enough to contact a fast pitch.

3. The graph in Figure 20.7 shows that the power that can be generated at any given velocity varies with the predominant fiber type. At any given velocity of movement, the power that results is higher in individuals with more than 50% FT fibers than in individuals with less than 50% FT fibers. Thus, individuals with high percentages of FT fibers would seem to be genetically predisposed (given sufficient training and practice) to be successful in power events such as sprinting, power lifting, and jumping, and in field events such as shot, javelin, and discus.

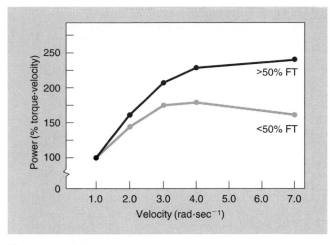

Figure 20.7
Influence of Fiber Type on Velocity-Power Relationship

Source: Coyle, et al. (1976).

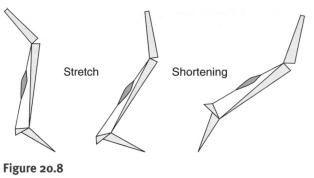

Figure 20.8
Stretch-Shortening Cycle

Source: P. V. Komi. Physiological and biomechanical correlates of muscle function: Effects of muscle structure and stretch-shortening cycle of force and speed. In R. Terjung (ed.), *Exercise and Sport Sciences Reviews* (Vol. 12). Lexington, MA: Collamore Press, 81–122 (1984). Reprinted by permission of Williams & Wilkins.

4. The power curve of the predominantly ST fiber individuals (those with less than 50% FT) not only levels off but also makes a downturn at the higher velocities. Although such a downturn is not evident at the tested speeds for the FT group, it is likely that there is an optimal speed of movement for the generation of power that is fiber-type specific.

Elasticity-Force Relationship   Elasticity is the third mechanical factor that must be considered in a description of the force development capabilities of muscles. Both the muscle fibers and their tendinous attachments contain elastic components. When a muscle fiber is stretched and then contracted, the resultant contraction is stronger than it would have been had there been no prestretching. In the intact human, the relationship between prestretch and force of contraction is expressed as a *stretch-shortening cycle* (SSC) (Komi, 1992). Stretch-shortening cycles do not occur in all human movements. They are most evident in activities such as running, jumping, and (to a lesser extent) bicycling. Figure 20.8 shows that the calf muscles and Achilles tendon are stretched while contracting eccentrically as the foot of a runner impacts the ground (Komi, 1992). The push-off, or concentric-shortening phase, is aided by the release of the potential energy stored during the stretch phase. To feel the impact of the SSC, stand up and see how high you can jump with a little flexion and then with moderate flexion at your hip, knee, and ankle joints. Then try a rebound jump from a small stool. This latter task is an example of a plyometric exercise. Plyometrics will be discussed more completely in

the neural flexibility chapter (Chapter 22), because more than just elasticity is involved in the physiological basis for their execution. As a result of additional power generation with increasing stretch-proceeding contraction, you should be able to jump successively higher in the three examples.

Not only does the stretch-shortening cycle lead to more powerful muscle contractions, but it also has an impact on mechanical efficiency. Efficiency is discussed at length in the unit on metabolism (Chapter 5). Here you simply need to be aware that more work can be done with less energy expenditure following a prestretch (Komi, 1992).

Cross-Sectional Area/Architectural Design   The maximal force that can be developed within a muscle fiber is related to its cross-sectional area. The force that can be developed by a whole muscle is also related to its cross-sectional area. However, this relationship is not as strong as the one within a single muscle fiber, largely owing to different arrangements of the muscle fiber within a muscle. Muscles that are designed for a high force generation (pennate, bipennate, and multipennate muscles) are arranged so as to maximize its cross-sectional area. Muscles that are designed for a high velocity of shortening have parallel fibers and are arranged in a fusiform manner (Goldspink, 1992).

Muscular Fatigue and Soreness

Despite all the benefits and enjoyment of exercise, there are also some unpleasant outcomes that can occur as a result of unaccustomed muscular activity. This section will deal with two of those consequences: muscular fatigue and muscular soreness.

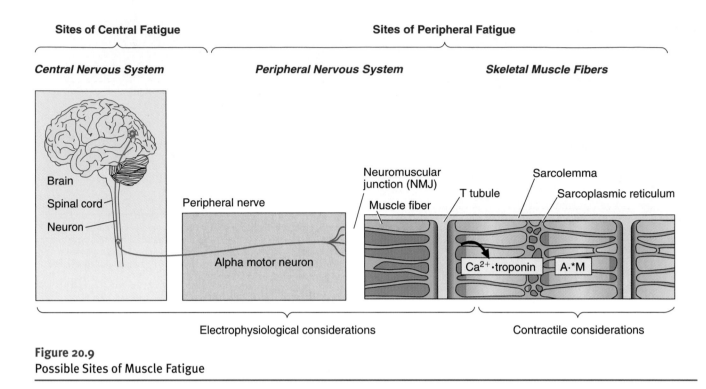

Figure 20.9
Possible Sites of Muscle Fatigue

Muscular Fatigue

Anyone who has participated in vigorous activity is familiar with muscular fatigue. Although exercise physiologists have studied fatigue for a long time, it is still to be precisely defined, and many questions remain regarding the basic causes of fatigue. Here is how one exercise physiologist summarizes the issue:

> Fatigue, generally defined as transient loss of work capacity resulting from preceding work, is one of the most fundamental problems both for research and for practical application. Fatigue limits performance in normal conditions and even more so in disease. It produces a general feeling of discomfort and frustration and interferes with well-being. (Simonson, 1971)

Fatigue results in the cessation of muscular work or the inability to maintain a given intensity of work. But what causes muscle fatigue? Muscle fatigue is a complex phenomenon that includes failure at one or more of the sites along the chain of events that leads to muscular contraction. As diagramed in Figure 20.9, fatigue can be classified as central and peripheral on the basis of the location of the site of fatigue.

Table 20.2 lists the possible sites of fatigue and summarizes the proposed mechanisms to explain muscle fatigue. Possible causes for central fatigue include a malfunction of the nerve cells or inhibition of voluntary effort in the central nervous system. Other factors that may influence central fatigue include psychological factors and motivation that influence

how much effort an individual will give, particularly if pain is associated with continuing an activity.

Peripheral fatigue refers to fatigue at a site beyond the central nervous system; this may include sites within the peripheral nervous system or within the skeletal muscle. Peripheral fatigue can occur at several sites: the neuromuscular junction, the sarcolemma–T tubules–sarcoplasmic reticulum system, and the myofilaments. Failure of neuromuscular transmission is a possible cause of fatigue. This failure could include inhibition of the axon terminal, depletion of the neurotransmitter, and/or problems with the binding of the neurotransmitter to the receptors on the motor end plate. Fatigue can also result from a failure of the electrical excitation along the sarcolemma and T tubules and an inability of the sarcoplasmic reticulum to release sufficient calcium. Likewise, fatigue could result from any alteration in the ability of calcium to bind to troponin and thereby remove tropomyosin from its blocking position on actin.

It is also possible that fatigue results from biochemical and metabolic changes within the contractile elements (myofilaments of the muscle cell). Notice in Figure 20.9 the categorizations of *electrophysiological considerations* and *contractile biochemical considerations* that relate to muscle fatigue. Electrophysiological considerations are concerned with steps within the central nervous system, the peripheral nervous system, or the muscle fiber leading up to the binding of the actin and myosin filaments. Contractile considerations involve the ability of actin and myosin to continue their cross-bridge attachment-detachment cycles, thus producing force and are therefore confined to the skeletal muscle fiber.

There are two primary hypotheses for the contractile causes of fatigue within muscle: the depletion (or exhaustion) hypothesis and the accumulation hypothesis (MacLaren, et al., 1989). The depletion hypothesis suggests that fatigue results from depletion of certain metabolites, specifically, ATP, phosphocreatine (PC), and glycogen. Hence, the muscle fibers are no longer able to produce force. The accumulation hypothesis suggests that fatigue is caused by the accumulation of certain metabolites that have been shown to impair force generation within muscles, specifically, lactate, hydrogen ions, ammonia, and phosphate.

Current research suggests that the most likely site of fatigue is within the muscle itself. The factors that contribute to fatigue are complex and interrelated and depend on the muscle fibers involved and the type of activity that is being performed. The depletion of PC leads to fatigue in FG fibers that rely on this substrate to regenerate ATP for explosive type events. The depletion of glycogen leads to fatigue in SO fibers that rely on this substrate to produce ATP aerobically during prolonged activity. The accumulation of lactate and the H^+ associated with lactic acid leads to fatigue by interfering with the contractile process in several places, decreasing the amount of calcium released, interfering with calcium-troponin binding, inhibiting anaerobic glycolysis (by inhibiting the rate-limiting enzyme PFK), and interfering with cross-bridging. The detrimental effects of H^+ accumulation are most evident in FOG fibers that produce large amounts of lactic acid. Because many types of activity involve more than one fiber type, several of these mechanisms may be involved in muscle fatigue for any given activity (Conley, 2000).

Type of Activity and Muscle Fatigue

It is now thought that fatigue results from different mechanisms for different types of activity. Furthermore, the fiber type involved in a given activity greatly influences the most probable mechanism of fatigue for that activity. Table 20.3 summarizes the most probable causes of fatigue for different types of activity. Note that any given activity may have several possible causes and that there is often an interaction among the proposed mechanisms.

Anaerobic (Sprint) Activities

Anaerobic (sprint) activities rely largely on FT fibers to produce ATP. Very short, explosive events rely more

Table 20.2
Site of Muscle Fatigue and Proposed Mechanism

Site of Fatigue	Proposed Mechanism
Central	
CNS	Malfunction of neurons
	Inhibition of voluntary effort (motor cortex)
	Psychological factors
Peripheral	
NMJ	Inhibition of axon terminal
	Depletion of neurotransmitter
	Altered neurotransmitter binding to receptors
T-tubule/SR	Inability to release Ca^{2+}
	Inability of Ca^{2+} to bind to troponin
Contractile elements	Depletion of ATP
	Depletion of PC
	Depletion of glycogen
	Accumulation of lactate, H^+, PO_4^-, etc.

heavily on FG, whereas activities that continue for 1–3 min rely more heavily on FOG fibers. For explosive type activities involving a predominance of FG fibers, it is most likely that fatigue results from a depletion of PC stores and the subsequent inability to regenerate ATP. For anaerobic activities that rely on anaerobic metabolism and utilize FOG fibers, it appears that the primary factor limiting performance is the accumulation of H^+ associated with an increase in lactic acid. The accumulation of H^+ interferes with the contractile process (see explanation above) and inhibits the production of ATP by anaerobic glycolysis (Conley, 2000).

Long-Term, Moderate to Heavy, Submaximal Aerobic Exercise

Steady-state activities that are performed at moderate workloads rely almost exclusively on SO fibers to produce ATP. As a result, lactic acid levels do not increase substantially during these activities. The most probable cause of fatigue in these types of activities is the depletion of glycogen stores. For prolonged activities that are performed at an intensity high enough to recruit FOG fibers, a significant amount of lactic acid is formed. In this case, the high levels of H^+ likely produce fatigue (Conley, 2000).

Table 20.3
Most Probable Causes of Muscle Fatigue

Type of Activity	Probable Causes of Fatigue
Anaerobic (sprint)	Depletion of PC stores
	Accumulation of H^+
	Inhibits glycolysis
	Decreases Ca^{2+} release from SR
	Interferes with Ca^{2+}-troponin binding
	La⁻ interferes with cross-bridging
Long-term, Moderate to Heavy, Submaximal Aerobic	Depletion of glycogen
	Accumulation of H^+
	Inhibits glycolysis
	Decreases Ca^{2+} release from SR
	Interferes with Ca^{2+}-troponin binding
	La⁻ interferes with cross-bridging
Incremental Aerobic Exercise to Maximum	Depletion of glycogen
	Accumulation of H^+
	Inhibits glycolysis
	Decreases Ca^{2+} release from SR
	Interferes with Ca^{2+}-troponin binding
	Depletion of PC
	La⁻ interferes with cross-bridging
Static	Depletion of PC
	Accumulation of H^+
	Inhibits glycolysis
	Decreases Ca^{2+} release from SR
	Interferes with Ca^{2+}-troponin binding
	Occlusion of blood flow
	Inhibition of motor cortex via sensory fibers in muscle
	La⁻ interferes with cross-bridging
Dynamic Resistance	
Low repetitions	Depletion of PC stores
High repetitions	Depletion of glycogen
	Accumulation of H^+
	Inhibits glycolysis
	Decreases Ca^{2+} release from SR
	Interferes with Ca^{2+}-troponin binding
	La⁻ interferes with cross-bridging

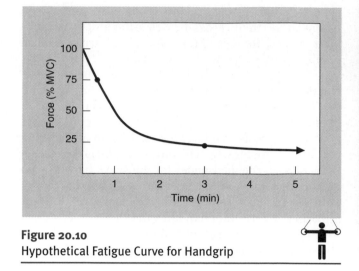

Figure 20.10
Hypothetical Fatigue Curve for Handgrip

Incremental Aerobic Exercise to Maximum

Incremental aerobic exercise to maximum involves recruiting all of the muscle fiber types in the order of SO, FOG, FG to correspond with the increasing intensity of effort. It is likely that all of the mechanisms described above play a role in fatigue during this type of exercise. Furthermore, the cardiovascular system may be unable to provide blood supply to the working muscle adequate to support aerobic energy production (Conley, 2000).

Static Exercise

If a person is asked to maintain a static contraction at a given intensity (expressed as a percentage of maximal voluntary contraction, % MVC), force decreases over time because of fatigue.

Figure 20.10 depicts graphically the force that a muscle can produce statically as a function of time. This figure suggests that if an individual is asked to sustain a static contraction (in this case, a handgrip exercise) at less than 20% MVC, the load can be maintained indefinitely. However, as the % MVC increases, the time that the contraction can be maintained decreases rapidly. A force equal to 50% MVC can be maintained only for approximately 1 min for a handgrip exercise. The precise shape of the fatigue curve varies among muscle groups, reflecting the differences in fiber-type distribution and architectural design.

Fatigue is likely the result of several factors: depletion of PC in FG fibers (if the intensity of effort is great enough to recruit them), the accumulation of H^+, and inhibition of the CNS by afferent fibers that are sensitive to the buildup of H^+ and other metabolites (Conley, 2000).

Dynamic Resistance Exercise

Dynamic resistance exercises that involve very few repetitions employ FG fibers. Hence, fatigue is likely due to a depletion of PC. In resistance exercise in which high repetitions or a high total volume of work is done, fatigue is more likely caused by an accumulation of H^+ associated with FOG fibers (Conley, 2000).

Muscular Soreness

Muscle soreness is a familiar consequence of overexertion. There are two generally recognized types of muscle soreness: immediate and delayed onset. *Immediate-onset soreness* is characterized by pain during and immediately after exercise, which may persist for several hours. This type of soreness is thought to be caused by stimulation of the pain receptors by metabolic by-products of cellular respiration, especially the H^+ associated with increased lactic acid levels. It is generally relieved by discontinuing exercise, or it subsides shortly thereafter.

Delayed-onset muscle soreness (DOMS) increases in intensity for the first 24 hr after activity, peaks from 24–48 hr postexercise, and then declines during the next 5–7 days (DeVries and Housh, 1994; Edington and Edgerton, 1976). Delayed-onset muscle soreness is generally considered to be an adult phenomenon, but some children also exhibit DOMS (Webber, et al., 1989).

DOMS is of concern to exercise professionals because it affects athletic performance and exercise participation. Despite its importance and considerable research attention, the causative factors and cellular mechanisms of DOMS remain elusive. There are, however, several theories that have attempted to integrate the findings of research on this topic. Two of the primary theories of DOMS are presented here: the mechanical trauma theory and the local ischemic theory. These theories are not mutually exclusive; on the contrary, they share many of the same elements.

Etiology and Mechanisms

The mechanical trauma model has been proposed by Armstrong (1984) to describe the mechanisms responsible for DOMS. As the name implies, this model suggests that the mechanical forces in the contractile

---

Delayed-Onset Muscle Soreness (DOMS)
Muscle soreness that increases in intensity for the first 24 hr after activity, peaks from 24–28 hr, and then declines during the next 5–7 days.

---

or elastic tissue result in structural damage to the muscle fibers. Damage to the sarcolemma of the cell leads to disruption in calcium homeostasis, which results in necrosis (death of tissue). The presence of cellular debris and immune cells (macrophages) leads to swelling and inflammation, which is responsible for the sensation of DOMS. The sequence of events whereby muscle trauma leads to inflammation and activation of the immune system is described fully in Chapter 17. In fact, the cytokine hypothesis of overtraining proposes that muscle damage, inflammation, and the immune response are central to explaining the symptoms of overtraining (Smith, 2000).

The local ischemic model has been proposed by DeVries and Housh (1994). This model suggests that exercise—even moderate, atraumatic activities—causes swelling in the muscle tissue, which increases tissue pressure. This increase in tissue pressure is thought to result in local ischemia (reduced blood flow), which causes pain and leads to tonic muscle constriction (spasm). This spasm causes additional swelling and perpetuates a cycle of swelling and ischemia that results in the painful sensation known as DOMS. DeVries also suggests that local ischemia can result in structural damage that leads to inflammation and swelling and, thus, exacerbates the cycle.

Figure 20.11 summarizes both the mechanical trauma and spasm models of DOMS. Note the considerable overlap in mechanisms that are proposed by the two models, which accounts for the considerable research evidence that supports each model. The major distinction between the models is the event that initiates the cycle. It is possible that both models are viable. On the one hand, DeVries points out that overexertion involving long-duration and moderate-intensity activities leads to DOMS. On the other hand, Armstrong concentrates on the manifestation of DOMS after activities that place considerable mechanical force on the muscle, specifically, eccentric contractions that are known to cause DOMS. Much of the research that supports the mechanical trauma model has used eccentric exercise as a means of eliciting DOMS.

One of the popular concepts (or rather misconceptions) regarding DOMS is that it is caused by the accumulation of lactic acid. Although this theory was originally proposed by researchers (Asmussen, 1956; Edington and Edgerton, 1976), its popularity now rests in the lay public. There is now considerable research evidence to argue against this theory, including the fact that individuals who have McArdle's syndrome and do not produce lactic acid also suffer from DOMS. Additional evidence against lactic acid as the cause of muscle soreness is that the type of activity that produces the greatest degree of soreness, namely

Figure 20.11
An Integrated Model to
Explain DOMS

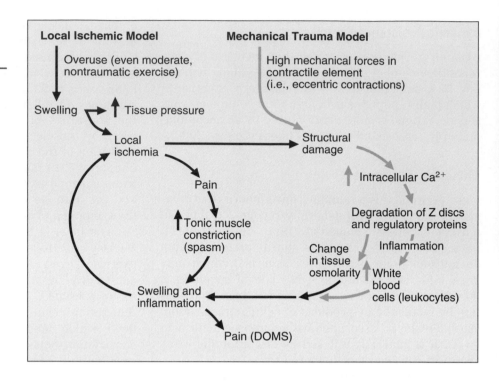

eccentric contractions, produces lower lactic acid levels than concentric contractions of the same power output (Armstrong, et al., 1983; Bonde-Petersen, et al., 1972; Davies and Barnes, 1972). Perhaps the most compelling evidence is that lactic acid has a half-life of 15–25 min and is fully cleared from muscle within an hour (see Chapter 4). Since lactic acid is not present (at least not at elevated levels) it cannot cause soreness 24–48 hr later.

Treatment for Relief and Prevention

The primary means of providing relief from muscular soreness appears to be static stretching of the sore muscle, acute exercise, and anti-inflammatory drugs. Muscular stretch is thought to initiate the inverse myotatic reflex (by stimulation of the Golgi tendon organ, GTO), which results in a relaxation of the stretched muscle (DeVries and Housh, 1994). (Reflexes will be discussed in detail in Chapter 22.) Although some research has demonstrated a reduction in soreness as a result of stretching (DeVries and Housh, 1994), other research has failed to demonstrate the same reduction in pain following static stretching (McGlynn, et al., 1979).

Acute exercise also diminishes DOMS (Armstrong, et al., 1983). Researchers suggest that this relief is due to an increased release of endorphins as a result of exercise (Kelly, 1982). The use of anti-inflammatory drugs has been suggested, too, since inflammation is clearly part of the DOMS cycle.

Although the use of aspirin and ibuprofin do help relieve DOMS, these drugs appear to be most effective if taken prior to exercise (Hasson, et al., 1990).

Assessing Muscular Function

Accurate assessment of the strength, endurance, and power a muscle is capable of generating is important for five reasons.

1. Assessment is an aid in *screening* to determine the extent of muscle weaknesses and/or imbalances. Both weakness and imbalance have been implicated as making an individual more prone to injury. Assessment also establishes baseline values for an individual.

2. Assessment can be used as a guide to *rehabilitation*. Assessment of the loss of function after an injury or accident is needed to determine rehabilitation workloads and to monitor progress.

3. Assessment is necessary for *exercise prescription*. Both athletes and fitness participants need realistic programs based on their own performance capabilities.

4. Assessment is an aid in *selection* of the best exercises for working on specific problems.

5. Assessment is a tool in *research* to study which types of training programs produce the greatest changes in muscle function.

A Question of Understanding

Listed below are the body weight (BW) and MVC for a handgrip task.

Name	Gender	BW (kg)	Absolute Strength MVC (kg)	Relative Strength kg·kg^{-1}	50% MVC
Jody	F	60.0	40.0		
Jill	F	68.0	60.0		
Pat	F	70.0	36.0		
Scott	M	63.0	50.0		
Tom	M	82.0	72.0		
Mike	M	70.0	71.0		

1. Calculate the relative strength for each individual (strength ÷ BW).

2. Calculate the load that would need to be held for each of the subjects to be working at 50% MVC (absolute strength × 0.5).

3. Who is the strongest person on an absolute basis? On a relative basis?

4. For whom would 50% MVC represent the most absolute force?

Check your answer in Appendix D.

Strength refers to the ability of a muscle or muscle group to exert force against a resistance. It is usually measured as one maximal effort. For dynamic resistance exercise, this is often called a one-repetition maximum (1-RM), whereas for static exercise it is referred to as a maximal voluntary contraction (MVC). *Torque* is the more correct term if movement is made through a range of motion, but *strength* is the more commonly used term. **Muscular endurance** is the ability of a muscle or muscle group to repeatedly exert force against a resistance; that is, the activity is typically performed at a given percentage of the 1-RM (for resistance exercise) or MVC (for static exercise). For example, an exerciser wishing to improve muscle endurance might lift a weight equal to 60% of her 1-RM for 12 repetitions. Similarly, a researcher wishing to study static muscle endurance may ask an individual to hold a handgrip dynamometer at 50% of MVC for 90 sec. **Power** is the amount of work done per unit of time and is the product of force and velocity ($P = F \times V$). Thus, it is the expression of strength exerted quickly.

Strength The ability of a muscle or muscle group to exert maximal force against a resistance in a single repetition.

Muscular Endurance The ability of a muscle or muscle group to repeatedly exert force against a resistance.

Power The amount of work done per unit of time; the product of force and velocity; the ability to exert force quickly.

Strength and muscular endurance can be expressed either as absolute values or as relative values. *Absolute values* represent the actual external load and are commonly measured in pounds (lb), kilograms (kg), newtons (N), or newton-meters (N·m). *Relative values* are expressed in relation to body weight. Both values are useful. For example, if two individuals are doing a two-arm curl and individual A can lift 70 kg and individual B can only lift 60 kg, you would probably conclude that individual A is stronger. However, if individual A weighs 55 kg and individual B weighs 47 kg, they both are lifting 1.27 kg per kg of body weight. Thus, on a relative basis, neither can be considered stronger. So if a comparison is to be made between individuals, a relative expression of strength is generally preferred. In contrast, absolute values are preferred for comparisons made on the same person.

In terms of muscular endurance, if individual A had a handgrip strength of 70 kg and individual B had a handgrip strength of 60 kg, and both were asked to hold a handgrip dynamometer at 40 kg, you would assume that individual A could do so for a longer period of time, because that load represents 57% MVC (40/70) for individual A and 67% MVC (40/60) for individual B. Thus, an absolute load puts the weaker individual at a disadvantage. However, if both were asked to hold a load that represented a 50% MVC (35 kg for individual A, 30 kg for individual B), and if they were equally motivated, you would expect that both individuals could hold that load for the same amount of time. To check that you understand the influence of body weight on the expression of strength, complete the Question of Understanding box above.

Laboratory Methods

In order to quantify the various aspects of muscular function just discussed, exercise physiologists use various laboratory and field methods. Laboratory methods are generally more accurate and precise than field methods in measuring different aspects of muscular function, but they have the disadvantage of being expensive and inaccessible to many people.

Electromyography

Electromyography (EMG) is the measurement of electrical activity, known as muscle action potentials, that brings about muscle contraction. Motor unit activity can be recorded by the use of needle electrodes, or whole-muscle activity can be recorded by the use of surface electrodes. The EMG voltage is proportional to the force of a static contraction, proportional to the tension developed in constant-velocity contractions (Lippold, 1952), and proportional to velocity in dynamic contractions (Bigland and Lippold, 1954). Therefore, one can obtain a reasonably valid estimation of tension development in a muscle by EMG.

EMG does not give an absolute value of force or torque; instead, it provides a direct functional indication of muscle activity. If it is plotted against incremental loads or values resulting from a submaximal hold, it can be used to predict strength or endurance, respectively. Such submaximal testing using EMG is particularly important in situations where an individual either cannot or is not motivated to perform maximally. In addition, because weak individuals produce a greater EMG signal than strong individuals for any absolute load (Fischer and Merhautova, 1961), EMG activity can be used to monitor rehabilitation or training progress.

Perhaps the most valuable contribution of EMG to muscle function assessment, however, is its ability to show which muscles are primarily responsible for specific actions. For example, when training or testing individuals for abdominal strength, one should select an exercise that maximizes the involvement of the abdominal muscles (the rectus abdominis and the external obliques) and that minimizes the involvement of the hip flexors and thigh muscles (rectus femoris). EMG helps in this selection.

The Question of Understanding box provides an example of the EMG activity of the muscles just mentioned during a sit-up with the feet supported and unsupported and the knees at various angles (Hall, et al., 1990; Halpern and Bleck, 1979). Work through the questions in the box to check on your understanding.

Isokinetic Machines

Isokinetic machines, such as a Cybex or MERAC (Figure 20.12), allow the velocity of limb movement

---

Electromyography (EMG) The measurement of the neural or electrical activity that brings about muscle contraction.

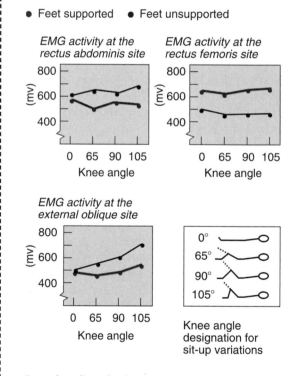

A Question of Understanding

Study the EMG data for each of the muscle groups with the feet supported (●) and with the feet unsupported (●), and answer the following questions.

● Feet supported   ● Feet unsupported

1. Does bending the knees eliminate the involvement of thigh muscles (rectis femoris) if the feet are held down? Which muscles are more active if the feet are held, the abdominal or thigh muscles?

2. Which muscle group does the angle of knee bend affect most?

3. Should the feet be held or not held to maximize the involvement of the abdominal muscles?

4. On the basis of your answers in 1–3, which sit-up form (feet held or not held) and which knee angle would you recommend?

Check your answers in Appendix D.

to be kept constant throughout a contraction. These devices provide accurate and reliable measurements of muscular strength, muscular endurance, and power while the speed of the limb is kept constant at a predetermined velocity. Any increase in muscular force results in increased resistance rather than increased acceleration of the limb (Heyward, 1991). Measurements obtained on isokinetic machines serve as a reference against which other methods of assessment can be compared. These devices can be configured to test the limbs of the upper or the lower body.

Force Transducers

Force transducers measure static strength and endurance. The displacement of the transducer sends an electrical signal to a computer, which displays the force output in digital form. By having the subject exert as much force as possible in a single maximal trial, these devices can be used to measure maximal strength during a maximal voluntary contraction. They can also be used to measure static muscular endurance by having the subject hold a given percentage of the predetermined maximal value (% MVC). Static muscular endurance is then calculated by determining either how long an individual can maintain the predetermined value or how long it takes the subject to drop to a specified percentage of his or her maximal contraction.

Laboratory and Field Methods

There are several other methods of assessing muscle function that require relatively simple testing devices. They may be encountered in a laboratory or in a field-testing environment.

Dynamometers

Dynamometers measure static strength and static muscular endurance. Two dynamometers are commercially available: the handgrip dynamometer and the back and leg dynamometer. Dynamometers use a spring device; as force is applied to the dynamometer, the spring is compressed and moves the needle to indicate force produced. Like the force transducer, these devices can be used to measure maximal strength by having the subject exert as much force as possible in a single maximal voluntary contraction (MVC). Because of its availability and ease of administration, the handgrip dynamometer has been extensively used to measure grip strength.

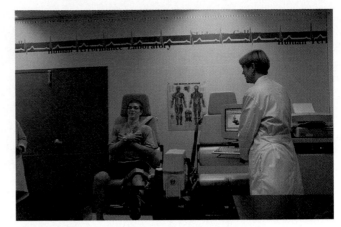

Figure 20.12
Isokinetic Exercise Equipment

The measurement of isokinetic strength of quadriceps is recorded throughout normal range of motion.

Dynamometers can also be used to measure static muscular endurance by having the subject perform at a given percentage of the predetermined maximal value. Muscular endurance is then calculated by determining how long an individual can maintain the predetermined (submaximal) value.

Constant-Resistance Equipment

The most common method of measuring dynamic strength is to determine the maximal amount an individual can lift in a single repetition using the constant resistance offered by free weight or weight machines. This is known as a one-repetition max (1-RM) and is a trial-and-error method of determining how much an individual can lift. If the selected weight is too heavy to be lifted, then a lower weight is used. If the weight is successfully lifted, then additional weight is added. Care must be taken in the use of this method, however, because too many trials will cause fatigue, thereby decreasing the true maximal strength value.

Constant-resistance equipment can also be used to measure dynamic muscular endurance by determining how many times an individual can lift a submaximal load. The submaximal load is usually a predetermined load (such as the 80-lb bench press test for males or the 35-lb test for females used in the YMCA assessment battery); or it may be expressed as a percentage of body weight or as a percentage of 1-RM.

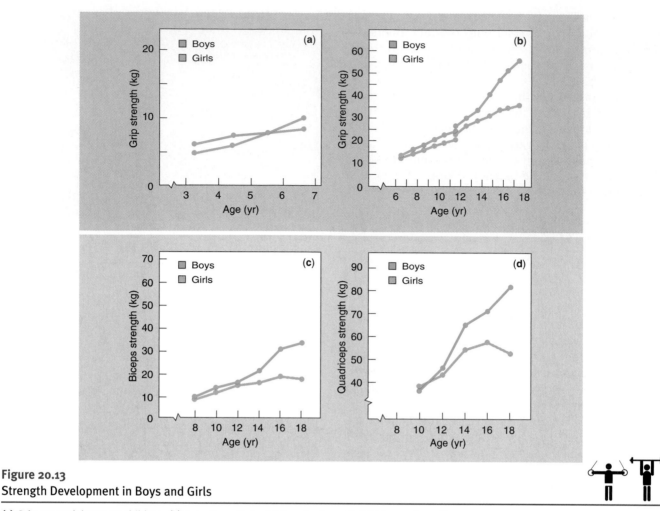

Figure 20.13
Strength Development in Boys and Girls

(a) Grip strength in young children. (b) Grip strength in children 6–18 yr old. (c) Biceps strength.
(d) Quadriceps strength.

Source: From *Growth, Maturation, and Physical Activity* (pp. 189, 191) by Robert M. Malina and Claude Bouchard.
   Champaign, IL: Human Kinetics. Copyright 1991 by Robert M. Malina and Claude Bouchard. Reprinted by
   permission.

Field Tests

There are several easily administered tests commonly used in the field to assess muscle function. Common field tests include calisthenic and jumping activities.

Calisthenic Activities

Calisthenic activities are often used in field settings to assess muscular endurance and, to a lesser extent, muscular strength. The most commonly administered tests include some version of sit-ups or curl-ups, push-ups, and pull-ups or flexed-arm hang. Although it is often reported that these tests measure strength, they are in fact usually endurance tests; that is, they measure the maximum number of times an individual can perform a given test (often within a specified time

period, such as the number of curl-ups per minute). If the participant is able to complete more than one repetition of the task, the result represents muscular endurance. If the subject is able to complete one repetition (or sometimes no repetitions), the result represents strength (or lack thereof). Note that these tests indicate relative strength or endurance, because the amount of resistance is determined by individual body size.

Vertical Jump/Standing Broad Jump

The jump tests are used to measure the explosive muscular power of the legs. Although they are easy to administer, they are also influenced by the weight of the individual. Furthermore, there may be a strong neural component and there is a definite alactic anaerobic metabolic component to these tests (see Chapter 4).

Although all of these calisthenic (performance) tests are commonly used, they have not been definitively validated as tests of strength, muscular endurance, and/or power. Therefore, it may be best just to call them what they are—that is, a push-up test, for example—rather than trying to say they are a substitute for a certain laboratory assessment.

The Influence of Age and Sex on Muscle Function

Children

Strength development in humans is evident from infancy through maturity. Figure 20.13 shows a common pattern of development. Strength increases rectilinearly from early childhood (3–7 yr) through early adolescence (13–14 yr) for both sexes. Then a marked increase in strength occurs during the rest of adolescence and into early adulthood (15–20 yr) for boys. Girls, however, do not show an accelerated increase in strength in late adolescence. They either maintain a slow rectilinear rise, as shown for grip strength (Figure 20.13b), or decline after age 16, as shown for both elbow flexion and knee extension (Figures 20.13c and 20.13d) (Malina and Bouchard, 1991). The increase in strength during childhood and adolescence, even without training, is more than can be accounted for just from growth in size.

During early childhood, there is virtually no difference in strength measurements between boys and girls. As puberty begins and progresses, though, the gap progressively widens. On the average, at 11–12 yr of age girls achieve approximately 90% of boys' strength; at 13–14 yr, this percentage has been reduced to 80%, and at 15–16 yr, to 75%. These percentages vary not only with age but also with the muscle group being measured.

Male-Female Differences

Adult females average only about 56% of the static strength values of adult males in upper-body locations, about 64% in trunk strength, and about 72% in lower-body locations (Lauback, 1976). As shown in Figure 20.14, the variation between upper- and lower-body strength has also been shown for the bench press and the leg press (Williams, 1994). Note that there is considerable overlap in the distribution of leg strength even in untrained males and females (Figure 20.14a), whereas virtually no overlap exists for the arm strength (bench press) distributions (Figure 20.14b).

Although field tests are not pure tests of muscle function, differences in these tests parallel those seen

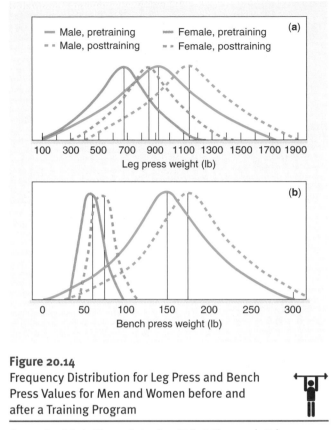

Figure 20.14

Frequency Distribution for Leg Press and Bench Press Values for Men and Women before and after a Training Program

Source: Reprinted with permission from Wells & Plowman (1983).

in strength with growth and maturation and between boys and girls. Figure 20.15 illustrates these relationships for the flexed-arm hang and the standing long jump. Adult performances also appear to parallel adolescent male-female strength differences. Part of what can be interpreted from Figure 20.16 is that throughout the adult age span men are able to perform more push-ups than women, even if the men are inactive. For leg lift exercise, however, the performance gap is smaller, with considerable overlap between inactive men and active women.

Why do these differences occur? Strength and other muscle functions increase as children grow because muscle mass increases parallel increases in body mass. The pubertal hormonal changes—particularly in the level of testosterone, which is involved with the anabolic process of muscle growth—favor the males. Whereas the young males are adding muscle mass under the influence of testosterone, the young females are adding fat under the influence of estrogen (Figure 20.17 on page 543) (Malina and Bouchard, 1991). The similarities among the graphic representations of fat-free mass (Figure 20.17a), strength (Figure 20.13), and muscle performance (Figure 20.15) are striking, leading to the conclusion

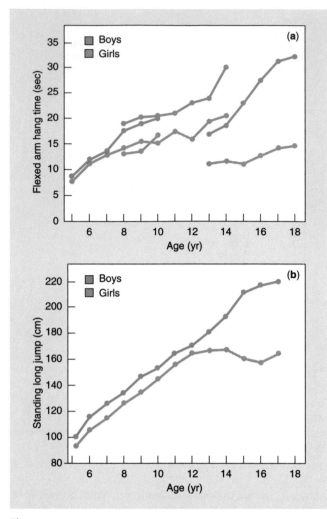

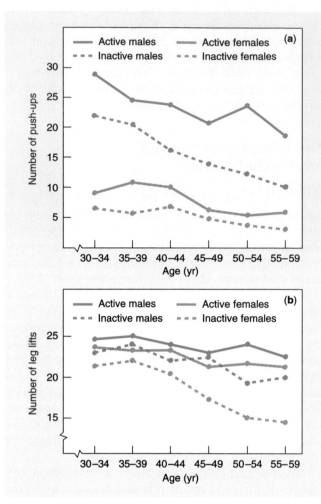

Figure 20.15

Performance on Field Tests of Muscular Function in Children

(a) Flexed-arm hang (muscular endurance). (b) Standing long jump (muscular power).

Source: From *Growth, Maturation, and Physical Activity* (pp. 192, 193) by Robert M. Malina and Claude Bouchard. Champaign, IL: Human Kinetics. Copyright 1991 by Robert M. Malina and Claude Bouchard. Reprinted by permission.

Figure 20.16

Performance on Field Tests of Muscular Function in Adults

(a) Push-up (muscular endurance). (b) Leg lifts.

Source: From "Age-Related Changes in Strength and Special Groups" by Siegfried Israel. In *Strength and Power in Sport* (p. 323) by P. V. Komi (ed.). Champaign, Il: Human Kinetics. Copyright 1992 by International Olympic Committee. Reprinted by permission.

that the quantity of muscle mass is what accounts for the difference in the expression of strength.

Another way to emphasize that it is the quantity of muscle and not the quality of muscle that is responsible for the male-female inequities is to calculate relative strength values (Wells and Plowman, 1983; Wilmore, 1974). In one study the percentage of handgrip strength exhibited by the females in relation to the males increased from 57%, when expressed in absolute strength terms, to 73% and to 83% when expressed on a relative basis, that is, absolute strength divided by total body weight and absolute strength divided by lean body mass, respectively (Wilmore,

1974). For the bench press the corresponding figures were 37%, 46%, and 53%; and for the leg press they were 73%, 92%, and 106%. Thus, in leg strength relative to lean body mass female performance actually exceeded that of males!

In addition, studies relating strength to cross-sectional area of muscle show no inequities between the sexes. From all these studies it must therefore be concluded that it is the larger size of males in general, their greater muscle mass, and their larger fiber size that are physiologically responsible for their greater strength, rather than any inherent difference in the potential or function of the muscle fibers per se.

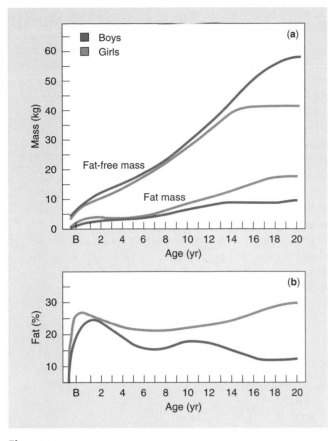

Figure 20.17
Growth Curves for Mass and Percent Fat in Children

Source: From *Growth, Maturation, and Physical Activity* (p. 97) by Robert M. Malina and Claude Bouchard. Champaign, IL: Human Kinetics. Copyright 1991 by Robert M. Malina and Claude Bouchard. Reprinted by permission.

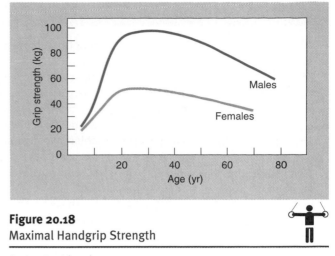

Figure 20.18
Maximal Handgrip Strength

Source: Komi (1992).

Another factor that cannot be ignored is cultural expectations. Many adolescent girls become less active as they grow up, detraining to some extent. Some detraining may be anatomically selective; that is, both males and females of all ages experience gravity equally in walking, climbing stairs, sitting down, and standing up. Yet individuals can selectively avoid upper-body activities, such as lifting heavy loads, opening jars, hammering, and weight lifting. Thus part of the reason for differences in upper-body versus lower-body activities in males and females may be cultural. Future studies may note a change in these relationships as more girls have the opportunity to enter sports at an early age and continue to be active into middle age and old age.

The Elderly

It is well documented that significant declines occur in muscular strength in both males and females from middle age to old age, but the rate of loss varies substantially among muscle groups (Rogers and Evans, 1993). Figure 20.18 represents a generalized change in strength (grip strength) over the normal life span for males and females. From the establishment of peak values in late adolescence or early adulthood, described previously, there is a maintenance of strength until approximately 45–50 yr and then a fairly gradual decline into and beyond the 70s. The decline in muscle strength, in general, amounts to about 15% in the sixth and seventh decades of life and 30% per decade after that (Rogers and Evans, 1993). Relative static endurance (at approximately 40–50% MVC) is similar between older and younger individuals. Figures 20.16 and 20.18 show parallel declines in performance and illustrate the fact that different muscle groups decline at different rates, even between the sexes.

What causes the age-related decline in strength? Three possibilities exist: (1) a loss of muscle mass, (2) a loss of mechanical or contractile properties (namely, fiber type changes, fiber size changes, fiber number changes), and (3) reduced activation of motor units or denervation.

There is no doubt that muscle mass is lost with age. Between the ages of 30 and 70 yr almost 25% of muscle mass is lost in both males and females (Rogers and Evans, 1993). This loss leads to a reduction in force production. There is, however, some evidence to support the contention that the decline in strength with aging is greater than can be accounted for just by the loss of muscle mass. The capacity to exert force per unit of cross-sectional area also declines (Rogers and Evans, 1993).

Early studies using traditional biopsy techniques seemed to show a preferential loss of FT and, especially, FG fibers. Since these fibers are the high-force fibers, this result was intuitively logical.

Focus on Application

✳ Effect of Different Training Programs on Muscle Size and Strength

The cross-sectional area of muscle is related to the force it can generate. This implies that if a training program brings about muscle hypertrophy (increase in size), it will also result in an increase in strength. However, there is considerable uncertainty about the optimal training program to bring out changes in muscle strength, and there has been some speculation that various populations may not experience muscle hypertrophy. Postmenopausal women who are estrogen deficient represent a group of individuals who have tremendous potential to benefit from increased strength because of the relationship between strength and independent living. Yet how this group of individuals would respond to different resistance training programs has not been established. Bemben and colleagues (2000) investigated the effects of a high load (80% of 1-RM; 8 reps) and a high

repetition (40% of 1-RM; 16 reps) resistance training protocols on the musculoskeletal system of early postmenopausal, estrogen-deficient women. The graphs below display changes in only two of the many variables investigated: rectus femoris muscle cross-sectional area (measured by ultrasound) and leg press strength.

These graphs reveal that both training protocols were effective in increasing muscle strength (as measured by the leg press) and increasing muscle cross-sectional area. Based on these data, and other data not presented here, the authors

concluded that both high-load and high-repetition resistance training programs are effective in improving muscular strength and size in post-menopausal women. This finding is important for exercise professionals because it indicates that postmenopausal women do adapt positively to exercise training and that a low-intensity, high-repetition training program can be beneficial for developing muscular fitness in women for whom a high-intensity program may not be appropriate. ✳

Source:

Bemben, et al. (2000)

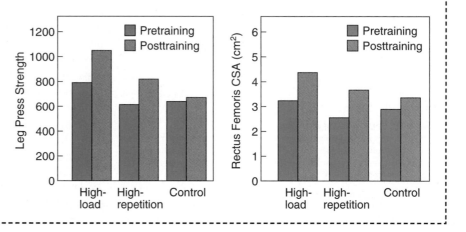

More recent studies utilizing whole-muscle cross-sectional techniques have shown that both ST and FT fibers are lost equally with aging.

As shown in Figure 20.19, the loss of muscle fibers begins at about age 30, and by age 80 a reduction of between 25% and 40% has occurred in females and males (Rogers and Evans, 1993). The genetically predetermined percentages of ST and FT fibers remain constant. The SO fibers appear to maintain their size longer than do FT fibers. Thus, although FT fibers are not lost at a faster rate than SO fibers, they do atrophy faster; and FG fibers atrophy faster than FOG fibers. Since FT fibers are generally the larger fibers, the preferential loss in size of these fibers accounts in large part for the overall decrease in muscle size and strength with aging.

Of great concern is the practical meaning of these changes. Weakened respiratory muscles restrict aerobic activity. Weakened muscles around joints lead to instability, difficulty in restoring balance, and, potentially, falls (Aoyagi and Shephard, 1992). Insufficient strength to get in and out of chairs, carry groceries, or take caps off medicine or food jars can lead to a loss of independent living. The most effective way to prevent these difficulties is by systematic exercise training. Aging of muscles cannot be prevented, but it can be delayed. Thus, maintaining and/or increasing muscular strength, endurance, and power is important for different reasons throughout the life span. However, muscles respond to exercise training in basically the same fashion at all ages; that is, trained muscles produce greater force.

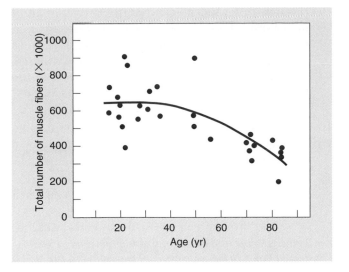

Figure 20.19
Loss of Muscle Fibers with Age

Source: M. A. Rogers & W. J. Evans. Changes in skeletal muscle with aging: Effects of exercise training. In J. O. Holloszy (ed.), *Exercise and Sport Science Reviews* (Vol. 21). Baltimore: Williams & Wilkins, 65–107 (1993). Reprinted by permission.

Heritability of Muscular Function

Many characteristics of an individual, including fitness measures, are partially determined by genetics. The precise extent to which measures of muscle fitness are determined by biological heritability is difficult to determine because of sampling and population variation, methodological differences, and variations in subjects' levels of physical activity (Malina and Bouchard, 1991). However, most studies suggest that genetics are an important determinant of muscle function, with heritability estimates of 20–40% being reported for muscular strength and endurance (Malina and Bouchard, 1991; Pérusse, et al., 1987).

The expression of muscular function is determined largely by the fiber type distribution and metabolic properties of muscle fibers. Both fiber type distribution and muscle content of enzymes that control metabolism have a significant genetic effect (Malina and Bouchard, 1991).

It also appears that genetic variation accounts for a substantial fraction of the individual differences in responses to exercise training (Bouchard, Dionne, et al., 1992; Bouchard, Chagnon, et al., 1989). Individual differences in sensitivity to exercise training are largely inherited, with some individuals being high responders and others being low responders (Bouchard, Dionne, et al., 1992; Bouchard, Chagnon, et al., 1989). These differences are the basis for the individualization principle of training, which states

in part that even when individuals engage in the same training program, different results should be expected.

Summary

1. The force developed when a contracting muscle acts on an object is called muscle tension, whereas the force exerted on the muscle by the object is called the load. In order for a muscle to move a load, the force of muscle tension must exceed the force of the load.

2. In isotonic contractions of muscle fibers, force production is constant as the muscle fiber contracts. In the intact human system such a contraction is practically impossible. Instead, the load is constant but the force produced to move it through the range of motion is not. Thus, the term *dynamic* more accurately describes contraction within the intact human.

3. If movement results from a contraction in which muscle shortening occurs, it is a concentric dynamic contraction. If movement results from a contraction in which muscle lengthening occurs, the contraction is referred to as an eccentric dynamic contraction.

4. In isokinetic contractions of muscle fibers the velocity of contraction is constant. In the intact human the velocity of movement varies with joint angle. Specialized equipment can be used to hold the rate of limb displacement constant, resulting in isokinematic contraction.

5. A muscle fiber contraction that does not result in a meaningful length change in the muscle fiber is termed isometric. An intact fiber has an elastic element, and so some fiber shortening actually occurs even though no limb displacement takes place. Thus, the term *static* is preferable to isometric to describe this type of contraction in humans.

6. The amount of force produced by muscles is affected by neural and mechanical factors. Important mechanical factors include length-tension-angle relationships, force-velocity relationships, elasticity-force relationships, and architectural design.

IP *Muscular–Contraction of Whole Muscles* (pages 1–18)

7. Muscular fatigue results in a loss of muscle function and may be caused by a variety of factors,

which can be described as central or peripheral, or as electrophysiological or biochemical in nature. The cause of muscle fatigue is determined largely by the muscle fiber type and therefore varies with different types of activity.

8. Muscular soreness may result from local ischemia, mechanical trauma, or some combination of these factors.

IP *Muscular–Muscle Metabolism* (pages 1–23)

9. Differences in strength between the sexes are largely due to the greater muscle mass of males. The magnitude of the difference in strength between males and females is influenced by the units used to express strength, the region of the body where strength is measured, and the training status of the individuals.

Review Questions

1. Define isotonic, isokinetic, and isometric contractions. Discuss how they relate to dynamic and static contractions.

2. Diagram the force-length relationship in a muscle fiber. Diagram a strength curve for biceps flexion, knee flexion, and knee extension. Discuss the relationship between the force-length relationship in the muscle fiber and in the whole muscle.

3. Graph the force-velocity relationship in (a) a muscle fiber and in (b) a whole muscle. Identify the eccentric contraction on graph (a) and identify a static contraction on graph (b).

4. Provide a schematic representation of the possible sites of muscular fatigue.

5. Indicate the most probable cause of muscle fatigue for the following categories of exercise: anaerobic sprint, long-term, moderate to heavy, submaximal aerobic, incremental aerobic exercise to maximum, static, and dynamic resistance.

6. Compare and contrast the two models proposed to explain delayed-onset muscle soreness. Is it possible that both models are correct? Why or why not?

7. What are the primary laboratory methods of assessing muscular function? What are the primary field tests to assess muscular function? What are the limitations of the various methods? What determines which is the appropriate test to administer?

8. Compare male and female strength development during childhood and adolescence.

9. Discuss differences in strength between adult males and females. How is the difference in strength affected by the units used to express strength (that is, absolute or relative values)? How does it vary among different regions of the body? What are the most likely causes of sex-related differences in muscular function?

10. What factors account for the age-related decline in muscular strength? Can this loss be minimized or slowed? If so, how?

11. What is the role of genetics in determining an individual's strength or an individual's response to a training program?

For further review and additional study tools, go to The Physiology Place (www.physiologyplace.com) and the Student Study Guide for Exercise Physiology for Health, Fitness, and Performance *by Sharon A. Plowman and Denise L. Smith.*

Passport to the Internet

Visit the following Internet sites to explore further topics and issues related to muscular contraction and human movement. To visit an organization's web site, go to www.physiologyplace.com and click on "Passport to the Internet."

The American College of Sports Medicine As the leading professional organization for individuals in sports medicine and exercise science, the ACSM issues position statements on a number of topics critical to the study of exercise physiology. Search through the ACSM's Position Statements and Current Comments to explore the organization's findings and beliefs on muscle injuries and their prevention and muscle development.

Masters Athlete Physiology & Performance This page is the jumping-off point for an ever-growing section on the physiological basis for endurance performance and training. Many exercise physiologists started out as athletes whose desire for better performance drove them to explore how the human machine worked. This site begins with the basics and allows the reader to explore topics in greater depth.

References

Aoyagi, Y., & R. J. Shephard: Aging and muscle function. *Sports Medicine.* 14(6):376–396 (1992).

Armstrong, R. B.: Mechanisms of exercise-induced delayed onset muscular soreness: A brief review. *Medicine and Science in Sports and Exercise.* 16(6):529–538 (1984).

Armstrong, R. B., M. H. Laughlin, L. Rome, & C. R. Taylor: Metabolism of rats running up and down an incline. *Journal of Applied Physiology.* 55:518–521 (1983).

Asmussen, E.: Observations on experimental muscular soreness. *Acta Rheumatologica Scandinavica.* 2:109–116 (1956).

Bemben, D. A., N. L. Fetters, M. G. Bemben, N. Nabavi, & E. T. Koh: Musculoskeletal responses to high- and low-intensity resistance in early menopausal women. *Medicine and Science in Sports and Exercise.* 32(11):1949–1957 (2000).

Bigland, B., & O. C. J. Lippold: The relation between force, velocity, and integrated electrical activity in human muscles. *Journal of Physiology.* 123:214–224 (1954).

Bonde-Petersen, F., H. G. Knuttgen, & J. Henriksson: Muscle metabolism during exercise with concentric and eccentric contractions. *Journal of Applied Physiology.* 33:792–795 (1972).

Bouchard, C., M. Chagnon, M. Thibault, M. Boulay, M. Marcotte, C. Cote, & J. Simoneau: Muscle genetic variants and relationship with performance and trainability. *Medicine and Science in Sports and Exercise.* 21(1):71–77 (1989).

Bouchard, C., F. T. Dionne, J. A. Simoneau, & M. R. Boulay: Genetics of aerobic and anaerobic performances. *Exercise and Sport Science Reviews.* 20:27–58 (1992).

Conley, M.: Bioenergetics of exercise training. In T. R. Baechle and R. W. Earle (eds.), *Essentials of Strength Training and Conditioning.* Champaign, IL: Human Kinetics, 73–90 (2000).

Coyle, E. F., D. L. Costill, & G. R. Lesmes: Leg extension power and muscle fiber composition. *Medicine and Science in Sports.* 11(1):12–15 (1976).

Davies, C. T. M., & C. Barnes: Negative (eccentric) work. II. Physiological responses to walking uphill and downhill on motor-driven treadmill. *Ergonomics.* 15:121–131 (1972).

DeLorme, T. L., & A. L. Watkins: Techniques of progressive resistance exercise. *Archives of Physical Medicine.* 29:263–273 (1948).

DeVries, H. A., & T. J. Housh: *Physiology of Exercise: For Physical Education, Athletics and Exercise Science.* Madison, WI: Brown & Benchmark (1994).

Edington, D. W., & V. R. Edgerton: *The Biology of Physical Activity.* Boston: Houghton Mifflin, 282 (1976).

Edman, K. A. P.: Contractile performance of skeletal muscle fibers. In P. V. Komi (ed.), *Strength and Power in Sport.* Boston: Blackwell Scientific, 96–114 (1992).

Enoka, R. M.: *Neuromechanical Basis of Kinesiology.* Champaign, IL: Human Kinetics, 31–64 (1988).

Fischer, A., & J. Merhautova: Electromyographic manifestations of individual stages of adapted sports technique. In *Health and Fitness in the Modern World.* Chicago: Athletic Institute, 134–147 (1961).

Goldspink, G.: Cellular and molecular aspects of adaptation in skeletal muscles. In P. V. Komi (ed.), *Strength and Power in Sport.* Boston, MA: Blackwell Scientific, 211–229 (1992).

Hall, S. J., J. Lee, & T. M. Wood: Evaluation of selected sit-up variations for the individual with low back pain. *Journal of Applied Sport Science Research.* 4(2):42–46 (1990).

Halpern, A. A., & E. E. Bleck: Sit-up exercises: An electromyographic study. *Clinical Orthopaedics and Related Research.* 145:172–178 (1979).

Hasson, S. M., J. C. Daniels, J. G. Divine, B. R. Niebuhr, S. Richmond, P. G. Stein, & J. Williams: Effect of ibuprofen use on muscle soreness, damage, and performance: A preliminary investigation. *Medicine and Science in Sports and Exercise.* 25(1):9–17 (1990).

Heyward, V. H.: *Advanced Fitness Assessment and Exercise Prescription.* Champaign, IL: Human Kinetics (1991).

Kelly, D. D.: The role of endorphins in stress-induced analgesia. *Annals of the New York Academy of Sciences.* 398:260–270 (1982).

Komi, P. V.: Physiological and biomechanical correlates of muscle function: Effects of muscle structure and stretch-shortening cycle of force and speed. In R. Terjung (ed.), *Exercise and Sport Sciences Reviews* (Vol. 12). Lexington, MA: Collamore Press, 81–122 (1984).

Komi, P. V.: Stretch-shortening cycle. In P. Komi (ed), *Strength and Power in Sport.* London: Blackwell Scientific, 169–180 (1992).

Kulig, K., J. G. Andrews, & J. G. Hay: Human strength curves. In R. Terjung (ed.), *Exercise and Sport Sciences Reviews* (Vol. 12). Lexington, MA: Collamore Press, 417–466 (1984).

Lauback, L. L.: Comparative muscle strength of men and women: A review of the literature. *Aviation, Space and Environmental Medicine.* 47:534–542 (1976).

Lippold, D. C. J.: The relation between integrated action potentials in a human muscle and its isometric tension. *Journal of Physiology.* 117:492–499 (1952).

MacLaren, D. P., H. Gibson, M. Parry-Billings, & R. H. T. Edwards: A review of metabolic and physiological factors in fatigue. *Exercise and Sport Sciences Reviews.* 17:29–66 (1989).

Malina, R. M., & C. Bouchard: *Growth, Maturation, and Physical Activity.* Champaign, IL: Human Kinetics (1991).

McGlynn, G. H., N. T. Laughlin, & V. Rowe: Effect of electromyographic feedback and static stretching on artificially induced muscle soreness. *American Journal of Physical Medicine.* 58:139–148 (1979).

Pérusse, L., G. Lortie, A. LeBlanc, A. Tremblay, G. Thériault, & C. Bouchard: Genetic and environmental sources of variation in physical fitness. *Annals of Human Biology.* 14:425–434 (198).

Powers, S. K., & E. T. Howley: *Exercise Physiology: Theory and Application to Fitness and Performance.* Dubuque, IA: Brown (1990).

Rogers, M. A., & W. J. Evans: Changes in skeletal muscle with aging: Effects of exercise training. In J. O. Holloszy (ed.), *Exercise and Sport Sciences Reviews* (Vol. 21). Baltimore: Williams & Wilkins, 65–102 (1993).

Sale, D. S.: Neural adaptations to strength training. In P. V. Komi (ed.), *Strength and Power in Sport*. Boston: Blackwell Scientific, 249–265 (1992).

Simonson, E.: *Physiology of Work Capacity and Fatigue*. Springfield, IL: Thomas (1971).

Smith, L. L.: Cytokine hypothesis of overtraining. *Medicine and Science in Sport and Exercise*. 32(2):317–331 (2000).

Stauber, W. T.: Eccentric action of muscles: Physiology, injury, and adaptation. *Exercise and Sport Sciences Reviews*. 17:157–186 (1989).

Thomas, C. L. (ed.): *Taber's Cyclopedia Medical Dictionary*. Philadelphia: Davis (1989).

Webber, L. M., W. C. Pyrnes, T. W. Rowland, & V. L. Foster: Serum creatine kinase activity and delayed onset muscle soreness in pre-pubescent children: A preliminary study. *Pediatric Exercise Science*. 1:351–359 (1989).

Wells, C. L., & S. A. Plowman: Sexual differences in athletic performance: Biological or behavioral? *The Physician and Sports Medicine*. 11(8):52–63 (1983).

Williams, J. H.: Normal musculoskeletal and neuromuscular anatomy, physiology and responses to training. In S. M. Hasson (ed.), *Clinical Exercise Physiology*. St. Louis: Mosby (1994).

Wilmore, J. H.: Alterations in strength, body composition, and anthropometric measurements consequent to a 10-week weight training program. *Medicine and Science in Sports*. 6:133–138 (1974).

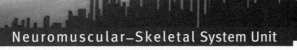
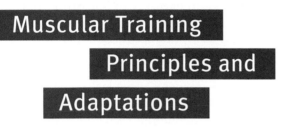

Chapter 21

Muscular Training Principles and Adaptations

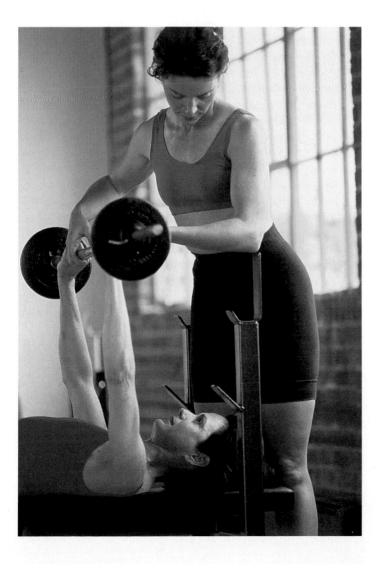

After studying the chapter, you should be able to

- Apply each of the training principles to the development of a resistance training program.
- Describe muscular adaptations to dynamic resistance training and dynamic aerobic endurance training programs.
- Discuss the relationship between muscle function and low-back pain.
- List the effects of anabolic steroid use, and summarize the position of the American College of Sports Medicine on the use of anabolic steroids in athletic competition.

Introduction

The previous chapters have provided a basis for understanding how isolated muscle fibers contract and how intact muscles contract to produce coordinated movements. This chapter discusses the specific applications of the training principles for the development of muscular fitness and the training adaptations that occur as a result of an exercise training program. The final section addresses the applications of this information to the problems of low-back pain and the use of anabolic steroids.

Although it is possible to develop a training program using static contractions, in reality such programs are rare. Therefore, this section will be limited to dynamic resistance and isokinetic training programs. The term *resistance training program* will be used as an inclusive term encompassing dynamic resistance and isokinetic training unless otherwise specified.

Overview of Resistance Training

Resistance training is a systematic program of exercises involving the exertion of force against a load used to develop strength, endurance, and/or hypertrophy of the muscular system (Davies and Barnes, 1972). It is commonly referred to as weight training. Resistance training is used by a wide range of individuals, including those seeking to improve overall health, improve athletic performance, rehabilitate an injury, change their physical appearance, or compete in power lifting or bodybuilding contests. Resistance training is a recommended component of a well-rounded fitness program for healthy adults. A resistance training program should be individualized, be progressive, and involve all of the major muscle groups (American College of Sports Medicine [ACSM], 1998b).

Resistance training—if done under skilled adult supervision with proper instruction in form, breathing, body mechanics, and prescription of loads—can be enjoyed by all individuals and carries relatively low risk of harm for prepubescent children (approximately 7–13 yr of age). However, the desire of the child should be taken into account, and, moreover, resistance training should be only one of a variety of activities and sports that the child participates in. Note that children should not participate in competitive

---

Resistance Training A systematic program of exercises involving the exertion of force against a load used to develop strength, endurance, and/or hypertrophy of the muscular system.

---

weight lifting, power lifting, and bodybuilding. It is also important to maintain realistic expectations.

Application of the Training Principles

The training principles that govern a safe and effective resistance training program are the same principles that guide other types of exercise programs.

Specificity

As in any training program, a plan for muscular fitness must be specific to the goals of the individual. These goals may include the development of muscular strength, muscular endurance, power, muscle hypertrophy, or any combination of the above.

Muscles respond specifically to the type of contraction being performed and to the load imposed. Many sports, including basketball, football, hockey, volleyball, etc., utilize dynamic resistance programs to increase muscle strength and mass. Other sports, including swimming, are more likely to utilize isokinetic training programs in an attempt to develop strength through a specified range of motion.

Resistance training is also specific to the muscle groups being trained. Therefore, a resistance training program should include at least one exercise for all the major muscle groups of the body (Fleck and Kraemer, 1987). To avoid fatigue, it is often recommended that exercises be arranged in a specific order, alternating lower-body exercises with exercises of the upper body. This tactic allows the muscles to recover between exercises or exercise sessions. Generally, large muscle groups should be exercised first, followed by smaller muscle groups. For example, if an exerciser is interested in working the latissimus dorsi (lats) and the biceps, the lats should be worked first (pull-downs), because they involve a larger muscle group. This schedule helps to ensure the fatigue of the smaller muscle group (the biceps), but it does not limit the work that can be performed by the larger muscle group (the lats).

The amount of stress, or load, applied to the muscle will determine, to a large extent, the response of the muscle. A muscle that is exposed to near-maximal load will develop greater strength than a muscle that is required to repeat many repetitions of a lighter load. In contrast, the muscle that performs many repetitions of a lighter load will develop relatively more muscular endurance than one exposed to a small number of near-maximal repetitions.

Specificity also appears to apply to the velocity of contraction for isokinetic exercises (Perrin, 1993). Exercise performed at slow velocities tends to produce increases in torque specific to the training velocity. Training at high velocities tends to increase strength at and below the exercise velocity and, thus, is not as specific as slow-velocity training. Furthermore, it is a misconception that the velocity of isokinetic exercise should be specific to athletic events (Perrin, 1993). In reality, the angular velocities of joint movements found in many athletic events (such as throwing) far exceed what can be performed during isokinetic exercise.

Overload

The successful application of the overload principle, as it applies to resistance training, necessitates the manipulation of intensity (load), frequency, and duration (number of repetitions, sets, and rest periods). Of these variables, intensity appears to have the greatest effect on the outcome of the program. There is an inverse relationship between the load (weight) that can be lifted and the number of repetitions that can be performed. By definition, the amount of weight that can be lifted one time is the one repetition maximum (1 rep max; 1-RM). Figure 21.1 provides some guidelines for estimating the number of repetitions that are possible at various loads, expressed as a percentage of 1-RM (Baechle, et al., 2000). When using Figure 21.1, keep in mind that the number of repetitions that can be performed at any given load is only an estimate. The actual number of repetitions that can be performed at any given load varies among individuals (resistance-trained athletes are commonly able to exceed the predicted repetitions) and among muscle groups.

Historically, the development of programs based on the overload principle began in 1948 when DeLorme and Watkins introduced *progressive resistance exercise*. The DeLorme and Watkins program uses 30 repetitions per training session for each muscle group exercised. The 30 repetitions are broken down into 3 sets of 10 repetitions (reps) each, as follows:

> set 1 = 10 repetitions at 50% of 10-RM
>
> set 2 = 10 repetitions at 75% of 10-RM
>
> set 3 = 10 repetitions at 100% of 10-RM

Since the 1950s, considerable research has been done to determine the optimal number of repetitions and sets, the workload, and the frequency necessary to develop muscular strength, endurance, and power. This research has resulted in the development of many training systems.

There is no single combination of repetitions and sets that produces the best results; rather, the ideal number of sets is determined by individual goals and differences. To elicit improvements in both muscular

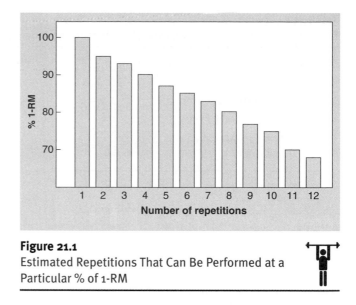

Figure 21.1
Estimated Repetitions That Can Be Performed at a Particular % of 1-RM

strength and endurance, the American College of Sports Medicine recommends that a minimum of one set of 8–12 repetitions be performed with each of the major muscle groups 2–3 d·wk^{-1}. It may be more appropriate for older or more frail individuals to perform 10–15 repetitions per muscle group. Although greater gains in strength may be obtained when more than one set of exercise is performed, for the general public, the incremental strength gains associated with additional sets is offset by the increased time required to complete the exercise and the increased risk of orthopedic injury. However, athletes and individuals wishing to optimize muscular fitness may benefit from performing more than one set.

Table 21.1 provides some guidelines for manipulating the overload variables to obtain different training goals. In general, if the primary goal is the development of muscular strength, it is advantageous to perform relatively few (≤6) repetitions at a high load (≥85%). Research indicates that 3–6 repetitions per set for 3–5 sets is probably best for developing muscular strength (Fleck and Kraemer, 1987). If the primary goal of the resistance training program is the development of power, then high loads and few repetitions should be performed. Power events can be categorized into those events requiring a single explosive effort and those requiring multiple efforts. If the goal is to produce as much power as possible in a single lift, then only 1–2 repetitions are recommended at a load equaling 80–90% of 1-RM. If the primary goal of training is muscle hypertrophy, then a relatively high number of repetitions should be performed (6–12) at 67–85% of 1-RM. If the primary goal is muscular endurance, a high number of repetitions (≥12) should be performed with a lesser load. Keep in mind that the muscle must still be "overloaded" in order to

Table 21.1
Guidelines for Manipulating Overload Variables for Athletic Training Goals

Training Goal	Load (%1-RM)	Repetitions	Sets	Rest Period (min)
Strength	≥85%	≤6	2–6	2–5
Power: Single-effort event	80–90	1–2	3–5	2–5
Power: Multiple-effort event	75–85	3–5	3–5	2–5
Hypertrophy	67–85	6–12	3–6	.5–1.5
Muscular endurance	≤67	≥12	2–3	≤.5

Source: Modified from Baechle, Earle, & Wathen (2000).

achieve a positive adaptation. If strength gains are sought, exercise intensity must be at least 60% of maximum. Gains in endurance can be achieved with an intensity of 30% of maximum if the muscle group is exercised until fatigued (Cureton, et al., 1988). Figure 21.2 depicts a theoretical continuum for the development of muscular strength and power, and muscular endurance (Fleck and Kraemer, 1987).

For isokinetic exercise, however, the duration of a single exercise bout appears to be more important than the total amount of work performed or the number of repetitions completed. Thus, isokinetic exercises are generally based on duration of exercise rather than the number of repetitions.

The length of rest periods between exercise sets is also related to the overload placed on the muscles. If the goal is maximal strength gains, relatively long (several minutes) rest periods should be used between sets. If endurance is the primary goal, shorter (less than 30 sec) rest periods should be used between sets (Baechle, et al., 2000; Fleck and Kraemer, 1987).

The frequency of resistance training varies with the goals and training status of the individual. Additionally, frequency of training will vary, depending on training stage (periodization). Obviously, a competitive bodybuilder will train more frequently than an adult fitness participant hoping to derive the health-related benefits of resistance training. The American College of Sports Medicine currently recommends that strengthening exercises should be done two to three times a week to achieve the health-related benefits of such exercises (ACSM, 1998b). Training between 2 and 4 days a week appears to be most popular with weight lifters. Twice a week is considered the minimum requirement necessary to improve muscular strength; training less than twice a week may predispose the individual to muscle soreness and injury. It is common for athletes who train 4 days a week to follow a program that alternates an upper-body workout day with a lower-body workout day, so that 2 days a week are devoted to the upper body and 2 days a week to the lower body.

Competitive resistance-trained athletes often follow a training program whereby they train 3–4 days consecutively and then take a day off. When utilizing this type of program, they follow a split routine: Each muscle group is exercised only twice a week. A split routine emphasizes a single muscle group in a workout. This muscle group is then rested for 48–72 hr. A variation of this program is the double-split routine in which two exercise sessions are performed on each workout day.

The frequency of training also depends on the periodization plan of the individual. An athlete may engage in resistance training four to six times per week in the general preparatory stage (off-season), three to four times per week in the specific preparatory stage (preseason), one to two times per week in the competitive season (in-season), and one to three times per week in the active-rest stage of periodization.

The duration—the amount of time spent in the weight room—will largely be determined by the number of repetitions, the sets, and the number of different exercises performed. The average duration is 20–30 min per session, although many people spend more time than that. The *training volume* for resistance exercise is equal to the total amount of weight lifted in the training session, and can be calculated as the number of sets multiplied by the number of repetitions multiplied by the load (Baechle, et al., 2000; Tesch, 1992). Larger volumes of training are important not only to individuals seeking greater strength gains but also to those seeking a decrease in percentage of body fat. Novice lifters, however, should avoid excessive volume in order to prevent injury, particularly early in the program. It is prudent to begin a program at a low intensity and a low volume and to increase the amount of training after the body has had time to adapt to the training stress.

Overloading for prepubescent children should involve the same factors as outlined for adults, with some modification. A beginning program should stress learning proper form, techniques, and safety considerations, such as spotting (National Strength and

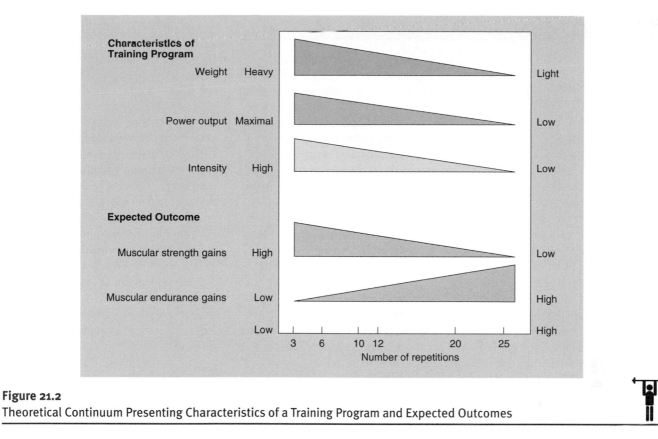

Figure 21.2
Theoretical Continuum Presenting Characteristics of a Training Program and Expected Outcomes

Conditioning Association, 1996). The equipment chosen should fit the child, which may mean that some exercise machines (designed primarily for adult males) should not be used. Exercises should include major muscle groups and work both agonist and antagonist muscles at each joint. Isolated eccentric training should be avoided (Blimkie, 1988). Children should be started on a program consisting of a single set for the first several (2–6) weeks while skill development is being emphasized. Rest periods should be between 2 and 3 min. Low-intensity work of 12–15 RM is best as a starting point. Maximal lifts should be avoided. A frequency of two to three times per week is recommended (Kraemer, et al., 1989). Virtually no information is available on a preferred order of the exercises for children.

Rest/Recovery/Adaptation

Muscles adapt to the stress placed on them. The most obvious changes that result from a resistance training program are increases in muscle strength and muscle size. However, the extent to which muscles adapt to training by becoming stronger and bigger depends on the training program that is followed. For example, at some point during a resistance training program, individuals will realize that their initial 10-repetition maximum can now be lifted more than 10 times. This result indicates that adaptation has occurred. The rate of adaptation depends on several factors, including rest periods and adequate diet, and it may not be the same for all muscle groups trained. The importance of rest (recovery) between exercise sessions to allow for the positive adaptations of exercise training cannot be overstressed. At least one day of rest should follow a day of training for a particular muscle group. Adequate rest periods and alternating heavy and light days are important to allow the training adaptations to occur and to prevent injury and soreness. As mentioned earlier, many competitive athletes who lift high volumes will allow 72-hr rest periods before training the same muscle group again.

Adaptation occurs in children as it does in adults. Careful monitoring of recovery between sessions is probably even more important for children to make sure that adequate rest (at least 48 hr) occurs.

Progression

Once the body has adapted to the current training level, exercise stress should be increased as dictated by the overload principle if further increases in strength are desired. This principle is the basis of progressive resistance exercise.

Focus on Application

✳ Does Supervision of a Strength Training Program Make a Difference?

Many individuals seek the assistance of an exercise professional to implement their training programs. A personal trainer may provide important information and advice and serve as a motivator. But does the supervision of a training program lead to improved performance? Mazzetti and colleagues (2000) performed a study that investigated the influence of direct supervision of resistance training on strength performance. Their results suggest that supervision does make a difference.

These researchers randomly assigned volunteers with 1–2 yr of lifting experience to a supervised group or an unsupervised group for a 12-week training period. The supervised group was trained one-on-one by a personal trainer. The unsupervised group attended one private fitness consultation at the beginning of the training and performed subsequent training without direct supervision, although the personal trainer was present at all training sessions (to answer questions concerning the program and to confirm the participants' adherence to the program). Both groups followed identical periodized resistance training programs consisting of preparatory (10–12-RM), hypertrophy (8–10-RM), strength (5–8-RM), and peaking (3–6-RM)

phases using free weights and variable resistance equipment. At the end of the 12 weeks there was no difference between the number of training sessions, sets, or repetitions performed per week for the squat and bench exercises. However, the supervised group had lifted more weight per set than the unsupervised. Both training groups experienced increases in strength, but the supervised group had greater increases than the unsupervised group. These results clearly show that personal training (one-on-one supervision) can affect the strength gains achieved by participants, even if they have been lifting on their own for 1–2 yr.   ✳

Source:

Mazetti, et al. (2000).

When indicated, progression should be done gradually. Progression can be accomplished by increasing the load, the repetitions, the number of sets, or the frequency of the workout, or by decreasing the rest period between sets. The variables that are most often manipulated are the load and the number of repetitions. Again, the choice will depend largely on the individual's goals. If strength is the primary goal, then a heavier weight should be used. If endurance is the goal, then the same weight should be lifted more times. It is not uncommon for a combination of these two variables to be used. For instance, many people will begin with a weight they can lift for 6 repetitions. As they adapt to this stress, they will progress to 7 repetitions, then 8 repetitions, and so on. Once they can perform 8–10 repetitions, they will increase the weight to something they can again only lift for 6 repetitions. As recommended earlier, a novice lifter should begin by doing more repetitions with a lighter load. Once the body has adapted, the individual can lift heavier weights.

Progression in prepubescent children should be done slowly, especially in terms of intensity. Moderate loads of 10–12-RM are recommended for the first 2 to 6 months of a program; after that, heavier intensities of 8–10-RM can be introduced. Loads heavier than 6-RM are never recommended for children, and the 8–10-RM load gives a safety zone. Shorter rest periods can be introduced, but frequency should be maintained at three times per week (Kraemer, et al., 1989).

Individualization

The first step in individualizing a resistance training program is to determine the individual goals of the participant. Once the individual's goals are established, the next step is to evaluate his or her current strength level. This assessment is usually done by determining the individual's one repetition maximum (1-RM). A 1-RM should be established for each muscle group exercised; it is then used to determine the work intensity. For example, a program may call for an individual to do 6 repetitions per set at 80% of the 1-RM.

The final step is determining the training cycle to be used. This technique is often referred to as the periodization of training (see Chapter 1), and it is a common step among athletes who use resistance training to supplement their training programs for athletic competition. For instance, a player who is using resistance training as part of conditioning for basketball would follow a different weight training program during the transition phase, general preparatory phase, and specific preparatory phase than during the competitive season. Periodization is also important to individuals who use weight training to maintain health-related muscular fitness; it prevents boredom by changing the training program on a regular basis. Competitive resistance-trained athletes also use periodization techniques to vary their training and to

Table 21.2
Developing a Resistance Training Program

Step	Special Considerations	Applicable Training Principles
1. Goal identification	Desired outcome	Specificity
	Component of muscular fitness to be stressed	Individualization
	Mode of contraction most appropriate	
	Muscle groups to be stressed	
2. Evaluation of initial strength or muscular endurance levels	Each muscle group to be used	Specificity
	Proper lifting techniques	
3. Determination of the training cycle (periodization)	Prevention of boredom	Adaptation
	Peaking	Progression
		Plateau/Retrogression
		Individualization
4. Determination of the training system (design of a single session)	Exercises to be included	Specificity
	Load	Overload
	Number of sets	Individualization
	Rest periods	Warm-up and cool-down
	Order in which exercises are to be done	
	Warm-up and cool-down	

prepare for a peak season. Table 21.2 provides an outline for developing a training program based on the individualization of the training principles.

Even if different individuals follow the same program, training effects should be expected to occur at different rates. The principle of individualization states that responses to exercise vary among individuals because of factors unique to the individual. In terms of resistance training, these factors include age, body size and type, initial strength, and, perhaps most importantly, genetic makeup (including fiber type distribution).

A coach or exercise leader must be sensitive to the differences in the rate of individual adaptation because it directly affects the progression of training. Unfortunately, it is a common mistake for a coach to design a program for the entire team and expect adaptations to occur at the same rate. The result is often frustration on the part of the coach and the athletes and sometimes even overtraining and/or injuries.

Individually prescribing a resistance training program is probably more important for the prepubescent child than for the adult. Children are growing both physiologically and psychologically, and the rate of growth varies greatly among children. Periodization can be used with children as well as adults (Tesch, 1992). Competition between individuals should be discouraged for children.

Maintenance

Once a desired level of muscular strength and endurance is achieved, it can be maintained by reduced amounts of work provided the intensity (workload) is maintained; that is, as long as the individual continues to lift the same weight, he or she can maintain strength with only one session per week. A reasonable program would allow individuals to train at a similar workload but with fewer days per week or at a lesser volume to maintain muscular strength and endurance.

Little information is available on maintenance in prepubescent children (Blimkie, 1988). One study that is available showed that 1 day of high-intensity training for 8 weeks was not sufficient to maintain gains achieved in a 20-week program.

Retrogression/Plateau/Reversibility

Despite the best laid plans of coaches, training improvements do not occur in a linear fashion. Even with progressively increasing workloads, there will be times when performance stays at the same level (plateau) or shows a decrease (retrogression). The causes may be overtraining or individual differences. If overtraining is suspected, it is wise to include more rest days or include light days in the training regimen. Additionally, it may be beneficial to consider altering the training program by using the periodization technique discussed earlier.

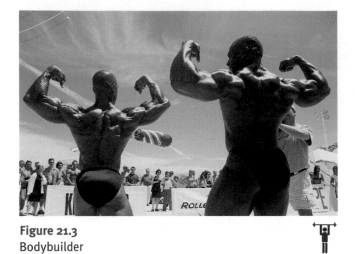

Figure 21.3
Bodybuilder

A goal of bodybuilding is to "sculpt" the body.

Detraining (reversibility) occurs when an individual ceases to train. The rate of detraining depends on the level of strength and endurance the individual has attained. Muscular strength is maintained to a greater degree during detraining than is muscular endurance. Although much of the individual's strength remains after discontinuation of a resistance program, detraining is evidenced on a cellular level. This evidence suggests that there are changes in the size and metabolic properties of the muscle fibers following detraining.

The impact of detraining in children is confounded by the concomitant effects of growth-related strength increases. The actual gains above this growth level do appear to be lost once training ceases (Blimkie, 1988).

Warm-Up and Cool-Down

A proper warm-up raises the body temperature and is often recommended to prevent injury and muscle soreness. Although it has not been conclusively proven that a warm-up will decrease the incidence of injury, there is evidence that is consistent with this theory. An increase in temperature decreases the viscosity of the joint capsule. Increased temperatures also increase the speed of muscle contraction and relaxation and enzymatic reactions (Enoka, 1988).

Warm-ups for resistance training may be considered either general or specific and are recommended for weight lifting and isokinetic exercises (Perrin, 1993). A general warm-up involves the major muscles of the body; it is similar to the warm-up used for aerobic activities and includes such activities as jumping rope or jogging. Specific warm-up activities for weight training involve performing the same lifts that are

part of the normal program but at a weight well below the training level. The duration and the intensity of the warm-up need to be suited to the individual and to the task to be performed. A proper warm-up should cause a rise in core body temperature of .5–1.0°C but should not be so strenuous that it causes fatigue. Generally, a warm-up is considered adequate when the individual begins to sweat.

A cool-down period, followed by stretching, is recommended after a training session. Cool-down may prevent muscle soreness and lead to an increase in flexibility, an aspect of muscular fitness that is often overlooked in resistance training programs. Cooling down is important in preventing venous pooling of blood in the lower extremities.

Warm-up and cool-down are just as important for children as for adults. The same pattern of activities should be followed to increase body temperature and to stretch the muscles.

Specific Application of Training Principles to Bodybuilding

The sport of competitive bodybuilding has gained great popularity in the past two decades. Furthermore, many individuals who initiate resistance training programs do so to enhance their physique. For many athletes weight lifting is not only about gaining strength but also about "sculpting" the body.

The goals of bodybuilding are to develop superior muscularity and mass, to develop symmetry and harmony between different body parts, and to enhance muscle density and visual separation of muscles (Tesch, 1992). The effect of such programs is shown in Figure 21.3. In order to achieve their goals, bodybuilders follow specific training strategies and a strict diet.

The training strategies of bodybuilders are designed to increase muscle hypertrophy. Muscle strength is not the primary goal, although strength undoubtedly increases as a result of training. Bodybuilders typically use loads that can be lifted 6–12 times, whereas power lifters lift heavier loads but complete fewer repetitions. Bodybuilders commonly end each set with muscular fatigue or failure; that is, the lifter performs the exercise until the muscles are no longer capable of lifting the weight. Bodybuilders typically use short rest periods (1–2 min) between sets and perform as many as 15–20 sets per muscle group per session for smaller muscle groups. As many as 6 repetitions may be performed with larger muscle groups. Therefore, bodybuilders use a very high volume of training.

The frequency of training for bodybuilders varies; however, split routines or double splits are most common among competitive bodybuilders. These programs typically allow for training on 3 or 4 consecutive days, followed by a day of rest. This schedule allows for more than 48 hr of recovery for each muscle group. Although this program is common, there is little scientific evidence to suggest it is the best training schedule. Furthermore, the overall cycle of training (periodization) is important to bodybuilders. Bodybuilders commonly do more strength training in the off-season in order to build muscle mass. As the season approaches, the load is reduced and more repetitions are performed in an attempt to gain muscle symmetry.

Diet is perhaps as important to the success of bodybuilders as is an appropriate training program. In order to enhance muscle definition and promote visual separation of the various muscle groups, bodybuilders maintain a low percentage of body fat through a combination of training and diet. Bodybuilders follow a strict low-fat diet, despite the large number of calories they consume. The practice of **cutting** *or ripping* refers to the bodybuilder's attempt to decrease body fat and body water to very low levels prior to competition in order to increase muscle definition.

Neuromuscular Adaptations to Training

This section addresses how skeletal muscles adapt as a result of resistance training and dynamic endurance training. Emphasis will be placed on the changes that occur within muscle tissue.

Neuromuscular Adaptations to Resistance Training Programs

The hallmark adaptations to resistance training are increases in muscle strength and muscle size (hypertrophy). There is a wide variation in strength gains following a resistance training program, owing largely to differences in initial strength and the training program followed. On average, formerly sedentary men and women achieve approximately a 25–30% improvement in strength after up to 6 months of training (ACSM, 1998b).

The initiation of a resistance training program typically results in strength gains within the first few weeks despite little or no change in muscle mass, suggesting that neural factors are largely responsible for early strength gains. Figure 21.4 provides a schematic representation of the relative roles of neural and muscular adaptations that contribute to strength

---

> **Cutting** Decreasing body fat and body water content to very low levels in order to increase muscle definition.

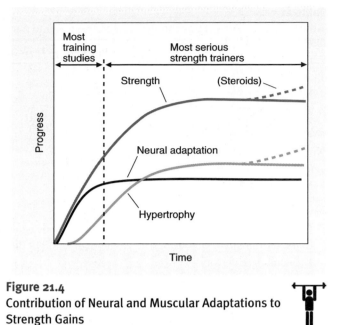

Figure 21.4
Contribution of Neural and Muscular Adaptations to Strength Gains

Source: D. G. Sale. Neural adaptation to resistance training. *Medicine and Science in Sports and Exercise.* 20(suppl.):S135–S145 (1988). Reprinted with permission of Williams & Wilkins.

gains. Neural adaptation is related to increased neural drive to the muscle, as indicated by EMG studies; increased synchronization of the motor units; and an inhibition of the protective mechanism of the Golgi tendon organs (Fleck and Kraemer, 1987).

Table 21.3 summarizes neuromuscular adaptations to resistance training and compares these adaptations to aerobic training. Participation in resistance training programs typically results in increased strength. The increased strength results from neural changes and increased muscle size. Resistance training increases the ability to activate motor units; thus, greater force can be produced. Resistance training is also associated with an inhibition of the muscle reflexes that inhibit muscle contraction in response to high-force production (see the discussion of Golgi tendon organ, Chapter 22). The increased cross-sectional area of muscle results primarily from an increase in the fiber area of both ST and FT muscle fibers. However, FT fiber area appears to be increased to a greater extent.

The magnitude of the changes seen in muscles is specific to the muscle group being tested and depends on the training program followed. The muscle hypertrophy that occurs is due to an increase in the total contractile protein, an increase in the size and number of the myofibrils per fiber, and an increase in the amount of connective tissue surrounding the muscle fibers (Rogers and Evans, 1993). Interestingly, there is some evidence that strength gains that result from

Table 21.3
Neuromuscular Adaptations to Resistance Training and Aerobic Training

Variable	Resistance Training	Aerobic Training
Performance		
Muscle strength	Increase	No change
Muscle power	Increase	No change
Aerobic power ($\dot{V}O_2$max)	No change or slight increase	Increase
Neural Adaptations		
Motor unit recruitment	Increase	No change
Neural inhibition	Decrease	No change
Muscle Structure Adaptations		
Fiber size	Increase	No change or slight increase
Capillary density	No change or slight decrease	Increase
Mitochondria density	Decrease	Increase

isokinetic training can occur in the absence of muscle hypertrophy (Perrin, 1993). This may be due to the absence of an eccentric mode of contraction during these training protocols.

In addition to an increase in strength and hypertrophy, metabolic adaptations occur within the muscle fibers that increase the ability of the muscle to generate ATP. These changes are characterized by an increased ability to generate ATP from anaerobic metabolism; hence, there is an increase in phosphocreatine (PC) and glycogen stores, an increase in the enzyme (creatine phosphokinase) that breaks down PC, and an increase in the rate-limiting enzyme (PFK) of glycolysis. Refer to Chapters 3 and 4 for a review of anaerobic metabolism if necessary.

Male-Female Comparisons

Although men are typically stronger than women, both sexes respond to resistance training in a similar fashion (Cureton, et al., 1988; Tesch, 1992; Wilmore, 1974). Typically, sedentary men and women who initiate a training program can attain strength gains of 25–30%, although the actual increase in strength varies among muscle groups and is affected by the initial strength of the individual (ACSM, 1998b). Figure 21.5 shows the percentage change in muscle strength for men and women for the elbow flexors, elbow extensors, knee flexor, and knee extensors after 16 weeks of participation in a weight training program (Cureton, et al., 1988). In addition to having similar patterns of strength gains, the men and women in this study both showed similar changes in muscle cross-sectional area (as determined from CT scans). The cross-sectional area of the upper arm

muscles for the men and women increased 15% and 23%, respectively, after the 16-week training program. Although the men had a greater cross-sectional area than the women, both before and after training, both sexes increased the muscle strength and the muscle cross-sectional area of the upper arm following training.

Children and Resistance Training

Resistance training produces strength gains in prepubescents and adolescents and is recognized as an important component of youth fitness programs (Falk and Tenenbaum, 1996; National Strength and Conditioning Association, 1996). Historically, exercise physiologists believed that resistance training programs would not increase strength in prepubescent children owing to their lack of testosterone. Results from early studies seemed to confirm this belief. However, these studies were based on low weights and low total volume of training. Newer studies that used higher-intensity loads, volumes, and duration have shown that children can increase strength, statically and isokinetically. The literature suggests that strength gains of approximately 30% are typical following short-term resistance training programs (up to 20 weeks) in children. Increases in strength appear to be relatively consistent between prepubescents and adolescents. There is no apparent difference in the relative strength increases between boys and girls (Falk and Tenenbaum, 1996; National Strength and Conditioning Association, 1996).

In one research study, fourteen 8–12-yr-old boys and girls trained twice a week for 8 weeks using 3 sets of 10–15 repetitions on 5 exercises with intensities

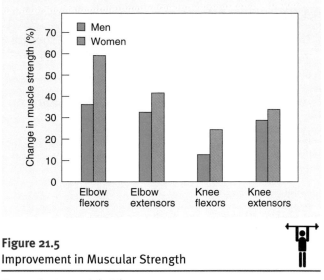

Figure 21.5
Improvement in Muscular Strength

Source: Cureton, et al. (1988).

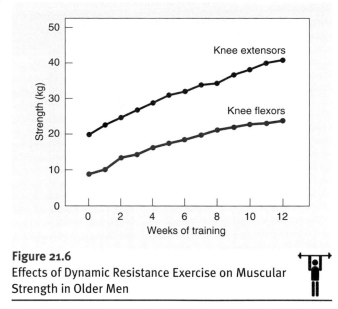

Figure 21.6
Effects of Dynamic Resistance Exercise on Muscular Strength in Older Men

Source: M. A. Rogers & W. J. Evans. Changes in skeletal muscle with aging: Effects of exercise training. In J. O. Holloszy (ed.), *Exercise and Sport Science Reviews* (Vol. 21). Baltimore: Williams & Wilkins, 65–102 (1993). Reprinted by permission.

varying between 50% and 100% of their 10-RM (Faigenbaum, et al., 1993). Following the training period these subjects increased their strength by 74.3%, whereas a control group increased their strength by 13%. The increase in strength reported in the control group was probably related to growth and maturation of the subjects.

Although the improvement in strength in this study is consistent with improvements documented in adults, the underlying physiological adaptations that account for increased strength appear to be somewhat different. It does not appear that resistance training induces muscle fiber hypertrophy in preadolescents. Changes do occur in the ability of the nervous system to activate motor units, as shown by increased EMG activity with training. Improved motor coordination is also thought to be a contributing neural factor. Thus, neurological factors rather than muscular factors are believed to be responsible for the strength changes in this age group (Blimkie, 1988).

The Elderly and Resistance Training

Resistance training is also safe and effective in increasing muscular strength and cross-sectional area in elderly individuals (Brown and Wilmore, 1974; Charette, et al., 1991; Frontera, et al., 1991; Larsson, 1982). In fact, older men and women show similar or even greater strength gains than young individuals after resistance training (Fleck and Kraemer, 1987). Resistance training is a recommended component of fitness programs for the elderly and is considered important for minimizing or reversing physical frailty, which is prevalent among the elderly (ACSM, 1998a;

Falk and Tenenbaum, 1996). Figure 21.6 shows the improvements in dynamic strength of the knee extensors (quadriceps) and the knee flexors (hamstrings) following the 12 weeks of training in older men (Frontera, et al., 1991). By the end of the training period, both muscle groups had increased by over 100%. Additionally, these men demonstrated an 11% increase in muscle cross-sectional area, which was accompanied by a 34% increase in ST fiber area and a 28% increase in FT fiber area. A similar response to resistance training has been shown in older women (Wilmore, 1974). For example, following a resistance training program of 12 weeks, elderly women had improved their strength from 28% to 115%, depending on the muscle group tested (Charette, et al., 1991).

In addition to being beneficial to healthy older individuals, resistance training is also beneficial for frail, institutionalized men and women (Fiatarone, et al, 1990). A group of 90–100-yr-old men and women who engaged in a resistance training program for 8 weeks increased their strength by 174% (from an average initial value of 8 kg to 21 kg). Additionally, these subjects increased the muscle cross-sectional area by 15%. These improvements demonstrate rather remarkably the capacity of the muscular system to adapt to progressive resistance exercise as long as a person is willing to participate in a program that utilizes an appropriate intensity of stimulus.

Figure 21.7 summarizes the changes in muscle strength (a) and cross-sectional area (b) that occurs in

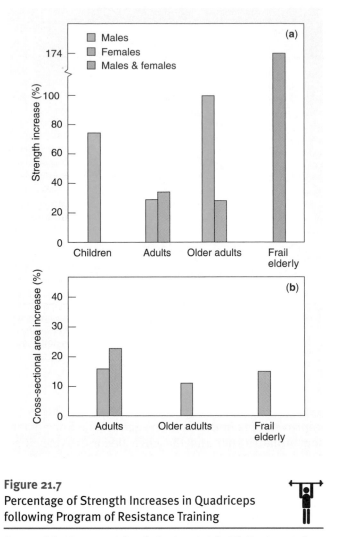

Figure 21.7
Percentage of Strength Increases in Quadriceps following Program of Resistance Training

Sources: Faigenbaum, et al. (1993); Cureton, et al. (1988); Frontera, et al. (1991); Charette, et al. (1991); Fiatarone, et al. (1990).

A Question of Understanding

The table gives data for initial strength and final strength in the biceps following a 16-week strength training program for older adults.

Name	Initial Strength (kg)	Final Strength (kg)
Mary	45	54
Dick	47	50
Jim	68	80
Ben	62	68
Ralph	84	88
Debbie	40	55

1. Calculate strength gain for each of the individuals (final − initial).
2. Calculate percentage improvement [(final − initial)/(initial) × 100].

Check your answer in Appendix D.

the quadriceps for males and females of various ages following a resistance training program. These values indicate a percentage change from initial values; thus, they imply neither that females are stronger than males as adults nor that the elderly are stronger than the younger subjects. In fact, those who are weakest initially may be in the best position to show a percentage improvement. Complete the Question of Understanding box to check your understanding of this concept.

Muscular Adaptations to Dynamic Aerobic Endurance Training Programs

Muscle fibers respond differently to aerobic training than they do to resistance training. Aerobic training is characterized by an increased aerobic power ($\dot{V}O_2$max) with little or no change in muscle strength or power. Similarly, the structural and metabolic

changes in muscle fibers facilitate the production of large quantities of ATP, primarily by aerobic means, following an aerobic training program.

Dynamic endurance training results in an increase in ST fiber size in adult males and no change in FT fiber size (Gollnick, et al., 1972). There is also evidence to suggest that dynamic endurance training can result in the transformation of FG muscle fibers to FOG muscle fibers (Fleck and Kraemer, 1987). Dynamic endurance training in older men and women also results in an increase in the cross-sectional area of the ST fibers (averaging 12%) and an increase in the percentage of FOG fibers (Coggan, et al., 1990).

Special Applications
Muscular Strength and Endurance and Low-Back Pain

At some point in their lives, 60–80% of all individuals experience low-back pain (LBP). The condition is disabling to 1–5% of the population. Most cases of LBP occur between the ages of 25 and 60 yr, but 12–26% of children and adolescents are LBP sufferers. Males and females are affected equally.

Neither exact causes nor established risk factors for LBP have been identified. However, there has been and still is great interest in the link between muscular fitness and the absence or occurrence of LBP. The interest is high enough that some tests of health-related physical fitness have included sit-and-reach, sit-ups or curl-ups, and trunk extension tests as means of testing low-back function. The theoretical

Table 21.4

Theoretical Relationship Between Physical Fitness Components and Healthy or Unhealthy Low-Back or Spinal Function

Physical Fitness Component (Neuromuscular)	Normal Anatomical Function in Low-Back: Healthy	Dysfunction	Results of Dysfunction: Unhealthy
Lumbar flexibility	Allows the lumbar curve to almost be reversed in forward flexion	Inflexible	Disrupts forward and lateral movement; places excessive stretch on hamstrings, leading to low-back and hamstring pain
Hamstring flexibility	Allows anterior rotation (tilt) of the pelvis in forward flexion and posterior rotation in the sitting position	Inflexible	Restricts anterior pelvic rotation and exaggerates posterior tilt; both cause increased disk compression; excessive stretching causes strain and pain
Hip flexor flexibility	Allows achievement of neutral pelvic position	Inflexible	Exaggerates anterior pelvic tilt if not counteracted by strong abdominal muscles, thereby increasing disk compression
Abdominal strength or endurance	Maintains pelvic position; reinforces back extensor fascia and pulls it laterally on forward flexion, providing support	Weak, easily fatigued	Allows abnormal pelvic tilt; increases strain on back extensor muscles
Back extensor strength or endurance	Provides stability for the spine; maintains erect posture; controls forward flexion	Weak, easily fatigued	Increases loading on the spine; causes increased disk compression

link between physical fitness and LBP is largely based on functional anatomy (Table 21.4), and at this time the anatomical logic is stronger than the research evidence.

In order to have a healthy, well-functioning back, an individual must have flexible low-back (lumbar) muscles, hamstrings, and hip flexors and strong, fatigue-resistant abdominal and back extensor muscles. The goal is to keep the vertebrae aligned properly without excessive disk pressure, allowing a full range of motion in all directions. In addition, the pelvis must freely rotate both posteriorly and anteriorly without strain on the muscle or fascia.

Research evidence shows that individuals suffering from LBP exhibit lower levels of strength in both abdominal and back extensors. EMG activity is also increased in the back muscles of individuals with LBP. These differences, however, are more likely to be the result of LBP rather than the cause. Studies that have attempted to predict who might get LBP, either for a first time or in recurrent episodes, from strength and muscular endurance measures have identified back extension endurance as the critical variable. That is, individuals with low levels of back extension endurance are more likely to develop LBP at a later date than individuals with high levels of back extensor endurance. Although high levels of back extensor

strength and abdominal flexion strength or endurance have not proven to offer this same predictive value, they have never been shown to be detrimental. Thus, a total body workout for strength and muscular endurance should include exercises for the back and abdominals. This program does not mean that individuals who follow it will be protected absolutely from LBP.

Anabolic Steroids

Despite warnings about the adverse effects of anabolic steroids, the use of these androgens appears to be widespread among athletes, particularly those involved in resistance training (Yesalis, et al., 1993). In fact, anabolic steroids have been used by professional athletes for decades in their attempt to become stronger, leaner, and more aggressive. Furthermore, the use of steroids extends to high school athletes and individuals wishing to enhance their physique.

Anabolic steroids are synthetic androgens that mimic the effects of the male hormone testosterone.

Anabolic Steroids Synthetic androgens that mimic the effects of the male hormone testosterone.

Focus on Research

Low-Back Strengthening

Carpenter, D. M., & B. W. Nelson: Low back strengthening for the prevention and treatment of low back pain. *Medicine and Science in Sports and Exercise.* 31(1):18–24 (1999).

This review article examines the effect of specific resistance training for back extension (lumbar extension) on the treatment of chronic low-back pain (CLBP). As Carpenter and Nelson point out, there is a great need for exercise leaders to understand the appropriate use of exercise to prevent and treat low-back pain because low-back pain is the fifth most frequent reason for hospitalization and third most frequent reason for surgical procedures. Acute low-back pain (defined as pain lasting less than 3 weeks) usually resolves itself without any intervention; by 3 weeks, 75% of individuals recover from acute low-back pain, and by 2 months 90% of individuals recover from low-back pain. However, patients with CLBP (defined as individuals with symptoms lasting more than 7 weeks) do not enjoy the same prognosis. In fact, CLBP is the number-one cause of disability in the United States. Furthermore, the longer an individual suffers from CLBP, the worse the prognosis. Patients with CLBP are characterized by the deconditioning syndrome, a cyclical pattern of pain, followed by avoidance of activity, followed by deconditioning, which leads to more pain. Therefore, the general consensus suggests that patients with CLBP need active reconditioning exercises that progressively apply overload to strengthen the back (lumbar) extensors. Research data reviewed by Carpenter and Nelson support the following exercise prescription for individuals who suffer from CLBP.

- Specific exercise — Resistance exercise of lumbar extensors with the pelvis stabilized
- Overload — 1 set of 6–15 repetitions to fatigue
- Frequency — 1 day per week

A rehabilitation program that utilized an exercise program similar to the one described above for patients who had suffered CLBP for an average of 26 months resulted in improved lumbar strength and range of motion and substantial improvements in low-back pain and leg pain. Furthermore, the patients who demonstrated the greatest gains in muscle strength also experienced the greatest decrease in pain. Exercise programs that apply progressive overload to strengthen the lumbar extensors have also been shown to prevent low-back pain. The graph summarizes the results of a study that examined the incidence of back injuries in a group of strip mine workers who participated in a program of isolated low-back muscle strengthening. Data are also presented for the industry average and the average incidence of low-back injury in this coal mine for the past 9 years.

This review article clearly shows that a progressive resistance training program aimed at strengthening the lumbar extensors can significantly help to prevent and treat low-back pain. Given the extremely high incidence of low-back pain, it is important for all exercise professionals to understand the potential beneficial effect of exercise. This information is applicable not only to individuals working in occupational settings but also to anyone who routinely recommends exercise to individuals — that is, to all exercise professionals.

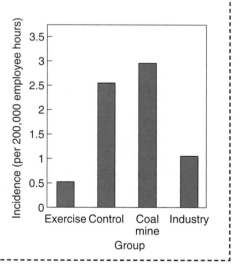

Although anabolic steroids are derived from testosterone, they have been altered to enhance their anabolic effect.

Although steroids build muscle mass, their use is dangerous, illegal, and unethical. After reviewing the available literature concerning anabolic steroids, the American College of Sports Medicine (ACSM) issued a position statement concerning the use of anabolic-androgenic steroids in sport (ACSM, 1987). This paper addresses the following adverse effects of steroid use:

- *Effects on the liver.* Anabolic steroids are associated with impaired excretory function (resulting in jaundice), blood-filled cysts (peliosis hepatis), and liver tumors.

- *Effects on the cardiovascular system.* The use of anabolic steroids results in hyperinsulinism and altered glucose tolerance, decreased levels of high-density lipoprotein, and elevated blood pressure.

- *Effects on the male reproductive system.* Anabolic steroid use has the effect of decreasing the number of sperm, decreasing testicular size, and reducing the levels of testosterone.

- *Effects on the female reproductive system.* The effects of anabolic steroids include a reduction in circulating levels of luteinizing hormone, follicle-stimulating hormone, estrogens and progesterone; inhibition of folliculogenesis and ovulation; and menstrual cycle changes.

- *Effects on psychological status.* The use of anabolic steroids decreases libido and causes mood swings and aggressive behavior.

- *Other effects.* Other side effects associated with anabolic steroids include premature closure of epiphyseal plates, acne, and hair loss.

Clearly, the use of anabolic steroids can have serious short-term and long-term effects. Exercise scientists thus have a responsibility to be involved in the ongoing educational efforts regarding the effects of steroid use.

Summary

1. Resistance training is used to improve overall health, improve athletic performance, rehabilitate an injury, and change physical appearance. It is also the primary activity of the sports of power lifting and bodybuilding.

   IP *Muscular–The Neuromuscular Junction* (pages 1–16)

2. A plan for muscular fitness is specific to the goals of the individual, which may include the development of muscular strength, muscular endurance, power, muscle hypertrophy, or any combination of these properties.

   IP *Muscular–Anatomy Review: Skeletal Muscle Tissue* (pages 1–13)

3. Overload of the muscular system is achieved by manipulating the intensity (load), frequency, and duration of training. The duration is determined by the number of repetitions and sets performed and the recovery period between lifts.

4. If the same training program is followed by different individuals, adaptation will occur at different rates owing to individual differences in age, body size and type, initial strength, and genetic makeup.

5. A coach or exercise leader must be sensitive to the differences in the rate of individual adaptation because it directly affects the progression of training. A common mistake is for coaches to design a program for the entire team and expect adaptations to occur at the same rate.

6. Adaptation to resistance training in children and the elderly is very similar to adaptations that occur in adults.

Review Questions

1. Give several reasons why an individual may engage in a resistance training program, and specify the different goals of a program.

2. Discuss how each of the training principles is applied in the development of a resistance training program. How do these applications vary if the exerciser is a child?

3. Is there an ideal number of repetitions and sets that should be performed by everyone? Defend your answer.

4. Discuss the importance of adequate recovery time in training adaptations to a resistance training program.

5. Do all individuals respond to a training program with the same adaptation (or magnitude of adaptation)? Why or why not?

6. What is the importance of a warm-up period prior to resistance training?

7. Compare and contrast the training adaptations that occur in skeletal muscle as a result of resistance training and endurance training.

8. What is the relationship between muscle function and low-back pain?

9. Why are anabolic steroids dangerous?

For further review and additional study tools, go to The Physiology Place (www.physiologyplace.com) and the Student Study Guide for Exercise Physiology for Health, Fitness, and Performance by Sharon A. Plowman and Denise L. Smith.

Passport to the Internet

Visit the following Internet sites to explore further topics and issues related to muscular training principles. To visit an organization's web site, go to www.physiologyplace.com and click on "Passport to the Internet."

The American College of Sports Medicine As the leading professional organization for individuals in sports medicine and exercise science, the ACSM issues position statements on a number of topics critical to the study of exercise physiology. Search for the ACSM position papers on "The Recommended Quantity and Quality of Exercise for Developing and Maintaining Cardiorespiratory and Muscular Fitness and Flexibility in Healthy Adults" and "Exercise and Physical Activity for Older Adults."

The American Orthopaedic Society for Sports Medicine The American Orthopaedic Society for Sports Medicine (AOSSM) is a national organization of orthopedic surgeons specializing in sports medicine. The AOSSM works closely with many other sports medicine specialists and clinicians, including family physicians, emergency physicians, pediatricians, athletic trainers, and physical therapists, to improve the identification, prevention, treatment, and rehabilitation of sports injuries.

National Strength & Conditioning Association Nonprofit association dedicated to facilitating the exchange of ideas in strength development as it relates to improvement of athletic performance and fitness.

References

American College of Sports Medicine: Position paper: The use of anabolic-steroids in sports. *Medicine and Science in Sports and Exercise.* 19(6):534–539 (1987).

American College of Sports Medicine: Position stand on exercise and physical activity for older adults. *Medicine and Science in Sports and Exercise.* 30:992–1008 (1998a).

American College of Sports Medicine: Position stand on the quantity and quality of exercise for developing and maintaining cardiorespiratory and muscular fitness and flexibility in healthy adults. *Medicine and Science in Sports and Exercise.* 30(6):975–991 (1998b).

Baechle, T. R., R. W. Earle, & D. Wathen: Resistance training. In T. R. Baechle and R. W. Earle (eds.), *Essentials of Strength Training and Conditioning.* Champaign, IL: Human Kinetics, 393–426 (2000).

Blimkie, C. J. R.: Resistance training during preadolescence: Issues and controversies. *Sports Medicine.* 15(6):389–407 (1988).

Brown, C. H., & J. H. Wilmore: The effects of maximal resistance training on the strength and body composition of women athletes. *Medicine and Science in Sports and Exercise.* 6:174–177 (1974).

Charette, S. L., L. McEvoy, G. Pyka, C. Snow-Harter, D. Guido, R. A. Wiswell, & R. Marcus: Muscle hypertrophy response to resistance training in older women. *Journal of Applied Physiology.* 70:1912–1916 (1991).

Coggan, A. R., R. J. Pina, D. S. King, M. A. Rogers, M. Brown, P. M. Nemeth, & J. O. Holloszy: Skeletal muscle adaptations to endurance training in 60- to 70-year-old men and women. *Journal of Applied Physiology.* 68:1896–1901 (1990).

Cureton, K. J., M. A. Collins, D. W. Hill, & F. M. McElhannon: Muscle hypertrophy in men and women. *Medicine and Science in Sports and Exercise.* 20(4):338–344 (1988).

Davies, C. T. M., & C. Barnes: Negative (eccentric) work. II. Physiological responses to walking uphill and downhill on motor-driven treadmill. *Ergonomics.* 15:121–131 (1972).

DeLorme, T. L., & A. L. Watkins: Techniques of progressive resistance exercise. *Archives of Physical Medicine.* 29:263–273 (1948).

Enoka, R. M.: *Neuromechanical Basis of Kinesiology.* Champaign, IL: Human Kinetics, 31–64 (1988).

Evans, W.: Exercise guidelines for the elderly. *Medicine and Science in Sports and Exercise.* 31(1):12–17 (1999).

Faigenbaum, A. D., L. D. Zaichkowsky, W. L. Westcott, L. J. Micheli, & A. F. Fehlandt: The effects of a twice-a-week strength training program on children. *Pediatric Exercise Science.* 5:339–346 (1993).

Falk, B., & G. Tenenbaum: The effectiveness of resistance training in children: A meta-analysis. *Sports Medicine.* 22(3):176–186 (1996).

Fiatarone, M. A., E. C. Marks, N. D. Ryan, C. N. Meredith, L. A. Lipsitz, & W. J. Evans: High intensity strength training in nonagenarians. Effects on skeletal muscle. *Journal of the American Medical Association.* 263:3029–3034 (1990).

Fleck, S. J., & W. J. Kraemer: *Designing Resistance Training Programs.* Champaign, IL: Human Kinetics (1987).

Frontera, W. R., V. A. Hughes, K. J. Lutz, & W. J. Evans: A cross-sectional study of muscle strength and mass in 45- to 78-yr-old men and women. *Journal of Applied Physiology.* 71:644–650 (1991).

Gollnick, P. D., R. B. Armstrong, C. W. Saubert IV, K. Piehl, & B. Saltin: Enzyme activity and fiber composition in skeletal muscle of untrained and trained men. *Journal of Applied Physiology.* 33(3):312–319 (1972).

Kraemer, W. J., A. D. Fry, P. N. Frykman, & B. Conroy: Resistance training and youth. *Pediatric Exercise Science.* 1:336–350 (1989).

Larsson, L.: Physical training effects on muscle morphology in sedentary males at different ages. *Medicine and Science in Sports and Exercise.* 14:203–206 (1982).

Mazzetti, S. A., W. J. Kraemer, J. S. Volek, N. D. Duncan, N. A. Ratamess, A. L. Gomez, R. U. Newton, K. Hakkinen, & S. J. Fleck: The influence of direct supervision of resistance training on strength performance. *Medicine and Science in Sports and Exercise.* 32(6):1175–1184 (2000).

McGlynn, G. H., N. T. Laughlin, & V. Rowe: Effect of electromyographic feedback and static stretching on artificially induced muscle soreness. *American Journal of Physical Medicine.* 58:139–148 (1979).

National Strength and Conditioning Association: Youth resistance training: Position statement paper and literature review. *Strength and Conditioning.* 18:32–75 (1996).

Perrin, D. H.: *Isokinetic Exercise and Assessment.* Champaign, IL: Human Kinetics (1993).

Rogers, M. A., & W. J. Evans: Changes in skeletal muscle with aging: Effects of exercise training. In J. O. Holloszy (ed.), *Exercise and Sport Sciences Reviews* (Vol. 21). Baltimore: Williams & Wilkins, 65–102 (1993).

Sale, D. G.: Neural adaptation to resistance training. *Medicine and Science in Sports and Exercise.* 20(suppl.): S135–S145 (1988).

Tesch, P. A.: Training for body building. In P. V. Komi (ed.), *Strength and Power in Sport.* London: Blackwell Scientific, 357–369 (1992).

Wilmore, J. H.: Alterations in strength, body composition, and anthropometric measurements consequent to a 10 week weight training program. *Medicine and Science in Sports.* 6:133–138 (1974).

Yesalis, C. E., S. P. Courson, & J. Wright: History of anabolic steroid use in sport and exercise. In C. E. Yesalis (ed.), *Anabolic Steroids in Sport and Exercise.* Champaign, IL: Human Kinetics (1993).

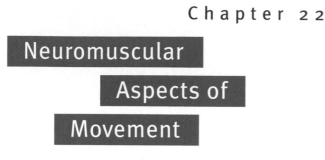

Chapter 22

Neuromuscular
Aspects of
Movement

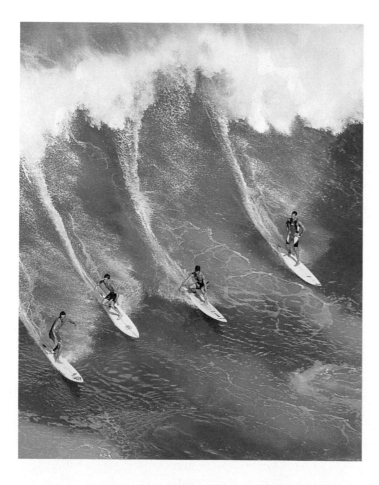

After studying the chapter, you should be able to

- Describe the nerve supply to muscle.

- Describe the sequence of events at the neuromuscular junction.

- Identify the components of a reflex arc.

- Describe the structure and innervation of the muscle spindle, and explain how the muscle spindle functions in the myotatic reflex.

- Describe the structure and innervation of the Golgi tendon organ, and explain how it functions in the inverse myotatic reflex.

- Provide research and clinical evidence that individual motor units can be volitionally controlled.

- Diagram the sequence of events involved in volitional control of movement.

- Differentiate between dynamic and static flexibility.

- Identify the anatomical factors that influence flexibility.

- Describe the basic methods of assessing flexibility.

- Discuss the relationship between flexibility and low-back pain.

- Differentiate among the different types of flexibility training.

- Apply the training principles to the development of a flexibility program.

Introduction

As spectators watching the Olympic games, we marvel at the grace and skill of figure skaters and stare in amazement at the incredible feats of gymnasts. As adults, we look on with wonder as a child learns a new task: rolling over, walking, tying a shoe. As coaches or fitness leaders, we experience the satisfaction of seeing individuals incorporate our suggestions to improve their skill. To understand the awe-inspiring accomplishments of athletes and the simple movements that are often taken for granted requires a knowledge of the nervous system.

The nervous system is made up of the brain, spinal cord, and nerves. It is the primary control and communication center for the entire body. As discussed in Chapter 2, the nervous system functions with the endocrine system to control and regulate the internal environment of the body; that is, it maintains homeostasis. All human movement depends on the nervous system; skeletal muscles will not contract unless they receive a signal from the nervous system.

This chapter will introduce some basic neuroanatomy and examine the role of the nervous system in controlling human movement. It will also discuss the influence of the nervous system on flexibility and flexibility training.

Neural Control of Muscle Contraction

Nerve Supply

All skeletal muscles require nervous stimulation to produce the electrical excitation in the muscle cells that leads to contraction. The neurons that carry information from the central nervous system to the muscle are called *efferent neurons*. Efferent neurons that innervate skeletal muscle are referred to as *motor neurons;* motor neurons may be classified as alpha motor neurons or gamma motor neurons. The *alpha* (α) *motor neurons* are relatively large motor neurons that innervate (connect to) skeletal muscle fibers and result in contraction of muscles. You should recall from Chapter 19 that α_1 motor neurons innervate FT muscle fibers, whereas α_2 motor neurons innervate ST muscle fibers. *Gamma* (γ) *motor neurons* innervate proprioceptors.

As a nerve enters the connective tissue of the muscle, it divides into branches, with each branch ending near the surface of a muscle fiber (cell). Because the axon of the motor neuron branches, each neuron is connected to several muscle fibers. As defined in Chapter 19, a motor neuron and the muscle fibers it innervates is called a *motor unit* (Figure 22.1). The motor unit is the basic unit of contraction.

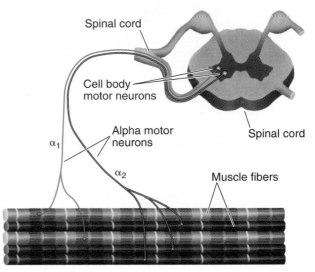

Figure 22.1
Motor Units

Two motor units are depicted. Notice that the muscle fibers of the two motor units are intermingled.

Because each muscle fiber in a motor unit is connected to the same neuron, the electrical activity in that neuron controls the contractile activity of all the muscle fibers in that motor unit. The number of muscle fibers controlled by a single neuron (that is, the number of muscle cells in a motor unit) varies tremendously, depending on the size and function of the muscle involved. Although a single neuron may innervate many muscle fibers, each muscle fiber is only innervated by a single motor neuron.

Figure 22.2 illustrates the relationship between the motor neuron (originating in the central nervous system) and the muscle fibers. The cell body of the motor neuron is located within the gray matter of the spinal cord [(2) in Figure 22.2], and the axon extends out through the ventral root of the spinal nerve [(3) in Figure 22.2] to carry the electrical signal to the muscle fiber [(4) in Figure 22.2]. Each branch of the motor neuron terminates in a slight bulge called the axon terminal, which lies very close to but does not touch the underlying muscle fiber [(4) in Figure 22.2].

The space between the membrane of the neuron and the muscle cell membrane at the motor end plate is called the neuromuscular (or synaptic) cleft. The entire region is referred to as the *neuromuscular junction*. The neuromuscular junction is important because it is here that the electrical signal from the motor neuron is transmitted to the surface of the muscle cell which is to contract.

Muscle cells are also supplied with afferent (sensory) nerve endings, which are sensitive to mechanical and chemical changes in the muscle tissue and

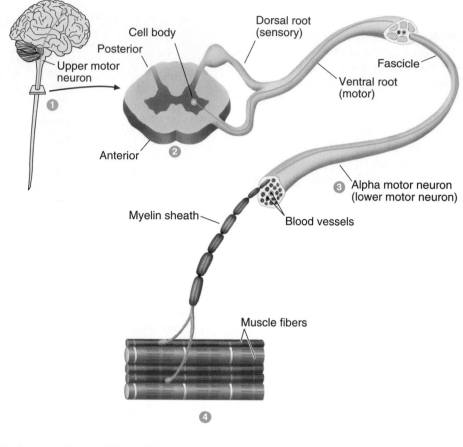

Figure 22.2

Functional Relationship between Motor (Efferent) Neurons and Muscle Cells

A motor neuron and the muscle cells it innervates is called a motor unit. (1) Schematic of central nervous system, (2) cross-sectional view of the spinal cord, (3) cross-sectional view of peripheral nerve emphasizing axon of motor neuron, and (4) the motor neuron branching near its terminal end where it forms the neuromuscular junction with the muscle fibers it innervates.

which relay this information back to the central nervous system. The information carried by afferent neurons is used by the central nervous system to make adjustments in muscular contractions.

The Neuromuscular Junction

The neuromuscular junction is a specialized synapse formed between a terminal end of a motor neuron and a muscle fiber. Figure 22.3 summarizes the events that occur at the neuromuscular junction. When an action potential reaches the axon terminal, the membrane of the neuron increases its permeability to calcium, and calcium is taken up into the cell (Figure 22.3a). The increased levels of calcium cause the synaptic vesicles to migrate to the cell membrane and release neurotransmitter (acetylcholine, ACh) into the synaptic cleft (by the process of exocytosis) (Figure 22.3b). The ACh then diffuses across the synaptic cleft and binds to receptors on the sarcolemma,

causing changes in the ionic permeability and leading to the depolarization of the sarcolemma (Figure 22.3c). This change in permeability and subsequent depolarization leads to the generation of an action potential in the sarcolemma of the muscle fiber. The action potential spreads in all directions from the neuromuscular junction, depolarizing the entire sarcolemma. The action potential is then spread into the interior of the cell through the T tubules (Figure 22.3d) as described in Chapter 19.

Although the neuromuscular junction functions much like other synapses, there are three important differences.

1. At a neuromuscular junction, a single presynaptic action potential leads to a postsynaptic action potential.

2. The synapse can only be excitatory.

3. A muscle fiber only receives synaptic input from one motor neuron.

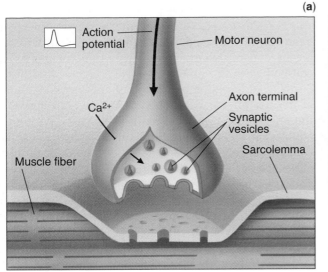

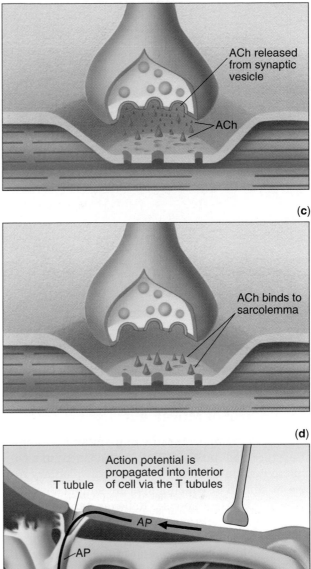

Figure 22.3

Events at the Neuromuscular Junction

(a) An action potential (AP) in the axon terminal causes the uptake of Ca^{2+} into the axon terminal and the subsequent release of the neurotransmitter. (b) The neurotransmitter (ACh) is released from the synaptic vesicles and diffuses across the synaptic cleft. (c) Generation of action potential: The binding of ACh to receptors on the sarcolemma causes a change in membrane permeability, causing an AP to be initiated in the sarcolemma. (d) The AP is propagated into the interior of the cells via the T tubules.

Note the two distinct roles that calcium plays in controlling muscular contraction. The first role is to facilitate the release of ACh from the synaptic vesicles in the motor neuron terminal. The second (and most often discussed) role of calcium is to control the position of the regulatory proteins troponin and tropomyosin on actin.

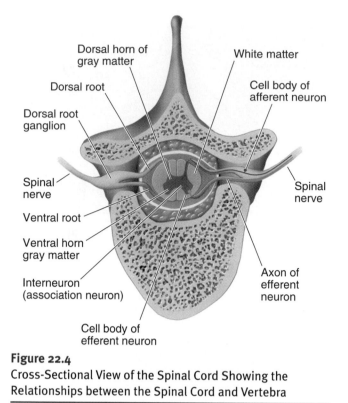

Figure 22.4
Cross-Sectional View of the Spinal Cord Showing the Relationships between the Spinal Cord and Vertebra

Reflex Control of Movement

Reflexes play an important role in maintaining an upright posture and in responding to movement in a coordinated fashion. A **reflex** is a rapid, involuntary response to stimuli in which a specific stimulus results in a specific motor response. Reflexes can be classified into two types: *Autonomic reflexes,* which activate cardiac and smooth muscle and glands, and *somatic reflexes,* which result in skeletal muscle contraction. This section will focus on somatic reflexes, which play an important role in movement.

Many spinal reflexes do not require the participation of higher brain centers to initiate a response. The higher brain centers, however, are often notified of the resultant movement by neurons that synapse with the afferent neuron.

Spinal Cord

The spinal cord is involved in both involuntary and voluntary movements. It performs two essential functions: It connects the peripheral nervous system with the brain, and it serves as the site of reflex integration.

> **Reflex** Rapid, involuntary response to stimuli in which a specific stimulus results in a specific motor response.

Figure 22.4 displays a cross-sectional view of the spinal cord; notice the spinal nerves extending from each side of the cord. Each spinal nerve contains afferent (sensory) fibers and efferent (motor) fibers. The cell bodies of the afferent neurons are located in the dorsal root ganglion of the spinal nerve, which is part of the peripheral nervous system. The cell bodies of the efferent neurons, however, are located within the central nervous system, and the axon exits through the ventral root of the spinal nerve. The most familiar efferent neurons are the alpha motor neurons that innervate skeletal muscles. The dorsal root and ventral root refer to the area of the spinal nerve that carries only afferent and efferent fibers, respectively. Once the two roots come together, it is referred to as a spinal nerve. Therefore, even though individual neurons have only sensory or motor functions, a nerve typically contains both afferent and efferent neurons, and hence has both sensory and motor functions.

Information is carried up and down the spinal cord by a series of tracts. A *tract* is a bundle of fibers in the central nervous system. The tracts that carry sensory (afferent) information are called ascending tracts. The tracts that carry motor (efferent) information are called descending tracts. There are specific tracts that are responsible for carrying different types of sensory information (such as pressure and temperature) and motor information (such as fine distal movement).

The descending pathways of the spinal cord can be divided into the pyramidal and extrapyramidal pathways, each of which includes several descending tracts that carry specific information. Voluntary motor impulses are transmitted from the motor area of the brain to somatic efferent neurons leading to skeletal muscles via the *pyramidal pathways* (Tortora and Anagnostakos, 1987).

Pyramidal System

The pyramidal (corticospinal) system is composed of neurons with cell bodies that originate in the cerebral cortex and axons that travel through the spinal cord. The neurons that extend from the brain down through the descending tract are called the upper motor neurons (see Figure 22.2). These neurons synapse with the lower motor neurons, also known as the alpha (α) motor neurons, in the anterior gray matter of the spinal cord. The lower motor neurons then carry the message to the skeletal muscles that specifically control precise, discrete movement (Tortora and Anagnostakos, 1987).

Both the lateral and anterior corticospinal (pyramidal) tracts decussate, or cross over, as they descend from the brain. Therefore, the motor cortex of the right side of the brain controls the muscles on the left side of the body, and vice versa. Thus, a patient who has had a cerebral vascular accident on the right side of the brain will lose the motor function of the left side of the body.

Extrapyramidal System

The extrapyramidal system consists of all descending tracts not included in the pyramidal system. Typically, the neurons found in these tracts have cell bodies located in the basal nuclei or reticular formation of the brain. The extrapyramidal system not only carries information that dictates muscle tone and posture but also controls head movements in response to visual stimuli and changes in equilibrium.

Components of a Reflex Arc

Many of the movements that individuals make daily depend upon spinal reflexes. The neural pathway over which a reflex occurs is called a *reflex arc*. The basic components of a reflex arc are described in the following list and are shown in Figure 22.5.

1. The *receptor* is the organ that responds to the stimulus by converting it into a neural (electrical) signal.
2. The *afferent* (sensory) *neuron* carries the signal to the central nervous system.
3. The *integration center* is located in the central nervous system. Here, the incoming neural signal is processed through the connection of the afferent neuron with *association neurons* (also called interneurons) and efferent neurons. The incoming afferent neuron may synapse directly with the efferent neuron or with association neurons, depending on the complexity of the reflex.
4. The *efferent* (motor) *neuron* carries the impulse from the central nervous system to the organ of the body that is to respond to the original stimulus.
5. The *effector organ* is the organ of the body that responds to the original stimulus. The effector organ may be a muscle or a gland.

Proprioceptors and Related Reflexes

Proprioceptive sensations provide an awareness of the activities of the muscles, tendons, and joints and provide a sense of equilibrium. Although all of the senses are important, this section emphasizes the role of the proprioceptive senses in order to explain the somatosensory system. Although the proprioceptive receptors will be emphasized, the other senses and receptors should not be forgotten; they too play a major role in human movement. For example, we use our

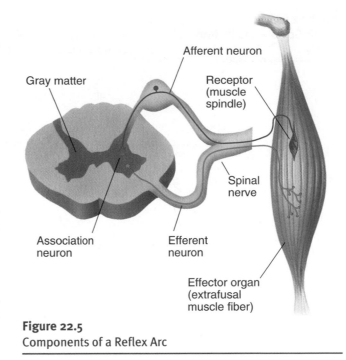

Figure 22.5
Components of a Reflex Arc

visual senses to provide important information regarding the speed and direction of a tennis ball during a tennis match. And we may listen to the sound created by the impact of the ball on the opponent's racket in order to judge the return. So keep in mind that human movement is not only extremely complex but also affected by a host of factors, including sensory receptors of all types.

Stimulation of the proprioceptors gives rise to kinesthetic perceptions. Historically, *kinesthesis* was defined as a person's perception of his or her own motion, specifically, the motion of the limbs with respect to one another and to the body as a whole. *Proprioception* was defined as the perception of movement of the body plus its orientation in space. Over the years these terms have become practically synonymous (Schmidt, 1988).

Vestibular Apparatus

Specialized equilibrium receptors in the inner ear, called the vestibular apparatus, provide important proprioceptive sensations. The primary function of the vestibular apparatus is to maintain equilibrium and to preserve a constant plane of head position by modifying muscle tone (Sage, 1971). Receptors of the vestibular apparatus can be divided into two categories: those located in the vestibule and those located in the semicircular canals.

The vestibule is comprised of two fluid-filled, saclike structures called the utricle and saccule. The

Figure 22.6
Muscle Spindle and Its Nerve Supply

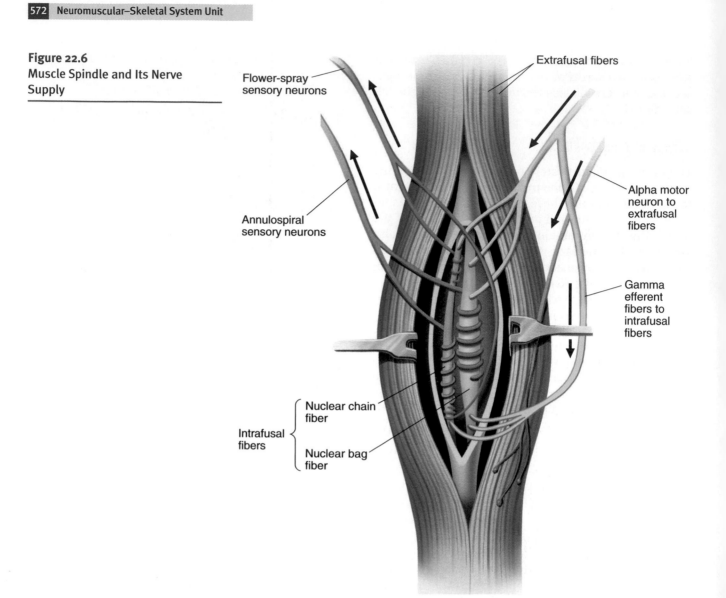

receptors in these structures, the maculae, sense information about the position of the head when the body is not moving and as a result of linear acceleration. The semicircular canals are oriented in three planes of space; that is, each of the semicircular canals is positioned at right angles to the other. This arrangement allows the equilibrium receptors in the semicircular canals, the crista ampullaris, to detect angular movement of the head in any plane. The receptors in the semicircular canals are sensitive to changes in the velocity of head movements—that is, to angular acceleration (Marieb, 2001; Sage, 1971).

Information from the vestibular apparatus is transmitted to the brain via the vestibulocochlear nerve. This information is carried to the vestibular nuclear complex and the cerebellum. Here, it is processed along with information from visual receptors and the somatic receptors of the muscles, tendons, and joints. Although the vestibular receptors are very important, they can be overruled by information from

other receptors. For example, the spotting technique (keeping the eyes focused on one spot) used by figure skaters allows them to perform spins without becoming dizzy.

Muscle Spindles and the Myotatic Reflex

Muscle spindles (sometimes called neuromuscular spindles, NMS) are located in skeletal muscle; they lie parallel to and are embedded in the muscle fibers. These receptors are stimulated by stretch, and they provide information to the central nervous system regarding the length and rate of length change in skeletal muscles. Stimulation of the muscle spindles results in reflex contraction of the stretched muscle via a myotatic reflex also known as a stretch reflex (Berne and Levy, 1988). Thus, the muscle spindle performs both a sensory and a motor function.

Figure 22.6 represents a muscle spindle and its nerve supply. The muscle spindle consists of a fluid-filled capsule composed of connective tissue; it is long and cylindrical with tapered ends. The typical spindle is 4–7 mm long and approximately ⅕ the diameter of a muscle fiber (extrafusal fiber) (Sage, 1971). The capsule contains specialized muscle fibers called *intrafusal muscle fibers*. Note that in contrast to intrafusal fibers, the muscle fibers that produce muscular movement are sometimes called *extrafusal fibers*. Each end of the spindle is attached to extrafusal muscle fibers.

There are two types of intrafusal fibers located within the muscle spindle: nuclear bag fibers and nuclear chain fibers. *Nuclear bag fibers* are thicker and contain many nuclei that are centrally located. These fibers extend beyond the spindle capsule and attach to the connective tissue of the extrafusal fibers. *Nuclear chain fibers* are shorter and thinner and have fewer nuclei in the central area of the fiber. Both types of intrafusal fibers contain contractile elements at their distal poles. The central region of the fibers do not contain contractile elements; this represents the sensory receptor area of the spindle.

A typical muscle spindle contains two nuclear bag fibers and approximately five nuclear chain fibers (Berne and Levy, 1988). The intrafusal fibers of the spindle are innervated by sensory nerves called annulospiral and flower-spray neurons. The branches of the *annulospiral neurons* wrap around the center of both types of intrafusal fibers. These annulospiral fibers are large, myelinated fibers (Berne and Levy, 1988).

The branches of the *flower-spray neurons* are located on either side of the annulospiral neurons (Tortora and Anagnostakos, 1987) and wrap around only the nuclear chain fibers. The flower-spray fibers are smaller than and conduct impulses slower than the annulospiral fibers. Both types of afferent fibers are stimulated when the central portion of the spindle is stretched. Since the intrafusal fibers are arranged in parallel with the extrafusal fibers, they are stretched or shortened with the whole muscle. The flower-spray nerve endings have a higher threshold of excitation than the annulospiral nerve endings. The flower-spray nerve endings provide information about relative muscle length; the annulospiral nerve endings are concerned primarily with the rate of length change.

The contractile intrafusal fibers also receive motor innervation from the central nervous system. The efferent fibers that terminate on the intrafusal fibers are called gamma efferents (γ motor neurons) or fusimotor neurons. The axons of the gamma motor neurons travel in the spinal nerve and terminate on the distal ends of the intrafusal fibers. Stimulation of the gamma motor neurons produces contraction of the intrafusal fiber, which causes the central region of the spindle to be stretched. Gamma motor neurons

are important enough to comprise almost a third of all motor neurons in the body.

Myotatic Reflex   The myotatic or stretch reflex is comprised of two separate components: a dynamic reaction and a static reaction. The dynamic reaction occurs in response to a sudden change in length of the muscle. When a muscle is quickly stretched, the annulospiral nerve endings (but not the flower-spray endings) transmit an impulse to the spinal cord, which results in an immediate strong reflex contraction of the same muscle from which the signal originated (Guyton, 1986). This is what happens in the knee jerk response, diagramed in Figure 22.7, or in the head jerk response when you fall asleep sitting up reading a book not nearly as interesting as this one.

Stretching of the skeletal muscle results in the stimulation of the muscle spindle fibers, which monitor changes in muscle length. In this example, the stretch is initiated by a tapping on the patellar tendon, thereby causing a deformation that will cause the quadriceps muscle group to be stretched [(1) in Figure 22.7]. Sudden stretching of the muscle spindle causes an impulse to be sent to the spinal cord by way of the annulospiral nerve fibers [(2) in Figure 22.7]. In the gray matter of the spinal cord this sensory fiber bifurcates, with one branch synapsing with an alpha motor neuron [(3a) in Figure 22.7]. The other branch synapses with an association neuron [(3b) in Figure 22.7]. The alpha motor neuron exits the spinal cord and synapses with the skeletal muscle, which was originally stretched [(4a) in Figure 22.7], resulting in a contraction that is roughly equal in force and distance to the original stretch [(5) in Figure 22.7]. The inhibitory association neuron synapses with another efferent neuron, which innervates the antagonist muscle (hamstring group in this example), where it causes inhibition; this reflex relaxation of the antagonist muscle in response to the contraction of the agonist is called **reciprocal inhibition**. This response facilitates contraction of the agonist muscle that was stimulated; the inhibited antagonist cannot resist the contraction of the agonist [(4b) in Figure 22.7]. The muscle spindle is also supplied with a gamma efferent neuron; for clarity, this neuron is shown on the opposite side of the spinal cord [(6) in Figure 22.7].

As soon as the lengthening of the muscle has ceased to increase, the rate of impulse discharge returns to its original level, except for a small static response that is maintained as long as the muscle is

---

Reciprocal Inhibition The reflex relaxation of the antagonist muscle in response to the contraction of the agonist.

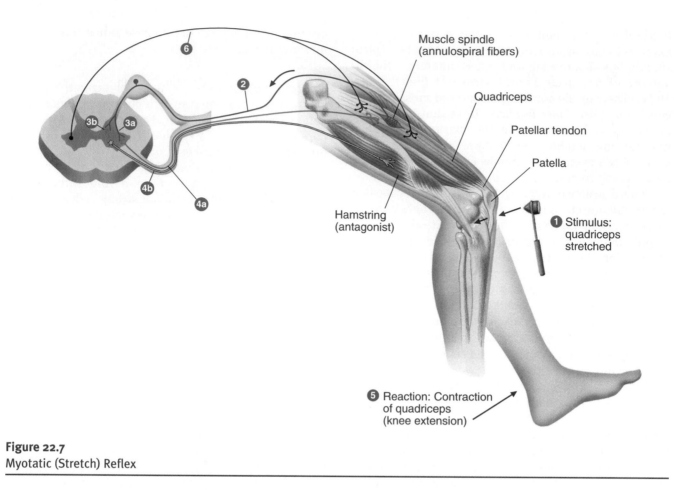

Muscle spindle
(annulospiral fibers)

Quadriceps

Patellar tendon

Patella

1 Stimulus:
quadriceps
stretched

Hamstring
(antagonist)

5 Reaction: Contraction
of quadriceps
(knee extension)

Figure 22.7
Myotatic (Stretch) Reflex

longer than its normal length. The static response is elicited by both the annulospiral and flower-spray nerve endings. The resultant low-level muscle contractions oppose the force that is causing the excess length, with the ultimate goal of returning to the resting length. A static response is also invoked if the sensory receptor portion of the neuromuscular spindle is stretched slowly.

Normally, the muscle spindles emit low-level sensory nerve signals that assist in the maintenance of muscle tonus and postural adjustments. **Muscle tonus** is a state of low-level muscle contraction at rest. Muscle spindles also respond to stretch by an antagonistic muscle, to gravity, or to a load being applied to the muscle. The head jerk is an example of the response to gravity, but other muscles such as the back extensors and quadriceps function the same way for unconscious postural adjustments. As an example of the load stimulus, think about what happens if you stand with your elbows at 90°, palms up, and someone places a 10-lb weight in your hands. Before you can consciously adjust

> **Muscle Tonus** A state of low-level muscle contraction at rest.

to this weight, and because the weight stretches your biceps, the muscle spindles will have caused a reflex contraction to stop your hands from dropping too far.

In addition to providing maintenance of muscle tone and adjustments for posture and load, the neuromuscular spindle serves as a damping mechanism that facilitates smooth muscle contractions. This is accomplished by a *gamma loop*.

In a gamma loop, the stretch reflex is activated by the gamma motor neurons [(6) in Figure 22.7]. Recall that the gamma motor neurons originate in the spinal cord and innervate the distal contractile portions of the intrafusal fibers. Pick up a rubber band and hold it at its maximal, unstretched length with your fingers. Now pull against both ends. What happens to the rubber band in the middle? Obviously, it is stretched. This is precisely what happens when the gamma motor neurons stimulate contractions at both ends of the intrafusal fibers. The central, noncontractile portion of the fibers is stretched, deforming the sensory nerve endings and eliciting the myotatic stretch response. The questions then are: What stimulates the gamma motor neurons, and why are they stimulated?

When signals are transmitted to the alpha motor neurons from the motor cortex or other areas of the brain, the gamma motor neurons are almost always simultaneously stimulated. This action is called *coactivation,* and it serves several purposes. First, it provides damping, as mentioned earlier. Sometimes, the alpha and gamma neural signals to contract arrive asynchronously. But because the response to the gamma motor neuron stimulation is contraction anyway, the gaps can be filled in by reflex contractions—hence smoothing out the force of contraction. Second, coactivation maintains proper load responsiveness regardless of the muscle length. If, for example, the extrafusal fibers contract less than the intrafusal fibers owing to a heavy external load, the mismatch would elicit the stretch reflex and the additional extrafusal fiber excitation would cause more shortening (Guyton, 1986). Similarly, because the intrafusal and extrafusal lengths are adjusted to each other, the neuromuscular spindle may be able to help compensate for fatigue by recruiting additional extrafusal fibers by reflex action. Finally, sensory information from the neuromuscular spindles is always carried to the higher brain centers, where it is unconsciously integrated with other sensory information. If the muscle spindles were not adjusted to the length of the extrafusal fibers during contraction, information on muscle length and the rate of change of that length could not be transmitted (Marieb, 2001). Since the gamma fibers do adjust the muscle spindle fibers, the gamma loop can assist voluntary motor activity, but it does not actually control voluntary motor activity.

Plyometrics   *Plyometrics,* also known as depth jumping or rebound training, is a training exercise that involves eccentric-concentric sequences of muscle activity. It involves such activities as jumping off a box with both feet together and then immediately performing a maximal jump back onto the box. While the training has proven effective in increasing jumping performance, the mechanisms responsible for the improved performance have not been fully elucidated, although the stretch-shortening cycle, which relies on the elastic properties of the muscle, is thought to be involved (see Chapter 18). It is also thought that the myotatic reflex plays a role. During the eccentric phase (lengthening) muscle spindles are believed to be activated, thus enhancing the contraction of the muscle during the concentric phase (Tortora and Anagnostakos, 1987).

Golgi Tendon Organ

Golgi tendon organs (GTOs) are receptors that are activated by stretch or active contraction of a muscle and that transmit information about muscle tension. Activation of these receptors results in a reflex inhibition

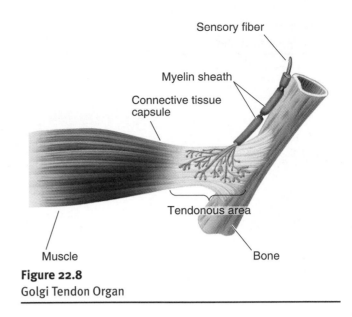

Figure 22.8
Golgi Tendon Organ

of the muscle via the inverse myotatic reflex (Berne and Levy, 1987). GTOs are located in the tendons, close to the point of muscular attachment. As shown in Figure 22.8, each Golgi tendon organ consists of a thin capsule of connective tissue that encloses collagenous fibers. The collagenous fibers within the capsule are penetrated by fibers of sensory neuron whose terminal branches intertwine with the collagenous fibers. This afferent neuron relays information about muscle tension to the spinal cord. The information is then transmitted to muscle efferents and/or to higher brain centers, particularly the cerebellum.

The Golgi tendon organ is in series with the muscle. Thus, the Golgi tendon organ can be stimulated by either stretch or contraction of the muscle. Because of elongation properties of the muscle during stretch, however, active contraction of a muscle is more effective in initiating action potentials within the Golgi tendon organ.

As with the myotatic reflex, the inverse myotatic reflex has both a static and dynamic component. When tension increases abruptly and intensely, the dynamic response is invoked. Within milliseconds this dynamic response becomes a lower-level static response within the GTO that is proportional to the muscle tension. The sequence of events in the inverse myotatic reflex is diagramed in Figure 22.9.

Contraction of a skeletal muscle (or stretching) results in tension that stimulates the Golgi tendon organs in the tendon attached to the skeletal muscle [(1) in Figure 22.9]. Stimulation of the Golgi tendon organ results in the transmission of impulses to the spinal cord by afferent neurons [(2) in Figure 22.9]. In the spinal cord, the afferent neuron synapses with an inhibitory association neuron and an excitatory motor

Figure 22.9
Inverse Myotatic Reflex

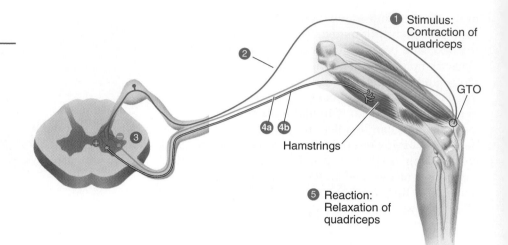

① Stimulus: Contraction of quadriceps

GTO

Hamstrings

⑤ Reaction: Relaxation of quadriceps

neuron [(3) in Figure 22.9]. In turn, the inhibitory association neuron synapses with a motor neuron that innervates the muscle attached to the tendon; the inhibitory impulses lead to the relaxation of the contracted muscle [(4a) in Figure 22.9]. The excitatory association neuron synapses with a motor neuron that innervates the antagonist muscle [(4b) in Figure 22.9].

Note that as the muscle group originally exhibiting the tension (the agonist) is relaxed, the opposing muscle group (or antagonist) is reciprocally activated. The relaxing action of the Golgi tendon organ serves several important functions (Guyton, 1986). First, excessive tension that might cause muscles and tendons to be torn or pulled away from their attachments is avoided. For example, a weight lifter who manages to get a heavier barbell off the ground than he or she can really handle may suddenly find that his or her muscle gives out. The Golgi tendon organs are responsible for the muscles giving out. It is speculated that increases in the amount of weight that can be lifted following resistance training are in part due to an inhibition of the Golgi tendon organ, allowing for a more forceful muscle contraction (Guyton, 1986).

The second important advantage of Golgi tendon organ–mediated relaxation is that muscle fibers that are relaxed can be stretched further without damage. This response is useful in the development of flexibility. Third, the sensory information regarding tension, which is provided to the cerebellum, allows for muscle adjustment so that only the amount of tension needed to complete the movement is produced. This feature ensures both a smooth beginning and a smooth ending to a movement and is particularly important in movements such as running that involve a rapid cycling between flexion and extension (Biering-Sorenseu, 1984).

Volitional Control of Movement

Although reflexes are important in controlling human movement, the volitional control of movement is more important in skilled movement. This section discusses the volitional control of motor units and of whole muscles.

Volitional Control of Individual Motor Units

Healthy people often take the ability to move for granted; they assume that if the proper signal is sent from their brain, the desired action will simply occur. An appreciation that it is not quite that simple occurs when one attempts to learn a new sport or when one has an illness or injury. Conscious control of single motor units is not something we normally think about. Most people think of reflex action as the most basic, albeit unconscious, form of muscle action. But even reflexes involve more than one motor unit and result in muscle activity that can be felt by the individual. In reality, motor unit control is really the most basic level of volitional control of movement that can be achieved.

Basmajian (1967) and his colleagues performed a series of experiments using intramuscular electrodes attached to a tape recorder and audio-amplifier for sound and an oscilloscope and camera for visual feedback. Initially, when subjects were asked to activate a motor unit, say, in the little finger, they moved the finger and got a typical EMG tracing such as the one shown in Figure 22.10d. Gradually, when movement was decreased to virtually nothing but neural signals continued to be sent, a single motor unit (identifiable by a characteristic sound and spike pattern) (Figure 22.10a) was isolated. Once one motor unit had been isolated, the frequency of its recruitment could be varied.

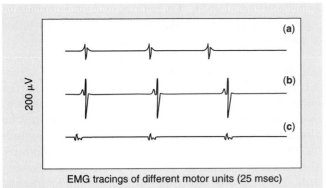

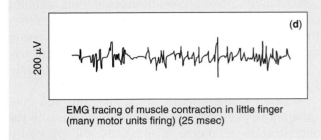

EMG tracing of muscle contraction in little finger
(many motor units firing) (25 msec)

Figure 22.10
Volitional Control of a Single Motor Unit

Source: J. V. Basmajian. Control of individual motor units. *American Journal of Physical Medicine.* (48)1:480–486 (1967). Reprinted by permission of Williams & Wilkins.

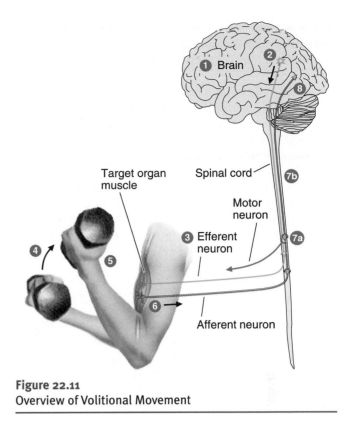

Figure 22.11
Overview of Volitional Movement

Additionally, other motor units could be isolated (Figures 22.10b and 22.10c), and firings could be varied between the motor units. Thus, it has been shown that motor units truly can be controlled. Precisely *how* this control is achieved is unclear both to the subjects doing it and the scientists observing it, although some type of proprioceptive feedback is suspected.

Such delicate, discrete control has obvious implications for the refinement of motor skills. Perhaps its greatest benefit, however, is in the area of therapeutic rehabilitation. For example, bioengineers have been able to utilize trained motor units to control myoelectric protheses and orthoses. Individuals disabled with conditions such as cerebral palsy can learn better motor control. And some individuals whose spinal cords have been injured but not totally destroyed can learn through such biofeedback to control first one motor unit and then another until muscle movement is regained.

Volitional Control of Muscle Movement

Figure 22.11 provides an overview of volitional movement. The brain initiates movement; [(1) in Figure 22.11]; that is, the plan for a desired movement, whether it be to lift a book or perform the high jump, originates in the brain. This information is then transmitted down the appropriate descending tract [(2) in Figure 22.11]. The neurons of the descending tract synapse with the motor neurons in the gray matter of the spinal cord. The efferent motor neuron then carries the impulse to the muscle, the effector organ [(3) in Figure 22.11].

Upon receiving the signal from the nervous system, the muscle contracts and produces movement [(4) in Figure 22.11]. Changes in muscle length, tension, and position stimulate receptors in the muscles and joints of surrounding muscles [(5) in Figure 22.11]. This information is transmitted to the central nervous system through afferent sensory neurons [(6) in Figure 22.11]. The afferent neurons synapse with various association neurons in the gray matter of the spinal cord. In some instances the neurons synapse with association neurons, which synapse with efferent motor neurons to reflexively control movement [(7a) in Figure 22.11]. In other cases, the association neurons synapse with neurons of the ascending tract, which will carry the information to the brain [(7b) in Figure 22.11].

The signals from the ascending pathway are transmitted to the brain, where the information is perceived, compared, evaluated, and integrated in light of past experience, desired outcome, and additional sensory information [(8) in Figure 22.11]. The brain then makes adjustments to its original message, which is again sent to the muscles via the descending pathway and the motor neuron.

This cycle continues throughout the duration of a given activity. The speed at which the information is transmitted is as remarkable as the degree of integration that occurs. What seems to be an instantaneous response on, say, a racquetball court (such as reaction to a powerful serve) actually requires a vast amount of communication within the neuromuscular system.

As already stated, many movements rely on both involuntary reflex action and volitional control of movement. An example is flexibility exercise. Although we decide to initiate stretches, the responses to them depend largely on reflexes.

Flexibility

Flexibility is defined as the range of motion (ROM) in a joint or series of joints that reflects the ability of the musculotendon structures to elongate within the physical limitations of the joint (Hubley-Kozey, 1991). There are two basic types of flexibility: static and dynamic. *Static flexibility* refers to the range of motion about a joint with no consideration of how easily or quickly the range of motion is achieved. *Dynamic flexibility* refers to the resistance to motion in a joint that will affect how easily and quickly a joint can move through the range of motion and, more recently, as the rate of increase in tension in a contracted or relaxed muscle as it is stretched. Thus, dynamic flexibility accounts for the resistance to stretch (Knudson, et al., 2000). Dynamic flexibility is undoubtedly the more important of the two when one considers athletic performances (especially speed events) and the health or diseased condition of the joints (such as arthritis). It is measured as *stiffness*. The opposite of stiffness is *compliance* (alteration in response to force). Stiffness is determined by the slope of a curve that plots the load (torque) against elongation (range of motion) for each individual tested. The steeper the line, the stiffer the muscle. This testing requires specialized laboratory equipment (Gleim and McHugh, 1997). No standardized measurement technique exists that can be used in practical settings for evaluating dynamic flexibility (Plowman, 1992). Thus, there is very little information available on dynamic flexibility (Shellock

and Prentice, 1985). Therefore, unless specifically stated otherwise, the discussion that follows is limited to static flexibility.

Several anatomical factors affect the range of motion in any given joint. The first is the actual structural arrangement of the joint—that is, the way the bones articulate. Each joint has a specific bony configuration that, in general, cannot and should not be altered. The soft tissue surrounding the joint, including the skin, ligaments, fascia, muscles, and tendons, also affects joint range of motion. The skin has very little influence on the range of motion under normal circumstances. The ligaments provide joint stability, and whatever restriction to the range of motion they provide is generally considered to be both necessary and beneficial. Thus, the muscles and their connective tissues are the critical factors that determine flexibility and that are altered by flexibility training.

Muscles actively resist elongation through contraction and passively resist elongation owing to the noncontractile elements of elasticity and plasticity. The difference between elastic and plastic properties can best be exemplified by thinking about a rubber band versus a balloon. If the rubber band is stretched and then let go, it should rebound to its original length—at least it should when it is new and has not been frequently stretched. That is elasticity. Blowing up a balloon also stretches it. However, if the air is let out of the previously fully inflated balloon, the balloon does not return to its original size. That is plasticity. What one is attempting to do in flexibility training is to influence the plastic deformation so that a degree of elongation remains when the force causing the stretch is removed (Plowman, 1992). Neuromuscular disorders characterized by spasticity and rigidity, any injuries resulting in scar tissue, or adaptive muscle shortening from casting will impact flexibility.

Flexibility and stretching are important for everyday living (putting on shoes, reaching the top shelf), for muscle relaxation and proper posture, and for relief of muscle soreness (discussed in Chapter 20). In relation to exercise it is advocated for two primary reasons: (1) as preparation for activity, which will enhance the performance of that activity, and (2) as a means of decreasing the likelihood of injury during physical activity.

There can be no doubt that flexibility is important to sport performance. The degree of importance differs, of course, with the sport. Table 22.1 gives a partial listing of popular sport and fitness activities according to the degree of flexibility required. The three degrees of flexibility listed are a normal range of motion, a slightly above average range of motion in one

---

Flexibility The range of motion in a joint or series of joints that reflects the ability of the musculotendon structures to elongate within the physical limits of the joint.

Table 22.1
Flexibility in Sport and Fitness Activities

Skills Requiring Extreme Range of Motion in Specific Joints	Skills Requiring Greater-Than-Normal Range of Motion in One or More Joints	Skills Requiring Only Normal Range of Motion in Involved Joints	
Figure skating	Jumping	Boxing	Bicycling
Gymnastics	Swimming	Long distance jogging or running	Stair stepping
Diving	Wrestling	Archery	Skating (in-line, roller)
Hurdles	Sprinting	Shooting	Horseback riding
Pitching	Racquet sports	Curling	Resistance training
Dancing (ballet, modern)	Most team sports	Basketball	
Karate		Cross-country skiing	
Yoga			

Note: Because the skills involved with a particular sport do not require greater-than-normal flexibility does not mean that stretching exercises should not be included in the exercise program.

Source: Modified from Hubley-Kozey (1991).

or more joints, and an extreme range of motion in specific joints.

It is obvious that the gymnast needs to be more flexible than long-distance runners and cyclists. However, there are no scientific studies that directly link selected flexibility values with performance if the athletes can move through the required range of motion (Gleim and McHugh, 1997; Plowman, 1992). For example, a bicyclist with normal range of motion in the ankle, knee, hip, and trunk will not become a better cyclist just by increasing her flexibility in those joints. But what about preventing injury?

Muscles, tendons, and ligaments are the tissues injured most frequently in work and in fitness and sport participation. Presently, however, there is no conclusive evidence that high levels of flexibility or improvements in flexibility either protect against injury or reduce the severity of injury (Plowman, 1992; Shellock and Prentice, 1985), including low-back pain. Indeed, there is some indication that hypermobility, or loose ligamentous structure, may predispose some individuals to injury or low-back pain (Gleim and McHugh, 1997; Plowman, 1992).

Nevertheless individuals with poor flexibility for the task they are expected to perform probably have an increased risk of exceeding the extensibility limits of the musculotendon unit. Such individuals should work on improving their flexibility. Likewise, individuals whose sports may cause maladaptive shortening in certain muscles should perform stretching exercises to counteract this tendency. Individuals who are shown to be hypermobile need to concentrate on strengthening the musculature around those joints.

Assessing Flexibility

The measurement of flexibility is not an exact, standardized procedure with a well-established criterion test. Direct measurement in the laboratory usually measures angular displacement (in degrees) between adjacent segments or from a reference point. Such measurements are usually obtained by a goniometer or flexometer. A goniometer resembles a protractor with two arms, one of which is movable. The center of the goniometer is placed over the joint about which movement will occur, and the arms are aligned with the body segments about the joint. Thus, for a measurement of the range of motion at the elbow joint, the center of the goniometer would coincide with the elbow, the stationary arm would be aligned with the upper arm, and the movable arm would be aligned with the forearm. The angle would be measured at the extreme range of motion for extension and flexion—that is, with the arm completely extended and completely flexed. The range of motion for this joint is the difference between the angles measured.

Flexibility measures can also be obtained by a flexometer. This instrument has a weighted 360° dial and pointer. Range of motion is measured relative to gravity. The instrument is attached to the body segment that is going to be moved, and the dial is locked at 0° at one extreme of the range of motion. The individual then performs the movement and the pointer is locked at the other extreme range of motion. Thus, the range of motion can be read from the dial.

Flexibility measurements can be made passively, in which case an external force causes the movement through the range of motion; or they can be made actively, in which case the individual being tested uses muscle action to produce the movement. One must indicate which technique is used because passive measurements generally give a higher value than active ones (Plowman, 1992).

The field methods of assessing flexibility typically involve linear measurements of distances between segments or from an external object. Some variation of the stand or sit-and-reach test is the most popular field test of flexibility. The sit-and-reach test is performed by having the individual being tested assume a sitting position with one (now recommended) or both (previously used) stocking feet flat against a testing box. The hands are positioned fully extended from the shoulders onto a scale on top of the testing box. The individual flexes as far forward as possible in a controlled fashion, sliding the fingertips along the scale. The point of maximum reach is recorded.

From the mid 1940s until the mid 1980s the stand or sit-and-reach test was described as a test of low-back (lumbar) and hip (hamstring) flexibility, mobility, or extensibility. In the mid to late 1980s several studies were published showing clearly that although the stand or sit-and-reach test is a valid test of hamstring flexibility, it is *not* a valid test of low-back flexibility (Biering-Sorenseu, 1984; Jackson and Baker, 1986; Jackson and Langford, 1989; Kippers and Parker, 1987; Nicolaisen and Jorgensen, 1985).

Because of its widespread use as the only flexibility test in physical fitness test batteries, the sit-and-reach test was often interpreted, although incorrectly, as a measure of total body flexibility. That is, if an individual was shown to have good flexibility using this test, equally good flexibility was assumed in other joint-muscle units. Although this idea is appealing in terms of simplicity and ease of testing, it is *not* accurate (Clarke, 1975; Shephard, et al., 1990). Joint flexibility is highly specific to individual locations; it is not a general trait common to all joints. Thus, if the goal of testing is to determine whether an individual is flexible, a profile of major joints must be compiled; one representative test does not indicate total body flexibility. Joint specificity for flexibility is true throughout the age span of childhood to old age.

The Influence of Sex and Age on Flexibility

Male-Female Comparisons

The specificity of flexibility to each joint makes generalizations regarding sex differences difficult. But as shown in one study, across the entire age spectrum from 10–75 yr, males exhibited greater anterior trunk flexion (also called lumbar mobility or low-back flexibility) than did females (Figure 22.12a). Conversely, across most of the same age span, females

exhibited greater right lateral trunk flexibility than males (Figure 22.12b). Although not shown in the figure, females had greater left lateral flexibility than males, at least in the adults.

The differences graphed in Figure 22.12a and 22.12b did not reach statistical significance at all ages and/or were not always tested for significance, so another possible interpretation is that there really aren't any differences in flexibility between the sexes. Either way, these observations are vastly different from the usual assumption that females are more flexible than males. Other data have shown that adult males are more flexible than adult females in trunk extension (Moll and Wright, 1971) and rotation, both left and right (Gomez, et al., 1991). However, adult males and females are not significantly different in trunk flexion; trunk extension; lateral trunk flexion, either left or right (Gomez, et al., 1991); head rotation, either left or right; external shoulder rotation; or ankle flexion, either plantar or dorsi. And adult males are less flexible than adult females in internal shoulder rotation and hip flexion (Sullivan, et al., 1992).

The often-stated, but apparently insupportable, assumption that females are more flexible than males is probably attributable to results from the sit-and-reach test. Because studies have shown that females have greater hip flexibility (Shephard, et al., 1990), it is expected that females would score better than males on the sit-and-reach test. Figure 22.13 on page 582 clearly shows that from 5–18 yr girls do have a higher sit-and-reach score than boys.

Despite the sit-and-reach results, it must be concluded from the results of many other studies that there is no consistent generalized pattern of sex differences in flexibility. Depending on which specific joint is being measured, females may have a larger, equal, or smaller range of motion than males.

Influence of Age

The impact of age on flexibility is only slightly less confusing. Again Figures 22.12a and 22.12b can be used to illustrate specificity through the pubertal growth years. The general trend is for lumbar flexibility to decrease between 10 and 15 yr of age, while lateral flexion generally increases during the same period. The sit-and-reach data (Figure 22.13) show an interaction of age and sex (Malina and Bouchard, 1991). Basically, the girls show a consistent improvement from age 5–18, while the boys show a U-shaped response—that is, a gradual decline from age 5–13 yr and then an improvement from 13–18 yr—so that they are more flexible in the hip and posterior thigh by adulthood. Thus, whether and how the range of motion changes through the growing years is joint specific.

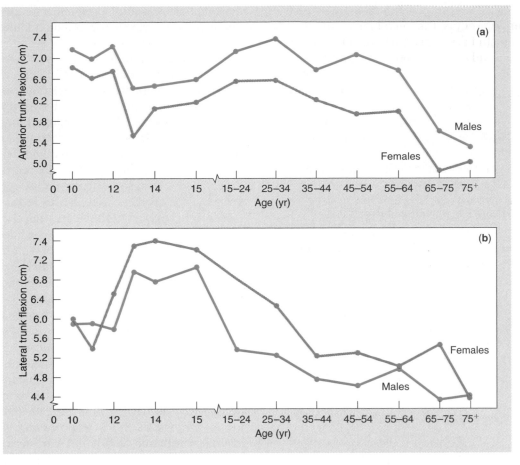

Figure 22.12
Flexibility in Males and Females

(a) Anterior trunk flexion (lumbar mobility). (b) Lateral trunk flexibility.

Source: Plotted from data of Moran et al., (1979); Moll & Wright (1971).

Although Figure 22.12 shows a pattern of declining flexibility as people progress from young adulthood through middle age and into old age, other studies investigating different joints suggest that flexibility does not change (Gomez, et al., 1991; Shephard, et al., 1990). What has not been shown is an increase, without training, in range of motion with age through the adult years. Therefore, it can be concluded that through the adult years flexibility either declines or stays the same. This is probably joint specific in terms of both direction and magnitude. Changes in flexibility with aging may also be confounded by the decreasing activity that often accompanies aging. Most of the information on flexibility is from cross-sectional rather than longitudinal studies, and this information has not been analyzed taking activity level into account.

All ages appear to be trainable in terms of flexibility (Clarke, 1975; Rider and Daly, 1991). This adaptation may be especially important to the elderly, where healthy, independent living is at stake.

Flexibility and Low-Back Pain

The theoretical link between muscle function and low-back pain (LBP) was described in Chapter 21 (Table 21.4), with particular emphasis at that time being placed on muscle strength and endurance. In this chapter emphasis is given to the flexibility needs for a healthy, well-functioning back. Flexibility of the low-back and hip area and strong and balanced lumbar, hamstrings, and hip flexor muscles are crucial for controlled pelvic movement. Controlled pelvic movement means having neither an exaggerated anterior tilt (lordotic curve) nor a restricted anterior tilt (no low-back curvature). Either an exaggerated or a restricted pelvic tilt can increase vertebral disc compression and cause pain and strain in the low-back area.

Research evidence shows that individuals suffering from LBP exhibit lower values for range of motion, particularly in the low-back and hamstring areas. As with the reduced strength and endurance values,

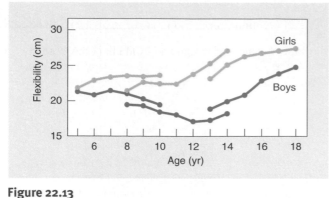

Figure 22.13
Flexibility as Measured by the Sit-and-Reach Test

Source: From *Growth, Maturation, and Physical Activity* (p. 196) by Robert M. Malina & Claude Bouchard. Champaign, IL: Human Kinetics. Copyright 1991 by Robert M. Malina and Claude Bouchard. Reprinted by permission.

however, these differences are more likely the result of LBP than a cause of it.

One study found that first-time low-back pain could be predicted from lumbar flexibility (Jackson and Baker, 1986). However, in this study high lumbar flexibility predicted LBP, not low flexibility, as might be expected; and it was predictive only in males. On the other hand, recurrent LBP has been found to be predictable from both low lumbar extension (not flexion) range of motion and low hamstring flexibility (Biering-Sorenseu, 1984).

Exactly what value constitutes too low or too high a range of motion is unknown. From the research that has been conducted, though, it can be recommended that flexibility of the hip, low back, and hamstrings be part of a general overall fitness program. Flexibility should be developed specifically for athletes as needed. However, flexibility should not be taken to extremes, nor should one expect that flexibility will mean absolute protection from LBP.

Stretching Techniques

The biggest decision in setting up a flexibility training program is determining which stretching technique to employ. There are three techniques used to increase flexibility: ballistic stretching, static stretching, and proprioceptive neuromuscular facilitation (PNF). **Ballistic stretching,** characterized by an action-reaction bouncing motion, is a form of stretching in which the joints involved are moved to the extremes of the joint range of motion by fast, active contractions of agonistic muscle groups. As a result, the antagonistic muscles are stretched quickly and forced to elongate. This quick stretch distorts the intrafusal fibers of the

neuromuscular spindle and activates the annulospiral nerve endings, which transmit an impulse to the spinal cord, resulting in an immediate strong reflex contraction (the myotatic reflex) of the muscles that had been stretched (Etnyre and Lee, 1987). This rebound bounce is proportional in force and distance to the original move. Although ballistic action is frequently seen in sport performance—for example, punting a football or a high kick in dance—and although ballistic stretching has been shown to be effective in increasing flexibility, this type of stretching is generally not recommended. Ballistic stretching may cause muscle soreness; and even though there is virtually no research or clinical evidence to support it, the fear is that the forces generated by the series of pulls will exceed the extensibility limits of the tissues involved and result in injury (Shellock and Prentice, 1985). Fortunately, there are alternative means of increasing flexibility that do not invoke this (real or imagined) fear of injury.

Static stretching is a form of stretching in which the muscle to be stretched (the antagonist) is slowly put into a position of controlled maximal or near-maximal stretch. The position is then held for 30–60 sec. Because the rate of change in muscle length is slow as the individual gets into position and then is nonexistent as the position is held, the annulospiral nerve endings of the neuromuscular spindle (NMS) are not stimulated to fire and a strong reflex contraction does not occur. That is, the dynamic phase of the NMS response is bypassed. Instead, if the stretch continues for at least 6 sec, the Golgi tendon organs (GTOs) respond, leading to the inverse myotatic reflex and causing relaxation in the stretched muscle group. This response is called *autogenic inhibition* (Etnyre and Lee, 1987). This relaxation is easily felt by the exerciser, and it allows the muscle to be elongated even further. The impulses from the GTO are able to override the weaker static response impulses coming from the NMS to allow this reflex relaxation and a continuous sustained stretch. If a maximal stretch is held long enough, the muscle being stretched will

Ballistic Stretching A form of stretching, characterized by an action-reaction bouncing motion, in which the joints involved are placed into an extreme range of motion by fast, active contractions of agonistic muscle groups.

Static Stretching A form of stretching in which the muscle to be stretched is slowly put into a position of controlled maximal or near-maximal stretch by contraction of the opposing muscle group and held for 30–60 sec.

Focus on Application

❊ Soreness and Flexibility

Ever wonder why some people get really sore—that is, experience delayed-onset muscle soreness, or DOMS, after an eccentric muscle workout or activity—whereas others don't? The key may be flexibility or, more specifically, dynamic muscle flexibility. Twenty subjects (both males and females) were divided into three groups (compliant, normal, or stiff) based on the measurement of passive muscle stiffness using the straight-leg-raise stretch. All subjects also performed 6 sets of 10 isokinetic eccentric contractions of the hamstring muscles at 60% of their individual maximal voluntary contractions. Stiff subjects experienced significantly greater strength loss, pain, muscle tenderness, and creatine kinase activity (which is a marker for muscle damage) than compliant subjects over the course of the next 3 days.

These results indicate that more flexible individuals are less susceptible to exercise-induced muscle damage. This is important not only because DOMS is unpleasant in daily life, but also because it can affect workouts following a highly eccentric event or training session. Muscle damage and DOMS limit the intensity and duration and increase metabolic costs of subsequent exercise bouts.

So, what can you do about this? The long-term choice is to include stretching exercises in your training program. The short-term option is to include fatiguing concentric exercise or cyclic passive activity prior to any future eccentric exercise bouts. It is unknown whether stretching to improve flexibility before eccentric exercise will limit muscle damage or DOMS. ❊

Source:

McHugh, et al. (1999).

---

ultimately reach a point of **myoclonus**—twitching or spasm in the muscle group—indicating the endpoint of an effective stretch.

Because no uncontrolled sudden forces are involved, injury is unlikely with this type of stretch (Shellock and Prentice, 1985). Indeed, static stretch has been touted as a means not only of avoiding injury but also of relieving muscle soreness. Static stretch done prior to or after dynamic activity involving eccentric muscle contractions does not appear to prevent muscle soreness, or the expression of delayed onset muscle soreness (DOMS) (High, et al., 1989; Knudson, 1998). However, the degree of dynamic flexibility may be related to DOMS (see the accompanying Focus on Application box).

Proprioceptive neuromuscular facilitation (PNF) is a stretching technique in which the muscle to be stretched is first contracted maximally. The muscle is then relaxed and is either actively stretched by contraction of the opposing muscle or is passively stretched. There are a number of different proprioceptive neuromuscular techniques currently being used for stretching, but the two most popular are the contract-relax (CR) and contract-relax-agonist-contract (CRAC) techniques. In both the CR and CRAC techniques the muscle to be stretched (the antagonist) is first placed in a position of maximal stretch by action of the agonist and then is contracted maximally, using either a dynamic concentric or static contraction. Both techniques also require the assistance of a partner or an implement that can provide resistance and elongation.

The contraction phase, which originates from the position of maximal stretch, typically lasts for at least 6 sec. Because of the slow rate of change of the muscle length as the individual gets to the maximal stretch position, the annulospiral nerve endings of the NMS are not stimulated to fire, and no reflex contraction occurs. As with a static stretch, the dynamic phase of the NMS response is bypassed. The exerciser then contracts the antagonists against the resistance provided by a partner. As tension is created in the muscle by the maximal contraction, the Golgi tendon organs respond and the inverse myotatic reflex is initiated, causing a relaxation in the stretched muscle group (Etnyre and Lee, 1987). At this point in the CR technique the partner who has been resisting the contraction moves the relaxed limb into a greater stretch. That is, the antagonist is further elongated passively until resistance to the stretch is again felt.

In the CRAC technique the exerciser actively contracts the agonist to assist the stretching of the antag-

---

Myoclonus A twitching or spasm in the muscle group that is maximally stretched.

Proprioceptive Neuromuscular Facilitation (PNF) A stretching technique in which the muscle to be stretched is first contracted maximally. The muscle is then relaxed and is either actively stretched by contraction of the opposing muscle or is passively stretched.

Table 22.2
Summary of Stretching Techniques

	Ballistic	**Static**	**PNF: CR**	**PNF: CRAC**
Action	Antagonist stretched by dynamic contraction of agonist	Antagonist moved slowly to limit of ROM and held	Antagonist moved slowly to limit of ROM by action of agonist, where it contracts maximally for about 6–10 sec	Antagonist moved slowly to limit of ROM by action of agonist, where it contracts maximally for about 6–10 sec
Reaction	Bounce back proportional to force of original contraction	Relaxation and further elongation, usually gravity assisted	Relaxation and further passive elongation by partner or implement, such as towel or jump rope	Relaxation and further passive elongation by active dynamic concentric contraction of agonist
Mechanism	Neuromuscular spindle (myotatic reflex)	Golgi tendon organ, autogenetic inhibition (inverse myotatic reflex)	Golgi tendon organ, autogenetic inhibition (inverse myotatic reflex)	Golgi tendon organ, autogenetic inhibition (inverse myotatic reflex) plus reciprocal inhibition
Advantages	Improves flexibility; may mimic action in sport performance	Improves flexibility and is safest; may provide relief from delayed-onset muscle soreness	Improves flexibility and is safe	Improves flexibility and is safe
Disadvantages	Muscle soreness or injury may result		Requires partner or implement, such as towel, jump rope, or sweats	Requires partner or implement

Note: ROM = range of motion.

onist. By reciprocal inhibition, the contraction of the agonist is thought to aid in the relaxation of the antagonist, allowing it to be stretched further. There is some danger of injury in PNF stretching if the partner attempts to push the relaxed limb too far. However, if the partner stops at the point of myoclonus, which can be easily felt with proper hand placement, injury is avoided.

The role of the Golgi tendon organ in bringing about an inhibitory relaxation of stretched muscle has generally been supported by research studies (Etnyre and Abraham, 1988; Etnyre and Lee, 1987; Hutton, 1992). When needle electrodes were implanted in the stretched muscles, very little EMG activity was recorded, indicating relaxation.

Table 22.2 summarizes the three stretching techniques. Although you have undoubtedly stretched using all three techniques before, try them again now using the stretches given next. Be very conscious of what you are feeling and why.

1. Stand up with your feet shoulder's width apart, legs straight, and quickly attempt to place your palms (or if that is easy, your elbows) on the floor. You should have bounced back up, but you probably didn't go down forcefully because you didn't want to pull your hamstring. Review the action of the NMS in your mind.

2. Stand up with your feet shoulder's width apart, legs straight, and bend over at the waist with your head and arms dangling down. Hold that position until you feel your hamstring muscles relax and allow you to bend even further. Repeat until your hamstring starts to quiver (myoclonus) or you can't go any further. If you can easily touch the floor initially, stand on a stable box that allows you to go beyond your feet. Think about the interaction of the GTO and NMS.

3. Lie supine on the floor and place a towel around the heel of one foot so that you can pull on it. Elevate that leg straight until resistance is felt. Statically, contract the hamstrings against the resistance being provided by your towel for 6 sec. Then pull on the towel with your arms to further stretch the hamstrings. This is the CR PNF technique. From the new position, repeat the isometric contraction for another 10 sec. This time, stretch the hamstrings by actively contracting the quadriceps of that leg. This is the CRAC PNF technique. Think about the interaction of the NMS, GTO, and reciprocal inhibition needed to perform these actions.

Work through the exercises provided in the Question of Understanding box to ensure that you understand these concepts.

Physiological Response to Stretching Techniques

The obvious and well-known response to an acute bout of stretching exercises is an increase in the range of motion. To achieve this, muscle relaxation actually occurs within the sarcomeres. Current evidence seems to suggest that this relaxation is the combined result of a decline in passive tension that results from the mechanical viscoelastic properties of the muscle and the neural actions for the inverse myotatic reflex (Gleim and McHugh, 1997; McHugh, Connolly, et al., 1999; Smith, 1994). The increased range of motion lasts for approximately 20–90 min.

Application of the Training Principles

The application of the training principles to flexibility development has not received a great deal of attention in the research literature. Some guidelines, however, can be suggested and are given in the following sections.

Specificity

Flexibility is joint specific (Marshall, et al., 1980; Shephard, et al., 1990). Hence, flexibility is also task or sport specific. Thus, the first step in developing a flexibility program is to analyze the task or sport to determine the degree of flexibility needed, the specific joint(s) involved, and the plane of action involved. For example, hurdling requires flexion and extension at both the hip and the knee joints and also hip adduction, abduction, and rotation. Swimming requires the same hip flexibility as hurdling; but instead of knee flexion and extension, swimming requires ankle flexion and extension plus inversion, eversion, and shoulder flexion and extension, adduction, abduction, and rotation (Hubley-Kozey, 1991). A general fitness participant should emphasize a total body workout of the major joints and muscle groups.

Specificity need not refer to the type of action the individual is planning on doing. How muscle and connective tissue are elongated does not matter as long as the elongation occurs. Because a movement will be done ballistically does not mean that ballistic flexibility work should be done (Etnyre and Lee, 1987; Hardy and Jones, 1986).

A Question of Understanding

Describe an exercise in each of the following techniques for the gastrocnemius (calf) muscle, and perform the exercise.

1. Ballistic
2. Static
3. CR PNF
4. CRAC PNF

Check your answers in Appendix D.

Overload

Overload in flexibility training is achieved by placing the muscle and connective tissue at or near the normal limits of extensibility and manipulating the NMS and GTO by holding the position or contracting the muscle to achieve an elongation. The duration of the static stretch hold should be between 15 and 30 sec (Knudson, 1998). PNF stretches with 6–10 sec of contraction followed by 6–10 sec of relaxation and elongation are repeated to myoclonus or extensibility limits.

Usually, two or three relaxation periods can be achieved in one repetition of static stretch. A high number of repetitions is not necessary. Two to five are frequently recommended for both the static and PNF flexibility techniques.

The intensity of the stretching exercises should be monitored by both myoclonus and pain. Stretched muscles that begin to twitch or spasm (myoclonus) are stretched too far and are fighting that stretch by reflexly trying to contract. Such a muscle should be shortened to the point where the myoclonus ceases before proceeding. Pain also means the stretch is too intense and should not be tolerated. Both the rate of stretch and amount of force should be minimized.

The frequency of the workout should be at least 3 days per week in the development phase. Reasonable daily stretching, however, should have no detrimental effects.

Rest/Recovery/Adaptation and Progression

Short-term improvements in flexibility have been shown to occur after as little as 1 week of daily sessions (Hardy and Jones, 1986). On the other hand, anecdotal evidence indicates that some people do not seem to improve at all. At any rate, since the individual begins both static and PNF stretching exercises at the limit of extensibility, progression will naturally follow whatever adaptation does occur. What is most

Focus on Research

Flexibility and Overuse Injuries

Hartig, D. E., & J. M. Henderson: Increasing hamstring flexibility decreases lower extremity overuse injuries in military basic trainees. *The American Journal of Sports Medicine.* 27(2): 173–176 (1999).

Although it has long been proposed that increased flexibility is associated with a decrease in injury rate, there has been limited scientific data to support this hypothesis. Decreasing the incidence of injury is important for obvious reasons, including the fact that injuries that occur with the initiation of a fitness program often cause participants to discontinue exercise. In the military, basic training is often interrupted because of injuries sustained during training. In order to test the hypothesis that increased hamstring flexibility would decrease lower extremity overuse injury in military basic trainees, Hartig and Henderson (1999) incorporated flexibility training into the scheduled fitness training of a company going through basic training. The change in flexibility and subsequent rate of lower extremity injury was compared to another group (control group) that went through basic training at the same time. Both the intervention and control groups participated in 13 weeks of basic training program with the normal routine of stretching before physical training, including hamstring stretching. The intervention group added three hamstring stretching sessions (before lunch, dinner, and bedtime) each day. The stretching routine involved having a partner hold the leg to be stretched at approximately 90° while the participant moved his trunk forward with an anterior tilt at the pelvis until he perceived a hamstring muscle stretching sensation without pain. Each stretch was performed 5 times for each extremity and held for 30 sec. At the completion of basic training, the control group had increased their hamstring flexibility by 3°, whereas the intervention group had increased their hamstring flexibility by 7°. Forty-three lower extremity overuse injuries occurred in the control group for an incidence rate of 29.1%, compared with 25 injuries in the intervention group for an incidence rate of 16.7%. These results are good news for military recruits and for all individuals initiating a fitness program. A simple stretching program, that requires little time, is effective in improving flexibility and decreasing the incidence of injury.

important is that, except in the case of specific athletic requirements, progression not continue to extreme flexibility.

Individualization

As stated previously, the most important consideration in flexibility training is that the goals and technique preferences of the individual be considered. In a school situation the maturity of the individuals might also need to be considered. For example, if a PNF technique with a partner is going to be used, the partner has to be able to detect the onset of myoclonus and not try to just push as far as possible. Otherwise, individualization is inherent in the flexibility exercises themselves. Each individual stretches to his or her own limits at his or her own rate. Joint looseness is an individual characteristic (Marshall, et al., 1980).

Maintenance

Once the appropriate or desired level of flexibility has been attained, it can be maintained by just one day per week of training at the same intensity level (Wallin, et al., 1985).

Retrogression/Plateau/Reversibility

Little is known about when or even if a plateau is achieved in a flexibility training program, although there will be a point, probably set by genetics, when further improvement ceases (Etnyre and Lee, 1987). Improvements in flexibility have been shown to continue for a least 8 weeks after the cessation of exercise (Clarke, 1975).

Warm-Up and Cool-Down

Considerable confusion exists about the relationship between warming up and stretching prior to an activity and flexibility training. A *flexibility training program* is a planned, deliberate, and regular program of exercises that can permanently and progressively increase the usable range of motion of a joint or set of joints over time (Alter, 1988). A *warm-up and cool-down stretching program* is a planned, deliberate, and regular program of exercises that are done immediately before and after an activity to improve performance and reduce the risk of injury (Alter, 1988).

Stretching does not cause an elevation in body temperature and therefore it is not a warm-up. In fact, a cardiovascular warm-up to elevate body temperature should precede flexibility exercises regardless of the reason for stretching. The cardiovascular warm-up will increase the body temperature and therefore make the muscles and joints more viscous and receptive to stretch. Furthermore, the value to performance of increased flexibility in a warm-up must be evaluated in relation to the demands of the performance. Stretching during a warm-up is clearly important and beneficial to individuals whose sport or activity requires greater than normal or extreme range of motion (see Table 22.1). However, recent research has indicated that maximal strength output is decreased after a warm-up that results in increased flexibility in the same muscle group (Kokkonen, et al., 1998). Therefore, intense stretching of the prime movers should probably be avoided when the expression of strength is of paramount importance (Knudson, 1999).

Despite the fact that an increase in body temperature should make stretching more effective, studies have not shown that flexibility gains after 3–4 min of warm-up are any different from flexibility gains after 3–4 min of warm-up plus 20–30 min of aerobic work (Cornelius, et al., 1988).

Adaptation to Flexibility Training

Flexibility exercises and flexibility training improve range of motion, whether the technique used is ballistic, static, or one of the PNF techniques (Etnyre and Lee, 1987; Hutton, 1992; Shellock and Prentice, 1985). Which technique brings about the greatest improvement has been the subject of a great number of studies. Results from these studies have occasionally shown that one type of athlete, or males as opposed to females, responds better to one stretching technique than another with a slight advantage overall to PNF stretching (Etnyre and Lee, 1987; Knudson, 1998; Osternig, et al., 1990). We can only conclude at this point that the question of which stretching method is most effective has not been definitively answered. Indeed, the exact position in which the stretching exercises are done may be more important than the method of stretching (Sullivan, et al., 1992). The physiological basis of training-induced changes in the range of motion is not well understood. It has been speculated that relatively permanent anatomical changes occur in connective tissue, but these changes have not been documented. It is possible that changes in neural sensitivity or simply an increase in "stretch tolerance" are involved (Gleim and McHugh, 1997; McHugh, Connolly, et al., 1999; Smith, 1994).

There is little scientific or empirical evidence to suggest that resistance training will decrease flexibility. In fact, studies have shown that heavy resistance training results in either an improvement or no change in flexibility (Massey and Chaudet, 1956). Furthermore, competitive weight lifters have average or above-average flexibility in most joints (Leighton, 1957). So that flexibility is not lost, those engaged in resistance training should stress the full range of motion of both the agonists and the antagonists.

Summary

1. The spinal cord performs the essential functions of connecting the peripheral nervous system with the brain and serving as a site of reflex integration.

IP *Muscular–The Neuromuscular Junction* (pages 1–16); *Muscular–Contraction of Motor Units* (pages 1–11)

2. Voluntary motor impulses are transmitted from the motor area of the brain to somatic efferent neurons leading to skeletal muscles via the pyramidal pathways.

3. Reflexes play an important role in maintaining an upright posture and responding to movement in a coordinated fashion. Reflexes are defined as rapid, automatic responses to stimuli in which a specific stimulus results in a specific motor response.

4. The myotatic reflex is initiated in response to a sudden change in length of the muscle. When a muscle is quickly stretched, the annulospiral nerve endings in the NMS transmit an impulse to the spinal cord, which results in an immediate strong reflex contraction of the same muscle from which the signal originated.

5. The inverse myotatic reflex is initiated when tension increases abruptly and intensely and stimulates Golgi tendon organs; it results in inhibition of the tensed muscle group, causing relaxation.

6. Volitional control of movement can be evidenced at the level of the motor unit as well as at the whole muscle level.

7. Flexibility is joint specific, and the degree or flexibility is specific to the individual. Static stretching or proprioceptive neuromuscular facilitation techniques are recommended to enhance flexibility.

8. There is little scientific evidence to suggest that resistance training will decrease flexibility. In fact, studies have shown that heavy resistance training results in either an improvement or no change in flexibility.

Review Questions

1. Describe the anatomical relationship between nerves and muscles. What is the functional significance of this relationship?

2. Diagram the sequence of events that occur at the neuromuscular junction.

3. Diagram the components of a generalized reflex arc.

4. Diagram the components of the myotatic reflex. Pay careful attention to the afferent and efferent neurons involved.

5. Diagram the components of the inverse myotatic reflex.

6. Outline the sequence of events involved in volitional control of movement.

7. Provide a rationale for incorporating a flexibility training program into an overall fitness program.

8. Critique the appropriateness of the sit-and-reach test to predict low-back pain.

9. What are the anatomical requirements of a healthy low back?

10. Describe static stretching, and explain the involvement of reflexes in providing for muscle elongation during this type of stretching.

11. Describe the proprioceptive neuromuscular facilitation technique, and explain the involvement of reflexes in providing for muscle elongation during this type of stretching.

12. Discuss the application of the individual training principles to the development of a flexibility program.

For further review and additional study tools, go to The Physiology Place (www.physiologyplace.com) and the Student Study Guide for Exercise Physiology for Health, Fitness, and Performance *by Sharon A. Plowman and Denise L. Smith.*

Passport to the Internet

Visit the following Internet sites to explore further topics and issues related to the neuromuscular aspects of movement. To visit an organization's web site, go to www.physiologyplace.com and click on "Passport to the Internet."

The American College of Sports Medicine As the leading professional organization for individuals in sports medicine and exercise science, the ACSM issues position statements on a number of topics critical to the study of exercise physiology. Search for the ACSM position statement on "The Recommended Quantity and Quality of Exercise for Developing and Maintaining Cardiorespiratory and Muscular Fitness and Flexibility in Healthy Adults."

Global Health and Fitness This online guide to healthy living and optimal fitness provides information on flexibility training, stretching exercises, and stretching programs. Information is aimed at beginners as well as advanced exercisers. The site is designed to help people interested in getting fit to become more efficient in their efforts.

InfoSports®.net The InfoSports web site is a portal for coaches, athletes, and parents to share ideas, training drills, game reports, announcements, and tournament information with others. Included is information on flexibility training (stretching), which helps balance muscle groups that might be overused during exercise or physical activity.

References

Alter, M. J.: *The Science of Stretching.* Champaign, IL: Human Kinetics (1988).

Basmajian, J. V.: Control of individual motor units. *American Journal of Physical Medicine.* 48(1):480–486 (1967).

Berne, R. M., & M. N. Levy: *Physiology.* St. Louis: Mosby (1988).

Biering-Sorenseu, F.: Physical measurements as risk indicators for low-back trouble over a one year period. *Spine.* 9(2):106–119 (1984).

Clarke, H. H.: Joint and body range of motion. In *Physical Fitness Research Digest* (series 5, no 4). Washington, DC: President's Council on Physical Fitness and Sports (1975).

Cornelius, W. L., R. W. Hagemann, & A. W. Jackson: A study on placement of stretching within a workout. *Journal of Sports Medicine and Physical Fitness.* 28:234–236 (1988).

Etnyre, B. R., & L. D. Abraham: Antagonist muscle activity during stretching: A paradox reassessed. *Medicine and Science in Sports and Exercise.* 20:285–289 (1988).

Etnyre, B. R., & E. J. Lee: Dialogue: Comments on proprioceptive neuromuscular facilitation stretching techniques. *Research Quarterly for Exercise and Sport.* 58:184–188 (1987).

Gleim, G. W., & M. P. McHugh: Flexibility and its effects on sports injury and performance. *Sports Medicine.* 24(5): 289–299 (1997).

Gomez, T. G., G. Beach, C. Cooke, W. Hrudey, & P. Goyert: Normative database for trunk range of motion, strength, velocity, and endurance with the isostation B-200 lumbar dynamometer. *Spine.* 16:15–21 (1991).

Guyton, A. C.: *Textbook of Medical Physiology.* Philadelphia: Saunders (1986).

Hardy, L., & D. Jones: Dynamic flexibility and proprioceptive neuromuscular facilitation. *Research Quarterly for Exercise and Sport.* 57:150–153 (1986).

High, D. M., E. T. Howley, & B. D. Franks: The effects of static stretching and warm-up on prevention of delayed-onset muscle soreness. *Research Quarterly for Exercise and Sport.* 60:356–361 (1989).

Hubley-Kozey, C. L.: Testing flexibility. In J. D. MacDougall, H. A. Weuger, & H. J. Green (eds.), *Physiological Testing of the High-Performance Athlete.* Champaign, IL: Human Kinetics (1991).

Hutton, R. S.: Neuromuscular basis of stretching exercises. In P. V. Komi (ed.), *Strength and Power in Sport.* London: Blackwell Scientific, 39–65 (1992).

Jackson, A. W., & A. A. Baker: The relationship of the sit and reach test to criterion measures of hamstring and back flexibility in young females. *Research Quarterly for Exercise and Sport.* 57:183–186 (1986).

Jackson, A. W., & N. J. Langford: The criterion-related validity of the sit and reach test: Replication and extension of previous findings. *Research Quarterly for Exercise and Sport.* 60:384–387 (1989).

Kippers, V., & A. W. Parker: Toe-touch test: A measure of its validity. *Physical Therapy.* 67:1680–1684 (1987).

Knudson, D.: Stretching during warm-up: Do we have enough evidence? *Journal of Physical Education Recreation and Dance.* 70(7):24–27 (1999).

Knudson, D.: Stretching: From science to practice. *Journal of Physical Education Recreation and Dance.* 69(3):38–42 (1998).

Knudson, D. V., P. Magnusson, & M. McHugh: Current issues in flexibility fitness. *President's Council on Physical Fitness and Sports Research Digest Series.* 3(10):1–8 (2000).

Kokkonen, J., A. G. Nelson, & A. Cornwell: Acute muscle stretching inhibits maximal strength performance. *Research Quarterly for Exercise and Sport.* 69(4):411–415 (1998).

Leighton, J.: Flexibility characteristics of three specialized skill groups of champion athletes. *Archives of Physical Medicine and Rehabilitation.* 36:580–583 (1957).

Malina, R. M., & C. Bouchard: *Growth, Maturation, and Physical Activity.* Champaign, IL: Human Kinetics (1991).

Marieb, E. N.: *Human Anatomy and Physiology* (5th edition) New York: Benjamin Cummings (2001).

Marshall, J. L., N. Johnson, T. L. Wickiewicz, H. M. Tischler, B. L. Koslin, S. Zeno, & A. Meyers: Joint looseness: A function of the person and joint. *Medicine and Science in Sports.* 12(3):189–194 (1980).

Massey, B. H., & N. L. Chaudet: Effects of heavy resistance exercise on range of joint movement in young male adults. *Research Quarterly.* 27:41–51 (1956).

McHugh, M. P., D. A. J. Connolly, R. G. Eston, I. J. Kreminic, S. J. Nichols, & G. W. Gleim: The role of passive muscle stiffness in symptoms of exercise-induced muscle damage. *The American Journal of Sports Medicine.* 27(5):594–599 (1999).

McHugh, M. P., I. J. Kreminic, M. B. Fox, & G. W. Gleim: The role of mechanical and neural restraints to joint range of motion during passive stretch. *Medicine and Science in Sports and Exercise.* 30(6):928–932 (1998).

Moll, J. M. H., & V. Wright: Normal range of spinal mobility: An objective clinical study. *Annals of Rheumatic Diseases.* 30:381–386 (1971).

Moran, H. M., M. A. Hall, A. Barr, & B. N. Ansell: Spinal mobility in the adolescent. *Rheumatology and Rehabilitation.* 18:181–185 (1979).

Nicolaisen, T., & K. Jorgensen: Trunk strength, back muscle endurance and low-back trouble. *Scandinavian Journal of Rehabilitation Medicine.* 17:121–127 (1985).

Osternig, L. R., R. N. Robertson, R. K. Troxel, & P. Hansen: Differential response to proprioceptive neuromuscular facilitation (PNF) stretch techniques. *Medicine and Science in Sports and Exercise.* 22:106–111 (1990).

Plowman, S. A.: Physical activity, physical fitness and low back pain. In J. O. Holloszy (ed.), *Exercise and Sport Science Reviews.* 20:221–242 (1992).

Rider, R. A., & J. Daly: Effects of flexibility training on enhancing spinal mobility in older women. *Journal of Sports Medicine and Physical Fitness.* 31:213–217 (1991).

Sage, G.: *Introduction to Motor Behavior: A Neurophysiological Approach.* Reading, MA: Addison-Wesley (1971).

Schmidt, R. A.: *Motor Control and Learning: A Behavioral Emphasis.* Champaign, IL; Human Kinetics (1988).

Shellock, F. G., & W. E. Prentice: Warming-up and stretching for improved physical performance and prevention of sports-related injuries. *Sports Medicine.* 2(4):267–278 (1985).

Shephard, R. J., M. Berridge, & W. Montelpare: On the generality of the "sit and reach" test: An analysis of flexibility data for an aging population. *Research Quarterly for Exercise and Sport.* 61:326–330 (1990).

Smith, C. A.: The warm-up procedure: To stretch or not to stretch. *Journal of Orthopedic Sports and Physical Therapy.* 19(1):12–17 (1994).

Sullivan, M. K., J. J. DeJulia, & T. W. Worrell: Effect of pelvic position and stretching method on hamstring muscle flexibility. *Medicine and Science in Sports and Exercise.* 24:1383–1389 (1992).

Tortora, G. J., & N. P. Anagnostakos: *Principles of Anatomy and Physiology* (5th edition). New York: Harper & Row, 280–305 (1987).

Wallin, D., B. Ekblom, R. Grahn, & T. Nordenborg: Improvement of muscle flexibility: A comparison between two techniques. *American Journal of Sports Medicine.* 13:263–268 (1985).

Appendix A

Units of Measure, the Metric System, and Conversions between the English and Metric Systems of Measurement

Table A.1
SI units (Système International) (Metric)

Physical Quantity	Unit	Symbol
Mass	kilogram	kg
Distance	meter	m
Volume (liquid or gas)	liter	L
Time	second	sec
Force	newton	N
Work	joule	J
Power	watt	W
Angle	radian	rad
Linear velocity	meters per second	$m \cdot sec^{-1}$
Angular velocity	radians per second	$rad \cdot sec^{-1}$
Temperature	degrees	°
Velocity	meters per second	$m \cdot sec^{-1}$
Torque	newton-meter	N-m
Acceleration	meters per second	$m \cdot sec^{-1}$
Amount of substance	mole	mol

Table A.2
SI Prefixes (Système International) (Metric)

Prefix*	Meaning	Scientific Notation	Symbol
Makes smaller			
deci-	one tenth of (0.1)	10^{-1}	d
centi-	one hundredth of (0.01)	10^{-2}	c
milli-	one thousandth of (0.001)	10^{-3}	m
micro-	one millionth of (0.000001)	10^{-6}	μm
Makes larger			
kilo-	a thousand times (1000)	10^{3}	k

* Most commonly used in this text

Table A.3

Conversions Between the English and Metric Systems of Measurement

Measurement	Unit and Abbreviation	Metric Equivalent	English-to-Metric Conversion Factor	Metric-to-English Conversion Factor
Length	1 kilometer (km)	= 1000 meters	1 mile = 1.61 km	1 km = 0.62 mile
	1 meter (m)	= 100 centimeters	1 yard = 0.914 m	1 m = 1.09 yards
		= 1000 millimeters	1 foot = 0.305 m	1 m = 3.28 feet
			1 foot = 30.5 cm	1 m = 39.37 inches
	1 centimeter (cm)	= 0.01 meter	1 inch = 2.54 cm	1 cm = 0.394 inch
	1 millimeter (mm)	= 0.001 meter		
	1 micrometer (μm)	= 0.000001 meter		
Mass	1 kilogram (kg)	= 1000 grams	1 pound = 0.454 kg	1 kg = 2.205 pounds
	1 gram (g)	= 1000 milligrams	1 ounce = 28.35 g	1 g = 0.035 ounce
	1 milligram (mg)	= 0.001 gram		
Volume (liquids and gases)	1 liter (L)	= 1000 milliliters	1 quart = 0.946 L 1 quart = 946 ml 1 gallon = 3.785 L	1 L = 0.264 gallon 1 L = 1.057 quarts
	1 milliliter (mL)	= 0.001 liter = 1 cubic centimeter	1 pint = 473 ml 1 fluid ounce = 29.57 ml	1 ml = 0.034 fluid ounce
	1 microliter (μL)	= 0.000001 liter		
Area	one square meter (m^2)	= 10000 square centimeters	1 square yard = 0.836 m^2	1 m^2 = 1.196 square yards
	one square centimeter (cm^2)	= 100 square millimeters	1 square inch = 6.452 cm^2	1 cm^2 = 0.155 square inch
Temperature	Degrees Celsius (°C)		°C = $\frac{5}{9}$(°F − 32)	°F = ($\frac{9}{5}$°C) + 32
Force	1 Newton (N)	= 0.1019 kilopond	1 ft-lb·sec[1] = 0.138 N	
Linear velocity	1 (m·sec^{-1})		1 mi·hr^{-1} = 26.m·min^{-1}	
Angular velocity	1 radian per second (rad·s^{-1})			1 radian^{-1} = 57.3°·s^{-1}
Work and energy	1 Joule (J)	= 1 N-m		1 J = 0.784 ft·lb
	1 kcal	= 426.85 kgm = 4.18 KJ		1 J = 0.239 cal
	1 kgm	= 1 kpm = 0.00234 kcal		
Power	1 watt (W)	1 W = 1 joule per sec (J·sec^{-1}) 1 W = 6.12 kgm·min^{-1}	1 hp = 745.7 W	1 W = 0.0013 hp
Pressure	1 Newton per square meter (N·m^2)		1 mmHg = 133.32 N·m^2 1 atmosphere = 760 mmHg	760 mmHg = 29.02 inches

Appendix B

Metabolic Calculations

This appendix describes three methods used to calculate oxygen consumption ($\dot{V}O_2$cons). The first series of equations are direct calculations using data obtained from open-circuit spirometry. This technique also allows for the calculation of carbon dioxide produced ($\dot{V}CO_2$prod), which the other two, because they are indirect techniques, do not. The second series of equations calculates submaximal oxygen consumption values for selected activities (walking, running, cycle ergometer riding, and stair stepping) using known rates of work. The third set of calculations estimates maximal oxygen consumption ($\dot{V}O_2$max) from selected field tests (the PACER, or 20-meter shuttle test, and the Rockport Fitness Walking Test).

The Calculation of Oxygen Consumed and Carbon Dioxide Produced from Data Obtained by Open-Circuit Spirometry

Basic Formulas

Theoretically, the amount of oxygen consumed is simply equal to the amount of oxygen in inspired air minus the amount of oxygen in the expired air. All values are expressed in $mL \cdot min^{-1}$ or $L \cdot min^{-1}$.

B.1 oxygen consumption ($L \cdot min^{-1}$) = amount of oxygen inspired ($L \cdot min^{-1}$) − amount of oxygen expired ($L \cdot min^{-1}$).

$$\dot{V}O_2\text{cons} = \dot{V}_IO_2 - \dot{V}_EO_2$$

In practice, there is no way to obtain $\dot{V}_IO_2$ or $\dot{V}_EO_2$ directly, so a working formula is used. The working formula is based on the fact that the amount of a gas depends on the fraction (F) of the gas and the volume of air containing that gas.

B.2 oxygen consumption ($L \cdot min^{-1}$) = [fraction of oxygen in inspired air × volume of inspired air ($L \cdot min^{-1}$)] − [fraction of oxygen in expired air × volume of expired air ($L \cdot min^{-1}$)]

$$\dot{V}O_2\text{cons} = (F_IO_2 \times \dot{V}_I) - (F_EO_2 \times \dot{V}_E)$$

Although the term *fraction* and the symbol *F* are always used in this equation, these values really represent the percentages of oxygen in inspired or expired air, and they are expressed mathematically as decimals. Thus, F_IO_2 is a constant 20.93%, or 0.2093. The inspired ventilation values either can be directly measured by a spirometer or pneumoscan, as described in Chapters 5 and 10, or can be calculated.

The F_EO_2 is measured by an oxygen analyzer, as described in Chapter 5. As with the inspired ventilation, expired ventilation can be either directly measured by a spirometer or pneumoscan or can be calculated. Either $\dot{V}_I$ or $\dot{V}_E$ must be directly measured. When the value from one of them is known, the other can be calculated.

Ventilation Conversions

As stated in Chapter 10, the volume of air (either inspired or expired) is collected under conditions known as ambient temperature and pressure saturated, or ATPS. To do metabolic calculations, air volumes must first be converted to standard temperature and pressure (STPD) values. This conversion is necessary so that the number of gas molecules in any given volume is equal. The equations vary slightly according to whether the measured volume is inspired or expired.

The conversion process is based on the impact of temperature, pressure, and water vapor molecules on volume. The effect of temperature on volume is described by Charles's Law. *Charles's Law* states that the volume of a gas is directly related to temperature assuming a constant pressure, that is,

$$\frac{T_1}{T_2} = \frac{V_1}{V_2}$$

Therefore, if the initial temperature (T_1) is increased (T_2), the initial volume (V_1) will also be increased (V_2). Conversely, if T_1 is decreased at T_2, then V_1 will also be decreased at V_2. In metabolic calculations, V_2 is the value that is unknown. Therefore, the working formula that takes into account the impact of temperature on volume becomes

$$V_2 \times T_1 = V_1 \times T_2 \quad \text{or} \quad V_2 = \frac{V_1 \times T_2}{T_1}$$

usually expressed as

$$V_2 = V_1 \left(\frac{T_2}{T_1} \right)$$

The effect of pressure on volume is primarily described by Boyle's Law. *Boyle's Law* states that the volume of a gas is inversely related to pressure assuming a constant temperature, that is

$$\frac{P_1}{P_2} = \frac{V_2}{V_1}$$

Table B.1
Water Vapor Pressure (PH$_2$O) at Selected Ambient Temperatures

Ambient Temperature (°C)	Ambient Temperature (°F)	PH$_2$O (mmHg)
20	68	17.5
21	70	18.7
22	72	19.8
23	73	21.1
24	75	22.4
25	77	23.8

Table B.2
Ventilation Conversion Factors

Volume	Pressure	Temperature
$\dot{V}_E$ATPS	$P_B - PH_2O$ at T°C	$273° + T°C$
$\dot{V}_I$ATPS	$P_B - [RH \times PH_2O$ at T°C]	$273° + T°C$
$\dot{V}_E$STPD	760	273°
$\dot{V}_E$BTPS	$P_B - 47$	$273° + 37°$

P_B = measured barometric pressure in mmHg

PH_2O = water vapor pressure in mmHg

T°C = measured temperature in degrees Celsius

RH = relative humidity as a fraction

273° Kelvin = 0° Celsius = standard temperature

37°C = normal body temperature

47 mmHg = water vapor pressure at 37°C

Therefore, if the initial pressure (P_1) is increased (P_2), the initial volume (V_1) will be decreased (V_2). Conversely, if P_1 is decreased at P_2, then V_1 will be increased at V_2. Because V_2 is again the value which is unknown, this formula rearranges to

$$V_2 \times P_2 = V_1 \times P_1 \quad \text{or} \quad V_2 = \frac{V_1 \times P_1}{P_2}$$

usually expressed as

$$V_2 = V_1 \left(\frac{P_1}{P_2}\right)$$

Water vapor molecules evaporate into air (or into other gases) and account for part of the pressure exerted by the gas. The amount of water vapor is related exponentially to temperature. If the temperature is constant and a gas goes from being saturated with water vapor (S) to dry (D), the volume of the gas decreases. Conversely, if a gas goes from D to S, the volume increases. Tables, such as the abbreviated version in Table B.1, are available to determine the water vapor pressure (PH$_2$O) at measured ambient temperatures.

In practice, the formulas just described are generally combined so that the effects of temperature and volume are calculated concurrently, as indicated in the following formula.

B.3 $V_2 = V_1 \left(\dfrac{T_2}{T_1}\right)\left(\dfrac{P_1}{P_2}\right)$

The order of the temperature and pressure components in this equation may be reversed. If necessary, pressure is adjusted for water vapor.

Table B.2 presents the factors that are used in converting ventilatory volumes from ATPS to BTPS or STPD using expired and inspired ventilation volumes. BTPS ventilations are not used in the calculation of $\dot{V}O_2$ consumed and $\dot{V}CO_2$ produced, but they are presented for completeness and because BTPS

values are used in determining ventilatory thresholds (Chapter 11) and lung volumes (Chapter 10).

The Conversion of $\dot{V}_E$ from ATPS to BTPS

When any ventilation volume is converted, it is first important to identify P_1, P_2, T_1, and T_2. Thus, in converting from $\dot{V}_E$ATPS to $\dot{V}_E$BTPS, P_1 is the ambient pressure; P_2 is body pressure, which equals barometric pressure; T_1 is the ambient temperature; and T_2 is body temperature. Second, the factor representing each of these components should then be identified from Table B.2: that is, $P_1 = P_B - PH_2O$ at T°C; $P_2 = P_B - 47$; $T_1 = 273 + T°C$; and $T_2 = 273 + 37°C$. This 273 is 273° Kelvin, to which either the measured temperature (T°C) or normal body temperature (37°C) is added. Ambient pressure is the measured barometric pressure at the data collection site corrected for the water vapor pressure at the ambient temperature. Table B.1 is used to determine the water vapor pressure. Body pressure is the measured barometric pressure corrected for water vapor pressure at body temperature. Normal body temperature is assumed to be 37°C. Water vapor pressure (PH$_2$O) at 37°C is 47 mmHg.

Based on Equation B.3, the conversion formula becomes

B.4 minute ventilation (L·min^{-1}) BTPS = minute ventilation (L·min^{-1}) ATPS × temperature correction (°Kelvin) × pressure correction (mmHg)

or

$$\dot{V}_E BTPS = \dot{V}_E ATPS \left(\frac{273° + 37°C}{273° + T°C}\right)\left(\frac{P_B - PH_2O \text{ at } T°C}{P_B - 47}\right)$$

For example, given the following information, we can correct $\dot{V}_E$ from ATPS to BTPS conditions.

$\dot{V}_E$ ATPS = 12 L·min^{-1}

T ATPS = 22°C

P_B = 745 mmHg

$\dot{V}_E$ BTPS =
$$12\ \text{L·min}^{-1}\left(\frac{273° + 37°C}{273° + 22°C}\right)\left(\frac{745\ \text{mmHg} - 19.8\ \text{mmHg}}{745 - 47\ \text{mmHg}}\right)$$

$\dot{V}_E$ BTPS = 13.1 L·min^{-1}

Under typical ambient conditions (without extremely high heat or altitude), BTPS values will be larger numerically than ATPS values because body temperature is usually higher than ambient temperature (which increases volume). Also, body pressure adjusted for water vapor pressure at body temperature is typically lower than ambient pressure adjusted for water vapor pressure at ambient temperature (which also increases volume).

The Conversion of $\dot{V}_E$ from ATPS to STPD

In converting from $\dot{V}_E$ ATPS to $\dot{V}_E$ STPD, we identify P_1 as ambient pressure; P_2 as standard pressure; T_1 as ambient temperature; and T_2 as standard temperature. Identifying each of these components from Table B.2 results in the following: $P_1 = P_B - PH_2O$ at T°C; $P_2 = 760$; $T_1 = 273° + T°C$; and $T_2 = 273°$. The body (barometric) pressure must be adjusted for the water vapor pressure at the ambient temperature so that the conversion goes from saturated or wet air to unsaturated or dry conditions. The formula for converting $\dot{V}_E$ ATPS to $\dot{V}_E$ STPD accounts for changes in temperature (T) and pressure (P) as follows:

B.5 minute ventilation (L·min^{-1}) STPD = minute ventilation (L·min^{-1}) ATPS × temperature correction (°Kelvin) × pressure correction (mmHg)

or

$$\dot{V}_E\ \text{STPD} = \dot{V}_E\ \text{ATPS}\left(\frac{273°}{273° + T°C}\right)\left(\frac{P_B - PH_2O\ \text{at T°C}}{760}\right)$$

In this equation, the 273 represents the standard temperature of 0°C, which equals 273° Kelvin. The T°C represents the ambient temperature in degrees Celsius. PH_2O represents the water vapor correction from Table B.1 to the body or barometric pressure (P_B), and 760 mmHg is standard pressure. Thus, given the following information, we can correct $\dot{V}_E$ from ATPS to STPD conditions.

$\dot{V}_E$ ATPS = 12 L·min^{-1}

T ATPS = 22°C

P_B = 745 mmHg

$\dot{V}_E$ STPD =
$$12\ \text{L·min}^{-1}\left(\frac{273°}{273° + 22°C}\right)\left(\frac{745\ \text{mmHg} - 19.8\ \text{mmHg}}{760\ \text{mmHg}}\right)$$

$\dot{V}_E$ STPD = 10.6 L·min^{-1}

The Conversion of $\dot{V}_I$ from ATPS to STPD

The conversion of $\dot{V}_I$ from ATPS to $\dot{V}_I$ STPD is the same as from $\dot{V}_E$ ATPS to $\dot{V}_E$ STPD, with one small addition: In most laboratory settings, the inspired air is not totally saturated; that is, the relative humidity is not 100%. The equation must therefore be modified to adjust for the measured relative humidity (RH), expressed as a decimal fraction at the ambient temperature. Thus, the conversion equation becomes

B.6 $\dot{V}_I$ STPD =
$$\dot{V}_I\ \text{ATPS}\left(\frac{273°}{273° + T°C}\right)\left(\frac{P_B - [RH \times PH_2O\ \text{at T°C}]}{760}\right)$$

Again, Table B.1 presents the water vapor pressures (PH_2O) at temperatures generally encountered in a laboratory (20–25°C or 67–77°F). Thus, under the conditions given in the previous example but with a RH of 46%, the calculations become

$\dot{V}_I$ STPD = 12 L·min^{-1}
$$\left(\frac{273°}{273° + 22°}\right)\left(\frac{745\ \text{mmHg} - [0.46 \times 19.8\ \text{mmHg}]}{760\ \text{mmHg}}\right)$$

$\dot{V}_I$ STPD = 10.8 L·min^{-1}

Under typical ambient conditions (without extreme high heat or altitude), STPD values, whether derived from expired or inspired ventilation volumes, are smaller numerically than ATPS values. The reason is that standard temperature is usually lower than ambient temperature (which decreases volume), and standard pressure is usually higher than ambient pressure (which decreases volume). The number of gas molecules depends on the volume they occupy. Therefore, STPD volumes are used when it is important to know the number of gas molecules, as in the calculation of O_2 consumed and CO_2 produced. The number of gas molecules and the volume they occupy under STPD conditions are constant and independent of the particular gas involved.

The Conversion of $\dot{V}_I$ from BTPS to STPD and Vice Versa

Occasionally it is necessary to convert between BTPS and STPD, often based on which values any particular software-driven printout is programmed to provide.

When BTPS is converted to STPD, P_1 is body or barometric pressure; P_2 is standard pressure; T_1 is body temperature; T_2 is standard temperature. From Table B.2, these factors are identified as: $P_1 = P_B - 47$; $P_2 = 760$; $T_1 = 273° + 37°C$; and $T_2 = 273°$. Substituting these into the generic Equation B.3,

$$V_2 = V_1 \left(\frac{T_2}{T_1}\right)\left(\frac{P_1}{P_2}\right)$$

we get

B.7 $\dot{V}_E$ STPD =

$$\dot{V}_E \text{ BTPS}\left(\frac{273°}{273° + 37°C}\right)\left(\frac{P_B - 47 \text{ mmHg}}{760 \text{ mmHg}}\right)$$

Using the values from our examples

$$\dot{V}_E \text{ BTPS} = 13.1 \text{ L·min}$$
$$P_B \text{ STPD} = 745 \text{ mmHg}$$

we can calculate $\dot{V}_E$ STPD as

$$\dot{V}_E \text{ STPD} =$$
$$13.1 \text{ L·min}\left(\frac{273°}{273° + 37°}\right)\left(\frac{745 \text{ mmHg} - 47 \text{ mmHg}}{760 \text{ mmHg}}\right)$$
$$\dot{V}_E \text{ STPD} = 10.6 \text{ L·min}$$

Conversely, when STPD is converted to BTPS, P_1 is standard pressure (760 mmHg); P_2 is body pressure ($P_B - 47$ mmHg); T_1 is standard temperature (0°C or 273°K); and T_2 is body temperature (assumed to be $273° + 37°C$). Substituting these values into the generic equation, we get

B.8 $\dot{V}_E$ BTPS =

$$\dot{V}_E \text{ STPD}\left(\frac{273° + 37°C}{273°}\right)\left(\frac{760 \text{ mmHg}}{P_B - 47 \text{ mmHg}}\right)$$

Again, using the values from our example:

$$\dot{V}_E \text{ STPD} = 10.6 \text{ L·min}^{-1}$$
$$P_B = 745 \text{ mmHg}$$
$$\dot{V}_E \text{ BTPS} =$$
$$10.6 \text{ L·min}^{-1}\left(\frac{273° + 37°}{273°}\right)\left(\frac{760 \text{ mmHg}}{745 \text{ mmHg} - 47 \text{ mmHg}}\right)$$
$$\dot{V}_E \text{ BTPS} = 13.1 \text{ L·min}$$

Calculation of the Unknown Ventilation Value

The Calculation of $\dot{V}_E$ from $\dot{V}_I$ and $\dot{V}_I$ from $\dot{V}_E$

Open-circuit metabolic systems measure either inspired or expired air, but not both. Typically the volume of expired air does not equal the volume of inspired air. The reason is that the number of oxygen molecules used from the inspired air is not replaced by the same number of carbon dioxide molecules, except when an individual is burning pure carbohydrate and has an RER of exactly 1.0. When fewer CO_2 molecules replace the O_2 molecules, the RER value is less than 1.0, and $\dot{V}_E$ will be smaller than $\dot{V}_I$. If the RER value is greater than 1.0, $\dot{V}_E$ will be larger than $\dot{V}_I$. This occurs when both metabolic and nonmetabolic CO_2 molecules (primarily from the buffering of lactic acid) are produced.

In order to solve Equation B.2 (that is, calculate $\dot{V}O_2$cons), we must have values for both $\dot{V}_E$ and $\dot{V}_I$. Fortunately, there is a way to convert $\dot{V}_E$ to $\dot{V}_I$ or $\dot{V}_I$ to $\dot{V}_E$ mathematically. This is called the *Haldane transformation* and is based on the fact that nitrogen (N_2) is an inert gas that does not participate in human metabolism nor easily combine with any blood constituents. The number of particles of nitrogen does not change, although the concentration or fraction of the nitrogen will change because the fractions of oxygen and carbon dioxide are changing. Thus, the amount (again defined as the fraction of the gas times the volume of air containing that gas) of gaseous nitrogen expired is exactly equal to the amount of gaseous nitrogen inspired. That is,

B.9 fraction of inspired nitrogen times the inspired minute ventilation = fraction of expired nitrogen times the expired minute ventilation

or

$$F_I N_2 \times \dot{V}_I = F_E N_2 \times \dot{V}_E$$

Rearranging the equation, it becomes

$$\dot{V}_I = \frac{F_E N_2 \times \dot{V}_E}{F_I N_2} \text{ or } \dot{V}_E = \frac{F_I N_2 \times \dot{V}_I}{F_E N_2}$$

B.10 $\dot{V}_I = \dot{V}_E\left(\dfrac{F_E N_2}{F_I N_2}\right)$ and $\dot{V}_E = \dot{V}_I\left(\dfrac{F_I N_2}{F_E N_2}\right)$

As usual in these formulas, the measurements are percentages, but they are expressed as decimal fractions. Both $F_I N_2$ and $F_E N_2$ are easily obtained from known and measured values. Air is composed of nitrogen, oxygen, and carbon dioxide, and the fractions of O_2 and CO_2 are known for room air (assumed to be the inspired air) and measured for expired air by the gas analyzers. Thus, N_2 can be calculated by simple subtraction:

$$F_I N_2 = 1 - [F_I O_2 + F_E CO_2] = .7904$$
$$.2093 + .0003$$

and

$$F_E N_2 = 1 - [F_E O_2 + F_E CO_2] = \text{variables measured by analyzers}$$

Therefore,

B.11 $\dot{V}_I = \dot{V}_E\left(\dfrac{1 - [F_E O_2 + F_E CO_2]}{.7904}\right)$

B.12 $\dot{V}_E = \dot{V}_I\left(\dfrac{.7904}{1 - [F_E O_2 + F_E CO_2]}\right)$

For example, given

$$\dot{V}_I \text{ STPD} = 10.8 \text{ L}^{-1}\cdot\text{min}^{-1}$$
$$O_2\% = 16.38$$
$$CO_2\% = 4.03$$

the computation becomes

$$\dot{V}_I \text{ STPD} = 10.8 \text{ L}^{-1}\cdot\text{min}^{-1}\left(\frac{0.7904}{1-[0.1638+0.0403]}\right)$$
$$= 10.73$$

Conversely, if we are given

$$\dot{V}_E \text{ STPD} = 10.6 \text{ L}^{-1}\cdot\text{min}^{-1}$$
$$O_2\% = 16.38$$
$$CO_2\% = 4.03$$

the computation becomes

$$\dot{V}_I \text{ STPD} = 10.6 \text{ L}^{-1}\cdot\text{min}^{-1}\left(\frac{1-[0.1638+0.0403]}{0.7904}\right)$$
$$= 10.67 \text{ L}^{-1}\cdot\text{min}^{-1}$$

Calculation of Oxygen Consumed

Now we are finally ready to go back to Equation B.2 and solve it.

$$\dot{V}O_2 \text{ L}^{-1}\cdot\text{min}^{-1} = (F_IO_2 \times \dot{V}_I) - (F_EO_2 \times \dot{V}_E)$$

The information we have available is as follows:

$$F_IO_2 = 0.2093 \text{ (assumed constant)}$$
$$\dot{V}_I \text{ STPD} = 10.8 \text{ L}^{-1}\cdot\text{min}^{-1} \text{ (measured as } \dot{V}_I \text{ ATPS}$$
by pneumoscan and converted by Eq. B.6)
$$F_EO_2 = 0.1638 \text{ (measured by oxygen analyzer)}$$
$$\dot{V}_E \text{ STPD} = 10.73 \text{ L}^{-1}\cdot\text{min}^{-1} \text{ (calculated by the}$$
Haldane transformation in Eq. B.12)

Inserting the given values into Equation B.2, we get

$$\dot{V}O_2 \text{ L}\cdot\text{min}^{-1} = (0.2093 \times 10.8 \text{ L}\cdot\text{min}^{-1})$$
$$- (0.1638 \times 10.73 \text{ L}\cdot\text{min}^{-1})$$
$$= 0.5 \text{ L}\cdot^{-1} \text{ or } 500 \text{ mL}\cdot\text{min}^{-1}$$

Calculation of Carbon Dioxide Produced

Theoretically, the amount of carbon dioxide produced is simply equal to the amount of carbon dioxide in expired air minus the amount of carbon dioxide in inspired air.

B.13 $\dot{V}_I CO_2$ prod $= \dot{V}_E CO_2 - \dot{V}_I CO_2$

Because there is no way to obtain $\dot{V}_E CO_2$ or $\dot{V}_I CO_2$ directly, a working formula must again be used. Thus, the calculation of the amount of carbon dioxide produced is very similar to the calculation of oxygen consumed.

B.14 carbon dioxide produced (L·min⁻¹) = [fraction of carbon dioxide in expired air × volume of expired air (L·min⁻¹)] − [fraction of inspired carbon dioxide × volume of inspired air (L·min⁻¹)].

$$\dot{V}_I CO_2 \text{ L}\cdot\text{min}^{-1} = (F_ECO_2 \times \dot{V}_E) - (F_ICO_2 \times \dot{V}_I)$$

The F_ICO_2 is a constant 0.0003 because the percentage of carbon dioxide in room air is assumed to be 0.03%. Because this number is so small and would have no meaningful effect on the calculation in Equation B.14, it is generally considered to be 0. As a result, only the expired portion of the equation needs to be computed. F_ECO_2 is measured by a carbon dioxide analyzer as described in Chapter 5. $\dot{V}_E$ either is directly measured by a spirometer or pneumoscan or is calculated as previously described.

Using the values of $CO_2\%$ and $\dot{V}_E$ given previously, the calculation example becomes

$$\dot{V}_I CO_2 \text{ L}\cdot\text{min}^{-1} = (0.0403 \times 10.73 \text{ L}\cdot\text{min}^{-1})$$
$$= 0.43 \text{ L}\cdot\text{min}^{-1} \text{ or } 430 \text{ mL}\cdot\text{min}^{-1}$$

Note that as mentioned in the section describing the calculation of $\dot{V}_E$ from $\dot{V}_I$, the oxygen consumed (500 mL·min⁻¹) is not equaled by the amount of carbon dioxide produced (430 mL·min⁻¹).

Complete the practice problems at the end of the appendix to determine your understanding of these concepts and calculations.

The Calculation of Oxygen Consumed using Mechanical Work or Speed of Movement

In exercise situations where an accurate assessment of mechanical work or speed of movement is possible but the actual measurement of oxygen consumed and carbon dioxide produced is not, the oxygen consumed can be estimated. These situations include walking, running, cycling on an ergometer, and bench stepping. Specific formulas recommended by the American College of Sports Medicine (2000) are available for each activity. The resulting oxygen consumption values will not be as accurate as the direct measurement of oxygen consumed, which was described in the last section. However, these estimated oxygen consumptions are much less difficult and much less expensive to obtain. They can be very useful in the practical field settings of health clubs, hospitals, and/or school gymnasia as the initial step in determining exercise prescriptions by MET level or determining the caloric cost of any activity. Because of differences in economy (Chapter 5), none of these equations should be used for children. Because no systematic differences in economy have been found between males and females, all of these equations can be used for both sexes.

The following computations show you how to determine the oxygen consumption values of the four activities specified earlier. Remember from Chapter 5 that converting to METs requires dividing the O_2 $mL \cdot kg^{-1} \cdot min^{-1}$ value by 3.5 $mL \cdot kg^{-1} \cdot min^{-1}$. Caloric cost (also discussed in Chapter 5) can be estimated by multiplying the O_2 $L \cdot min^{-1}$ value by 5 $kcal \cdot L \cdot min^{-1}$, because 5 $kcal \cdot L \cdot min^{-1}$ is the estimated caloric equivalent if the RER is unknown.

Oxygen Consumed during Horizontal (Level) and Vertical (Graded) Walking

Level Walking

To determine the oxygen consumed while walking on level ground or on a treadmill at zero percent elevation, it is necessary to determine the walking speed in meters per minute ($m \cdot min^{-1}$). It is known that for speeds between 1.9 and 3.7 $mi \cdot hr^{-1}$ (or 50–100 $m \cdot min^{-1}$; 26.8 $m \cdot min^{-1} = 1$ $mi \cdot hr^{-1}$), the net oxygen cost of level walking is 0.1 $mL \cdot kg^{-1} \cdot min^{-1}$ per $m \cdot min^{-1}$. Because this oxygen consumption constant is a net value, the oxygen consumed during rest (1 MET or 3.5 $mL \cdot kg^{-1} \cdot min^{-1}$) is added to obtain the total amount of oxygen consumed. Therefore, the equation can be stated as follows:

B.15 oxygen consumed during horizontal walking ($mL \cdot kg^{-1} \cdot min^{-1}$) =
horizontal component ($mL \cdot kg^{-1} \cdot min^{-1}$) +
resting component ($mL \cdot kg^{-1} \cdot min^{-1}$)

or

$$\dot{V}O_2cons \ (mL \cdot kg^{-1} \cdot min^{-1}) = [speed \ (m \cdot min^{-1})$$
$$\times \frac{0.1 \ mL \cdot kg^{-1} \cdot min^{-1}}{m \cdot min^{-1}}] + 3.5 \ mL \cdot kg^{-1} \cdot min^{-1}$$

For example, if an individual were walking on a treadmill at 0% grade and 3 $mi \cdot hr^{-1}$, it would first be necessary to convert the speed to meters per minute (3 $mi \cdot hr^{-1} \times 26.8$ $m \cdot min^{-1}/mi \cdot hr^{-1} = 80.4$ $m \cdot min^{-1}$). Then, substituting this value into Equation B.15 we get

$$\dot{V}O_2cons \ (mL \cdot kg^{-1} \cdot min^{-1}) = [80.4 \ m \cdot min^{-1}$$
$$\times \frac{0.1 \ mL \cdot kg^{-1} \cdot min^{-1}}{m \cdot min^{-1}}] + 3.5 \ mL \cdot kg^{-1} \cdot min^{-1}$$
$$\dot{V}O_2cons = 11.54 \ mL \cdot kg^{-1} \cdot min^{-1}$$

Graded Walking

To determine the oxygen consumed during uphill walking or walking on a treadmill at a grade, a verti-

cal component is added to Equation B.15. The vertical component is determined by the percent grade expressed as a decimal. Each $m \cdot min^{-1}$ of vertical rise consumes an additional 1.8 $mL \cdot kg^{-1} \cdot min^{-1}$ for each $m \cdot min^{-1}$ of speed. The following formula incorporates the vertical component in Equation B.15.

B.16 oxygen consumed during vertical walking ($mL \cdot kg^{-1} \cdot min^{-1}$) =
horizontal component ($mL \cdot kg^{-1} \cdot min^{-1}$) +
resting component ($mL \cdot kg^{-1} \cdot min^{-1}$) +
vertical component ($mL \cdot kg^{-1} \cdot min^{-1}$)

or

$$\dot{V}O_2cons \ (mL \cdot kg^{-1} \cdot min^{-1}) = [speed \ (m \cdot min^{-1})$$
$$\times \frac{0.1 \ mL \cdot kg^{-1} \cdot min^{-1}}{m \cdot min^{-1}}] + 3.5 \ mL \cdot kg^{-1} \cdot min^{-1}$$
$$+ [decimal \ grade \times speed \ (m \cdot min^{-1})$$
$$\times \frac{1.8 \ mL \cdot kg^{-1} \cdot min^{-1}}{m \cdot min^{-1}}]$$

If we change the percent grade in the previous example from 0% to 5%, we now have only to calculate the vertical component.

$$Vertical \ component = [0.05 \times 80.4 \ m \cdot min^{-1}$$
$$\times \frac{1.8 \ mL \cdot kg^{-1} \cdot min^{-1}}{m \cdot min^{-1}}] = 7.24 \ mL \cdot kg^{-1} \cdot min^{-1}$$

The vertical component is then added to the horizontal and resting components to get the total amount of oxygen consumed while walking at a speed of 3 $mi \cdot hr^{-1}$ with a 5% grade on a treadmill.

Horizontal component	= 8.04 $mL \cdot kg^{-1} \cdot min^{-1}$
Resting component	= 3.50 $mL \cdot kg^{-1} \cdot min^{-1}$
Vertical component	= 7.24 $mL \cdot kg^{-1} \cdot min^{-1}$
Total $\dot{V}O_2cons$	= 18.78 $mL \cdot kg^{-1} \cdot min^{-1}$

Oxygen Consumed during Horizontal (Level) and Vertical (Graded) Running

The formulas for estimating the amount of oxygen consumed during running differ from those for walking only in two factors. The first is that the net oxygen cost of level running is 0.2 $mL \cdot kg^{-1} \cdot min^{-1}$ per $m \cdot min^{-1}$, or double the same cost for walking. Conversely, the additional cost for the vertical components is only half as much as for walking, because of differences in the biomechanics of the two gaits, especially the greater forefoot pushoff in running. This difference necessitates multiplying the vertical component by 0.5. Thus, 1.8 $mL \cdot kg^{-1} \cdot min^{-1} \times 0.5 = 0.9$ $mL \cdot kg^{-1} \cdot min^{-1}$.

Running is defined as speeds greater than 5 $mi \cdot hr^{-1}$ (134 $m \cdot min^{-1}$). This leaves a gap between the top walking speeds (3.7 $mi \cdot hr^{-1}$ or 100 $m \cdot min^{-1}$) and the lowest running speed. The best formula for these intermediate speeds depends on whether the individual is actually running or walking.

The formula for determining the oxygen consumed while running on level ground or a treadmill is as follows:

B.17 $\dot{V}O_2$cons (mL·kg^{-1}·min^{-1}) = [speed (m·min^{-1})

$$\times \frac{0.2 \text{ mL·kg}^{-1} \cdot \text{min}^{-1}}{\text{m·min}^{-1}}] + 3.5 \text{ mL·kg}^{-1} \cdot \text{min}^{-1}$$

Graded running adds a vertical component to Equation B.17:

B.18 $\dot{V}O_2$cons (mL·kg^{-1}·min^{-1}) = [speed (m·min^{-1})

$$\times \frac{0.2 \text{ mL·kg}^{-1} \cdot \text{min}^{-1}}{\text{m·min}^{-1}}] \, 3.5 \text{ mL·kg}^{-1} \cdot \text{min}^{-1}$$

+ [decimal grade × speed (m·min^{-1})

$$\times \frac{.9 \text{ mL·kg}^{-1} \cdot \text{min}^{-1}}{\text{m·min}^{-1}}]$$

If the individual in the previous example switches from walking at 3 $mi \cdot hr^{-1}$ up a 5% grade to running the same grade at 7 $mi \cdot hr^{-1}$ (188 $m \cdot min^{-1}$), this example works out as follows:

$\dot{V}O_2$cons (mL·kg^{-1}·min^{-1}) = [188 m·min^{-1}

$$\times \frac{0.2 \text{ mL·kg}^{-1} \cdot \text{min}^{-1}}{\text{m·min}^{-1}}] + 3.5 \text{ mL·kg}^{-1} \cdot \text{min}^{-1}$$

+ [0.05 × 188 m·min^{-1}]

Horizontal component	= 37.60 mL·kg^{-1}·min^{-1}
Resting component	= 3.50 mL·kg^{-1}·min^{-1}
Vertical component	= 8.46 mL·kg^{-1}·min^{-1}
Total $\dot{V}O_2$cons	= 49.56 mL·kg^{-1}·min^{-1}

Oxygen Consumed during Cycling Using Either the Legs or the Arms

The formulas for calculating the amount of oxygen consumed during cycling are intended only for cycling on an ergometer, which permits the actual measurement of the workload. The mechanical work completed (as described in Chapter 5) is determined by multiplying the force exerted, in the form of the load or resistance overcome, in kilograms, by the distance traveled (m·min^{-1}) using the following equation.

B.19 work rate (kgm·min^{-1}) = kg of resistance × m·rev^{-1} × rev·min^{-1}

The distance traveled per revolution is the circumference off the flywheel. On many ergometers, including the often-used Monark friction ergometers, this distance is 6 m. The pedaling rate, or revolutions per minute value, is typically displayed on the console of the ergometer and can vary from 30–110 rev·min^{-1}, with 50 or 60 rev·min^{-1} being the most common.

Leg Cycling

Oxygen consumed during leg cycling can be estimated using the following equation. This formula is most accurate when the work rate is between 300 and 1200 kgm·min^{-1}, but it may be used up to rates of 4200 kgm·min^{-1}. The oxygen cost against the external load is equal to that of vertical walking, or 1.8 mL·kg^{-1}·min^{-1} per m·min^{-1}.

B.20 oxygen consumed during leg cycling (mL·kg^{-1}·min^{-1}) = [oxygen consumed during the resistance component (mL·kg^{-1}·min^{-1}) divided by body weight (kg)] + oxygen consumed during the resting component (mL·kg^{-1}·min^{-1}) + oxygen associated with unloaded cycling

or

$\dot{V}O_2$cons (mL·kg^{-1}·min^{-1})

$$= [\frac{1.8 \text{ mL·kg}^{-1} \cdot \text{min}^{-1}}{\text{m·min}^{-1}} \text{ work rate (kgm·min}^{-1}\text{)}$$

$$\div \text{ body weight (kg)}] + 7 \text{ mL·kg}^{-1} \cdot \text{min}^{-1}$$

For example, if a 50-kg individual pedals a Monark bike at 60 rev·min^{-1} at a load of 2 kg (denoted as 2 kp on the ergometer itself; 1 kg = 1 kp), she consumes 32.92 mL·kg^{-1}·min^{-1}, which is calculated as follows:

$$\dot{V}O_2 \text{ (mL·kg}^{-1} \cdot \text{min}^{-1}\text{)} = [\frac{1.8 \text{ mL·kg}^{-1} \cdot \text{min}^{-1}}{\text{m·min}^{-1}}$$

(2 kg × 6·m rev^{-1} × 60 rev·min^{-1}) ÷ 50 kg]

+ 7 mL·kg^{-1}·min^{-1}

Resistance component	= 25.92 mL·kg^{-1}·min^{-1}
Rest + unloaded component	= 7.00 mL·kg^{-1}·min^{-1}
Total $\dot{V}O_2$cons	= 32.92 mL·kg^{-1}·min^{-1}

Arm Cranking

Cycling with the arms is more properly referred to as arm cranking. The formula for arm cranking differs from leg cycling in the constant for oxygen use per kilogram of resistance. The arm musculature used in cranking is smaller than the leg musculature used in cycling; hence there is no need for the addition of an unloaded cycling cost. However, additional muscles in the shoulders, back, and chest are recruited to stabilize the arms, elevating the oxygen cost. Thus, instead of a constant 1.8 $mL \cdot kg^{-1} \cdot min^{-1}$ per $m \cdot min^{-1}$, the value used is 3 $mL \cdot kg^{-1} \cdot min^{-1}$ per $m \cdot min^{-1}$. This is appropriate for power outputs between 150 and 750 $kgm \cdot min^{-1}$.

B.21 oxygen consumed during arm cranking ($mL \cdot kg^{-1} \cdot min^{-1}$) = [oxygen consumed during the resistance component ($mL \cdot kg^{-1} \cdot min^{-1}$ per $m \cdot min^{-1}$) divided by body weight] + oxygen consumed during rest

$$\dot{V}O_2 cons \ (mL \cdot kg^{-1} \cdot min^{-1}) = [\frac{3 \ mL \cdot kg^{-1} \cdot min^{-1}}{m \cdot min^{-1}}$$
$$\text{work rate} \ (kgm \cdot min^{-1}) \div \text{body weight (kg)}]$$
$$+ \ 3.5 \ mL \cdot kg^{-1} \cdot min^{-1}$$

If the individual in the previous example switches from leg cycling to arm cranking, she now consumes 46.7 $mL \cdot kg^{-1} \cdot min^{-1}$ of oxygen, calculated as follows:

$$\dot{V}O_2 cons \ (mL \cdot kg^{-1} \cdot min^{-1}) = [\frac{3 \ mL \cdot kg^{-1} \cdot min^{-1}}{m \cdot min^{-1}}$$
$$(2 \ kg \times 6 \ m \cdot rev^{-1} \times 60 \ rev \cdot min^{-1}) \div 50 \ kg]$$
$$+ \ 3.5 \ mL \cdot kg^{-1} \cdot min^{-1}$$

Resistance component	$= 43.2 \ mL \cdot kg^{-1} \cdot min^{-1}$
Resting component	$= 3.5 \ mL \cdot kg^{-1} \cdot min^{-1}$
Total $\dot{V}O_2 cons$	$= 46.7 \ mL \cdot kg^{-1} \cdot min^{-1}$

The Oxygen Consumed During Bench Stepping

Like cycling, bench stepping allows for the exact computation of the work being done if the height of the step, the rate of stepping, and the body weight of the stepper are known.

B.22 oxygen consumption during bench stepping ($mL \cdot kg^{-1} \cdot min^{-1}$) = oxygen consumed during the horizontal component ($mL \cdot kg^{-1} \cdot min^{-1}$) + oxygen consumed during the vertical component ($mL \cdot kg^{-1} \cdot min^{-1}$) + oxygen consumed at rest

or

$$\dot{V}O_2 cons \ (mL \cdot kg^{-1} \cdot min^{-1}) =$$
$$[\frac{0.2 \ mL \cdot kg^{-1} \cdot min^{-1}}{steps \cdot min^{-1}} \ (\text{stepping rate}) \ (steps \cdot min^{-1})]$$
$$+ [1.33 \times \frac{1.8 \ mL \cdot kg^{-1} \cdot min^{-1}}{m \cdot min^{-1}} \ (\text{step height}) \ (m \cdot step^{-1})$$
$$\times \ (\text{stepping rate}) \ (steps \cdot min^{-1})]$$
$$+ \ 3.5 \ mL \cdot kg^{-1} \cdot min^{-1}$$

In the first component, 0.2 $mL \cdot kg^{-1} \cdot min^{-1}$ is the oxygen cost of stepping back and forth along the horizontal plane. In the second component, as with walking or running, each $m \cdot min^{-1}$ of vertical rise requires 1.8 $mL \cdot kg^{-1} \cdot min^{-1}$ of oxygen. The 0.33 in the constant 1.33 accounts for the fact that bench stepping has both a positive (up) and a negative (down) action. Negative work in this situation requires one-third as much oxygen as positive work.

For an individual stepping up and down on a 10-inch (0.254-m) bench at 24 $steps \cdot min^{-1}$, oxygen consumption is calculated as follows:

$$\dot{V}O_2 cons \ (mL \cdot kg^{-1} \cdot min^{-1}) = [24 \ steps \cdot min^{-1}$$
$$\times \frac{0.2 \ mL \cdot kg^{-1} \cdot min^{-1}}{steps \cdot min^{-1}}] + [0.254 \ m \cdot step^{-1}$$
$$\times 24 \ steps \cdot min^{-1} \times \frac{1.8 \ mL \cdot kg^{-1} \cdot min^{-1}}{m \cdot min^{-1}} \times 1.33]$$
$$+ \ 3.5 \ mL \cdot kg^{-1} \cdot min^{-1}$$

Horizontal component	$= 4.8 \ mL \cdot kg^{-1} \cdot min^{-1}$
Vertical component	$= 14.6 \ mL \cdot kg^{-1} \cdot min^{-1}$
Resting component	$= 3.5 \ mL \cdot kg^{-1} \cdot min^{-1}$
Total $\dot{V}O_2 cons$	$= 22.9 \ mL \cdot kg^{-1} \cdot min^{-1}$

The Calculation of Maximal Oxygen Consumption from Cardiovascular Endurance Field Tests

The direct measurement of maximal oxygen consumption ($\dot{V}O_2 max$) is the best indicator of cardiovascular respiratory fitness. However, the direct measurement of $\dot{V}O_2 max$ requires expensive equipment, trained technicians, and considerable time. This makes it unsuitable for mass testing. Therefore, as indicated in Chapter 12, field tests are often used to estimate $\dot{V}O_2 max$. The calculation of $\dot{V}O_2 max$ from the 1-mi run/walk is explained in Chapter 12. This section details the calculation of $\dot{V}O_2 max$ from the PACER and from the Rockport Fitness Walking Test (RFWT).

PACER $\dot{V}O_2 max$

Several different formulas are available to determine $\dot{V}O_2 max$ from the results of the PACER test. Two have been included here to cover as wide an age span as possible. The first equation should be used for both male and female children and adolescents (Léger, et al., 1988). It requires knowing only the final speed at which the individual ran and the age of the individual.

B.23 $\dot{V}O_2 max = 31.025 + 3.238$ (final speed in $km \cdot hr^{-1}$) $- 3.248$ (age in yr) $+ 0.1536$ (final speed $\times$ age).

For example, if a 9-yr-old boy had a final speed of 11 km·hr^{-1}, we would substitute into the equation as follows:

$$\dot{V}O_2max = 31.025 + 3.238\ (11) - 3.248\ (9)$$
$$+ 0.1536\ (11 \times 9) = 52.62\ mL·kg^{-1}·min^{-1}$$

The second equation should be used for young adult males and females (Ramsbottom, et al., 1988). It requires knowing only the total number of minutes the individual completed.

B.24 $\dot{V}O_2max = 14.4 + 3.48$ (minutes completed)

Thus if a 20-yr-old college student ran for 10 min, the calculation would be

$$\dot{V}O_2max = 14.4 + 3.48\ (10) = 49.2\ mL·kg^{-1}·min^{-1}$$

RFWT $\dot{V}O_2$max

The RFWT can be used to estimate $\dot{V}O_2max$ in male and female adults from approximately age 30–70 yr (Kline, et al., 1987) and adolescents 14–18 yr (McSwegin, et al., 1998), but not young adults.

Five variables are needed to estimate $\dot{V}O_2max$: body weight in pounds, age in years, sex (females are coded as 0 and males are coded as 1), time for completion of the mile walk (in minutes, including a decimal) and heart rate in beats per minute (recorded by a heart rate monitor during the final quarter mile or manually in the 15 sec immediately postexercise).

B.25 $\dot{V}O_2max = 132.853 - 0.0769$ (body weight)
$- 0.3877$ (age) $+ 6.3150$ (sex) $- 3.2649$ (walk time) $- 0.1565$ (heart rate)

For example, if a 64-yr-old, 195-lb male completed the mile walk in 19.01 min with a last quarter heart rate of 113 b·min^{-1}, the calculation would be as follows:

$$\dot{V}O_2max = 132.853 - 0.0769(195) - 0.3877(64)$$
$$+ 6.3150(1) - 3.2649(19.01) - 0.1565(113)$$
$$= 19.61\ mL·kg^{-1}·min^{-1}$$

Standard Error of the Estimate

Because all of these formulas are estimates, knowing the accuracy of the estimate is helpful. Accuracy is determined during the development of the equations when the estimated values are compared to the actual values statistically and a standard error of the estimate (SEE) is obtained. The PACER equation for children and adolescents (Eq. B.23) has a SEE of 5.9 mL·kg^{-1}·min^{-1}. The PACER equation for young

adults (Eq. B.24) has a SEE of 3.5 mL·kg^{-1}·min^{-1}. The RFWT equation (Eq. B.25) has a SEE of 5.0 mL·kg^{-1}·min^{-1}. Each SEE means that the calculated $\dot{V}O_2max$ could differ from an actual measured value by one or two times the amount of the SEE. Most scores (68%) should vary only plus or minus one SEE from the calculated estimated value.

Thus, the $\dot{V}O_2max$ 49.2 mL·kg^{-1}·min^{-1} calculated for the college student from Equation B.24 could actually be anywhere from 45.7 to 52.7 mL·kg^{-1}·min^{-1}. Obviously, the smaller the SEE, the greater the equation's accuracy (Jackson, 1989). All of these estimation equations are deemed to have acceptable accuracy.

Practice Problems

Us the data in Table B.3 to work the problems that follow. Answers are provided at the end of the section.

1. Correct the expired minute ventilations from ATPS to STPD.

2. Correct the expired minute ventilations from ATPS to STPD.

3. Calculate the inspired minute ventilations from the expired minute ventilations using the Haldane transformation.

4. Calculate the expired minute ventilations from the inspired minute ventilations using the Haldane transformation.

5. Calculate $\dot{V}O_2cons$ substituting the information given and computed from the maximal treadmill results in Equation B.2. Present your answer in both relative (mL·kg^{-1}·min^{-1}) and absolute (L·min^{-1}) oxygen units.

6. Calculate the $\dot{V}CO_2$ produced using the information given and computed from the maximal treadmill results in L·min^{-1}.

7. Calculate the oxygen consumed during submaximal walking.

8. Calculate the oxygen consumed during submaximal running.

9. Calculate the oxygen consumed during submaximal cycling, assuming that subject 3 is doing leg work and subject 4 is doing arm cranking.

10. Calculate the oxygen consumed during bench stepping.

11. Calculate the estimated $\dot{V}O_2max$ for each subject using the appropriate formula for the information presented.

Table B.3
Practice Problem Data

	Subjects			
VARIABLES	No. 1	No. 2	No. 3	No. 4
Descriptive Information				
Sex	Female	Female	Male	Male
Age (yr)	15	24	32	58
Weight (lb)	108	132	175	201
Maximal Treadmill Data				
$\dot{V}_E$ATPS (L·min^{-1})	45		130	
P_B (mmHg)	740	742	738	739
T (°C)	20	23	21	24
$F_E O_2$ (%)	16.08	16.2	16.04	16.75
$F_E CO_2$ (%)	4.94	5.01	5.12	4.73
$\dot{V}_I$ATPS (L·min^{-1})		70		75
RH (%)		50		25
Submaximal Exercise Data				
Speed (m·min^{-1})	90	161		
Grade	11	0		
Ergometer load (kp)			4	3
Pedaling rate (rev·min^{-1})			80	50
Flywheel circumference (m)			6	3
Step height (m)		.305		
Step rate (steps·min^{-1})		30		
Field Test Data				
PACER speed (km·hr^{-1})	10			
PACER time (min)		9	16	
1-mi walk time (min)				17.6
HR (b·min^{-1})				108

Solutions and Answers

1. **Subject No. 1**

$\dot{V}_E$ STPD =
$45 \text{ L·min}^{-1}\left(\dfrac{273°}{273° + 20°}\right)\left(\dfrac{740 - 17.5 \text{ mmHg}}{760}\right)$

$= 39.86 \text{ L·min}^{-1}$

Subject No. 3

$\dot{V}_E$ STPD =
$130 \text{ L·min}^{-1}\left(\dfrac{273°}{273° + 21°}\right)\left(\dfrac{738 - 18.7 \text{ mmHg}}{760}\right)$

$= 114.25$

2. **Subject No. 2**

$\dot{V}_I$ STPD =
$70 \text{ L·min}^{-1}\left(\dfrac{273°}{273° + 23°}\right)\left(\dfrac{742[0.5 \times 21.1] \text{ mmHg}}{760 \text{ mmHg}}\right)$

$= 62.13 \text{ L·min}^{-1}$

Subject No. 4

$\dot{V}_I$ STPD =
$75 \text{ L·}^{-1}\left(\dfrac{273°}{273° + 24°}\right)\left(\dfrac{739[0.25 \times 22.4] \text{ mmHg}}{760}\right)$

$= 66.52 \text{ L·min}^{-1}$

3. **Subject No. 1**

$\dot{V}_I$ STPD $= 39.86 \text{ L·min}^{-1}\left(\dfrac{1 - [0.1608 + 0.0494]}{0.7904}\right)$

$= 39.83$

Subject No. 3

$\dot{V}_I$ STPD $= 114.25 \text{ L·min}^{-1}\left(\dfrac{1 - [0.1604 + 0.0512]}{0.7904}\right)$

$= 113.96$

4. **Subject No. 2**

$\dot{V}_E$ STPD $= 62.13 \text{ L·min}^{-1}\left(\dfrac{0.7904}{1 - [0.1620 + 0.0510]}\right)$

$= 61.93$

Subject No. 4

$$\dot{V}_E \text{ STPD} = 66.52 \text{ L·min}^{-1} \left(\frac{0.7904}{1 - [0.1675 + 0.0473]} \right)$$

$$= 66.96 \text{ L·min}^{-1}$$

5. **Subject No. 1**

$$\dot{V}O_2\text{cons} = (0.2093 \times 39.83 \text{ L·min}^{-1})$$
$$- (0.1609 \times 39.86 \text{ L·min}^{-1}) = 1.93 \text{ L·min}^{-1}$$
$$= 1930 \text{ mL·min}^{-1} \div 49.1 \text{ kg}$$
$$= 39.31 \text{ mL·kg}^{-1}\text{·min}^{-1}$$

Subject No. 2

$$\dot{V}O_2\text{cons} = (0.2093 \times 62.13 \text{ L·min}^{-1})$$
$$- (0.1620 \times 61.93 \text{ L·min}^{-1}) = 2.97 \text{ L·min}^{-1}$$
$$= 2970 \text{ mL·min}^{-1} \div 60 \text{ kg}$$
$$= 49.52 \text{ mL·kg}^{-1}\text{·v}^{-1}$$

Subject No. 3

$$\dot{V}O_2\text{cons} = (0.2093 \times 113.96 \text{ L·min}^{-1})$$
$$- (0.1604 \times 114.25 \text{ L·min}^{-1}) = 5.53 \text{ L·min}^{-1}$$
$$= 5530 \text{ mL·min}^{-1} \div 79.55 \text{ kg}$$
$$= 69.52 \text{ mL·kg}^{-1}\text{·min}^{-1}$$

Subject No. 4

$$\dot{V}O_2\text{cons} = (0.2093 \times 66.52 \text{ L·min}^{-1})$$
$$- (0.1675 \times 66.96 \text{ L·min}^{-1}) = 2.71 \text{ L·min}^{-1}$$
$$= 2710 \text{ mL·min}^{-1} \div 91.36 \text{ kg}$$
$$= 29.66 \text{ mL·kg}^{-1}\text{·min}^{-1}$$

6. **Subject No. 1**

$$\dot{V}CO_2 \text{ prod} = (0.0494 \times 39.86 \text{ L·min}^{-1})$$
$$= 1.97 \text{ L·min}^{-1}$$

Subject No. 2

$$\dot{V}CO_2 \text{ prod} = (0.0501 \times 61.93 \text{ L·min}^{-1})$$
$$= 3.10 \text{ L·min}$$

Subject No. 3

$$\dot{V}CO_2 \text{ prod} = (0.0512 \times 114.25 \text{ L·min}^{-1})$$
$$= 5.85 \text{ L·min}$$

$$\dot{V}CO_2 \text{ prod} = (0.0473 \times 66.96 \text{ L·min}^{-1})$$
$$= 3.17 \text{ L·min}^{-1}$$

7. **Subject No. 1**

$$\dot{V}O_2\text{cons} = 90 \text{ m·min}^{-1} \times \frac{0.1 \text{ mL·kg}^{-1}\text{·min}^{-1}}{\text{m·min}^{-1}}$$
$$+ 3.5 \text{ mL·kg}^{-1}\text{·min}^{-1} + 0.11 \times 90 \text{ m·min}^{-1}$$
$$\times \frac{1.8 \text{ mL·kg}^{-1}\text{·min}^{-1}}{\text{m·min}^{-1}} = 30.32 \text{ mL·kg}^{-1}\text{·min}^{-1}$$

8. **Subject No. 2**

$$\dot{V}O_2\text{cons} = 161 \text{ m·min}^{-1} \times \frac{0.2 \text{ mL·kg}^{-1}\text{·min}^{-1}}{\text{m·min}^{-1}}$$
$$+ 3.5 \text{ mL·kg}^{-1}\text{·min}^{-1} = 35.7 \text{ mL·kg}^{-1}\text{·min}^{-1}$$

9. **Subject No. 3**

$$\dot{V}O_2\text{cons} = [\frac{1.8 \text{ mL·kg}^{-1}\text{·min}^{-1}}{\text{m·min}^{-1}} \times (4 \text{ kg} \times 6 \text{ m·rev}^{-1}$$
$$\times 80 \text{ rev·min}^{-1}) \div 79.55 \text{ kg}]$$
$$+ 7 \text{ mL·kg}^{-1}\text{·min}^{-1}$$
$$= 50.44 \text{ mL·kg}^{-1}\text{·min}^{-1}$$

Subject No. 4

$$\dot{V}O_2\text{cons} = [\frac{3 \text{ mL·kg}^{-1}\text{·min}^{-1}}{\text{m·min}^{-1}} \times (3 \text{ kg} \times 3 \text{ m·rev}^{-1}$$
$$\times 50 \text{ rev·min}^{-1}) \div 91.4 \text{ kg}]$$
$$+ 3.5 \text{ mL·kg}^{-1}\text{·min}^{-1}$$
$$= 18.27 \text{ mL·kg}^{-1}\text{·min}^{-1}$$

10. **Subject No. 2**

$$\dot{V}O_2\text{cons} = [\frac{0.2 \text{ mL·kg}^{-1}\text{·min}^{-1}}{\text{m·min}^{-1}} \times 30 \text{ steps·min}^{-1}]$$
$$+ [1.33 \times \frac{1.8 \text{ mL·kg}^{-1}\text{·min}^{-1}}{\text{m·min}^{-1}} \times .305 \text{ m·step}$$
$$\times 30 \text{ steps·min}^{-1}] + 3.5 \text{ mL·kg}^{-1}\text{·min}^{-1}$$
$$= 31.41 \text{ mL·kg}^{-1}\text{·min}^{-1} =$$

11. **Subject No. 1** PACER $\dot{V}O_2$max (Eq. B.17)

$$\dot{V}O_2\text{max} = 31.025 + 3.238 (10) - 3.248 (15)$$
$$+ 0.1536 (10 \times 15)$$
$$= 37.73 \text{ mL·kg}^{-1}\text{·min}^{-1}$$

Subject No. 2 PACER $\dot{V}O_2$max (Eq. B.18)

$$\dot{V}O_2\text{max} = 14.4 - 3.48 (9) = 48.72 \text{ mL·kg}^{-1}\text{·min}^{-1}$$

References

American College of Sports Medicine: *Guidelines for Exercise Testing and Prescription* (6th edition). Baltimore: Williams & Williams (2000).

Jackson, A. S.: Application of regression analysis to exercise science. In M. J. Safrit & T. M. Wood (eds.), *Measurement Concepts in Physical Education and Exercise Science.* Champaign, IL: Human Kinetics (1989).

Kline, G. M., J. P. Porcari, R. Huntermeister, P. S. Freedson, A. Ward, R. F. McCarron, J. Ross, & J. M. Rippe: Estimation of $\dot{V}O_2$max from a one mile track walk, gender, age, and body weight. *Medicine and Science in Sports and Exercise.* 19:253–259 (1987).

Leger, L. A., D. Mercier, C. Gadoury, & J. Lambert: The multistage 20 metre shuttle run test for aerobic fitness. *Journal of Sport Sciences.* 6:93–101 (1988).

McSwegin, P. J., S. A. Plowman, G. M. Wolff, & G. L. Guttenburg: The validity of a one-mile walk test for high school age individuals. *Measurement in Physical Education and Exercise Science.* 2(1):47–63 (1998).

Ramsbottom, R., J. Brewer, & C. Williams: A progressive shuttle run test to estimate maximal oxygen uptake. *British Journal of Sports Medicine.* 22(4):141–144 (1988).

Physical Activity and Health: A Report of the Surgeon General Executive Summary*

Introduction

This is the first Surgeon General's report to address physical activity and health. The main message of this report is that Americans can substantially improve their health and quality of life by including moderate amounts of physical activity in their daily lives. Health benefits from physical activity are thus achievable for most Americans, including those who may dislike vigorous exercise and those who may have been previously discouraged by the difficulty of adhering to a program of vigorous exercise. For those who are already achieving regular moderate amounts of activity, additional benefits can be gained by further increases in activity level.

This report grew out of an emerging consensus among epidemiologists, experts in exercise science, and health professionals that physical activity need not be of vigorous intensity for it to improve health. Moreover, health benefits appear to be proportional to amount of activity; thus, every increase in activity adds some benefit. Emphasizing the amount rather than the intensity of physical activity offers more options for people to select from in incorporating physical activity into their daily lives. Thus, a moderate amount of activity can be obtained in a 30-minute brisk walk, 30 minutes of lawn mowing or raking leaves, a 15-minute run, or 45 minutes of playing volleyball, and these activities can be varied from day to day. It is hoped that this different emphasis on moderate amounts of activity, and the flexibility to vary activities according to personal preference and life circumstances, will encourage more people to make physical activity a regular and sustainable part of their lives.

The information in this report summarizes a diverse literature from the fields of epidemiology, exercise physiology, medicine, and the behavioral sciences. The report highlights what is known about physical activity and health, as well as what is being learned about promoting physical activity among adults and young people.

*Appendix C has been adapted from *Physical Activity and Health: A Report of the Surgeon General Executive Summary*, U.S. Department of Health and Human Services, Centers for Disease Control and Prevention, National Center for Chronic Disease Prevention and Health Promoting, The President's Council on Physical Fitness and Sports.

Development of the Report

In July 1994, the Office of the Surgeon General authorized the Centers for Disease Control and Prevention (CDC) to serve as lead agency for preparing the first Surgeon General's report on physical activity and health. The CDC was joined in this effort by the President's Council on Physical Fitness and Sports (PCPFS) as a collaborative partner representing the Office of the Surgeon General. Because of the wide interest in the health effects of physical activity, the report was planned collaboratively with representatives from the Office of the Surgeon General, the Office of Public Health and Science (Office of the Secretary), the Office of Disease Prevention (National Institutes of Health [NIH]), and the following institutes from the NIH: the National Heart, Lung, and Blood Institute; the National Institute of Child Health and Human Development; the National Institute of Diabetes and Digestive and Kidney Diseases; and the National Institute of Arthritis and Musculoskeletal and Skin Diseases. CDC's nonfederal partners—including the American Alliance for Health, Physical Education, Recreation, and Dance; the American College of Sports Medicine; and the American Heart Association—provided consultation throughout the development process.

The major purpose of this report is to summarize the existing literature on the role of physical activity in preventing disease and on the status of interventions to increase physical activity. Any report on a topic this broad must restrict its scope to keep its message clear. This report focuses on disease prevention and therefore does not include the considerable body of evidence on the benefits of physical activity for treatment or rehabilitation after disease has developed. This report concentrates on endurance-type physical activity (activity involving repeated use of large muscles, such as in walking or bicycling) because the health benefits of this type of activity have been extensively studied. The importance of resistance exercise (to increase muscle strength, such as by lifting weights) is increasingly being recognized as a means to preserve and enhance muscular strength and endurance and to prevent falls and improve mobility in the elderly. Some promising findings on resistance exercise are presented here, but a comprehensive review of resistance training is beyond the scope of this report. In addition, a review of the special concerns regarding physical activity for pregnant women and for people with disabilities is not undertaken here, although these important topics deserve more research and attention.

Finally, physical activity is only one of many everyday behaviors that affect health. In particular, nutritional habits are linked to some of the same aspects of health as physical activity, and the two may be related lifestyle characteristics. This report deals solely with physical activity; a Surgeon General's Report on Nutrition and Health was published in 1988.

Chapters 2 through 6 of this report address distinct areas of the current understanding of physical activity and health.* Chapter 2 offers a historical perspective: after outlining the history of belief and knowledge about physical activity and health, the chapter reviews the evolution and content of physical activity recommendations. Chapter 3 describes the physiologic responses to physical activity—both the immediate effects of a single episode of activity and the long-term adaptations to a regular pattern of activity. The evidence that physical activity reduces the risk of cardiovascular and other disease is presented in Chapter 4. Data on patterns and trends of physical activity in the U.S. population are the focus of Chapter 5. Lastly, Chapter 6 examines efforts to increase physical activity and reviews ideas currently being proposed for policy and environmental initiatives.

Major Conclusions

1. People of all ages, both male and female, benefit from regular physical activity.

2. Significant health benefits can be obtained by including a moderate amount of physical activity (e.g., 30 minutes of brisk walking or raking leaves, 15 minutes of running, or 45 minutes of playing volleyball) on most, if not all, days of the week. Through a modest increase in daily activity, most Americans can improve their health and quality of life.

3. Additional health benefits can be gained through greater amounts of physical activity. People who can maintain a regular regimen of activity that is of longer duration or of more vigorous intensity are likely to derive greater benefit.

4. Physical activity reduces the risk of premature mortality in general, and of coronary heart

*Conclusions reached from these chapters are included in this appendix, although the chapters themselves are not.

disease, hypertension, colon cancer, and diabetes mellitus in particular. Physical activity also improves mental health and is important for the health of muscles, bones, and joints.

5. More than 60 percent of American adults are not regularly physically active. In fact, 25 percent of all adults are not active at all.

6. Nearly half of American youths 12–21 years of age are not vigorously active on a regular basis. Moreover, physical activity declines dramatically during adolescence.

7. Daily enrollment in physical education classes has declined among high school students from 42 percent in 1991 to 25 percent in 1995.

8. Research on understanding and promoting physical activity is at an early stage, but some interventions to promote physical activity through schools, worksites, and health care settings have been evaluated and found to be successful.

Summary

The benefits of physical activity have been extolled throughout western history, but it was not until the second half of this century that scientific evidence supporting these beliefs began to accumulate. By the 1970s, enough information was available about the beneficial effects of vigorous exercise on cardiorespiratory fitness that the American College of Sports Medicine (ACSM), the American Heart Association (AHA), and other national organizations began issuing physical activity recommendations to the public. These recommendations generally focused on cardiorespiratory endurance and specified sustained periods of vigorous physical activity involving large muscle groups and lasting at least 20 minutes on 3 or more days per week. As understanding of the benefits of less vigorous activity grew, recommendations followed suit. During the past few years, the ACSM, the CDC, the AHA, the PCPFS, and the NIH have all recommended regular, moderate-intensity physical activity as an option for those who get little or no exercise. The *Healthy People 2000* goals for the nation's health have recognized the importance of physical activity and have included physical activity goals. The 1995 *Dietary Guidelines for Americans,* the basis of the federal government's nutrition-related programs, included physical activity guidance to maintain and improve weight—30 minutes or more of moderate-intensity physical activity on all, or most, days of the week.

Underpinning such recommendations is a growing understanding of how physical activity affects physiologic function. The body responds to physical activity in ways that have important positive effects on musculoskeletal, cardiovascular, respiratory, and endocrine systems. These changes are consistent with a number of health benefits, including a reduced risk of premature mortality and reduced risks of coronary heart disease, hypertension, colon cancer, and diabetes mellitus. Regular participation in physical activity also appears to reduce depression and anxiety, improve mood, and enhance ability to perform daily tasks throughout the life span.

The risks associated with physical activity must also be considered. The most common health problems that have been associated with physical activity are musculoskeletal injuries, which can occur with excessive amounts of activity or with suddenly beginning an activity for which the body is not conditioned. Much more serious associated health problems (i.e., myocardial infarction, sudden death) are also much rarer, occurring primarily among sedentary people with advanced atherosclerotic disease who engage in strenuous activity to which they are unaccustomed. Sedentary people, especially those with preexisting health conditions, who wish to increase their physical activity should therefore gradually build up to the desired level of activity. Even among people who are regularly active, the risk of myocardial infarction or sudden death is somewhat increased during physical exertion, but their overall risk of these outcomes is lower than that among people who are sedentary.

Research on physical activity continues to evolve. This report includes both well-established findings and newer research results that await replication and amplification. Interest has been developing in ways to differentiate between the various characteristics of physical activity that improve health. It remains to be determined how the interrelated characteristics of amount, intensity, duration, frequency, type, and pattern of physical activity are related to specific health or disease outcomes.

Attention has been drawn recently to findings from three studies showing that cardiorespiratory fitness gains are similar when physical activity occurs in several short sessions (e.g., 10 minutes) as when the same total amount and intensity of activity occurs in one longer session (e.g., 30 minutes). Although, strictly speaking, the health benefits of such intermittent activity have not yet been demonstrated, it is reasonable to expect them to be similar to those of continuous activity. Moreover, for people who are unable to set aside 30 minutes for physical activity, shorter episodes are clearly better than none. Indeed, one study has shown greater adherence to a walking program among those walking several times per day than

among those walking once per day, when the total amount of walking time was kept the same. Accumulating physical activity over the course of the day has been included in recent recommendations from the CDC and ACSM, as well as from the NIH Consensus Development Conference on Physical Activity and Cardiovascular Health.

Despite common knowledge that exercise is healthful, more than 60 percent of American adults are not regularly active, and 25 percent of the adult population are not active at all. Moreover, although many people have enthusiastically embarked on vigorous exercise programs at one time or another, most do not sustain their participation. Clearly, the processes of developing and maintaining healthier habits are as important to study as the health effects of these habits.

The effort to understand how to promote more active lifestyles is of great importance to the health of this nation. Although the study of physical activity determinants and interventions is at an early stage, effective programs to increase physical activity have been carried out in a variety of settings, such as schools, physicians' offices, and worksites. Determining the most effective and cost-effective intervention approaches is a challenge for the future. Fortunately, the United States has skilled leadership and institutions to support efforts to encourage and assist Americans to become more physically active. Schools, community agencies, parks, recreational facilities, and health clubs are available in most communities and can be more effectively used in these efforts.

School-based interventions for youth are particularly promising, not only for their potential scope—almost all young people between the ages of 6 and 16 years attend school—but also for their potential impact. Nearly half of young people 12–21 years of age are not vigorously active; moreover, physical activity sharply declines during adolescence. Childhood and adolescence may thus be pivotal times for preventing sedentary behavior among adults by maintaining the habit of physical activity throughout the school years. School-based interventions have been shown to be successful in increasing physical activity levels. With evidence that success in this arena is possible, every effort should be made to encourage schools to require daily physical education in each grade and to promote physical activities that can be enjoyed throughout life.

Outside the school, physical activity programs and initiatives face the challenge of a highly technological society that makes it increasingly convenient to remain sedentary and that discourages physical activity in both obvious and subtle ways. To increase physical activity in the general population, it may be necessary to go beyond traditional efforts. This report highlights some concepts from community initiatives that are being implemented around the country. It is hoped that these examples will spark new public policies and programs in other places as well. Special efforts will also be required to meet the needs of special populations, such as people with disabilities, racial and ethnic minorities, people with low income, and the elderly. Much more information about these important groups will be necessary to develop a truly comprehensive national initiative for better health through physical activity. Challenges for the future include identifying key determinants of physically active lifestyles among the diverse populations that characterize the United States (including special populations, women, and young people) and using this information to design and disseminate effective programs.

Chapter Conclusions

Chapter 2: Historical Background and Evolution of Physical Activity Recommendations

1. Physical activity for better health and well-being has been an important theme throughout much of western history.

2. Public health recommendations have evolved from emphasizing vigorous activity for cardiorespiratory fitness to including the option of moderate levels of activity for numerous health benefits.

3. Recommendations from experts agree that for better health, physical activity should be performed regularly. The most recent recommendations advise people of all ages to include a minimum of 30 minutes of physical activity of moderate intensity (such as brisk walking) on most, if not all, days of the week. It is also acknowledged that for most people, greater health benefits can be obtained by engaging in physical activity of more vigorous intensity or of longer duration.

4. Experts advise previously sedentary people embarking on a physical activity program to start with short durations of moderate-intensity activity and gradually increase the duration or intensity until the goal is reached.

5. Experts advise consulting with a physician before beginning a new physical activity program for people with chronic diseases, such as cardiovascular disease and diabetes mellitus, or for those who are at high risk for these diseases. Experts also advise men over age 40 and women over age 50 to consult a physician before they begin a vigorous activity program.

6. Recent recommendations from experts also suggest that cardiorespiratory endurance activity should be supplemented with strength-developing exercises at least twice per week for adults, in order to improve musculoskeletal health, maintain independence in performing the activities of daily life, and reduce the risk of falling.

Chapter 3: Physiologic Responses and Long-Term Adaptations to Exercise

1. Physical activity has numerous beneficial physiologic effects. Most widely appreciated are its effects on the cardiovascular and musculoskeletal systems, but benefits on the functioning of metabolic, endocrine, and immune systems are also considerable.

2. Many of the beneficial effects of exercise training—from both endurance and resistance activities—diminish within 2 weeks if physical activity is substantially reduced, and effects disappear within 2 to 8 months if physical activity is not resumed.

3. People of all ages, both male and female, undergo beneficial physiologic adaptations to physical activity.

Chapter 4: The Effects of Physical Activity on Health and Disease

Overall Mortality

1. Higher levels of regular physical activity are associated with lower mortality rates for both older and younger adults.

2. Even those who are moderately active on a regular basis have lower mortality rates than those who are least active.

Cardiovascular Diseases

1. Regular physical activity or cardiorespiratory fitness decreases the risk of cardiovascular disease mortality in general and of coronary heart disease mortality in particular. Existing data are not conclusive regarding a relationship between physical activity and stroke.

2. The level of decreased risk of coronary heart disease attributable to regular physical activity is similar to that of other lifestyle factors, such as keeping free from cigarette smoking.

3. Regular physical activity prevents or delays the development of high blood pressure, and exercise reduces blood pressure in people with hypertension.

Cancer

1. Regular physical activity is associated with a decreased risk of colon cancer.

2. There is no association between physical activity and rectal cancer. Data are too sparse to draw conclusions regarding a relationship between physical activity and endometrial, ovarian, or testicular cancers.

3. Despite numerous studies on the subject, existing data are inconsistent regarding an association between physical activity and breast or prostate cancers.

Non–Insulin-Dependent Diabetes Mellitus

1. Regular physical activity lowers the risk of developing noninsulin-dependent diabetes mellitus.

Osteoarthritis

1. Regular physical activity is necessary for maintaining normal muscle strength, joint structure, and joint function. In the range recommended for health, physical activity is not associated with joint damage or development of osteoarthritis and may be beneficial for many people with arthritis.

2. Competitive athletics may be associate with the development of osteoarthritis later in life, but sports-related injuries are the likely cause.

Osteoporosis

1. Weight-bearing physical activity is essential for normal skeletal development during childhood and adolescence and for achieving and maintaining peak bone mass in young adults.

2. It is unclear whether resistance- or endurance-type physical activity can reduce the accelerated rate of bone loss in postmenopausal women in the absence of estrogen replacement therapy.

Falling

1. There is promising evidence that strength training and other forms of exercise in older adults preserve the ability to maintain independent living status and reduce the risk of falling.

Obesity

1. Low levels of activity, resulting in fewer kilocalories used than consumed, contribute to the high prevalence of obesity in the United States.

2. Physical activity may favorably affect body fat distribution.

Mental Health

1. Physical activity appears to relieve symptoms of depression and anxiety and improve mood.

2. Regular physical activity may reduce the risk of developing depression, although further research is needed on this topic.

Health-Related Quality of Life

1. Physical activity appears to improve health-related quality of life by enhancing psychological well-being and by improving physical functioning in persons compromised by poor health.

Adverse Effects

1. Most musculoskeletal injuries related to physical activity are believed to be preventable by gradually working up to a desired level of activity and by avoiding excessive amounts of activity.

2. Serious cardiovascular events can occur with physical exertion, but the net effect of regular physical activity is a lower risk of mortality from cardiovascular disease.

Chapter 5: Patterns and Trends in Physical Activity

Adults

1. Approximately 15 percent of U.S. adults engage regularly (3 times a week for at least 20 minutes) in vigorous physical activity during leisure time.

2. Approximately 22 percent of adults engage regularly (5 times a week for at least 30 minutes) in sustained physical activity of any intensity during leisure time.

3. About 25 percent of adults report no physical activity at all in their leisure time.

4. Physical inactivity is more prevalent among women than men, among blacks and Hispanics than whites, among older than younger adults, and among the less affluent than the more affluent.

5. The most popular leisure-time physical activities among adults are walking and gardening or yard work.

Adolescents and Young Adults

1. Only about one-half of U.S. young people (ages 12–21 years) regularly participate in vigorous physical activity. One-fourth report no vigorous physical activity.

2. Approximately one-fourth of young people walk or bicycle (i.e., engage in light to moderate activity) nearly every day.

3. About 14 percent of young people report no recent vigorous or light-to-moderate physical activity. This indicator of inactivity is higher among females than males and among black females then white females.

4. Males are more likely than females to participate in vigorous physical activity, strengthening activities, and walking or bicycling.

5. Participation in all types of physical activity declines strikingly as age or grade in school increases.

6. Among high school students, enrollment in physical education remained unchanged during the first half of the 1990s. However, daily attendance in physical education declined from approximately 42 to 25 percent.

7. The percentage of high school students who were enrolled in physical education and who reported being physically active for at least 20 minutes in physical education classes declined from approximately 81 percent to 70 percent during the first half of this decade.

8. Only 19 percent of all high school students report being physically active for 20 minutes or more in daily physical education classes.

Chapter 6: Understanding and Promoting Physical Activity

1. Consistent influence on physical activity patterns among adults and young people includes confidence in one's ability to engage in regular physical activity (e.g., self-efficacy), enjoyment of physical activity, support from others, positive beliefs concerning the benefits of physical activity, and lack of perceived barriers to being physically active.

2. For adults, some interventions have been successful in increasing physical activity in communities, worksites, and health care settings, and at home.

3. Interventions targeting physical education in elementary school can substantially increase the amount of time students spend being physically active in physical education class.

Appendix D

Answers to "A Question of Understanding" Boxes

Chapter 1, p. 15

Pattern (c) is the best. This incorporates step loading with recovery/rejuvenation microcycles programmed into the overload progression. Pattern (b) remains for too long at one level and makes too large a jump between levels. Pattern (a) progresses in small increments but does not plan for any rest or recovery cycles. Overtraining is most likely to occur in individuals when large increases in training occur abruptly and when the rest and recovery periods included in the periodization program are insufficient.

Chapter 3, p. 69

The number of ATP produced in heart muscle from glucose:

1. Stage I $\qquad$ $+ 4 - 2 = 2$
2. Stage III $\qquad$ $= 2$
3. Stage IV 2NADH + H$^+$ (from Stage I) $= 6$
$\qquad$ 2NADH + H$^+$ (from Stage II) $= 6$
$\qquad$ 6NADH + H$^+$ (from Stage III) $= 18$
$\qquad$ 2FADH$_2$ (from Stage III) $\underline{= 4}$
$\qquad$ Total $= 38$

The number of ATP produced in skeletal muscle from glycogen:

1. Stage I $\qquad$ $+ 4 - 1 = 3$
2. Stage III $\qquad$ $= 2$
3. Stage IV 2NADH + H$^+$ (from Stage I) $\rightarrow$
$\qquad$ 2FADH$_2$ $= 4$
$\qquad$ 2NADH + H$^+$ (from Stage II) $= 6$
$\qquad$ 6NADH + H$^+$ (from Stage III) $= 18$
$\qquad$ 2FADH$_2$ (from Stage III) $\underline{= 4}$
$\qquad$ Total $= 37$

The number of ATP produced in heart muscle from glycogen:

1. Stage I $\qquad$ $+ 4 - 1 = 3$
2. Stage III $\qquad$ $= 2$
3. Stage IV 2NADH + H$^+$ (from Stage I) $= 6$
$\qquad$ 2NADH + H$^+$ (from Stage II) $= 6$
$\qquad$ 6NADH + H$^+$ (from Stage III) $= 18$
$\qquad$ 2FADH2 (from Stage III) $\underline{= 4}$
$\qquad$ Total $= 39$

Chapter 3, p. 72

The number of ATP produced from the 18-carbon fatty acid stearate.

1. $n/2 - 1 = 18/2 - 1 = 8$ cycles of beta oxidation
2. FADH$_2$ = 8×2 ATP = 16 ATP
$\qquad$ NADH$_2$ = $8 \times \underline{3 \text{ ATP}} = \underline{24 \text{ ATP}}$
$\qquad\qquad$ 8×5 ATP = 40 ATP
3. Acetyl CoA = 9:
$\qquad\qquad$ 9×12 ATP = 108 ATP
4. Activation energy = -2 ATP
5. Total: $\quad$ 108 ATP
$\qquad\qquad$ $\underline{+ \text{ 40 ATP}}$
$\qquad\qquad$ 148 ATP
$\qquad\qquad$ $\underline{- \text{ 2 ATP}}$
$\qquad\qquad$ 146 ATP

Chapter 5, p. 129

Yes, this is a true max. RER = 1.34 (greater than 1.1 criterion level); HR = 200 b·min^{-1} (predicted 220 − 22 = 198 ± 12 = 186 − 210); $\dot{V}O_2$ mL·kg^{-1}·min^{-1} difference minutes 27 − 28 = 2.07 (less than half the expected 5.8 mL·kg^{-1}·min^{-1}); $\dot{V}O_2$ reaches a plateau.

Chapter 5, p. 133

Minute 2:	RER = 0.99; CHO = 96.6%; FAT = 3.4%
Minute 14:	RER = 0.96; CHO = 86.4%; FAT = 13.6%
Minute 28:	RER = 1.34; CHO = 100%

Chapter 5, p. 135

RER = 0.96
$\dot{V}O_2$ L·min^{-1} = 2.36
kcal·L O$_2$$^{-1}$ = 4.988 (from Table 5.4)
4.998 kcal·L O$_2$$^{-1}$ × 2.36 L O$_2$·min^{-1}
= 11.79 kcal·min^{-1}
11.79 kcal·min^{-1} × 4.18 kJ·kcal^{-1}
− 49.28 kJ·min^{-1}

Chapter 5, p. 137

$$\frac{35.75 \text{ mL·kg}^{-1}\text{·min}^{-1}}{3.5 \text{ mL·kg}^{-1}\text{·min}^{-1}} = 10.21 \text{ METs}$$

Chapter 5, p. 138

$1200 \text{ mL·min}^{-1} \text{ O}_2 = 1.2 \text{ L·min}^{-1} \text{ O}_2$

$1.2 \text{ L·min}^{-1} \times 5 \text{ kcal·L}^{-1} = 6 \text{ kcal·min}^{-1}$

$300 \text{ kcal} \div 6 \text{ kcal·min}^{-1} = 50 \text{ min}$

Chapter 5, p. 146

Computing the % $\dot{V}O_2$max values for the given oxygen costs of each individual at each speed, we get:

Oxygen Cost	Daughter	Son	Mother	Father	Grand-mother
10 min·mi^{-1}	77	78	60	62	83
9 min·mi^{-1}	83	86	64	65	90
8 min·mi^{-1}	94	98	76	79	100
7 min·mi^{-1}	100	100	86	88	—

Therefore, the family could probably stay together easily at a 10 min·mi^{-1} pace, a little less easily because of the grandmother's 9 min·mi^{-1} pace. Perhaps grandmother and the kids should run together somewhere between 9 min·mi^{-1} and 10 min·mi^{-1} and let mom and dad go faster.

Chapter 6, p. 155

	7:39	7:04	4:37.32	4:25.57
ATP-PC	2.5%	2.5%	~3.5%	~3.5%
LA	~15%	~15%	~22%	~22%
O$_2$	~82.5%	~82.5%	~75%	~75%

Although there is undoubtedly some real difference between the contributions for the 4:37.32 and 4:25.57 times, this cannot be discerned from the graph in Figure 4.2. What can be seen is the greater LA contribution after puberty, when more glycogen and less fat is burned and the anaerobic (glycolytic) contribution to exercise approaches the adult level.

Chapter 7, p. 194

1. Training replenishment and carbohydrate loading

Drink	Support
Gatorlode	High CHO; some Na
Nutrament	
Gator Pro	

2. Pre-event meal (3–4 hr)

Drink	Support
Gatorlode	Light meal
Nutrament	50–100 g CHO
Gator Pro	200–500 kcal

3. The drinks to be used during training runs and competition

Drink	Support
All Sport	Water (~ 240 mL)
Body Fuel 450	2.5–10% concentration of CHO
Exceed	as G, GP, S, or F combination
Gatorade	(not F alone); 4–8% is optimal
Power Ade	30–110 mg Na

Chapter 8, p. 208

1. $M_A = 112 \text{ lb} \div 2.2 \text{ lb·kg}^{-1} = 50.91 \text{ kg}$

2. Selected weight from underwater trials. 8.35 kg (trial 4) is the highest weight, but it was only obtained once, not more than twice as listed in the selection criteria, so it cannot be used. 8.325 kg is the second-highest obtained weight and it is observed more than once (trials 6 and 8), so it is the selected representative weight. 8.325 kg − 7.06 kg = 1.265 kg M_W.

3. $D_B =$

$$\frac{50.91 \text{ kg}}{\left(\dfrac{50.91 \text{ kg} - 1.265 \text{ kg}}{0.9941}\right) - (1.2274 \text{ L} + 0.1 \text{ L})}$$

$D_B = 1.0473$

$$\%\text{BF} = \frac{4.570}{1.0473} - 4.142 \times 100 = 22.2\%$$

4. $\text{FFW} = 112 \text{ lb} \times \left(\dfrac{100 - 22.2}{100}\right) = 87.14 \text{ lb}$

$$\text{WT}_2 = \frac{100 \times 87.14}{100\% - 19\%} = 107.58 \text{ lb}$$

$\Delta\text{WT} = 107.58 \text{ lb} - 112 \text{ lb} = -4.42 \text{ lb}$

Phyllis needs to lose approximately 4.5 lb to have 19% BF, assuming she maintains her muscle mass (FFW).

Chapter 9, p. 250

Zachary's weight should be 132 lb. He needs to lose 6 lb. These results are computed as follows using Equation 9.2.

$D_B = 1.0982 - [0.000815 (8 + 9 + 12)$
$+ 0.0000084 (8 + 9 + 12)^2$
$= 1.0982 - [0.023635 + 0.0070644]$
$= 1.0982 - 0.0306994 = 1.0675 \text{ g·cc}^{-1}$

For a 14-yr-old male the %BF formula from Table 8.1 is

$$\%BF = \left(\frac{5.07}{1.0675} - 4.64\right) \times 100 = 10.9$$

Using Equation 8.4

$$FFW = 138 \text{ lb} \times \left(\frac{100\% - 10.9\%}{100}\right) = 123 \text{ lb}$$

Zachary should wrestle at no less than 7%BF with a weight loss not exceeding 7% of body weight. Using Equation 8.5

$$WT_2 = \frac{100\% \times 123 \text{ lb}}{100\% - 7\%} = 132.26 \text{ lb}$$

Using Equation 8.6

$$132 \text{ lb} - 138 \text{ lb} = -6 \text{ lb}$$

Chapter 10, p. 264

1. Pattern A:

   $[(600 \text{ mL·br}^{-1}) - (150 \text{ mL·br}^{-1})] \times$
   $(10 \text{ br·min}^{-1}) = (450 \text{ mL·br}^{-1}) \times$
   $(10 \text{ br·min}^{-1}) = 4500 \text{ mL·min}^{-1}$

   Pattern B:

   $[(200 \text{ mL·br}^{-1}) - (150 \text{ mL·br}^{-1})] \times$
   $(30 \text{ br·min}^{-1}) = (50 \text{ mL·br}^{-1}) \times$
   $(30 \text{ br·min}^{-1}) = 1500 \text{ mL·min}^{-1}$

   At identical minute ventilations, alveolar ventilation is greatly reduced as the depth (tidal volume) of the ventilation decreases. Increasing the frequency of breathing does not compensate for a small tidal volume at the alveolar level. Shallow, frequent breathing is not as effective as deep, infrequent breathing.

2. Both situations decrease alveolar ventilation. When tidal volume is low, as in trying to inhale without exhaling first or in taking short, quick gulps of air, the volume of the dead space has a negative impact on the amount of air available for exchange (the alveolar ventilation). This result is exemplified by the calculations in problem 1. Inadequate alveolar ventilation can lead to dizziness or unconsciousness, which are dangerous situations, especially in water.

3. A snorkel extends the dead space. Thus, the tidal volume must be increased sufficiently to compensate for that volume as well as the anatomical dead space to maintain an effective alveolar ventilation.

Chapter 10, p. 276

Site	PO_2	PCO_2
Alveoli	104 mmHg	
Pulmonary capillary	40 mmHg; arterial end; 104 mmHg, venous end	
Left side of heart	95 mmHg	
Systemic arteries	95 mmHg	40 mmHg
Tissue (resting)	40 mmHg	45 mmHg
Systemic capillary	95 mmHg, arterial end; 40 mmHg, venous end	40 mmHg, arterial end; 45 mmHg, venous end
Systemic veins	40 mmHg	45 mmHg
Right side of heart	40 mmHg	45 mmHg
Pulmonary artery	40 mmHg	45 mmHg
Alveoli		40 mmHg
Pulmonary capillary		45 mmHg, arterial end; 40 mmHg, venous end
Left side of heart		40 mmHg

Chapter 12, p. 328

1. LVEDV = 150; SV ~ 80 mL·b^{-1}
   LVEDV = 200; SV ~ 100 mL·b^{-1}
   LVEDV = 250; SV ~ 105 mL·b^{-1}
   LVEDV = 300; SV ~ 95 mL·b^{-1}

2. $EF = \dfrac{80}{150} = 53\%$

   $EF = \dfrac{100}{200} = 50\%$

   $EF = \dfrac{105}{250} = 42\%$

   $EF = \dfrac{95}{300} = 31.6\%$

Chapter 12, p. 329

	HR (b·min^{-1})	SV (mL·b^{-1})	$\dot{Q}$ (L·min^{-1})
Mike	80	90	7.20
Keiko	60	120	7.20
Kirk	122	146.5	17.87
Don	72	88.05	6.34
Nora	58	98	5.68

Chapter 12, p. 336

$$PP = SBP - DBP = 150 - 90 = 60 \text{ mmHg}$$

$$MAP = \frac{PP}{3} + DBP = \frac{60}{3} + 90 = 110 \text{ mmHg}$$

$$TPR = \frac{MAP}{\dot{Q}} = \frac{110 \text{ mmHg}}{5.1 \text{ L·min}^{-1}} = 21.57$$

Chapter 12, p. 340

The calculation is

$$y = 3.66 + (6.81)(2.0 \text{ L·min}^{-1}) = 17.28 \text{ L·min}^{-1}$$

Chapter 13, p. 354

Condition	MAP (mmHg)	TPR (units)	RPP (units)
Rest	102*	17.0	107
Light aerobic	118†	11.8	195
Heavy aerobic	129†	9.9	263
Maximal aerobic	144†	9.6	360
Sustained static	155†	19.4	284

* Use Equation 12.5a.
† Use Equation 12.5b.

Chapter 14, p. 389

% HRmax Method

Lisa:

estimated HRmax = $220 - 50 = 170$ b·min^{-1}
training HR = $170 \times 0.35 = 60$ b·min^{-1}
training HR = $170 \times 0.54 = 92$ b·min^{-1}

On the basis of the % HRmax method, a light exercise for Lisa elicits a heart rate between 60* and 92 b·min^{-1}.

Susie:

estimated HRmax = $220 - 50 = 170$ b·min^{-1}
training HR = $170 \times 0.35 = 60$ b·min^{-1}
training HR = $170 \times 0.54 = 92$ b·min^{-1}

On the basis of the % HRmax method, a light exercise for Susie elicits a heart rate between 60* and 92 b·min^{-1}.

---

* Obviously a person cannot be working at less than his or her RHR, but this means that any activity above the resting level to the upper level can be done and would be beneficial for health for this person.

% HRR Method

Lisa:

estimated HRmax = $220 - 50 = 170$ b·min^{-1}
training HHR = $[(170 - 62) \times 0.20] + 62$
$\qquad\qquad = 84$ b·min^{-1}
training HHR = $[(170 - 62) \times 0.39] + 62$
$\qquad\qquad = 105$ b·min^{-1}

On the basis of the % HHR method, a light exercise for Lisa elicits a heart rate between 84 and 105 b·min^{-1}.

Susie:

estimated HRmax = $220 - 50 = 170$ b·min^{-1}
training HHR = $[(170 - 82) \times 0.20] + 82$
$\qquad\qquad = 100$ b·min^{-1}
training HHR = $[(170 - 82) \times 0.39] + 82$
$\qquad\qquad = 116$ b·min^{-1}

On the basis of the % HHR method, a light exercise for Susie elicits a heart rate between 100 and 116 b·min^{-1}.

Chapter 14, p. 391

1. A moderate workout represents 40–59% $\dot{V}O_2R$ or HRR.

Individual	40%	59%
Janet	52 mL·kg^{-1}·min^{-1} − 3.5 mL·kg^{-1}·min^{-1} 48.5 mL·kg^{-1}·min^{-1} × 0.4 19.4 mL·kg^{-1}·min^{-1} + 3.5 mL·kg^{-1}·min^{-1} 22.9 mL·kg^{-1}·min^{-1}	52 mL·kg^{-1}·min^{-1} − 3.5 mL·kg^{-1}·min^{-1} 48.5 mL·kg^{-1}·min^{-1} × 0.59 28.6 mL·kg^{-1}·min^{-1} + 3.5 mL·kg^{-1}·min^{-1} 32.1 mL·kg^{-1}·min^{-1}
Juan	64 mL·kg^{-1}·min^{-1} − 3.5 mL·kg^{-1}·min^{-1} 60.5 mL·kg^{-1}·min^{-1} × 0.4 24.2 mL·kg^{-1}·min^{-1} + 3.5 mL·kg^{-1}·min^{-1} 27.7 mL·kg^{-1}·min^{-1}	64 mL·kg^{-1}·min^{-1} − 3.5 mL·kg^{-1}·min^{-1} 60.5 mL·kg^{-1}·min^{-1} × 0.59 35.7 mL·kg^{-1}·min^{-1} + 3.5 mL·kg^{-1}·min^{-1} 39.2 mL·kg^{-1}·min^{-1}
Mark	49 mL·kg^{-1}·min^{-1} − 3.5 mL·kg^{-1}·min^{-1} 45.5 mL·kg^{-1}·min^{-1} × 0.4 18.2 mL·kg^{-1}·min^{-1} + 3.5 mL·kg^{-1}·min^{-1} 21.7 mL·kg^{-1}·min^{-1}	49 mL·kg^{-1}·min^{-1} − 3.5 mL·kg^{-1}·min^{-1} 45.5 mL·kg^{-1}·min^{-1} × 0.59 26.9 mL·kg^{-1}·min^{-1} + 3.5 mL·kg^{-1}·min^{-1} 30.4 mL·kg^{-1}·min^{-1}
Gail	56 mL·kg^{-1}·min^{-1} − 3.5 mL·kg^{-1}·min^{-1} 52.5 mL·kg^{-1}·min^{-1} × 0.4 21 mL·kg^{-1}·min^{-1} + 3.5 mL·kg^{-1}·min^{-1} 24.5 mL·kg^{-1}·min^{-1}	56 mL·kg^{-1}·min^{-1} − 3.5 mL·kg^{-1}·min^{-1} 52.5 mL·kg^{-1}·min^{-1} × 0.59 31.0 mL·kg^{-1}·min^{-1} + 3.5 mL·kg^{-1}·min^{-1} 34.5 mL·kg^{-1}·min^{-1}

4 mph is too low for Juan. 7, 8, and 9 mph are too high for everyone. 6 mph is moderate only for Juan. 5 mph falls within the moderate range for all runners.

2. In order to determine the anticipated heart rate during the 5 mph run, you must first determine what percent $\dot{V}O_2$max (as a fraction) each individual is working at. Refer back to the box in the chapter to find the $\dot{V}O_2$max for each individual and the oxygen cost of running 5 mph.

Rearrange the $TE \times \dot{V}O_2$ equation to solve for %$\dot{V}O_2$R.

$$\%\dot{V}O_2R = \frac{Ex\dot{V}O_2 - \dot{V}O_2rest}{\dot{V}O_2R}$$

Janet:

$$\frac{30.3 \text{ mL·kg}^{-1}\text{·min}^{-1} - 3.5 \text{ mL·kg}^{-1}\text{·min}^{-1}}{52 \text{ mL·kg}^{-1}\text{·min}^{-1} - 3.5 \text{ mL·kg}^{-1}\text{·min}^{-1}} = \frac{26.8}{48.5} = 0.553$$

Juan:

$$\frac{30.3 \text{ mL·kg}^{-1}\text{·min}^{-1} - 3.5 \text{ mL·kg}^{-1}\text{·min}^{-1}}{64 \text{ mL·kg}^{-1}\text{·min}^{-1} - 3.5 \text{ mL·kg}^{-1}\text{·min}^{-1}} = \frac{26.8}{60.5} = 0.443$$

Mark:

$$\frac{30.3 \text{ mL·kg}^{-1}\text{·min}^{-1} - 3.5 \text{ mL·kg}^{-1}\text{·min}^{-1}}{49 \text{ mL·kg}^{-1}\text{·min}^{-1} - 3.5 \text{ mL·kg}^{-1}\text{·min}^{-1}} = \frac{26.8}{45.5} = 0.589$$

Gail:

$$\frac{30.3 \text{ mL·kg}^{-1}\text{·min}^{-1} - 3.5 \text{ mL·kg}^{-1}\text{·min}^{-1}}{56 \text{ mL·kg}^{-1}\text{·min}^{-1} - 3.5 \text{ mL·kg}^{-1}\text{·min}^{-1}} = \frac{26.8}{48.5} = 0.511$$

These percentages (as fractions) can then be used in the HRR equation.

Janet	Juan	
220	220	
− 23	− 35	(Age (yr)
197	185	Predicted HRmax (b·min^{-1})
− 60	− 48	RHR (b·min^{-1})
137	137	
× 0.553	× 0.443	% $\dot{V}O_2$R = % HRR (b·min^{-1})
76	61	
+ 60	+ 48.0	RHR (b·min^{-1})
136	109	Exercise HR (b·min^{-1})

Mark	Gail	
220	220	
− 22	−28	Age (yr)
198	192	Predicted HRmax (b·min^{-1})
− 64	− 58	RHR (b·min^{-1})
134	134	
× 0.589	× 0.511	% $\dot{V}O_2$R = % HRR (b·min^{-1})
79	69	
+ 64	+ 58	RHR (b·min^{-1})
143	127	Exercise HR (b·min^{-1})

Chapter 18, p. 482

		37-yr-old		69-yr-old	
		BMD	% Young Adult	BMD	% Young Adult
1.	a. arms	.977	116	.631	75
	b. pelvis	1.217	110	.717	65
	c. spine	1.289	113	.718	63
	d. total body	1.197	106	.847	75

2. Based on the low BMD of this individual and the fact that she has BMD values well below average for her age (her BMD is only 63–75% of the BMD of young women), the likelihood of suffering a fracture from minimal force is high.

Chapter 18, p. 487

1. Low-to-moderate impact loading activities are recommended, including hiking, cross-country skiing, stair climbing activities on commercially available machines, and weight lifting. These are activities that promote bone health while minimizing the risk of injury.

2. High-impact-loading activities, such as sprinting, jumping, and soccer, would be recommended in order to promote the attainment of a high peak bone mass. High-impact activities increase the likelihood that an individual will attain her genetic potential for peak bone mass. She should also be careful to ensure adequate calcium intake in her diet.

Chapter 19, p. 517

To determine the percentage of ST fibers, divide the number of ST fibers (approximately 12) by the total number of fibers (approximately 41) and multiply by 100. The percentage of FT fibers can also be determined by subtracting the percentage of ST fibers from 100. [Some staining techniques also permit the calculation of the percentage of the subcategories of FT (FOG and FG) using the same procedure as above, although this is not possible in this example.]

Total number of fibers = 41

Number of FT fibers = 12

Number of ST fibers = 29

% of FT = (Number of FG/total fiber count) × 100

29% = (12/41) × 100

% of ST = (Number of ST/total fiber count) × 100

71% = (29/41) × 100

Chapter 20, p. 537

Name	Absolute Strength MVC (kg)	Relative Strength kg·kg^{-1}	50% MVC
Jody	40.0	0.66	20.0
Jill	60.0	0.88	30.0
Pat	36.0	0.51	18.0
Scott	50.0	0.79	25.0
Tom	72.0	0.88	36.0
Mike	71.0	1.01	35.5

3. Tom; Mike
4. Tom

Chapter 20, p. 538

1. No, bending the knees (changing knee angle) does not eliminate the involvement of the thigh muscles. If the feet are supported (held down), the thigh muscles are more active than the rectus abdominis.

2. External obliques

3. Not held

4. From the available choices, you should have selected feet unsupported and knees bent at a 105° position in order to maximize the use of the abdominal muscles. These results indicate the best form of the sit-up from the standpoint of hip angle and foot support, but they do not take into account arm position. Also, they do not permit comparison with a curl-up or crunch (in which the head, shoulders, and trunk are lifted off the floor only about 30°). Other research has actually shown that the abdominal muscles are responsible for only the first 30–45° of the sit-up motion, and it is easier on the spinal discs if only a partial sit-up and not a full sit-up is performed. Combining this information, it must be concluded that on the basis of currently available information, a curl-up test with knees bent and feet unsupported is the exercise of choice for the abdominal muscles for most individuals.

Chapter 21, p. 560

strength gain = final strength − initial strength

for Mary: 9 kg = 54 − 45 kg

% improvement = [(final strength − initial strength) ÷ initial strength] × 100

for Mary: $\frac{9 \text{ kg}}{45 \text{ kg}} \times 100 = 20\%$

	Strength Gain	% Improvement
Mary	9	20
Dick	3	6
Jim	12	18
Ben	6	10
Ralph	4	5
Debbie	15	38

Chapter 22, p. 585

1. A ballistic technique is to stand on a step and bounce on your toes so that your heal goes below step height and then above it. This exercise will not work on a level surface.

2. A static technique is the wall stretch. Extend one leg straight back and stretch it, with the other bent at the knee and forward. Hold the position.

3. A CR PNF technique is to assume the long sitting position, a jump rope (or a towel or sweats) around your foot in a neutral position. Resist a maximal isometric contraction of foot, attempting to plantarflex. Relax and pull your foot into dorsiflexion with the implement. Repeat.

4. A CRAC PNF technique is the same as the CR technique, except that you actively contract the shin muscles (dorsiflex). Repeat.

Glossary

Absolute Submaximal Workload A set exercise load performed at any intensity from just above resting to just below maximum.

Acclimatization The adaptive changes that occur when an individual undergoes prolonged or repeated exposure to a stressful environment; these changes reduce the physiological strain produced by such an environment.

Action Potential Reversal of polarity or change in electrical potential.

Acute Phase Proteins (APPs) Blood proteins produced in the liver that function in the innate immune response. APPs are important in the response to infection and inflammation.

Adenosine Triphosphate (ATP) Stored chemical energy that links the energy-yielding and energy-requiring functions within all cells.

Aerobic In the presence of, requiring, or utilizing oxygen.

Afterload Resistance presented to the contracting ventricle.

All-or-None Principle When a motor neuron is stimulated, all of the muscle fibers in that motor unit contract to their fullest extent or they do not contract at all.

Alveolar Ventilation ($\dot{V}_A$) The volume of air available for gas exchange; calculated as tidal volume minus dead space volume times frequency.

Amenorrhea The absence of menses.

Anabolic Steroids Synthetic androgens that mimic the effects of the male hormone testosterone.

Anaerobic In the absence of, not requiring, nor utilizing oxygen.

Anorexia Athletica An eating disorder occurring primarily in young female athletes that is characterized by a food intake less than that required to support the training regimen and by body weight no more than 95% of normal.

Anorexia Nervosa An eating disorder characterized by marked self-induced weight loss accompanied by an intense fear of fatness and reproductive hormonal changes.

Antibodies Proteins produce by B cells to attack antigens.

Antigens Substances capable of provoking an immune response.

Apolipoprotein The protein portion of lipoproteins.

Archimedes' Principle The principle that a partially or fully submerged object will experience an upward buoyant force equal to the weight or the volume of fluid displaced by the object.

Arteriosclerosis The natural aging changes that occur in blood vessels—namely, thickening of the walls, loss of elastic connective tissue, and hardening of the vessel wall.

Arteriovenous Oxygen Difference (a-vO$_2$ diff) The difference between the amount of oxygen returned in venous blood and the amount originally carried in arterial blood.

Atherosclerosis A pathological process that results in the buildup of plaque inside the blood vessels.

Ballistic Stretching A form of stretching characterized by an action-reaction bouncing motion, in which the joints involved are placed into an extreme range of motion by fast, active contractions of agonistic muscle groups.

Basal Metabolic Rate (BMR) The level of energy required to sustain the body's vital functions in the waking state, when the individual is in a fasted condition, at normal body and room temperature, and without psychological stress.

B Cells Lymphocytes that are part of the adaptive immune response and are responsible for the production of antibodies to a specific antigen.

Beta Oxidation A cyclic series of steps that breaks off successive pairs of carbon atoms from FFA, which are then used to form acetyl CoA.

Blood Pressure (BP) The force exerted on the wall of the blood vessel by the blood as a result of contraction of the heart (systole) or relaxation of the heart (diastole).

Body Composition The partitioning of body mass into fat-free mass (weight or percentage) and fat mass (weight or percentage).

Bone Modeling The process of altering the shape of bone by bone resorption and bone deposition.

Bone Remodeling The continual process of bone breakdown (resorption) and formation (deposition of new bone).

Bradycardia A heart rate less than 60 b·min^{-1}.

Bulimia Nervosa An eating disorder marked by an unrealistic appraisal of body weight and/or shape that is manifested by alternating bingeing and purging behavior.

Caloric Balance Equation The mathematical summation of the caloric intake (+) and energy expenditure (−) from all sources.

Caloric Cost Energy expenditure of an activity performed for a specified period of time. It may be expressed as total calories (kcal), calories or kjoules per minute (kcal·min^{-1} or kJ·min^{-1}), or relative to body weight (kcal·kg^{-1}·min^{-1} or kJ·kg^{-1}·min^{-1}).

Caloric Equivalent The number of kilocalories produced per liter of oxygen consumed.

Calorimetry The measurement of heat energy liberated or absorbed in metabolic processes.

Capacitance Vessels Another name for veins, owing to their distensibility, which enables them to pool large volumes of blood and become reservoirs for blood.

Carbohydrate Loading (Glycogen Supercompensation) A process of nutritional modification that results in an additional storage of glycogen in muscle fiber that can be approximately three to four times the normal levels.

Carbon Dioxide Produced ($\dot{V}CO_2$) The amount of carbon dioxide generated during metabolism.

Cardiac Cycle One complete sequence of contraction and relaxation of the heart.

Cardiac Output The amount of blood pumped per unit of time, in liters per minute.

Cardiorespiratory Fitness The ability to deliver and use oxygen under the demands of intensive, prolonged exercise or work.

Cardiovascular Drift The changes in observed cardiovascular variables that occur during prolonged, heavy submaximal exercise without a change in workload.

Cellular Respiration The process by which cells transfer energy from food to ATP in a stepwise series of reactions; relies heavily upon the use of oxygen.

Central Cardiovascular Adaptations Adaptations that occur in the heart and contribute to an increased ability to deliver oxygen.

Cholesterol A derived fat that is essential for the body but may be detrimental in excessive amounts.

Coenzyme A A nonprotein substance derived from a vitamin that activates an enzyme.

Complement Group of approximately 20 plasma proteins. When activated, they lyse microorganisms, enhance phagocytosis, and enhance the inflammatory response. Complement may be activated and function in either the innate or adaptive immune response.

Concentric Contraction A dynamic muscle contraction that produces tension during shortening.

Contractility The force of contraction of the heart. Also the ability of a muscle to respond to a stimulus by shortening.

Contraction Initiation of the tension-producing process of the contractile elements within muscle.

Coupled Reactions Linked chemical processes in which a change in one substance is accompanied by a change in another.

Criterion Test The standard against which other tests are judged.

Cross-Bridging Cycle The sequence of events that are necessary for the generation of force or tension exerted by the myosin heads during muscle contraction.

Cross Training The development or maintenance of cardiovascular fitness by alternating between or concurrently training in two or more modalities.

Cutting Decreasing body fat and body water content to very low levels in order to increase muscle definition.

Cytokines Chemicals release from sensitized T cells (lymphokines) and activated macrophages (monokines) to help regulate the immune response.

Delayed-Onset Muscle Soreness (DOMS) Muscle soreness that increases in intensity for the first 24 hr after activity, peaks from 24–28 hr, and then declines during the next 5–7 days.

Densitometry The measurement of mass per unit volume.

Diet (a) The food regularly consumed during the course of normal living; (b) a restriction of caloric intake.

Diffusion The tendency of gaseous, liquid, or solid molecules to move from areas of high concentration to areas of low concentration by constant random action.

Doppler Echocardiography A technique that calculates stroke volume from measurements of aortic cross-sectional area and time-velocity integrals in the ascending aorta.

Dynamic Contraction A muscle contraction in which the force exerted varies as the muscle shortens to accommodate change in muscle length and/or joint angle throughout the range of motion while moving a constant external load.

Dyspnea Labored or difficult breathing.

Eccentric Contraction A dynamic muscle contraction that produces tension (force) while lengthening.

Economy The oxygen cost of walking or running at varying speeds.

Ejection Fraction (EF) The percentage of LVEDV that is ejected from the heart.

Elasticity The ability of a muscle to return to resting length after being stretched.

Electromyography (EMG) The measurement of the neural or electrical activity that brings about muscle contraction.

Electron Transport System (ETS) The final metabolic pathway; it proceeds as a series of chemical reactions in the mitochondria that transfer electrons from the hydrogen atom carriers NAD and FAD to oxygen; water is formed as a by-product; the electrochemical energy released by the hydrogen ions is coupled to the formation of ATP from ADP and P_i.

Energy System Capacity The total amount of energy that can be produced by an energy system.

Energy System Power The maximal amount of energy that can be produced per unit of time.

Entrainment The synchronization of limb movement and breathing frequency that accompanies rhythmical exercise.

Enzyme A protein that accelerates the speed of a chemical reaction without itself being changed by the reaction.

Eupnea Normal respiration rate and rhythm.

Excess Postexercise Oxygen Consumption (EPOC) Oxygen consumption during recovery that is above normal resting values.

Excitation-Contraction Coupling The sequence of events by which an action potential in the sarcolemma initiates the sliding of the myofilaments, resulting in contraction.

Exercise A single acute bout of bodily exertion or muscular activity that requires an expenditure of energy above resting level and that in most, but not all, cases results in voluntary movement.

Exercise-Induced Hypoxemia (EIH) A condition found in elite male endurance athletes in which the amount of oxygen carried in arterial blood is severely reduced.

Exercise Modality or Mode The type of activity or sport; usually classified by energy demand or type of muscle action.

Exercise Physiology A basic and an applied science that describes, explains, and uses the body's response to exercise and adaptation to exercise training to maximize human physical potential.

Exercise Response The pattern of homeostatic disruption or change exhibited by physiological variables during a single acute bout of physical exertion.

Extensibility The ability of a muscle to be stretched or lengthened.

External Respiration The exchange of gases between the lungs and the blood.

Fartlek Workout A type of training session, named from the Swedish word meaning "speed play," that combines the aerobic demands of a continuous run with the anaerobic demands of sporadic speed intervals.

Fast Glycolytic (FG) Fibers Fast-twitch muscle fibers that perform primarily under glycolytic conditions.

Fast Oxidative Glycolytic (FOG) Fibers Fast-twitch muscle fibers that have the ability to work under oxidative and glycolytic conditions.

Fat-Free Weight The weight of body tissue excluding extractable fat.

Fatigue Index (FI) Percentage of peak power drop-off during high-intensity, short-duration work.

Fick Equation An equation used to calculate cardiac output from oxygen consumption and arteriovenous oxygen difference (a-vO_2 diff).

Field Test A test that can be conducted anywhere; is performance-based and estimates the values measured by the criterion test.

First Law of Thermodynamics or the Law of Conservation of Energy Energy can neither be created nor destroyed but only changed in form.

Flavin Adenine Dinucleotide (FAD) A hydrogen carrier in cellular respiration.

Flexibility The range of motion in a joint or series of joints that reflects the ability of the musculotendon structures to elongate within the physical limits of the joint.

Food Efficiency An index of the amount of calories an individual needs to ingest in order to maintain a given weight or percent body fat.

Gluconeogenesis The creation of glucose in the liver from noncarbohydrate sources, particularly glycerol, lactate or pyruvate, and alanine.

Glycemic Index A measure that compares the elevation in blood glucose caused by the ingestion of 50 g of any carbohydrate food with the elevation caused by the ingestion of 50 g of white bread.

Glycogen Stored form of carbohydrate composed of chains of glucose molecules chemically linked together.

Glycogenolysis The process by which stored glycogen is broken down (hydrolyzed) to provide glucose.

Glycolysis The energy pathway responsible for the initial catabolism of glucose in a 10- or 11-step process that begins with glucose or glycogen and ends with the production of pyruvate (aerobic/slow glycolysis) or lactate (anaerobic/fast glycolysis).

Health-Related Physical Fitness That portion of physical fitness directed toward the prevention of or rehabilitation from disease as well as the development of a high level of functional capacity for the necessary and discretionary tasks of life.

Heart Rate (HR) The number of cardiac cycles per minute, expressed as beats per min (b·min^{-1}).

Heat Illness A spectrum of disorders that range in intensity and severity from mild cardiovascular and central nervous system disruptions to severe cell damage, including the brain, kidney, and liver.

Heat Stress Index A scale used to determine the risk of heat stress from measures of ambient temperature and relative humidity.

Hematocrit The ratio of blood cells to total blood volume, expressed as a percentage.

Hemoglobin (Hb) The protein portion of the red blood cell that binds with oxygen, consisting of four iron-containing pigments called *hemes* and a protein called *globin.*

High-Density Lipoprotein (HDL) A lipoprotein in blood plasma composed primarily of protein and a minimum of cholesterol or triglyceride whose purpose is to transport cholesterol from the tissues to the liver.

Hormone Chemical substance originating in glandular tissue (or cells) that is transported though body fluids to a target cell to influence its physiological activity.

Hydrolysis A chemical process in which a substance is split into simpler compounds by the addition of water.

Hydrostatic Weighing Criterion measure for determining body composition through the calculation of body density.

Hydroxyapatite Calcium and phosphate salts that are responsible for the hardness of the bone matrix.

Hyperplasia Growth in a tissue or organ through an increase in the number of cells.

Hyperpnea Increased pulmonary ventilation that matches an increased metabolic demand, as in an exercise situation.

Hypertension High blood pressure, defined as values equal to or greater than 140/90 mmHg.

Hyperventilation Increased pulmonary ventilation, especially ventilation that exceeds metabolic requirements; carbon dioxide is blown off, leading to a decrease in its partial pressure in arterial blood.

Hypokinetic Diseases Diseases caused by and/or associated with lack of physical activity.

Immune System A precisely ordered system of cells, hormones, and chemicals that regulates susceptibility to, severity of, and recovery from infection and illness.

Impulse An electrical charge transmitted through certain tissue that results in the stimulation or inhibition of physiological activity.

Inflammation Bodily response to an injury, infection, or antigen; prevents the spread of damaging agents, disposes of pathogens and cellular debris, and sets the stage for tissue repair.

Intercalated Discs The junction between cardiac muscle cells that forms the mechanical and electrical connection between the two cells.

Internal Respiration The exchange of gases at the cellular level.

Interval Training An aerobic and/or anaerobic workout that consists of three elements: a selected work interval (usually a distance), a target time for that distance, and a predetermined recovery period before the next repetition of the work interval.

Irritability The ability of a muscle to receive and respond to stimuli.

Isokinematic Contraction A muscle contraction in which the rate of limb displacement or joint rotation is held constant with the use of specialized equipment.

Isokinetic Contraction A muscle fiber contraction in which the velocity of the contraction is kept constant.

Isometric Contraction A muscle fiber contraction that does not result in a length change in muscle fiber.

Isotonic Contraction A muscle fiber contraction in which the tension generated by the muscle fiber is constant through the range of motion.

Kilocalorie The amount of heat needed to raise the temperature of 1 kg of water 1°C.

Krebs Cycle A series of eight chemical reactions that begins and ends with the same substance; energy is liberated for direct substrate phosphorylation of ATP from ADP and P_i; carbon dioxide is formed and hydrogen atoms removed and carried by NAD and FAD to the electron transport system; does not directly utilize oxygen but requires its presence.

Laboratory Test Precise, direct measurement of physiological functions for the assessment of exercise responses or training adaptations; usually involves monitoring, collection, and analysis of expired air, blood, or electrical signals.

Lactate Thresholds Points on the linear-curvilinear continuum of lactate accumulation that appear to indicate sharp rises, often labeled as the first (LT1) and second (LT2) lactate threshold.

Left Ventricular End–Diastolic Volume (LVEDV) The volume of blood in the left ventricle at the end of diastole.

Left Ventricular End–Systolic Volume (LVESV) The volume of blood in the left ventricle at the end of systole.

Lipoprotein Water-soluble compound composed of apolipoprotein and lipid components that transport fat in the bloodstream.

Load Force exerted on the muscle by an object.

Long Slow Distance (LSD) Workout A continuous aerobic training session performed at a steady-state pace for an extended period of time or distance.

Low-Density Lipoprotein (LDL) A lipoprotein in blood plasma composed of protein, a small portion of triglyceride, and a large portion of cholesterol whose purpose is to transport cholesterol to the cells.

Lysis The filling of a cell via destruction of the cell membrane.

Macrophages Immune cells that (1) phagocytize pathogens, (2) present parts of the engulfed antigen on its plasma membrane to activate the T cell response, and (3) secretes cytokines. They are important in both the innate and adaptive immune responses.

Maximal Exercise The highest intensity, greatest load, or longest duration exercise of which an individual is capable.

Maximal Lactate Steady State The highest workload that can be maintained over time without a continual rise in blood lactate; it indicates an exercise intensity above which lactate production exceeds clearance.

Maximal Oxygen Consumption ($\dot{V}O_2$max) The highest amount of oxygen an individual can take in and utilize to produce ATP aerobically while breathing air during heavy exercise.

Maximal Voluntary Contraction The maximal force (100%) that a muscle can exert.

Mean Power (MP) The average power (force times distance divided by time) exerted during short- (typically 30 sec) duration work.

Mechanical Efficiency The percentage of energy input that appears as useful external work.

MET A unit that represents the metabolic equivalent in multiples of the resting rate of oxygen consumption of any given activity.

Metabolic Pathway A sequence of enzyme-mediated chemical reactions resulting in a specified product.

Metabolism The total of all energy transformations that occur in the body.

Minerals Elements not of animal or plant origin which are essential constituents of all cells and of many functions in the body.

Minute Ventilation (Minute Volume) ($\dot{V}_I$ or $\dot{V}_E$) The amount of air inspired or expired each minute; the pulmonary ventilation rate per minute; calculated as tidal volume times frequency of breathing.

Mitochondria Cell organelles in which the Krebs cycle, electron transport, and oxidative phosphorylation take place.

Motor Unit A motor neuron and the muscle fibers it innervates.

Muscle Tension Force developed when a contracting muscle acts on an object.

Muscle Tonus A state of low-level muscle contraction at rest.

Muscular Endurance The ability of a muscle or muscle group to repeatedly exert force against a resistance.

Myoclonus A twitching or spasm in the muscle group that is maximally stretched.

Myofibril Contractile structures composed of myofilaments.

Myofilaments Contractile (thick and thin) proteins that are responsible for muscle contraction.

Natural Killer (NK) Cells Innate immune cells that destroy virus-infected and cancerous body cells by cell lysis.

Neurotransmitter Chemical released from axon terminals.

Neutralization A process that occurs when antibodies block the binding site on antigens so that they cannot bind to tissues and cause damage.

Neutrophils Innate immune cells that phagocytize pathogens.

Nicotinamide Adenine Dinucleotide (NAD) A hydrogen carrier in cellular respiration.

Non–Weight-Bearing Exercise A movement performed in which the body weight is supported or suspended and thereby not working against the pull of gravity.

One Repetition Maximum (1-RM) The most weight an individual can lift once during a dynamic resistance exercise.

Opsinization The process of coating the membrane of an antigen, making it easier for phagocytes to adhere to and engulf the antigen.

Osteoblasts Bone cells that cause the deposition of bone tissue (bone-forming cells).

Osteoclasts Bone cells that cause the resorption of bone tissue (bone-destroying cells).

Osteocytes Mature osteoblasts surrounded by calcified bone that help regulate the process of bone remodeling.

Osteopenia A condition of decreased bone mineral density (BMD), diagnosed when BMD is greater than one standard deviation (SD) below (but not more than 2.5 SD below) values for young, normal adults.

Osteoporosis A condition of porosity and decreased bone mineral density that is defined as a BMD greater than 2.5 standard deviations (SD) below values for young, normal adults.

Overtraining A state of overstress or failure to adapt to an exercise training load.

Overtraining Syndrome (OTS) A state of chronic decrement in performance and ability to train in which restoration may take several weeks, months, or even years.

Oxidation A gain of oxygen, a loss of hydrogen, or the direct loss of electrons by an atom or substance.

Oxidative Phosphorylation (OP) The process in which NADH + H$^+$ and FADH$_2$ are oxidized in the electron transport system and the energy released is used to synthesize ATP from ADP and P$_i$.

Oxygen Consumption ($\dot{V}O_2$) The amount of oxygen taken up, transported, and used at the cellular level.

Oxygen Deficit The difference between the oxygen required during exercise and the oxygen supplied and utilized. Occurs at the onset of all activity.

Oxygen Dissociation The separation or release of oxygen from the red blood cells to the tissues.

Oxygen Drift A situation that occurs in submaximal activity of long duration, or above 70% $\dot{V}O_2$max, or in hot and humid conditions where the oxygen consumption increases, despite the fact that the oxygen requirement of the activity has not changed.

Partial Pressure of a Gas (P$_G$) The pressure exerted by an individual gas in a mixture; determined by multiplying the fraction of the gas by the total barometric pressure.

Peak Power (PP) The maximum power (force times distance divided by time) exerted during very short (5 sec or less) duration work.

Percent Saturation of Hemoglobin (SbO$_2$%) The ratio of the amount of hemoglobin combined with oxygen to the total hemoglobin capacity for combining with oxygen, expressed as a percentage; indicated generally as SbO$_2$% or specifically as SaO$_2$% for arterial blood or as SvO$_2$% for venous blood.

Perfusion of the Lung Pulmonary circulation, especially capillary blood flow.

Periodization Plans for training based on a manipulation of the fitness components with the intent of peaking the athlete for the competitive season or varying health-related fitness training in cycles of harder or easier training.

Peripheral Cardiovascular Adaptations Adaptations that occur in the vasculature or the muscles that contribute to an increased ability to extract oxygen.

Phagocytosis The process of engulfing and digesting an antigen.

Phosphorylation The addition of a phosphate (P$_i$).

Physical Fitness A physiological state of well-being that provides the foundation for the tasks of daily living, a degree of protection against hypokinetic disease, and a basis for participation in sport.

Power The amount of work done per unit of time; the product of force and velocity; the ability to exert force quickly.

Preload Volume of blood returned to the heart.

Pressor Response The rapid increase in both systolic pressure and diastolic pressure during static exercise.

Proprioceptive Neuromuscular Facilitation (PNF) A stretching technique in which the muscle to be stretched is first contracted maximally. The muscle is then relaxed and is either actively stretched by contraction of the opposing muscle or is passively stretched.

Pulmonary Ventilation The process by which air is moved into the lungs.

Rating of Perceived Exertion A subjective impression of overall physical effort, strain, and fatigue during acute exercise.

Reciprocal Inhibition The reflex relaxation of the antagonist muscle in response to the contraction of the agonist.

Reduction A loss of oxygen, a gain of electrons, or a gain of hydrogen by an atom or substance.

Reflex Rapid, involuntary response to a stimulus in which a specific stimulus results in a specific motor response.

Relative Humidity The moisture in the air relative to how much moisture, or water vapor, can be held by the air at any given ambient temperature.

Relative Submaximal Workload A workload above resting but below maximum that is prorated to each individual; typically set as some percentage of maximum.

Residual Volume (RV) The amount of air left in the lungs following a maximal exhalation.

Resistance The factors that oppose air or blood flow.

Resistance Training A systematic program of exercises involving the exertion of force against a load used to develop strength, endurance, and/or hypertrophy of the muscular system.

Resistance Vessels Another name for arterioles due to their ability to vasodilate and vasoconstrict; changing diameter allows them to control the flow of blood.

Respiratory Cycle Inspiration and expiration.

Respiratory Exchange Ratio (RER) The ratio of the volume of CO_2 produced divided by the volume of O_2 consumed on a total body level.

Respiratory Quotient (RQ) The ratio of the amount of carbon dioxide produced divided by the amount of oxygen consumed at the cellular level.

Resting Metabolic Rate (RMR) The energy expended while an individual is resting quietly in a supine position.

Risk Factor An aspect of personal behavior or lifestyle, an environmental exposure, or an inherited characteristic that has been shown by epidemiological evidence to predispose an individual to the development of a specific disease.

Sarcomere The functional unit (contractile unit) of muscle fibers.

Sarcoplasmic Reticulum (SR) The specialized muscle cell organelle that stores calcium.

Skinfolds The double thickness of skin plus the adipose tissue between the parallel layers of skin.

Sliding Filament Theory of Muscle Contraction The theory that explains muscle contraction as the result of the myofilaments sliding over one another.

Slow Oxidative (SO) Fibers Slow-twitch muscle fibers that rely primarily on oxidative metabolism to produce energy.

Spirometry An indirect calorimetry method for estimating heat production or calorimetry in which expired air is measured and analyzed for the amount of oxygen consumed and carbon dioxide produced.

Sport-Specific Physical Fitness That portion of physical fitness which is directed toward optimizing athletic performance.

Sports Anemia A transient decrease in red blood cells and hemoglobin levels (grams per deciliter of blood).

Static Contraction A muscle contraction that produces an increase in muscle tension but does not cause meaningful limb displacement or joint displacement and therefore does not result in movement of the skeleton.

Static Stretching A form of stretching in which the muscle to be stretched is slowly put into a position of controlled maximal or near-maximal stretch by contraction of the opposing muscle group and held for 30–60 sec.

Steady State A condition in which the energy expenditure provided during exercise is balanced with the energy required to perform that exercise and factors responsible for the provision of this energy reach elevated levels of equilibrium.

Strength The ability of a muscle or muscle group to exert maximal force against a resistance in a single repetition.

Stress The state manifested by the specific syndrome that consists of all the nonspecifically induced changes within a biological system; a disruption in body homeostasis and all attempts by the body to regain homeostasis.

Stress Fracture A fine hairline break in bone that occurs in the absence of acute trauma, is clinically symptomatic, and is detectable by X rays or bone scans.

Stress Reactions Maladaptive areas of bone hyperactivity where the balance between resorption and deposition is progressively lost such that resorption exceeds deposition.

Stroke Volume (SV) Amount of blood ejected from the ventricles with each beat of the heart.

Substrate A substance acted upon by an enzyme.

Substrate-Level Phosphorylation The transfer of P_i directly from a phosphorylated intermediate or substrates to ADP without any oxidation occurring.

Supramaximal Exercise An exercise bout in which the energy requirement is greater than that which can be supplied aerobically at $\dot{V}O_2$max.

Syncytium The individual cells of the myocardium that function collectively as a unit during depolarization.

T cells Lymphocytes that are responsible for cell-mediated responses of the adaptive immune system. There are two classes of T cells: cytotoxic T cells (CD8), which destroy virus-infected and cancer cells directly via cell lysis; and helper T cells (CD4 cells), regulatory cells that influence the activity of cytotoxic T cells, B cells, NK, and macrophages; both may slow or stop the T and C cells once the infection is controlled.

Thermic Effect of a Meal (TEM) The increased heat production as a result of food ingestion.

Thermogenesis The production of heat.

Tidal Volume (V_T) The amount of air that is inspired or expired in a normal breath.

Torque The capability of a force to produce rotation of a limb around a joint.

Total Lung Capacity (TLC) The greatest amount of air that the lungs can contain.

Tracking A phenomenon in which a characteristic is maintained, in terms of relative rank, over a long time span or even a lifetime.

Training A consistent or chronic progression of exercise sessions designed to improve physiological function for better health or sport performance.

Training Adaptations Physiological changes or adjustments resulting from an exercise training program that promote optimal functioning.

Training Principles Fundamental guidelines that form the basis for the development of an exercise training program.

Training Taper A reduction in training prior to important competitions that is intended to allow the athlete to recover from previous hard training, maintain physiological conditioning, and improve performance.

Training Volume The total amount of work done, usually expressed as mileage or load.

Transamination The transfer of the NH_2 amino group from an amino acid to a keto acid.

Transverse Tubules (T tubules) Organelles that carry the electrical signal from the sarcolemma into the interior of the cell.

Type A Behavior Pattern (TABP) Behavior that is characterized by hard-driving competitiveness; time urgency, haste, and impatience; a workaholic lifestyle; and hostility.

Type B Behavior Pattern (TBBP) Behavior associated with characteristics of relaxation without guilt and no sense of time urgency.

Valsalva Maneuver Breath-holding that involves closing of the glottis and contraction of the diaphragm and abdominal musculature.

Velocity at $\dot{V}O_2max$ The speed at which an individual can run when working at his or her maximal oxygen consumption; based both on submaximal running economy and $\dot{V}O_2max$.

Ventilatory Thresholds Points where the rectilinear rise in minute ventilation breaks from linearity during an incremental exercise to maximum.

Vital Capacity (VC) The greatest amount of air that can be exhaled following a maximal inhalation.

Vitamins Organic substances of plant or animal origin that are essential for normal growth, development, metabolic processes, and energy transformations.

Voluntary Dehydration Exercise-induced dehydration that develops despite an individual's access to unlimited water.

Weight Cycling Repeated bouts of weight loss and regain.

Weight-Bearing Exercise A movement performed in which the body weight is supported by muscles and bones.

Index

Page references followed by *fig* indicate illustrated figures; page references followed by *t* indicate tables.

Photo Credits

p. xx: Sharon Ann Plowman and Denise L. Smith
p. 1: PhotoResearchers
p. 2: Denise L. Smith
p. 19: Tony Neste
p. 22: Gary Walts/The Image Works
p. 53: Photo Researchers
p. 54: Superstock
p. 58: Dian Molsen, Northern Illinois University
p. 62: K. R. Porter/Photo Researchers
p. 70 (top photo): Cross and Mercer/
© 1993 W. H. Freeman and Co.
p. 70 (bottom photo): Professor P. Motta/Department of
Anatomy, University "La Sapienza" Rome/Science
Photo Library/Photo Researchers
p. 85: Steven Starr/Stock Boston
p. 92 (top photo): Will Hart
p. 92 (bottom photos): Northern Illinois University
Media Services
p. 94: Taylor (Hunt) Conard
p. 110: Bob Daemmrich/The Image Works
p. 112: Robert Daemmrich/Tony Stone Images
p. 121: Linc Cornell/Stock Boston
p. 123: Pat Yen/PARVO Medics/Concentius
p. 139: Northern Illinois University Media Services
p. 154: CORBIS (Competitive Sports CD, vol.20)
p. 176: Bob Daemmrich/Stock Boston
p. 203: Bob Daemmrich/The Image Works
p. 206: Yoav Levy/Phototake NY
p. 210: Tony Neste
p. 212: Northern Illinois University Media Services
p. 220: Jody Clasey/Arthur Weltman

p. 228: Stone/GettySource
p. 236: Bettmann/CORBIS
p. 238: Spencer Grant/Photo Edit
p. 249: Will Hart
p. 255: Sharon Ann Plowman/Kathleen Cunningham
p. 256: Tony Freeman/PhotoEdit
p. 267: Northern Illinois University Media Services
p. 276: CNRI/SPL/Photo Researchers
p. 284: Bohemian Nomad Picturemakers/CORBIS
p. 319: Doug Pensinger/Allsport
p. 351: Dugald Bremner/Tony Stone Images
p. 383: Robert Harbison
p. 450: C. H. Petit Nikon/Vandystadt/Photo
Researcher, Inc.
p. 475: Jason Brandenburg/Dave Docherty/Aaron
Randell/Kathleen Cunningham
p. 476: Will Hart
p. 482: GE Medical Systems Lunar
p. 483 (both images): GE Medical Systems Lunar
p. 484 (both images): Patricia Fehling
p. 490 (both images): Custom Medical Stock
p. 499: Tony Neste
p. 500: Lewis Portney/The Stock Market
p. 504: Biology Media/Science Source/Photo
Researchers
p. 516: Michael Jensen/Mayo Clinic
p. 517: G. W. Willis/Visuals Unlimited
p. 521: Sohm/Chromosohn/Stock Market
p. 539: Taylor (Hunt) Conard
p. 549: David Madison/Tony Stone Images
p. 556: Jeff Greenbert/Visuals Unlimited
p. 566: Warren Bolster/Tony Stone Images